✴ PRIORITY CONCEPT

Sherpath Vantage provides everything you need in **one integrated course solution**

Comprehensive digital lessons offer multimedia, confidence indicators, adaptive remediation, mini assessments throughout the lesson, and a final assessment to gauge understanding of the material.

Assignment analytics give both faculty and students a comprehensive performance dashboard to help gauge strengths, weaknesses, confusion, and confidence throughout the course.

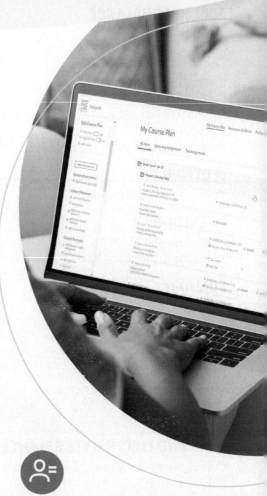

An **Elsevier eBook** provides expert health education content in a convenient and interactive format.

Elsevier Adaptive Quizzing (EAQ) delivers dynamic, personalized quizzes based on each student's performance, and allows you to choose relevant topics on which to quiz students.

Osmosis® helps actively engage students through bite-sized, illustrated health education videos that simplify complex concepts and promote active learning. A carefully curated collection of Osmosis videos are seamlessly integrated into your Sherpath Vantage course.

Course-Based SimChart® combines practical, real-world experience in electronic documentation with powerful, fully integrated educator support to help you incorporate electronic health record (EHR) practice into your course.

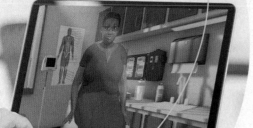

Shadow Health® Digital Clinical Experiences™ deliver high-fidelity, state-of-the-art, screen-based simulations that allow students to demonstrate and perfect their clinical reasoning skills through lifelike interactions with virtual patients.

CONTACT *your*
Elsevier Sales Representative
today to learn more!

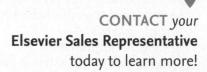

23-NHPjezgunter-0117
TM/AF 2/23

ELSEVIER

MEDICAL-SURGICAL NURSING

Concepts for Clinical Judgment and Collaborative Care

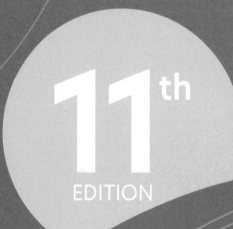

11th EDITION

DONNA D. IGNATAVICIUS, MS, RN, CNE, CNEcl, ANEF, FAADN
Speaker and Nursing Education Consultant;
Founder, Boot Camp for Nurse Educators;
President, DI Associates, Inc.
Littleton, Colorado

CHERIE R. REBAR, PhD, MBA, RN, CNE, CNEcl, COI, FAADN
Subject Matter Expert and Nursing Education Consultant
Beavercreek, Ohio;
Professor of Nursing, Galen College of Nursing
Louisville, Kentucky

NICOLE M. HEIMGARTNER, DNP, RN, CNE, CNEcl, COI, FAADN
Subject Matter Expert and Nursing Education Consultant;
Associate Professor of Nursing, Galen College of Nursing
Louisville, Kentucky

ELSEVIER

Elsevier
3251 Riverport Lane
St. Louis, Missouri 63043

MEDICAL-SURGICAL NURSING: CONCEPTS FOR CLINICAL
JUDGMENT AND COLLABORATIVE CARE, ELEVENTH EDITION

ISBN (single volume): 978-0-323-87826-5
ISBN (2-volume set): 978-0-323-87827-2

Copyright © 2024 by Elsevier Inc. All rights reserved.

Notice

Previous editions copyrighted 2021, 2018, 2016, 2013, 2010, 2006, 2002, 1999, 1995, 1991.

International Standard Book Number (single volume): 978-0-323-87826-5
International Standard Book Number (2-volume set): 978-0-323-87827-2

Executive Content Strategist: Lee Henderson
Director, Content Development: Laurie Gower
Senior Content Development Specialist: Rebecca Leenhouts
Publishing Services Manager: Julie Eddy
Senior Project Manager: Jodi Willard
Design Direction: Amy Buxton

Printed in Canada

Last digit is the print number: 9 8 7 6 5 4 3 2 1

Working together
to grow libraries in
developing countries

www.elsevier.com • www.bookaid.org

Marie Bashaw, DNP, RN, NEA-BC
Professor and Director of Nursing
Department of Nursing
Wittenberg University
Springfield, Ohio

Meg Blair, PhD, MSN, RN, CEN
Professor
Nursing
Nebraska Methodist College
Omaha, Nebraska

Julia E. Blanchette, PhD, RN, BC-ADM, CDCES
Nurse Scientist
Department of Medicine, Endocrinology
University Hospitals Cleveland Medical
    Center;
Diabetes Care and Education
    Specialist
Center for Diabetes and Obesity
University Hospitals Cleveland Medical
    Center;
Clinical Assistant Professor
School of Medicine
Case Western Reserve University
Cleveland, Ohio

Ardette Creeks, DNP, MSN-Ed, RN, HP
Professor of Nursing
Health & Human Services
Lone Star College
Houston, Texas

Keelin Cromar, MSN, RN
Adjunct Faculty
Department of Nursing
Midwestern State University
Wichita Falls, Texas

Charity Lynn Hacker, MSN-Ed, RN
Registered Nurse—Case Manager
Geriatric Extended Care—Nursing
Veterans Affairs Medical Center
Louisville, Kentucky

Katherine Hendricks, MSN, FNP, AGACNP
Critical Care Nurse Practitioner
Critical Care Medicine
Atrium Health Wake Forest Baptist
Winston-Salem, North Carolina

Jennifer Heisleman Ingalls, MSN, RN, OCN, CNL
Full-Time Faculty
Nursing
Olympic College
Bremerton, Washington

Linda Laskowski-Jones, MS, APRN, ACNS-BC, CEN, NEA-BC, FAWM, FAAN
Editor-in-Chief
Nursing: The Journal of Clinical Excellence
Philadelphia, Pennsylvania;
Clinical Nurse Specialist
Laskowski-Jones New Frontiers Health
    Consulting, LLC
Newark, Delaware;
Executive Director
Appalachian Center for Wilderness Medicine
Morganton, North Carolina

Michelle L. Litchman, PhD, FNP-BC, FAAN, FAANP, FADCES
Assistant Professor
College of Nursing
University of Utah
Salt Lake City, Utah

Hannah M. Lopez, MSN, RN, OCN, CBCN
Clinical Nurse Manager
Hematology/Oncology, Chemo Infusion,
    Neuro-Oncology
Baylor Scott & White Health
Round Rock, Texas

Melanie N. Luttrell, DNP, APRN, AGPCNP-BC
Certified Nurse Practitioner
Internal Medicine
The Christ Hospital Medical Associates
Cincinnati, Ohio

Robyn Mitchell, DNP, ACNPC-AG, CCRN-CSC-CMC, E-AEC
Critical Care Nurse Practitioner
Lovelace Medical Group
Albuquerque, New Mexico

Casey Moebius, DNP, RN
Assistant Chair, Associate Professor
Department of Nurse Education
Del Mar College
Corpus Christi, Texas

Donna Mower-Wade, DNP, MS, APRN, ACNS-BC, CNRN
Director of Advanced Practice
    Clinicians
The Medical Group
ChristianaCare Health System
Newark, Delaware

Michael Joseph Rebar, DO, DPM; Board Certified by ABIM
Internal Medicine/Hospitalist
Miami Valley Hospitalist Group
Premier Health/Miami Valley
    Hospital
Dayton, Ohio

Karen L. Toulson, DNP, MBA, CEN, NE-BC
Director, Clinical Operations
Emergency Department
ChristianaCare Health System
Newark, Delaware

Lisa Vaira, MSN, RN, CNE, CHSE
Assistant Professor II
BSN Nursing
Unitek Learning—Provo College,
    Remote
Lakeside, Montana

CONTRIBUTORS TO TEACHING/LEARNING RESOURCES
PowerPoint Slides

Cherie R. Rebar, PhD, MBA, RN, CNE, CNEcl, COI, FAADN
Subject Matter Expert and Nursing
    Education Consultant
Beavercreek, Ohio;
Professor of Nursing
Galen College of Nursing
Louisville, Kentucky

Nicole M. Heimgartner, DNP, RN, CNE, CNEcl, COI, FAADN
Subject Matter Expert and Nursing
    Education Consultant;
Associate Professor of Nursing
Galen College of Nursing
Louisville, Kentucky

TEACH® for Nurses Lesson Plans

Nicole M. Heimgartner, DNP, RN, CNE, CNEcl, COI, FAADN
Subject Matter Expert and Nursing
    Education Consultant;
Associate Professor of Nursing
Galen College of Nursing
Louisville, Kentucky

Cherie R. Rebar, PhD, MBA, RN, CNE, CNEcl, COI, FAADN
Subject Matter Expert and Nursing
    Education Consultant
Beavercreek, Ohio;
Professor of Nursing
Galen College of Nursing
Louisville, Kentucky

Test Bank

Donna D. Ignatavicius, MS, RN, CNE, CNEcl, ANEF, FAADN
Speaker and Nursing Education Consultant;
Founder, Boot Camp for Nurse Educators;
President, DI Associates, Inc.
Littleton, Colorado

Linda Turchin, MSN, CNEr
Professor Emeritus
Fairmont State University
Fairmont, West Virginia

Review Questions for the NCLEX® Examination

Donna D. Ignatavicius, MS, RN, CNE, CNEcl, ANEF, FAADN
Speaker and Nursing Education Consultant;
Founder, Boot Camp for Nurse Educators;
President, DI Associates, Inc.
Littleton, Colorado

Cherie R. Rebar, PhD, MBA, RN, CNE, CNEcl, COI, FAADN
Subject Matter Expert and Nursing
    Education Consultant
Beavercreek, Ohio;
Professor of Nursing
Galen College of Nursing
Louisville, Kentucky

Nicole M. Heimgartner, DNP, RN, CNE, CNEcl, COI, FAADN
Subject Matter Expert and Nursing
    Education Consultant;
Associate Professor of Nursing
Galen College of Nursing
Louisville, Kentucky

The first edition of this textbook, entitled *Medical-Surgical Nursing: A Nursing Process Approach,* was a groundbreaking work in many ways. The following nine editions built on that achievement and further solidified the book's position as a major trendsetter for the practice of evidence-based adult health nursing. Now in its eleventh edition, "Iggy" again provides a cutting-edge approach for the future of adult nursing practice, as reflected in its current title: *Medical-Surgical Nursing: Concepts for Clinical Judgment and Collaborative Care.* This new edition continues to help students learn how to build clinical judgment skills to provide safe, quality nursing care that is patient-centered, evidence-based, and interprofessionally collaborative. In addition to print formats, this edition is available in a variety of electronic formats.

KEY COMPONENTS OF THE ELEVENTH EDITION

Similar to the previous edition's conceptual learning approach, the eleventh edition organizes the content in each chapter by the most important *professional nursing and/or health concepts* and then presents commonly occurring *exemplars* for each concept. The key components for this edition that strengthen the text's conceptual focus are consistent with the Quality and Safety Education for Nurses' (QSEN) competencies and the 2021 AACN *Essentials* and include *clinical judgment, safety, evidence-based practice, quality care, patient-centeredness, teamwork and collaboration, and use of informatics.* Further information about these components is described below.

- **Enhanced Emphasis on Professional Nursing and Health Concepts.** This edition uniquely balances a focus on nursing concepts with a conceptual approach to teaching and learning. Prelicensure programs that embrace a concept-based nursing curriculum, system-focused curriculum, or a hybrid or modified approach will find this edition easy to use. To help students connect previously learned concepts with new information in the text, Chapters 1 and 3 review the main concepts used in this edition, giving a working definition upon which students can reflect and build as they learn new material. These unique features build on basic concepts learned in nursing fundamentals courses, such as gas exchange and safety, to help students make connections between foundational concepts and interprofessional care for patients with medical-surgical conditions. For continuity and reinforcement, a list of specific Priority and Interrelated Nursing Concepts is highlighted at the beginning of each chapter. This placement is specifically designed to help students better understand the priority and associated needs that the nurse will address when providing safe, evidence-based, patient-centered care for individuals with selected health conditions.
- **Emphasis on Common Exemplars.** For each priority concept listed in the beginning of the Nursing Care chapters, the authors have identified common or major exemplars. The nursing and interprofessional collaborative care for patients experiencing these exemplar diseases and illnesses is discussed through the lens of the priority and interrelated concepts. Patient problems are presented as a collaborative problem list to assist with prioritized needs.
- **Focus on Clinical Judgment.** Stressing the importance of clinical judgment helps to prepare students for professional nursing practice and the Next-Generation NCLEX® (NGN) Examination for nursing licensure. Chapter 2, entitled *Clinical Judgment and Systems Thinking,* focuses on how nurses use clinical judgment in practice. Systems thinking allows the nurse to look beyond an individual action for additional or enhanced methods to promote safety and increase quality of care, which drives more favorable patient outcomes. Inversely, the nurse looks at evidence-based interventions that have served populations and then navigates ways to bring those to individual patient care.

  The Nursing Care chapters in this edition present **Next-Generation NCLEX® Examination Challenges** that require students to use clinical judgment skills based on the NCSBN's Clinical Judgment Measurement Model (CJMM). Answers and rationales for these questions are provided on the companion Evolve website (http://evolve.elsevier.com/Iggy/).

  In the eleventh edition, the six cognitive skills of the NCSBN's CJMM are aligned with each nursing process step. The authors use this alignment to help students and faculty use critical thinking and clinical reasoning required for clinical judgment, in alignment with the nursing process steps, as follows:

  - Recognize Cues: Assessment
  - Analyze Cues and Prioritize Hypotheses: Analysis
  - Generate Solutions and Take Actions: Planning and Implementation
  - Evaluate Outcomes: Evaluation
- **Emphasis on Patient Safety.** Patient safety is emphasized throughout this edition and is highlighted in the **Nursing Safety Priority boxes** that enable students to immediately identify the most important care needed for patients with specific health problems. These highlighted features are further classified as an Action Alert, Drug Alert, or Critical Rescue. We also continue to include our leading-edge **Best Practice for Patient Safety & Quality Care boxes** to emphasize the most important nursing care.
- **Highlight on Quality Care.** The QSEN Institute has set the standard for clinical agencies requiring that nurses have *quality improvement* knowledge, skills, attitudes, and abilities. To help prepare students for that role, **Systems Thinking and Quality Improvement boxes** summarize a quality improvement project published in the literature and discusses the implications of the project's success in improving nursing care. The inclusion of these boxes disseminates information

and research. It also helps students understand that quality improvement begins at the bedside as the nurse identifies potential evidence-based solutions to practice problems and that external evidence is brought to the bedside to improve patient care and outcomes.

- **Enhanced Focus on Patient-Centered Care.** Patient-centered care is enhanced in this eleventh edition in numerous ways. This edition continues to use the term "patient" instead of "client" throughout. Although the use of these terms remains a subject of discussion among nurse educators, we have not defined the patient as a dependent person. Rather, the patient can be an individual, a family, or a group—all of whom have rights that are respected in a mutually trusting nurse–patient relationship. Most health care agencies and professional organizations use "patient" in their practice and publications, and most professional nursing organizations support the term. To illustrate the importance of Patient-Centered Care, this text incorporates the following special boxes:
  - Patient-Centered Care: Older Adult Health
  - Patient-Centered Care: Veteran Health
  - Patient-Centered Care: Culture and Spirituality
  - Patient-Centered Care: Genetics/Genomics
  - Patient-Centered Care: Gender Health
  - Patient-Centered Care: Health Equity (new to this edition)

  An emphasis on *health equity* is highlighted in this latest edition with the addition of Patient-Centered Care: Health Equity boxes. These boxes draw the student's attention to the nurse's role in promoting health equity, "the state in which everyone has a fair and just opportunity to attain their highest level of health" (Centers for Disease Control and Prevention, 2022 Health equity. https://www.cdc.gov/nchhstp/healthequity/index.html).

  Unique health needs of transgender and nonbinary patients are addressed in **Chapter 5.** Along with other individuals in the LGBTQIA2S+ population, the health needs of this population are included in *Healthy People 2030* and in The Joint Commission's Standards. This chapter, first introduced in the eighth edition, continues to provide evidence-based tools to prepare students and faculty to provide safe, evidence-based, patient-centered care for transgender and nonbinary patients. This edition also integrates content on the care of patients with physical disabilities where appropriate, especially in units about musculoskeletal and neurologic conditions.
- **Emphasis on Evidence-Based Practice.** The eleventh edition focuses again on the importance of *using best current evidence in nursing practice* and how to locate and use this information to improve patient care. **Evidence-Based Practice boxes** offer a solid foundation in this essential component of nursing practice. Each box summarizes a useful research article, explains the implications of its findings for nursing practice and further research, and rates the level of evidence based practice on a well-respected scale.
- **Emphasis on Preparation for the Next-Generation NCLEX® Examination.** An enhanced emphasis on the NCLEX® Examination and consistency with the 2023 NCLEX-RN® Test Plan has been refined in this edition. The eleventh edition emphasizes "readiness"—readiness for the NCLEX® Examination, readiness for disaster and mass casualty events, readiness for safe drug administration, and readiness for implementation of actions that promote health equity. An increased number of new **NCLEX Examination Challenges** are interspersed throughout the text to allow students the opportunity to practice test taking and decision making. **NCLEX Mastery Questions** are at the end of each chapter. Answers and rationales for the NCLEX Examination Challenges and the NCLEX Mastery Questions are provided on the Evolve website (http://evolve.elsevier.com/Iggy).

  In a world that needs more nurses than ever before, it is critical that students be ready to pass the licensure examination on the first try. To help students achieve that goal, **Learning Outcomes** at the beginning of each chapter continue to be consistent with the competencies outlined in the 2023 NCLEX-RN® Test Plan. The eleventh edition continues to include an innovative end-of-chapter feature called **Get Ready for the Next-Generation NCLEX® Examination!** In Assessment chapters, this unique and effective learning aid consists of a list of **Essential Assessment Points.** In care chapters, **Essential Nursing Care Points**, which are in alignment with the American Association of Colleges of Nursing's *2021 Essentials: Core Competencies for Professional Nursing*, are presented in a visually appealing table format for ease of use and understanding.
- **Focus on Care Coordination and Transition Management.** Similar to the tenth edition, the eleventh edition includes a priority focus on continuity of care via a Care Coordination and Transition Management section in each Nursing Care chapter. Literature continues to emphasize the importance of care coordination and transition management between acute care and community-based care. To help students prepare for this role, this edition of our text provides content focusing on Self-Management Education and Health Care Resources. A new feature, Home Health Care, helps students to understand how nursing care is continued in the home setting following discharge.

CLINICAL CURRENCY AND ACCURACY

To ensure currency and accuracy, we listened to students and faculty who have used the previous editions, hearing their impressions of and experiences with the book. We conducted ongoing, thorough literature searches of current best evidence regarding nursing education and clinical practice to validate best practices and health care trends that have shaped the focus of the eleventh edition. Further cumulative efforts are reflected in this edition:

- Strong, consistent focus on Next-Generation NCLEX-RN® Examination preparation, clinical judgment, safe patient-centered interprofessional care, pathophysiology, drug therapy, quality improvement, evidence-based clinical practice, and care coordination and transition management
- Inclusion of relevant current research and best practice guidelines

- Emphasis on critical "need-to-know" information that entry-level nurses must possess to provide safe patient care

With the amount of information that continues to evolve in health care practice and education, it is easy for a book to become larger with each new edition. The reality is that today's nursing students have limited time to absorb and apply essential information to provide safe medical-surgical nursing care. Materials in this edition were carefully scrutinized to determine the essential information that students will actively *use* when providing safe, patient-centered, interprofessional, evidence-based, quality nursing care for adults.

OUTSTANDING READABILITY

Today's students must maximize their study time to read information and quickly understand it. In the United States, 50% of citizens cannot read beyond the 8th grade level (The Literacy Project, 2022, https://literacyproj.org/). To ensure readability without reducing the quality or depth of material that students need to know, this text uses a direct-address style (where appropriate) that speaks directly to the reader. Sentences are as short as possible without sacrificing essential material. The new edition has continued to improve within consistency among chapters. The result of our efforts is a medical-surgical text of consistently outstanding readability in which content is clear, focused, and accessible.

EASE OF ACCESS

To make this text as easy to use as possible, we have maintained our approach of having smaller chapters of more uniform length. Consistent with our focus on "need-to-know" material, we chose exemplars to illustrate concepts of care versus detailing every health disorder. The focused eleventh edition contains 65 chapters. To decrease the number of chapters and stay focused on essential "need-to-know" content, several changes were made, including:

- Combining essential information from the former chapter on HIV into the current chapter on Immunity (Chapter 16: Concepts of Inflammation and Immunity)
- Deleting the chapter on cancer development but moving essential content into a chapter regarding Concepts of Care for Patients With Cancer (Chapter 18)
- Placing information about oxygen therapy and tracheostomy in chapters in Unit VI, Interprofessional Collaboration for Patients With Respiratory System Conditions, where these therapies are most used.

The overall presentation of the eleventh edition has been updated, including more current, high-quality photographs and artistic renderings for realism. Careful attention was given to representation of adults of various races and ethnicities. Design changes have been made to improve accessibility of material. There is appropriate placement of display elements (e.g., figures, tables, and boxes) for a chapter flow that enhances text reading without splintering content or confusing the reader. Key terms are defined at the beginning of the chapters for quick reference. To increase the smoothness of flow and reader concentration,

side-turned tables and charts or tables and charts that span multiple pages are infrequently used.

We have maintained the unit structure of previous editions, with larger vital body systems appearing earlier in the book. However, complex care content is found in separate critical care chapters for patients with acute coronary syndrome, severe respiratory conditions, and emergent neurologic health conditions.

To break up long blocks of text and highlight key information, we continue to include streamlined yet eye-catching headings, bulleted lists, tables, boxes, and in-text highlights. Current references at the end of each chapter include research articles, nationally accepted clinical guidelines, and other sources of evidence when available for each chapter. Classic or definitive works on a subject are noted with an asterisk (*).

A PATIENT-CENTERED, INTERPROFESSIONAL COLLABORATIVE CARE APPROACH

As in previous editions, we maintain in this edition a collaborative, interprofessional care approach to patient care. In the world of health care, nurses and all other providers who are part of the interprofessional team *share* responsibility with patients for the management of health conditions. Thus, we present information in a collaborative framework with an increased emphasis on the interprofessional nature of care. In this framework we make no *artificial* distinctions between medical treatment and nursing care. Instead, under each Interprofessional Collaborative Care heading we discuss how the nurse coordinates care and transition management while interacting with members of the interprofessional team. **Interprofessional Collaboration boxes** present helpful content on how nurses collaborate with the interprofessional health care team to help meet optimal patient outcomes. Each box identifies the Interprofessional Education Collaborative (IPEC) Expert Panel's Competency of Roles and Responsibilities that aligns with its content.

Although our approach has a focus on interprofessional care, this book is first and foremost a *nursing* text. We therefore use a nursing process/clinical judgment approach to organize discussions of patient health conditions and their management. Discussions of *major* health problems follow a full nursing process format using this structure:

[Health problem]
Pathophysiology Review
    Etiology (and Genetic Risk when appropriate)
    Incidence and Prevalence
Health Promotion/Disease Prevention (when appropriate)
Interprofessional Collaborative Care
    Recognize Cues: Assessment
    Analyze Cues and Prioritize Hypotheses: Analysis
    Generate Solutions and Take Actions: Planning and Implementation:
        [Collaborative Intervention Statement (based on priority patient problems)]
        Planning: Expected Outcomes
        Interventions

Care Coordination and Transition Management
  Home Care Management (when appropriate)
  Self-Management Education (when appropriate)
  Health Care Resources (when appropriate)
Evaluate Outcomes: Evaluation

Discussions of less common (but important) or less complex disorders follow a similar yet abbreviated format: a discussion of the condition itself (including a pertinent pathophysiology review) followed by a section on interprofessional collaborative care. To demonstrate our commitment to providing the content foundational to nursing education, and consistent with the recommendations of Benner and colleagues through the Carnegie Foundation for the Future of Nursing Education, we highlight essential pathophysiologic concepts that are key to understanding the basis for collaborative management.

Integral to the interprofessional care approach is a narrative of who on the health care team is involved in the care of the patient. When a responsibility is primarily the nurse's, the text says so. When a decision must be made collaboratively by various members of the team (e.g., by the patient, nurse, primary health care provider, and physical therapist), this is clearly stated. When health care practitioners in different care settings are involved in the patient's care, this is noted.

ORGANIZATION

The 65 chapters of *Medical-Surgical Nursing: Concepts for Interprofessional Collaborative Care* are grouped into 15 sections. Unit I, Essential Concepts of Medical-Surgical Nursing, provides fundamental information for the health care concepts incorporated throughout the text. Unit II consists of three chapters on concepts of emergency care and disaster preparedness.

Unit III consists of three chapters on the management of patients with fluid, electrolyte, and acid-base imbalances. Chapters 13 and 14 review key assessments associated with fluid and electrolyte balance, acid-base balance, and related patient care in a clear, concise discussion. The chapter on infusion therapy (Chapter 15) is supplemented with an online Fluids & Electrolytes Tutorial on the companion Evolve website.

Unit IV contains four chapters that address normal immunity and health problems related to immunity. This material includes information on inflammation and the immune response, altered cell growth and cancer development, and interventions for patients with autoimmune conditions, infections, other immunologic disorders, and cancer.

The remaining 11 units focus on medical-surgical information grouped by body system. Each of these units begins with an Assessment chapter and continues with one or more Nursing Care chapters for patients with selected health conditions, highlighted via exemplars, in that body system. This framework is familiar to students who learn the body systems in preclinical foundational science courses such as anatomy and physiology.

MULTINATIONAL, MULTICULTURAL, MULTIGENERATIONAL FOCUS

To reflect the increasing diversity of our society, *Medical-Surgical Nursing: Concepts for Clinical Judgment and Collaborative Care* values a multinational, multicultural, and multigenerational focus. Addressing the needs of U.S. and Canadian readers, we have included U.S. and international units for normal values of selected laboratory tests. When appropriate, we identify specific Canadian health care resources, including their websites. In many areas, Canadian health statistics are combined with those of the United States to provide an accurate picture of North American information.

To help nurses provide quality, evidence-based care for patients with diverse beliefs and values, numerous **Patient-Centered Care: Culture and Spirituality** and **Patient-Centered Care: Gender Health boxes** highlight important aspects of culturally congruent care. Chapter 5 is dedicated to the special health care needs of transgender and nonbinary patients.

Increases in life expectancy and aging of the baby boom generation contribute to a steadily increasing older adult population. To help nurses care for this population, the eleventh edition continues to provide thorough coverage of the care of older adults. Chapter 4 offers information on the role of the nurse and interprofessional team in promoting health for this population, with coverage of common health conditions that older adults may experience, such as falls and inadequate nutrition. **Patient-Centered Care: Older Adult Health boxes** that specify normal physiologic changes to expect in the older population are found throughout the text. These boxes present key points for the student to consider when caring for these patients. Boxes entitled **Patient-Centered Care: Veterans Health** continue to include emphasis on the special health needs of this population. An increasing number of veterans have multiple physical and mental health concerns that require special attention in today's environment of care.

AN INTEGRATED MULTIMEDIA RESOURCE BASED ON PROVEN STRATEGIES FOR STUDENT ENGAGEMENT AND LEARNING

Medical-Surgical Nursing: Concepts for Clinical Judgment and Collaborative Care, 11th edition, is the centerpiece of a comprehensive package of electronic and print learning resources that break new ground in the application of proven strategies for student engagement, learning, and evidence-based educational practice. This integrated multimedia resource actively engages the student in problem solving and using clinical judgment to make important clinical decisions.

Resources for Instructors

For the convenience of faculty, all Instructor Resources are available on a streamlined, secure instructor area of the Evolve website (http://evolve.elsevier.com/Iggy/). All ancillaries for this edition were developed with **direct involvement of the** textbook authors. Included among these Instructor Resources are the *TEACH® for Nurses* **Lesson Plans.** These Lesson Plans focus on the most important material within each chapter and provide innovative, active learning strategies for student engagement. *TEACH for Nurses* for the eleventh edition incorporates numerous interprofessional activities that give students an opportunity to practice as an integral part of the health care team. Lesson Plans are provided for each chapter and are categorized into several parts:

> Chapter Objectives
> Student Resources
> Clinical Judgment Classroom Tools
> Instructor Resources
> Teaching Strategies
> Nursing Curriculum Standards
> > Nursing Concepts
> > 2021 AACN *Essentials* Domains and QSEN Competencies
> > Interprofessional Collaborative Core Competencies

Additional Instructor Resources provided on the Evolve website include:

- A completely revised, updated, high-quality **Test Bank** consisting of traditional multiple-choice and NCLEX-RN® "alternate-item" types, written to better prepare students for the Next-Generation NCLEX®. Each question is coded for correct answer, rationale, cognitive level, NCLEX Integrated Process, NCLEX Client Needs Category, and key words to facilitate question searches. (Questions at the Applying [Application] and above cognitive level require the student to draw on an understanding of multiple or broader concepts from multiple textbook pages, so page cross references are not provided for these higher-level critical thinking questions.) The Test Bank is provided in the Evolve Assessment Manager and in ExamView and ParTest formats. 150 Next-Generation NCLEX® Examination Review questions are provided within an interactive application for further testing options. An additional 75 questions are NGN-style and help students develop clinical judgment skills.
- An electronic **Image Collection** containing all images from the book (approximately 550 images), delivered in a format that makes incorporation into lectures, presentations, and online courses easier than ever.
- A completely revised collection of more than 2000 **PowerPoint slides** corresponding to each chapter in the text and highlighting key materials with integrated images and Unfolding Case Studies. Audience Response System Questions (discussion-oriented questions at the end of each chapter's slide presentation) are included for use with audience response systems. Answers and rationales to the Audience Response System Questions and Unfolding Case Studies are found in the "Notes" section of each slide.

Resources for Students

Resources for students include a revised and updated Study Guide, a Clinical Companion, and Evolve Learning Resources.

The *Study Guide* has been completely revised and updated featuring a fresh emphasis on clinical judgment. Correct responses with rationales are provided to allow students the opportunity to enhance their understanding of materials, which ultimately increases their clinical judgment and test-taking abilities.

The pocket-sized *Clinical Companion* is a handy clinical resource that retains its easy-to-use alphabetical organization and streamlined format, with thoroughly revised content for ease of use and on-the-go care. New to this edition of the Clinical Companion is a color layout with improved images that support bedside nursing care. The bulleted format is integrated with key elements of the NCSBN Clinical Judgment Measurement Model. It includes "Critical Rescue," "Drug Alert," and "Action Alert" highlights throughout based on the Nursing Safety Priority features in the textbook. Additional features include National Patient Safety Goals as well as specific Patient-Centered Care boxes. This "pocket-sized Iggy" has been tailored to the special needs of students preparing for clinicals and clinical practice.

Also available for students is a dynamic collection of Evolve Student Resources, available at http://evolve.elsevier.com/Iggy/. The Evolve Student Resources include the following:

- Review Questions—NCLEX® Examination
- Review Questions—Next-Generation NCLEX® Examination
- Answers and Rationales for Next-Generation NCLEX® Challenges
- Answers and Rationales for NCLEX® Examination Challenges
- Answers and Rationales for NCLEX® Mastery Questions
- Concept Maps
- Concept Map Creator (a handy tool for creating customized Concept Maps)
- Fluid & Electrolyte Tutorial (a complete self-paced tutorial on this perennially difficult content)
- Key Points (downloadable expanded chapter reviews for each chapter)
- Audio Glossary
- Audio Clips and Video Clips

In summary, *Medical-Surgical Nursing: Concepts for Clinical Judgment and Collaborative Care,* 11th edition, together with its fully integrated multimedia ancillary package, provides the tools needed to equip nursing students to meet the opportunities and challenges of nursing practice now and in an evolving health care environment. The only elements that remain to be added to this package are those that you uniquely provide—your passion, your commitment, your innovation, *your nursing expertise.*

Donna D. Ignatavicius
Cherie R. Rebar
Nicole M. Heimgartner

We are dedicating the eleventh edition of this publication to three wonderful men. They have walked alongside us for many years and through countless long days and nights, providing unconditional support and love during our shared professional and personal journeys.

It is with love and gratitude that we honor:

Donna's husband, Charles Ignatavicius

Cherie's husband, Dr. Michael Joseph Rebar

Nicole's husband, Jeremy Heimgartner

We also wish to recognize the nursing students, nurse educators, and nurses who answered the call during COVID-19. For your service and commitment to the patients and families who needed you most during the pandemic, thank you for being there.

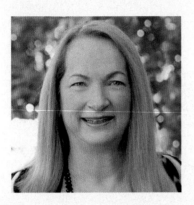

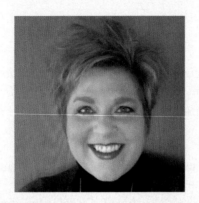

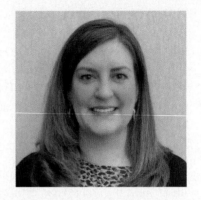

Donna D. Ignatavicius received her diploma in nursing from the Peninsula General School of Nursing in Salisbury, Maryland. After working as a charge nurse in medical-surgical nursing, she became an instructor in staff development at the University of Maryland Medical Center. She then received her BSN from the University of Maryland School of Nursing. For 5 years she taught in several schools of nursing while working toward her MS in Nursing, which she received in 1981. Donna then taught in the BSN program at the University of Maryland, after which she continued to pursue her interest in gerontology and accepted the position of Director of Nursing of a major skilled-nursing facility in her home state of Maryland. Since that time, she has served as an instructor in several associate degree nursing programs. Through her consulting activities, faculty development workshops, and international nursing education conferences (such as Boot Camp for Nurse Educators®), Donna is nationally recognized as an expert in nursing education. She is currently the President of DI Associates, Inc. (http://www.diassociates.com/), a company dedicated to improving health care through education and consultation for faculty. In recognition of her contributions to the field, she was inducted as a charter Fellow of the prestigious Academy of Nursing Education in 2007, received her Certified Nurse Educator credential in 2016, and obtained her Academic Clinical Nurse Educator certification in 2020. Additionally, Donna was inducted as a fellow into the Academy of Associate Degree Nursing in 2021.

Cherie R. Rebar has spent most of her life inside a classroom, whether as a student or a professor. She earned her first degree in education from Morehead State University in Morehead, Kentucky. She returned to school to earn an Associate of Science degree in Nursing from Kettering College, MSN and MBA degrees from the University of Phoenix, a post-masters certificate in Family Nurse Practitioner studies from the University of Massachusetts—Boston, a Psychiatric-Mental Health Nurse Practitioner post-masters certificate from the University of Cincinnati College of Nursing, and a PhD in Psychology (Health Behaviors) from Northcentral University. Combining her loves of nursing and education, Cherie continues to teach students in prelicensure and graduate nursing programs. She has served in numerous leadership positions over the years, including Chair of ASN, BSN Completion, and BSN Prelicensure Nursing Programs and Director of Nursing. She currently is a Professor of Nursing at Galen College of Nursing and is certified as an academic nurse educator, academic clinical nurse educator, and online instructor. Cherie was inducted as a fellow into the Academy of Associate Degree Nursing in 2021. Her years of clinical practice include medical-surgical, acute care, ear/nose/throat surgery, allergy, community, and psychiatric–mental health nursing. A frequent presenter at national and state nursing conferences, Cherie serves as a consultant to nursing programs and faculty nationwide and in Canada, contributes regularly to professional publications, and holds student success at the heart of all she does.

Nicole M. Heimgartner received her BSN from Spalding University in Louisville, Kentucky, her MSN with an emphasis in education from the University of Phoenix, and her Doctorate of Nursing Practice in Educational Leadership from American Sentinel University in Aurora, Colorado. Nicole is certified in both online education and nursing education. She has a very diverse clinical background, with extensive clinical practice experience in cardiovascular, medical-surgical, and community nursing. As her love for the nursing profession grew, Nicole started teaching in undergraduate and graduate degree programs. Nicole now has over 20 years of experience as an educator, focusing on innovative educational strategy and nursing leadership and incorporating online learning into nursing education. She is currently an Associate Professor of Nursing at Galen College of Nursing. Her expertise includes currency in clinical practice as well as teaching and designing curriculum at the undergraduate and graduate levels of nursing education. Nicole also presents at the state and national level on best nursing practice, serves as a consultant with nursing programs and faculty, contributes regularly to professional publications, and is passionate about current practice and engaging the adult learner. Connecting students with the nursing profession and empowering growth within the profession is her passion.

ACKNOWLEDGMENTS

Publishing a textbook and ancillary package of this magnitude would not be possible without the combined efforts of many people. With that in mind, we would like to extend our deepest gratitude to many people who were such an integral part of this journey.

Our contributing authors once again provided excellent manuscripts to underscore the clinical relevancy of this publication.

The staff of Elsevier has, as always, provided us with meaningful guidance and support throughout every step of the planning, writing, revision, and production of the eleventh edition. Executive Content Strategist Lee Henderson worked closely with us from the early stages of this edition to help us focus our revision plan while coordinating the project from start to finish. The Content Development team of Laura Goodrich, Jennifer Wade, and Rebecca Leenhouts then worked with us to bring the logistics of the eleventh edition from vision to publication. The development team also held the reins of our complex ancillary package and worked with the authors and content experts to provide an outstanding library of resources to complement and enhance the text.

Senior Project Manager Jodi Willard was, as always, an absolute joy with whom to work. If the mark of a good editor is that their work is invisible to the reader, then Jodi is the consummate editor. Her unwavering attention to detail, flexibility, and conscientiousness helped to make the eleventh edition consistently readable while making the production process incredibly smooth. Also, a special thanks to Publishing Services Manager Julie Eddy.

Designer Amy Buxton is responsible for the beautiful cover and the new interior design of the eleventh edition. Amy's work on this edition has cast important features in exactly the right light, contributing to the readability and colorful beauty of this edition.

Our acknowledgments would not be complete without recognizing our dedicated team of Educational Solutions Consultants and other key members of the Sales and Marketing staff who helped to put this book into your hands.

Donna D. Ignatavicius
Cherie R. Rebar
Nicole M. Heimgartner

CONTENTS

Asterisk (*) denotes a Concept Exemplar.

GUIDE TO SPECIAL FEATURES

PATIENT-CENTERED CARE: VETERAN HEALTH

BEST PRACTICE FOR PATIENT SAFETY AND QUALITY CARE

COMMON EXAMPLES OF DRUG THERAPY

EVIDENCE-BASED PRACTICE

HOME HEALTH CARE

KEY FEATURES

LABORATORY PROFILE

PATIENT AND FAMILY EDUCATION

SYSTEMS THINKING/QUALITY IMPROVEMENT

Assessment of the Nervous System

Donna D. Ignatavicius

http://evolve.elsevier.com/Iggy/

LEARNING OUTCOMES

1. Use knowledge of anatomy and physiology to perform a focused assessment of the nervous system.
2. Teach evidence-based health promotion activities to help prevent neurologic health problems or trauma.
3. Demonstrate clinical judgment to interpret assessment findings in a patient with a neurologic health problem.
4. Identify factors that affect health equity for patients with neurologic health problems.
5. Explain how genetic implications and physiologic aging of the nervous system affect *mobility.*
6. Interpret assessment findings for patients with a suspected or actual neurologic problem.
7. Plan evidence-based care and support for patients undergoing diagnostic testing of the nervous system.

KEY TERMS

Bell's palsy A peripheral nervous system disorder in which the patient has paralysis of all facial muscles on the affected side (also called *facial paralysis*). The patient cannot close the eye on the affected side or wrinkle the forehead, smile, whistle, or grimace. Tearing may stop or become excessive. The face appears masklike and sags.

decerebration Abnormal movement with rigidity characterized by extension of the arms and legs, pronation of the arms, plantar flexion, and opisthotonos (body spasm in which the body is bowed forward).

decortication Abnormal motor movement seen in the patient with lesions that interrupt the corticospinal pathways.

electroencephalography (EEG) A diagnostic test that records the electrical activity of the cerebral hemispheres of the brain. The frequency, amplitude, and characteristics of the brain waves are recorded.

electromyography (EMG) A diagnostic test used to identify nerve and muscle disorders, such as myasthenia gravis, as well as spinal cord disease.

Glasgow Coma Scale (GCS) A tool used in many acute care settings to establish baseline data in each of these areas: eye opening, motor response, and verbal response. The patient is assigned a numeric score for each of these areas. The lower the score, the lower the patient's neurologic function.

Guillain-Barré syndrome (GBS) A rare acute inflammatory disorder that affects the axons and/or myelin of the peripheral nervous system resulting in ascending muscle weakness or paralysis.

level of consciousness (LOC) The degree of alertness or amount of stimulation needed to engage a patient's attention and can range from alert to comatose.

magnetoencephalography (MEG) A noninvasive imaging technique used to measure the magnetic fields produced by electrical activity in the brain via extremely sensitive devices such as superconducting quantum interference devices.

myasthenia gravis A rare progressive autoimmune disease characterized by muscle weakness as a result of impaired acetylcholine receptors.

neurotransmitter A chemical (e.g., acetylcholine and serotonin) within the nervous system that can either enhance or inhibit the neurologic impulse but not do both.

nystagmus Involuntary eye movement that may cause the eyes to rapidly move from side to side, up and down, or in a circle.

PERRLA *P*upils are *e*qual in size, *r*ound and *r*egular in shape, and react to *l*ight and *a*ccommodation (a desired normal finding for most individuals).

physical disability A limitation in mobility or activity that can affect one or more ADLs, such as walking, transferring, bathing, toileting, or dressing; the limitation often requires the use of special equipment such as a cane or wheelchair.

single-photon emission computed tomography (SPECT) A diagnostic imaging study that uses a radiopharmaceutical agent to enable radioisotopes to cross the blood-brain barrier.

trigeminal neuralgia A persistently painful and debilitating disorder that involves the trigeminal cranial nerve (CN V) and affects women more often than men.

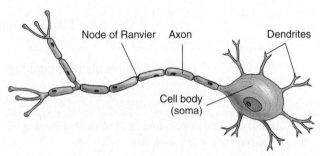

FIG. 35.1 Structure of a typical neuron.

The major divisions of the nervous system are the central nervous system (CNS) (brain and spinal cord), peripheral nervous system (PNS), and autonomic nervous system (ANS). The divisions of the nervous system work together to control *cognition, mobility,* and *sensory perception*. See Chapter 3 for a review of these health concepts. Health problems usually affect the CNS more often than other divisions of the nervous system and are the primary focus of this textbook unit.

ANATOMY AND PHYSIOLOGY REVIEW

Nervous System Cells: Structure and Function

The basic unit of the nervous system, the neuron, transmits impulses, or "messages." Some neurons are *motor* (causing purposeful physical movement or *mobility*), and some are *sensory* (resulting in the ability to perceive stimulation through one's sensory organs or *sensory perception*). Some process information and some retain information (*cognition*). When a neuron receives an impulse from another neuron, the effect may be excitation (increasing action) or inhibition (decreasing action). Each neuron has a *cell body,* or *soma;* short, branching processes called *dendrites;* and a single *axon* (Fig. 35.1).

Afferent neurons, also known as *sensory neurons,* are specialized to send impulses toward the CNS, away from the PNS. *Efferent* neurons are motor nerve cells that carry signals away from the CNS to the cells in the PNS. Each dendrite synapses with another cell body, axon, or dendrite and sends impulses along the efferent and afferent neuron pathways.

Many axons are covered by a myelin sheath—a white, lipid covering. Myelinated axons appear whitish and therefore are also called white matter. Nonmyelinated axons have a grayish cast and are called gray matter. Myelinated axons have gaps in the myelin called nodes of Ranvier. The nodes of Ranvier play a major role in impulse conduction (see Fig. 35.1). When the myelin is impaired, the impulses cannot travel from the brain to the rest of the body, such as in patients with multiple sclerosis (see Chapter 37).

The enlarged distal end of each axon is called the synaptic or terminal knob. Within the synaptic knobs are the mechanisms for manufacturing, storing, and releasing a transmitter substance. Each neuron produces a specific neurotransmitter chemical (e.g., acetylcholine and serotonin) that can either enhance or inhibit the impulse, but it cannot do both (Rogers, 2023).

Impulses are transmitted to their eventual destination through synapses, or spaces between neurons. There are two distinct types of synapses: *neuron to neuron* and *neuron to muscle* (or gland). Between the terminal knob and the next cell is a small space called the *synaptic cleft.* The knob, the cleft, and the portion of the cell to which the impulse is being transmitted make up the *synapse.*

Neuroglia cells (sometimes referred to as *glial cells*), which vary in size and shape, provide protection, structure, and nutrition for the neurons. They are classified into four types: astroglial cells, ependymal cells, oligodendrocytes, and microglial cells. These cells are also part of the blood-brain barrier and help regulate cerebrospinal fluid (CSF) (Rogers, 2023). Malignant tumors that affect glial cells are very aggressive and typically have a poor outcome.

Central Nervous System: Structure and Function

The central nervous system (CNS) is composed of the *brain,* which directs the regulation and function of the nervous system and all other systems of the body, and the *spinal cord,* which starts reflex activity and transmits impulses to and from the brain.

Brain

The meninges form the protective covering of the brain and the spinal cord. The outside layer is the dura mater. The subdural space is located between the *dura mater* and the middle layer, the *arachnoid.* The *pia mater* is the most inner layer. Situated between the arachnoid and pia mater is the *subarachnoid space,* where CSF circulates. The *epidural space* is located between the skull and the outer layer of the dura mater. This area also extends down the spinal cord and is used for the delivery of epidural analgesia and anesthesia.

The dura mater also lies between the cerebral hemispheres and the cerebellum and is called the *tentorium.* It helps decrease or prevents the transmission of force from one hemisphere to another and protects the lower brainstem when head trauma occurs. Clinical references may be made to a lesion (e.g., a tumor) as being supratentorial (above the tentorium) or infratentorial (below the tentorium).

Major Parts of the Brain

The brain consists of three main areas—the forebrain, cerebellum, and brainstem (Fig. 35.2). The *forebrain* lies above the brainstem and cerebellum and is the most advanced in function complexity. This area of the brain is further divided into three areas—the diencephalon, cerebrum, and cerebral cortex.

The *diencephalon,* which lies below the cerebrum, includes the thalamus, hypothalamus, and epithalamus. The *thalamus* is

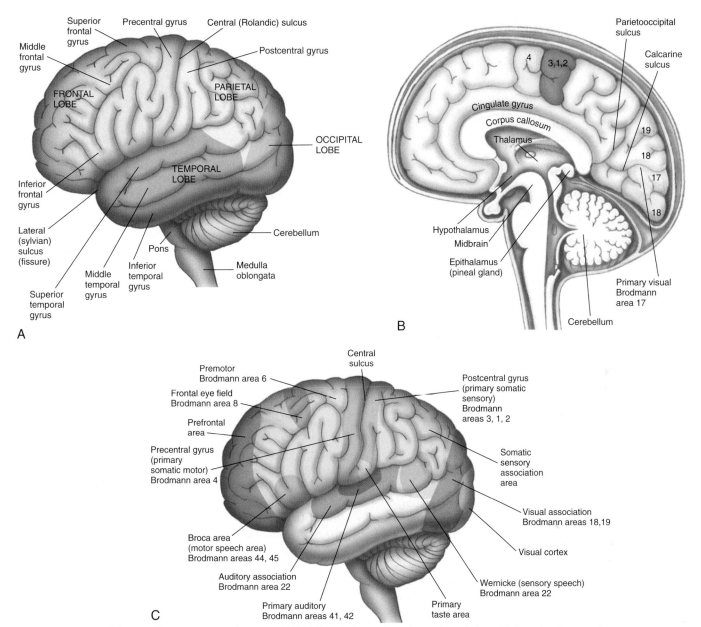

FIG. 35.2 The cerebral hemispheres. (A) Left hemisphere of cerebrum, lateral view. (B) Functional areas of the cerebral cortex, midsagittal view. (C) Functional areas of the cerebral cortex, lateral view. (From Rogers, J.L. [2023]. *McCance and Huether's Pathophysiology: The biologic basis for disease in adults and children* [9th ed.]. St. Louis: Mosby.)

the major "relay station," or "central switchboard," for the CNS. The *hypothalamus* plays a major role in autonomic nervous system control (controlling temperature and other functions) and **cognition**. The *epithalamus* connects the pathways to regulate emotion and contribute to smooth voluntary motor function.

The *cerebrum* is the largest part of the brain and controls intelligence, creativity, and memory. The "gray matter" of the cerebrum is the central cortex—the center that receives information from the thalamus and all the lower areas of the brain. The cerebrum consists of two halves, referred to as the *right hemisphere* and the *left hemisphere,* which are joined by the corpus callosum. The *left* hemisphere is the dominant hemisphere in most people (even in many left-handed people). Within the

deeper structures of the cerebrum are the right and left lateral ventricles. At the base of the cerebrum near the ventricles is a group of neurons called the *basal ganglia,* which help regulate motor function.

The *cerebral cortex* is part of the cerebrum and is involved with almost all of the higher functions of the brain. This part of the brain processes and communicates all information coming from the peripheral nervous system (PNS). It also translates the impulses into understandable feelings and thoughts. The cerebral cortex is so complex that it is further divided into four lobes: the frontal lobe, parietal lobe, temporal lobe, and occipital lobe (see Fig. 35.2). Box 35.1 summarizes the major functions of each cerebral lobe.

BOX 35.1   Cerebral Lobe Main Functions

Frontal Lobe
- Primary motor area (also known as the motor "strip" or cortex) *(mobility)*
- Broca speech center on the dominant side
- Voluntary eye movement
- Access to current sensory data *(sensory perception)*
- Access to past information or experience
- Affective response to a situation
- Behavior regulation
- Cognition
  - Judgment
  - Ability to develop long-term goals
  - Reasoning, concentration, abstraction

Parietal Lobe
- Understanding sensory input such as texture, size, shape, and spatial relationships
- Three-dimensional (spatial) perception
- Needed for singing, playing musical instruments, and processing nonverbal visual experiences
- Perception of body parts and body position awareness
- Taste impulses for interpretation

Temporal Lobe
- Auditory center for sound interpretation
- Complicated memory patterns
- Wernicke area for language comprehension

Occipital Lobe
- Primary visual center

BOX 35.2   Brainstem Functions

Medulla
- Cardiac-slowing center
- Respiratory center
- Cranial nerve nuclei IX (glossopharyngeal), X (vagus), XI (accessory), and XII (hypoglossal) and parts of cranial nerves VII (facial) and VIII (vestibulocochlear)

Pons
- Cardiac acceleration and vasoconstriction centers
- Pneumotaxic center that helps control respiratory pattern and rate
- Cranial nerve nuclei V (trigeminal), VI (abducens), VII (facial), and VIII (vestibulocochlear)

Midbrain
- Contains the cerebral aqueduct or aqueduct of Sylvius
- Location of periaqueductal gray, which may abolish pain when stimulated
- Cranial nerve nuclei III (oculomotor) and IV (trochlear)

The *cerebellum* receives immediate and continuous information about the condition of the muscles, joints, and tendons. Cerebellar function enables a person to:
- Keep an extremity from overshooting an intended target
- Move from one skilled movement to another in an orderly sequence
- Predict distance or gauge the speed with which one is approaching an object
- Control voluntary movement
- Maintain equilibrium (balance)

Unlike the motor cortex, cerebellar control of the body is ipsilateral (situated on the same side). The right side of the cerebellum controls the right side of the body, and the left side of the cerebellum controls the left side of the body.

The *brainstem* includes the midbrain, pons, and medulla. The functions of these structures are presented in Box 35.2. Throughout the brainstem are special cells that constitute the reticular activating system (RAS), which controls awareness and alertness. For example, this tissue awakens a person from sleep when presented with a stimulus such as loud noise or pain or when it is time to awaken. The RAS has many connections with the cerebrum, the rest of the brainstem, and the cerebellum.

Circulation in the Brain. Circulation in the brain originates from the carotid and vertebral arteries. The internal carotid arteries branch into the anterior cerebral artery (ACA) and middle cerebral artery (MCA), the largest ones. The two posterior vertebral arteries become the basilar artery, which then divides into two posterior cerebral arteries. The anterior, middle, and posterior cerebral arteries are joined together by small communicating arteries to form a ring at the base of the brain known as the *circle of Willis.*

The *middle* cerebral artery supplies the lateral surface of the cerebrum from about the mid-temporal lobe upward (i.e., the area for hearing and upper body motor and sensory neurons). The *anterior* cerebral artery supplies the midline, or medial, aspect of the same area (i.e., the lower body motor and sensory neurons). The *posterior* cerebral arteries supply the area from the mid-temporal region down and back (occipital lobe), as well as much of the brainstem. When blood flow is interrupted in any of these arteries (e.g., by a clot), perfusion to the area of the brain being supplied is affected and may not function as it should.

The *blood-brain barrier (BBB)* seems to exist because the endothelial cells of the cerebral capillaries are joined tightly together. This barrier keeps some substances in the bloodstream out of the cerebrospinal circulation and out of brain tissue. Substances that can pass through the BBB include oxygen, glucose, carbon dioxide, alcohol, anesthetics, and water. Large molecules such as albumin, any substance bound to albumin, and many antibiotics are prevented from crossing the barrier.

Cerebrospinal fluid (CSF) also circulates, surrounds, and cushions the brain and spinal cord. While moving through the subarachnoid space, the fluid is continuously produced by the choroid plexus, reabsorbed by the arachnoid villi, and then channeled into the superior sagittal sinus.

Spinal Cord

The spinal cord controls **mobility;** regulates organ function; processes **sensory perception** information from the extremities, trunk, and many internal organs; and transmits information to and from the brain. It contains H-shaped *gray matter* (neuron cell bodies) that is surrounded by *white matter* (myelinated axons). Groups of cells in the white matter (ascending and descending tracts) have been fairly well identified. These tracts carry impulses from the spinal cord to the brain (ascending

TABLE 35.1 Origins, Types, and Functions of Cranial Nerves

Cranial Nerve	Origin	Type	Function
I: Olfactory	Olfactory bulb	Sensory	Smell
II: Optic	Midbrain	Sensory	Central and peripheral vision
III: Oculomotor	Midbrain	Motor to eye muscles	Eye movement via medial and lateral rectus and inferior oblique and superior rectus muscles; lid elevation via the levator muscle
		Parasympathetic-motor	Pupil constriction; ciliary muscles
IV: Trochlear	Lower midbrain	Motor	Eye movement via superior oblique muscles
V: Trigeminal	Pons	Sensory	Sensory perception from skin of face and scalp and mucous membranes of mouth and nose
		Motor	Muscles of mastication (chewing)
VI: Abducens	Inferior pons	Motor	Eye movement via lateral rectus muscles
VII: Facial	Inferior pons	Sensory	Pain and temperature from ear area; deep sensations from the face; taste from anterior two-thirds of the tongue
		Motor	Muscles of the face and scalp
		Parasympathetic-motor	Lacrimal, submandibular, and sublingual salivary glands
VIII: Vestibulocochlear	Pons-medulla junction	Sensory	Hearing
			Equilibrium
IX: Glossopharyngeal	Medulla	Sensory	Pain and temperature from ear; taste and sensations from posterior one-third of tongue and pharynx
		Motor	Skeletal muscles of the throat
		Parasympathetic-motor	Parotid glands
X: Vagus	Medulla	Sensory	Pain and temperature from ear; sensations from pharynx, larynx, thoracic and abdominal viscera
		Motor	Muscles of the soft palate, larynx, and pharynx (swallowing)
		Parasympathetic-motor	Thoracic and abdominal viscera; cells of secretory glands; cardiac and smooth muscle innervation to the level of the splenic flexure
XI: Accessory	Medulla (anterior gray horn of the cervical spine)	Motor	Skeletal muscles of the pharynx and larynx and sternocleidomastoid and trapezius muscles (swallowing)
XII: Hypoglossal	Medulla	Motor	Skeletal muscles of the tongue (swallowing)

tracts, such as the spinothalamic tract) or from the brain to the spinal cord (descending tracts, such as the corticospinal tract). Spinal nerves connect the spinal cord with the rest of the body and consist of motor, sensory, and autonomic nerve fibers.

Peripheral Nervous System: Structure and Function

The peripheral nervous system (PNS) is composed of the spinal nerves, cranial nerves, and autonomic nervous system. There are 31 pairs of spinal nerves (8 cervical, 12 thoracic, 5 lumbar, 5 sacral, and 1 coccygeal) exiting from the spinal cord. Each of the nerves has a posterior and an anterior branch. The posterior branch carries **sensory perception** information to the cord (*afferent pathway*). The anterior branch transmits motor impulses to the muscles of the body to allow **mobility** (*efferent pathway*).

Each spinal nerve is responsible for the muscle innervation and sensory reception of a given area of the body. The cervical and thoracic spinal nerves are relatively close to their areas of responsibility, whereas the lumbar and sacral spinal nerves are some distance from theirs. Because the spinal cord ends between L1 and L2, the axons of the lumbar and sacral cord extend downward before exiting at the appropriate intervertebral foramen.

Sensory receptors throughout the body monitor and transmit impulses of pain, temperature, touch, vibration, pressure, visceral sensation, and proprioception. Sensory receptors also monitor and transmit the sensory perceptions of the special senses (i.e., vision, taste, smell, and hearing).

The cell bodies of the anterior spinal nerves are located in the anterior gray matter (anterior horn) of each level in the spinal cord. The anterior motor neurons are also referred to as *lower motor neurons.* As each nerve axon leaves the spinal cord, it joins other spinal nerves to form plexuses (clusters of nerves). Plexuses continue as trunks, divisions, and cords and finally branch into individual peripheral nerves.

The reflex arc is a closed circuit of spinal and peripheral nerves and therefore requires no control by the brain. *Reflexes* consist of sensory input from:

- Skeletal muscles, tendons, skin, organs, and special senses
- Small cells in the spinal cord lying between the posterior and anterior gray matter (interneurons)
- Anterior motor neurons, along with the muscles they innervate

There are 12 *cranial nerves.* Their number, name, origin, type, and function are summarized in Table 35.1. Cranial nerve function is an important part of the comprehensive neurologic examination performed by health care providers (Jarvis & Eckhardt, 2024).

Autonomic Nervous System: Structure and Function

The autonomic nervous system (ANS) is composed of two parts: the sympathetic nervous system (SNS) and the parasympathetic nervous system. ANS functions are not usually under conscious control but may be altered in some people by using biofeedback and other methods.

The SNS cells originate in the gray matter of the spinal cord from T1 through L2 or L3. This part of the ANS is considered *thoracolumbar* because of its anatomic location. The SNS stimulates the functions of the body needed for "fight or flight" (e.g., heart and respiratory rate). It also inhibits certain functions not needed in urgent and stressful situations.

The parasympathetic cells originate in the gray matter of the sacral area of the spinal cord (from S2 through S4) plus portions of cranial nerves III, VII, IX, and X *(craniosacral)*. The parasympathetic nervous system can slow body functions when needed and contribute to digestion and reproduction ("feed and breed").

Parasympathetic fibers to the organs have some sensory ability in addition to motor function. Sensory perceptions of irritation, stretching of an organ, or a decrease in tissue oxygen are transmitted to the thalamus through pathways not yet fully understood. Because pain from internal organs is often felt below the body wall innervated by the spinal nerve, it is presumed that there are connections between the viscera and body structure that relay pain sensation.

Neurologic Changes Associated With Aging

Neurologic changes associated with aging often affect *mobility* and *sensory perception*. Mobility changes in late adulthood can cause slower movement and response time and a decrease in sensory perception as outlined in the Patient-Centered Care: Older Adult Health box (Jarvis & Eckhardt, 2024). Any problems that affect the nerves and muscles affect motor and ADL ability. Determining functional status is a recommended quality indicator for patients with complex chronic conditions.

Sensory changes in older adults can also affect their ADLs. Pupils decrease in size, which restricts the amount of light entering the eye, and adapt more slowly. Older adults need increased lighting to see. Chapter 40 describes collaborative care for people with hearing loss. Touch sensation decreases, which may lead to falls because the older person may not feel small objects or a step underfoot (Touhy & Jett, 2022). (See the discussion on fall prevention in Chapter 4.)

Cognitive functions of perceiving, registering, storing, and using information often change as a normal part of aging. *Intellect does not decline as a result of aging.* However, a person with certain health problems may have a decrease in **cognition.** Acute cognitive decline is frequently caused by drug interactions or toxicity or by an inadequate oxygen supply to the brain (hypoxia). Some older adults may need more time than a younger person to process questions, learn and process new information, solve problems, or complete analogies.

Subtle memory changes can occur for many older people. Long-term memory often seems better than recall (recent) or immediate (registration) memory. Older adults may need more time to retrieve information. These changes may be partly caused by the loss of cerebral neurons, which is associated with the aging process.

PATIENT-CENTERED CARE: OLDER ADULT HEALTH

Changes in the Nervous System Related to Aging

Physiologic Change	Nursing Implication	Rationale
Slower cognitive processing time	Provide sufficient time for the affected older adult to respond to questions and/or direction.	Allowing adequate time for processing helps differentiate normal findings from neurologic deterioration.
Recent memory loss	Reinforce teaching by repetition, using written reminders or electronic memory aids, such as electronic alarms or smartphone applications that provide alerts or alarms.	Greatest loss of brain weight is in the white matter of the frontal lobe. Repetition helps the patient learn new information and recall it when needed.
Decreased sensory perception of touch	Remind patients to look where their feet are placed when walking. Instruct patients to wear shoes that provide good support when walking. If patients are unable to change their position frequently (every hour) while in a bed or chair, assist them to change position. Teach patients to check water temperature with a thermometer due to decreased lower extremity sensation caused by decreased circulation.	Decreased sensory perception may cause patients to fall. Decreased lower extremity sensation can cause burns if water is too hot.
Possible change in perception of pain	Ask the patient to describe the nature and specific characteristics of pain. Monitor additional assessment variables to detect possible health problems.	Accurate and complete nursing assessment ensures that the interventions will be appropriate for the older adult (see Chapters 4 and 6).
Change in sleep patterns	Ascertain sleep patterns and preferences. Ask if sleep pattern interferes with ADLs. Adjust patients' daily schedules to their personal sleep patterns and preferences as much as possible (e.g., evening vs. morning bath).	Older adults require as much sleep as younger adults. It is more common for older adults to fall asleep early and arise early. Daytime napping is especially common in older adults of advanced age.
Altered balance and/or decreased coordination	Instruct the patient to move slowly when changing positions. If needed, advise the patient to hold on to handrails when ambulating. Assess the need for an ambulatory aid, such as a cane or walker.	The patient may fall if moving too quickly. Assistive and adaptive aids provide support and prevent falls.
Increased risk for infection	Monitor the patient carefully for signs and symptoms of infection.	Older adults often have structural deterioration of microglia, the cells responsible for cell-mediated immune response in the central nervous system (CNS).

Mental status may be impaired in the older adult as a result of infection, hypoxia, hypoglycemia, or hyperglycemia. These conditions are usually easily assessed and managed. During an acute change in mental status, assess the adult for peripheral oxygenation saturation level (SpO_2), serum glucose value, and potential infection.

Health Promotion/Disease Prevention

Prevention of neurologic health problems includes avoiding risky behaviors and practicing a healthy lifestyle. Young adults, especially men, are particularly at risk for engaging in risky physical activities, such as motorcycle or car racing without wearing a helmet or diving into shallow water. Unfortunately, these activities often lead to serious spinal cord or traumatic brain injuries and should be avoided. Remind adults of any age to avoid excessive alcohol or other substances that can impair judgment and cause an accident. Teach adults who enjoy outdoor time to protect against mosquitoes and ticks that can cause West Nile encephalitis or other vector-borne infections. These infections are increasing due to climate change, which has led to increased flooding and global temperatures.

PATIENT-CENTERED CARE: VETERAN HEALTH

Traumatic Brain Injury

Active military men and women who are in or near combat areas are also at risk for neurologic problems, especially traumatic brain injury (TBI). The most common cause of TBI in this population is a blast from an improvised explosive device (IED). Continued improvements in IED detection and protective headgear may help decrease these injuries. TBI in veterans is discussed later in Chapter 38.

Practicing a healthy lifestyle can help promote nervous system health. For example, smoking constricts blood vessels and can lead to decreased perfusion to the brain, resulting in a brain attack or stroke. Teach these patients the importance of smoking cessation as discussed elsewhere in this text.

Sleep deprivation at any age can lead to significant changes in *cognition*. Interrupted sleep and sleep deprivation can also impair physical function and self-management. Sleep and rest are both necessary to promote health. Teach patients that proper nutrition and regular exercise are also important to prevent neurologic impairment. For example, the brain requires adequate glucose to function properly. Decreased blood glucose can cause light-headedness and dizziness, leading to falls, especially among older adults. Skipping meals or poor nutrition can affect the function of the body's neurons.

NCLEX Examination Challenge 35.1

Health Promotion and Maintenance

The nurse performs an initial baseline neurologic assessment on an older client. Which of the following findings would the nurse expect for this client?

A. Long-term memory loss
B. Altered balance
C. Inability to ambulate
D. Acute confusion

RECOGNIZE CUES: ASSESSMENT

Patient History

Obtain information from the patient about health problems, drug therapy history, smoking and substance abuse history, occupation, and current lifestyle. During your introduction, note the patient's appearance and assess speech ability, affect, and movement. If the patient seems to have *cognition* deficits or has trouble speaking or hearing, ask a family member or significant other to stay during the interview to help obtain an accurate history. If the patient is not English-speaking, obtain an interpreter to ensure accuracy of patient information. Be sure that glasses, contact lenses, and hearing aids are available if the patient wears any of these devices.

Document if the patient has a physical disability or mental health disability, such as paralysis from a stroke or spinal cord injury or a neurocognitive disorder such as dementia or traumatic brain injury. *Mobility* limitation requires many individuals to use ambulatory aids or wheelchairs, especially middle-aged and older adults.

PATIENT-CENTERED CARE: HEALTH EQUITY

Physical Disability

As discussed in Chapter 41, physical disability occurs most commonly in older adults from Hispanic, American Indian/Alaska Native, and other racial groups when compared to White groups due to a number of social determinants of health (SDOH) (Smeltzer, 2021). Assess patients and their families for SDOH that may affect health equity, such as lack of housing or food insecurity. Inquire if they have access to health care services and transportation.

Patients who are physically disabled may also have difficulty with one or more functional activities, such as bathing, toileting, and dressing. Inquire about the ability to perform ADLs. Knowing the level of daily activity helps establish a baseline for later comparison as the patient improves or worsens.

Ask patients to provide a detailed medical history. Many chronic health conditions, including diabetes mellitus, hypertension, and kidney disease, place patients at risk for neurologic health problems. Assess the use of alcohol, tobacco, recreational drugs, and other medications, especially for older adults who often experience adverse drug events. Also for older adults, inquire about any history of falls and, if so, when the falls occurred.

Nutrition History

Like all body systems, the nervous system functions at its optimal level when a person's nutritional intake is adequate to meet cellular needs. In addition to glucose and the amino acids needed to promote adequate neurologic function, vitamin B (especially vitamin B_{12}) helps promote nerve health. Ask patients about their intake of foods high in vitamin B, including eggs, beef, organ meats, and fish. Patients who consume a vegan diet can get adequate vitamin B from fortified grain cereals or bread.

Family History and Genetic Risk

Ask about family neurologic history, such as stroke. Some diseases occur more often in certain groups of people and may be caused by a genetic influence or other reason. Many neurologic diseases have a genetic basis, such as migraine headaches and epilepsy. These genetic risks are described with specific neurologic health problems found later in this unit.

Current Health Problems

The most common reports of people with a neurologic problem are pain, weakness, numbness, or cognitive impairment. Collect data pertinent to the patient's presenting health symptom(s):

- Date and time of onset
- Factors that cause or exacerbate (worsen) the problem
- Course of the problem (e.g., intermittent or continuous)
- Signs and symptoms (as expressed by the patient), pattern of their occurrence, and location of pain, weakness, or numbness
- Measures that improve symptoms, if any (e.g., heat, ice, over-the-counter (OTC) medications or supplements)

Assessment of pain can present many challenges. Pain is most often related to peripheral nerve damage or dysfunction. It may be acute or persistent, depending on the onset and duration. Assess the intensity of pain by using a pain scale and asking the patient to rate the level experienced. Quality of pain may be described as burning, aching, or stabbing. Determine the location of pain and areas to which it radiates. With any assessment, it is always best if patients describe the pain in their own words and point to its location, if possible. Chapter 6 describes acute and persistent pain in detail.

Weakness may be related to individual muscles or muscle groups due to lack of adequate innervation. Determine whether weakness occurs in proximal or distal muscles or muscle groups. Distal weakness and impaired *sensory perception* (especially in lower extremities) may indicate neuropathy (a problem in nerve tissue). Muscle weakness and/or numbness in the lower extremities may increase the risk for falls and injury. Weakness and/or numbness in the upper extremities may interfere with *mobility* and functional ability.

Impaired *cognition* may occur suddenly as a result of acute trauma to the brain or more slowly over years as a result of dementia or other disorder. Patients with impaired cognition may not be able to provide information about their symptoms. In that case, gather information from a family member who can provide the data needed prior to the physical assessment.

Physical Assessment

Two types of neurologic assessments may be performed: a complete (comprehensive) assessment and a focused assessment. Bedside staff nurses perform focused neurologic assessments; primary health care providers and neuroscience ICU nurses perform complete neurologic examinations as needed. Banzon et al., 2023 found that neurologic assessment and documentation varies among nurses and health care providers in non-neuroscience ICU units. The focused assessment should vary only depending on whether the patient is awake and alert or has altered consciousness.

Consciousness is the ability to be aware of the environment, an object, and oneself; it is often documented as one's level of consciousness. Level of consciousness (LOC) refers to the degree of alertness or amount of stimulation needed to engage a patient's attention and can range from *alert* to *comatose*. The patient who is described as *alert* is awake, engaged, and responsive. A patient may be alert but not oriented to person, place, or time. Patients who are less than alert are labeled *lethargic, stuporous,* or *comatose*. A *lethargic* patient is drowsy but easily awakened. One who is arousable only with vigorous or painful stimulation is *stuporous*. The *comatose* patient is unconscious and cannot be aroused despite vigorous or noxious simulation.

Another way to assess a patient's LOC is to use this AVPU method:

- **A**lert
- **V**oice responsive
- **P**ain responsive
- **U**nresponsive

Neurologic Assessment of the Awake and Alert Patient

The nurse includes five components in a baseline-focused assessment, which includes the following (Bell et al., 2021):

- Level of consciousness
- Language and speech
- Cranial nerve status
- Movement and sensation
- Vital signs

A more detailed assessment may be conducted by the nurse generalist or advanced practice nurse if neurologic deficits are present.

Assessment of Level of Consciousness. Assessing patients who are alert and awake allows the nurse to perform several components of the exam, such as ***mobility***, language and speech, and ***cognition***. To evaluate *alertness*, call patients by their name or touch them gently. Do not use painful stimuli unless the patient's LOC decreases (Bell et al., 2021).

After determining alertness, the next step is to evaluate *awareness*. Once the patient's attention is engaged, ask questions to determine orientation. Varying the sequence of questioning on repeated assessments prevents the patient from memorizing the answers. Responses that indicate orientation include the ability to answer questions about person, place, time, and situation, such as:

- The patient's ability to relate the onset of symptoms
- The name of the primary health care provider or nurse
- The year and month
- Home address
- The name of the health care agency

The nurse documents findings for a patient who is fully alert and oriented as "alert and oriented x 4," or "AAO x 4." Fully conscious patients should be able to respond coherently unless they have dementia or delirium. Ask patients to follow a few simple and complex commands to assess their memory, comprehension, and judgment. *Loss of memory, especially recent memory, tends to be an early sign of neurologic problems, especially in older adults.* Be aware that patients' literacy level, sensory ability (hearing and vision), and age/generation can affect their responses (Bell et al., 2021).

✚ NURSING SAFETY PRIORITY

Critical Rescue

A decrease in LOC and orientation is the earliest and most reliable indication that central neurologic function has declined! Be alert to both *sudden* and *subtle* changes, particularly when changes are noted by family members or others who know the patient. If a decline in LOC occurs, contact the Rapid Response Team or primary health care provider immediately.

Assessment of Language and Speech. Language and speech skills can be assessed during the initial interview. *Language* skills include understanding the spoken or written word and being able to coherently speak or write. Patients may demonstrate understanding by following directions on admission (e.g., getting undressed). If patients hesitate, it may be that they do not understand the vocabulary or word, or that they usually converse in a language that is different from the nurse's primary language.

Speech is assessed as being normal, slow, garbled (nonsensical), difficult to find words, or other impairments. If the change in speech is new and represents a deterioration from a previous ability to communicate, this change must be urgently reported to the primary health care provider because it may indicate a stroke, new onset of confusion, or other serious neurologic condition.

Assessment of Cranial Nerve Status. Cranial nerves are typically tested to establish a baseline from which to compare progress or deterioration. Cranial nerve examination assesses the function of the cerebrum and brainstem (see Table 35.1). Damage or malfunction of cranial nerves can cause either unilateral or bilateral dysfunction. In a baseline-focused assessment of an alert patient, include evaluation of (Bell et al., 2021):

- Vision, visual fields, and pupil reaction (CN II and III) by having patients read text, checking for peripheral vision, and assessing pupil response.
- Facial symmetry (CN VII) by observing the patient's entire face and comparing sides.
- Swallowing (CN IX and X) by observing the patient swallow unless the patient is NPO.
- Extraocular movements (EOMs) (CN III, IV, and V) by observing for unusual eye movements such as strabismus (inward or outward deviation of eye).

Pupil constriction is a function of cranial nerve III, the oculomotor nerve. **P**upils should be **e**qual in size, **r**ound and **r**egular in shape, and react to **l**ight and **a**ccommodation (**PERRLA**). Estimate the size of both pupils using a millimeter scale or a pupillometer (Jarvis & Eckhardt, 2024). Patients who have had eye surgery for cataracts or glaucoma often have irregularly shaped pupils. Those using eyedrops for either cataracts or glaucoma may have unequal pupils if only one eye is being treated, and the pupillary response may be altered.

To test for pupil constriction, dim the room lights and ask the patient to close both eyes. Bring a penlight in from the side of the patient's head and shine the light in the eye being tested as soon as the patient opens both eyes. The pupil being tested should constrict (direct response). The other pupil should also constrict slightly (consensual response). To test accommodation, relight the room and ask the patient to focus on a distant object and then immediately look at an object 4 to 5 inches from the nose. The eyes should converge, and the pupils should constrict. Pinpoint or severely dilated nonreactive pupils are usually late signs of neurologic deterioration (Jarvis & Eckhardt, 2024).

During the cranial nerve assessment, look for asymmetry, such as unequal movement in the facial muscles. For example, patients with Bell's palsy, a peripheral nervous system (PNS) disorder, have paralysis of all facial muscles on the affected side (also called *facial paralysis*). The patient cannot close the eye on the affected side, wrinkle the forehead, smile, whistle, or grimace. Tearing may stop or become excessive; the face appears masklike and sags. Taste is usually impaired to some degree, but this symptom seldom persists beyond the second week of paralysis.

Ask patients about the presence of facial pain. Severe, intermittent facial pain is consistent with trigeminal neuralgia, a persistently painful and debilitating disorder that involves the trigeminal cranial nerve (CN V).

Assessment of Movement and Sensation. If possible, assess the patient's gait and balance. An altered gait or balance may be an indication of cerebellar dysfunction. Certain medical conditions, especially hypertension, dysrhythmias, and heart failure, can also cause these problems. Determine if the patient has any of these conditions (Bell et al., 2021).

Throughout the neurologic assessment, observe the patient for involuntary tremors or movements. Describe these movements as accurately as possible, such as "pill-rolling with the thumbs and fingers at rest" or "intention tremors of both hands" (tremors that occur when the patient tries to do something). These abnormalities can indicate certain conditions, such as multiple sclerosis, or the effects of selected psychotropic drugs. In addition, assess the patient for movements that indicate irritability, hyperactivity, or slowed movements.

Measure the patient's hand *strength* by asking the patient to grasp and squeeze two fingers of each of your hands. Compare the grasps for equality of strength. As another means of evaluating strength, try to withdraw the fingers from the patient's grasp and compare the ease or difficulty. The patient should release the grasps on command—another assessment of consciousness and the ability to follow commands.

The acuity level of the patient determines how often the *sensory assessment* is done. For example, patients with acute spinal cord trauma or ascending Guillain-Barré syndrome are assessed every hour until stable and then every 4 hours. Guillain-Barré syndrome (GBS) is a rare acute inflammatory disorder that affects the axons and/or myelin of the PNS, resulting in ascending muscle weakness or paralysis. As the condition improves, neurologic assessment may be needed only once each shift. Findings are documented according to agency protocol. A special spinal cord assessment flow sheet may be used to document sensory and/or motor findings for the patient with a spinal cord injury. If GBS does not improve, respiratory failure may result in death.

Light touch discrimination is likely to be normal if pain and temperature sensory tracts are intact. For testing *touch discrimination*, patients first close their eyes. The nurse touches the patient with a finger and asks that the patient point to the area touched. This procedure is repeated on each extremity at random rather than at sequential points. Next, the nurse touches the patient on each side of the body on corresponding sites at the same time. The patient should be able to point to both sites (Jarvis & Eckhardt, 2024).

Pain and other abnormal sensory findings may have a CNS or a PNS cause. For example, the neuropathies of diabetes mellitus, malnutrition, and vascular problems have a PNS cause. For patients who report neuropathic pain, perform a complete pain assessment as described in Chapter 6. Ask the patient about numbness or tingling and where those sensations are felt and when they occur.

Assessment of the Patient With Altered Consciousness

Although the patient may be unable to actively participate in the neurologic assessment, a number of functions should be tested for patients who have altered consciousness. If the patient is sedated, the neurologic assessment will probably be unreliable (Bell et al., 2021).

For a baseline-focused assessment the nurse includes four components, which include the following (Bell et al., 2021):

- Level of consciousness
- Cranial nerve status
- Motor response
- Vital signs

Assessment of Level of Consciousness. Assess the patient with altered consciousness for the depth or degree of alertness by using a standardized tool like the Glasgow Coma Scale (GCS) (Fig. 35.3). The GCS is used in many acute care settings to establish baseline data in each of these areas: eye opening, motor response, and verbal response. The patient is assigned a numeric score for each of these areas. The lower the score, the lower the patient's neurologic function. A fully alert patient has a total score of 15; a total score of 7 or less indicates the patient is comatose (Jarvis & Eckhardt, 2024). For patients who are intubated and cannot talk, record their score with a "t" after the number for verbal response.

If the patient does not follow commands or is unresponsive to voice, the nurse proceeds to increasingly noxious (painful) stimuli to elicit an eye and motor response. Failure to apply painful stimuli appropriately may lead to an incorrect conclusion about the patient's neurologic status.

Start with the least noxious irritation or pressure and proceed to more painful stimulation if the patient does not respond. Begin each phase of the assessment by speaking in a normal voice. If no response is obtained, use a loud voice. If you still see no response, gently shake the patient. The shaking should be similar to that used in attempting to wake up a child. If that is unsuccessful, apply painful stimuli by squeezing the trapezius muscle (shoulder) or applying nail bed pressure on one finger or toe on the right and left (Bell et al., 2021).

GLASGOW COMA SCALE*

Eye Opening
Spontaneous	4
To sound	3
To pain	2
Never	1

Motor Response
Obeys commands	6
Localizes pain	5
Normal flexion (withdrawal)	4
Abnormal flexion	3
Extension	2
None	1

Verbal Response
Oriented	5
Confused conversation	4
Inappropriate words	3
Incomprehensible sounds	2
None	1

* The highest possible score is 15.

FIG. 35.3 The Glasgow Coma Scale.

✚ NURSING SAFETY PRIORITY

Critical Rescue

A decrease of 2 or more points in the Glasgow Coma Scale total is clinically significant and should be communicated to the primary health care provider immediately. Other findings requiring urgent communication with the primary health care provider include a new finding of abnormal flexion or extension, particularly of the upper extremities (decerebrate or decorticate posturing); pinpoint or dilated nonreactive pupils; and sudden or subtle changes in mental status. *Remember, a change in level of consciousness is the earliest sign of neurologic deterioration and should be treated as an emergency!* Communicate early recognition of neurologic changes to the Rapid Response Team or primary health care provider for the best opportunity to prevent complications and preserve CNS function.

The patient may respond to painful stimuli in several ways. Although the initial response to pain may be abnormal flexion or extension, continued application of pain for no more than 20 to 30 seconds may demonstrate that the patient can localize or withdraw. If the patient does not respond after 20 to 30 seconds, stop applying the painful stimulus.

Assessment of Cranial Nerve Status. In a focused assessment of a patient with altered consciousness, include evaluation of the following (Bell et al., 2021):

- Pupil reaction, size, and shape (CN II and III)
- Corneal reflex (CN V and VII)
- Gag/cough reflex (CN IX and X)

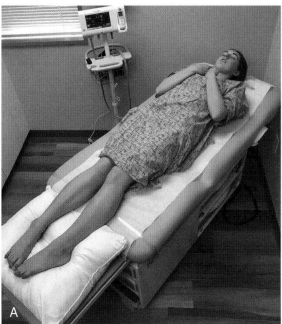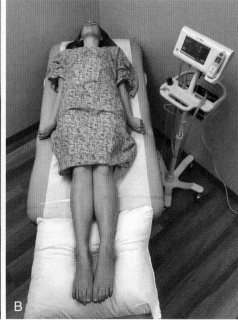

FIG. 35.4 Types of abnormal posturing. (A) Decorticate posturing. (B) Decerebrate posturing. (From Hollen, C. J., & Melton Stein, L. N. (2021). *Concept-based clinical nursing skills: Fundamental to advanced.* St. Louis: Elsevier.)

To assess the patient's *pupils,* open the eyes and observe for any abnormal eye movements, such as nystagmus. Nystagmus is involuntary eye movement that may cause the eyes to rapidly move from side to side, up and down, or in a circle. Assess the size and shape of the pupil. The pupils should be equal and round, as described earlier. An oval pupil indicates progressive damage to the oculomotor nerve (CN III). Assess the pupils' reaction to light, and measure size using a pupillometer, if available, or use a millimeter scale.

If the patient is comatose, assess for *corneal reflex* to ensure that eyes are protected to prevent corneal abrasions (Bell et al., 2021). Use a small piece of cotton on the eyelid and observe for blinking. Avoid making direct contact with the cornea to prevent abrasion.

If unsure about whether the patient has a *gag/cough reflex,* assess the patient by lightly touching the back of the tongue with a tongue blade. The patient with an intact reflex will have immediate elevation of the palate and constriction of the muscles of the pharynx.

Assessment of Motor Response. Observe the patient for movement, being sure to compare the right and left sides. Note any asymmetry or abnormal positions of the head, extremities, and trunk of the body. If the patient has no spontaneous movement, lift the patient's arms one at a time and let them drop to the bed. A weak or paralyzed arm falls more freely than one that has intact muscle innervation (Bell et al., 2021).

Abnormal posturing may occur in patients who are comatose. Decortication is abnormal motor movement seen in the patient with lesions that interrupt the corticospinal pathways (Fig. 35.4A). The patient's arms, wrists, and fingers are flexed with internal rotation and plantar flexion of the legs. Decerebration is abnormal movement with rigidity characterized by extension of the arms and legs, pronation of the arms, plantar flexion, and opisthotonos (body spasm in which the body is bowed forward) (Fig. 35.4B). Decerebration is usually associated with brainstem dysfunction.

Assessment of Vital Signs. The brainstem regulates blood pressure, heart rate, and respirations. When intracranial pressure (ICP) increases, the Cushing reflex is triggered, causing hypertension with a widened pulse pressure, bradycardia, and irregular respiratory rate. Therefore, assessing vital signs frequently in patients with altered consciousness is a vital part of the neurologic assessment.

Psychosocial Assessment

Patients vary in their responses to a suspected or actual health problem, often depending on whether it is acute or chronic. Response is also influenced by the patient's **mobility**, **sensory perception,** and/or **cognition.** These abilities can be temporarily or permanently altered as a result of neurologic disease or injury. For example, patients who have a mild stroke and no lasting neurologic deficits are less likely to be severely depressed than patients who experience a loss of independent movement or impaired communication as a result of a stroke. Cultural and spiritual factors affecting response to neurologic health problems are described in the Patient-Centered Care: Culture and Spirituality box.

PATIENT-CENTERED CARE: CULTURE AND SPIRITUALITY

Patient Response to Neurologic Health Problems

Age may also be a factor in how a patient accepts the illness. For instance, a young adult who has a motorcycle crash causing a traumatic brain injury (TBI) may react differently from an older adult who has a spinal injury. In some cases, the patient's emotional responses result from the health problem itself, especially for TBI patients.

Regardless of what the health problem is, do not assume that everyone reacts the same way to illness or injury. Consider the cultural and spiritual backgrounds of patients because these factors may influence their reactions. Patients experiencing the grieving process may fluctuate among denial, anger, and depression. Encourage patients to express their feelings and have hope. Assess the patient's support systems, including family members and friends, if available. Be sure to document your assessment in the electronic health record.

Depression can result in cognitive and behavioral changes that are similar to delirium or dementia. Depression is a common mental health disorder that is often missed in a variety of health care settings, especially in settings that care for older adults (Touhy & Jett, 2022). Consider using a depression screening tool such as the Center for Epidemiological Studies Depression-Revised (CESD-R) or the Geriatric Depression Scale (short form) to identify patients with depressive symptoms. Refer patients to the appropriate provider (both primary care and mental health care) if the screening is positive. Chapter 4 briefly discusses depression in older adults. More information on depression can be found in mental/behavioral health resources.

Diagnostic Assessment

Laboratory Assessment

Fluid, electrolyte, and glucose abnormalities can cause neurologic impairment. The basic metabolic panel (BMP) and serum calcium, phosphorus, and magnesium are evaluated. Both anemia and malnutrition can contribute to neurologic disorders, so a complete blood count and serum levels of prealbumin, albumin, and minerals/vitamins (particularly B vitamins) may be collected.

For patients with a neurologic problem resulting from an infection, cultures are necessary to identify the pathogen. Although the cause of infection must be determined for any patient, this is especially true for those with existing CNS disease. The blood-brain barrier (BBB) is often not intact in neurologic disease; and the patient is more likely to get an infection of the nervous system, such as meningitis or encephalitis.

Imaging Assessment

Radiography. Plain *x-rays* of the skull and spine are used to determine bony fractures, curvatures, bone erosion, bone dislocation, and possible calcification of soft tissue, which can damage the nervous system. Several views are taken (i.e., anteroposterior, lateral, oblique, and, when necessary, special views of the facial bones). *In head trauma and multiple injuries, after assessing the ABCs (airway, breathing, and circulation), one of the first priorities is to rule out cervical spine fracture.* Explain that the x-ray procedure for the skull and spine is similar to that for a chest x-ray. The patient must remain still during the procedure.

Computed tomography (CT) scanning is accurate, quick, easy, noninvasive, painless, and the least expensive method of diagnosing neurologic problems. Using x-rays (i.e., ionizing radiation), pictures are taken at many horizontal levels, or slices, of the brain or spinal cord. A computer then generates three-dimensional detailed anatomic pictures of tissues, typically the brain, spinal cord, or peripheral neuromuscular system in neurologic testing. A contrast medium may be used to enhance the image. CT scans distinguish bone, soft tissue (e.g., the brain, vascular system, ventricular system), and fluids such as cerebrospinal fluid (CSF) or blood. Tumors, infarctions, hemorrhage, hydrocephalus, and bone malformations can also be identified.

The patient is placed on a movable table in a head-holding device and is instructed to remain completely still during the test. Most patients with new cranial neurologic symptoms have both a precontrast and postcontrast study of the head. Contrast-enhanced CT is especially useful in locating and identifying tumor types and abscesses. For situations in which bleeding is the only concern (e.g., in trauma patients), contrast scans are not usually required.

After a standard CT scan, imaging software digitally removes images of soft tissue so that only images of bone remain. Through the use of this technology, bone deformities, trauma, and birth defects are more easily identified.

CT angiography involves administering contrast dye IV before the CT scan. It is used to identify blockages or narrowing of blood vessels, aneurysms, and other blood vessel abnormalities. A *CT perfusion study* is an important tool in the evaluation of patients with acute strokelike symptoms. These symptoms have several causes, and the cause must be determined as quickly as possible so that the correct treatment can begin for optimal outcomes. Perfusion CT is performed using an advanced CT scanner with a special software system. For the patient, though, it will seem like a standard CT examination.

An intrathecal contrast-enhanced CT scan is performed to diagnose disorders of the spine and spinal nerve roots. A lumbar puncture (LP) is performed so that a small amount of spinal fluid can be removed and mixed with contrast dye and injected. The patient is positioned to allow for the contrast medium to move around the spinal cord and nerve roots as needed. The patient may have a headache after the procedure. Follow facility policy regarding patient positioning after the procedure.

NCLEX Examination Challenge 35.2

Physiological Integrity

The nurse assesses a nonresponsive client using the Glasgow Coma Scale and determines the client's total score is 6. How would the nurse interpret this finding?

A. The client is alert and awake.
B. The client is drowsy and lethargic.
C. The client is stuporous.
D. The client is comatose.

Magnetic Resonance Imaging. Magnetic resonance imaging (MRI or MR) has advantages over CT in the diagnostic imaging of the brain, spinal cord, and nerve roots. It does not use ionizing radiation but instead relies on magnetic fields. Multiple sets of images are taken to determine normal and abnormal anatomy. Images may be enhanced with the use of gadolinium, a non–iodine-based contrast medium. MRIs of the spine have largely replaced CT scans and myelography for evaluation. Bony structures cannot be viewed with MRI; CT scans are the best way to see bones. Some facilities have a *functional MRI (fMRI)* machine that can assess blood flow to the brain rather than merely show its anatomic structure.

In addition to the traditional MRI, *magnetic resonance angiography (MRA), magnetic resonance spectroscopy (MRS),* or *diffusion imaging (DI)* may be requested. MRA is used to evaluate perfusion and blood vessel abnormalities such as an arterial blockage, intracranial aneurysms, and arteriovenous (AV) malformations. MRS is used to detect abnormalities in the brain's biochemical processes, such as that which occurs in epilepsy, Alzheimer's disease, and brain attack (stroke). Diffuse imaging uses MRI techniques to evaluate ischemia in the brain to determine the location and severity of a stroke.

Open-sided units ("open MRI") produce adequate images for patients who are claustrophobic or do not want standard MRI scanners. However, image quality from these scanners is not as good as that from long-bore traditional scanners. Traditional scanners have higher magnetic field strength and provide better resolution, especially for patients with neurologic health problems (Fig. 35.5).

In the past, MRI has been contraindicated for patients with cardiac pacemakers, other implanted pumps or devices, and ion-containing metal aneurysm clips. However, newer pacemakers and internal defibrillators may be scanned, depending on the type of device. Other implanted devices, such as vascular stents, intravascular catheter (IVC) filters, and metal antiembolic devices, may be scanned immediately or after a certain period of time, depending on manufacturer recommendations. MRI may also be contraindicated in patients who are confused or agitated, have unstable vital signs, are on continuous life support, or have older tattoos (which contain lead). New physiologic monitoring systems made specifically for the scanner allow some patients who are unstable to be scanned. A comprehensive online list of medical devices tested for MRI safety and compatibility can be found at www.mrisafety.com. Medical personnel must remove any medical devices they are carrying or wearing and ensure that only approved devices are allowed in the MRI room.

Computed Tomography–Positron Emission Tomography. Combination CT-PET scanners fuse images together to produce detailed information about the type and location of neurologic dysfunction. They are particularly useful in staging brain, spinal cord, and other primary cancers. The physician or nuclear medicine technologist injects the patient with IV deoxyglucose, which is tagged to an isotope. The isotope emits activity in the form of positrons, which are scanned and converted into a color image by computer. The more active a given part of the brain, the greater the glucose uptake. This test is used to evaluate drug

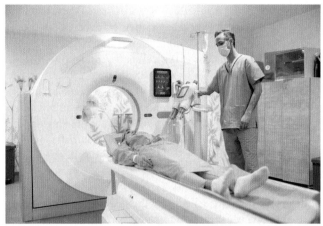

FIG. 35.5 Radiologist preparing a patient for a magnetic resonance imaging (MRI) machine scan. (Used with permission from istockphoto.com, 2022, andresr.)

metabolism and detect areas of metabolic alteration that occur in dementia, epilepsy, psychiatric and degenerative disorders, neoplasms, and Alzheimer's disease. The level of radiation is equivalent to that of five or six x-rays but much less than exposure during CT.

Teach patients that they will be NPO the night before morning testing and 4 hours before afternoon testing. Patients with diabetes have their test in the morning before taking their antidiabetic drugs. During this 2- to 3-hour procedure, the patient may be blindfolded and have earplugs inserted for all or part of the test. Patients are asked to perform certain mental functions to activate different areas of the brain. Older adults and patients with mental health/behavioral health problems may be too anxious to have a CT-PET scan.

Single-Photon Emission Computed Tomography. Single-photon emission computed tomography (SPECT) uses a radiopharmaceutical agent to enable radioisotopes to cross the BBB. The agent is administered by IV injection. Gamma-emitting radionuclides have longer half-lives, therefore eliminating the need for a cyclotron near the scanner. Although SPECT is less expensive than PET, the resolution of the images is limited. SPECT is particularly useful in studying cerebral blood flow, neoplasms, head trauma, or persistent vegetative state. The test is contraindicated in women who are breast-feeding.

The patient is injected with the material about 1 hour before the actual scan by the radiologist, certified nuclear medicine technologist, or specially trained RN. The patient is positioned on an x-ray table in a quiet dark room for the actual scans. Several gamma cameras scan the patient's head. When completed, the images are downloaded to a computer.

Magnetoencephalography. Magnetoencephalography (MEG) is a noninvasive imaging technique used to measure the magnetic fields produced by electrical activity in the brain via extremely sensitive devices such as superconducting quantum interference devices (SQUIDs). MEG is somewhat similar to electroencephalography (EEG). The advantage is greater accuracy because of the minimal distortion of the signal. This allows for more usable and reliable localization of brain function. The brain can be observed "in action" rather than just from viewing a still magnetic resonance image. These machines are not widely available because of their extremely high cost.

Cerebral Angiography. Cerebral angiography (arteriography) may be done to visualize the cerebral circulation to detect blockages in the arteries or veins in the brain, head, or neck that impair **perfusion**. It remains the gold standard for the diagnosis of intracranial vascular disease and is required for any transcatheter therapy or for surgical intervention. Angiography may be used to identify aneurysms, traumatic injuries, strictures/occlusions, tumors, blood vessel displacement from edema, and AV malformations.

Patient Preparation. Risk factors for adverse events must be determined before scheduling the test. Patients sensitive to iodine may be sensitive to iodinated contrast agents. Patients with a history of hypersensitivity in general (e.g., multiple food allergies or asthma) are more likely than the general population to have an adverse reaction. Seafood allergies are no longer considered an indicator of iodinated contrast allergy. Patients with known contrast sensitivity are pretreated with steroids. Box 35.3 summarizes the precautions that must be taken for patients having any test using contrast agents.

To minimize the risk for aspiration during the procedure, assess for the presence of nausea or recent vomiting and medicate as needed before the test. Ensure that the patient is NPO 4 to 6 hours before the test. Assess and document neurologic signs, vital signs, and neurovascular checks.

Reinforce these important points:
- Your head is immobilized during the procedure.
- Do not move during the procedure.
- Contrast dye is injected through a catheter placed in the femoral artery. You will feel a warm or hot sensation when the dye is injected; this is normal.
- You will be able to talk to health care professionals during the procedure; let them know if you are in pain or have any concerns.

Procedure. The patient is placed on an examining table and made as comfortable as possible. At this time, dentures and hearing aids must be removed. The patient is then connected to cardiac monitoring throughout the procedure. Deep or moderate sedation is usually not used, although the patient may be given medication for relaxation.

The interventional radiologist or other specially trained physician numbs the area at the groin and inserts a catheter into the femoral artery. Under fluoroscopic guidance, the catheter is advanced into a carotid or vertebral artery. Then the physician injects contrast material into each vessel while recording images from different angles over the head and neck. After all the vessels have been imaged, the radiologist reviews all the images and consults with the referring physician to decide whether the patient could benefit from a therapeutic radiologic procedure or surgery. An arterial closure device is typically used to seal the artery and prevent bleeding.

The x-ray images are stored on a computer. With older equipment, a two-dimensional picture of the vessels is produced. Most radiographic systems now come with software to create three-dimensional images of the blood vessels in the head and/or neck. These systems can also display a "subtracted

---

BOX 35.3 Best Practice for Patient Safety and Quality Care

Precautions for Use of Contrast for Neurologic Diagnostic Testing

Special precautions are taken for patients who will receive an iodinated or high-osmolar contrast agent (e.g., gadolinium) as part of their diagnostic test. These measures include:

- Following agency guidelines regarding informed consent.
- Screening patients at risk for developing contrast-induced kidney damage:
  - Ask the patient about all allergies (food, drug, environmental antigens), asthma, and prior reaction to contrast agents.
  - Review for the presence of these conditions:
    - Preexisting renal disease such as a diagnosis of chronic kidney disease
    - Diabetic nephropathy
    - Heart failure
    - Dehydration
    - Older age
    - Drugs that interfere with renal perfusion such as metformin or NSAIDs
    - Administration of contrast media in the previous 72 hours
- Evaluating current kidney function. Patients with a serum creatinine greater than or equal to 1.5 mg/dL *or* a calculated glomerular filtration rate (GFR) of less than 60 mL/min are at highest risk for kidney damage from contrast media.
- Communicating with the primary health care provider before diagnostic testing when risk factors and allergic reaction to iodinated contrast are present:
  - Consider including a discussion of the patient's serum creatinine as a component of the "time-out" process before a diagnostic procedure.
  - Document the date, time, and name of the primary health care provider with whom communication of risk occurred and which actions were prescribed, if any.
  - Hold drugs that are associated with kidney damage for 24 to 48 hours before *and* after the test.
- Providing adequate hydration before and after contrast administration:
  - Collaborate with the primary health care provider to determine whether hydration before the diagnostic test, typically with IV normal saline, is needed. Bicarbonate with normal saline or an IV dose of *N*-acetylcysteine may be used in a high-risk patient.
  - Determine the optimal postdiagnostic intake and output. Provide sufficient hydration to flush out the contrast with oral or IV fluids over the 4 to 5 hours following the test.
- Reevaluating serum creatinine and glomerular filtration rate (GFR) 24 to 48 hours after the diagnostic test. Report an increase of serum creatinine 0.5 mg/dL above baseline and a decrease in GFR greater than 25% to the primary health care provider. Document SBAR communication and follow-up interventions, if any. The peak creatinine rise is typically at 48 to 72 hours after the administration of contrast.

---

image" made from two images—one just before the contrast was injected and one with the contrast in the artery.

Follow-up Care. Follow agency policy regarding nursing care of the injection entry site, which may include the following:
- Check the dressing for bleeding and swelling around the site.
- Apply an ice pack to the site.
- Keep the extremity straight and immobilized.
- Maintain the pressure dressing for 2 hours.

Check the extremity for adequate circulation to include skin color and temperature, pulses distal to the injection site, and capillary refill. Monitor blood pressure and pulse frequently for indications of internal bleeding; if bleeding occurs, the client's blood pressure would decrease and the pulse would increase. Assess neurologic status for changes, including a decrease in LOC or a new onset of weakness or paralysis.

✚ NURSING SAFETY PRIORITY

Critical Rescue

Be sure to monitor for the risks of the procedure, including contrast reaction (usually manifested by hives and flushing), thrombosis (clotting), and bleeding from the entry site. A contrast reaction usually occurs during the procedure, but thrombosis and bleeding occur after the procedure. *If bleeding occurs at the injection entry site, maintain manual pressure on the site and notify the primary health care provider or Rapid Response Team immediately!* Increase IV fluid rate unless contraindicated. Document all nursing assessments and interventions.

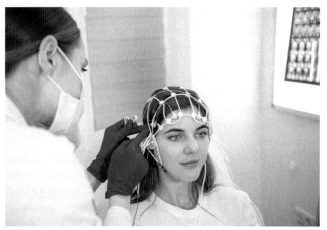

FIG. 35.6 Patient having an electroencephalogram to detect seizure activity. (Used with permission from istockphoto.com, 2021, romaset.)

Electromyography

Electromyography (EMG) is used to identify nerve and muscle disorders, as well as spinal cord disease. During EMG, recording electrodes are placed onto skeletal muscles to monitor their electrical activity. A progressive decrease in the amplitude of the electric waveform is a classic sign of several neuromuscular diseases, such as myasthenia gravis, a rare progressive autoimmune disease characterized by muscle weakness as a result of impaired acetylcholine receptors. EMG and electroneurography, or nerve-conduction studies, are usually used together and are referred to as *electromyoneurography.*

Electroencephalography

Electroencephalography (EEG) records the electrical activity of the cerebral hemispheres. The frequency, amplitude, and characteristics of the brain waves are recorded. Certain illnesses or health problems can cause changes in brain waves. For example, a cerebral tumor or infarct may have abnormally slow waveforms.

Fasting is avoided before EEG testing because hypoglycemia can alter the test results. Ensure that hair is clean and without conditioners, hair creams, lotions, sprays, or styling gels. Teach the patient to avoid the use of sedatives or stimulants in the 12 to 24 hours preceding the EEG. Ensure a quiet room with signage to inform visitors of EEG recording in progress. Instruct the patient or family members about the reasons for periodic or continuous monitoring. The reasons for EEG monitoring include:

- Determining the general activity of the cerebral hemispheres
- Determining the origin of seizure activity (such as epilepsy)
- Determining cerebral function in epilepsy and other pathologic conditions such as tumors, abscesses, cerebrovascular disease, hematomas, injury, metabolic diseases, degenerative brain disease, and drug intoxication
- Differentiating between organic and hysterical blindness or deafness
- Monitoring cerebral activity during surgical anesthesia or sedation in the intensive care unit
- Diagnosing sleep disorders (If the EEG is related to a sleep disorder diagnosis, the patient may be asked to sleep less the night before the EEG.)
- Assisting in the determination of brain death

The patient is placed on a reclining chair or bed. Multiple electrodes are applied to the scalp with a jellylike substance and connected to the machine. The physician or EEG technician places glue over the electrodes to prevent slippage (Fig. 35.6). The patient must lie still with both eyes closed during the initial recording. The rest of the test engages the patient in certain activities: hyperventilation, photic stimulation, and sleep. A portable EEG may be performed at the bedside if necessary, but the preference is for the EEG to be done in a very quiet room.

Hyperventilation produces cerebral vasoconstriction and alkalosis, which increase the likelihood of seizure activity. The patient is asked to breathe deeply 20 times per minute for 3 minutes. In *photic stimulation,* a flashing bright light is placed in front of the patient. Frequencies of 1 to 20 flashes per second are used with the patient's eyes open and then closed. If the patient's seizures are photosensitive in origin, seizure activity may be seen on the EEG. A *sleep* EEG may be performed to aid in the detection of abnormal brain waves that are seen only when the patient is sleeping, such as with frontal lobe epilepsy.

During an EEG test, which takes 45 to 120 minutes, the recording can be stopped about every 5 minutes to allow the patient to move. If the patient moves during the recording, movement creates a change in the brain waves and the technician will note movements on the graph. Examples of unintentional movement that can affect the recordings are tongue movement, eye blinking, and muscle tensing. The technician may induce or request certain movements or sensory stimulation and record these events on the EEG record to link changes in brain waves with motor activity or sensory stimulation; these intentional movements are also documented on the EEG recording.

The gel and glue used for placing electrodes can be washed out immediately after the test ends. Acetone or witch hazel will dissolve the paste. Advise the patient who is scheduled for a sleep-deprived EEG to arrange for someone else to drive the patient home.

Evoked Potentials

Evoked potentials (also called *evoked response*) measure the electrical signals to the brain generated by sound, touch, or light. These tests are used to assess sensory nerve problems and confirm neurologic conditions, including multiple sclerosis, brain tumor, acoustic neuroma (small tumors of the inner ear), and spinal cord injury. Evoked potentials are also used to monitor brain activity in comatose patients and confirm brain death. During evoked potentials, a second set of electrodes is attached to the part of the body that will experience sensation. A stimulus is applied, and the amount of time it takes for the impulse generated by the stimulus to reach the brain is recorded. Under normal circumstances, the process of signal transmission is instantaneous.

Auditory evoked potentials (also called *brainstem auditory evoked response*) are used to assess high-frequency hearing loss, diagnose any damage to the acoustic nerve and auditory pathways in the brainstem, and detect acoustic neuromas. The patient sits in a soundproof room and wears headphones. Clicking sounds are delivered one at a time to one ear while a masking sound is sent to the other ear.

Visual evoked potentials detect loss of vision from optic nerve damage (in particular, damage caused by multiple sclerosis). The patient sits close to a screen and is asked to focus on the center of a shifting checkerboard pattern. Only one eye is tested at a time. The other eye is either kept closed or covered with a patch.

Somatosensory evoked potentials measure response from stimuli to the peripheral nerves and can detect nerve or spinal cord damage or nerve degeneration from multiple sclerosis and other degenerating diseases. Tiny electrical shocks are delivered by electrode to a nerve in an arm or leg.

Lumbar Puncture

Lumbar puncture (spinal tap) is the insertion of a spinal needle into the subarachnoid space between the third and fourth (sometimes the fourth and fifth) lumbar vertebrae. A lumbar puncture (LP) is used to:
- Obtain cerebrospinal fluid (CSF) pressure readings with a manometer
- Obtain CSF for analysis
- Check for spinal blockage caused by a spinal cord lesion
- Inject contrast medium or air for diagnostic study
- Inject selected drugs

Because of the danger of sudden release of CSF pressure, an LP is not done for patients with symptoms indicating severely increased intracranial pressure (ICP). The procedure is also not performed in patients with skin infections at or near the puncture site because of the danger of introducing infective organisms into the CSF.

> ### ⚠ NURSING SAFETY PRIORITY
> #### *Action Alert*
>
> It is very important that the patient not move during a lumbar puncture. If the patient is restless or cannot cooperate, two people may need to assist instead of one. The patient may need a sedative to reduce movement. Consider patient needs for additional assistance or sedation before beginning the procedure.

In preparation for the procedure, position the patient in a fetal side-lying position to separate the vertebrae and move the spinal nerve roots away from the area to be accessed. The primary health care provider then cleans the skin site thoroughly. The injection site is determined, and a local anesthetic is injected. In a few minutes, a spinal needle is inserted between the third and fourth lumbar vertebrae. Instruct the patient to inform the primary health care provider if there is shooting pain or a tingling sensation. After determining proper placement in the subarachnoid space by removing the stylet and seeing CSF, the patient is asked to relax as much as possible so that the pressure reading will be accurate. Opening and closing pressure readings are taken and recorded. The normal opening pressure should be no more than 20 cm H_2O; the CSF should be clear and colorless and contain only a few cells. Three to five test tubes of CSF are usually collected and numbered sequentially. After specimen collection, the needle is withdrawn, slight pressure is applied, and an adhesive bandage strip is placed over the insertion site.

Examination of CSF has been a useful diagnostic tool for some time. Recent technical advances are increasing the number of analyses that can be done on CSF. Gram stain smears can test for particular types of meningitis, such as tubercular meningitis. CSF can be cultured, and sensitivity studies determine the best choice of antibiotic if an infection is diagnosed. A specific test for neurosyphilis is the fluorescent treponemal antibody absorption (FTA-ABS) test. Cytologic studies of CSF can identify tumor cells.

Obtain vital signs and perform frequent neurologic checks as directed by agency protocol. Follow agency policy regarding how long the patient should be on bed rest and remain flat. Encourage the patient to increase fluid intake unless contraindicated. Monitor for complications, especially increased ICP (severe headache, nausea, vomiting, photophobia, and change in level of consciousness). Serious complications of LP, although not common, include brainstem herniation (discussed in Chapter 38), infection, CSF leakage, and hematoma formation. Observe the needle insertion site for leakage and notify the primary health care provider if it occurs. Provide the prescribed medication for patient report of headache. Be sure to notify the health care provider if the medication does not relieve pain.

Transcranial Doppler Ultrasonography

Intracranial hemodynamics can be evaluated through the use of transcranial Doppler (TCD), which uses sound waves to measure blood flow through the arteries. The test is particularly valuable in evaluating cerebral vasospasm or narrowing of arteries. TCD is safe, can be used repeatedly for the same patient, and is an inexpensive alternative to angiography.

GET READY FOR THE NEXT-GENERATION NCLEX® EXAMINATION!

Essential Assessment Points

- The nervous system is comprised of the central nervous system (brain and spinal cord), peripheral nervous system (extremities), and autonomic nervous system (cranial nerves and organ innervation).
- Older adults typically experience neurologic changes associated with aging, including recent memory loss, decreased sensation, and altered balance, increasing their risk for falls.
- Nurses should assess for and document any preexisting physical disability or neurocognitive disorder such as dementia.
- Patients with neurologic problems often report neuropathic (nerve) pain, weakness, abnormal sensations, and/or cognitive changes.
- A focused neurologic assessment of patients who are alert and awake includes LOC, language and speech, selected cranial nerve status, movement and sensation, and vital signs.
- A focused neurologic assessment of patients with altered consciousness includes LOC, selected cranial nerve status, motor response, and vital signs.
- The Glasgow Coma Scale (GCS) is a commonly used tool for evaluating LOC. A fully alert and oriented patient will have a total score of 15; a score of 7 or less indicates the patient is comatose.
- Patients vary in their psychosocial response to neurologic disorders or trauma, often based on cultural and spiritual factors.
- Imaging procedures are commonly used to diagnose neurologic deficits or disorders, including plain x-rays, computed tomography (CT) scans, and a variety of magnetic resonance imaging (MRI) techniques.
- Cerebral angiography involves the use of contrast media to visualize cerebral circulation; nurses need to ensure that the patient's kidney function is adequate before the test and monitor the patient carefully for bleeding at the entry site.
- If bleeding occurs after cerebral angiography, apply manual pressure and contact the Rapid Response Team and health care provider immediately for this emergency.

Mastery Questions

1. The nurse is caring for a client who recently had a traumatic brain injury but has been alert and oriented all day. Which of the following assessments would the nurse carefully monitor to detect early changes in the client's condition?
   A. Level of consciousness
   B. Cranial nerve status
   C. Movement
   D. Sensation

2. The nurse is caring for a client who returned from the interventional radiology suite after cerebral angiography. Which of the following is the **most** important assessment for the nurse to monitor?
   A. Pain level
   B. Allergic response to contrast medium
   C. Blood pressure and pulse
   D. Cranial nerve status

REFERENCES

Banzon, P. C., Vashisht, A., Euckert, M., Nairon, E., Aiyagari, V., et al. (2023). Practice variations in documenting neurologic examinations in non-neuroscience ICUs, *American Journal of Nursing*, *123*(1), 24–31.

Bell, S. D., Lee, C.-C. T., Zeeman, J., Kearney, M., Macko, L., & Cartwright, C. C. (2021). *Neurological assessment of the adult hospitalized patient.* Chicago: American Association of Neuroscience Nurses.

Jarvis, C., & Eckhardt, A. (2024). *Physical examination & health assessment* (9th ed.). St. Louis: Elsevier.

Rogers, J. L. (2023). *McCance and Huether's Pathophysiology: The biologic basis for disease in adults and children* (9th ed.). St. Louis: Elsevier.

Smeltzer, S. C. (2021). Delivering quality healthcare for people with disability. Indianapolis. In *Sigma Theta Tau International Honor Society of Nursing*.

Touhy, T. A., & Jett, K. F. (2022). *Gerontological nursing and healthy aging* (6th ed.). St. Louis: Elsevier.

36

Concepts of Care for Patients With Conditions of the Central Nervous System: The Brain

Meg Blair

http://evolve.elsevier.com/Iggy/

PRIORITY AND INTERRELATED CONCEPTS

The priority concepts for this chapter are:
- *Cognition*
- *Mobility*

The *Cognition* concept exemplar for this chapter is Alzheimer's Disease.
The *Mobility* concept exemplar for this chapter is Parkinson's Disease.

The interrelated concepts for this chapter are:
- *Pain*
- *Infection*

Neurologic disorders can interfere with self-management and functional ability; many of them cause impaired *cognition,* decreased *mobility,* and persistent *pain. Infection* can also cause neurologic problems. For example, many individuals who had COVID-19 infections during the pandemic have persistent cognitive deficits. Chapter 3 briefly reviews these health concepts. Care of patients with health problems affecting the brain requires coordination by nurses and interprofessional collaboration.

COGNITION CONCEPT EXEMPLAR: ALZHEIMER'S DISEASE

Pathophysiology Review

Dementia, sometimes referred to as a *chronic confusional state* or *syndrome,* is a general term for progressive loss of brain function and impaired *cognition*; there are many types of dementia. Alzheimer's disease (AD) is clinically considered the most common type of dementia that affects people older than 65 years. Vascular dementia, such as *multi-infarct dementia,* results from strokes or other vascular disorders that decrease blood flow to

parts of the brain (Rogers, 2023). Table 36.1 compares AD with vascular dementia, another common type of dementia.

Recent research has focused on AD as a pathophysiologic process rather than a type of dementia. Biomarkers, especially abnormal levels of beta amyloid and tau proteins, can be used to diagnose AD in the preclinical phase before dementia symptoms occur. Not every individual with preclinical AD develops dementia, but they are at an increased risk for the disease (Smedinga et al., 2021).

Dementia is not a normal physiologic change of aging. The brain of the older adult usually weighs less and occupies less space in the cranium than does the brain of a younger person. Other age-related changes in the brain include widening of the cerebral sulci, narrowing of the gyri, and enlargement of the ventricles. In the presence of AD and other types of dementia, these normal changes are greatly accelerated, causing further reductions in brain weight. COVID-19 infection also accelerated AD pathology and symptoms during the pandemic. Marked atrophy of the cerebral cortex and loss of cortical neurons result in the classic symptoms associated with AD dementia (Rogers, 2023).

Microscopic changes of the brain found in people with AD include neurofibrillary tangles, amyloid-rich neuritic plaques, and vascular degeneration. *Neurofibrillary tangles* are composed of twisted fibrous tissue containing abnormal amounts of the tau protein. They impair the ability of impulses to be transmitted from neuron to neuron (Rogers, 2023).

Neuritic plaques are composed of degenerating nerve terminals and are found particularly in the hippocampus, an important part of the limbic system. Deposited within the plaques are increased amounts of an abnormal protein called *beta amyloid.* These proteins have a tendency to accumulate and form the neurotoxic plaques found in the brain that impair neuronal transmission (Rogers, 2023).

Although *vascular degeneration* occurs in the normally aging brain, its presence is significantly increased in patients with

TABLE 36.1	Comparison of the Two Major Types of Dementia: Alzheimer's Disease and Vascular Dementia	
	Alzheimer's Disease	**Vascular Dementia**
Cause	Genetic and environmental factors; possibly viral	Strokes or other vascular disorders that decrease blood flow to the brain
Pathophysiologic changes	Chronic, terminal disease that is characterized by formation of neuritic plaques, neurofibrillary tangles, and vascular degeneration in the brain	Impaired blood flow to the brain, causing ischemia or necrosis of brain neurons
Course of dementia	Steady and gradual decline of cognitive, mobility, and ADL function from mild through severe stages; patients usually die from complications of immobility	Stepwise progression of dementia symptoms that get significantly worse after each vascular event, such as a stroke or series of ministrokes; symptoms may improve as collateral circulation to vital neurons develops
Risk factors	Female Over 65 years of age Down syndrome Traumatic brain injury	Male Over 65 years of age History of diabetes mellitus (DM), high cholesterol, myocardial infarction, atherosclerosis, hypertension, smoking, obesity
Management	Safety measures to prevent injury, wandering, or falls Cholinesterase inhibitors Behavior management ADL and mobility assistance as needed based on stage	Identification of risk factors and management of the risk for or actual vascular event (e.g., antidiabetes drugs for DM, antihypertensive drugs, low-fat diet, smoking cessation, weight loss) Safety measures to prevent injury or falls Behavior management

dementia. Vascular degeneration accounts for at least partial loss of the ability of nerve cells to function properly. This pathologic change contributes to the cognitive decline and mortality associated with AD.

In addition to the structural changes in the brain associated with this disorder, abnormalities in the neurotransmitters (acetylcholine [ACh], norepinephrine, dopamine, and serotonin) may occur. High levels of beta amyloid can reduce the amount of acetyltransferase in the hippocampus. This loss is important because the decrease in ACh interferes with cholinergic innervation to the cerebral cortex. This change results in impaired *cognition,* recent memory, and the ability to acquire new memories.

Etiology and Genetic Risk

The exact cause of AD is unknown. Age, gender, and genetics are the most studied risk factors. Age is strongly linked to the incidence of AD for people older than 65, and women are more likely to develop the disease than men (Rogers, 2023). As older adults age further, they become more at risk for the disease.

Recent research has demonstrated that during menopause, increased serum follicle-stimulating hormone (FSH) binds to FSH receptors on neurons in the brain, activating the pathway that accelerates formation of amyloid plaques and tau protein (Xiong et al., 2022). These abnormal proteins impair neuronal transmission as described in the Pathophysiology Review section.

Common risk factors for AD and other dementias include cardiovascular disease, decreased hearing, smoking, and depression. Other risk factors for AD have been studied, including traumatic brain injury (TBI), environmental agents, inflammation, immunologic changes, excessive stress, and sleep deprivation. There is also a high incidence of AD in people who have Down syndrome (Alzheimer's Association, 2022; Denning & Aldridge, 2021).

 PATIENT-CENTERED CARE: VETERAN HEALTH

Relationship of Traumatic Brain Injury and Alzheimer's Disease

Veterans who have experienced a traumatic brain injury (TBI) and those with posttraumatic stress disorder (PTSD) are more likely to develop dementia than veterans without these risk factors. Research has demonstrated high levels of tau protein accumulation in the brains of many veterans, making them at high risk for early-onset Alzheimer's disease (AD) (Mohamed et al., 2019). Veterans exposed to chemical weapons have shown decreases in brain volume in areas that correspond to similar findings in patients with AD (Chao, 2020).

 PATIENT-CENTERED CARE: GENETICS/ GENOMICS

Alzheimer's Disease

There is little doubt that there are genetic factors that increase the risk for developing Alzheimer's disease (AD). The most well-established genetic factor for AD in Whites is apolipoprotein E *(APOE),* a protein that transports cholesterol. Individuals who have one or more of the e4 forms of the protein are at higher risk for AD; however, they may not actually develop the disease (Alzheimer's Association, 2022).

Incidence and Prevalence

There is a significant increase in both the incidence and prevalence of AD after 65 years of age, although the disease may affect anyone older than 40 years. Although not common, when AD is diagnosed in people in their 40s and 50s, it is referred to as *younger/early-onset Alzheimer's disease.*

One in nine people in the United States over 65 years of age has AD; 72% are age 75 years or older. It is the sixth leading cause of death and one of the major causes of mental health disability in older adults (Navia & Constantine, 2022).

 PATIENT-CENTERED CARE: HEALTH EQUITY

Dementia and Social Determinants of Health

Black individuals have twice the risk of developing AD or other dementias compared with Whites; Hispanics have about a 1½ times higher risk (Alzheimer's Association, 2022). Recent research indicates that selected social determinants of health (SDOH) lead to the higher risk of AD and other dementias in these minority populations when compared with Whites, including (Majoka & Schimming, 2021):
- Lower socioeconomic status
- Low educational level
- Performance of manual labor jobs
- Lack of food security
- Decreased social interaction or social isolation
- Increased stress

Lack of access to health care may also contribute to differences in health equity. Nurses need to assess for the presence of these social determinants of health (SDOH) and incorporate them into the patient's plan of care, as discussed later.

Health Promotion/Disease Prevention

There are no proven ways to prevent AD; however, research is ongoing. Many patients with AD have other chronic health problems, such as diabetes mellitus, strokes, and atherosclerosis. Maintaining a healthy lifestyle helps prevent these conditions and can assist in controlling them. Eating a well-balanced diet and exercising not only increase muscle tone and strength but also may decrease cognitive decline. Potentially harmful lifestyle habits that increase the individual's risk of stroke and cardiovascular disease should be avoided, such as smoking and excessive alcohol intake. Be aware that some patients may not be able to consume a well-balanced diet due to food insecurity. Other patients may not engage in exercise or other self-care strategies due to high stress about the ability to meet basic needs such as housing or food. Teach patients about community resources that can assist individuals who are struggling to meet these needs.

Interprofessional Collaborative Care
Recognize Cues: Assessment

History. A thorough history and physical assessment are necessary to differentiate AD from other, possibly reversible, causes of impaired *cognition.* Some patients experience cognitive impairment as acute confusion (delirium). Table 3.1 in Chapter 3 compares dementia and delirium. Patients who have dementia are at an increased risk of delirium when hospitalized or admitted to an assisted-living or long-term care (LTC) setting.

Obtain information from family members or significant others because the patient may be unaware of cognitive changes, deny their existence, or cover them up. Some family members often do not recognize or may deny early changes in their loved one as well. Others may recognize subtle changes early in the disease process.

The most important information to be obtained is the onset, duration, progression, and course of the symptoms. Question the patient and the family about changes in memory or increasing forgetfulness and about the ability to perform ADLs or instrumental activities of daily living (IADLs). Ask about current employment status; work history; military history; and ability to fulfill household responsibilities, including cleaning, grocery shopping, and preparing meals. Inquire about changes in driving ability, ability to handle routine financial transactions, and language and communication skills. In addition, document any changes in personality and behavior. Assessing functional status for complex chronic conditions such as dementia is a recommended core measure by the Centers for Medicare and Medicaid Services.

Physical Assessment/Signs and Symptoms

Stages of Alzheimer's Disease. The Alzheimer's Association (2022) in the United States recognizes an asymptomatic preclinical phase during which changes are occurring in the brain, followed by three clinical phases of AD:

- Early stage (mild)
- Moderate stage (moderate)
- Late stage (severe)

When assessing the patient, recall that AD is a chronic, progressive disease that has an overall predictable course. However, the patient does not necessarily progress from one stage to the next in an orderly fashion. A stage may be bypassed, or patients may exhibit symptoms of one or several stages. Each patient exhibits different disease stages and signs and symptoms. Consequently, most authorities recognize AD as a continuum (Haney, 2020). The typical symptoms and behaviors associated with the three clinical phases are outlined in Box 36.1 (Rogers, 2023).

Changes in Cognition. As defined in Chapter 3, *cognition* is the complex integration of mental processes and intellectual function for the purposes of reasoning, learning, and memory. Therefore assess the patient for deficits in these abilities:

- Attention and concentration
- Judgment and perception
- Learning and memory
- Communication and language
- Speed of information processing

One of the first symptoms of AD is short-term memory impairment. New memory and defects in information retrieval result from dysfunction in the hippocampal, frontal, or parietal region. Alterations in communication abilities, such as apraxia (inability to form words or use objects correctly), aphasia (inability to speak or understand), anomia (inability to find words), and agnosia (loss of sensory comprehension, including

---

BOX 36.1 Key Features
Stages of Alzheimer's Disease (AD)

Early-Stage AD
- Independent in ADLs
- May deny presence of symptoms
- Forgets names; misplaces household items
- Has short-term memory loss and difficulty recalling new information
- Shows subtle changes in personality and behavior
- Loses initiative and is less engaged in social relationships
- Has mild impaired **cognition** and problems with judgment
- Demonstrates decreased performance, especially when stressed
- Unable to travel alone to new destinations
- Often has decreased sense of smell

Moderate-Stage AD
- Has impairment of all cognitive functions
- Demonstrates problems with handling or is unable to handle money and finances
- Is disoriented to time, place, and event
- Is possibly depressed and/or agitated
- Is increasingly dependent in ADLs
- Has visuospatial deficits: has difficulty driving and gets lost
- Has speech and language deficits: less talkative, decreased use of vocabulary, increasingly nonfluent, and eventually aphasic
- Incontinent of urine and stool
- Psychotic behaviors, such as delusions, hallucinations, and paranoia
- Has episodes of wandering; trouble sleeping

Late-Stage AD (Severe)
- Completely incapacitated; bedridden
- Totally dependent in ADLs
- Has loss of **mobility** and verbal skills
- Possibly has seizures and tremors
- Has agnosia

---

facial recognition), are due to dysfunction of the temporal and parietal lobes. Frontal lobe impairment causes problems with judgment, an inability to make decisions, decreased attention span, and a decreased ability to concentrate.

As the disease progresses to a later stage, the patient loses all cognitive abilities, is totally unable to communicate, and becomes less aware of the environment. Assess patients for memory loss, communication problems, and issues with judgment and concentration.

To more clearly identify the nature and extent of the patient's impaired **cognition,** the neurologist or clinical psychologist administers several neuropsychological tests. The tests selected depend on clinician preference and the ability of the patient to participate in testing. All of the tests focus on cognitive ability and may be repeated over time to measure changes. Folstein's Mini-Mental State Examination (MMSE) is a classic example of a tool used to determine the onset and severity of cognitive impairment. The MMSE is also known as the "mini-mental exam." The MMSE assesses five major areas—orientation, registration, attention and calculation, recall, and speech-language (including reading). The patient performs certain cognitive tasks that are scored and added together for a total score of 0 to

30. The lower the score is, the greater the severity of the dementia. It is not unusual for a patient with advanced AD to score below 5.

Another sensitive tool used by health professionals to screen for dementia is the Montreal Cognitive Assessment Test (MoCA). Although the MMSE and MoCA are used frequently, they require that the patient be able to read. For the patient who cannot read or for a quicker screening test, the "set test" can be used. The patient is asked to name 10 items in each of four sets or categories: fruits, animals, colors, and towns (FACT). Other categories can be used, if needed. The patient receives 1 point for each item for a possible maximum score of 40. Patients who score above 25 do not have dementia. Although this assessment is easy to administer, it should not be used for patients with hearing impairments or speech and language problems.

The Clock Drawing Test does not require that the patient be able to read and is nonthreatening to perform. In LTC settings, the federally required Brief Interview for Mental Status (BIMS) is included as part of the Minimum Data Set 3.0 for Nursing Homes.

Several U.S. Food and Drug Administration (FDA)–approved computer-based tests, such as the Cognigram, can be used to assess cognitive function while eliminating variations in clinical technique or interpretation. These modalities can detect even very small changes in cognition (Alzheimer's Association, 2022).

Changes in Behavior and Personality. One of the most difficult aspects of AD and other types of dementia with which families and caregivers cope is the behavioral changes that can occur in advanced disease. Assess the patient for:

- Aggressiveness, especially verbal and physical abusive tendencies
- Rapid mood swings
- Increased confusion at night or when light is not adequate ("sundowning") or in excessively fatigued patients

The patient may wander and become lost or may go into other rooms to rummage through another's belongings. Hoarding or hiding objects is also common. For example, patients may hoard washcloths in the long-term care setting.

For some patients with dementia, emotional and behavioral problems occur with the primary disease. They may experience paranoia (suspicious behaviors), delusions, hallucinations, and depression. Document these behaviors and ensure the patient's safety. (Refer to a mental health/behavior health nursing textbook for a complete discussion of these psychotic disorders.)

Changes in Self-Management Skills. Observe for changes in the patient's self-management skills that decline over time, such as:

- Decreased interest in personal appearance
- Selection of clothing that is inappropriate for the weather or event
- Loss of bowel and bladder control
- Decreased appetite or ability to eat (often due to forgetting how to chew food and swallow in late dementia)

Over time, the patient becomes less mobile, and complications of impaired *mobility* develop. Examples of these potential complications are listed in Table 3.2 in Chapter 3 of this textbook. In late-stage AD, the patient eventually becomes immobile (bedridden) and requires total physical care 24 hours a day until death (Navia & Constantine, 2022).

Psychosocial Assessment. In people with dementia, the cognitive changes and biochemical and structural dysfunctions affect personality and behavior. In the early stage, patients often recognize that they are experiencing memory or cognitive changes and may attempt to hide the problems. Recognize that they begin the grieving process because of anticipated loss, experiencing denial, anger, bargaining, and depression at varying times.

Assess patients who recently received a diagnosis of dementia for suicide risk. Establishing a therapeutic patient-centered relationship and asking patients if they currently have or have had thoughts of suicide is an important part of nursing assessment (Smeltzer, 2021). If the patient is considering suicide, ask if there is a plan and determine if the patient has the means to commit suicide, including firearms. Older men with dementia or other neurocognitive disorders are most at risk for suicide because they are often depressed and anxious (Smeltzer, 2021).

When the patient and family receive an AD diagnosis, one or more family members may desire genetic testing. Support the patient's/family's decisions regarding testing and help them find credible resources for testing and professional genetic counseling.

As the disease progresses, patients begin to display major changes in emotional and behavioral affect. Of particular importance is the need for an assessment of the patients' reactions to changes in routine or environment. For example, a hospital admission is very traumatic for most patients with dementia. It is not unusual for them to exhibit a catastrophic response or overreact to any change by becoming excessively aggressive or abusive.

Sexual disinhibition is one of the most challenging symptoms for both family and staff members. Sexually inappropriate behaviors may include masturbating publicly, attempting sexual acts on staff or other patients, disrobing or exposing the genital area, and/or making sexualized comments to staff or other patients. Assess a history of or current manifestation of these behaviors to include into the patient's plan of care.

Neuropsychiatric symptoms are common in patients with AD and increase as the disease progresses and aphasia increases. The patient's emotions are often displayed as nonverbal behaviors, including hitting, yelling, and agitation. Any emergency department (ED) visit, hospital admission, or medical procedure can cause anxiety and fear as a trigger for these behaviors.

As patients become unaware of their behavior, the focus of the psychosocial assessment shifts to the family or significant others. Millions of informal caregivers, most often spouses/partners or other family members, provide care at home for years for most patients with AD. Many of these individuals are at risk for physical and psychosocial problems as a result of the burden of caregiving (Alzheimer's Association, 2022).

Laboratory and Imaging Assessment. An AD diagnosis is made based on patient history, clinical presentation, and imaging assessment. The most sensitive diagnostic tool to detect biomarkers for the disease is amyloid positron emission tomography

(PET) imaging. The patient is injected with a radioactive tracer that can highlight amyloid protein in the brain. Individuals who are at high risk for developing AD have high amounts of this biomarker. Although this test could positively change the diagnostic process and management of AD, Medicare currently does not pay for amyloid PET imaging (Smedinga et al., 2021).

An MRI may be performed to rule out other treatable causes of cognitive impairment. The CT scan typically shows cerebral atrophy, vascular degeneration, ventricular enlargement, wide sulci, and shrunken gyri in the later stages of the disease.

Genetic testing, specifically for *apolipoprotein E4 (APOE-e4)*, is available but controversial for public use. The presence of the APOE-e4 only indicates increased risk of developing the disease. Tests for the genes that cause "familial" AD are also available (Alzheimer's Association, 2022). *Amyloid beta protein precursor (soluble)* (sBPP) may be measured in patients in order to diagnose AD. A decrease in the patient's sBPP in the cerebrospinal fluid (CSF) supports the diagnosis because the amyloid protein tends to deposit in the brain and is not circulating in the CSF (Pagana et al., 2022).

NCLEX Examination Challenge 36.1

Psychosocial Integrity

The nurse assesses a client with a diagnosis of Alzheimer's disease (AD). Which of the following assessment findings would demonstrate the client has progressed to the moderate stage? **Select all that apply.**

A. Unable to dress self
B. Forgets neighbors' names
C. Is unable to balance the checkbook
D. Demonstrates agnosia
E. Gets lost when traveling to familiar places
F. Cannot identify time, place, and event
G. Unable to find the new grocery store

Analyze Cues and Prioritize Hypotheses: Analysis

The priority collaborative problems for patients with Alzheimer's disease (AD) include:

1. Decreased memory and *cognition* due to neuronal changes in the brain
2. Potential for injury or falls due to wandering or inability to ambulate independently
3. Potential for elder abuse by caregivers due to the patient's prolonged progression of disability and increasing care needs
4. Potential need for symptom management at end of life

Generate Solutions and Take Actions: Planning and Implementation

The priority for interprofessional care for patients in the early and moderate stages of AD is safety! Chronic confusion and physical deficits place the patient with AD at a high risk for injury, accidents, and elder abuse. In late-stage AD, patients usually need 24-hour palliative care to promote comfort (Navia & Constantine, 2022).

Managing Memory and Cognitive Dysfunction

Planning: Expected Outcomes. In the very early stages of the disease, the patient with AD is expected to maintain the ability to perform basic mental processes. As the disease progresses, patients cannot meet this outcome. Instead, the desired outcome is to maintain memory and **cognition** for as long as possible to keep patients safe and increase their quality of life.

Interventions. Although drug therapy may be used for patients with AD, nonpharmacologic interventions are the main focus of nursing teamwork and interprofessional collaboration. Teach family members and significant others about the importance of being consistent in following the patient-centered plan of care.

Nonpharmacologic Management. Nonpharmacologic management of patients who have AD include managing a variety of behaviors, maintaining a structured environment, and using selective integrative modalities.

Behavioral management in a structured environment. The primary health care provider should answer the patient's questions truthfully concerning the diagnosis of AD. In this way, the patient and family can more fully participate in the interprofessional plan of care. Interventions are the same whether the patient is cared for at home, in an adult day-care center, in an assisted-living center, in an LTC facility, or in a hospital. *The patient with memory problems benefits best from a structured and consistent environment.*

Many factors, including physical illness and environmental factors, can exacerbate (worsen) the signs and symptoms of AD. The patient with dementia frequently has other health conditions; changes in vision and hearing also may be present. Managing these problems often improves the patient's functional ability.

Approaches to managing the patient who has AD include:

- Cognitive stimulation and memory training
- Structuring the environment
- Orientation or validation therapy
- Promoting self-management
- Promoting bowel and bladder continence
- Promoting communication

The purpose of *cognitive stimulation and memory training* is to reinforce or promote desirable cognitive function and facilitate memory. Cognitive-stimulation therapy programs and mindfulness provide some benefit for patients. An example of cognitive stimulation is to show a video of family members to the patient with dementia to manage behaviors or help improve memory.

As the disease progresses, patients may lose the ability to recognize familiar faces, including their own. Encourage the family to provide pictures of family members and close friends that are labeled with the person's name on the picture. In addition, advise the family to reminisce with the patient about pleasant experiences from the past. Use *reminiscence therapy* while assisting the patient with ADLs or performing a treatment or assessment. Refer to personal items in the room to help the patient begin to talk about their meaning in the present and in the past.

It is not unusual for patients to talk to their image in the mirror. This behavior should be allowed as long as it is not harmful. If the patient becomes frightened by the mirror image, remove or cover the mirror. In some long-term care or memory care units, a picture of the patient is placed on the room door to help with facial recognition and to help patients locate their room. This picture also helps the staff locate the patient in case of wandering or elopement.

Teach the family to keep environmental distractions and noise to a minimum. The patient's home, hospital room, or nursing home room should not have pictures on the wall or other decorations that could be misinterpreted as people or animals that could harm the patient. An abstract painting or wallpaper might look like a fire or an explosion and scare the patient. The room should have adequate, nonglare lighting and no potentially frightening shadows.

In addition to disturbed sleep, other negative effects of high noise levels include decreased nutritional intake, changes in blood pressure and pulse rates, and feelings of increased stress and anxiety. The patient with AD is especially susceptible to these changes and needs to have as much undisturbed sleep at night as possible. Fatigue increases confusion and behavioral manifestations such as agitation and aggressiveness.

! NURSING SAFETY PRIORITY

Action Alert

When a patient with Alzheimer's disease is in a new setting or environment, collaborate with the staff and admitting department to select a room that is in the quietest area of the unit and away from obvious exits, if possible. A private room may be needed if the patient has a history of agitation or wandering. The television should remain off unless the patient turns it on or requests that it be turned on.

Objects such as furniture, a hairbrush, and eyeglasses should be kept in the same place. Establish a daily routine and follow it as much as possible. Arrange for a communication board or digital handheld device for scheduled activities and other information to promote orientation such as the day of the week, the month, and the year. Pictures of people familiar to the patient can also be placed on this board.

Explain changes in routine to the patient before they occur, repeating the explanation immediately before the changes take place. Clocks and single-date calendars also help the patient maintain day-to-day orientation to the environment in the early stages of the disease process. *For the patient with early disease, reality orientation is usually appropriate.* Teach family members and health care staff to frequently reorient the patient to the environment. Remind patients what day and time it is, where they are, and who you are.

For the patient in the later stages of AD or dementia, reality orientation does not work and often increases agitation. The interprofessional health care team uses validation therapy for the patient with moderate or severe AD. In validation therapy, the staff member recognizes and acknowledges the patient's feelings and concerns. For example, if the patient is looking for "Mother," ask about what Mother looks like and what she might be wearing. This response does not argue with the patient but also does not reinforce the patient's belief that Mother is still living.

As the disease progresses, altered thought processes affect the *ability to perform ADLs.* Encourage the patient to perform as much self-care as possible and to maintain independence in daily living skills for as long as possible. For example, in the home setting, complete clothing outfits placed on a single hanger allow patient selection. When possible, the patient should participate in meal preparation, grocery shopping, and other household routines.

INTERPROFESSIONAL COLLABORATION

Care of Patients With Alzheimer's Disease

Collaborate with the occupational and physical therapists to provide a complete evaluation and assistance in helping the patient remain as independent as possible. Adaptive devices, such as grab bars in the bathtub or shower area, an elevated commode, and adaptive eating utensils, may enable the patient to maintain independence in grooming, toileting, and feeding in the early and moderate stages of the disease. The physical therapist prescribes an exercise program to improve physical health and functionality.

According to the Interprofessional Education Collaborative (IPEC) Expert Panel's Competency of Roles and Responsibilities, using the unique and complementary abilities of other team members optimizes health and patient care (IPEC, 2016; Slusser et al., 2019).

NCLEX Examination Challenge 36.2

Psychosocial Integrity

A client with moderate-stage Alzheimer's disease (AD) in a memory care unit appears to be frightened at the assigned dining room table. What would be the nurse's most appropriate action?
A. Explain to the client that there is no cause for alarm.
B. Move the client to another table.
C. Encourage active conversation at the table.
D. Assess surroundings for sensory stimuli.

The patient may remain continent of bowel and bladder for long periods if taken to the bathroom every 2 hours. Toileting may be needed more often during the day and less frequently at night. Assistive personnel (AP) or home caregivers should encourage the patient to drink adequate fluids to promote optimal voiding. A patient may refuse to drink enough fluids because of a fear of incontinence. Ensure that patients are toileted on a regular schedule to prevent incontinence episodes. The patient who is totally bedridden requires the use of a bedpan or urinal.

When patients with dementia are in the hospital or another unfamiliar place, avoid the use of restraints, including side rails. Serious injury can occur when a patient with dementia attempts to get out of bed with either limb restraints or raised side rails. Use frequent surveillance, toileting every 1 to 2 hours, and other strategies to prevent falls. In some cases, sitters or family members may be used to help prevent patient injury. Chapter 4 discusses fall prevention in detail.

Maintain a clear path between the bed and bathroom at all times. For patients who are too weak to walk to the bathroom, a bedside commode may be used. Some patients may void in unusual places, such as the sink or a wastebasket. As a reminder of where they should toilet, place a picture of the commode on the bathroom door.

BOX 36.2 Best Practice for Patient Safety and Quality Care

Promoting Communication With the Patient Who Has Alzheimer's Disease

- Ask simple, direct questions that require only a "yes" or "no" answer if the patient can communicate.
- Provide instructions with pictures in a place that patients will see if they can read them.
- Use simple, short sentences and one-step instructions.
- Use gestures to help the patient understand what is being said.
- Validate the patient's feelings as needed.
- Limit choices; too many choices cause frustration and increased confusion.
- Never assume that the patient is totally confused and cannot understand what is being communicated.
- Try to anticipate the patient's needs and interpret nonverbal communication.

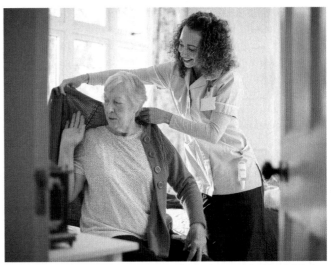

FIG. 36.1 Home care worker helping older woman get dressed in her bedroom. (Used with permission from iStockphoto.com, 2019, sturti.)

Complementary and integrative health. Many types of complementary and integrative health modalities for AD have been studied. If culturally appropriate and if the patient allows being touched by staff, teach AP to provide a massage before bedtime to promote sleep or at other times to reduce stress and promote relaxation. Aromatherapy, animal-assisted therapy, art, and group activities are important parts of behavior management. Music has shown strong results in overcoming apathy and improving cognitive outcomes (Aarskog et al., 2019; Tomaino, 2021).

Use redirection by attracting the patient's attention to promote communication. Keep the environment as free from distractions as possible. Speak directly to the patient in a distinct manner. Sentences should be clear and short. Remind the patient to perform one task at a time and allow sufficient time for completion. It may be necessary to break each task down into many small steps and limit choices. Box 36.2 lists other tips for communicating with patients who have AD.

As the disease progresses, the patient is unable to perform tasks when asked. Show the patient what needs to be done, or provide cues as reminders of how to perform the task. When possible, explain and demonstrate the task that the patient is asked to perform (Fig. 36.1).

Patients with dementia disorders typically have specific speech and language problems. Recognize that emotional and physical behaviors may be a form of communication. Interpret the meaning of these behaviors to address them. For example, restlessness may indicate urinary retention, pain, infection, or hypoxia (lack of oxygen to the brain). Collaborate with the speech-language pathologist (SLP) to assist with communication ability.

Pharmacologic Management. At this time there are no available drugs that can cure or slow the progression of Alzheimer's disease, but a few drugs may improve symptoms associated with the disease for some patients. Psychotropic drugs may be prescribed to help control the signs and symptoms of associated mental/behavioral health problems (e.g., depression, anxiety, paranoia).

Cholinesterase inhibitors are drugs approved for treating AD symptoms. They work to improve cholinergic neurotransmission in the brain by delaying the destruction of acetylcholine (ACh) by the enzyme cholinesterase. This action may slow the onset of cognitive decline in some patients, but none of these drugs alters the course of the disease. In some cases, cholinesterase inhibitors can improve functional ADL ability. Examples include donepezil, galantamine, and rivastigmine (Burchum & Rosenthal, 2022).

NURSING SAFETY PRIORITY

Drug Alert

Teach the family to monitor the patient's heart rate and report dizziness or falls because cholinesterase inhibitors can cause bradycardia. Therefore they are used cautiously in patients who have a history of heart disease.

Memantine is the first of a newer class of drugs that is a low to moderate affinity N-methyl-D-aspartate (NMDA) receptor antagonist. Overexcitation of NMDA receptors by the neurotransmitter *glutamate* may play a role in AD. This drug blocks excess amounts of glutamate that can damage nerve cells. It is indicated for advanced AD and has been shown in some patients to slow the pace of deterioration (Burchum & Rosenthal, 2022). Memantine may help maintain patient function for a few months longer. Some patients also have improved memory and thinking skills. This drug can be given with donepezil, a cholinesterase inhibitor.

In 2022 the U.S. Food and Drug Administration (FDA) gave fast track approval for aducanumab, the first new drug for AD in 20 years. It is an amyloid beta–directed monoclonal antibody that is proposed to treat AD by reducing amyloid plaques (FDA, 2022). Controversy surrounded the FDA approval based on clinical data being less than robust and the exorbitant cost of the drug.

Some patients with AD develop depression and may be treated with *antidepressants*. Selective serotonin reuptake inhibitors (SSRIs), such as paroxetine and sertraline, are typically prescribed. Managing depression may improve cognitive function.

Psychotropic drugs, also called *antipsychotic* or *neuroleptic drugs,* should be reserved for patients with psychoses that sometimes accompany dementia, such as hallucinations and delusions. However, in clinical practice these drugs are sometimes incorrectly used for agitation, combativeness, or restlessness. Psychotropic drugs are considered chemical restraints because they decrease **mobility** and patients' self-management ability. Therefore, most geriatricians recommend that they be used as a last resort and with caution in low doses for a specific mental/behavioral health problem. The specific drug prescribed depends on side effects, the condition of the patient, and expected outcomes. *Follow agency policy and The Joint Commission standards concerning the use of chemical restraints.*

Preventing Injuries or Falls

Planning: Expected Outcomes. The patient with dementia is expected to remain free from physical harm and not injure anyone else.

Interventions. Many patients with dementia tend to wander and may easily become lost. Teach the family the importance of a patient identification badge or bracelet. The badge should include how to contact the primary caregiver. In an inpatient setting, check patients frequently and place them in a room that can be monitored easily. The room should be away from exits and stairs. Some health care agencies place large stop signs or red tape on the floor in front of exits. Others have installed alarm systems to indicate when a patient is opening the door or getting out of a bed or chair.

Restlessness may be decreased if patients are taken for frequent walks. If patients begin to wander, redirect them. For example, if patients insist on going shopping for clothes, redirect them to their closet to select clothing that they will not recognize as their own. This type of activity can be repeated a number of times because the patient has lost short-term memory. Interventions for preventing and managing wandering are listed in Box 36.3.

BOX 36.3 Best Practice for Patient Safety and Quality Care

Approaches to Prevent and Manage Wandering in Hospitalized Patients

- Identify the patients most at risk for wandering through observation and history provided by family.
- Provide appropriate supervision, including frequent checks (especially at shift-change times).
- Place the patient in an area that provides maximum observation but not in the nurses' station.
- Use family members, friends, volunteers, and sitters as needed to monitor the patient.
- Keep the patient away from stairs and elevators.
- Do not change rooms to prevent increasing confusion.
- Avoid physical or chemical restraints.
- Assess and treat pain.
- Use reorientation methods or validation therapy, as appropriate.
- Provide frequent toileting and incontinence care as needed.
- Use bed and/or chair alarms, as available.
- If possible, prevent overstimulation, such as excessive noise.
- Use soft music and nonglare lighting if possible.

In any setting, keep the patient busy with structured activities. In a health care agency, an activity therapist or volunteer may work with patients as a group or individually to determine the type of activity that is appropriate for the stage of the disease. Puzzles, board games, art supplies, and computer games are often appropriate. Music and art therapy are also helpful activities to keep patients with AD busy while stimulating **cognition.** These activities allow patients to be engaged and promote their creativity.

Patients with dementia may be injured because they cannot recognize objects or situations as harmful. Remove or secure all potentially dangerous objects (e.g., knives, drugs, cleaning solutions). Patients are often unaware that their driving ability is impaired and usually want to continue this activity even if their driver's license has been suspended or they are unsafe. Automobile keys must be secured, but the patient should be told why they were taken.

Patients in the community or in an institution may also experience falls as their disease progresses. Assistive technology can assist in keeping patients safe (see the Evidence-Based Practice box). Chapter 4 discusses best practices for fall reduction and prevention in older adults.

📄 EVIDENCE BASED PRACTICE

Do Assistive Technologies Keep Patients With Dementia Safe in the Home?

Brims, L., & Oliver, K. (2019). Effectiveness of assistive technology in improving the safety of people with dementia: a systematic review and meta-analysis. *Aging & Mental Health, 23*(8), 942–951.

The authors conducted a systematic review and meta-analysis of the literature to determine if assistive technologies could prevent falls and reduce nursing home admissions in community-dwelling adults living with dementia. After conducting their search, the authors selected three randomized controlled trials for review inclusion. Assistive technologies included low-tech items, such as grab bars, and high-tech items, such as hallway lights set to a sensor and telehealth packages. Research findings included:

- Use of a comprehensive fall package including a sensor-activated nightlight and a telehealth assistance package reduced falls by 50%.
- Use of a caregiver-supported fall prevention program including grab bars and sensor lights and a support booklet led to fewer accidents and episodes of "risky behavior."
- Use of a fall prevention program including a sensor-activated nightlight, grab bars, and an individualized exercise program resulted in no significant difference in falls.
- No intervention reduced nursing home admission.

Level of Evidence: 1
This research was a systematic review of randomized controlled trials.

Implications for Nursing Practice and Research
Although only three studies were included, the evidence for using high-tech assistive technologies to prevent falls is compelling. Recurring falls are often the driving factor that leads to nursing home placement. Telehealth and telehealth technologies is a growing area of research and development and interest, particularly for those living in rural areas who have limited access to support. Nurses should advocate for technologies that promote independence and should continue to research the best practices for maintaining safety in the home for people living with dementia.

Late in the disease process, the patient may experience seizure activity. If the patient is cared for at home, teach caregivers what action to take when a seizure occurs to prevent injury. (See the discussion of Interventions in the Seizures and Epilepsy section.)

In later stages of the disease, some patients may also become severely agitated and physically or verbally abusive to others. Talking calmly and softly and attempting to redirect the patient to a more positive behavior or activity are effective strategies when the patient is agitated. For example, some patients refuse to take a bath or are unable to bathe. Bathing disability predicts decline for patients with dementia and, combined with safety issues, often leads the family to place them in long-term care (LTC) settings. LTC staff may label these patients as "difficult" when they aggressively refuse to bathe.

Use calm, positive statements and reassure patients that they are safe. Statements such as "I'm sorry that you are upset," "I know it's hard," and "I will have someone stay with you until you feel better" may help. Actions to *avoid* when the patient is agitated include raising the voice, confronting, arguing or reasoning, taking offense, or explaining. Teach the caregiver to not show alarm or make sudden movements out of the person's view. If patients remain agitated, ensure their safety and the safety of others; leave the room after explaining that you will return later. Conduct frequent visual checks during this time. If patients are connected to any type of tubing or other device, they may try to disconnect it or pull it out. These devices should be used cautiously in the patient with dementia. For example, if IV access is needed, the catheter or cannula is placed in an area that the patient cannot easily see, or it should be covered.

Another way to manage this problem is to provide a diversion. For example, if the patient is doing an activity or holding an item such as a stuffed animal or other special item, less attention might be paid to medical devices.

Preventing Elder Abuse

Planning: Expected Outcomes. The family or other caregivers of the patient with dementia are expected to plan time to care for themselves to promote a reasonable quality of life and satisfaction, which should help prevent patient abuse.

Interventions. AD is a chronic, progressive condition that eventually leaves the patient completely dependent on others for all aspects of care. The patient with moderate or severe dementia requires continual 24-hour supervision and caregiving. Severe cognitive changes leave the patient unable to manage finances, property, or personal care. The family needs to seek legal counsel regarding the patient's competency and the need to obtain guardianship or a durable medical power of attorney when necessary.

Patients who are cared for at home are at high risk for neglect or abuse. *The Joint Commission requires all patients to be assessed for neglect and abuse on admission to a health care facility.* Patients with early dementia may not report these concerns for fear of retaliation. Asking questions such as "Who cooks for you?" "Do you get help when you need it?" or "Do you wait long for help to the bathroom?" may be less stressful for the patient to answer.

Millions of family caregivers provide direct care for patients with impaired **cognition.** Family caregivers include relatives, significant others, and neighbors who provide the majority of home health care. These individuals often report negative impacts on their health from their role as caregivers, including anxiety. A 2020 study showed that providing caregivers with education on promoting their physical and emotional health had several positive outcomes, including decreased anxiety (Zarepour et al., 2020).

Teach family caregivers to be aware of their own health and stress levels. Signs of stress include anger, social withdrawal, anxiety, depression, lack of concentration, sleepiness, irritability, and physical health problems. When signs of stress and strain occur, the caregiver should be referred to the primary health care provider or seek one independently. It is not unusual for the caregiver to refuse to accept help from others, even for a few brief hours. Initially the caregiver may be more comfortable accepting help for just a few minutes a day in order to shower, enjoy a cup of tea, or take a brief walk. Some caregivers find that eventually they need to place their loved one into a respite setting or unit so they can reenergize and prevent or manage spiritual distress.

🧍 PATIENT-CENTERED CARE: CULTURE AND SPIRITUALITY

Alzheimer's Disease

Both religion and spirituality can help family caregivers give meaning to the work they provide for patients with Alzheimer's disease (AD). Spirituality is considered an important part of holistic patient care; it may or may not include religion. Spirituality and religion may decrease the incidence of caregiver depression and anxiety. Assess the patient's and family caregiver's cultural beliefs and values related to spirituality and religion. Box 36.4 lists strategies for reducing caregiver stress and includes interventions to promote spirituality and prevent spiritual distress.

BOX 36.4 **Patient and Family Education**

Reducing Family/Informal Caregiver Stress

- Maintain realistic expectations for the person with Alzheimer's disease (AD).
- Take each day one at a time.
- Try to find the positive aspects of each incident or situation.
- Use humor with the person who has AD.
- Use the resources of the Alzheimer's Association in the United States (or Alzheimer Society of Canada, or Alzheimer's Disease International), including attending local support group meetings and using AD toll-free hotlines when needed and where available.
- Explore alternative care settings early in the disease process for possible use later.
- Establish advance directives with the patient who has AD early in the disease process.
- Set aside time each day for rest or recreation away from the patient, if possible.
- Seek respite care periodically for longer periods of time.
- Take care of yourself by watching your diet, exercising, and getting plenty of rest.
- Be realistic about what you or they can do, and accept help from family, friends, and community resources.
- Use relaxation techniques, including meditation and massage.
- Seek out clergy or other spiritual counselor as needed.

As stated earlier, Black and Hispanic individuals have a greater risk for developing AD and often it develops earlier. These groups are known to be very family centered and tend to care for their family members more at home when compared with Whites. As a result of these values and beliefs, an increase in family caregivers is expected as the number of older minority adults increases dramatically within the next 20 to 30 years. More research that focuses on older adults from these populations is needed to better provide essential care and support.

Managing Symptoms at End of Life

Planning: Expected Outcomes. AD is a terminal illness that can cause pain and other symptoms requiring palliative care (Navia & Constantine, 2022). Therefore the expected outcome is that the patient achieves adequate pain management and is as comfortable as possible during the end of life (EOL).

Interventions. When caring for patients who have dementia, the nurse considers many legal/ethical issues related to care, especially at EOL (see the Legal/Ethical Considerations box). As AD progresses, patients and families need assistance with advance care planning for each stage. Patients in the late stage of AD usually require 24-hour total care by family or other caregivers. Nurses need to help families make EOL decisions that include hospice and/or palliative care. Medicare supports and pays for hospice for patients who are terminally ill and need pain and symptom management (Navia & Constantine, 2022).

🔍 LEGAL/ETHICAL CONSIDERATIONS

Common Legal/Ethical Issues Associated With Care of Patients Who Have Alzheimer's Disease (AD)

Legal and ethical considerations for care of patients who have AD depend on the stage of the disease process. For example, in the *early stage* of the disease, nurses need to educate patients and families that patients should be involved with decision making about advance care planning, even though they have memory loss and impaired judgment at times. To determine the patient's decision-making capacity, nurses and other health care professionals need to assess these four cognitive processes (Chiong et al., 2021):

- Does the patient understand the situation?
- Does the patient appreciate the situation?
- Does the patient have adequate reasoning ability?
- Can the patient make appropriate choices?

If the answer to these four questions is "yes," patients are able to make their own health care and other decisions.

Patients in the *moderate stage* of the disease often display agitation and disruptive behaviors that lead families or other surrogate decision makers to explore patient placement in a memory care or long-term care facility or make other caregiver decisions. Nurses or other health care professionals need to help families work through the decision-making process by providing support and recommending resources. To the extent possible, patients should be involved in all decisions about their care.

Patients in the *late stage* of AD cannot report their pain or other symptoms and therefore may not receive adequate care to meet their needs (Chiong et al., 2021). Nurses need to educate family caregivers about the patient's need for palliative care to promote comfort and quality of life during the end of life.

About half of all patients who have AD experience **pain** in the last few months of life but are not able to verbalize their experience. Many older adults have arthritis or other chronic diseases that cause persistent pain. Other commonly occurring problems include (Navia & Constantine, 2022):

- Dyspnea
- Behavioral issues
- Infections
- Cachexia

Several tools are available to assess *pain* in noncommunicative patients, including the Pain Assessment in Advance Dementia instrument (PAINAD). Ensure that patients receive around-the-clock acetaminophen for mild to moderate pain. Patients who have more severe pain may need opioids such as oral concentrated morphine administered sublingually. Chapter 6 discusses pain management in more detail.

Collaborate with the respiratory therapist for patients who develop *dyspnea* at EOL. Opioids and oxygen therapy can be helpful in managing dyspnea for some patients. Teach caregivers to monitor for and report symptoms associated with *infections*, especially urinary tract infection and pneumonia.

Patients in the late stage of AD often display *aggressive and psychotic behaviors*, including delirium and hallucinations. If possible, antipsychotic drugs should be used as a last resort. Teach caregivers to use music therapy, massage, and other soothing methods to calm patients.

Patients in the late stage of AD forget how to chew and swallow, and therefore giving them food and fluids is often not possible. However, use of feeding tubes to supply hydration and nutrition is contraindicated at EOL, even if the patient has cachexia, due to life-threatening complications (Navia & Constantine, 2022). Withholding food and fluids is not painful or uncomfortable, and is discussed in more detail in Chapter 8 on EOL care.

Care Coordination and Transition Management

Home Care Management. Assess the patient for factors (e.g., social determinants of health) that may prevent or hinder safe, high-quality care, including food insecurity, lack of housing, lack of transportation, lack of family or caregiver support, and financial issues. Refer families to appropriate community resources to obtain basic needs. Whenever possible, the patient and family should have a case manager who can assess their needs for health care resources and help with advance care planning throughout the course of the disease.

In the early stages of AD, patients may be cared for at home with little need for outside intervention. As the disease progresses, the need for assistance with care usually increases. Some health care agencies have adult medical day-care centers or memory care units for patients with AD. In the day-care center, patients spend all or part of the day at the facility and participate in activities as their condition permits. Although these centers are usually open only on weekdays, this arrangement allows the caregiver to work or participate in other activities. If patients require 24-hour care, they may be placed in a memory care unit of a long-term care or assisted-living facility.

The patient usually begins to withdraw from friends and social events as memory impairment and personality and behavior changes progress. The family may begin to decrease their own social activities as the demands of the patient's care take more of their time. Emphasize to the family the importance of maintaining their own social contacts and leisure activities.

In most areas of the United States and Canada, respite care is available for families. The patient may be placed in a respite facility or nursing home for the weekend or for several weeks to give the family a rest from the constant care demands. The family may also be able to obtain respite care in the home through a home care agency or assisted-living facility. Remind the family that respite care is for a short period; it is not permanent placement.

Self-Management Education. Patients with AD or other types of dementia are typically cared for in the home until late in the disease process unless they can afford private-pay care. Because health insurance coverage in the United States and family finances may not be sufficient to cover the services of a home care aide, family members typically provide the care. The patient plan of care developed by the nurse or case manager, in conjunction with the family, must be reasonable and realistic for the family to implement.

Provide information to the family on what to do in the event of a seizure and how to protect the patient from injury. Instruct them to notify the primary health care provider if the seizure is prolonged or if the patient's seizure pattern changes.

Review with the family or other caregiver the name, time, and route of administration; the dosage; and the side effects of all drugs. Remind the family to check with the health care provider before using any over-the-counter (OTC) drugs or herbs because they may interact with prescribed drug therapy.

Emphasis is placed on the need for the patient to have an established exercise program to maintain *mobility* for as long as possible and to prevent complications of immobility. In collaboration with the family, the physical therapist (PT) may develop an individualized exercise program. The PT may continue to work with the patient at home until goals are achieved, depending on the payer source.

Remind the family or other caregiver to take special precautions to maintain the patient safely at home. The environment must be uncluttered, consistent, and structured. All hazardous items (e.g., cooking range and oven, power tools) are removed, secured, or "locked out." All electrical sockets not in use should be covered with safety plugs. Box 36.5 lists additional best practices for care of patients who have AD at home.

Health Care Resources. Refer all families to their local chapter of the Alzheimer's Association (www.alz.org) in the United States, the Alzheimer Society of Canada (www.alzheimer.ca), or Alzheimer's Disease International (https://www.alzint.org). These organizations provide information and support services to patients and their families, including seminars, audiovisual aids, and publications. In most locations, caregiver telephone or email support is available. Encourage the family to explore telehealth services designed for people living with dementia.

Teach the family to enroll the patient in the Safe Return Program, a U.S. government–funded program of the Alzheimer's Association that assists in the identification and safe, timely return of people with dementia. The program

---

BOX 36.5 Best Practice for Patient Safety and Quality Care

Managing Behaviors for Patients With Alzheimer's Disease at Home

- Carefully evaluate the patient's environment to ensure it is safe:
  - Remove small area rugs.
  - Consider replacing tile floors with nonslip floors.
  - Arrange furniture and room decorations to maximize the patient's safety when walking.
  - Minimize clutter in all rooms in and outside of the house.
  - Install nightlights in patient's bedroom, bathroom, and hallway.
  - Install and maintain smoke alarms, fire alarms, and natural gas detectors.
  - Install safety devices in the bathroom such as handles for changing position (sitting to standing).
  - Install alarm system or bells on outside doors; place safety locks on doors and gates.
  - Ensure that door locks cannot be easily opened by the patient.
  - Enroll the patient in the Safe Return Program
- Help the patient with mild-stage disease remain oriented to the extent possible:
  - Place single-date calendars in patient's room and in kitchen.
  - Use large-face clocks with a neutral background.
- Communicate with the patient based on the ability to understand:
  - Explain activity immediately before the patient needs to carry it out.
  - Break complex tasks down to simple steps.
- Allow and encourage the patient to be as independent as possible in ADLs:
  - Place complete outfits for the day on hangers; have the patient select one to wear.
  - Develop and maintain a predictable routine (e.g., meals, bedtime, morning routine).
- When a problem behavior occurs, divert patient to another activity; minimize excessive stimulation:
  - Take the patient on outings when crowds are small.
  - If crowds cannot be avoided, minimize the amount of time the patient is present in a crowd. For example, at family gatherings, provide a quiet room for the patient to rest throughout the visit.
  - Arrange for a day-care program to maintain interaction and provide respite for home caregiver.
- In the United States, register the patient with the Alzheimer's Association (www.alz.org); in Canada, register the patient with the Alzheimer Society of Canada Medic Alert Safely Home program (www.alzheimer.ca).

---

includes registration of the patient and a 24-hour hotline to be called to assist in finding a lost patient. If a patient wanders and becomes lost, the family (or health care institution) should immediately notify the police department. An up-to-date picture of the patient makes it easier for local authorities, the public, and neighbors to identify the missing patient. Devices using radio-wave beacons and the Global Positioning System (GPS) have been developed to help families and law enforcement officials find a lost patient more easily. These devices include shoes with a GPS unit implanted, jewelry that is hard to remove, and bracelets. Caution families that these devices are not foolproof. Just like cell phones, there are some areas where the signal from the patient may not be picked up easily, if at all.

When the patient can no longer be cared for at home, referral to an assisted-living or long-term care facility may be needed. Early in the course of the disease, advise the family that placement might be needed at some point in the disease. This allows the family to begin to search for an appropriate facility before a crisis develops and immediate placement is needed. The national office of the Alzheimer's Association publishes an outline of criteria for a memory care unit. In the advanced stage of the disease, the patient may need referral to palliative and possibly hospice services for total care. (See the discussion of end-of-life and hospice care in Chapter 8.)

Evaluate Outcomes: Evaluation

Evaluate the care of the patient with AD based on the identified priority patient problems. The expected outcomes include that the patient and/or family will:

- Maintain memory and *cognition* for as long as possible and increase their quality of life
- Remain free from injury and accidents and have a safe environment
- Manage caregiver stress and strain to prevent elder abuse
- Manage pain and other symptoms at the end of life to promote comfort and quality of life

✳ MOBILITY CONCEPT EXEMPLAR: PARKINSON'S DISEASE

Parkinson's disease (PD), also referred to as *Parkinson disease* and *paralysis agitans,* is a progressive neurodegenerative disease that is one of the most common neurologic disorders of older adults. Most people have *primary,* or idiopathic, disease. A few patients have *secondary* parkinsonian symptoms from conditions such as brain tumors and certain antipsychotic drugs.

Pathophysiology Review

PD is a debilitating disease affecting *mobility* and is characterized by four cardinal symptoms: tremor, muscle rigidity, bradykinesia/akinesia (slow movement/no movement), and postural instability. Changes in *cognition,* including dementia and psychoses, can occur in some patients with late-stage PD. Nonmotor signs such as constipation, soft voice, micrographia (small handwriting), loss of smell, sexual dysfunction, and sleep disturbances can appear years before the cardinal signs (Vacca, 2019; Vice & Tenhunen, 2020).

Normally, motor activity occurs as a result of integrating the actions of the cerebral cortex, basal ganglia, and cerebellum. The basal ganglia are a group of neurons located deep within the cerebrum at the base of the brain near the lateral ventricles. When the basal ganglia are stimulated, muscle tone in the body is inhibited and voluntary movements are refined. The secretion of two major neurotransmitters accomplishes this process: dopamine and acetylcholine (ACh).

Dopamine is produced in the substantia nigra and the adrenal glands and is transmitted to the basal ganglia along a connecting neural pathway for secretion when needed. *ACh* is produced and secreted by the basal ganglia and in the nerve endings in the periphery of the body. ACh-producing neurons transmit *excitatory* messages throughout the basal ganglia. Dopamine *inhibits* the function of these neurons, allowing control over voluntary movement. This system of checks and balances usually allows for refined, coordinated movement, such as picking up a pencil and writing.

In PD, widespread degeneration of the *substantia nigra* leads to a decrease in the amount of dopamine in the brain. An abnormal protein, alpha synuclein, has been found in the brain and body cells and is thought to be the major cause for this degeneration. When dopamine levels are decreased to 70% to 80% of usual levels, a person becomes symptomatic and loses the ability to refine voluntary movement (Vacca, 2019). The large numbers of excitatory ACh-secreting neurons remain active, creating an imbalance between excitatory and inhibitory neuronal activity. The resulting excessive excitation of neurons prevents a person from controlling or initiating voluntary movement (Rogers, 2023).

PD interferes with movement as a result of dopamine loss in the brain, but it also reduces the sympathetic nervous system influence on the heart, blood vessels, and other areas of the body. This loss results in the orthostatic hypotension, drooling, nocturia (voiding at night), and other autonomic symptoms frequently seen in the patient with PD.

PD is separated into stages according to the symptoms and degree of disability. Stage 1 is mild disease with unilateral limb involvement, whereas the patient with Stage 5 disease is completely dependent in all ADLs. Other classifications refer simply to mild, moderate, and severe disease (Box 36.6).

Etiology and Genetic Risk

Although the exact cause of PD is not known, it is probably the result of environmental and genetic factors. Exposure to pesticides, herbicides, and industrial chemicals and metals and being older than 40 years are known risk factors for the development of PD.

Primary Parkinson's disease (PD) often has a familial tendency. The disease is associated with a variety of mitochondrial DNA (mtDNA) variations that often involve deletions in the genetic sequences that are used in central nervous system

---

🔲 BOX 36.6 Key Features

Stages of Parkinson's Disease

Stage 1: Initial Stage
- Unilateral limb involvement
- Minimal weakness
- Hand and arm trembling

Stage 2: Mild Stage
- Bilateral limb involvement
- Masklike face
- Slow, shuffling gait

Stage 3: Moderate Disease
- Postural instability
- Increased gait disturbances

Stage 4: Severe Disability
- Akinesia
- Rigidity

Stage 5: Complete ADL Dependence

(CNS) mitochondria, the energy powerhouses of cells. These variations ultimately cause destruction of neurons that produce dopamine in the substantia nigra (Rogers, 2023).

Patients with traumatic brain injury (TBI) experience a higher incidence of PD when compared with those who do not have TBI. Therefore, teach amateur athletes (especially those participating in contact sports) that they should wear protective headgear such as a helmet. Veterans are also at high risk for developing PD as a result of TBI from combat experiences. Lewy bodies (abnormal proteins) deposit in the brains of patients with PD, which causes problems with body movement. Some patients develop Lewy body dementia later in the course of the disease.

Incidence and Prevalence

In the United States, about 60,000 new cases of PD are diagnosed each year, most in people older than 50 years. More than 1 million patients live with the disease. As the population ages, the number of people affected by PD is expected to dramatically increase. About 50% more men than women currently have the disease, but the exact reason for this difference is not known (Parkinson's Foundation, 2022).

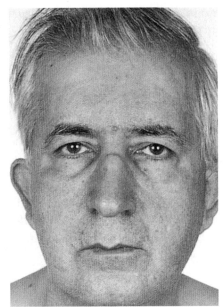

FIG. 36.2 The masklike facial expression typical of patients with Parkinson's disease.

👤 PATIENT-CENTERED CARE: VETERAN HEALTH

Parkinson's Disease in Veterans

About 110,000 veterans have Parkinson's disease (PD). Exposure to Agent Orange and other herbicides and chemicals during the Vietnam War and other military deployments is a major risk factor. Veterans may be entitled to disability compensation if their disease can be linked to such exposure (VA Office of Research and Development, 2022). When interviewing veterans, ask about their deployment(s) and whether they are aware of any chemical or herbicide exposures.

Interprofessional Collaborative Care

Recognize Cues: Assessment

History. Collect data related to the time and progression of symptoms noticed by the patient or family. The older adult may assume that these behaviors are normal changes associated with aging and therefore ignore early signs and symptoms such as *resting* tremors, bradykinesia, fatigue, and problems with muscular rigidity.

Physical Assessment/Signs and Symptoms. In Stage 1 of Parkinson's disease (PD), unilateral resting tremors are usually noticed in one arm. Slow voluntary movements and reduced automatic movements may also occur. In Stage 2, signs and symptoms begin to worsen and become bilateral. In mid-stage PD (Stage 3), loss of balance and slow movement (bradykinesia) occur and the patient is at higher risk for falls (Vacca, 2019). Some patients report "freezing" because they feel that they are stuck to the floor. Assess the patient for *rigidity,* or resistance to passive movement of the extremities. Rigidity is present early in the disease process and progresses over time. Observe the patient's ability to relax a muscle or move a selected muscle

group. Observe the patient's gait, posture (often unstable), and ability to ambulate with or without ambulatory aids.

Due to increased muscle stiffness, patients in Stage 4 require a walker to ambulate and assistance with ADLs (Vacca, 2019). Changes in facial expression or a *masklike face* with wide-open, fixed, staring eyes is caused by rigidity of the facial muscles (Fig. 36.2). In late-stage advanced disease, or Stage 5, this rigidity can lead to difficulties in chewing and swallowing, particularly if the pharyngeal muscles are involved. As a result, the patient may have inadequate nutrition. Uncontrolled drooling may occur. Some patients develop dementia later as the disease progresses and can experience psychotic events, such as delusions, paranoia, and/or hallucinations. Patients can also develop emotional changes such as depression, irritability, apathy, anxiety, and insecurity. In addition to changes in voluntary movement, many patients experience autonomic nervous system symptoms, such as excessive perspiration and orthostatic hypotension. Orthostatic hypotension is likely related to loss of sympathetic innervation in the heart and blood vessel response.

Changes in speech pattern are common in PD patients. They may speak very softly, slur or repeat their words, use a monotone voice or a halting speech, hesitate before speaking, or exhibit a rapid speech pattern.

Bowel and bladder problems are commonly seen in PD as a result of malfunction of the autonomic nervous system, which regulates smooth muscle activity. Patients can exhibit symptoms of either urinary incontinence or difficulty urinating. Constipation can occur because of slow motility of the GI tract, lack of adequate nutritional and fluid intake, and/or impaired *mobility.*

Laboratory and Imaging Assessment. The diagnosis of PD is made based on clinical findings after other neurologic diseases have been eliminated as possibilities. There are no specific diagnostic tests for PD. Analysis of cerebrospinal fluid (CSF) may show a decrease in dopamine levels, although the results of other studies are usually normal. Some diagnostic tests may be done, such as single-photon emission computed tomography (SPECT), to rule out other CNS health problems. SPECT can also reveal a loss of dopamine-producing neurons. Diffusion-weighted imaging is a type of MRI that can differentiate PD from other types of neurodegenerative disorders (Vacca, 2019).

A newer imaging test called a *dopamine transporter (DaT) scan* may be performed via SPECT to confirm abnormalities in dopamine transmission in the basal ganglia. This scan uses a radioactive agent that binds to DaT proteins in the substantia nigra and is used to monitor neuronal degeneration (Vacca, 2019). However, imaging is usually done when the diagnosis is not certain (American Parkinson Disease Association, 2023).

Analyze Cues and Prioritize Hypotheses: Analysis

The priority collaborative problems for patients with PD include:
1. Decreased *mobility* (and possible self-care deficit) due to muscle rigidity, resting tremors, and postural/gait changes
2. Impaired *cognition* due to neurotransmitter and neuronal changes in the brain

Generate Solutions and Take Actions: Planning and Implementation

The priority for care of patients who have PD is to maintain *mobility* and ADL independence for as long as possible. The needs of the patient change depending on which stage of the disease the patient is experiencing.

Promoting Mobility

Planning: Expected Outcomes. The expected outcome is that the patient will maintain optimal *mobility* to promote safety and not experience complications of impaired *mobility.*

Interventions. Interventions for PD are usually nonsurgical, but surgery may be performed as a last resort.

Nonsurgical Management. Nonsurgical care for the patient with PD includes drug therapy, exercise programs or physical therapy, and interprofessional collaboration to promote *mobility* and self-care and to prevent falls or other injuries. Box 36.7 summarizes best practices for nursing management of the patient with PD.

Drug therapy. Drugs are prescribed to treat the symptoms of PD with the purpose of increasing the patient's *mobility* and self-care abilities. An equally important desired outcome is that drugs used for the disease have minimal long-term side effects. Many controversies remain about which drugs to use, when to start therapy, and how to prevent complications. Drug administration is closely monitored, and the primary health care provider adjusts the dosage or changes therapy as the patient's condition requires. Teach the patient and family how to monitor for and report adverse effects of drug therapy.

Dopamine agonists mimic dopamine by stimulating dopamine receptors in the brain. They are typically the most effective during the first 3 to 5 years of use. The benefit of these agents is fewer incidents of dyskinesias (problems with movement) and "wearing off" phenomenon (loss of response to the drug) when compared with other drugs (Burchum & Rosenthal, 2022). This problem is characterized by periods of good mobility ("on" periods) alternating with periods of altered *mobility* ("off" periods). Patients report that their most distressing symptom is the "off time."

BOX 36.7   Best Practice for Patient Safety and Quality Care

Care of the Patient With Parkinson's Disease

- Allow the patient extra time to respond to questions.
- Administer medications promptly on the patient's individualized schedule to maintain continuous therapeutic drug levels.
- Provide drug therapy for pain and/or tingling in limbs, as needed.
- Monitor for drug side effects, especially orthostatic hypotension, hallucinations, and acute confusional state (delirium).
- Place the patient on Fall Precautions according to agency protocol.
- Collaborate with physical and occupational therapists to keep the patient as mobile and independent as possible in ADLs.
- Allow the patient time to perform ADLs and *mobility* skills; provide assistance only as needed.
- Implement interventions to prevent complications of impaired *mobility,* such as constipation, pressure injuries, and contractures.
- Schedule appointments and activities late in the morning to prevent rushing the patient, or schedule them at the time of the patient's optimal level of functioning.
- Teach the patient to speak slowly and clearly. Use alternative communication methods, such as a communication board or handheld mobile device. Refer to the speech-language pathologist.
- Monitor the patient's ability to eat and swallow. Monitor actual food and fluid intake.
- Collaborate with the registered dietitian nutritionist to provide high-protein, high-calorie foods or supplements to maintain weight.
- Recognize that Parkinson's disease can affect the patient's self-esteem. Focus on the patient's strengths.
- Assess for depression, anxiety, and impaired *cognition.*
- Assess for insomnia or sleeplessness.

Examples of dopamine agonists are apomorphine (a morphine derivative), pramipexol, and ropinirole. Another drug in

🔔 NURSING SAFETY PRIORITY

Drug Alert

Dopamine agonists are associated with adverse effects, such as orthostatic (postural) hypotension, hallucinations, sleepiness, and drowsiness, which can be mistaken for signs and symptoms of Parkinson's disease (PD). Remind patients to avoid operating heavy machinery or driving if they have any of these symptoms. Teach them to change from a lying or sitting position to standing by moving slowly. The primary health care provider should not prescribe drugs in this class to older adults because of their severe adverse drug effects.

this class, rotigotine, is available as a continuous transdermal patch to maintain a consistent level of dopamine.

Almost all patients are on levodopa or a combination *levodopa/carbidopa* drug at some point in their disease. It may be the initial drug of choice if the patient's presenting symptoms are severe or interfere with daily life. Both an immediate-release (IR) and a controlled-release (CR) form in varying doses are available. It can also be administered enterally through a percutaneous gastrostomy tube into the small intestine as an infusion. Levodopa agents are less expensive than dopamine agonists and are better at improving motor function. An inhaled form of levodopa has been approved for "off" periods (Parkinson's

Foundation, 2022). Safinamide is an adjunct drug to levodopa combination agents when these drugs do not work alone.

Long-term use of levodopa preparations can lead to **dyskinesia** (inability to perform voluntary movement). Teach the patient and family to give the drug before meals to increase absorption and transport across the blood-brain barrier. Keep in mind that long-term use of levodopa preparations can cause the same adverse effects as dopamine agonists, including orthostatic hypotension and psychotic episodes.

Catechol-O–methyltransferases (COMTs) are enzymes that inactivate dopamine. Therefore COMT *inhibitors* block this enzyme activity, thus prolonging the action of levodopa. One example is entacapone, which is often used in combination with levodopa. The benefit of these combinations is that the disease is treated in several ways. However, they are not beneficial for patients who need more specific dosages of individual drugs.

Monoamine oxidase type B inhibitors (MAOI-Bs) are more popular for use in patients with early or mild symptoms of PD. Entacapone and selegiline are often given with levodopa for early or mild disease. A newer MAOI-B for PD is rasagiline mesylate, which can be given as a single drug or with levodopa. The MAOI-B drugs work by slowing the main type (B) of monoamine oxidase in the brain, increasing dopamine concentrations, and helping reduce the signs and symptoms of PD. They may also protect neurons in the brain. Nonselective MAOs should not be taken within 2 weeks of inhaled levodopa (Burchum & Rosenthal, 2022).

🖊 NURSING SAFETY PRIORITY

Drug Alert

> Teach patients taking monoamine oxidase inhibitors (MAOIs) about the need to avoid foods, beverages, and drugs that contain tyramine, including cheese and aged, smoked, or cured foods and sausage. Remind them to also avoid red wine and beer to prevent severe headache and life-threatening hypertension (Burchum & Rosenthal, 2022). Patients should continue these restrictions for 14 days after the drug is discontinued.

When other drugs are no longer effective, bromocriptine mesylate, a *dopamine receptor agonist,* may be prescribed to promote the release of dopamine. It may be used alone or in combination with carbidopa/levodopa. Some providers may prescribe bromocriptine early in the course of treatment. It is especially useful in the patient who has experienced side effects such as dyskinesias or orthostatic hypotension while receiving levodopa or a combination drug.

Amantadine is an *antiviral drug* that has anti-Parkinson benefits. It may be given early in disease to reduce symptoms. It is also prescribed with levodopa/carbidopa preparations to reduce dyskinesias. Rivastigmine is a *cholinesterase inhibitor* that is used only when patients with PD have dementia. This drug works to improve the transmission of acetylcholine in the brain by delaying its destruction by the enzyme acetylcholinesterase.

A recently approved drug for PD during "off times" is istradefylline, an adenosine A2A antagonist. This drug blocks the release of adenosine in the brain, triggering dopamine signals, and is used when other drug classes are ineffective in controlling PD signs and symptoms.

For the patient on any long-term drug therapy regimen, drug tolerance or *drug toxicity* often develops. Drug toxicity may be evidenced by changes in **cognition** such as delirium (acute confusion) or hallucinations and decreased effectiveness of the drug. Delirium may be difficult to assess in the patient who is already experiencing chronic dementia as a result of PD or another disease. If possible, compare the patient's current cognitive and behavioral status with the baseline before drug therapy begins.

When drug tolerance is reached, the drug's effects do not last as long as previously. The treatment of PD drug toxicity or tolerance includes:

- A reduction in drug dosage
- A change of drug or in the frequency of administration
- A drug holiday (particularly with levodopa therapy)

During a *drug holiday,* which typically lasts up to 10 days, the patient receives no drug therapy for PD. Carefully monitor the patient for symptoms of PD during this time and document assessment findings.

Many patients are on additional drugs to help relieve symptoms associated with the disease. For example, muscle spasms may be relieved by baclofen, drooling can be minimized by sublingual atropine sulfate, and insomnia may require a sleeping aid such as zolpidem tartrate.

GLP-1 receptor agonists (used in the treatment of diabetes mellitus type 2) are being investigated and may have a disease-modifying effect. GLP-1 receptors have been found in the brain. Insulin has a role in neuron metabolism and repair and in the ability of synapses to function effectively. The brain of the patient with PD becomes desensitized to this effect. A Cochrane review found possible improvements in motor movement, but more research is needed (Dix et al., 2020; Mulvaney et al., 2020).

Medical marijuana. Medical marijuana, also called *cannabis,* has been legalized in Canada. In the United States, most states and territories permit medical cannabis (National Conference of State Legislatures, 2023). Although there is inadequate evidence that medical marijuana is effective in managing symptoms associated with PD, many patients report its ability to help relieve tremors, dyskinesias, pain, insomnia, fatigue, and depression (Yenilmez et al., 2020). Side and adverse effects of cannabis are minimal for most patients (Clark, 2021). Large studies are needed to provide strong evidence that marijuana is an appropriate drug to prescribe to patients with PD. Nurses should stay up-to-date on legislation in their states and remain nonjudgmental regarding their patients' choice to use this product (Theisen & Koneyczny, 2019).

Other interventions. A freezing gait and postural instability are major problems for patients with PD. Suggested interventions for freezing gait include attempting to step sideways then forward, shifting the weight side-to-side then attempting a step, and visualizing an object on the ground to step over (Ellis & DeAngelis, n.d.). Nontraditional exercise programs, such as yoga and tai chi, may improve **mobility** in the early stage of the disease. Early in the disease process, collaborate with physical and occupational therapists to plan and implement a program to keep the patient flexible, prevent falling, and retain mobility by incorporating active and passive range-of-motion (ROM) exercises, muscle stretching, and out-of-bed activity. *If the patient is hospitalized for any reason, be sure that fall risk precautions are applied according to agency policy.*

In collaboration with the rehabilitation team, encourage the patient to participate as much as possible in self-management, including ADLs. The team makes the environment conducive to independence in activity and as stress free and safe as possible. Occupational therapists (OTs) and PTs provide training in ADLs and the use of adaptive devices, as needed, to facilitate independence. The OT evaluates the patient for the need for adaptive devices (e.g., special utensils for eating).

Patients with PD tend to not sleep well at night because of drug therapy and the disease itself. Some patients nap for short periods during the day and may not be aware that they have done so. This sleep misperception may put the patient at risk for injury. For example, patients may fall asleep while driving an automobile. Therefore teach patients and families to monitor the patient's sleeping pattern and discuss whether they can operate machinery or perform other potentially high-risk tasks safely.

Collaborate with the registered dietitian nutritionist, if needed, to evaluate the patient's food intake and ability to eat. The patient's intake of nutrients is evaluated, especially in the patient who has difficulty swallowing or is susceptible to injury from falling. The dietitian considers the patient's bowel habits and adjusts the diet if constipation occurs. If the patient has trouble swallowing, collaborate with the speech-language pathologist (SLP) for an extensive swallowing evaluation. Based on these findings and the patient interview, a patient-centered nutritional plan is developed. Usually a soft diet and thick, cold fluids, such as milkshakes, are tolerated more easily.

Small, frequent meals or a commercial powder, such as Thick-It, added to liquids may assist the patient who has difficulty swallowing. Elevate the patient's head to allow easier swallowing and prevent aspiration. Remind AP and teach the family to be careful when serving or feeding the patient. The SLP can be very helpful in recommending specific feeding strategies. Be sure that AP record food intake daily or as needed. The patient often experiences unintended weight loss, which is most likely due to disease progress but may be attributed to increased calories used because of muscle spasm/rigidity (Vacca, 2019). Teach the family to weigh the patient once a week and make adjustments to the diet as indicated. As the disease progresses and swallowing becomes more of a problem, supplemental feedings become the main source of nutrition to maintain weight, with meals and other foods taken as the patient can tolerate.

Collaborate with the SLP if the patient has speech difficulties. Together with the interprofessional health care team, patient, and family, develop a communication plan. The SLP teaches exercises to strengthen muscles used for breathing, speech, and swallowing. Remind the patient to speak slowly and clearly and to pause and take deep breaths at times during each sentence. Teach the family the importance of reducing environmental noise to increase the listener's ability to hear and understand the patient. Ask the patient to repeat words that the listener does not understand. Have the listener watch the patient's lips and nonverbal expressions for cues to the meaning of conversation. Remind the patient to organize thoughts before speaking and use facial expression and gestures, if possible, to assist with communication. In addition, the patient should exaggerate words to increase the listener's ability to understand. If the patient cannot communicate verbally, alternative methods of communication may be used, such as a communication board, mechanical voice synthesizer, computer, or handheld mobile device. The SLP assesses the ability and desire to use these devices before a decision is made about which method, if any, to use.

NCLEX Examination Challenge 36.3
Physiological Integrity

The nurse is preparing to teach a client who has been prescribed ropinirole for Parkinson's disease. Which of the following statements would the nurse include when teaching the client and family? **Select all that apply.**

A. "Move slowly when changing positions from sitting to standing."
B. "Change the patch every 24 hours to a new site on your arm."
C. "This drug causes sleepiness, so do not drive or operate machinery while taking it."
D. "Be sure to report if this drug causes worse trouble with motor movements."
E. "Do not eat cheese, wine, or cured or smoked foods while taking ropinirole."
F. "Have someone take your blood pressure every day."

Surgical Management. Surgery is a last resort when drugs are not effective in symptom management. The most common surgeries are stereotactic pallidotomy and deep brain stimulation (DBS), although newer surgical procedures are being tried. DBS has largely replaced the older thalamotomy procedure.

Stereotactic pallidotomy (opening into the pallidum within the corpus striatum) can be a very effective treatment for controlling the dyskinesias associated with PD. The procedure destroys the pallidum, improving stiffness, dyskinesia, and tremors. It may improve the "off" state; however, it is rarely performed today. Focused ultrasound destruction of specific areas of brain tissue is another uncommon, but approved, procedure (Eisenberg et al., 2020; Parkinson's Foundation, n.d.).

Deep brain stimulation (DBS) is approved as a treatment for PD. In DBS, electrodes are implanted into the brain and connected to a small electrical device called a *pulse generator* that delivers electrical current. The generator is placed under the skin similar to a cardiac pacemaker device. It is externally programmed to deliver an electrical current to decrease involuntary movements known as dyskinesias, resulting in a reduced need for levodopa and related drugs. DBS also helps to alleviate fluctuations of symptoms and reduce tremors, slowness of movements, and gait problems (National Institute of Neurological Disorders and Stroke [NINDS], 2022). This is typically not an option while medications are working.

Fetal tissue transplantation is an experimental and highly controversial ethical and political treatment. Fetal substantia nigra tissue, either human or pig, is transplanted into the caudate nucleus of the brain. Preliminary reports suggest that patients show clinical improvement in motor symptoms without dyskinesias after receiving the transplanted tissue. Long-term results are yet to be seen or studied (NINDS, 2022).

Managing Cognitive Dysfunction

Planning: Expected Outcomes. The expected outcome is that the patient with PD will maintain memory and *cognition* for as long as possible. For patients experiencing cognitive dysfunction, the expected outcome is to keep them safe and increase their quality of life.

Interventions. About 50% of patients with PD have cognitive dysfunction, which usually develops later in the disease process. Pimavanserin is a drug that is used only for Parkinson's disease–related hallucinations and delusions (psychoses).

⚕ NURSING SAFETY PRIORITY

Drug Alert

Patients who have been diagnosed with cardiac dysrhythmias should not take pimavanserin because it can prolong the Q-T interval. Teach patients and their families to report any irregular heart rhythm to their primary health care provider immediately. In addition, the concurrent use of strong CYP3A4 inhibitors, such as ketoconazole, clarithromycin, and itraconazole, can increase the activity of pimavanserin. In this case the health care provider should prescribe pimavanserin in a very low dose (Burchum & Rosenthal, 2022).

Although not all patients with PD have dementia, impaired *cognition* and memory deficits are common. Some patients also experience changes in gait and tremors that are uncontrollable. In the late stages of the disease, they cannot move without assistance, have difficulty talking, have minimal facial expression, and may drool. Patients often state that they are embarrassed and tend to avoid social events or groups of people. They should not be forced into situations in which they feel ashamed of their appearance. Many patients become depressed as a result of their disease. If patients are moderately to severely depressed, an antidepressant such as short-acting venlafaxine may be prescribed.

Teach the family to emphasize the patient's abilities or strengths and provide positive reinforcement when expected outcomes are met. The patient, family or significant other, and rehabilitation team mutually set realistic expected outcomes that can be achieved.

Care Coordination and Transition Management

Home Care Preparation. The long-term management of PD presents a special challenge in the home care setting. A case manager may be required to coordinate interprofessional care and provide support for the patient and family. Impaired *mobility* and *cognition* can affect the patient's daily lifestyle and self-concept, including sexuality. The case manager or other health care professional uses a holistic approach to ensure that both psychosocial and physical needs are addressed.

Self-Management Education. Teach patients and their families about the need to follow instructions regarding the safe administration of drug therapy. Remind them to immediately report adverse effects of medication such as dizziness, falls, acute confusion (delirium), and hallucinations. For patients who had surgery, review discharge instructions about when to resume activity and contact the surgeon.

Teach family members or other caregivers the importance of maintaining or improving the patient's quality of life by helping to alleviate or manage symptoms. For example, constipation can be prevented or managed by encouraging adequate fluids, a high-fiber diet, and a regular bowel-training program with suppositories and bulk-forming laxatives. Sleep disorders may be managed with a good sleep-hygiene program, including avoiding alcohol and caffeine, darkening the bedroom, and performing bedtime rituals.

Neuropsychiatric health problems, such as impulse control disorders, altered *cognition*, anxiety, and depression, can be very difficult for both the patient and family. Remind families and other caregivers that the patient cannot control these symptoms. Caregiver role strain can be a major problem when caring for patients with PD (see earlier discussion under Alzheimer's disease for caregiver stress management).

Health Care Resources. Collaborate with the social worker or case manager to help the family with financial and health insurance issues, as well as respite care or permanent placement if needed. Refer the patient and family to social and state agencies, support groups, and information as needed. Examples in the United States are the National Parkinson Foundation (www.parkinson.org), American Parkinson Disease Association (www.apdaparkinson.org), and Parkinson Disease Foundation (www.pdf.org). The Michael J. Fox Foundation for Parkinson's Research (www.michaeljfox.org) provides an extensive list of resources about living with PD. Patients and families in Canada can access Parkinson Canada (www.parkinson.ca) for information about the disease and support groups.

As the disease progresses and drug effectiveness decreases, refer the family to a palliative care organization or hospice for end-of-life care. Referral sources can be obtained from the Center to Advance Palliative Care (www.capc.org), which advocates applying the principles of palliative care to chronic disease. Chapter 8 discusses palliative and hospice care in detail.

Evaluation: Evaluate Outcomes

Evaluate the care of the patient with PD based on the identified priority patient problems. The expected outcomes include that the patient and/or family will:

- Improve *mobility* to provide self-care and not experience complications of impaired mobility
- Maintain safety and an acceptable quality of life

MIGRAINE HEADACHE

Most individuals experience some type of headache during their lifetime from a variety of causes, such as low blood sugar, sinus infection, alcohol, and stress. These headaches are acute and temporary and often resolve by managing the cause of the headache and/or with mild analgesics such as acetaminophen. Some adults have specific types of headaches that cause severe, debilitating *pain* and recur. The most common type is migraine headache. This type of headache is most likely to affect quality of life when compared with other, less common types.

Pathophysiology Review

A migraine headache is a common clinical syndrome characterized by recurrent episodic attacks of head pain that serve no protective purpose. Migraine headache *pain* is usually described as throbbing and unilateral. Migraines are often accompanied by associated symptoms such as nausea or sensitivity to light, sound, or head movement and can last 4 to 72 hours. They tend to be familial, and women are affected more commonly than men. Women diagnosed with migraines are more likely to have major depressive disorder. Migraine sufferers are also at risk for stroke and epilepsy (Rogers, 2023).

The cause of migraine headaches is not clear. Currently, the most widely accepted theory includes a process that both activates and sensitizes the trigeminovascular system (TVS). When the TVS is activated, a signal is produced and travels to the neurons in the trigeminal complex, mediated by the neurotransmitter calcitonin gene–related peptide (CGRP). CGRP is a potent vasodilator released during a migraine and is thought to play a major role in the sensation of migraine-related *pain* (Schellack et al., 2019). Genetic, hormonal, and environmental factors may play a role as well.

Activation of the trigeminal nerve pathways contributes to the cascade of events that activate nociceptors. Substances that increase sensitivity to *pain* such as glutamate are synthesized through the trigeminal pathway (Rogers, 2023). As cerebral arteries dilate, prostaglandins (chemicals that cause inflammation and swelling) are released. Vasodilation, in turn, allows prostaglandins and other intravascular molecules to leak (extravasate), contributing to widespread tissue swelling and the sensation of throbbing *pain.*

Many patients find that certain factors, or *triggers,* such as caffeine, red wine, and monosodium glutamate (MSG), tend to cause migraine headache attacks. Other triggers include:

- High-intensity light
- Stress
- Excessive fatigue
- Change in weather
- Tyramine-containing products (such as pickled products, aged cheeses, smoked sausages, and beer)
- Preservatives
- Artificial sweeteners

Each patient is different regarding which environmental factors trigger headaches. These stimuli are thought to initiate the cascade of events that cause migraines by activating hyperexcitable neurons, which become increasingly susceptible to these triggers and to the cascade of events that culminate in migraine *pain.* Therefore, interprofessional care includes not only managing *pain* but also disrupting the migraine cascade to decrease sensitization and recurrent attacks.

Interprofessional Collaborative Care

Recognize Cues: Assessment

Migraines fall into two major categories: migraines with aura and migraines without aura. They can also be classified as

chronic or episodic (International Headache Society, 2022). An aura is a temporary symptom in the central nervous system (e.g., visual changes) that signals the onset of a migraine headache. If accompanied by an aura, it will occur immediately before the migraine episode, although an aura can occur without a headache. *Most headaches are migraines without aura.* Migraines are classified as chronic if they occur on at least 15 days of the month and episodic if they occur less frequently (International Headache Society, 2022). Some people have a prodrome that occurs 1 to 2 days before a migraine. The key features of migraines are listed by stage in Box 36.8.

The diagnosis of migraine headache is based on the patient's history and on physical, neurologic, and psychological assessment. Patients tend to have the same signs and symptoms each time they have a migraine headache. Some may have to refrain from regular activities for several days if they cannot control or relieve the *pain* in its early stage.

Neuroimaging such as MRI may be indicated if a migrainous infarction is suspected or if the patient has other neurologic findings, a history of seizures, findings not consistent with a

 BOX 36.8   Key Features

Migraine Headaches

Phases of Migraine With Aura (Classic Migraine)
Prodromal Phase
- Occurs 1–2 days prior to onset of migraine
- Subtle changes such as yawning excessively, constipation, emotional alterations, and food cravings
- Aura, which includes two or more of the following temporary central nervous system symptoms that last 5–60 minutes. Symptoms are generally unilateral. Visual disturbances include:
  - Flashing lights
  - Lines or spots
  - Shimmering or zigzag lights
- A variety of other neurologic changes may occur, including:
  - Numbness, tingling of the lips or tongue
  - Acute confusional state
  - Aphasia
  - Vertigo
  - Unilateral weakness
  - Drowsiness

Migraine Phase
- Headache accompanied by nausea and/or vomiting
- Unilateral, frontotemporal, throbbing *pain* in the head that is often worse behind one eye or ear; also includes photophobia and or phonophobia

Migraine Without Aura (Common Migraine)
- Migraine beginning without an aura before the onset of the headache
- *Pain* aggravated by performing routine physical activities
- *Pain* that is unilateral and pulsating
- One of these symptoms is present:
  - Nausea and/or vomiting
  - Photophobia (light sensitivity)
  - Phonophobia (sound sensitivity)
  - Headache lasting 4 to 72 hours
  - Migraine often occurring in the early morning, during periods of stress, or in those with premenstrual tension or fluid retention

migraine, or a change in the severity of the symptoms or frequency of the attacks. Neuroimaging is also recommended in patients older than 50 years with a new onset of headaches, especially women. Women with a history of migraines with visual symptoms may have an increased risk for stroke, particularly if a migraine with visual symptoms occurred in the past year. Teach women older than 50 years who have migraines about the risk factors for cardiovascular disease. *Encourage them or their family to call 911 if they experience symptoms such as facial drooping, arm weakness, or difficulties with speech!*

Take Actions: Interventions

*The priority for care of the patient having migraines is **pain** management.* This outcome may be achieved by abortive and/or preventive therapy. Drug therapy, trigger management, and complementary and integrative therapies are the major approaches to care. Provide detailed patient and family education regarding the collaborative plan of care. Effective health care provider-patient communication is increasingly important in managing the symptoms of migraines.

Abortive Drug Therapy. Abortive drug therapy is aimed at alleviating *pain* during the aura phase (if present) or soon after the headache has started. Some of the drugs used have major side effects, contraindications, and nursing implications. The primary health care provider must consider any other medical conditions that the patient has when prescribing drug therapy. In general, the patient is started on a low dose that is increased until the desired clinical effect is obtained. Many new drugs are being investigated for this painful and often debilitating health problem.

Mild migraines may be relieved by acetaminophen. NSAIDs such as ibuprofen and naproxen may also be prescribed. In the United States and Canada, several over-the-counter (OTC) NSAID drugs combined with caffeine for migraines are available. Caffeine narrows blood vessels by blocking adenosine, which dilates vessels and increases inflammation. Antiemetics may be prescribed to relieve nausea and vomiting. Metoclopramide may be administered with NSAIDs to promote gastric emptying and decrease vomiting.

For more severe migraines, drugs such as triptans, ditans, ergotamine derivatives, and isometheptene combinations are often needed. A potential side effect of these drugs is rebound headache, also known as medication overuse headache, in which another headache occurs after the drug relieves the initial migraine.

Triptan preparations relieve the headache and associated symptoms by activating the 5-HT (serotonin) receptors on the cranial arteries, the basilar artery, and the blood vessels of the dura mater to produce a vasoconstrictive effect. Examples are sumatriptan, eletriptan, naratriptan, and almotriptan. The older drug sumatriptan is available as an oral agent, injection, and nasal spray (Burchum & Rosenthal, 2022). For many patients, these drugs are highly and quickly effective for pain, nausea, vomiting, and light and sound sensitivity with few side effects. However, sumatriptan may cause chest pain. Therefore most triptans are contraindicated in patients with actual or suspected ischemic heart disease,

cerebrovascular ischemia, hypertension, and peripheral vascular disease and in those with Prinzmetal angina because of the potential for coronary vasospasm. Patients respond differently to drugs, and several types or combinations may be tried before the headache is relieved (Burchum & Rosenthal, 2022).

> ### NURSING SAFETY PRIORITY
> *Drug Alert*
>
> Teach patients taking triptan drugs to take them as soon as migraine symptoms develop. Instruct patients to report angina (chest pain) or chest discomfort to their primary health care provider immediately to prevent cardiac damage from myocardial ischemia. Remind them to use contraception (birth control) while taking the drugs because they may not be safe for women who are pregnant. Teach patients to expect common side effects that include flushing, tingling, and a hot sensation. These annoying sensations tend to subside after the patient's body gets used to the drug. Triptan drugs should not be taken with selective serotonin reuptake inhibitor (SSRI) antidepressants or St. John's wort, an herb used commonly for depression (Burchum & Rosenthal, 2022).

Ditans, such as the recently approved lasmiditan, are a newer group of abortive drugs that block only one specific serotonin receptor without constricting blood vessels. Therefore this class of drugs tends to be safer and work more effectively than triptans.

Ergotamine preparations may be taken at the start of the headache. The patient may take tablets or use a rectal suppository. Dihydroergotamine (DHE) may be given intravenously, intramuscularly, or as a nasal spray with an antiemetic if pain control and relief of nausea are not achieved with other drugs. It should not be given within 24 hours of a triptan drug.

A combination drug containing acetaminophen, isometheptene, and dichloralphenazone is the most common *isometheptene combination* given for treating migraines and is an excellent option when ergotamine preparations are not tolerated or do not work.

Preventive Drug Therapy. Prevention drugs and other strategies are used when a migraine occurs more than twice per month, the duration of headache is greater than 24 hours, the headache interferes with ADLs for 3 or more days, abortive medications are used more than twice a week, or the headache is not relieved with acute treatment. Unless otherwise contraindicated, the primary health care provider may initially prescribe an NSAID, a beta-adrenergic blocker, a calcium channel blocker, or an antiepileptic drug (AED). Propranolol and timolol are common *beta blockers* approved for migraine prevention. Verapamil, a *calcium channel blocking agent,* may also be used for some patients. The calcium channel and beta blockers are thought to reduce the activity of hyperexcitable neurons and act on the neurogenic causes of migraine. Both calcium channel blockers and beta blockers interfere with vasodilation, a contributing cause of migraine pain. Both beta-adrenergic blockers and calcium channel blocking drugs can lower blood pressure and decrease pulse rate (Burchum & Rosenthal, 2022).

Topiramate is one of the most common *antiepileptic drugs (AEDs)* used for migraines, but it should be used in low doses. The mechanism of action is not clear, but this drug may inhibit the sodium channels, channels that may be hyperexcitable in patients with migraine. Reports of suicides have been associated with this drug when it is used in larger doses most often in patients who have bipolar disorder.

Nortriptyline is a tricyclic *antidepressant* that is often effective as a drug to prevent or reduce migraine episodes. The drug is started in a low dose and may be increased depending on the patient's needs. Side effects include dry mouth, urinary retention, and constipation. This anticholinergic drug is not used in older adults because it can also cause delirium (acute confusion) (Burchum & Rosenthal, 2022).

Some patients experience chronic migraine, which is defined as having 15 or more migraine headaches in a month. For chronic migraine, *onabotulinumtoxinA* was approved in 2010. Monthly treatments for up to five treatment cycles are considered safe and effective.

The newest drugs for chronic migraine are in a monoclonal antibody drug class known as *calcitonin gene–related peptide receptor (CGRP-R) antagonists.* Examples of these drugs administered by injection subcutaneously every 1 to 3 months include erenumab, fremanezumab, and, most recently, galcanezumab (Dix et al., 2020). Side effects of this class of drugs are not common, but teach the patient receiving any of them to report pain, redness/hyperpigmentation, or swelling at the injection site.

Encourage patients to keep a headache diary to help identify the type of headache they are experiencing and the response to preventive medication or other intervention. Teach them to notify their primary health care provider if the quality, intensity, or nature of the headache increases or changes. Encourage them to report whether the headache is associated with new or unusual visual changes and if the prescribed drug is no longer effective.

In addition to drug therapy, *trigger avoidance* and *management* are important interventions for preventing migraine episodes. Help patients identify triggers that could cause migraine episodes and teach them to avoid them once identified. For example, at the beginning of a migraine attack, the patient may be able to reduce pain by lying down and darkening the room. The patient may want both eyes covered and a cool cloth on the forehead and to be undisturbed until awakening.

Medical Marijuana. Some patients get relief of pain or have fewer migraine episodes each month by smoking marijuana, also known as cannabis. Cannabis contains two natural compounds called cannabinoids: tetrahydrocannabinol (THC) and cannabidiol (CBD). THC is a mind-altering and intoxicating substance; CBD does not alter the mind or cause intoxication. CBD is the more effective in easing the pain of migraines. Inhaled cannabis has been shown to reduce migraine severity by 50% in one study and in more than 60% of treated patients in another, although tolerance did develop over time (Aviram et al., 2020).

External Trigeminal Nerve Stimulator. A certified medical device called the Cefaly is available in the United States, Europe, and Canada without a prescription to prevent and treat migraines. This *external trigeminal nerve stimulator (E-TNS)* is a wearable headband that stimulates several branches of the trigeminal nerve associated with migraine attacks and pain. Teach the patient to use the device for no more than 20 minutes per day as recommended by its manufacturer. For more information, teach the patient to visit either www.cefaly.us or www.cefaly.ca for a video about how to use this nondrug alternative to preventive medications (Saleh, 2022).

Complementary and Integrative Health. Many patients use complementary and integrative therapies as adjuncts to drug therapy. Yoga, meditation, massage, exercise, and biofeedback are helpful in preventing or treating migraines for some patients. Vitamin B_{12} (riboflavin) and magnesium supplements to maintain normal serum values may have a role in migraine prevention (National Center for Complementary and Integrative Health [NCCIH], 2022). A number of herbs are also used for headaches, for both prevention and pain management. Teach patients that all herbs and nutritional remedies should be approved by their primary health care provider before use because they could interact with prescribed medication.

Acupuncture and acupressure may be effective in relieving pain for some patients (NCCIH, 2022). Some plastic surgeons have resected the trigeminal nerve to relieve chronic migraine pain.

SEIZURES AND EPILEPSY

A **seizure** is an abnormal, sudden, excessive, uncontrolled electrical discharge of neurons within the brain that may result in a change in level of consciousness (LOC), motor or sensory ability, and/or behavior. A single seizure may occur for no known reason. Some seizures are caused by a pathologic condition of the brain, such as a tumor. In this case, once the underlying problem has been treated, the patient is often asymptomatic.

Pathophysiology Review

Epilepsy is defined by the National Institute of Neurological Disorders and Stroke (NINDS) as a chronic disorder in which repeated unprovoked seizure activity occurs. It may be caused by an abnormality in electrical neuronal activity; an imbalance of neurotransmitters, especially gamma-aminobutyric acid (GABA); or a combination of both (Rogers, 2023).

Types of Seizures

The International League Against Epilepsy recognizes several broad categories of seizure disorders: generalized seizures, partial seizures (focal), combined generalized and partial seizures, and unclassified or unknown seizures.

Five types of *generalized seizures* may occur in adults and involve *both* cerebral hemispheres. The *tonic-clonic seizure* lasting 2 to 5 minutes begins with a tonic phase that causes stiffening or rigidity of the muscles, particularly of the arms and legs, and immediate loss of consciousness. *Clonic* or rhythmic jerking (clonus) of all extremities follows. The patient may bite the tongue and become incontinent of urine or feces. Fatigue, acute confusion, and lethargy may last up to an hour after the seizure (*postictal state*, or "after the seizure" state).

Occasionally only tonic or clonic movement may occur. A *tonic seizure* is an abrupt increase in muscle tone, loss of consciousness, and autonomic changes lasting from 30 seconds to several minutes. The *clonic seizure* lasts several minutes and causes muscle contraction and relaxation.

The *myoclonic seizure* causes a brief jerking or stiffening of the extremities that may occur singly or in groups. Lasting for just a few seconds, the contractions may be symmetric (both sides) or asymmetric (one side).

In an *atonic (akinetic) seizure,* the patient has a sudden loss of muscle tone, lasting for seconds, followed by postictal confusion. In most cases, these seizures cause the patient to fall, which may result in injury. This type of seizure tends to be most resistant to drug therapy.

Partial seizures, also called *focal* or *local* seizures, begin in a part of *one* cerebral hemisphere. They are further subdivided into two main classes: complex partial seizures and simple partial seizures. In addition, some partial seizures can become generalized tonic-clonic, tonic, or clonic seizures. Partial seizures are most often seen in adults and generally are less responsive to medical treatment when compared with other types.

Complex partial seizures may cause loss of consciousness (syncope), or "blackout," for 1 to 3 minutes. Characteristic automatisms may occur as in absence seizures. The patient is unaware of the environment and may wander at the start of the seizure. In the period after the seizure, the patient may have amnesia (loss of memory). Because the area of the brain most often involved in this type of epilepsy is the temporal lobe, complex partial seizures are often called *psychomotor* seizures or *temporal lobe* seizures.

Seizures

Complex partial seizures are most common among older adults. These seizures are difficult to diagnose because symptoms appear similar to those of dementia, psychosis, or other neurobehavioral disorders, especially in the postictal stage (after the seizure). New-onset seizures in older adults typically are associated with conditions such as hypertension, cardiac disease, diabetes mellitus, stroke, dementia, and recent brain injury (Rogers, 2023).

Patients with a *simple partial seizure* remain conscious throughout the episode. They often reports an aura (unusual sensation) before the seizure takes place. This may consist of a "déjà vu" (already seen) phenomenon, perception of an offensive smell, or sudden onset of pain. During the seizure, the patient may have one-sided movement of an extremity, experience unusual sensations, or have autonomic symptoms. Autonomic changes include a change in heart rate, skin flushing, and epigastric discomfort.

Unclassified (unknown) or idiopathic seizures account for about half of all seizure activity. They occur for no known reason and do not fit into the generalized or partial classifications.

Etiology and Genetic Risk

Primary or *idiopathic epilepsy* is not associated with any identifiable brain lesion or other specific cause; however, genetic factors most likely play a role in its development. *Secondary seizures* result from an underlying brain lesion, most commonly a tumor or trauma. They may also be caused by:

- Metabolic disorders
- Acute alcohol withdrawal
- Electrolyte disturbances (e.g., hyperkalemia, water intoxication, hypoglycemia)
- High fever
- Stroke
- Head injury
- Substance abuse
- Heart disease

Seizures resulting from these problems are not considered epilepsy. Various risk factors can trigger a seizure, such as increased physical activity, emotional stress, excessive fatigue, alcohol or caffeine consumption, or certain foods or chemicals.

Interprofessional Collaborative Care

Recognize Cues: Assessment

Question the patient or family about how many seizures the patient has had, how long they last, and any pattern of occurrence. Ask the patient or family to describe the seizures that the patient has had. Signs and symptoms vary, depending on the type of seizure experienced, as described earlier. Ask about the presence of an aura before seizures begin (*preictal phase*). Question whether the patient is taking any prescribed drugs or

TABLE 36.2 Common Examples of Drug Therapy

Drug Therapy Used to Treat Seizures and Epilepsy

Drug Category	Selected Nursing Implications
Hydantoins Common examples of hydantoins: • Phenytoin • Fosphenytoin	When given IV for status epilepticus, dilute in 0.9% normal saline (NS). Teach patients to expect side effects such as headache and drowsiness, especially when starting drug therapy. Teach patients to perform frequent oral care and have regular dental exams, if possible, due to the development of gingival hyperplasia. Check if patients starting phenytoin are on warfarin therapy; patients should not be prescribed both drugs to prevent excessive bleeding and phenytoin toxicity. Be aware that the desired therapeutic drug level of phenytoin = 10–20 mcg/mL. Be aware that the desired therapeutic drug level of fosphenytoin = 1.0–2.5 mcg/mL.
Iminostilbenes Common examples of iminostilbenes: • Carbamazepine • Eslicarbazepine • Oxcarbazepine	Teach patients that drug may cause dizziness and drowsiness. Monitor for a rash in patients starting carbamazepine. Be aware that carbamazepine is also used for chronic neuropathic pain.
Succinimides Common example of succinimides: • Ethosuximide	Teach patients that drug may cause dizziness, drowsiness, impaired cognition, ataxia, and gingival hyperplasia.
Benzodiazepines Common examples of benzodiazepines: • Lorazepam • Clorazepate	Recognize that lorazepam is most often given intravenously to manage status epilepticus. Be aware that clorazepate is used to prevent patient seizures; monitor for multiple side/adverse effects including hypotension and respiratory depression.
Miscellaneous Common examples of miscellaneous drugs: • Gabapentin • Lamotrigine • Topiramate • Pregabalin • Valproic acid • Ezogabine	Teach patients that any of these drugs can cause drowsiness and dizziness, especially when first starting them. Recognize that some of these drugs can also be used to manage neuropathic pain, especially gabapentin and pregabalin. Remind patients that topiramate can cause weight loss.

herbs or has had head trauma or high fever. Assess any alcohol and/or illicit drug history. Ask about any other medical condition such as a previous stroke or hypertension.

If the seizure is a new symptom, ask the patient or family if any loss of consciousness or brain injury has occurred, in both the recent and distant past. Often patients may have had a head or brain injury sufficient to cause a loss of consciousness but may not remember this at the time of the seizure, especially if it was during their childhood.

Diagnosis is based on the history and physical examination. A variety of diagnostic tests are performed to rule out other causes of seizure activity and to confirm the diagnosis of epilepsy. Typical diagnostic tests include an electroencephalogram (EEG), CT scan, MRI, and/or SPECT/PET scan. These tests are described in Chapter 35 of this textbook.

Take Actions: Interventions

Removing or treating the underlying condition or cause of the seizure manages *secondary* epilepsy and seizures that are not considered epileptic. In most cases, primary epilepsy is successfully managed through drug therapy.

Nonsurgical Management. Most seizures can be completely or almost completely controlled through the administration of *antiepileptic drugs (AEDs),* sometimes referred to as *anticonvulsants,* for specific types of seizures.

Drug Therapy. Drug therapy is the major component of seizure management (Table 36.2). The primary health care provider introduces one antiepileptic drug (AED) at a time to achieve control for the type of seizure that the patient has. If the chosen drug is not effective, the dosage may be increased, or another drug introduced. At times, seizure control is achieved only through a combination of drugs. The dosages are adjusted to achieve therapeutic blood levels without causing major side effects. Because of these potential side effects, teach patients to:

- Follow up on laboratory test appointments to monitor the patient's complete blood count (CBC) and liver enzymes and assess for therapeutic drug levels. Most AEDs can cause leukopenia and liver dysfunction.
- Some drugs, especially the hydantoins, can cause gingival hyperplasia. Observe for and report beginning gingival changes and perform frequent oral care to prevent permanent damage. If possible, have regular dental checkups.

PATIENT-CENTERED CARE: GENDER HEALTH

Seizures in Women

Management of women with epilepsy is often challenging. Hormonal changes from menstrual cycling and the interaction of oral contraceptives with antiepileptic drugs (AEDs) require the primary health care provider and patient to be aware of a variety of guidelines and to monitor drug effectiveness more frequently. AEDs can also contribute to osteoporosis in menopausal women. As a result, coordination among the neurologist, the woman's primary health care provider, and the patient is required for safe, effective care. Nurses can facilitate patient education, communication, and collaboration to promote safe, effective care.

Teach patients to take their drugs on time and as prescribed to maintain therapeutic blood levels and maximum effectiveness. Instruct patients that they can build up sensitivity to the drugs as they age. If sensitivity occurs, tell them they will need to have blood levels of this drug checked frequently to adjust the dose. In some cases, the antiseizure effects of drugs can decline and lead to an increase in seizures. Because of this potential for "drug decline and sensitivity," patients need to keep their scheduled laboratory appointments to check serum drug levels.

Be aware of drug-drug and drug-food interactions. For instance, phenytoin should not be given with warfarin (Burchum & Rosenthal, 2022). Document side and adverse effects of the prescribed drugs and report to the health care provider. Teach patients that some citrus fruits, such as grapefruit juice, can interfere with the metabolism of these drugs. This interference can raise the blood level of the drug and cause the patient to develop drug toxicity.

Seizure Precautions. Precautions are taken to prevent the patient from injury if a seizure occurs. Specific seizure precautions vary, depending on health care agency policy.

! NURSING SAFETY PRIORITY

Action Alert

Seizure precautions include ensuring that oxygen and suctioning equipment with an airway are readily available. If the patient does not have IV access, insert a saline lock, especially if the patient is at significant risk for generalized tonic-clonic seizures. The saline lock provides ready access if IV drug therapy must be given to stop seizure activity.

Side rails are rarely the source of significant injury, and the effectiveness of the use of padded side rails to maintain safety is debatable. Padded side rails may embarrass the patient and the family. Follow agency policy about the use of side rails because they may be classified as a restraint device.

Seizure Management. The actions taken during a seizure should be appropriate for the type of seizure, as outlined in Box 36.9.

It is not unusual for the patient to become cyanotic during a generalized tonic-clonic seizure. The cyanosis is generally self-limiting, and no treatment is needed. Some primary health care providers prefer to give the high-risk patient (e.g., older adult, critically ill, or debilitated patient) oxygen by nasal

BOX 36.9 Best Practice for Patient Safety and Quality Care

Care of the Patient During a Tonic-Clonic or Complex Partial Seizure

- Protect the patient from injury.
- Do not force anything into the patient's mouth.
- Turn the patient to the side to prevent aspiration and to keep the airway clear.
- Remove any objects that might injure the patient.
- Suction oral secretions, if possible, without force.
- Loosen any restrictive clothing the patient is wearing.
- Do not restrain or try to stop the patient's movement; guide movements if necessary.
- Record the time the seizure began and ended.
- At the completion of the seizure:
  - Take the patient's vital signs.
  - Perform neurologic checks.
  - Keep the patient lying on the side.
  - Allow the patient to rest.
- Document the seizure:
  - How often the seizures occur: date, time, and duration of the seizure
  - Whether more than one type of seizure occurs
- Observations during the seizure:
  - Changes in pupil size and any eye deviation
  - Level of consciousness
  - Presence of apnea, cyanosis, and salivation
  - Incontinence of bowel or bladder during the seizure
  - Eye fluttering or blinking
  - Movement and progression of motor activity
  - Lip smacking or other automatism
  - Tongue or lip biting
  - How long the seizure lasts
  - When the last seizure took place
  - Whether the seizure was preceded by an aura
  - What the patient does after the seizure
  - How long it takes for the patient to return to preseizure status

cannula or facemask during the postictal phase. For any type of seizure, carefully observe the seizure and document assessment findings.

Emergency Care: Acute Seizure and Status Epilepticus Management. Seizures occurring in greater intensity, number, or length than the patient's usual seizures are considered *acute*. They may also appear in clusters that are different from the patient's typical seizure pattern. Treatment with lorazepam or diazepam may be given to stop the clusters to prevent the development of status epilepticus. IV phenytoin or fosphenytoin may be added (Burchum & Rosenthal, 2022).

Status epilepticus is a medical emergency and is a prolonged seizure lasting longer than 5 minutes or repeated seizures over the course of 30 minutes. It is a potential complication of all types of seizures. Any one seizure lasting longer than 10 minutes can cause death! Common causes of status epilepticus include:

- Sudden withdrawal from antiepileptic drugs
- Infection
- Acute alcohol or drug withdrawal
- Traumatic brain injury
- Cerebral edema
- Metabolic disturbances

NURSING SAFETY PRIORITY

Critical Rescue

Convulsive status epilepticus must be treated promptly and aggressively! Establish an airway and notify the primary health care provider or Rapid Response Team immediately if this problem occurs. *Establishing an airway is the priority for this patient's care.* Intubation by an anesthesia provider or respiratory therapist may be necessary. Administer oxygen as indicated by the patient's condition. If not already in place, establish IV access with a large-bore catheter and start 0.9% sodium chloride. The patient is usually placed in the ICU for continuous monitoring and management.

Brain damage and death may occur in the patient with tonic-clonic status epilepticus. Left untreated, metabolic changes result, leading to hypoxia, hypotension, hypoglycemia, cardiac dysrhythmias, or lactic (metabolic) acidosis. Further harm to the patient occurs when muscle breaks down and myoglobin accumulates in the kidneys, which can lead to acute kidney injury and electrolyte imbalance. *This is especially likely in the older adult.*

The drugs of choice for treating status epilepticus are IV-push lorazepam or diazepam. Diazepam rectal gel may be used instead. Lorazepam is usually given as over a 2-minute period; this may be repeated, if necessary.

NURSING SAFETY PRIORITY

Drug Alert

To prevent additional tonic-clonic seizures or cardiac arrest, a loading dose of IV phenytoin is given and oral doses are administered as a follow-up after the emergency is resolved. Initially give phenytoin using an infusion pump. If the drug is piggybacked into an existing IV line, use only normal saline (0.9% NS) as the primary IV fluid to prevent drug precipitation. Be sure to flush the line with normal saline before and after phenytoin administration (Burchum & Rosenthal, 2022).

An alternative to phenytoin is fosphenytoin, a water-soluble phenytoin prodrug. It is compatible with most IV solutions. It also causes fewer cardiovascular complications than phenytoin and can be given in an IV dextrose solution. After administration, fosphenytoin converts to phenytoin in the body. Therefore the FDA requires the dosage to be written as a phenytoin equivalent (PE).

Teach the patient and family that serum drug levels are checked every 6 to 12 hours after the loading dose and then 2 weeks after oral phenytoin has started. The desired serum therapeutic range is 10 to 20 mcg/mL (Burchum & Rosenthal, 2022).

Surgical Management. Patients who cannot be managed effectively with drug therapy may be candidates for surgery, including vagal nerve stimulation (VNS). VNS has been very successful for many patients with epilepsy and is sometimes referred to as being similar to a cardiac pacemaker.

VNS may be performed for control of continuous simple or complex partial seizures. Patients with generalized seizures are not candidates for surgery because VNS may result in severe neurologic deficits. The stimulating device (much like a cardiac pacemaker) is surgically implanted in the left chest wall. An electrode lead is attached to the left vagus nerve, tunneled under the skin, and connected to a generator. The procedure usually takes 2 hours with the patient under general anesthesia. The stimulator is activated by the primary health care provider either in the operating room or, more commonly, 2 weeks after surgery. Programming is adjusted gradually over a period of time. The pattern of stimulation is individualized to the patient's tolerance. The generator runs continuously, stimulating the vagus nerve according to the programmed schedule.

The patient can activate the VNS with a handheld magnet when experiencing an aura, thus aborting the seizure. Patients experience a change in voice quality, which signifies that the vagus nerve has been stimulated. They usually report a relief in intensity and duration of seizures and an improved quality of life (Chandra et al., 2020).

Observe for complications after the procedure such as hoarseness (most common), cough, dyspnea, neck pain, or dysphagia (difficulty swallowing). Teach the patient to avoid MRIs, microwaves, shortwave radios, and ultrasound diathermy (a physical therapy heat treatment).

Care Coordination and Transition Management

Provide self-management education for the patient and family (Box 36.10). Ask them what they understand about the disorder and correct any misinformation. As new information is presented, be sure that the patient and family can understand it.

Emphasize that AEDs must not be stopped even if the seizures have stopped. Discontinuing these drugs can lead to the recurrence of seizures or the life-threatening complication of status epilepticus (discussed earlier). Some patients may stop therapy because they do not have the money to purchase the drugs. Refer limited-income patients to the social services department for assistance or to a case manager to locate other resources.

BOX 36.10 **Patient and Family Education**

Health Teaching for the Patient With Epilepsy

- Know and understand drug therapy information:
  - Name, dosage, time of administration
  - Actions to take if side effects occur
  - Importance of taking drugs as prescribed and not missing a dose
  - What to do if a dose is missed or cannot be taken
- Understand the importance of having blood drawn for therapeutic or toxic levels as requested by the primary health care provider.
- Do not take any drug, including over-the-counter drugs, without asking your primary health care provider.
- Wear a medical alert bracelet or necklace or carry an identification card indicating epilepsy.
- Follow up with your neurologist or other primary health care provider as directed.
- Be sure that a family member or significant other knows how to help you in the event of a seizure and knows when your primary health care provider or emergency medical services should be called.
- Investigate and follow state laws concerning driving and operating machinery.
- Avoid alcohol and excessive fatigue.
- Contact the Epilepsy Foundation (www.epilepsy.com) or other organized epilepsy group for additional information. Epilepsy Canada (www.epilepsy.ca) also provides resources and support.

A balanced diet, proper rest, and stress-reduction techniques usually minimize the risk for breakthrough seizures. Encourage the patient to keep a seizure diary to determine whether there are factors that tend to be associated with seizure activity.

All states prohibit discrimination against people who have epilepsy. Having appropriate employment has been recognized as a major burden of epilepsy (Mlinar et al., 2021). Patients who work in occupations in which a seizure might cause serious harm to themselves or others (e.g., construction workers, operators of dangerous equipment, pilots) may need other employment. They may need to decrease or modify strenuous or potentially dangerous physical activity to avoid harm, although this varies with each person. Various local, state, and federal agencies can help with finances, living arrangements, and vocational rehabilitation.

MENINGITIS

Meningitis is an **infection** of the meninges of the brain and spinal cord, specifically the pia mater and arachnoid mater. Bacterial and viral organisms are most often responsible for meningitis, although fungal and protozoal meningitis also occur. Cancer and some drugs, notably NSAIDs, antibiotics, and IV immunoglobulins, can also cause sterile meningitis. Regardless of cause of meningitis, the symptoms are similar.

Pathophysiology Review

The organisms responsible for meningitis enter the central nervous system (CNS) via the bloodstream or are directly introduced into the CNS. Direct routes of entry occur as a result of penetrating trauma, surgical procedures on the brain or spine, or a ruptured brain abscess. A basilar skull fracture may lead to meningitis as a result of the direct communication of cerebrospinal fluid (CSF) with the ear or nasal passages, manifesting with otorrhea (ear discharge) or rhinorrhea (nasal discharge, or "runny nose") that is actually CSF. The infecting organisms follow the tract created by skull damage to enter the CNS and circulate in the CSF. The patient with an infection in the head (i.e., eye, ear, nose, mouth) or neck/throat has an increased risk for meningitis because of the proximity of anatomic structures. Infections linked to meningitis include otitis media, acute or chronic sinusitis, and tooth abscess; there are also reports of rare cases from tongue piercing. The immunocompromised patient (e.g., one without a spleen receiving treatment for cancer, a patient taking immunosuppressant drugs to manage autoimmune disease or solid organ transplant, and older adults) is also at increased risk for meningitis. The infecting organism may spread to both cranial and spinal nerves, causing irreversible neurologic damage. Increased intracranial pressure (ICP) may occur as a result of blockage of the flow of CSF, change in cerebral blood flow, or thrombus (blood clot) formation (Rogers, 2023).

Viral meningitis, the most common type, is sometimes referred to as *aseptic meningitis* because no organisms are typically isolated from culture of the CSF. Common viral organisms causing meningitis are enterovirus, herpes simplex virus 2 (HSV-2), varicella zoster virus (VZV) (also causes shingles),

mumps virus, and human immunodeficiency virus (HIV) (Rogers, 2023). The severity of symptoms can vary according to the infecting viral agent. For example, the herpes simplex virus alters cellular metabolism, which quickly results in necrosis of the cells. HSV-2 meningitis may be accompanied by genital infections. Other viruses cause an alteration in the production of enzymes or neurotransmitters. Although these alterations result in cell dysfunction, neurologic defects are more likely to be temporary, and a full recovery occurs as the inflammation resolves.

Cryptococcus neoformans meningitis is the most common fungal infection that affects the CNS of patients with human immunodeficiency virus (HIV) stage 3. Fulminant invasive fungal sinusitis is also a recognized cause of fungal meningitis. The signs and symptoms vary because the compromised immune system affects the inflammatory response. For example, some patients have fever and others do not.

The most frequently involved organisms responsible for bacterial meningococcal meningitis are *Streptococcus pneumoniae* (pneumococcal disease) and *Neisseria meningitidis*. *N. meningitidis* meningitis is also known as meningococcal meningitis. Meningococcal meningitis is a medical emergency with a fairly high mortality rate, often within 24 hours. Unlike other types, this disorder is highly contagious. Outbreaks of meningococcal meningitis are most likely to occur in areas of high population density, such as college dormitories, military barracks, and crowded living areas.

! **NURSING SAFETY PRIORITY**

Action Alert

People ages 16 to 21 years have the highest rates of infection from life-threatening *Neisseria meningitidis* meningococcal infection. The Centers for Disease Control and Prevention (CDC) recommends an initial meningococcal vaccine between ages 11 and 12 years with a booster at age 16 years (www.cdc.gov). Adults are advised to get an initial or a booster vaccine if living in a shared residence (college residence hall, military barracks, group home) or traveling or residing in countries in which the disease is common or if they are immunocompromised as a result of a damaged or surgically removed spleen. If the patient's baseline vaccination status is unclear and the immediate risk for exposure to *N. meningitidis* infection is high, the CDC recommends vaccination. It is safe to receive a booster as early as 8 weeks after the initial vaccine.

Interprofessional Collaborative Care

Recognize Cues: Assessment

Perform a complete neurologic and neurovascular assessment to detect signs and symptoms associated with a diagnosis of meningitis or suspected meningitis as outlined in Box 36.11.

Although the classic nuchal rigidity (stiff neck) and positive Kernig and Brudzinski signs have been traditionally used to diagnose meningitis, these findings occur in only a small percentage of patients with a definitive diagnosis. Older adults, patients who are immunocompromised, and those who are receiving antibiotics may not have fever. Assess the patient

BOX 36.11 Key Features

Meningitis

- Decreased level of consciousness
- Disorientation to person, place, and time
- Pupil reaction and eye movements:
  - Photophobia (sensitivity to light)
  - Nystagmus (involuntary condition in which the eyes make repetitive uncontrolled movements)
- Motor response:
  - Normal early in disease process
  - Hemiparesis (weakness on one side of the body), hemiplegia (paralysis on one side of the body), and decreased muscle tone possible later
  - Cranial nerve (CN) dysfunction, especially CN III, IV, VI, VII, VIII
- Memory changes:
  - Attention span (usually short)
  - Personality and behavior changes
- Severe, unrelenting headaches
- Generalized muscle aches and pain (myalgia)
- Nausea and vomiting
- Fever and chills
- Tachycardia
- Red macular rash (meningococcal meningitis)

for complications, including increased ICP. Left untreated, increased ICP can lead to herniation of the brain and death (see Chapter 38).

Seizure activity may occur when meningeal inflammation and *infection* spreads to the cerebral cortex. Inflammation can also result in abnormal stimulation of the hypothalamic area where excessive amounts of antidiuretic hormone (ADH) (vasopressin) are produced. Excess vasopressin results in water retention and dilution of serum sodium caused by increased sodium loss by the kidneys. This syndrome of inappropriate antidiuretic hormone (SIADH; see discussion in Chapter 54) may lead to further increases in ICP.

Meningitis may be misdiagnosed as encephalitis, an *infection* (usually viral) of brain tissue and often the surrounding meninges. Diagnostic testing is needed to differentiate these two diseases.

The most significant laboratory test used in the diagnosis of meningitis is the analysis of the *cerebrospinal fluid (CSF)*. Patients older than 60 years, those who are immunocompromised, or those who have signs of increased ICP usually have a CT scan before the lumbar puncture (LP). If there will be a delay in obtaining the CSF, blood is drawn for culture and sensitivity. A broad-spectrum antibiotic should be given immediately after the LP, unless the LP will be delayed. The CSF is analyzed for cell count, differential count, and protein. Glucose concentrations are determined, and culture, sensitivity, and Gram stain studies are performed.

Counterimmunoelectrophoresis (CIE) may be performed to determine the presence of viruses or protozoa in the CSF. CIE is also indicated if the patient has received antibiotics before the CSF was obtained. To identify a bacterial source of infection, specimens for Gram stains and culture are obtained from the urine, throat, and nose when indicated.

A complete blood count (CBC) is performed. The white blood cell (WBC) count is usually elevated well above the normal value. Serum electrolyte values are also checked to assess and maintain fluid and electrolyte balance.

X-rays of the chest, air sinuses, and mastoids are obtained to determine the presence of *infection.* A CT or MRI scan may be performed to identify increased ICP, hydrocephalus, or the presence of a brain abscess.

Take Actions: Interventions

Prevent meningitis by teaching people to obtain vaccination. Vaccines are available to protect against *Haemophilus influenzae* type B (Hib), pneumococcal, mumps, varicella, and meningococcal organisms. Although many of these vaccines were developed to prevent respiratory illness, they have also reduced CNS infections. Mandatory vaccination programs for school enrollment and proof of vaccination that are prerequisites for group home or dormitory experiences have significantly reduced the incidence of meningitis.

The most important nursing interventions for patients with meningitis are accurate monitoring and documenting of their neurologic status.

! NURSING SAFETY PRIORITY

Action Alert

For the patient with meningitis, assess the neurologic status and vital signs at least every 2 to 4 hours or more often if clinically indicated. *The priority for care is to monitor for early neurologic changes that may indicate increased intracranial pressure (ICP), such as decreased level of consciousness (LOC).* The patient is also at risk for seizure activity. Care should be provided as discussed under Interventions in the Seizures and Epilepsy section.

Cranial nerve testing is included as part of the routine neurologic assessment because of possible cranial nerve involvement. *A sixth cranial nerve defect (inability to move the eyes laterally) may indicate the development of* hydrocephalus *(excessive accumulation of CSF within the brain's ventricles).* Other indicators of hydrocephalus include signs of increased ICP and urinary incontinence. Urinary incontinence can result from decreasing LOC.

To avoid life-threatening complications from bacterial meningitis, the primary health care provider prescribes a broad-spectrum antibiotic until the results of the culture and Gram stain are available. After this information is available, the appropriate antiinfective drug to treat the specific type of meningitis is given. Treatment of bacterial meningitis generally requires a 2-week course of IV antibiotics. Drug therapy should begin within 1 to 2 hours after it is prescribed. Monitor and document the patient's response.

Drugs may be used to treat increased ICP or seizures, including mannitol, a hyperosmolar agent for ICP, and antiepileptic drugs (AEDs). Controversy exists as to whether adjuvant steroids are helpful in the treatment of adults with acute bacterial meningitis. However, they may be used for some patients with *S. pneumoniae* meningitis.

People who have been in close contact with a patient with *N. meningitidis* should have prophylaxis (preventive) treatment with rifampin, ciprofloxacin, or ceftriaxone. Preventive treatment with rifampin may be prescribed for those in close contact with a patient with *H. influenzae* meningitis (Burchum & Rosenthal, 2022).

⚠ NURSING SAFETY PRIORITY

Action Alert

Place the patient with bacterial meningitis that is transmitted by droplets on Droplet Precautions *in addition to* Standard Precautions. When possible, place the patient in a private room. Stay at least 3 feet from the patient unless wearing a mask. Patients who are transported outside of the room should wear a mask (see Chapter 19). Teach visitors about the need for these precautions and how to follow them.

Perform a complete vascular assessment every 4 hours or more often, if indicated, to detect early vascular compromise. Thrombotic or embolic complications are most often seen in circulation to the hand. Assess the patient's temperature, color, pulses, and capillary refill in the fingernails. If vascular compromise is not noticed and is left untreated, gangrene can develop quickly, possibly leading to loss of the involved arm. The health care team monitors the patient for other complications, including septic shock, coagulation disorders, acute respiratory distress syndrome, and septic arthritis. These health problems are discussed elsewhere in this textbook.

Standard Precautions are appropriate for all patients with meningitis unless the patient has a bacterial type that is transmitted by droplets, such as *N. meningitides* and *H. influenzae*. Best practices for general nursing care of patients who have meningitis are listed in Box 36.12.

BOX 36.12 Best Practice for Patient Safety and Quality Care

Nursing Care of the Patient With Meningitis

- Prioritize care to maintain airway, breathing, and circulation.
- Take vital signs and perform neurologic checks every 2 to 4 hours, as needed.
- Perform cranial nerve assessment, with particular attention to cranial nerves III, IV, VI, VII, and VIII, and monitor for changes.
- Manage pain with drug and nondrug methods.
- Perform vascular assessment and monitor for changes.
- Give drugs and IV fluids as prescribed and document the patient's response.
- Record intake and output carefully to maintain fluid balance and prevent fluid overload.
- Monitor body weight to identify fluid retention early.
- Monitor laboratory values closely; report abnormal findings to the physician or nurse practitioner promptly.
- Position carefully to prevent pressure injuries.
- Perform range-of-motion exercises every 4 hours as needed.
- Decrease environmental stimuli:
  - Provide a quiet environment.
  - Minimize exposure to bright lights from windows and overhead lights.
- Maintain bed rest with head of bed elevated 30 degrees.
- Maintain Transmission-Based Precautions per hospital policy (for bacterial meningitis).
- Monitor for complications:
  - Increased intracranial pressure
  - Vascular dysfunction
  - Fluid and electrolyte imbalance
  - Seizures
  - Shock

GET READY FOR THE NEXT-GENERATION NCLEX® EXAMINATION!

Essential Nursing Care Points

Health Promotion/Disease Prevention

- Maintaining a healthy lifestyle can help prevent Alzheimer's disease (AD) and other dementias; assess whether individuals have adequate housing, food, and access to health care.
- Patients with traumatic brain injury (TBI) experience a higher incidence of Parkinson's disease (PD) when compared with those who do not have TBI. Therefore athletes participating in contact sports should wear helmets because they are at high risk for developing PD, often at a young age.
- The Centers for Disease Control and Prevention (CDC) recommends an initial meningococcal vaccine between ages 11 and 12 years with a booster at age 16 years. Adults are advised to get an initial or a booster vaccine if living in a shared residence (college residence hall, military barracks, group home) or traveling or residing in countries in which the disease is common or if they are immunocompromised as a result of a damaged or surgically removed spleen.

Chronic Disease Care

- AD is a chronic, progressive disease affecting **cognition**.
- The clinical phase of AD includes three disease stages: early stage, moderate stage, and late stage. Nursing care for patients who have AD depends on the stage of their disease.
- AD occurs more commonly in people of color (Black and Hispanic individuals) when compared with Whites due to social determinants of health such as lower socioeconomic status and educational level.
- The priority outcome for patients who have AD or PD is safety.
- Patients who have AD should be involved in advance care planning in the early and moderate stages of the disease process, if possible.
- In late-stage AD or PD, patients usually die from complications of immobility.

Regenerative or Restorative Care

- A migraine headache is a common clinical syndrome characterized by recurrent episodic attacks of head pain that serve no protective purpose.
- Patients who have migraines use both preventive and abortive drug therapy to reduce pain and the frequency of migraine episodes.
- Status epilepticus is a medical emergency and is a prolonged seizure lasting longer than 5 minutes or repeated seizures over the course of 30 minutes.
- The priority for interprofessional care of patients who experience seizure activity is to prevent injury.
- For patients who are diagnosed with meningitis, the priority for nursing care is to monitor for early neurologic changes that may indicate increased intracranial pressure (ICP), such as decreased level of consciousness (LOC).

Hospice/Palliative/Supportive Care

- Nurses and other health care professionals should assess patients with AD who require caregivers for signs of abuse and neglect; assess caregivers for their stress level and coping skills.
- Nurses need to educate families about the need for patients with late-stage AD and PD to have hospice and/or palliative care at the end of life to promote comfort and quality of life.

Mastery Questions

1. The nurse is planning health teaching for a client who has late-stage Alzheimer's disease (AD). Which of the following statements would be **most appropriate** for the nurse to include for the client and family?
   A. "The client should have input into advance care planning with the health care team."
   B. "The client may need placement in a memory care unit in the local assisted-living facility."
   C. "The client likely needs palliative care to manage pain and other symptoms to promote comfort."
   D. "The client would be an ideal candidate to attend adult day care while you are working during the day."

2. The nurse is assessing an ambulatory client who was recently diagnosed with early Parkinson's disease. Which of the following client findings would the nurse anticipate during the assessment?
   A. Lewy body dementia
   B. Resting tremors of the arms
   C. Inability to chew or swallow food
   D. Urinary incontinence

3. A hospitalized client experiences a tonic-clonic seizure that is observed by the nurse. Which of the following actions by the nurse would be **most appropriate** during the seizure? **Select all that apply.**
   A. Lower the client gently to the floor.
   B. Insert an oropharyngeal airway.
   C. Gently suction any excess oral secretions if possible.
   D. Take the client's vital signs.
   E. Move any objects that might harm the patient.
   F. Administer diazepam or lorazepam immediately.

NGN Challenge 36.1

The nurse is caring for a 54-year-old client admitted to an acute care unit.

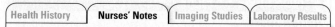

| Health History | **Nurses' Notes** | Imaging Studies | Laboratory Results |

0935: Had 3 tonic-clonic seizures lasting 2–3 minutes during the past hour. Given IVP lorazepam per protocol. IV infusion of fosphenytoin in 0.9% NS started. Continuous oxygen at 2 L/min via NC initiated. SpO_2 99%. Neurologic status returned to preseizure status. Alert and oriented × 4; moves all extremities; PERRLA; CNs intact. VS: T 99°F (37.2°C); HR 78 BPM; RR 16 bpm; BP 120/72 mm Hg.

Complete the diagram by selecting from the choices below to specify what potential condition the client is likely experiencing, **2** nursing actions that are appropriate to take, and **2** parameters the nurse should monitor to assess the client's progress.

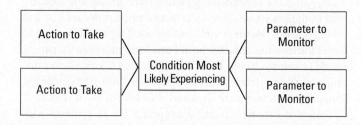

Actions to Take	Potential Conditions	Parameters to Monitor
Give IV push diazepam or lorazepam	Cerebral edema	Level of consciousness
Start IV antibiotics	Encephalitis	Serum glucose level
Administer IVP osmotic diuretic	Hypoglycemia	Client's airway
Plan transfer to critical care unit	Status epilepticus	Body temperature
Monitor kidney function		Kidney function tests

NGN Challenge 36.2

The nurse is caring for a 21-year-old client admitted last night. Highlight the findings that require **immediate** follow up.

NURSING FLOW SHEET

Time	0400 (ED)	0600 (Admission)	0700
Temperature	101.6°F (38.7°C)	102.4°F (39.1°C)	100.8°F (38.2°C)
Heart rate	82 beats/min	85 beats/min	86 beats/min
Respiratory rate/Sp0₂	18 breaths/min/97%	20 breaths/min/96%	16 breaths/min/96%
Blood pressure	118/70 mm Hg	122/74 mm Hg	116/66 mm Hg

0600: Alert and oriented × 4; CN check normal; PERRLA; moves all 4 extremities. Reports headache at 8/10. Analgesic administered per protocol. No seizure activity since admission. Seizure Precautions initiated; placed on Standard and Droplet Precautions. Had lumbar puncture; awaiting stat CSF lab analysis. WBC count 18,000/mm³ (18 × 10⁹/L).

0700: Drowsy but easily awakened; oriented × 2, not sure of day and time. PERRLA, moves all extremities. Reports feeling very sleepy. Headache 5/10. No seizure activity since admission.

REFERENCES

Asterisk(*) indicates a classic or definitive work on this subject.

Aarskog, N. K., Hunskår, I., & Bruvik, F. (2019). Animal-assisted interventions with dogs and robotic animals for residents with dementia in nursing homes: A systematic review. *Physical and Occupational Therapy in Geriatrics, 37*(2), 77–93.

Alzheimer's Association. (2022). *Facts and Figures. 2021 Alzheimer's Disease Facts and Figures.* https://www.alz.org/media/Documents/alzheimers-facts-and-figures.pdf.

American Parkinson Disease Association. (2023). *Diagnosing Parkinson's.* https://www.apdaparkinson.org/what-is-parkinsons/diagnosing/.

Aviram, J., Vysotski, Y., Berman, P., Lewitus, G. M., Eisenberg, E., & Meiri, D. (2020). Migraine frequency decrease following prolonged medical cannabis treatment: A cross-sectional study. *Brain Science, 10*(6), Article 360 https://www.ncbi.nlm.nih.gov/pmc/articles/PMC7348860/.

Brims, L., & Olivera, K. (2019). Effectiveness of assistive technology in improving the safety of people with dementia: a systematic review and meta-analysis. *AGING & MENTAL HEALTH 2019, 23*(8), 942–951.

Burchum, J. L. R., & Rosenthal, L. D. (2022). *Lehne's pharmacology for nursing care* (11th ed.). St. Louis: Elsevier.

Chandra, P. S., Samala, R., Agrawal, M., Doddamani, R. S., Ramanujam, B., & Tripathi1, M. (2020). Vagal nerve stimulation for drug refractory epilepsy. *Neurology India, 68*(Supplement 2), S325–327.

Chao, L. L. (2020). The prevalence of mild cognitive impairment in a convenience sample of 202 Gulf War veterans. *International Journal of Environmental Research and Public Health, 17*, 7158–7178.

Chiong, W., Tsou, A. Y., Simmons, Z., Bonnie, R. J., & Russell, J. A. (2021). Ethical considerations in dementia diagnosis and care: AAN position paper. *Neurology, 97*(2), 80–89.

Clark, C. S. (2021). *Cannabis: A handbook for nurses.* Philadelphia, PA: Wolters Kluwer.

Denning, K. H., & Aldridge, Z. (2021). Dementia: Recognition and cognitive testing in primary care settings. *Journal of Clinical Nursing, 35*(1), 43–49.

Dix, A. L., Barton, L. J., & Hunter, S. F. (2020, June). Anti-CGRP: A novel class of preventive treatments for adults with migraine. *The Clinical Advisor*, 12–20.

Eisenberg, H. M., Krishna, V., Elias, W. J., Cosgrove, G. R., Gandhi, D., Aldrich, C. E., et al (2020). *MR-guided focused ultrasound pallidotomy for Parkinson's disease: Safety and feasibility.* https://doi.org/10.3171/2020.6.JNS192773.

Ellis, T. & DeAngelis, T. (n.d.). Freezing. https://www.apdaparkinson.org/what-is-parkinsons/symptoms/freezing/.

Haney, A. A. (2020). Update on Alzheimer dementia spectrum: diagnosis and management. *The Clinical Advisor, 23*(10), 6–12.

International Headache Society. (2022). *International Classification of Headache Disorders* (3rd ed.). https://ichd-3.org/.

*Interprofessional Education Collaborative Expert Panel. (2016). *Core competencies for interprofessional collaborative practice: Report of an expert panel* (2nd ed.). Washington, D.C: Interprofessional Education Collaborative.

Majoka, M. A., & Schimming, C. (2021). Effect of social determinants of health on cognition and risk of Alzheimer's disease and related dementias. *Clinical Therapeutics, 43*(6), 922–929.

Mlinar, S., Rener Primec, Z., & Petek, D. (2021). Psychosocial factors in the experience of epilepsy: A qualitative analysis of narratives. *Behavioural Neurology*, Article 9976110. https://doi.org/10.1155/2021/9976110.

Mohamed, A. Z., Cumming, P., Götz, J., & Nasrallah, F. (2019). Tauopathy in veterans with long-term posttraumatic stress disorder and traumatic brain injury. *European Journal of Nuclear Medicine and Molecular Imaging, 46*, 1139–1151.

Mulvaney, C. A., Duarte, G. S., Handley, J., Evans, D. J., Menon, S., Wyse, R., et al. (2020). *GLP-1 receptor agonists for Parkinson's disease Cochrane Database of Systematic Reviews.* https://www.ncbi.nlm.nih.gov/pmc/articles/PMC7390475/pdf/CD012990.pdf.

National Center for Complementary and Integrative Health (NCCIH). (2022). Headaches: In depth. https://nccih.nih.gov/health/pain/headachefacts.htm#hed3.

National Conference of State Legislatures. (2023). *State medical marijuana laws.* https://www.ncsl.org/research/health/state-medical-marijuana-laws.aspx.

National Institute of Neurological Disorders and Stroke (NINDS). (2022). *Parkinson's disease.* www.ninds.nih.gov/disorders/parkinsons_disease/parkinsons_disease.htm.

Navia, R. O., & Constantine, L. A. (2022). Palliative care for patients with advanced dementia. *Nursing, 52*(3), 19–25.

Pagana, K. D., Pagana, T. J., & Pagana, T. N. (2022). *Mosby's Manual of diagnostic and laboratory tests* (7th ed.). St. Louis: Elsevier.

Parkinson's Foundation. (2022). *Understanding Parkinson's disease.* https://www.parkinson.org/understanding-parkinson-disease.

Parkinson's Foundation. (n.d.) Understanding surgical options. https://www.parkinson.org/Understanding-Parkinsons/Treatment/Surgical-Treatment-Options/Other-Surgical-Options.

Rogers, J. L. (2023). *McCance and Huether's Pathophysiology: The biologic basis for disease in adults and children* (9th ed.). St. Louis: Elsevier.

Saleh, N. (2022). *Using Cefaly for Migraine Prevention and Treatment.* Verywellhealth. https://www.verywellhealth.com/cefaly-migraine-prevention-and-treatment-4156863.

Schellack, N., Mogole, O., Magongwa, N., & Makola, F. (2019). Migraine headache: A brief overview. *Professional Nursing Today*, *23*(3), 9–12.

Slusser, M. M., Garcia, L. I., Reed, C.-R., & McGinnis, P. Q. (2019). *Foundations of interprofessional collaborative practice in health care*. St. Louis: Elsevier.

Smedinga, M., Bunnik, E. M., Richard, E., & Schermer, M. H. N. (2021). The framing of "Alzheimer's disease" differences between scientific and lay literature and their ethical implications. *The Gerontologist*, *61*(5), 746–755.

Smeltzer, S. C. (2021). Delivering quality healthcare for people with disability. Indianapolis. In *Sigma Theta Tau International Honor Society of Nursing*.

Theisen, E., & Koneyczny, E. (2019). Medical cannabis: What nurses need to know. *American Nurse Today*, *14*(11), 6–10.

Tomaino, C. M. (2021). Music therapy: Evidence-based practice to benefit people with neurologic issues. *Journal of Nurse Life Care Planning*, *21*(1), 24–28.

U.S. Food and Drug Administration. (2022). *FDA's Decision to Approve New Treatment for Alzheimer's Disease*. https://www.fda.gov/drugs/news-events-human-drugs/fdas-decision-approve-new-treatment-alzheimers-disease.

VA Office of Research and Development. (2022). *VA research on Parkinson's disease*. https://www.research.va.gov/topics/parkinsons.cfm.

Vacca, V. M. (2019). Parkinson's disease: Enhance nursing knowledge. *Nursing2019*, *49*(11), 24–32.

Xiong, J., Kang, S. S., Wang, Z., Liu, X., Kuo, T.-C., Korkmaz, F., et al. (2022). FSH blockade improves cognition in mice with Alzheimer's disease. *Nature*. https://doi.org/10.1038/s41586-022-04463-0.

Vice, K., & Tenhunen, M. L. (2020). Parkinson's Disease: A clinical review. *MEDSURG Nursing*, *29*(5), 327–332.

Yenilmez, F., Fründt, O., Hidding, U., & Buhmann, C. (2020). Cannabis shown to relieve Parkinson Disease symptoms. *Journal of Parkinson's Disease*. https://doi.org/10.3233/JPD-202260.

Zarepour, A., Hazrati, M., & Kadivar, A. (2020). The impact of educational intervention on the anxiety of family caregivers of the elderly with dementia: A randomized controlled trial. *International Journal of Community Based Nursing & Midwifery*, *8*(3), 234–242.

37

Concepts of Care for Patients With Conditions of the Central Nervous System: The Spinal Cord

Meg Blair

http://evolve.elsevier.com/Iggy/

LEARNING OUTCOMES

1. Plan collaborative care with the interprofessional team to promote *mobility, sensory perception,* and *cognition* in patients with multiple sclerosis.
2. Teach adults how to decrease the risk for low back pain and spinal cord injury.
3. Teach the patient and caregiver(s) about common drugs and other management strategies used for multiple sclerosis affecting *immunity.*
4. Plan patient- and family-centered nursing interventions to decrease the psychosocial impact caused by living with common spinal cord conditions.
5. Apply knowledge of anatomy, physiology, and pathophysiology to provide evidence-based care for patients with spinal cord injury.
6. Analyze assessment and diagnostic findings to generate solutions and prioritize nursing care for patients who have multiple sclerosis.
7. Organize care coordination and transition management for patients living with spinal cord injury.
8. Use clinical judgment to plan evidence-based nursing care to promote *sexuality* and decrease complications in patients with common spinal cord conditions.
9. Incorporate factors that affect health equity into the plan of care for patients with common spinal cord conditions.

KEY TERMS

amyotrophic lateral sclerosis (ALS) A progressive neurodegenerative disease that affects neurons in the brain and spinal cord that is likely caused by genetic mutations.

autonomic dysreflexia (AD) (sometimes referred to as *autonomic hyperreflexia*) A potentially life-threatening condition in which noxious visceral or cutaneous stimuli cause a sudden, massive, uninhibited reflex sympathetic discharge in people with high-level spinal cord injury.

cough assist A technique in which an assistant places both hands on the patient's upper abdomen over the diaphragm and below the ribs. Hands are placed one over the other, with fingers interlocked and away from the skin while the patient takes a breath and coughs during expiration. The assistant locks elbows and pushes inward and upward as the patient coughs.

diplopia Double vision.

dysarthria Difficulty speaking due to slurred speech.

dysmetria The inability to direct or limit movement.

dysphagia Difficulty swallowing.

ergonomics An applied science in which the workplace is designed to increase worker comfort (thus reducing injury) while increasing efficiency and productivity.

heterotopic ossification (HO) Bony overgrowth, often into muscle; a complication of immobility.

hyperesthesia Increased *sensory perception.*

hypoalgesia A decreased sensitivity to pain.

hypoesthesia Decreased *sensory perception.*

intention tremor A tremor, usually of the arm and hand, that occurs while performing an activity.

log rolling A position change in which the patient turns as a unit while the back is kept as straight as possible.

multiple sclerosis (MS) A chronic disease caused by immune, genetic, and/or infectious factors that affects the myelin and nerve fibers of the brain and spinal cord.

neurogenic shock A type of shock that can occur in clients who have severe spinal cord injury; dilation of blood vessels leads to decreased perfusion to vital body organs.

nystagmus An involuntary condition in which the eyes make repetitive uncontrolled movements.

paraparesis Weakness that affects only the lower extremities, as seen in lower thoracic and lumbosacral injuries or lesions.

paraplegia Paralysis that affects only the lower extremities, as seen in lower thoracic and lumbosacral injuries or lesions.

progressive multifocal leukoencephalopathy (PML) An opportunistic viral infection of the brain that leads to death or severe disability.

KEY TERMS

quadriparesis Weakness involving all four extremities, as seen with cervical cord and upper thoracic injury.

radiculopathy Spinal nerve root involvement.

scotomas Changes in peripheral vision, often in patients with multiple sclerosis.

spinal cord stimulation An invasive technique that provides pain relief by applying an electrical field over the spinal cord.

spinal shock A syndrome that occurs immediately as the cord's response to injury in which the patient has complete but temporary loss of motor, sensory, reflex, and autonomic function. It typically lasts less than 48 hours but may continue for several weeks.

spinal stenosis Narrowing of the spinal canal, nerve root canals, or intervertebral foramina typically seen in people older than 50 years of age.

tetraplegia (also called *quadriplegia*) Paralysis of all four extremities, as seen with cervical cord and upper thoracic cord injury.

tinnitus Ringing in the ears.

vertigo Dizziness.

✴ PRIORITY AND INTERRELATED CONCEPTS

The priority concepts for this chapter are:
- *Immunity*
- *Mobility*

The *Immunity* concept exemplar for this chapter is Multiple Sclerosis.
The *Mobility* concept exemplar for this chapter is Spinal Cord Injury.

The interrelated concepts for this chapter are:
- *Sensory Perception*
- *Cognition*
- *Sexuality*
- *Pain*

The spinal cord relays messages to and from the brain. Besides injuries, the spinal cord can develop inflammatory and autoimmune diseases, such as multiple sclerosis (MS) and tumors, both benign and malignant. The spinal cord itself may be damaged, or the spinal nerves leading from the cord to the extremities may be affected. In some cases, both the spinal cord and the nerves are involved. Adult spinal health conditions may be acute or chronic and often can be managed in the community. End-of-life care is not needed unless the patient has a large, inoperable cancerous spinal cord tumor or spinal metastatic disease.

Signs and symptoms of spinal cord health conditions vary but often include problems with *immunity, mobility, sensory perception, cognition,* and *sexuality.* Interprofessional health care team members with expertise in symptom management collaborate to improve quality of life, promote a safe environment, and prevent complications from spinal cord health conditions. Chapter 3 briefly reviews each of these nursing and health concepts in detail.

✴ IMMUNITY CONCEPT EXEMPLAR: MULTIPLE SCLEROSIS

Multiple sclerosis (MS) is a chronic disease caused by immune, genetic, and/or infectious factors that affects the myelin and nerve fibers of the brain and spinal cord. It is one of the leading causes of neurologic disability in young and middle-age adults.

Pathophysiology Review

Multiple sclerosis is characterized by periods of remission and exacerbation (flare). Patients progress at different rates and over different lengths of time. However, as the severity and duration of the disease progress, the periods of exacerbation become more frequent. Patients with MS can have a normal life expectancy as long as the effects of the disease are managed effectively.

As described in Chapter 35, myelin is responsible for the electrochemical transmission of impulses between the brain and spinal cord and the rest of the body; demyelination can result in slowed or stopped impulse transmission. MS is characterized by demyelination (loss of myelin sheaths). Diffuse random or patchy areas of *plaque* in the white matter of the central nervous system (CNS) are the definitive findings (Rogers, 2023). Initially, remyelination takes place to some degree, and clinical symptoms decrease. However, over time, new lesions develop and neuronal injury and muscle atrophy occur. The areas particularly affected include optic nerves, spinal pyramidal tracts, spinal posterior columns, brainstem nuclei, and the ventricular region of the brain. The four major types of MS include (National Multiple Sclerosis Society, 2020.):

- Clinically isolated syndrome (CIS)
- Relapsing-remitting
- Primary progressive
- Secondary progressive

The CIS is an episode of neurologic symptoms often attributed to MS that lasts for at least 24 hours. An MRI may or may not show evidence of MS, so a diagnosis is not yet possible. A little over half of patients diagnosed with CIS develop MS within 10 years, and disease-modifying therapies are often started to prevent or delay the onset. Radiologically isolated syndrome (RIS) is often diagnosed incidentally in a person having an MRI for another problem, such as headache or head trauma. It is characterized by isolated lesions that are similar to those of MS in a person who does not have a past or current history of symptoms of the disease (National Multiple Sclerosis Society, 2020).

Relapsing-remitting multiple sclerosis (RRMS) occurs in most cases of MS. The course of the disease may be mild or moderate, depending on the degree of disability. Symptoms develop and resolve in a few weeks to months, and the patient returns to baseline. During the relapsing phase, the patient reports loss of function and the continuing development of new symptoms. The majority of patients are diagnosed with this type initially (Rogers, 2023).

Primary progressive multiple sclerosis (PPMS) involves a steady and gradual neurologic deterioration without remission of symptoms. The patient has progressive disability with no acute attacks. Patients with this type of MS tend to be between 40 and 60 years of age at onset of the disease.

Secondary progressive multiple sclerosis (SPMS) begins with a relapsing-remitting course that later becomes steadily progressive. Many people with RRMS develop SPMS within 10 years. The current addition of disease-modifying drugs as part of disease management may decrease the development of SPMS.

Progressive-relapsing multiple sclerosis (PRMS) is an older label for an uncommon type of MS characterized by frequent relapses with partial recovery but not a return to baseline. This type of MS is seen in only a small percentage of patients. Progressive, cumulative symptoms and deterioration occur over several years (Rogers, 2023).

Etiology and Genetic Risk

The cause of MS is very complex and involves multiple immune, genetic, and/or infectious factors, although changes in **immunity** are the most likely etiology. The environment may also contribute to its development. For example, the disease is seen more often in the colder climates of the northeastern, Great Lakes, and Pacific northwestern states and in Canada (National Multiple Sclerosis Society, 2020).

👤 PATIENT-CENTERED CARE: GENETICS/ GENOMICS

Familial Patterns of Multiple Sclerosis

Large genome studies of families have helped identify familial patterns of multiple sclerosis (MS). For example, having a first-degree relative such as a parent or sibling with MS increases a person's risk for developing the disease. Research also confirms the association of MS with over 100 gene variants, including interleukin (IL)-7 and IL-2 receptor genes (Rogers, 2023; National Multiple Sclerosis Society, 2020). These findings have helped guide the development of targeted drug therapies that are important in current disease management.

Incidence and Prevalence

MS usually occurs in people between the ages of 20 and 50 years, but cases may occur at any age. Nearly 1 million people in the United States have MS. The disease affects over 2.3 million people worldwide (National Multiple Sclerosis Society, 2020). About 90,000 Canadians have MS (MS Society of Canada, 2020).

👤 PATIENT-CENTERED CARE: GENDER HEALTH

Women and Multiple Sclerosis

MS affects women two to three times more often than men, suggesting a possible hormonal role in disease development. Some studies show that the disease occurs up to four times more often in women than men. However, the exact reason for this difference is not known (National Multiple Sclerosis Society, 2020).

Interprofessional Collaborative Care

Recognize Cues: Assessment

History. Multiple sclerosis (MS) often presents like other neurologic diseases, such as amyotrophic lateral sclerosis (ALS), which can make the diagnosis difficult and prolonged. ALS is also a progressive neurodegenerative disease that affects neurons in the brain and spinal cord and that is likely caused by genetic mutations. Unlike MS, there is no established treatment or cure for ALS, which is 100% fatal. Recently, a combination drug, sodium phenylbutyrate and taurursodiol, has been approved to slow physical function decline for patients who have ALS. Table 37.1 compares these two neurologic health conditions.

Patients often visit many primary health care providers and undergo a variety of diagnostic tests and treatments to obtain the correct diagnosis. Obtaining a thorough history is essential for accurate diagnosis. Ask the patient about a history of vision, *mobility,* and *sensory perception* changes, all of which are *early* indicators of MS. Symptoms are often vague and nonspecific in the early stages of the disease and may disappear for months or years before returning. Many patients have a single isolated clinical episode that lasts for 24 hours or more. These neurologic symptoms then disappear and occur later.

Ask about the progression of symptoms. Pay particular attention to whether they are intermittent or are becoming progressively worse. Document the date (month and year) when the patient first noticed these changes.

Next, ask about factors that aggravate the symptoms, such as fatigue, stress, overexertion, temperature extremes, or a hot shower or bath. Ask the patient and the family about any personality or behavioral changes that have occurred (e.g., euphoria [very elated mood], poor judgment, attention loss). In addition, determine whether there is a family history of MS or autoimmune disease.

👤 PATIENT-CENTERED CARE: CULTURE AND SPIRITUALITY

Race and Multiple Sclerosis

MS has historically been thought to occur most often in White individuals. However, a recent study shows that MS is nearly as prevalent in the Black population as in the White population. A study of 3863 people in Southern California diagnosed with MS showed estimated prevalence rates (based on census and study data) to be very similar at 226/100,000 for Blacks and at 238/100,000 in Whites (Langer-Gould et al., 2022).

TABLE 37.1	Comparison of Multiple Sclerosis and Amyotrophic Lateral Sclerosis	
	Multiple Sclerosis (MS)	**Amyotrophic Lateral Sclerosis (ALS)**
Pathophysiology and etiology	Chronic neurologic disease that affects the brain and spinal cord due to immune-mediated demyelination and nerve injury; characterized by remissions and exacerbations	Chronic neurologic disease of unknown cause (genetic and environmental factors identified), causing progressive muscle weakness and wasting and leading to paralysis of respiratory muscles
Populations affected	Commonly occurring disease that affects people (women twice as often as men) between the ages of 20 and 50 yr; most often affects Whites	Uncommon disease that affects people (more men than women) between the ages of 40 and 60 yr; incidence increases with each decade of life
Signs and symptoms	Fatigue Muscle spasticity Blurred or double vision (diplopia) Scotomas Nystagmus Paresthesias Areflexic (flaccid) or spastic bladder Decreased sexual function Intention tremors Gait changes	Fatigue Muscle atrophy (including tongue) Muscle weakness Twitching of face and tongue Dysarthria Dysphagia Stiff and clumsy gait Abnormal reflexes
Interprofessional collaborative care	Multiple immunomodulating and antineoplastic drugs available Collaborative care to promote and maintain optimal functioning Symptom management to achieve maximal function Psychosocial support	Supportive care to promote optimal function Palliative care for symptom management at end of life Psychosocial support

Physical Assessment/Signs and Symptoms. MS produces a wide variety of signs and symptoms, as listed in Box 37.1. Therefore, each patient may present differently. Some patients with RRMS also report *pain*. Perform a complete pain assessment as described in Chapter 6 for all patients with MS.

Psychosocial Assessment. A major concern reported by most patients is how long it takes to establish a diagnosis of MS. Many patients go to several primary health care providers, are given varying diagnoses and treatment, and/or are told that their symptoms are related to stress and anxiety. Often, young adults present with weakness, fatigue, or changes in vision and are diagnosed with exhaustion and advised to get more sleep. The patient and family are relieved to have a definite diagnosis but may express anger and frustration that it took a long time to start appropriate treatment. Therefore, establish open and honest communication with patients and allow them to share frustrations, anger, and anxiety.

After the initial diagnosis of MS, the patient is often anxious. Apathy and emotional lability are common problems that occur later. Depression may occur at the time of diagnosis and can also occur later with disease progression. The patient may be euphoric either as a result of the disease itself or because of the drugs used to treat it. Assess the patient's previously used coping and stress-management skills in preparing for a chronic, potentially debilitating disease. Secondary depression is the most frequent mental health disorder diagnosed in patients with MS.

Assess the patient for mental status changes. Changes in *cognition* are usually seen late in the course of the disease and can include decreases in short-term memory, concentration, and the ability to perform calculations; inattentiveness; and impaired judgment.

Assess the impact of bowel and bladder problems. Managing urinary or fecal incontinence or constipation can be time consuming and embarrassing.

BOX 37.1   Key Features

Multiple Sclerosis

Common Symptoms and Conditions
- Muscle weakness and spasticity
- Fatigue (usually with continuous sensitivity to temperature)
- Flexor muscle spasms
- Numbness or tingling sensations (paresthesia)
- Visual changes such as diplopia, nystagmus (involuntary eye movements), decreased visual acuity, scotomas (changes in peripheral vision)
- Bowel and bladder dysfunction (flaccid or spastic)
- Alterations in sexual function, such as erectile dysfunction
- Cognitive changes, such as memory loss, impaired judgment, and decreased ability to solve problems or perform calculations
- Depression
- Dysesthesia ("MS hug") squeezing sensation around the torso, often one of the first symptoms of the disease or a relapse
- Difficulty walking (including dysmetria [inability to direct or limit movement and ataxia])
- Vertigo (dizziness)
- Pain and itching
- Emotional changes

Less Common Symptoms and Conditions
- Intention tremor (tremor when performing an activity)
- Hypoalgesia (decreased sensitivity to pain)
- Dysarthria (difficulty speaking due to slurred speech)
- Dysphagia (difficulty swallowing)
- Decreased hearing acuity
- Tinnitus (ringing in the ears)
- Loss of taste
- Seizures

Sexuality can be affected in people with MS, and sexual dysfunction can have a major impact on quality of life. Assess the patient's fatigue level and pattern, since fatigue contributes to sexual dysfunction. Be sensitive when asking about the patient's sexual practices and orientation. Women often report impaired genital sensation, diminished orgasm, and loss of sexual interest. Men most often report difficulty in achieving and maintaining an erection and delayed ejaculation.

Laboratory Assessment. No single specific laboratory test is definitively diagnostic for MS. However, the collective results of a variety of tests are usually conclusive. Abnormal cerebrospinal fluid (CSF) findings include elevated proteins (oligoclonal bands) and an increase in the white blood cell (WBC) count. CSF electrophoresis reveals an increase in the myelin basic protein and the presence of increased immunoglobulins, especially immunoglobulin G (IgG) (Pagana et al., 2022). Newer tests are being developed to identify biomarkers for MS.

Other Diagnostic Assessments. An *MRI* of the brain and spinal cord that demonstrates the presence of plaques in at least two areas is considered diagnostic for MS. MRIs with contrast may show active plaques and reveal older lesions not associated with current symptoms (Fig. 37.1).

Evoked potential testing, usually the visual evoked response (VER), may be performed for patients suspected of having MS. This noninvasive test can identify impaired transmission along the optic nerve pathway. Chapter 35 discusses this test in more detail.

NCLEX Examination Challenge 37.1

Physiological Integrity

The nurse is caring for a client recently diagnosed with multiple sclerosis. Which of the following common client findings would the nurse expect? **Select all that apply.**

A. Muscle weakness
B. Memory loss
C. Visual changes such as diplopia
D. Hallucinations
E. Muscle spasticity
F. Fatigue

Analyze Cues and Prioritize Hypotheses: Analysis

The priority collaborative problems for patients with multiple sclerosis include:

1. Impaired *immunity* due to the disease and drug therapy for disease management
2. Decreased or impaired *mobility* due to muscle spasticity, intention tremors, and/or fatigue
3. Decreased visual acuity and *cognition* due to dysfunctional brain neurons

Generate Solutions and Take Actions: Planning and Implementation

The purpose of management is to modify the disease's effects on the immune system, prevent exacerbations, manage symptoms, improve function, and maintain quality of life. As with other spinal cord conditions, care of the patient with MS requires the collaborative efforts of the interprofessional health care team.

Managing Impaired Immunity

Planning: Expected Outcomes. The patient with MS is expected to be free from episodes of secondary infection due to impaired *immunity* from the disease or from drug therapy used to manage the illness.

Interventions. As with any chronic disease, clients who have been diagnosed with MS are at an increased risk for infection. Teach these patients to avoid large crowds and anyone who is sick. Remind them to wash their hands frequently and use hand sanitizer when soap and water are not readily available.

Drug Therapy. The patient with MS is treated with a variety of drugs to treat and control disease progression. Medications can be administered orally, by injection, or by infusion. Many of these drugs are immunomodulators or antiinflammatory medications that can alter *immunity* and place patients at risk for secondary infection. Teach patients receiving drug therapy for MS to avoid crowds and anyone with an infection. If signs and symptoms of an infection occur, remind them to contact their primary health care provider for prompt management and medical observation. Other medications are used to control symptoms, such as bladder or bowel dysfunction, fatigue, itching, pain, sexual problems, spasticity, tremors, or gait disturbances.

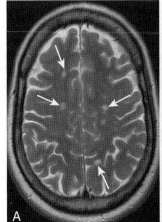 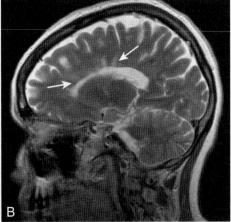

FIG. 37.1 Typical plaques *(arrows)* seen in brain CT images of patient with multiple sclerosis. (From Herring, W. [2020]. *Learning radiology.* [4th ed.]. St. Louis: Elsevier.)

Examples of drugs used for treatment of relapsing types of MS include (Burchum & Rosenthal, 2022):

- Interferon-beta preparations (interferon beta-1a and beta-1b drugs), immunomodulators that *modify* the course of the disease and also have antiviral effects
- Glatiramer acetate, a synthetic protein that is similar to myelin-based protein
- Mitoxantrone, an IV antineoplastic antiinflammatory agent used to resolve relapses but with risks for leukemia and cardiotoxicity
- Natalizumab, the first IV monoclonal antibody approved for MS that binds to white blood cells (WBCs) to prevent further damage to the myelin
- Fingolimod, teriflunomide, ponesimod, and diroximel fumarate, *oral* immunomodulating drugs

NURSING SAFETY PRIORITY

Drug Alert

> The interferons and glatiramer acetate are subcutaneous injections that patients can self-administer. Teach patients how to give and rotate the site of injections because local injection site (skin) reactions are common. The first dose of these drugs is given under medical supervision to monitor for allergic response, including anaphylactic shock. Teach patients receiving them to avoid crowds and people with infections because these drugs can cause bone marrow suppression. Remind them to report any sign or symptom associated with infection immediately to their primary health care provider.
>
> Instruct patients about flulike reactions that are very common for patients receiving any of the interferons. These symptoms can be minimized by starting at a low drug dose and giving acetaminophen or ibuprofen. Adverse effects of glatiramer are not common (Burchum & Rosenthal, 2022).

Natalizumab, a humanized monoclonal antibody, can cause many adverse events. It is usually given as an IV infusion in a specialty clinic under careful supervision. The patient is monitored carefully for allergic or anaphylactic reaction when each dose is given because the drug tends to build up in the body. *Patients receiving this drug are at risk for* progressive multifocal leukoencephalopathy (PML). This opportunistic viral infection of the brain leads to death or severe disability. Monitor for neurologic changes, especially changes in mental state, such as disorientation or acute confusion. PML is confirmed by MRI and by examining the cerebrospinal fluid for the causative pathogen (Burchum & Rosenthal, 2022). Natalizumab can also damage hepatic cells. Carefully monitor liver enzymes, and teach patients to have frequent laboratory tests to assess for changes.

Mitoxantrone, a chemotherapy drug, has been shown to be effective in reducing neurologic disability. It also decreases the frequency of clinical relapses in patients with secondary progressive, progressive-relapsing, or worsening relapsing-remitting MS.

Fingolimod was the first oral immunomodulator approved for the management of MS. The capsules may be taken with or without food. Teach patients to monitor their pulse every day because the drug can cause bradycardia, especially within the first 6 hours after taking it. Several other immunomodulating drugs have been approved for MS. Like fingolimod, these drugs inhibit

immune cells and have antioxidant properties that protect brain and spinal cord cells. Teach the patient that the two most common side effects of all the oral drugs are facial flushing and GI disturbances (Burchum & Rosenthal, 2022). Remind the patient to keep follow-up appointments for laboratory monitoring of the WBC count because the oral drugs can cause a decrease in WBCs, which can predispose the patient to infection.

PATIENT-CENTERED CARE: HEALTH EQUITY

Health Equity Issues for Patients Who Have Multiple Sclerosis

> MS is an expensive disease to treat. Bebo et al. (2022) found that the average annual cost for an individual living with MS is $88,487. Medications, particularly disease-modifying drugs, account for the largest amount of that cost. When compared to White patients who have MS, Black patients have a lower median income and less coverage for health insurance. These social determinants of health may explain the higher mortality rate of Black patients who have MS when compared to White patients because Black patients may be unable to afford the most effective drugs (Amezcua et al., 2021). All nurses should advocate for policy changes that make drugs needed for MS affordable for all those who have the disease (Bebo et al., 2022).

Medical Marijuana (Cannabis). The National Multiple Sclerosis Society supports the use of medical marijuana (cannabis) for symptom management. Studies have shown that cannabis can reduce neuropathic *pain*, muscle stiffness, and spasticity for some patients with MS (Clark, 2021). Consistent availability of quality cannabis in a legalized-use state gives patients more options about the type of product that may be effective.

Stem Cell Therapy. Stem cell therapy is being researched as a promising treatment to manage MS (Cona, 2021; Drillinger, 2021). Stem cells may be derived from adults or embryonic tissue, although embryonic stem cells are preferred because they are often more effective. This therapy may slow the progression of the disease and decrease symptoms. (See the Legal/Ethical Considerations box.)

LEGAL/ETHICAL CONSIDERATIONS

Stem Cell Research

> Human embryonic stem cell research remains ethically and politically controversial because human embryos are destroyed. The embryos, which are obtained through the in vitro fertilization (IVF) process, are between 3 and 5 days old (blastocysts), and are no longer needed for transfer into the uterus to create a pregnancy. Individuals who believe that life begins at conception oppose stem cell therapy when embryos are terminated. Nurses must respect the beliefs, morals, and values of all individuals regardless of their own personal feelings about the research and use of stem cells as regenerative therapy.

Improving Mobility

Planning Expected Outcomes. The patient with MS is expected to have optimal *mobility* as a result of successful interprofessional management and self-care interventions.

Interventions. The symptoms of MS that affect *mobility* include spasticity, tremor, pain, and fatigue. Referral to rehabilitative services, such as physical and occupational therapy, can help manage functional deficits from MS symptoms. An interprofessional team approach is important to attain patient-centered outcomes for care.

To lessen muscle spasticity (which often contributes to *pain*), the primary health care provider may prescribe baclofen or tizanidine (Burchum & Rosenthal, 2022). Severe muscle spasticity may also be treated with intrathecal baclofen (ITB) administered through a surgically implanted pump. Paresthesia may be treated with carbamazepine or tricyclic antidepressants. Propranolol hydrochloride and clonazepam have been used to treat cerebellar ataxia.

In collaboration with physical and occupational therapists, plan an exercise program that includes range-of-motion (ROM) exercises and stretching and strengthening exercises to manage spasticity and tremor. If needed as a last resort, neurosurgery (e.g., thalamotomy or deep brain stimulation) may provide some relief from tremors.

Emphasize the importance of avoiding rigorous activities that increase body temperature. Increased body temperature may lead to increased fatigue, diminished motor ability, and decreased visual acuity resulting from changes in the conduction abilities of the injured axons.

In collaboration with the case manager and occupational therapist, assess the patient's home before discharge for any hazards. Any items that might interfere with *mobility* (e.g., scatter rugs) are removed. In addition, care must be taken to prevent injury resulting from vision problems. Teach the patient and family to keep the home environment as structured and free from clutter as possible. As the disease progresses, the home may need to be adapted for wheelchair accessibility. Adaptation in the kitchen, bedroom, and bathroom may also be needed to promote self-management. Any necessary assistive-adaptive device should be readily available before discharge from the hospital.

The patient with MS is often weak and easily fatigued. Teach the patient the importance of planning activities and allowing sufficient time to complete activities. For example, patients should check that all items needed for work are gathered before leaving the house. Items used on a daily basis should be easily accessible. A recent study showed beneficial effects of brief mindfulness training for hospitalized patients to manage their fatigue (Sauder et al., 2021).

If the patient experiences dysarthria as a result of muscle weakness, refer the patient to the speech-language pathologist (SLP) for evaluation and treatment. It is not unusual for the patient with dysarthria also to have dysphagia. The SLP performs a swallowing evaluation, but further diagnostic testing may be indicated. Monitor the patient to determine whether there are problems swallowing at mealtime that increase the risk of aspiration. In some cases, thickened liquids may be necessary.

Managing Decreased Visual Acuity and Cognition

Planning: Expected Outcomes. The patient with MS is expected to maintain optimal visual acuity and *cognition* with use of available drug treatment and supportive services.

Interventions. Alterations in visual acuity and cognition can occur at any time during the course of the disease process. Areas affected include attention, memory, problem solving, auditory reasoning, handling distractions, and visual perception.

> **! NURSING SAFETY PRIORITY**
> *Action Alert*
>
> For the patient with MS who has impaired *cognition,* assist with orientation by using a single-date calendar. Give or encourage the patient to use written lists or recorded messages. To maintain an organized environment, encourage the patient to keep frequently used items in familiar places. Applications for handheld devices such as mobile phones and electronic tablets can also be used for reorientation, reminders, and behavioral cues.

An eye patch that is alternated from eye to eye every few hours usually relieves diplopia (double vision). For peripheral visual deficits, teach scanning techniques by having the patient move the head from side to side. Changes in visual acuity may be helped by corrective lenses.

Complementary and Integrative Health. Patients with MS often report that complementary therapies are successful in decreasing their symptoms and managing anxiety and/or depression. Some of the integrative therapies used by patients with MS are:

- Reflexology
- Massage
- Yoga
- Relaxation and meditation
- Acupuncture
- Aromatherapy

Care Coordination and Transition Management

Patients usually are able to live independently with their disease, but some may need assistance. To help the patient maintain maximum strength, function, and independence, continuity of care by an interprofessional team in the rehabilitation and/or home setting may be needed. In severe disease, placement in an assisted-living or long-term care facility may be the best alternative. The population of young and middle-age residents in these settings is increasing as people with physical disabilities live longer.

The primary health care provider explains to the patient and family the development of MS and the factors that may exacerbate the symptoms. Emphasize the importance of avoiding overexertion, stress, extremes of temperatures (fever, hot baths, use of sauna baths and hot tubs, overheating, and excessive chilling), humidity, and people with infections. Explain all medications to be taken on discharge, including the time and route of administration, dosage, purpose, and side effects. Teach the patient how to differentiate expected side effects from adverse or allergic reactions, and provide the name of a resource person to call if questions or problems occur. Provide written instructions as a resource for the patient and caregivers at home.

The physical therapist develops an exercise program appropriate for the patient's tolerance level at home. The patient is instructed in techniques for self-care, daily living skills, and the use of required adaptive equipment such as walkers and electric carts. Include information related to bowel and bladder management, skin care, nutrition, and positioning techniques. Chapter 7 describes in detail these aspects of chronic illness and rehabilitation.

Teach patients about conservation strategies that balance periods of rest and activity, including regular social interactions. Remind them to use assistive devices and modify the environment to avoid fatigue. Explore strategies to manage stress and avoid undue stress. Often patients are anxious and worry about how long the remission will last or when the disease will progress.

MS affects the entire family because of the unpredictability and uncertainty of the course of the disease. Chronic fatigue may also prevent the patient from participating in family and community activities. Assess coping strategies of family members or other caregivers, and help them identify support systems that can assist them as they live with the patient with MS.

Because personality changes are not unusual, teach the family or significant others strategies to enable them to cope with these changes. For example, the family may develop a nonverbal signal to alert the patient to potentially inappropriate behavior. This action avoids embarrassment for the patient.

Sexual dysfunction may occur as a result of fatigue, nerve involvement, and/or psychological reasons. Therefore, some patients may benefit from counseling. If able, answer the patient's questions or refer the patient to a counselor or urologist with experience in the field of *sexuality,* intimacy, and disability.

Prostaglandin-5 inhibitors (sildenafil, vardenafil, tadalafil) can be used to help men with erectile dysfunction. Penile prostheses are also used for men. The EROS Clitoral Therapy Device is a U.S. Food and Drug Administration (FDA)–approved therapy for women with impaired sexual response.

Refer the patient and family members or significant others to the local chapter of the National Multiple Sclerosis Society (www.nationalmssociety.org) or the MS Society of Canada (https://mssociety.ca). Other community resources include meal-delivery services (e.g., Meals on Wheels), transportation services for the disabled, and homemaker services.

Evaluate Outcomes: Evaluation

Evaluate the care of the patient with MS on the basis of the identified priority problems. The expected outcomes are that the patient:

- Remains free of infection as a result of drug therapy affecting *immunity* or the disease process
- Maintains optimal *mobility* and function as a result of managing fatigue and pain
- Maintains adequate visual acuity and *cognition* to function independently

✳ MOBILITY CONCEPT EXEMPLAR: SPINAL CORD INJURY

Spinal cord injury (SCI) can occur at any level of the spine. Potential survivors of acute SCI experience injury below the third cervical level (C3). SCI is the leading cause of paralysis and results in a physical disability. Many health issues experienced by patients who live with SCI are related to impaired *mobility* (Smeltzer, 2021).

Pathophysiology Review

Spinal cord injuries can be classified as complete or incomplete. A *complete* SCI is one in which the spinal cord has been damaged in a way that eliminates all innervation below the level of the injury. Injuries that allow some function or movement below the level of the injury are described as an *incomplete* SCI. Incomplete SCIs are more common than complete injuries. Loss of or decreased *mobility, sensory perception,* and bowel and bladder control often result from an SCI.

Mechanisms of Injury

When enough force is applied to the spinal cord, the resulting damage causes many neurologic deficits. Sources of force include direct injury to the vertebral column (fracture, dislocation, and subluxation [partial dislocation]) or penetrating injury from violence (gunshot or knife wounds). Although in some cases the cord itself may remain intact, at other times it undergoes a destructive process caused by a contusion (bruise), compression, laceration, or transaction (severing of the cord, either complete or incomplete).

The causes of SCI can be divided into primary and secondary mechanisms of injury. Five *primary* mechanisms may result in an SCI (Rogers, 2023):

- *Hyperflexion:* a sudden and forceful acceleration (movement) of the head forward, causing extreme flexion of the neck (Fig. 37.2). This is often the result of a head-on motor vehicle collision or diving accident. Flexion injury to the lower thoracic and lumbar spine may occur when the trunk is suddenly flexed on itself, such as occurs in a fall on the buttocks.
- *Hyperextension* occurs most often in vehicle collisions in which the vehicle is struck from behind or during falls when the patient's chin is struck (Fig. 37.3). The head is suddenly accelerated and then decelerated. This stretches or tears the anterior longitudinal ligament, fractures or subluxates the vertebrae, and perhaps ruptures an intervertebral disk. As with flexion injuries, the spinal cord may easily be damaged.
- *Axial loading or vertical compression* injuries resulting from diving accidents, falls on the buttocks, or a jump in which a person lands on the feet can cause many of the injuries attributable to *axial loading* (vertical compression) (Fig. 37.4). A blow to the top of the head can cause the vertebrae to shatter. Pieces of bone enter the spinal canal and damage the cord.
- *Excessive rotation* results from injuries that are caused by turning the head beyond the normal range.
- *Penetrating trauma* is classified by the speed of the object (e.g., knife, bullet) causing the injury. Low-speed or low-impact injuries cause damage directly at the site or local damage to the spinal cord or spinal nerves. In contrast, high-speed injuries that occur from gunshot wounds (GSWs) cause both direct and indirect damage.

Secondary Injury

Secondary injury worsens the primary injury and may result in death. Secondary injuries include (Rogers, 2023):

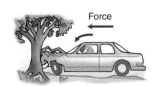

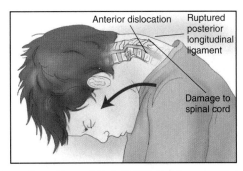

FIG. 37.2 Hyperflexion injury of the cervical vertebrae. (From Leonard, P. C. [2022]. *Building a medical vocabulary: With Spanish translations.* [11th ed.]. St. Louis: Elsevier.)

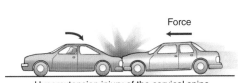

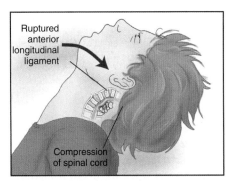

FIG. 37.3 Hyperextension injury of the cervical vertebrae. (From Leonard, P. C. [2022]. *Building a medical vocabulary: With Spanish translations.* [11th ed.]. St. Louis: Elsevier.)

- Hemorrhage
- Ischemia (lack of oxygen, typically from reduced/absent blood flow)
- Hypovolemia (decreased circulating blood volume)
- Impaired tissue perfusion from neurogenic shock *(a medical emergency)*
- Local edema

Hemorrhage into the spinal cord may manifest with contusion or petechial leaking into the central gray matter and later into the white matter. Systemic hemorrhage can result in shock and decreased perfusion to the spinal cord. Edema occurs with both primary and secondary injuries, contributing to capillary compression and cord ischemia. In neurogenic shock, loss of blood vessel tone (dilation) after *severe* cord injury may result in hypoperfusion (Rogers, 2023).

Patients who have SCI have a decreased life expectancy, owing to complications of immobility or, more often, some type of infection. The major causes of death are pneumonia and septicemia.

Etiology and Genetic Risk

Trauma is the leading cause of spinal cord injuries (SCIs), with more than a third resulting from vehicle crashes. Other leading causes are falls, acts of violence (usually gunshot wounds [GSWs]), and sports- or recreation-related accidents. SCIs from falls are particularly likely among older adults. Spinal cord damage in older adults can also result from nontraumatic vertebral fracture and diseases such as tumors or degenerative conditions (Rogers, 2023).

Incidence and Prevalence

About 18,000 *new* SCIs occur every year in the United States. However, an estimated 300,000 or more individuals live with an SCI as a physical disability. Almost 80% of all SCIs occur in young males, with the majority being White. Cervical cord injuries are more common than thoracic or lumbar cord injuries (Rogers, 2023). The most common neurologic level of injury is C5. For patients with paraplegia, T12 and L1 are the most common levels. The average age of patients who have SCI is 43 years (Rogers, 2023).

PATIENT-CENTERED CARE: VETERAN HEALTH

Veterans and Spinal Cord Injury

SCI is more prevalent among veterans who served in combat in Iraq and Afghanistan when compared to those who served in previous wars. Most of those SCIs resulted from blunt trauma caused by blast injuries. Be aware that veterans who experience an SCI from blast injury typically have other polytraumatic injuries, including traumatic brain injury and amputation of one or more limbs (Elliott et al., 2021). These additional injuries may take priority over attending to the problems related to the SCI and present a major challenge in managing care.

Health Promotion/Disease Prevention

Because trauma is the leading cause of SCI, teach people to avoid taking risks, if possible, by ensuring adequate protective measures (e.g., padding and helmets) for sports and recreational

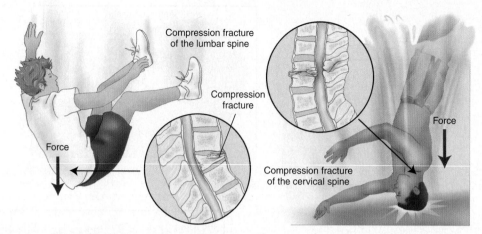

FIG. 37.4 Vertical compression of the cervical spine and the lumbar spine. (From Leonard, P. C. [2022]. *Building a medical vocabulary: With Spanish translations.* [11th ed.]. St. Louis: Elsevier.)

activities. Remind them to wear seat belts at all times when driving and to avoid impaired driving caused by alcohol, marijuana, and other substances. Instruct them on the danger of diving into shallow pools or other water when the depth is unknown. Water should be at least 9 feet deep before diving is attempted.

Interprofessional Collaborative Care
Recognize Cues: Assessment

History. When obtaining a history from a patient with an acute SCI, gather as much data as possible once the patient is stabilized about how the accident occurred and the probable mechanism of injury. Important data include:

- Location and position of the patient immediately after the injury
- Symptoms that occurred immediately with the injury
- Changes that have occurred subsequently
- Type of immobilization devices used and whether any problems occurred during stabilization and transport to the hospital
- Treatment given at the scene of injury or in the emergency department (ED) (e.g., medications, IV fluids)
- Medical history, including osteoporosis or arthritis of the spine, congenital deformities, cancer, and previous injury or surgery of the neck or back
- History of any respiratory problems, especially if the patient has experienced a cervical SCI

Physical Assessment/Signs and Symptoms

Initial Assessment. *The initial and priority assessment focuses on the patient's ABCs (**a**irway, **b**reathing, and **c**irculation).* After an airway is established, assess the patient's breathing pattern. The patient with a cervical SCI is at high risk for respiratory compromise because cervical spinal nerves (C3-5) innervate the phrenic nerve controlling the diaphragm.

Evaluate pulse, blood pressure, and peripheral perfusion such as pulse strength and capillary refill. Multiple injuries may contribute to circulatory compromise from hemorrhagic hypovolemic shock. Assess for indications of *hemorrhage*. All symptoms of circulatory compromise or hypovolemic shock must be treated aggressively to preserve tissue perfusion to the spinal cord. Shock is discussed in detail in Chapter 31.

Use the Glasgow Coma Scale (see Chapter 35) or other agency-approved assessment tool to assess the patient's *level of consciousness (LOC).* Cognitive impairment as a result of an associated traumatic brain injury (TBI) or substance use disorder can occur in patients with traumatic SCIs.

Spinal shock, also called *spinal shock syndrome,* occurs immediately as the cord's response to the injury. The patient has complete but temporary loss of motor, sensory, reflex, and autonomic function that often lasts less than 48 hours but may continue for several weeks. Common symptoms include decreased heart rate, increased blood pressure, and pale/ash gray or flushed skin (Rogers, 2023). Spinal shock is *not* the same as neurogenic shock.

Sensory Perception and Mobility Assessment. Perform a detailed assessment of the patient's **mobility** and **sensory perception** status to determine the level of injury and establish baseline data for future comparison. The level of injury is the lowest neurologic segment with intact or normal motor and sensory function. Tetraplegia, also called *quadriplegia* (paralysis), and quadriparesis (weakness) involve all four extremities, as seen with cervical cord and upper thoracic injury. Paraplegia (paralysis) and paraparesis (weakness) involve only the lower extremities, as seen in lower thoracic and lumbosacral injuries or lesions.

Neurologic level defined by the American Spinal Injury Association (ASIA) refers to the highest neurologic level of normal function and is not the same as the *anatomic* level of injury. The neurologic level is determined by evaluating the zones of sensory and motor function, known as *dermatomes* (area of skin in which sensory nerves derive from a single spinal nerve root) and *myotomes* (set of muscles innervated by a spinal nerve). The patient may report a complete sensory loss, hypoesthesia (decreased **sensory perception**), or hyperesthesia (increased **sensory perception**).

✚ NURSING SAFETY PRIORITY

Critical Rescue

In *acute* SCI, monitor for a decrease in **sensory perception** from baseline, especially in a proximal (upward) dermatome and/or new loss of motor function and **mobility.** The presence of these changes is considered an emergency and requires immediate communication with the Rapid Response Team or primary health care provider, using SBAR or other agency-approved protocol for notification. Document these assessment findings in the electronic health record.

The primary health care provider may also test deep tendon reflexes (DTRs), including the biceps (C5), triceps (C7), patella (L3), and ankle (S1). It is not unusual for these reflexes, as well as all *mobility* or *sensory perception,* to be absent immediately after the injury because of spinal shock. After spinal shock has resolved, the reflexes may return.

Cardiovascular and Respiratory Assessment. *Cardiovascular* dysfunction results from disruption of sympathetic fibers of the autonomic nervous system (ANS), especially if the injury is above the sixth thoracic vertebra. Bradycardia, hypotension, and hypothermia occur because of loss of sympathetic input. These changes may lead to cardiac dysrhythmias. *A systolic blood pressure below 90 mm Hg requires treatment because lack of perfusion to the spinal cord could worsen the patient's condition.*

A patient with a cervical SCI is at risk for *breathing* problems resulting from an interruption of spinal innervation to the respiratory muscles. In collaboration with the respiratory therapist (RT), if available, perform a complete respiratory assessment, including pulse oximetry for arterial oxygen saturation, at least every 8 to 12 hours, more often in the acute stage. An oxygen saturation of 92% or less and adventitious breath sounds may indicate a complication such as atelectasis or pneumonia.

Autonomic dysreflexia (AD), sometimes referred to as *autonomic hyperreflexia,* is a potentially life-threatening condition in which noxious visceral or cutaneous stimuli cause a sudden, massive, uninhibited reflex sympathetic discharge in people with high-level SCI. The signs and symptoms of AD are listed in Box 37.2. Severely elevated blood pressure can cause a hemorrhagic stroke, discussed in Chapter 38.

🔹 BOX 37.2   Key Features

Autonomic Dysreflexia

- Sudden, significant rise in systolic and diastolic blood pressure, accompanied by bradycardia
- Profuse sweating above the level of lesion—especially in the face, neck, and shoulders; rarely occurs below the level of the lesion because of sympathetic cholinergic activity
- Goose bumps above or possibly below the level of the lesion
- Flushing of the skin above the level of the lesion—especially in the face, neck, and shoulders
- Blurred vision
- Spots in the patient's visual field
- Nasal congestion
- Onset of severe, throbbing headache
- Feeling of apprehension

The causes of AD are typically GI, gynecologic-urologic (GU), and vascular stimulation. Specific risk factors are bladder distention, urinary tract infection, epididymitis or scrotal compression, bowel distention or impaction from constipation, or irritation of hemorrhoids. Pain; circumferential constriction of the thorax, abdomen, or an extremity (e.g., tight clothing); contact with hard or sharp objects; and temperature fluctuations can also cause AD. Patients with altered *sensory perception* are at great risk for this complication (Rogers, 2023).

Gastrointestinal and Genitourinary Assessment. Assess the patient's *abdomen* for symptoms of internal bleeding, such as abdominal distention, pain, or paralytic ileus. Hemorrhage may result from the trauma, or it may occur later from a stress ulcer or the administration of steroids. Monitor for abdominal *pain* and changes in bowel sounds. Paralytic ileus may develop within 72 hours of hospital admission. During the period of spinal shock, peristalsis decreases, leading to a loss of bowel sounds and to gastric distention. This disruption of the autonomic nervous system may lead to a hypotonic bowel.

After the first few days, when edema subsides, the spinal reflexes that innervate the bowel and bladder usually begin to establish function, depending on the level of the injury. Patients with cervical or high thoracic SCIs have upper motor neuron damage that spares lower spinal reflexes, causing a *spastic* bowel and bladder. Patients with lower thoracic and lumbosacral injuries usually have damage to their lower spinal nerves and therefore have a *flaccid* bowel and bladder.

Assessment of Patients for Long-Term Complications. Patients with complete SCI are at a high risk for complications that result from prolonged impaired *mobility,* including *pressure injuries* and *venous thromboembolism (VTE).* Assess skin integrity with each turn or repositioning. Monitor for signs of VTE with vital signs, including lower extremity deep vein thrombosis (DVT). More detailed information on prevention and management of these complications may be found elsewhere in this text.

Bones can become *osteopenic* and *osteoporotic* without weight-bearing exercise, placing the long-term SCI patient at risk for fractures. Another complication of prolonged immobility is heterotopic ossification (HO) (bony overgrowth, often into muscle). Assess for swelling, redness/hyperpigmentation, warmth, and decreased range of motion (ROM) of the involved extremity. The hip is the most common place where HO occurs. Changes in the bony structure are not visible until several weeks after initial symptoms appear.

Psychosocial Assessment. Patients experiencing an SCI may have significant behavioral and emotional reactions as a result of changes in functional ability, body image, role performance, and self-concept. Many of these patients are young men who may feel guilty for engaging in high-risk behaviors such as diving into shallow water or racing a vehicle that caused the injury. Some patients with SCI are war veterans. Assess patients for their reaction to the injury and provide opportunities to listen to their concerns. Be realistic about their abilities and projected function, but offer hope and encouragement. Aggressive rehabilitation can help most patients live productive and independent lives.

Laboratory and Imaging Assessment. The primary health care provider may request basic laboratory studies for the patient with an SCI to establish baseline data. A spine CT and MRI are performed to determine the degree and extent of damage to the spinal cord and detect the presence of blood and bone within the spinal column. In addition, patients may have a series of x-rays of the spine to identify vertebral fractures, subluxation, or dislocation.

Analyze Cues and Prioritize Hypotheses: Analysis

The priority collaborative problems for patients with an *acute* spinal cord injury (SCI) include:

1. Potential for respiratory distress/failure due to aspiration, decreased diaphragmatic innervation, and/or decreased *mobility*
2. Potential for cardiovascular instability (e.g., shock and autonomic dysreflexia) due to loss or interruption of sympathetic innervation or hemorrhage
3. Potential for secondary spinal cord injury due to hypoperfusion, edema, or delayed spinal column stabilization
4. Decreased *mobility* and *sensory perception* due to spinal cord damage and edema

In addition, the patient with a long-term SCI is at risk for multiple problems caused by prolonged immobility or impaired *mobility.* These problems are discussed in fundamentals textbooks and reviewed in Chapter 7.

Generate Solutions and Take Actions: Planning and Implementation

Caring for a patient with an SCI requires both a patient- and family-centered collaborative approach and involves every health care team member to help meet the patient's expected outcomes. Optimally, patients with a new SCI are quickly transported to an SCI Model System Center. Because of the complexity of an SCI, discharge planning, including the rehabilitation team, needs to begin on the day of admission.

The desired outcomes of patient-centered collaborative care following acute SCI are to stabilize the vertebral column, manage damage to the spinal cord, and prevent secondary injuries.

Managing the Airway and Improving Breathing

Planning: Expected Outcomes. The patient with an SCI is expected to not experience respiratory distress as evidenced by a patent airway and adequate ventilation.

Interventions. *Airway management is the priority for a patient with cervical spinal cord injury!* Patients with injuries at or above T6 are especially at risk for respiratory distress and pulmonary embolus during the first 5 days after injury. These complications are caused by impaired functioning of the intercostal muscles and disruption in the innervation to the diaphragm. Depending on the level of injury, intubation or tracheotomy with mechanical ventilation may be needed.

> **! NURSING SAFETY PRIORITY**
>
> ### Action Alert
>
> Assess breath sounds every 2 to 4 hours during the first few days after SCI, and document and report any adventitious or diminished sounds. Monitor vital signs with pulse oximetry. Watch for changes in respiratory pattern or airway obstruction. Intervene per agency or primary health care provider protocol when there is a decrease in oxygen saturation (Spo₂) to below 95%.

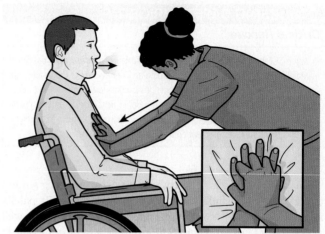

FIG. 37.5 "Cough assist" technique for patient with high spinal cord injury.

Respiratory secretions are managed with manually assisted coughing, pulmonary hygiene, and suctioning. Implement strategies to prevent ventilator-associated pneumonia (VAP) when the patient needs continuous mechanical ventilation as discussed in Chapter 26. Encourage the non–mechanically ventilated patient to use an incentive spirometer. The nurse and respiratory therapist perform a respiratory assessment at least every 8 hours to determine the effectiveness of these strategies. In some cases, it may be necessary to perform oral or nasal suctioning if the patient cannot effectively clear the airway of secretions.

Teach the patient who is tetraplegic to coordinate cough effort with an assistant. The nurse, or other assistant, places both hands on the upper abdomen over the diaphragm and below the ribs. Hands are placed one over the other, with fingers interlocked and away from the skin (Fig. 37.5). If the patient is obese, an alternate hand placement is one hand on either side of the rib cage. Have the patient take a breath and cough during expiration. The assistant locks the elbows and pushes inward and upward as the patient coughs. This technique is sometimes called *assisted coughing, quad cough,* or cough assist. Repeat the coordinated effort, with rest periods as needed, until the airway is clear.

Monitoring for Cardiovascular Instability

Planning: Expected Outcomes. The patient is expected to not develop neurogenic or hypovolemic shock due to hemorrhage and is expected to be free from episodes of autonomic dysreflexia (AD). If any of these potentially life-threatening complications occur, the patient is expected to receive prompt interventions with positive outcomes.

Interventions. Maintain adequate hydration through IV therapy and oral fluids as appropriate, depending on the patient's overall condition. Carefully observe for manifestations of *neurogenic shock,* which may occur within 24 hours after injury, most commonly in patients with injuries above T6. This potentially life-threatening problem results from disruption in the communication pathways between upper motor neurons and lower motor neurons.

Dextran, a plasma expander, may be used to increase capillary blood flow within the spinal cord and prevent or treat hypotension. *Atropine sulfate* is used to treat bradycardia if the pulse rate falls below 50 to 60 beats/min. Hypotension, if severe, is treated with continuous IV sympathomimetic agents such as phenylephrine, dopamine, or other vasoactive agent. Chapter 31 discusses in detail the care of patients experiencing or at risk for shock.

✚ NURSING SAFETY PRIORITY

Critical Rescue

Monitor the patient with acute spinal cord injury at least hourly for indications of neurogenic shock:

- Temperature dysregulation, including warm, flushed skin
- Symptomatic bradycardia, including reduced level of consciousness and deceased urine output
- Hypotension with systolic blood pressure (SBP) <90 or mean arterial pressure (MAP) <65 mm Hg

Notify the Rapid Response Team or primary health care provider immediately if these symptoms occur because this is an emergency! Similar to interventions for any type of shock, neurogenic shock is treated symptomatically by providing fluids to the circulating blood volume, adding vasopressor IV therapy, and providing supportive care to stabilize the patient. In addition, respiratory compromise (pulse oximetry [Spo$_2$] <95% or symptoms of aspiration [e.g., stridor, garbled speech, or inability to clear airway]) may be treated with intubation or bronchial endoscopy.

In addition to observing the patient for shock or hypotension, monitor the patient who has a high-level SCI injury for the additional risk of autonomic dysreflexia (AD). *AD is a neurologic emergency and must be promptly treated to prevent a hypertensive stroke!* Be sure to reduce potential causes for this complication by preventing bladder and bowel distention, managing pain and room temperature, and monitoring for infections (Harmison et al., 2023).

✚ NURSING SAFETY PRIORITY

Critical Rescue

If the patient experiences AD, raise the head of the bed *immediately* to help reduce the blood pressure as the first action. Notify the Rapid Response Team or primary health care provider immediately for drug therapy to quickly reduce blood pressure as indicated. Determine the cause of AD, and manage it promptly as described in Box 37.3.

NCLEX Examination Challenge 37.2

Safe and Effective Care Environment

A client who experienced a recent T1 spinal cord injury appears flushed and diaphoretic in the face and neck and is reporting "seeing spots." Which action would the nurse take **first**?

A. Notify the primary health care provider.
B. Perform a bedside bladder scan.
C. Raise the head of the client's bed.
D. Obtain and document vital signs.

Preventing Secondary Spinal Cord Injury

Planning: Expected Outcomes. The patient with an *acute* SCI is expected to have adequate spinal cord stabilization as evidenced by no further deterioration in neurologic status.

Interventions. During the immediate care of the patient with a suspected or confirmed *cervical* spine injury, a hard

---

BOX 37.3 Best Practice for Patient Safety and Quality Care

Emergency Care of the Patient Experiencing Autonomic Dysreflexia: Immediate Interventions

- Place patient in a sitting position (first priority!), or return to a previous safe position.
- Assess for and remove/manage the cause:
  - Check for urinary retention or catheter blockage.
  - Check the urinary catheter tubing (if present) for kinks or obstruction.
  - If a urinary catheter is not present, check for bladder distention, and catheterize immediately if indicated. (Consider using anesthetic ointment on the tip of the catheter before catheter insertion to reduce urethral irritation.)
- Determine if a urinary tract infection or bladder calculi (stones) are contributing to genitourinary irritation.
- Check the patient for fecal impaction or other colorectal irritation, using anesthetic ointment at rectum; disimpact if needed.
- Examine skin for new or worsening pressure injury symptoms.
- Monitor blood pressure every 10 to 15 minutes.
- Give nifedipine or nitrate as prescribed to lower blood pressure as needed. (Patients with recurrent autonomic dysreflexia may receive clonidine or another centrally acting alpha-agonist agent prophylactically [Burchum & Rosenthal, 2022].)

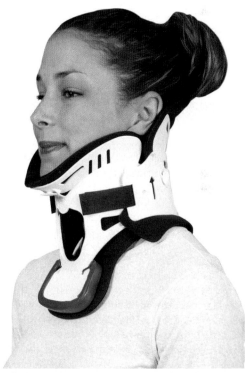

FIG. 37.6 Patient with spinal cord injury wearing a hard cervical (Miami J) collar. (Found in Ostendork, W. R., Perry, A. G., & Potter, P. A. [2020.] *Nursing interventions & clinical skills.* [7th ed.] St. Louis: Elsevier. From Össur Americas.)

cervical collar, such as the Miami J or Philadelphia collar, is placed to stabilize the spine until a specific order indicates that it can be removed (Fig. 37.6). Padding at pressure points beneath and at the edges of the collar, particularly at the occiput, may be necessary to maintain skin integrity. Until the spinal column is stabilized, a jaw-thrust maneuver is preferable to a head-tilt maneuver to open the airway should the patient need an airway intervention. Maintain spinal alignment at all times, with log rolling to change position from supine to side-lying.

If the patient has a fractured vertebra, the primary concern of the health care team is to reduce and immobilize the fracture to prevent further damage to the spinal cord from bone fragments. Nonsurgical techniques include external fixation or orthotic devices, but surgery is often needed to better stabilize the spine and prevent further spinal cord damage. Typical surgical procedures include spinal fusion to manage cervical injuries. Metal wiring is used to secure bone chips taken from the patient's hip or other source of bone grafting, such as donor bone tissue. Chapter 9 discusses general postoperative nursing care.

After surgical spinal fusion, assess the patient's neurologic status and vital signs at least every hour for the first 4 to 6 hours and then, if the patient is stable, every 4 hours. Assess for complications of surgery, including worsening of motor or sensory function at or above the site of surgery. *Document your assessments carefully and in detail. Failure to do so may prevent other staff members from quickly recognizing deterioration in neurologic status.*

The patient may be placed in fixed skeletal traction to maintain vertebral alignment, facilitate bone healing, and prevent further injury, often after surgical stabilization. The most commonly used device for immobilization of the cervical spine is the *halo fixator* device, also called a *halo crown,* which is worn for 6 to 12 weeks. This static device is affixed by four pins (or screws) into the outer aspect of the skull and is connected to a vest or jacket (Fig. 37.7). For patients not having surgery, the addition of traction helps reduce the fracture.

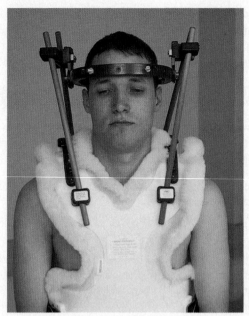

FIG. 37.7 Halo fixation device with jacket.

IV or orally. Oral doses may be taken with or without food (Burchum & Rosenthal, 2022). An anticoagulant may be given as part of the VTE prevention protocol. Bulk-forming laxatives or stool softeners are given to prevent constipation.

Other drugs to prevent or treat complications of immobility may be needed *later* during the rehabilitative phase. For example, celecoxib may be prescribed to prevent or treat heterotopic ossification (bony overgrowth). However, recall that the adverse effects of this drug include an increased risk of myocardial infarction and stroke. Calcium and bisphosphonates may prevent the osteoporosis that results from lack of weight-bearing or resistance activity. Osteoporosis can cause fractures in later years. Early and continued exercise may help decrease the incidence of these complications.

Centrally acting skeletal muscular relaxants may help control muscle spasticity. Intrathecal baclofen (ITB) therapy may be prescribed to treat muscle spasms without incurring the drowsiness and sedation often seen with oral medications (Burchum & Rosenthal, 2022). This drug is administered through a programmable, implantable infusion pump and intrathecal catheter directly into the cerebrospinal fluid. The pump is surgically placed in a subcutaneous pouch in the lower abdomen. Monitor for common adverse effects, which include sedation, fatigue, headache, hypotension, and changes in mental status (Burchum & Rosenthal, 2022). *Seizures and hallucinations may occur if ITB is suddenly withdrawn.*

⚠ NURSING SAFETY PRIORITY

Action Alert

Never move or turn the patient by holding or pulling on the halo device. Do not adjust the screws holding it in place. Check the patient's skin frequently to ensure that the jacket is not causing pressure. Pressure is avoided if one finger can be inserted easily between the jacket and the patient's skin. Monitor the patient's neurologic status for changes in movement or decreased strength. A special wrench is needed to loosen the vest in emergencies such as cardiopulmonary arrest. Tape the wrench to the vest for easy and consistent accessibility. Do not use sharp objects (e.g., coat hangers, knitting needles) to relieve itching under the vest; skin damage and infection will slow recovery.

Common complications of the halo device are pin loosening, local infection, and scarring. More serious but less common complications include osteomyelitis (cranial bone infection), subdural abscess, and instability. Hospital policy is followed for pin-site care, which may specify the use of solutions such as saline. Vaseline dressings may also be used. *Monitor the patient for indications of possible infection (e.g., fever, purulent drainage from the pin sites), and report any changes to the primary health care provider immediately.*

For thoracic and lumbar fusions, metal or steel rods (e.g., Harrington rods) are used to keep the bone ends in alignment after fracture reduction. After surgery the patient usually wears a molded plastic support (cervical or thoracic-lumbar or both) to keep the injured and operative areas immobilized during recovery. Postoperative care is similar to that described in Chapter 9.

Because SCI is a physical trauma, the patient is started on a proton pump inhibitor, such as pantoprazole, to help prevent the development of stress ulcers. This drug may be administered

NCLEX Examination Challenge 37.3

Safety and Infection Control

A nurse is caring for a client with a spinal cord injury being treated with a halo fixator with vest. Which action by the nurse is **most important** for client safety?

A. Assess the pin sites daily.
B. Ensure that the wrench is taped to the vest.
C. Provide straws for ease of drinking.
D. Keep the client in a sitting position.

Managing Decreased Mobility

Planning: Expected Outcomes. The patient with an SCI is expected to be free from complications of decreased *mobility* and perform ADLs as independently as possible with or without assistive-adaptive devices.

Interventions. Patients with an SCI are especially at risk for pressure injuries due to altered *sensory perception* of pressure areas on skin below the level of the injury. They are also at risk for venous thromboembolism (VTE), contractures, orthostatic hypotension (especially in patients with high SCI), and fractures related to osteoporosis due to impaired *mobility*. Frequent and therapeutic positioning not only helps prevent complications but also provides alignment to prevent further SCI or irritability. Reposition patients frequently (every 1 to 2 hours). Assess the condition of the patient's skin, especially over pressure points, with each turn or repositioning. Turning may be performed manually, or the patient may be placed on an automatic rotating bed. Reduce pressure on any reddened area, and monitor it with the next turn. When sitting in a chair, patients are repositioned or taught to reposition themselves more often than every hour. Paraplegic patients usually perform frequent "wheelchair push-ups" to relieve skin pressure. Use a pressure-reducing mattress and wheelchair or chair pad to help prevent skin breakdown. Prevent pressure injuries by using best practices as described in Chapter 21. The prevention of VTE includes the interventions of intermittent pneumatic compression stockings and low–molecular-weight heparin (LMWH).

Patients with cervical cord injuries especially are at high risk for orthostatic (postural) hypotension, but anyone who is immobilized may have this problem. If the patient changes from a lying position to a sitting or standing position too quickly, the patient may experience hypotension, which could result in dizziness and falls. Because of interrupted sympathetic innervation caused by the SCI, the blood vessels do not constrict quickly enough to push blood up into the brain. The resulting vasodilation causes dizziness or light-headedness and possible falls with syncope ("blackout").

In collaboration with the rehabilitation team, teach or reinforce teaching for bed *mobility* skills and bed-to-chair transfers. Patients with paraplegia are usually able to transfer from the bed to chair or wheelchair with minimal or no assistance unless balance is a problem (seen in patients with high thoracic injuries). Techniques to improve balance are usually taught by occupational or physical therapists. Tetraplegic patients may learn how to transfer using a slider, also called a *sliding board*. This simple boardlike device allows the patient to move from the bed to chair or vice versa by creating a bridge. When using the slider, remind patients to lift the buttocks while moving incrementally and slowly across the board. Patients with severe muscle spasticity have more challenges when learning transfer skills, and contractures are common. Contractures may be prevented or minimized with splints and range-of-motion exercises. Managing decreased *mobility* requires communication and coordination among multiple members of the health care team, as described in Box 37.4.

Care of Patients With Spinal Cord Injury

Consult with the physical therapist (PT) and occupational therapist (OT) to ensure positive patient outcomes. Coordinate care with the rehabilitative team to ensure collaborative care. According to the Interprofessional Education Collaborative (IPEC) Expert Panel's Competency of Interprofessional Communication, be sure to use language that is easily understood by the patient when coordinating care. Avoid discipline-specific terminology when possible (IPEC, 2016; Slusser et al., 2019).

All patients with an SCI require bowel and bladder retraining, including adequate fluids (1.5 to 2 L each day) and stool softeners to prevent constipation from immobility and the injury itself. Those with *upper* motor neuron lesions (usually cervical and high thoracic injuries) have *spastic* bowel and bladder function with an intact spinal reflex for elimination. However, voiding patterns may be uncontrollable and require long-term indwelling or external catheters, leading to frequent urinary tract infections (Elliott et al., 2021). An implanted intraurethral device may be an option for some female SCI patients (Schimke & Connolly, 2020). Rectal suppositories are often successful to promote regular bowel elimination.

The patient with a *lower* motor neuron lesion has a *flaccid* bowel and bladder. Intermittent urinary catheterizations, manual pressure over the bladder area, and bowel disimpaction on a regular basis help to establish a routine. Chapter 7 describes bowel and bladder training in more detail.

In patients with established or long-term SCI, assess baseline ability, and encourage their participation in self-care and management. Encourage family members' participation in care, and support their effort to keep the patient engaged in family life.

Care Coordination and Transition Management

Rehabilitation Phase. Rehabilitation after an acute SCI begins in the acute or critical care unit when patients are hemodynamically stable. They are usually transferred from the acute care setting to a rehabilitation setting, where they learn more about self-care, mobility skills, and bladder and bowel retraining. The primary purpose of rehabilitation for a SCI is to enable patients to function independently in their communities. However, physical barriers still exist in some communities that prevent the patient in a wheelchair from finding a parking place, using sidewalks, and attending activities or accessing resources (Smeltzer, 2021) (Fig. 37.8). Chapter 7 describes nursing care and the role of rehabilitative services in detail.

One new but promising therapy in rehabilitation is functional electrical stimulation (FES). FES uses small electrical pulses to paralyzed muscles to restore or improve their function. It is commonly used for exercise, but it is also used to assist with breathing, grasping, transferring, standing, and walking. The occupational therapist instructs the patient in the correct use of all adaptive equipment and therapies.

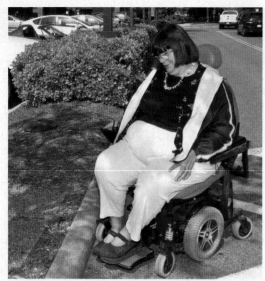

FIG. 37.8 Community physical barrier example: A curb prevents the patient in a wheelchair from getting onto the sidewalk.

Wearable robotic exoskeletons have also shown promise in improving quality of life in patients with spinal cord injury (Chis et al., 2020). These battery-powered devices typically fit over the hips and lower extremities, allowing clients to "walk" at home and in the community.

Living with a Spinal Cord Injury in the Community. A full-time caregiver or personal assistant is sometimes required when the patient with tetraplegia returns home from rehabilitation. The caregiver may be a family member or a nursing assistant employed to help provide care and companionship. A patient who is paraplegic is usually able to provide self-care without assistance after an appropriate rehabilitation program. Abu-Baker et al. (2021) conducted a study to determine which specific factors contribute to high self-care ability and quality of life for patients with SCI living in the community (see the Evidence-Based Practice box).

In addition to self-care ability, sexual function after SCI also depends on the level and extent of injury. Incomplete lesions allow some control over ***sensory perception*** and ***mobility.*** Complete lesions disconnect the messages from the brain to the rest of the body and vice versa. However, men with injuries above T6 are often able to have erections by stimulating reflex activity. For example, stroking the penis will cause an erection. Ejaculation is less predictable and may be mixed with urine. However, urine is sterile, so the patient's partner will not get an infection. To prevent autonomic dysreflexia (AD), prophylactic administration of a vasodilator may be needed before intercourse.

Women with an SCI have a different challenge because they have indwelling urinary catheters more commonly than men. Some women do become pregnant and have full-term children. For others, ovulation stops in response to the injury. In this case, alternate methods for pregnancy, such as *in vitro* fertilization, may be an option. Some women

EVIDENCE-BASED PRACTICE

What Factors Predict a High Quality of Life for Patients Who Have a Spinal Cord Injury?

Abu-Baker, N. N., Al-Zyoud, N. H., & Alshraifeen, A. (2021). Quality of life and self-care ability among individuals with spinal cord injury. *Clinical Nursing Research, 30*(6), 883–891.

The researchers studied a convenience sample of 152 individuals living with a spinal cord injury in the community to identify their self-care ability, quality of life, and related factors. Two tools were used to collect data—the Modified Barthel Index of ADL and the World Health Organization Quality of Life—BRIEF. The results showed that 55.3% of the sample reported moderate dependence on others to support self-care, 48% reported a good quality of life, and 65.8% were satisfied with their health. Having paraplegia or an incomplete SCI at any level significantly predicted the highest self-care ability. The highest quality of life was reported by males who had a high educational level, paraplegia, an incomplete spinal injury, and no pressure injuries.

Level of Evidence: 4

This was a descriptive study that used a convenience sample.

Implications for Nursing Practice and Research

Nurses need to recognize that many patients with spinal cord injury can enjoy a high level of independence and quality of life. This research indicates that educated men who have incomplete paraplegia and no complications of mobility would likely have the best quality of life when compared to other individuals who have SCI. More research is needed to determine what factors prevent women from having the same quality of life as their male counterparts. Research is also needed using a larger study sample.

About 25% of the U.S. population lives with a disability, including those who have an SCI. Research has shown that disabled individuals are less likely than those without a disability to seek preventive health care services.

MEETING *HEALTHY PEOPLE 2030* OBJECTIVES

Preventive Health and Disability

One major goal of *Healthy People 2030* is to increase the health and well-being of people living with disabilities. Barriers such as difficulty in obtaining health care access or inadequate financial ability to pay for preventive services contribute to the lack of health promotion. Nurses should help patients locate affordable local community resources for preventive health to improve their overall health and well-being.

also report vaginal dryness. Recommend a water-soluble lubricant for both partners to promote comfort during intercourse.

Many individuals have had their SCI for many years and continue to function successfully as productive members of the community. Teach patients what they need to know about health and aging, especially when living with an SCI (see Patient-Centered Care: Older Adult Health box).

PATIENT-CENTERED CARE: OLDER ADULT HEALTH

What Patients Need to Know About Aging With Spinal Cord Injury

Health Teaching	Rationale
Follow guidelines for adult vaccination, particularly influenza and pneumococcus vaccination recommendations.	Respiratory complications are the most common cause of death after spinal cord injury (SCI).
For women, have Papanicolaou (Pap) smears and mammograms as recommended by the American Cancer Society or your primary health care provider.	Limitations in movement may make breast self-awareness difficult.
Take measures to prevent osteoporosis, such as increasing calcium and vitamin D intake, avoiding caffeine, and not smoking. Exercise against resistance can maintain muscle strength and slow bone loss.	Women older than 50 years often lose bone density, which can result in fractures. Men can also have osteoporotic fractures as a result of immobility.
Practice meticulous skin care, including frequent repositioning, using pressure-reduction surfaces in bed and chairs/wheelchairs, and applying skin protective products.	As a person ages, skin becomes dry and less elastic, predisposing the patient to pressure injuries.
Take measures to prevent constipation, such as drinking adequate fluids, eating a high-fiber diet, adding a stool softener or bowel stimulant daily, and establishing a regular time for bowel elimination.	Constipation is a problem for most patients with SCI, and bowel motility can slow, contributing to constipation later in life.
Modify activities if joint *pain* occurs; use a powered rather than a manual wheelchair. Ask the primary health care provider about treatment options.	Arthritis occurs in more than half of people older than 65 years. Patients with SCI are more likely to develop arthritis as a result of added stress on the upper extremities when using a wheelchair.

Unfortunately, some patients living with SCIs living in the community are periodically admitted to the acute care or long-term care setting for complications of immobility, such as pressure injuries or fractures resulting from osteoporosis. Pressure injuries contribute to local or systemic infection, including osteomyelitis and septicemia. Priorities in care may need to be reevaluated as complications occur and resolve.

Refer patients and their families to local, state or province, and national organizations for more information and support for patients with SCI. These organizations include the United Spinal Association (www.unitedspinal.org) in the United States and Spinal Cord Injury Canada (www.sci-can.ca). Many excellent consumer-oriented books, journals, and DVDs are also available. Support groups may help the patient and family adjust to a changed lifestyle and provide solutions to commonly encountered problems.

PATIENT-CENTERED CARE: VETERAN HEALTH

Health Care Resources for Veterans With Spinal Cord Injury

The U.S. Veterans Health Administration services is the largest provider of SCI care in the world (Elliott et al., 2021). The Paralyzed Veterans of America (PVA) (www.pva.org) can assist with educational materials, caregiver services, medical equipment, and support groups. The PVA also sponsors spinal cord research and raises money to help veterans with a variety of needs. It also supports wheelchair-sports teams composed of veterans with an SCI or diseases that affect the spinal cord.

The Independence Program of the Wounded Warriors Project is designed to help veterans with neurologic health conditions such as SCI and traumatic brain injury to progress toward independent living. This nonprofit program offers services such as wellness, life skills, and social and recreational activities (Elliott et al., 2021).

Evaluate Outcomes: Evaluation

Evaluate the care of the patient with an SCI based on the identified priority patient problems. The expected outcomes are that the patient:

- Exhibits no deterioration in neurologic status
- Maintains a patent airway, a physiologic breathing pattern, and adequate ventilation
- Does not experience a cardiovascular event (e.g., shock, hemorrhage, autonomic dysreflexia) or receives prompt treatment if an event occurs
- Does not experience secondary complications, including VTE and heterotopic ossification
- Is free from complications of decreased *mobility*
- Performs *mobility* skills and basic ADLs as independently as possible with or without the use of assistive-adaptive devices

LOW BACK PAIN (LUMBOSACRAL BACK PAIN)

Back *pain* affects most adults at some time in their life. It can be recurrent, and subsequent episodes tend to increase in severity. The lumbosacral (lower back) and cervical (neck) vertebrae are most commonly affected because these are the areas where the vertebral column is the most flexible. *Acute* back pain is usually self-limiting and lasts less than 12 weeks. If the *pain* continues for 12 weeks (3 months) or more, the patient has *chronic* back pain (National Institute of Neurologic Disorders and Stroke, 2021).

Pathophysiology Review

Low back pain (LBP) occurs along the lumbosacral area of the vertebral column. Acute *pain* is caused by muscle strain or spasm, ligament sprain, disk (also spelled "disc") degeneration (osteoarthritis), or herniation of the center of the disk, the nucleus pulposus. A herniated nucleus pulposus (HNP) in the lumbosacral area can press on the adjacent spinal nerve (usually the sciatic nerve), causing burning or stabbing

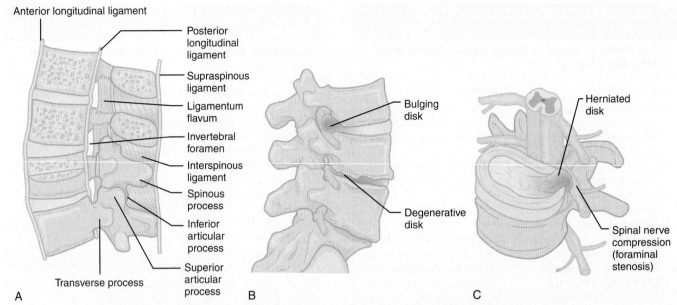

FIG. 37.9 Spinal ligaments, degenerative disk, and herniated disk. (A) Ligaments of the spine. (B) Bulging disk with spinal nerve compression and degenerative disk showing collapse of vertebral body. (C) Herniated disk with spinal nerve compression. (From Rogers, J. L. [2023]. *McCance & Huether's Pathophysiology: The biologic basis for disease in adults and children.* [9th ed.]. St. Louis: Elsevier.)

pain down into the leg or foot, which in some cases can be severe (Fig. 37.9). Herniated disks occur most often between the fourth and fifth lumbar vertebrae (L4-L5) but may occur at other levels. The specific area of symptoms depends on the level of herniation.

In addition to acute or persistent *pain,* there may be both muscle spasm and numbness and tingling (paresthesia) in the affected leg because spinal nerves have both motor and sensory fibers. The HNP may press on the spinal cord itself, causing leg weakness. Bowel and bladder incontinence or retention may occur with motor nerve involvement because sacral spinal nerves have parasympathetic fibers that help control bowel and bladder function (Rogers, 2023).

Back pain may also be caused by spinal stenosis, which is a narrowing of the spinal canal, nerve root canals, or intervertebral foramina typically seen in people older than 50 years. This narrowing may be caused by infection, trauma, herniated disk, arthritis, and disk degeneration. Most adults older than 50 years have some degree of degenerative disk disease, although they may not be symptomatic.

LBP is most prevalent during the third to sixth decades of life but can occur at any time. Women have a higher incidence of LBP compared to men (Pfieffer, 2020). *Acute* back *pain* usually results from injury or trauma, such as during a fall or vehicular crash or when lifting a heavy object. The mechanisms of injury include repetitive flexion and/or extension and hyperflexion or hyperextension with or without rotation. Obesity places increased stress on the vertebral column and back muscles, contributing to risk for injury. Smoking has been linked to disk degeneration, possibly caused by constriction of blood vessels that supply the spine. Congenital spinal conditions such as scoliosis (an abnormal lateral curvature of the spine) can also lead to LBP at any age.

PATIENT-CENTERED CARE: OLDER ADULT HEALTH

Older Adults and Low Back Pain

Older adults are at high risk for acute and chronic LBP. Vertebral fracture from osteoporosis contributes to LBP. Petite, older White women are at high risk for both bone loss and subsequent vertebral fractures. Specific factors that can cause LBP in the older adult include (Touhy & Jett, 2022):

- Spinal stenosis
- Hypertrophy of the intraspinal ligaments
- Osteoarthritis
- Osteoporosis
- Changes in vertebral support structures and malalignment with deformity
- Scoliosis
- Lordosis (an inward abnormal curvature of the lumbar spinal area)
- Vascular changes
- Diminished blood supply to the spinal cord or cauda equina caused by arteriosclerosis
- Blood dyscrasias
- Intervertebral disk degeneration

Vertebral compression fractures are discussed in Chapter 42.

Health Promotion/Disease Prevention

Many of the problems related to back pain can be prevented by recognizing the factors that contribute to tissue injury and taking appropriate preventive measures to prevent *pain.* For example, proper posture and exercise can significantly decrease the incidence of LBP. Box 37.5 summarizes various ways to help prevent LBP.

The U.S. Occupational Safety and Health Administration (OSHA) has mandated that all industries develop and implement plans to decrease musculoskeletal injuries among their workers. One way to meet this requirement is to develop an

BOX 37.5 Patient and Family Education

Prevention of Low Back Pain and Injury

- Use safe manual handling practices, with specific attention to bending, lifting, and sitting.
- Assess the need for assistance with your household chores or other activities.
- Participate in a regular exercise program, especially one that promotes back strengthening, such as swimming and walking.
- Do not wear high-heeled shoes.
- Use good posture when sitting, standing, and walking.
- Avoid prolonged sitting or standing. Use a footstool and ergonomic chairs and tables to lessen back strain. Be sure that equipment in the workplace is ergonomically designed to prevent injury.
- Keep weight within 10% of ideal body weight.
- Ensure adequate calcium intake. Consider vitamin D supplementation if serum levels are low.
- Stop smoking. If you are not able to stop, cut down on the number of cigarettes or decrease the use of other forms of tobacco.

ergonomic plan for the workplace. Ergonomics is an applied science in which the workplace is designed to increase worker comfort (thus reducing injury) while increasing efficiency and productivity. An example is a ceiling lift designed to help nurses assist patients to get out of bed. A variety of equipment can be used to decrease injury related to moving patients. Professional guidelines and legislative rules promote safe patient handling and mobility for health care workers (ANA, 2022).

NURSE WELL-BEING REMINDER!

Remember: Avoid lifting patients or equipment to prevent back injury. Be sure that every patient area is equipped with an appropriate mechanical or electric lift. Follow best practices for safe patient handling and mobility, including ensuring that agency furniture is ergonomically designed to promote comfort while reducing injury.

Interprofessional Collaborative Care

Recognize Cues: Assessment

Physical Assessment/Signs and Symptoms. The patient's *primary concern is continuous pain*. Some patients have so much *pain* that they walk in a stiff, flexed posture, or they may be unable to bend at all. They may walk with a limp, indicating possible sciatic nerve impairment. Walking on the heels or toes often causes severe pain in the affected leg, the back, or both.

Conduct a complete *pain* assessment as discussed in Chapter 6. Record the patient's current pain score and the worst and best score since the pain began. Ask about precipitating or relieving factors, such as symptoms at night or during rest. Determine whether a recent injury to the back has occurred. It is not unusual for the patient to say, "I just moved to do something and felt my back go out."

Inspect the patient's back for vertebral alignment and tenderness. Examine the surrounding anatomy and lower extremities for secondary injury. Patients will often describe *pain* as stabbing and continuous in the muscle closest to the affected disk. They often describe a sharp, burning posterior thigh or calf pain that may radiate to the ankle or toes along the path of one or more spinal nerves. Pain usually does not extend the entire length of the limb. Patients may also report the same type of pain in the middle of one buttock or hip. The pain is often aggravated by sneezing, coughing, or straining. Driving a vehicle is particularly painful.

Ask whether *paresthesia* (tingling sensation) or numbness is present in the involved leg. Both extremities may be checked for **sensory perception** by using a cotton ball and a paper clip for comparison of light or dull and sharp touch. The patient may feel sensation in both legs but may experience a stronger sensation on the unaffected side. Ask about urinary and fecal continence and difficulty with urination or having new-onset constipation.

If the sciatic nerve is compressed, severe *pain* usually occurs when the patient's leg is held straight and lifted upward. Foot, ankle, and leg weakness may accompany LBP. To complete the neurologic assessment, evaluate the patient's muscle tone and strength. Muscles in the extremity or lower back can atrophy as a result of severe persistent back pain. The patient has difficulty with movement, and certain movements create more pain than others.

Ask patients whether they have frequent feelings of sadness or have considered suicide. For many patients, persistent pain can cause depression and/or suicidal ideation.

Imaging Assessment. Imaging studies for patients who report mild nonspecific back *pain* may not be done, depending on the nature of the pain. Patients with severe or progressive motor or **sensory perception** deficits or who are thought to have other underlying conditions (e.g., cancer, infection) require complete diagnostic assessment. To determine the exact cause of the pain, a number of diagnostic tests may be used, including:

- Plain x-rays (show general arthritis changes and bony alignment)
- CT scan (shows spinal bones, nerves, disks, and ligaments)
- MRI (provides images of the spinal tissue, bones, spinal cord, nerves, ligaments, musculature, and disks)
- Bone scan (shows bone changes after injection of radioactive tracers, which attach to areas of increased bone production or show increased vascularity associated with tumor or infection)

Electrodiagnostic testing, such as electromyography (EMG) and nerve-conduction studies, may help distinguish motor neuron diseases from peripheral neuropathy and radiculopathy (spinal nerve root involvement). These tests are especially useful in chronic diseases of the spinal cord or associated nerves. Chapter 35 describes these tests in more detail.

Take Actions: Interventions

Management of patients with low back *pain* varies with the severity and chronicity of the problem. If acute pain is not treated or managed effectively, persistent *pain* may occur. Most patients with acute LBP experience spontaneous resolution of pain and other symptoms in less than 3 months.

Some patients need only a brief treatment regimen of at-home exercise or physical therapy to manage *pain*. In general, return to work, if safe, is beneficial for recovery and well-being. Some patients have continuous or intermittent chronic pain that must be managed for an extended period. Referral to an interprofessional team that specializes in *pain* or back pain can provide expert long-term management.

Nonsurgical Management. For patients with acute, nonspecific LBP, nonpharmacologic measures are often the first-line treatment, although a recent clinical guideline published by the North American Spine Society (NASS, 2020) found insufficient evidence to support many of the most commonly recommended treatments. A short period of back rest with heat or ice may be prescribed; heat has been shown to offer some short-term benefits. Physical therapy can help strengthen surrounding muscles, and the therapist can educate the patient on preventing further injury. The NASS work groups could not find conclusive evidence to endorse ultrasound treatments, transcutaneous electrical nerve stimulation (TENS), laser therapy, traction, dry needling or acupuncture, bracing, or massage therapy, although individual patients may get relief from any of these modalities.

The patient should begin stretching exercises and resume normal daily activities as soon as possible, including returning to work, if safe to do so. Aerobic exercise has good evidence to support its use when the patient is able (NASS, 2020). Most patients also find that they need to change position frequently. Prolonged standing, sitting, or lying down increases back pain. If the patient must stand for a long time for work or other reasons, shoe insoles or special floor pads may help decrease pain.

The Williams position is typically more comfortable and therapeutic for the patient with *acute* LBP from a bulging or herniated disk. In this position, the patient lies in semi-Fowler's position with a pillow under the knees to keep them flexed or sits in a recliner chair. This position relaxes the muscles of the lower back and relieves pressure on the spinal nerve root.

Many patients worry that their back *pain* will not resolve, and in some cases the pain can convert to a chronic condition. Other patients will have no further reoccurrences. The nurse should provide honest information and reassure patients that with care, another episode might never occur. NASS (2020) recommends that psychosocial and workplace factors, pain severity, prior episodes of back pain, and functional impairment be considered when assessing risk of chronicity. NASS was unable to find conclusive evidence that sleep quality, smoking, or obesity were predictive of a chronic condition.

Patients with chronic LBP are also initially managed with nonpharmacologic interventions. In addition to the measures described earlier, patients may benefit from complementary and integrative therapies, such as stress reduction, mindfulness, progressive muscle relaxation, and yoga. Pain catastrophizing has been shown to cause increased distress (Conti et al., 2020). Cognitive-behavioral therapy in addition to physical therapy had strong evidence to support its use in patients whose pain continues beyond 12 months (NASS, 2020).

If medications are needed, nonselective NSAIDs, such as aspirin, ibuprofen, and naproxen, are helpful. Although antidepressants and antiepileptics such as gabapentin are often prescribed, NASS does not recommend them in the treatment of LBP. On the

other hand, patients with chronic pain may become depressed; in that case, antidepressants are appropriate. NASS also found insufficient evidence for treatment with steroids, either oral or IV. Opioids have a very limited role in the treatment of back pain; they are used sparingly and for a very short time if needed for acute *pain*. Topical capsicum provides good pain relief on a short-term basis; there is no evidence that lidocaine patches provide significant relief (NASS, 2020). Ziconotide is a potent analgesic sometimes used for patients who have severe persistent pain.

Muscle spasms can occur for which the provider may prescribe centrally acting muscle relaxants. Commonly used medications include diazepam, cyclobenzaprine, metaxalone, carisoprodol, and tizanidine.

⚕ NURSING SAFETY PRIORITY

Drug Alert

All centrally acting muscle relaxants can cause sedation, dizziness, or light-headedness. Most muscle relaxants have anticholinergic properties (dry mouth, urinary retention, blurred vision, constipation, and tachycardia). These side effects, plus sedation, increase an older adult's fall risk and should, therefore, be avoided in this population. All patients taking these medications should be advised to avoid driving or other potentially hazardous activities, drinking alcohol, or taking other CNS depressants. Metaxalone can cause liver damage (Burchum & Rosenthal, 2022).

Ziconotide should not be given to patients with severe mental health/behavioral health problems because it can cause psychosis. If symptoms such as hallucinations and delusions occur, teach patients to stop the drug immediately and notify their primary health care provider (Burchum & Rosenthal, 2022).

A physical therapist (PT) works with the patient to develop an individualized exercise program. The type of exercises prescribed depends on the location and nature of the injury and the type of pain. McKenzie exercises are often utilized to help reposition the misaligned vertebral disks, strengthen surrounding muscles, and teach the patient how to manage back (or neck) pain themselves (Mann et al., 2021). These exercises include extension and flexion positions to centralize the back pain. The patient does not begin exercises until acute pain is reduced by other means. Water therapy combined with exercise is helpful for some patients with chronic pain. The water also provides muscle resistance during exercise to prevent atrophy.

Weight reduction may help reduce persistent LBP by decreasing the strain on the vertebrae caused by excess weight. If the patient's weight exceeds the ideal by more than 10%, caloric restriction is considered, although NASS found insufficient evidence that BMI is a predictor of recurrent back *pain* (NASS, 2020). Health care professionals must be sensitive when discussing weight reduction and include behavioral approaches to weight loss and positive reinforcement as part of the plan.

Surgical Management. Surgery may be performed if conservative measures fail to relieve persistent back pain or if neurologic deficits continue to progress. An orthopedic surgeon and/or neurosurgeon perform these surgeries. Two general surgical methods are used, depending on the severity and exact location of pain: minimally invasive surgery (MIS) and conventional open surgical procedures. MIS is not done if the disk is pressing into the spinal cord (central cord involvement).

Preoperative Care. Preoperative care for the patient preparing for lumbar spinal surgery is similar to that for any patient undergoing surgery (see Chapter 9). Teach the patient about postoperative expectations, depending on surgical method, including:

- Techniques to get into and out of bed
- Turning and moving in bed
- Immediately reporting new **sensory perception,** such as numbness and tingling, or new motor impairment that may occur in the affected leg or in both legs
- Home care activities and restrictions, if any

As part of preoperative teaching, make sure that patients understand the type of procedure they are having and the postoperative care that will be needed. A recent randomized controlled trial found that the knowledge of patients about their surgical procedures was inadequate. There was no significant difference between the knowledge of patients who had routine preoperative education and of patients who had specific preoperative education on their spinal surgical procedures (Kesänen et al., 2019).

Newer surgical procedures allow many patients to have same-day surgery. Other patients are discharged to home within 23 to 48 hours after surgery. Therefore, teach family members or other caregivers how to assist the patient and what restrictions the patient must follow at home before surgery occurs.

Operative Procedures. *Minimally invasive surgery (MIS)* using endoscopy or percutaneous instrumentation results in minimal muscle injury, decreased blood loss, and decreased postoperative pain. Therefore, the primary advantages of MIS procedures are a shortened hospital stay, less pain, and the possibility of an ambulatory care (same-day) procedure. Spinal cord and nerve complications are also less likely. Several specific procedures are commonly performed.

A *microdiskectomy* involves microscopic surgery directly through a 1-inch incision using an endoscope. This procedure allows easier identification of anatomic structures, improved precision in removing small fragments, and decreased tissue trauma and pain. A special cutting tool or laser probe is threaded through the cannula for removal or destruction of the *disk pieces* that are compressing the nerve root. This process is also called a *percutaneous endoscopic diskectomy (PED)*. A newer procedure combines the PED with *laser thermodiskectomy* to also shrink the herniated disk before removal. Inpatient hospitalization is not necessary for this procedure.

Laser-assisted laparoscopic lumbar diskectomy combines a laser with modified standard disk instruments inserted through the laparoscope using an umbilical ("belly button") incision. The procedure may be used to treat herniated disks that are bulging but do not involve the vertebral canal. The primary risks of this surgery are infection and nerve root injury. The patient is typically discharged in 23 hours but may go home sooner.

The newest addition to MIS procedures is robot-assisted spinal surgery. This procedure requires additional training and

experience for the surgeon and is currently limited to assistance with hardware placement (Staub & Sadrameli, 2019).

The most common *open surgical procedures* are diskectomy, laminectomy, and/or spinal fusion. Artificial disk replacement may also be part of this type of surgery. These procedures involve a surgical incision to expose anatomic landmarks for extensive muscle and soft-tissue dissection. The location and length of incision depends on the procedure and on surgeon preference and training.

As the name implies, a *diskectomy* is removal of a herniated disk. A *laminectomy* involves removal of part of the laminae and facet joints to obtain access to the disk space. A *spinal fusion* connects two or more vertebrae to stabilize the spine and release compression on spinal nerves. In an *interbody cage fusion surgery*, a titanium mesh device is implanted into the space where the disk was removed, and several screws ensure stabilization.

When repeated laminectomies are performed or the spine is unstable, the surgeon may perform a spinal fusion (arthrodesis) with bone graft to stabilize the affected area. Chips of cadaver bone are ground and grafted between the vertebrae for support and to strengthen the back. Metal implants (usually titanium pins, screws, plates, or rods) may be required to ensure the fusion of the spine. The surgeon may give an intrathecal (spinal) or epidural dose of long-acting morphine to decrease postoperative pain.

Postoperative Care. Postoperative care depends on the surgical method and procedure that was performed. In the postanesthesia care unit (PACU), vital signs and level of consciousness are monitored frequently, as for any surgery. Best practices for PACU nursing care are discussed in Chapter 9. Patients who have a *minimally invasive spinal surgery* go home the same day or the day after surgery with one or more wound closure tapes over the small incision. Those having a microdiskectomy may also have a clear or gauze dressing over the bandage. Most patients notice less pain immediately after surgery, but mild oral analgesics are needed while nerve tissue heals over the next few weeks to promote patient comfort. Teach the patient to follow the prescribed exercise program, which begins immediately after discharge. Patients should start walking routinely every day. Complications of MIS are rare.

Early postoperative nursing care focuses on preventing and assessing complications that might occur in the first 24 to 48 hours for patients having conventional open surgeries. Major complications for open traditional lumbar spinal surgery include nerve injuries, diskitis (disk inflammation), and dural tears (tears in the dura covering the spinal cord). Table 37.2 highlights major complications of open conventional back surgery, nursing assessment, and interventions to manage each complication.

As for any patient undergoing surgery, take vital signs at least every 4 hours during the first 24 hours to assess for fever, hypotension, or severe pain. Perform a neurologic assessment every 4 hours. Of particular importance are movement, strength, and **sensory perception** in the lower extremities.

Carefully check the patient's ability to void after urinary catheter removal. Acute back **pain** and a flat position in bed make voiding difficult, especially for men. An inability to

TABLE 37.2 **Assessing and Managing the Patient With Major Complications of Open Traditional Lumbar Spinal Surgery**

Complication	Assessment and Interventions
Cerebrospinal fluid (CSF) leakage	Observe for clear fluid on or around the dressing. If leakage occurs, place patient flat. Report CSF leakage immediately to the surgeon. (The patient is usually kept on flat bed rest for several days while the dural tear heals.)
Fluid volume deficit	Monitor intake and output; assess for dehydration, including vital signs and skin turgor. Monitor vital signs carefully for hypotension and tachycardia.
Acute urinary retention	Assist the patient to the bathroom or a bedside commode as soon as possible after surgery or urinary catheter removal. Help male patients stand at the bedside as soon as possible after surgery or urinary catheter removal.
Paralytic ileus	Monitor for flatus or stool. Assess for abdominal distention, nausea, and vomiting.
Fat embolism syndrome (more common in people with traditional open spinal fusion)	Observe for and report chest pain, dyspnea, anxiety, and mental status changes (more common in older adults). Note petechiae around the neck, upper chest, buccal membrane, and conjunctiva. Monitor arterial blood gas values for decreased Pao_2.
Persistent or progressive lumbar radiculopathy (nerve root pain)	Report pain not responsive to analgesics. Document the location and nature of pain. Administer analgesics as prescribed.
Infection (e.g., wound, diskitis, hematoma)	Monitor the patient's temperature carefully (a slight elevation is normal). Increased temperature elevation or a spike after the second postoperative day may indicate infection. Report increased pain or swelling at the wound site or in the legs. Give antibiotics as prescribed if infection is confirmed.

✚ NURSING SAFETY PRIORITY

Critical Rescue

For the patient after back surgery, inspect the surgical dressing for blood or any other type of drainage. Clear drainage may mean cerebrospinal fluid (CSF) leakage. Blood and CSF may be mixed on the dressing, with the CSF being visible as a "halo" around the outer edges of the dressing. The loss of a large amount of CSF may cause the patient to report having a sudden headache. *If a CSF leak is suspected, keep the patient on bed rest and lower the head of the bed immediately to slow the loss of fluid! Report signs of any drainage on the dressing to the surgeon or Rapid Response Team. Bulging at the incision site may be due to a CSF leak or a hematoma, both of which should also be reported immediately.*

◎ CORE MEASURES

Prevention of VTE

Follow best practices to avoid venous thromboembolism (VTE) after surgery with early *mobility,* intermittent sequential compression or pneumatic devices, and an anticoagulant/antiplatelet drug per The Joint Commission's Core Measures.

void may indicate damage to the sacral spinal nerves, which control the detrusor muscle in the bladder. The patient with an open traditional diskectomy, laminectomy, and/or traditional open spinal fusion typically gets out of bed with assistance on the evening of surgery, which may help with voiding.

Correct turning of the patient in bed who is recovering from open traditional lumbar spinal injury is especially important. Do not place an overhead trapeze on the bed to assist the patient with *mobility* skills. This apparatus can cause more back pain and damage the surgical area. Teach the patient to log roll every 2 hours from side to back and vice

versa. In **log rolling,** the patient turns as a unit while the back is kept as straight as possible. A turning sheet may be used for obese patients. Either turning method may require additional assistance, depending on how much the patient can assist. Instruct the patient to keep the back straight when getting out of bed. The patient should sit in a straight-back chair with the feet resting comfortably on the floor. As with all surgical patients, prevent atelectasis and hypostatic pneumonia with deep breathing and incentive spirometry.

When a lumbar spinal fusion is performed in addition to an open laminectomy, more care is taken with positioning. The nurse or assistive personnel (AP) assist with log rolling the patient every 2 hours while in bed. Remind the patient to avoid prolonged sitting or standing. Be sure to check with the surgeon or surgeon's prescription regarding whether to place the orthotic device or brace on the patient before or after getting the patient out of bed.

Care Coordination and Transition Management

The patient with back pain who does not undergo surgery is typically managed at home. If back surgery is performed, the patient is usually discharged to home with support from family or significant others. For older adults without a community support system, a short-term stay in a nursing home or transitional care unit may be needed. Collaborate with the case manager or discharge planner, patient, and family to determine the most appropriate placement.

Patients having any of the *MIS procedures* or a lumbar interbody fusion may resume normal activities within a few days up to 3 weeks after surgery, depending on the specific procedure and the condition of the patient. The patient may take a shower on the third or fourth day after surgery. Teach the patient to leave the wound closure tapes in place for removal by the surgeon or until they fall off. Instruct the patient to contact the primary health care provider immediately if clear drainage seeps from the incision. Clear drainage usually indicates a dural tear and that cerebrospinal fluid is leaking.

After *conventional open lumbar surgery,* the patient may have activity restrictions and recommendations for the first 4 to 6 weeks, such as:

- Limit daily stair climbing.
- Restrict or limit driving.
- Do not lift objects heavier than 5 lb.
- Restrict pushing and pulling activities (e.g., dog walking).
- Avoid bending and twisting at the waist.
- Take a daily walk.

While the bone graft heals for an open spinal fusion, the patient may wear a back orthotic device for 4 to 6 weeks or longer after surgery. Provide information about the importance of wearing the brace as instructed during the healing process, how to take it off and put it on while maintaining spinal alignment, and how to clean it.

The duration of home-based recovery depends on the nature of the patient's job and the extent and type of surgery. Most patients return to work after 2 to 6 weeks; some patients having more complex open spinal procedures may not return for several months if their jobs are physically strenuous.

The primary health care provider may want the patient to continue taking antiinflammatory drugs or, if muscle spasm is present, to take muscle relaxants. Remind the patient and family about the possible side effects of drugs and what to do if they occur.

In a few patients, back surgery is unsuccessful. This situation, referred to as *failed back surgery syndrome (FBSS),* is a complex combination of organic, psychological, and socioeconomic factors. Repeated surgical procedures often discourage these patients, who must continue aggressive pain management after multiple operations. Nerve blocks, implantable spinal cord stimulators (neurostimulators), and other modalities may be needed on a long-term basis to help with persistent *pain.* A newer alternative is lysis of epidural adhesions, if present, through a minimally invasive technique (Geudeke et al., 2021).

NURSING SAFETY PRIORITY

Critical Rescue

For patients who have a spinal cord stimulator implanted in the epidural space, assess neurologic status below the level of insertion frequently. Monitor for early changes in **sensory perception,** movement, and muscle strength. Ensure that the patient can void without difficulty. *If any changes occur, document and report them immediately to the surgeon!*

Spinal cord stimulation is an *invasive* technique that provides persistent pain relief by applying an electrical field over the spinal cord. A trial with a percutaneous spinal cord stimulator is conducted to determine whether permanent placement is appropriate. If the trial is successful, electrodes are surgically placed internally in the epidural space and connected to an external or implanted programmable generator. The patient is taught to program and adjust the device to maximize comfort. Spinal cord stimulation can be extremely effective in select patients, but it is reserved for intractable (unrelenting and continuous) neuropathic pain syndromes that have been unresponsive to other treatments.

CERVICAL NECK PAIN

Cervical neck pain most often results from a bulging or herniation of the nucleus pulposus (HNP) in a cervical intervertebral disk, illustrated in Fig. 37.1. The disk tends to herniate laterally where the annulus fibrosus is weakest and the posterior longitudinal ligament is thinned.

Pathophysiology Review

The result of cervical HNP is spinal nerve root compression with motor and sensory manifestations and moderate to severe *pain,* typically in the neck, upper back (over the shoulder), and down the affected arm. The disk between the fifth and sixth cervical vertebrae (C5-C6) is affected most often.

If the disk does not herniate, nerve compression may be caused by osteophyte (bony spur) formation from osteoarthritis. The osteophytes press on the intervertebral foramen, which results in a narrowing of the disk and pressure on the nerve root. As with sciatic nerve compression, the patient with cervical nerve compression may have either continuous or intermittent chronic pain. When the disk herniates centrally, pressure on the spinal cord occurs and requires prompt surgery to prevent paresis or paralysis.

Cervical *pain*—acute or persistent— can also occur from muscle strain, ligament sprain resulting from aging, poor posture, lifting, tumor, rheumatoid arthritis, osteoarthritis, or infection. The typical history of the patient includes a report of pain and numbness or tingling when moving the neck, which radiates to the shoulder and down the arm. The *pain* may interrupt sleep and may be accompanied by a headache or numbness and tingling in the affected arm. To determine the exact cause, plain x-rays and imaging studies may be used. Electromyography/ nerve conduction studies are used to help differentiate cervical radiculopathy, ulnar or radial neuropathy, carpal tunnel syndrome, or other peripheral nerve problems.

Interprofessional Collaborative Care

Conservative treatment for acute neck *pain* is the same as described for low back pain except prescribed exercises focus on the shoulders and neck. The physical therapist teaches the patient the correct techniques for performing "shoulder shrug," "shoulder squeeze," and "seated rowing." Some primary health care providers prescribe a soft collar to stabilize the neck, especially at night. Using the collar for longer than 10 days can lead to decreased muscle strength and range of motion. For that reason, many providers do not recommend collars for cervical disk problems. Therapeutic manipulation (chiropractic interventions) alone or in combination with other interventions does not appear to cause harm for most patients but does not consistently reduce pain or disability.

If conservative treatment is ineffective, surgery may be required—either *minimally invasive surgery* or *conventional open surgery*. A neurosurgeon usually performs this surgery because of the complexity of the nerves and other structures in that area of the spine. For open procedures and depending on the cause and the location of the disk herniation, either an anterior or a posterior surgical approach is used.

One of the most commonly performed procedures is the anterior or lateral interbody cervical fusion (AICF or LICF). In these procedures, a titanium mesh device is implanted into the space where the cervical disk was removed, and several screws ensure stabilization. For clients who have multiple cervical disk herniations, a traditional anterior cervical diskectomy and fusion (ACDF) with bone grafting may be performed. This surgery is much more complex and causes more postoperative complications than the AICF or LICF. The patient having traditional ACDF usually wears a soft collar for about 2 to 3 weeks after surgery. Other general preoperative

---

➕ NURSING SAFETY PRIORITY

Critical Rescue

The priority for care in the immediate postoperative period after an ACDF is maintaining an airway and ensuring that the patient has no problem with breathing. Swelling from the surgery can narrow the trachea, causing a partial obstruction. Surgery can also interfere with cranial innervation for swallowing, resulting in a compromised airway or aspiration. If these changes occur, open the patient's airway, sit the patient upright, suction if needed, and provide supplemental oxygen. Promptly notify the surgeon or Rapid Response Team using SBAR, and document your assessment and interventions. Box 37.6 summarizes best practices for postoperative care and discharge planning.

BOX 37.6   Best Practice for Patient Safety and Quality Care

Care of the Patient After a Traditional Anterior Cervical Diskectomy and Fusion

Postoperative Interventions

- Assess *a*irway, *b*reathing, and *c*irculation (first priority!).
- Check for bleeding and drainage at the incision site.
- Monitor vital signs and neurologic status frequently.
- Check for swallowing ability.
- Monitor intake and output.
- Assess the patient's ability to void (may be a problem secondary to opiates or anesthesia).
- Manage *pain* adequately.
- Assist the patient with ambulation within a few hours of surgery, if able.

Discharge Teaching

- Be sure that someone stays with the patient for the first few days after surgery.
- Review drug therapy.
- Teach care of the incision.
- Review activity restrictions:
  - No lifting
  - No driving until surgeon permission received
  - No strenuous activities
- Walk every day.
- Call the surgeon if symptoms of pain, numbness, and tingling worsen or if swallowing becomes difficult.
- Wear collar per the primary health care provider's prescription.

---

and postoperative care nursing interventions are the same as described in Chapter 9.

Some patients are candidates for minimally invasive surgery (MIS), such as percutaneous cervical diskectomy (PCD) through an endoscope, with or without laser thermodiskectomy, to shrink the herniated portion of the disk. The care for these patients is very similar to that for the patient with low back pain who has MIS (see the discussion of surgical management of patients with low back pain earlier in this chapter).

Many patients have positive clinical outcomes after interbody fusion (ADIF or LDIF) procedures, reducing the need for more complex fusions with bone grafting (ACDF). The patient has a small incision and is able to return to work in a few weeks. Complications of these procedures are not common.

Patients may also benefit from the placement of an artificial disk, a surgical option that preserves movement of the vertebrae. Artificial disks are approved by the FDA. Although there is evidence of their safety, the long-term effects on patient health are not yet established.

GET READY FOR THE NEXT-GENERATION NCLEX® EXAMINATION!

Essential Nursing Care Points

Health Promotion/Disease Prevention

- Because trauma is the leading cause of SCI, nurses should teach people to avoid taking risks, if possible, and to use adequate protective measures (e.g., padding and helmets) for sports and recreational activities.
- Many of the problems related to low back pain (LBP) can be prevented by recognizing the factors that contribute to injury and taking appropriate preventive measures to prevent *pain.* For example, proper posture, exercise, ergonomic work furniture, and not wearing high-heeled shoes can significantly decrease the incidence of LBP.
- One major goal of *Healthy People 2030* is to increase the health and well-being of people living with disabilities, such as spinal cord injury.

Chronic Disease Care

- **Multiple sclerosis** is a chronic neurologic disease caused by immune, genetic, and/or infectious factors that affect the myelin and nerve fibers of the brain and spinal cord.
- Many of the drugs used to manage multiple sclerosis are immunomodulators that effectively control disease progression; these drugs decrease immune activity, which can place the patient at risk for infection.
- Drug therapy for MS is very expensive and may not be ordered for patients who are underinsured or cannot afford the medication.
- In a few patients with low back pain, back surgery is unsuccessful. This situation, referred to as *failed back surgery syndrome (FBSS)*, is a complex combination of organic, psychological, and socioeconomic factors.
- **Spinal cord stimulation** is an *invasive* technique that provides persistent low back pain relief by applying an electrical field over the spinal cord.
- A full-time caregiver or personal assistant is sometimes required when the patient with tetraplegia returns home from rehabilitation.
- A patient who is paraplegic is usually able to provide self-care without assistance after an appropriate rehabilitation program.
- Some patients with SCI develop complications of impaired *mobility,* including osteoporosis and pressure injuries.

Regenerative or Restorative Care

- *The initial and priority assessment of the patient who has a cervical spinal cord injury (SCI) focuses on the patient's ABCs (**a**irway, **b**reathing, and **c**irculation).*
- The patient with a cervical SCI is at high risk for respiratory compromise because cervical spinal nerves (C3-5) innervate the phrenic nerve controlling the diaphragm.
- **Autonomic dysreflexia (AD),** sometimes referred to as autonomic *hyperreflexia,* is a potentially life-threatening condition in which noxious visceral or cutaneous stimuli cause a sudden, massive, uninhibited reflex sympathetic discharge in people with high-level SCI. The signs and symptoms of AD are listed in Box 37.2.
- If an SCI is caused by vertebral fractures, the vertebral column must be immobilized and stabilized, often using a surgical procedure. For a cervical fracture, an external fixator such as the halo with vest is applied after surgery until the fracture heals.
- *Acute* low back pain is usually self-limiting and lasts less than 12 weeks.
- Minimally invasive surgery, such as a diskectomy, is performed most often for patients who have a herniated nucleus pulposus with central cord compression.
- Open laminectomies with spinal fusions are sometimes needed for patients who have multiple HNP herniations or cord compression; bone grafts are usually from donor bone tissue.

Hospice/Palliative/Supportive Care

- End-of-life or hospice care is not needed for patients who have spinal health conditions unless they have a large inoperable malignant tumor or metastatic disease.
- Clients who have spinal cord injury require aggressive rehabilitation. The primary purpose of rehabilitation for a SCI is to enable patients to function independently in their communities.

Mastery Questions

1. A client with a C6 fracture recently underwent external fixation with a halo device. What statement by the client indicates the need for the nurse to provide **immediate** follow-up?
   A. "This device feels as if it will be too heavy to get up."
   B. "My arms and shoulders feel different than they did earlier."
   C. "I don't know if I want to wear this thing as long as they say I should."
   D. "My feet and toes still feel numb, even after this was put on."

2. The nurse is teaching a client who will be taking an interferon beta-1a drug for multiple sclerosis. Which of the following instructions would the nurse include in the teaching for the client? **Select all that apply.**
   A. "Take your pulse once a day."
   B. "Avoid crowds and people who are sick."
   C. "Notify your provider immediately if you get confused."
   D. "Rotate the injection site daily."
   E. "Take acetaminophen if you get body aches."
   F. "Monitor your weight daily."

3. The nurse is providing education to a community group on preventing back injury. Which of the following recommendations would the nurse provide? **Select all that apply.**
   A. "If you smoke, try to cut down or quit altogether."
   B. "Ask if your workplace has ergonomic evaluations."
   C. "Maintain a healthy weight."
   D. "Use good posture when sitting or standing."
   E. "Turn yourself in bed by log rolling."
   F. "Avoid prolonged sitting or standing."

NGN Challenge 37.1

37.1.1

The nurse is caring for a 21-year-old client who was admitted for a C7 spinal cord injury.

History and Physical	**Nurses' Notes**	Imaging Studies	Laboratory Results

1315: Client admitted to rehabilitation unit this morning with cervical SCI after spinal fusion and halo fixator with vest. Alert and oriented × 4; lung sounds clear; S_1S_2 present; BS present × 4; indwelling urinary catheter draining large amount of yellow clear urine. Vital signs: T 98.2°F (36.8°C); HR 76 beats/min; RR 20 breaths/min; BP 146/82 mm Hg; Spo₂ 97% on RA. Client's goals are to increase mobility skills, control bowel and bladder, participate in self-care, and remain sexually active.
1435: Reports new-onset throbbing frontal headache with blurred vision and feeling very sleepy. Skin on face and neck flushed with profuse sweating. Vital signs: T 99°F (37.2°C); HR 58 beats/min; RR 22 breaths/min; BP 184/95 mm Hg; Spo₂ 95% on RA.

Select the 5 client findings that would require **immediate** follow-up.
- ○ Placement of a halo fixator with vest
- ○ New-onset throbbing frontal headache
- ○ Flushed skin on face and neck
- ○ Profuse sweating
- ○ Temperature of 99°F (37.2°C)
- ○ HR 58 beats/min
- ○ RR 22 breaths/min
- ○ BP 184/95 mm Hg
- ○ Spo₂ 95% on RA

37.1.2

The nurse is caring for a 21-year-old client who was admitted for a C7 spinal cord injury.

History and Physical	**Nurses' Notes**	Imaging Studies	Laboratory Results

1315: Client admitted to rehabilitation unit this morning with cervical SCI after spinal fusion and halo fixator with vest. Alert and oriented × 4; lung sounds clear; S_1S_2 present; BS present × 4; indwelling urinary catheter draining large amount of yellow clear urine. Vital signs: T 98.2°F (36.8°C); HR 76 beats/min; RR 20 breaths/min; BP 146/82 mm Hg; Spo₂ 97% on RA. Client's goals are to increase mobility skills, control bowel and bladder, participate in self-care, and remain sexually active.
1435: Reports new-onset throbbing frontal headache with blurred vision and feeling very sleepy. Skin on face and neck flushed with profuse sweating. Vital signs: T 99°F (37.2°C); HR 58 beats/min; RR 22 breaths/min; BP 184/95 mm Hg; Spo₂ 95% on RA

For each client finding listed below, determine if the finding is consistent with the health conditions of spinal shock, neurogenic shock, or autonomic dysreflexia. Each finding may support more than 1 condition.

Client Findings	Spinal Shock	Neurogenic Shock	Autonomic Dysreflexia
Profuse sweating			
Flushed skin			
Drowsiness			
Elevated blood pressure			
Bradycardia			
Frontal headache			
Blurred vision			

37.1.3

The nurse is caring for a 21-year-old client who was admitted for a C7 spinal cord injury.

History and Physical	**Nurses' Notes**	Imaging Studies	Laboratory Results

1315: Client admitted to rehabilitation unit this morning with cervical SCI after spinal fusion and halo fixator with vest. Alert and oriented × 4; lung sounds clear; S_1S_2 present; BS present × 4; indwelling urinary catheter draining large amount of yellow clear urine. Vital signs: T 98.2°F (36.8°C); HR 76 beats/min; RR 20 breaths/min; BP 146/82 mm Hg; Spo₂ 97% on RA. Client's goals are to increase mobility skills, control bowel and bladder, participate in self-care, and remain sexually active.
1435: Reports new-onset throbbing frontal headache with blurred vision and feeling very sleepy. Skin on face and neck flushed with profuse sweating. Vital signs: T 99°F (37.2°C); HR 58 beats/min; RR 22 breaths/min; BP 184/95 mm Hg; Spo₂ 95% on RA.

Complete the following sentence by selecting from the list of word choices below.

The *priority* at this time is to manage the client's **[Word Choice]** to prevent **[Word Choice]**.

Word Choices
Tachypnea
Elevated blood pressure
Fever
Stroke
Infection

37.1.4

The nurse is caring for a 21-year-old client with a C7 spinal cord injury.

History and Physical	**Nurses' Notes**	Imaging Studies	Laboratory Results

1315: Client admitted to rehabilitation unit this morning with cervical SCI after spinal fusion and halo fixator with vest. Alert and oriented × 4; lung sounds clear; S_1S_2 present; BS present × 4; indwelling urinary catheter draining large amount of yellow clear urine. Vital signs: T 98.2°F (36.8°C); HR 76 beats/min; RR 20 breaths/min; BP 146/82 mm Hg; Spo$_2$ 97% on RA. Client's goals are to increase mobility skills, control bowel and bladder, participate in self-care, and remain sexually active.

1435: Reports new-onset frontal headache with blurred vision and feeling very sleepy. Skin on face and neck flushed with profuse sweating. Vital signs: T 99°F (37.2°C); HR 58 beats/min; RR 22 breaths/min; BP 184/95 mm Hg; Spo$_2$ 95% on RA.

1450: Checked urinary catheter—no kinks and draining large amount of yellow clear urine. Notified primary health care provider. Vital signs: T 98.8°F (37.7°C); HR 56 beats/min; RR 20 breaths/min; BP 192/98 mm Hg; Spo$_2$ 95% on RA. Headache pain 8/10 and "feeling worse."

The nurse begins to plan care for the client. Determine whether the following potential nursing actions are indicated or not indicated for the client at this time.

Potential Nursing Actions	Indicated	Not Indicated
Assess skin for new or worsening pressure injury		
Monitor blood pressure every hour		
Administer supplemental oxygen		
Check for fecal impaction		
Place the client in a flat supine position		
Remove the client's urinary catheter		

37.1.5

The nurse is caring for a 21-year-old client with a C7 spinal cord injury.

History and Physical	**Nurses' Notes**	Imaging Studies	Laboratory Results

1315: Client admitted to rehabilitation unit this morning with cervical SCI after spinal fusion and halo fixator with vest. Alert and oriented × 4; lung sounds clear; S_1S_2 present; BS present × 4; indwelling urinary catheter draining large amount of yellow clear urine. Vital signs: T 98.2°F (36.8°C); HR 76 beats/min; RR 20 breaths/min; BP 146/82 mm Hg; Spo$_2$ 97% on RA. Client's goals are to increase mobility skills, control bowel and bladder, participate in self-care, and remain sexually active.

1435: Reports new-onset frontal headache with blurred vision and feeling very sleepy. Skin on face and neck flushed with profuse sweating. Vital signs: T 99°F (37.2°C); HR 58 beats/min; RR 22 breaths/min; BP 184/95 mm Hg; Spo$_2$ 95% on RA.

1450: Checked urinary catheter—no kinks and draining large amount of yellow clear urine. Notified physician. Vital signs: T 98.8°F (37.7°C); HR 56 beats/min; RR 20 breaths/min; BP 192/98 mm Hg; Spo$_2$ 95% on RA. Headache pain 8/10 and "feeling worse."

1515: BP 188/92 mm Hg; headache starting to throb and reports pain of 9/10. Physician in to evaluate client.

The nurse plans interventions to manage the client's condition. Which of the following nursing actions would the nurse plan to implement? **Select all that apply.**

○ Place the client in a sitting position.
○ Administer nifedipine per protocol.
○ Monitor the client's headache pain intensity.
○ Observe client for any neurologic changes.
○ Monitor the client's blood pressure every 10 to 15 minutes.

37.1.6

The nurse is caring for a 21-year-old client with a C7 spinal cord injury.

History and Physical	**Nurses' Notes**	Imaging Studies	Laboratory Results

1315: Client admitted to rehabilitation unit this morning with cervical SCI after spinal fusion and halo fixator with vest. Alert and oriented × 4; lung sounds clear; S_1S_2 present; BS present × 4; indwelling urinary catheter draining large amount of yellow clear urine. Vital signs: T 98.2°F (36.8°C); HR 76 beats/min; RR 20 breaths/min; BP 146/82 mm Hg; Spo$_2$ 97% on RA. Client's goals are to increase mobility skills, control bowel and bladder, participate in self-care, and remain sexually active.

1435: Reports new-onset frontal headache with blurred vision and feeling very sleepy. Skin on face and neck flushed with profuse sweating. Vital signs: T 99°F (37.2°C); HR 58 beats/min; RR 22 breaths/min; BP 184/95 mm Hg; Spo$_2$ 95% on RA.

1450: Checked urinary catheter—no kinks and draining large amount of yellow clear urine. Notified physician. Vital signs: T 98.8°F (37.7°C); HR 56 beats/min; RR 20 breaths/min; BP 192/98 mm Hg; Spo$_2$ 95% on RA. Headache pain 8/10 and "feeling worse."

1515: BP 188/92 mm Hg; headache starting to throb and reports pain of 9/10. Physician in to evaluate client.

1550: Client reports headache pain of 5/10 after fecal disimpaction and nifedipine. Vital signs: T 98°F (36.7°C); HR 68 beats/min; RR 18 breaths/min; BP 132/82 mm Hg; Spo$_2$ 97% on RA. Skin remains slightly flushed.

Based on the Nurses' Note entry at 1550, complete the following sentence by selecting from the lists of options below.

The most recent assessment findings indicate that the client's condition has **1[Select]** as evidenced by **2[Select]** and **3[Select]**.

Options for 1	Options for 2	Options for 3
Worsened	Continued headache pain	Less headache pain
Improved	Decreased temperature	Increased oxygen saturation
Not changed	Decreased blood pressure	Continued skin flushing

REFERENCES

Abu-Baker, N. N., Al-Zyoud, N. H., & Alshraifeen, A. (2021). Quality of life and self-care ability among individuals with spinal cord injury. *Clinical Nursing Research, 30*(6), 883–891.

American Nurses Association (ANA). (2022). *Safe patient handling and mobility* (2nd Ed.). Washington, DC: Author.

Amezcua, L., Rivira, V. M., Vasquez, T. C., Baezconde-Garbanati, L., & Langer-Gould, A. (2021). Health disparities, inequities, and social determinants of health in multiple sclerosis and related disorders in the United States. *JAMA Neurology, 78*(12), 1515–1524.

Bebo, B., Cintina, I., LaRocca, N., Ritter, L., Talente, B., Hartung, D., et al (2022, April 13). Economic burden of Multiple sclerosis in the United States: Estimate of direct and indirect costs. *Neurology.* https://doi.org/10.1212/WNL.0000000000200150.

Burchum, J. L. R., & Rosenthal, L. D. (2022). *Lehne's pharmacology for nursing care* (11th ed.). St. Louis: Elsevier.

Chis, L. C., Copotoio, M., & Moldovan, L. (2020). Different Types of Exoskeletons can Improve the Life of Spinal Cord Injury's Patients – a Meta-Analysis. *Procedia Manufacturing, 46,* 844–849. https://www.sciencedirect.com/science/article/pii/S2351978920310015.

Clark, C. S. (2021). *Cannabis: A handbook for nurses.* Philadelphia, PA: Wolters Kluwer.

Cona, L. S. (2021). *Stem cell therapy: A new multiple sclerosis breakthrough in 2022? DVCSTEM (blog).* https://www.dvcstem.com/post/stem-cell-therapy-for-ms.

Conti, Y., Jean-Jacques, V., Levy, S., Meltz, Y. L., Hamdan, S., & Elkana, O. (2020). Pain catastrophizing mediates the association between mindfulness and psychological distress in chronic pain syndrome. *Pain Practice, 20*(7), 714–723.

Drillinger, M. (2021). FAD has approved a new MS medication: What to know. *Healthline.* https://www.healthline.com/health-news/fda-has-approved-a-new-ms-medication-what-to-know.

Elliott, B., Chargualaf, K. A., & Patterson, B. (2021). *Veteran-centered care in education and practice.* New York, NY: Springer Publishing.

Geudeke, M. W., Krediet, A. C., Bilecen, S., Huygen, F., J. P. M., & Rijsdijk, M. (2021). Effectiveness of epiduroscopy for patients with failed back surgery syndrome: A systematic review and metanalysis. *Pain Practice, 21*(4), 468–481.

Harmison, L. E., Beckham, J. W., & Adelman, D. S. (2023). Autonomic dysreflexia in patients with spinal cord injury. *Nursing 2023, 53*(1), 21–27.

*Interprofessional Education Collaborative Expert Panel. (2016). *Core competencies for interprofessional collaborative practice: Report of an expert panel* (2nd ed.). Washington, D.C: Interprofessional Education Collaborative.

Kesänen, J., Leino-Kilpi, H., Lund, T., Montin, L., Puukka, P., & Valkeapää, K. (2019). Spinal stenosis patients' visual and verbal description of the comprehension of their surgery. *Orthopaedic Nursing, 38*(4), 253–261.

Langer-Gould, A. M., Gonzales, E. G., Smith, J. B., Li, B. H., & Nelson, L. M. (2022). Racial and ethnic disparities in Multiple Sclerosis prevalence. *Neurology.* https://doi.org/10.1212/WNL.0000000000200151.

Mann, S. J., Lam, J. C., & Singh, P. (2021). *McKenzie Back Exercises.* StatPearls [Internet]. StatPearls Publishing. https://www.ncbi.nlm.nih.gov/books/NBK539720/.

MS Society of Canada. (2020). *What is multiple sclerosis?.* https://mssociety.ca/about-ms-what-is-ms.

National Institute of Neurologic Disorders and Stroke. (2021). *Low back pain fact sheet.* National Institutes of Health. https://www.ninds.nih.gov/Disorders/Patient-Caregiver-Education/Fact-Sheets/Low-Back-Pain-Fact-Sheet.

National Multiple Sclerosis Society. (2020). *Who gets MS.* www.nationalmssociety.org/about-multiple-sclerosis/what-we-know-about-ms/index.aspx.

North American Spine Society (NASS). (2020). *Evidence based clinical guidelines for multidisciplinary spine care: Diagnosis and treatment of low back pain.* Author. https://www.spine.org/Portals/0/assets/downloads/ResearchClinicalCare/Guidelines/LowBackPain.pdf.

Pagana, K. D., Pagana, T. J., & Pagana, T. N. (2022). *Mosby's manual of diagnostic and laboratory tests* (7th ed.). St. Louis: Elsevier.

Pfieffer, M. L. (2020). How to care for adults with low back pain in the primary care setting. *Nursing 2020, 50*(2), 48–53.

Rogers, J. L. (2023). *McCance and Huether's Pathophysiology: The biologic basis for disease in adults and children* (9th ed.). St. Louis: Elsevier.

Sauder, T., Hansen, S., Bauswein, C., Müller, R., Jaruszowic, S., Keune, J. et al., (2021). Mindfulness training during brief periods of hospitalization in multiple sclerosis (MS): Beneficial alterations in fatigue and the mediating role of depression. *BMC Neurology, 390*(21), 1–15.

Schimke, L., & Connolly, K. M. (2020). First report: U.S. patient and clinician experiences with the inFlow™ Urinary Prosthesis for permanent urinary retention in women. *UROLOGIC NURSING, 40*(2), 61–84.

Slusser, M. M., Garcia, L. I., Reed, C.-R., & McGinnis, P. Q. (2019). *Foundations of interprofessional collaborative practice in health care.* St. Louis: Elsevier.

Smeltzer, S. C. (2021). *Delivering quality healthcare for people with disability.* Indianapolis, IN: Sigma Theta Tau International Honor Society of Nursing.

Staub, B. N., & Sadrameli, S. S. (2019). The use of robotics in minimally invasive spinal surgery. *Journal of Spine Surgery, 5*(Suppl. 1), S31–S40.

Touhy, T. A., & Jett, K. (2022). *Ebersole and Hess' Gerontological nursing and health aging* (6th Ed.). St. Louis: Elsevier.

38

Critical Care of Patients With Neurologic Emergencies

Donna Mower-Wade

http://evolve.elsevier.com/Iggy/

LEARNING OUTCOMES

1. Plan collaborative care with the interprofessional team to promote *mobility, sensory perception, perfusion*, and *cognition* in patients with neurologic emergencies.
2. Teach adults how to decrease the risk for traumatic brain injury and stroke.
3. Teach the patient and caregiver(s) about common drugs and other management strategies used for brain tumors affecting *mobility* and *cognition.*
4. Plan patient- and family-centered nursing interventions to decrease the psychosocial impact caused by living with traumatic brain injury and stroke.
5. Apply knowledge of anatomy, physiology, and pathophysiology to provide evidence-based care for patients with neurologic emergencies.
6. Analyze assessment and diagnostic findings to generate solutions and prioritize nursing care for patients who have neurologic emergencies.
7. Organize care coordination and transition management for patients living with neurologic emergencies.
8. Use clinical judgment to plan evidence-based nursing care to promote *perfusion* and decrease complications in patients with neurologic emergencies.
9. Incorporate factors that affect health equity into the plan of care for patients with stroke.

KEY TERMS

acalculia The inability to perform math calculations.

acute ischemic stroke (AIS) A stroke caused by the occlusion (blockage) of a cerebral or carotid artery by either a thrombus or an embolus.

agnosia The inability to use an object correctly.

agraphia The inability to write.

alexia The inability to read.

amnesia Loss of memory.

aphasia Problems with speech (expressive aphasia) and/or language (receptive aphasia).

apraxia Inability to perform previously learned motor skills or commands; may be verbal or motor.

arteriovenous malformation (AVM) An angled collection of malformed, thin-walled, dilated vessels without a capillary network.

ataxia Lack of muscle control and coordination that affects gait, balance, and the ability to walk.

atherosclerotic plaque A buildup of fat and other substances that adhere to the arterial wall and obstruct or restrict blood flow.

bruit A sound heard over an artery through a stethoscope that indicates turbulent blood flow, usually due to a narrowed or partially obstructed blood vessel.

carotid stenosis The hardening and narrowing of the artery, which decreases blood flow to the brain.

chronic traumatic encephalopathy (CTE) An uncommon degenerative brain disease that occurs most often in military veterans, athletes, and others who have experienced repetitive trauma to the brain.

concussion A traumatic injury to the brain caused by a blow to the head or from vigorous shaking of the head; may or may not result in some period of unconsciousness.

craniotomy Surgical incision to open the cranium and allow access to the brain.

Cushing triad A classic but late sign of increased intracranial pressure that manifests with severe hypertension, a widened pulse pressure (increasing difference between systolic and diastolic values), and bradycardia.

diplopia A condition in which the client has double vision.

dysarthria Slurred speech caused by muscle weakness or paralysis.

dysphagia Difficulty swallowing.

embolectomy Surgical blood clot (thrombosis) removal.

embolic stroke A stroke caused by an embolus (dislodged clot).

emotional lability An uncontrollable emotional state that can occur in patients who have had a stroke or other brain injury.

epidural hematoma An accumulation of blood (clot) that results from arterial bleeding into the space between the dura and the inner skull.

KEY TERMS—cont'd

expressive (Broca or motor) aphasia Aphasia that is the result of damage in the Broca area of the frontal lobe. It is a motor speech problem in which the patient generally understands what is said but cannot speak.

hemianopsia A condition in which the vision of one or both eyes is affected.

hemiparesis One-sided weakness of the body affecting the arm and/or leg.

hemiplegia One-sided paralysis of the body affecting the arm and/or leg.

homonymous hemianopsia Blindness in the same side of both eyes.

hydrocephalus A condition in which there is increased cerebrospinal fluid in the brain.

hyperbaric oxygen therapy (HBOT) An intervention that is used to provide high-dose oxygen to treat ischemia and hypoxia.

impaired airway defense An inability to clear one's airway.

infratentorial tumor A tumor that is located beneath the tentorium (the area of the brainstem structures and cerebellum).

intracerebral hemorrhage (ICH) The accumulation of blood within the brain tissue caused by the tearing of small arteries and veins in the subcortical white matter.

nystagmus Involuntary movements of the eyes that can be vertical or horizontal.

organ procurement The process of donating an organ from a person who is designated as an organ donor and has been declared brain dead.

papilledema Edema and hyperemia (increased blood flow) of the optic disc; a sign of increasing intracranial pressure.

photophobia Sensitivity to light.

postconcussion syndrome The most common secondary injury resulting from mild traumatic brain injury (TBI) in which the patient reports that headaches, impaired cognition, and dizziness continue to occur for weeks to months after the initial brain injury.

proprioception Body position sense.

ptosis Eyelid drooping.

receptive (Wernicke or sensory) aphasia Aphasia that is caused by injury involving the Wernicke area in the temporoparietal area. The patient cannot understand the spoken or written word. Although perhaps able to talk, the language is often meaningless.

second-impact syndrome Occurs when a second TBI occurs before the first concussion has resolved; the brain rapidly swells shortly after insult.

spine precautions Interventions that protect the spinal cord from a new or secondary injury through special positioning of the patient.

stroke A neurologic health problem caused by an interruption of perfusion to any part of the brain that results in infarction (cell death).

stroke center An agency that is designated by The Joint Commission (TJC) or other body for its ability to rapidly recognize and effectively treat strokes.

subdural hematoma (SDH) An accumulation of blood (clot) that results from venous bleeding into the space beneath the dura and above the arachnoid.

supratentorial tumor A tumor that is within the cerebral hemispheres above the tentorium (dural fold).

thrombotic stroke A stroke that is caused by a thrombus (clot).

transient ischemic attack (TIA) A temporary neurologic dysfunction resulting from a brief interruption in cerebral blood flow.

trauma-informed care An approach to health care involving understanding, acceptance, and support for victims of trauma through positive adaptation and healing.

traumatic brain injury (TBI) Damage to the brain from an external mechanical force and not caused by neurodegenerative or congenital conditions.

unilateral neglect (or inattention) A patient's inability to recognize own physical impairment, especially on one side of the body.

vertigo A feeling of spinning or dizziness.

✳ PRIORITY AND INTERRELATED CONCEPTS

The priority concepts for this chapter are:
- *Perfusion*
- *Cognition*

The *Perfusion* concept exemplar for this chapter is Stroke.
The *Cognition* concept exemplar for this chapter is Traumatic Brain Injury.

The interrelated concepts for this chapter are:
- *Mobility*
- *Sensory Perception*

Acute neurologic emergencies are often associated with high mortality and severe morbidity and can create a significant and enduring impact on patients, their families, and society. Early recognition and comprehensive care of adult patients with acute neurologic compromise by the nurse and interprofessional health care team can reduce mortality. However, many patients who survive neurologic emergencies experience physical disability and possibly mental health disability for the rest of their lives.

Be aware that individuals with disability find hospitalization for any reason very frightening because they anticipate poor quality care, negative attitudes by nursing staff, and negative clinical outcomes. Box 38.1 lists essential interventions

BOX 38.1 Best Practice for Patient Safety and Quality Care

Patient-Centered Care for Hospitalized Patients With Physical Disability

- Ask patients what their goals are for care, and assist them in meeting those goals.
- Assess patient preferences, values, and beliefs, and incorporate them into care.
- Recognize that patients are experts in their disability.
- Communicate effectively with the patient and family, keeping them informed at all times.
- Maintain mobility, if possible, by providing assistance while ensuring patient safety.
- Ensure that patients have access to devices and aids to assist with mobility and ADL performance.
- Collaborate with physical and occupational therapy as needed to ensure that the patient's disability needs are met.

BOX 38.2 Key Features

Transient Ischemic Attack

Visual Symptoms
- Blurred vision
- Diplopia (a condition in which the client has double vision)
- Hemianopsia (a condition in which the vision of one or both eyes is affected)
- Tunnel vision

Mobility (Motor) Symptoms
- Weakness (facial droop, arm or leg drift, hand grasp)
- **Ataxia** (lack of muscle control and coordination that affects gait, balance, and the ability to walk)

Sensory Perception Symptoms
- Numbness (face, hand, arm, or leg)
- **Vertigo** (a feeling of spinning or dizziness)

Speech Symptoms
- **Aphasia** (problems with speech and/or language)
- **Dysarthria** (slurred speech caused by muscle weakness or paralysis)

that nurses and other health staff need to implement to provide patient-centered care for patients with physical disability (Smeltzer, 2021).

Acute neurologic problems from stroke, brain trauma, and malignancy cause varying degrees of impaired *perfusion, cognition, mobility,* and *sensory perception.* Chapter 3 reviews each of these health concepts for nursing practice.

TRANSIENT ISCHEMIC ATTACK

Pathophysiology Review

Acute ischemic strokes often follow warning signs such as a transient ischemic attack (TIA). A TIA is a temporary neurologic dysfunction resulting from a *brief* interruption in cerebral blood flow. The symptoms of TIA are easy to ignore or miss, particularly if symptoms resolve by the time the patient reaches the emergency department (ED). Typically, symptoms of a TIA resolve within 30 to 60 minutes but may last as long as 24 hours (Box 38.2).

Interprofessional Collaborative Care

On admission to the ED, a complete neurologic assessment is performed. The interprofessional health care team administers the National Institutes of Health Stroke Scale (NIHSS; see later discussion under Stroke) and other agency-specific assessment tools. Routine laboratory tests, including coagulation tests (prothrombin time [PT], international normalized ratio [INR], activated partial thromboplastin time [aPTT]) and lipids, ECG, and imaging scans are performed. The initial scan is typically a head CT, followed by MRI brain scan without contrast. Depending on agency protocol and the patient's assessment, computed tomography angiography (CTA) or magnetic resonance angiography (MRA) of the brain and neck is also performed to determine the patency of the carotid arteries, which provide *perfusion* to the brain, and arterial circulation within the brain.

Common causes of a TIA or stroke are carotid stenosis (hardening and narrowing of the artery, which decreases blood flow to the brain), often with atherosclerotic plaque buildup,

and atrial fibrillation. Atherosclerotic plaque consists of fat and other substances that adhere to the arterial wall and obstruct or restrict blood flow (Rogers, 2023).

In addition to the NIH score, patients are often evaluated using the ABCD2 assessment tool to determine their risk of having a stroke in the days and weeks after the TIA. The following factors are scored:

- **A**ge greater than or equal to 60 (stroke risk increases with age)
- **B**lood pressure (BP) greater than or equal to 140/90 mm Hg (either systolic or diastolic or both)
- **C**linical TIA features (unilateral [one-sided] weakness increases stroke risk)
- **D**uration of symptoms (the longer the TIA symptoms last, the greater the risk of stroke) and history of **D**iabetes.

Patients diagnosed with TIA may or may not be admitted to the acute care hospital, depending on their neurologic and cardiovascular status. For example, a patient who has a new onset of atrial fibrillation with the TIA or a TIA and carotid artery stenosis of greater than 70% will most likely be admitted, depending on agency protocol. Some agencies have a dedicated TIA unit. Management of the patient who had a TIA includes treating the cause, if determined. Depending on the patient, collaborative interventions may include:

- Performing traditional or minimally invasive surgery to remove atherosclerotic plaque buildup within the carotid artery and increase *perfusion* to the brain
- Performing a carotid angioplasty with stenting to increase *perfusion* to the brain (see discussion of arterial stenting under Endovascular Interventions discussion for stroke later in this chapter)
- Prescribing antiplatelet drugs, typically aspirin or clopidogrel, to prevent thrombotic or embolic strokes (may be placed on a combination of both drugs)
- Reducing high blood pressure (the most common risk factor for stroke) by adding or adjusting drugs to lower blood pressure

- Controlling diabetes (if present) and keeping glucose levels within a target range, typically 100 to 180 mg/dL
- Promoting lifestyle changes, such as smoking cessation, eating more heart-healthy foods, and increasing *mobility* and physical activity

In collaboration with the interprofessional health team, teach patients about how to achieve a healthier lifestyle to prevent more TIAs or a major stroke. Provide them with information about community resources that can help them meet this desired outcome.

 PERFUSION CONCEPT EXEMPLAR: STROKE

A stroke is caused by an interruption of *perfusion* to any part of the brain that results in infarction (cell death). Stroke is a leading cause of death, disability, dementia, and depression in the United States and throughout the world. While many improvements have been made in acute stroke care, the management of patients in stroke care transitions is lagging behind (Camicia et al., 2021).

Pathophysiology Review

The National Stroke Association uses the term "brain attack" to convey the urgency for acute stroke care similar to the urgency provided for acute myocardial infarction (MI; heart attack). *A stroke is a medical emergency and should be treated immediately to reduce or prevent permanent disability.*

The brain cannot store oxygen or glucose and therefore must receive a constant flow of blood to provide these substances for normal function. In addition, blood flow is important for the removal of metabolic waste (e.g., carbon dioxide, lactic acid). If *perfusion* to any part of the brain is interrupted for more than a few minutes, infarction occurs. Brain metabolism and blood flow after a stroke can be affected around the infarction and in the contralateral (opposite side) hemisphere. Effects of a stroke on the *nonaffected* side may be the result of brain edema or global changes in brain *perfusion.* As a result of brain edema, patients may develop increased intracranial pressure (ICP) and secondary brain injury. These secondary changes most commonly occur following a severe traumatic brain injury (TBI) and are discussed in that section of this chapter in detail.

Types of Strokes

Strokes are generally classified as ischemic (occlusive) or hemorrhagic (Fig. 38.1). Acute ischemic strokes are either thrombotic or embolic in origin (Table 38.1). Most strokes are ischemic.

Acute Ischemic Stroke. An acute ischemic stroke (AIS) is caused by the occlusion (blockage) of a cerebral or carotid artery by either a thrombus or an embolus. A stroke that is caused by a *thrombus* (clot) is referred to as a thrombotic stroke, whereas a stroke caused by an *embolus* (dislodged clot) is referred to as an embolic stroke.

Thrombotic strokes account for more than half of all strokes and are commonly associated with the development of atherosclerosis in either intracranial or extracranial arteries (usually

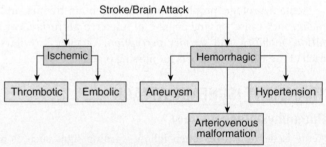

FIG. 38.1 Types of stroke or brain attack.

TABLE 38.1	**Differential Features of the Types of Stroke**		
ISCHEMIC STROKE			
Stroke Feature	**Thrombotic**	**Embolic**	**Hemorrhagic Stroke**
Evolution	Intermittent or stepwise improvement between episodes of worsening symptoms Completed stroke	Abrupt development of completed stroke Steady progression	Usually abrupt onset
Onset	Gradual (minutes to hours)	Sudden	Sudden; may be gradual if caused by hypertension
Level of consciousness	Preserved (patient is awake)	Preserved (patient is awake)	Deepening lethargy/stupor or coma
Contributing associated factors	Hypertension Atherosclerosis	Cardiac disease	Hypertension Vessel disorders Genetic factors
Prodromal symptoms	Transient ischemic attack (TIA)	TIA	Headache
Neurologic deficits	May be deficits during the first few weeks Slight headache Speech deficits Visual problems Confusion	Maximum deficit at onset Paralysis Expressive aphasia	Focal deficits Severe, frequent
Cerebrospinal fluid	Normal; possible presence of protein	Normal	Bloody
Seizures	No	No	Usually
Duration	Improvements over weeks to months Permanent deficits possible	Usually rapid improvements	Variable Permanent neurologic deficits possible

the carotid arteries). Atherosclerosis is the process by which fatty plaques develop on the inner wall of the affected arterial vessel. Chapter 30 describes this health problem in detail.

Rupture of one or more atherosclerotic plaques can promote clot formation. When the clot is of sufficient size, it interrupts blood flow to the brain tissue supplied by the vessel, causing an ischemic (occlusive) stroke. The bifurcation (point of division) of the common carotid artery with the internal carotid artery and the vertebral arteries at their junction with the basilar artery are the most common sites involved in atherosclerotic plaque formation because of turbulent blood flow. Because of the gradual nature of clot formation when atherosclerotic plaque is present, thrombotic strokes tend to have a slow onset, evolving over minutes to hours (Rogers, 2023).

An embolic stroke is caused by a thrombus or a group of thrombi that breaks off from one area of the body and travels to the cerebral arteries via the carotid artery or vertebrobasilar system. The usual source of emboli is the heart. Emboli can occur in patients with atrial fibrillation, heart valve disease, mural thrombi after a myocardial infarction (MI), a prosthetic heart valve, or endocarditis (infection within the wall of the heart). Another source of emboli may be an atherosclerotic clot that breaks off from the carotid sinus or internal carotid artery. Emboli tend to become lodged in the smaller cerebral blood vessels at their point of bifurcation or where the lumen narrows.

As the emboli block the vessel, ischemia develops, and the patient experiences the signs and symptoms of the stroke. The occlusion (blockage) may be temporary if the embolus breaks into smaller fragments, enters smaller blood vessels, and is absorbed. For these reasons, embolic strokes are characterized by the sudden development and rapid occurrence of neurologic deficits. The symptoms may resolve over a few days. Conversion of an occlusive stroke to a hemorrhagic stroke may occur because the arterial vessel wall is also vulnerable to ischemic damage from blood supply interruption. Sudden hemodynamic stress may result in vessel rupture, causing bleeding directly within the brain tissue (Rogers, 2023).

Hemorrhagic Stroke. The second major classification of stroke is hemorrhagic stroke. In this type of stroke, vessel integrity is interrupted, and bleeding occurs into the brain tissue or into the subarachnoid space.

Intracerebral hemorrhage (ICH) describes bleeding into the brain tissue generally resulting from severe or sustained hypertension. Elevated blood pressure (BP) leads to changes within the arterial wall that leave it likely to rupture. Damage to the brain occurs from bleeding, causing edema, inflammation, and displacement, which cause pressure on brain tissue. Cocaine use is one example of a trigger for sudden, dramatic BP elevation, leading to hemorrhagic stroke.

Subarachnoid hemorrhage (SAH) is much more common and results from bleeding into the subarachnoid space—the space between the pia mater and arachnoid layers of the meninges covering the brain. This type of bleeding is usually caused by a ruptured aneurysm or arteriovenous malformation (AVM) (Rogers, 2023).

An aneurysm is an abnormal ballooning or blister along a normal artery, commonly developing in a weak spot on the artery wall. Larger aneurysms are more likely to rupture than smaller

ones (see Chapter 30). An arteriovenous malformation (AVM) is an angled collection of malformed, thin-walled, dilated vessels without a capillary network. This uncommon abnormality occurs during embryonic development. Vasospasm may occur as a result of a sudden and periodic constriction of a cerebral artery, often following an SAH or bleeding from an aneurysm or AVM rupture. This constriction interrupts blood flow to distal areas of the brain. Reduced *perfusion* from vasospasm contributes to secondary cerebral ischemia and further neurologic dysfunction.

Etiology and Genetic Risk

As with many health problems, the causes of stroke are likely a combination of genetic and environmental risk factors. The leading causes of stroke include smoking, obesity, hypertension, diabetes mellitus, and elevated cholesterol. One in three U.S. adults has at least one of these conditions or lifestyle habits (Centers for Disease Control and Prevention [CDC], 2021a). Many of these risk factors have a familial or genetic predisposition and are discussed elsewhere in this text.

For example, first-degree relative (mother, father, sister, brother) stroke risk increases with a strong family history of hypertension, atherosclerotic disease, and a diagnosis of aneurysm (Rogers, 2023). Relatives of a patient with an aneurysm, regardless of vessel location, may be at higher risk for intracranial aneurysms and should consider diagnostic testing and follow-up. Other risk factors for stroke include substance use disorder (especially cocaine and heavy alcohol consumption) and the use of oral contraceptives by women who are at risk for cardiovascular adverse effects.

Incidence and Prevalence

Stroke is the fifth leading cause of death and the leading cause of long-term disability in the United States. According to the U.S. Centers for Disease Control and Prevention (CDC), more than 795,000 people experience a stroke each year with 610,000 being a new stroke. Almost 150,000 Americans die each year from stroke (CDC, 2021a). Women have a higher incidence of strokes than men, most likely because they tend to live longer.

Eight southeastern states in the United States are known as the "stroke belt" because they have a mortality rate that is 20% to 50% higher than the rest of the nation (Washington et al., 2021). Possible factors influencing these differences include income, education, dietary habits, and access to health care.

It is estimated that there are more than 7 million stroke survivors in the United States (Stroke Awareness Foundation, 2021). Deaths from stroke have declined over the past few decades as a result of advances in prompt and effective acute medical management. However, the number of strokes occurring in the younger-adult and middle-age population is increasing (CDC, 2021a). In this group, strokes are associated with illicit drug use because many "street" drugs cause hypercoagulability, vasospasm, or hypertensive crisis (Rogers, 2023).

Health Promotion/Disease Prevention

Most strokes are preventable. The *Healthy People 2030* initiative addresses the need to improve cardiovascular outcomes (Office of Disease Prevention and Health Promotion, n.d.).

Improving Stroke Outcomes

A major goal of the *Healthy People 2030* initiative is to improve cardiovascular health and reduce deaths from heart disease and stroke. Specific objectives to help meet this goal include:
- Increase the proportion of adult stroke survivors who participate in rehabilitation services
- Reduce stroke death

Another objective addresses the need to increase blood pressure and cholesterol control to help reduce the incidence of stroke and therefore reduce stroke death. Nurses have a vital role in helping to meet these objectives through patient and family education and coordinating transitions in care.

The CDC and other cardiovascular professional organizations recommend applying the ABCS of heart health *under medical supervision* to prevent strokes:
- **A**spirin use when appropriate
- **B**lood pressure control
- **C**holesterol management
- **S**moking cessation

Lifestyle changes include smoking cessation, if needed; a heart-healthy diet rich in fruits and vegetables and low in saturated fats (including red meats); and regular physical activity, including planned exercise. Teach patients about the importance of identifying and managing risk factors such as hypertension, obesity, substance use disorder, and diabetes mellitus, which contribute to the potential for a major stroke.

PATIENT-CENTERED CARE: HEALTH EQUITY

Stroke Prevalence and Outcomes

American Indian and Alaskan Native groups have the highest prevalence of stroke when compared with other populations. Black men and women have strokes twice as often as White men and women, especially hemorrhagic strokes caused by hypertension. Hispanic or Latino men have more strokes than non-Hispanic men. All of these groups tend to be at a higher risk for hypertension than the White population and have a higher death rate (Towfighi et al., 2020).

Socioeconomic factors, such as lifestyle (e.g., diet), health care disparities, and genetic or familial factors, may play a role in stroke risk among these minority groups (CDC, 2021a). For example, Blacks are twice as likely to smoke and have poorly controlled diabetes mellitus and hypertension when compared to Whites. Blacks are also more likely to have less access to high-quality health care (Towfighi et al., 2020).

Nurses need to be aware of these determinants of health and incorporate them into the plan of care for people of color. First, determine whether basic needs for housing, comfort, and food are being met. If basic needs are not being met, recognize that these needs are the priority concern for the patient. If the patient is ready for stroke prevention education, teach patients about the risk factors and consequences of stroke. Provide information about community resources that are easily accessible to help patients avoid these risks. Assess whether the patient has transportation and Internet access, if needed, to use these resources. For example, for those who smoke, provide information on convenient, cost-free, or low-cost smoking-cessation resources.

Interprofessional Collaborative Care
Recognize Cues: Assessment

History. Although an accurate history is important in the diagnosis of a stroke, *the first priority is to ensure that the patient is transported to a stroke center.* A **stroke center** is designated by The Joint Commission (TJC) or other organization for its ability to rapidly recognize and effectively treat strokes. TJC designates two distinct levels of stroke-center certification. The *primary certified* stroke center is required to provide diagnostic testing (imaging), stroke therapy with IV fibrinolytic therapy, and a stroke team. The *comprehensive* stroke center provides timely and advanced diagnostics and lifesaving measures, such as endovascular interventions and decompressive hemicraniectomy, which can prevent long-term disability. Obtaining a history should not delay the patient's arrival to either the stroke center or interventional radiology within the comprehensive stroke center. A focused history to determine whether the patient has had a recent bleeding event or is taking an anticoagulant is an important part of the *rapid stroke assessment* protocol.

Several important parts of the history should be collected:
- When did symptoms begin? The time of onset of symptoms is essential for making treatment decisions.
- What was the patient doing when the stroke began? Hemorrhagic strokes tend to occur during activity. Ischemic strokes tend to occur early in the morning.
- How did the symptoms progress? Symptoms of a hemorrhagic stroke tend to occur abruptly, whereas thrombotic strokes generally have a more gradual progression.
- Did the symptoms worsen after the initial onset, or did they begin to improve? Improvement of symptoms could signify a warning TIA, or a waxing and waning of symptoms could signify an incomplete stroke dependent on *perfusion.*
- What is the patient's medical history (with specific attention directed toward a history of head trauma, diabetes, hypertension, heart disease, anemia, and obesity)?
- What are the patient's current medications, including prescribed drugs, over-the-counter (OTC) drugs, herbal and nutritional supplements, and recreational (illicit) drugs?
- What is the patient's social history, including education, employment, travel, leisure activities, and personal habits (e.g., smoking, diet, exercise pattern, drug and alcohol use)?

During the interview, observe the patient's level of consciousness (LOC) and assess for indications of impaired *cognition, mobility,* and *sensory perception.* Question the patient or family member about the presence of sensory deficits or motor changes, visual problems, problems with balance or gait, communication problems, and changes in reading or writing abilities.

When LOC is suddenly decreased or altered, immediately determine whether hypoglycemia or hypoxia is present because these conditions may mimic emergent neurologic disorders! Hypoglycemia and hypoxia are easily treated and reversed, unlike brain injury from inadequate *perfusion* or trauma.

The patient with an SAH, particularly when the hemorrhage is from a ruptured (leaking) aneurysm, often reports the onset of a sudden, severe headache described as "the worst headache of my life." Additional symptoms of SAH or cerebral aneurysmal and AVM bleeding are nausea and vomiting, photophobia (sensitivity to light), cranial nerve deficits, stiff neck, and change in mental status. There may also be a family history of aneurysms (see Chapter 30).

Physical Assessment/Signs and Symptoms. First-responder personnel (e.g., paramedics, emergency medical technicians) perform an initial neurologic examination using well-established stroke assessment tools.

✚ NURSING SAFETY PRIORITY

Critical Rescue

In the ED, assess the stroke patient within 10 minutes of arrival. This same standard applies to patients already hospitalized for other medical conditions who have a stroke. The priority is assessment of the ABCs—airway, breathing, and circulation. Many hospitals have designated stroke teams and centers that are expert in acute stroke assessment and management.

Nurses also perform a complete neurologic assessment on arrival to the ED. The National Institutes of Health Stroke Scale (NIHSS) is a commonly used valid and reliable assessment tool that nurses complete as soon as possible after the patient arrives in the ED. This tool is used as one assessment to determine eligibility for IV fibrinolytics (Table 38.2).

Although the NIHSS is the standard tool for assessing neurologic status after an acute stroke, there is no standard for when and how often to use the tool. Wells-Pittman and Gullicksrud (2020) implemented a quality improvement (QI) project to determine the minimum use of the NIHSS across their large health care system (see the Systems Thinking/Quality Improvement box).

▷▷ SYSTEMS THINKING/QUALITY IMPROVEMENT

Is There a Standard for Using the NIHSS After Acute Stroke?

Wells-Pittman, J., & Gullicksrud, A. (2020). Standardizing the frequency of neurologic assessment after acute stroke. *American Journal of Nursing, 120*(3), 48–54.

The authors of this QI project were employed in a large health care system that has four Joint Commission–certified primary stroke centers and two Joint Commission–certified comprehensive stroke centers. Each center determined when and how often to assess stroke patients using the National Institutes of Health Stroke Scale (NIHSS). A QI nursing team was formed to review the literature and collect data on national best practices regarding the use of the NIHSS. A six-item questionnaire was sent to 22 stroke centers across the United States. Examples of questions included:

- Do you use the full NIHSS or the modified NIHSS?
- How frequently is the NIHSS being completed?
- Do you do other neurologic assessment on your stroke patients as well?

The QI nursing team analyzed the data and developed guidelines that allowed nurses to use clinical judgment about when the NIHSS would be used for patient assessment. These guidelines were based on national best practices, available evidence, and nursing expertise.

Commentary: Implications for Practice and Research
The system in this QI project was the health system stroke centers. The QI team worked to develop standardized guidelines to establish consistency but still allow nurses to use clinical judgment about when and how often to assess stroke patients using the NIHSS.

As the patients are transitioned from the ED to other settings, the most important area to assess is the patient's LOC. Use the Glasgow Coma Scale (GCS; see Chapter 35) or a modified NIHSS to frequently monitor for changes in LOC throughout the patient's acute care.

Strokes and other neurologic injuries, including brain tumors or traumatic brain injury, can cause an impaired airway defense, or an inability to clear one's airway. This impairment can cause inadequate cough and dysphagia (difficulty swallowing), which can lead to aspiration (causing aspiration pneumonia) or death. Therefore, assess the client's ability to effectively cough. Some agencies also allow nurses to use one of a variety of screening tools to assess for the presence of dysphagia (Green et al., 2021).

Stroke symptoms can appear at any time of the day or night. In general, the five most common symptoms are (CDC, 2021b):
- Sudden confusion or trouble speaking or understanding others
- Sudden numbness or weakness of the face, arm, or leg
- Sudden trouble seeing in one or both eyes
- Sudden dizziness, trouble walking, or loss of balance or coordination
- Sudden severe headache with no known cause

More specific stroke symptoms depend on the extent and location of the ischemia and the arteries and parts of the brain affected, as described in Box 38.3.

The *right* cerebral hemisphere is more involved with visual and spatial awareness and proprioception (sense of body position). A person who has a stroke involving the right cerebral hemisphere is often unaware of any deficits and may be disoriented to time and place. Personality changes include impulsivity (poor impulse control) and poor judgment. The *left* cerebral hemisphere, the dominant hemisphere in people who are right-handed (70% of the population), is the center for speech, language, mathematic skills, and analytic thinking. Therefore, problems in these areas are expected for patients who have a left-sided stroke.

Patients with *embolic* strokes may have a heart murmur, dysrhythmias (most often atrial fibrillation), heart failure, endocarditis, and/or hypertension (Washington et al., 2021). It is not unusual for patients to be admitted to the hospital with a blood pressure greater than 180 to 200/110 to 120 mm Hg, especially if they have hypertensive bleeding. Although a somewhat higher blood pressure of 150/100 mm Hg is needed to maintain cerebral **perfusion** after an acute *ischemic* stroke, pressures above this reading may lead to extension of the stroke.

Psychosocial Assessment. Assess the patient's reaction to the illness, especially in relation to changes in body image, self-concept, and ability to perform ADLs. In collaboration with the patient's family and friends, identify any problems with coping or personality changes. Screening and treatment for depression should be initiated and is a best practice guideline (Washington et al., 2021).

Ask about the patient's financial status and occupation because they may be affected by the residual neurologic deficits of the stroke and the potential long recovery. Patients who do

TABLE 38.2   **National Institutes of Health Stroke Scale (NIHSS)**

Category and Measurement	Score[a]

1a. Level of Consciousness (LOC) _____

0 = Alert; keenly responsive

1 = Not alert; but arousable by minor stimulation to obey, answer, or respond

2 = Not alert; requires repeated stimulation to attend or is obtunded and requires strong or painful stimulation to make movements (not stereotyped)

3 = Responds only with reflex motor or autonomic effects or totally unresponsive, flaccid, and areflexic

1b. LOC Questions _____

0 = Answers two questions correctly

1 = Answers one question correctly

2 = Answers neither question correctly

1c. LOC Commands _____

0 = Performs two tasks correctly

1 = Performs one task correctly

2 = Performs neither task correctly

2. Best Gaze _____

0 = Normal

1 = Partial gaze palsy; gaze abnormal in one or both eyes, but forced deviation or total gaze paresis not present

2 = Forced deviation, or total gaze paresis not overcome by the oculocephalic maneuver

3. Visual _____

0 = No visual loss

1 = Partial hemianopia

2 = Complete hemianopia

3 = Bilateral hemianopia (blind, including cortical blindness)

4. Facial Palsy _____

0 = Normal symmetric movements

1 = Minor paralysis (flattened nasolabial fold, asymmetry on smiling)

2 = Partial paralysis (total or near-total paralysis of lower face)

3 = Complete paralysis of one or both sides (absence of facial movement in the upper and lower face)

5. Motor (Arm)   Right arm: _____

0 = No drift; limb holds 90 (or 45) degrees for full 10 seconds

1 = Drift; limb holds 90 (or 45) degrees, but drifts down before full 10 seconds; does not hit bed or other support   Left arm: _____

2 = Some effort against gravity; limb cannot get to or maintain (if cued) 90 (or 45) degrees; drifts down to bed but has some effort against gravity

3 = No effort against gravity; limb falls

4 = No movement

Untestable = Amputation or joint fusion

6. Motor (Leg)   Right leg: _____

0 = No drift; leg holds 30-degree position for full 5 seconds

1 = Drift; leg falls by the end of the 5-second period but does not hit bed   Left leg: _____

2 = Some effort against gravity; leg falls to bed by 5 seconds but has some effort against gravity

3 = No effort against gravity; leg falls to bed immediately

4 = No movement

Untestable = Amputation or joint fusion

7. Limb Ataxia _____

0 = Absent

1 = Present in one limb

2 = Present in two limbs

Untestable = Amputation or joint fusion

8. Sensory _____

0 = Normal; no sensory loss

1 = Mild to moderate sensory loss; patient feels pinprick less sharp or dull on the affected side; or loss of superficial pain with pinprick, but patient aware of being touched

2 = Severe to total sensory loss; patient not aware of being touched in the face, arm, and leg

9. Best Language _____

0 = No aphasia; normal

1 = Mild to moderate aphasia; some obvious loss of fluency or facility of comprehension without significant limitation on ideas expressed or form of expression

2 = Severe aphasia; all communication is through fragmentary expression; great need for inference, questioning, and guessing by the listener

3 = Mute, global aphasia; no usable speech or auditory comprehension

TABLE 38.2 National Institutes of Health Stroke Scale (NIHSS)—cont'd

Category and Measurement	Score[a]
10. Dysarthria	_____
0 = Normal	
1 = Mild to moderate dysarthria; patient slurs at least some words and, at worst, can be understood with some difficulty	
2 = Severe dysarthria; patient's speech so slurred as to be unintelligible in the absence of or out of proportion to any dysphasia or is mute/anarthric	
Untestable = Intubated or other physical barrier	
11. Extinction and Inattention (Neglect)	_____
0 = No abnormality	
1 = Visual, tactile, auditory, spatial, or personal inattention or extinction to bilateral simultaneous stimulation in one of the sensory modalities	
2 = Profound hemi-inattention or extinction to more than one modality; does not recognize own hand or orients to only one side of space	

[a]The patient can have a score of 0 to 40, with 0 indicating no neurologic deficits and 40 indicating the most deficits.
Adapted from *National Institutes of Health Stroke Scale (NIHSS), 2013*. www.stroke.nih.gov/documents/NIH_Stroke_Scale.pdf.

BOX 38.3 Key Features

Stroke

Middle Cerebral Artery Strokes (Most Common)
- Contralateral (opposite side) hemiparesis (one-sided weakness) or hemiplegia (one-sided paralysis); typically, the arm is flaccid and the leg is spastic if both extremities are affected
- Dysphagia
- Contralateral sensory perception deficit (numbness, tingling, unusual sensations)
- Ptosis
- Nystagmus
- Homonymous hemianopsia
- Unilateral neglect or inattention
- Dysarthria
- Aphasia
- Anomia
- Apraxia
- Agnosia
- Alexia, agraphia, and/or acalculia
- Impaired vertical sensation
- Visual and spatial deficits
- Memory loss (amnesia)
- Altered level of consciousness: drowsy to comatose

Posterior Cerebral Artery Strokes
- Perseveration (word or action repetition)
- Aphasia, amnesia, alexia, agraphia, visual agnosia, and ataxia
- Loss of deep sensation
- Decreased touch sensation
- Increased lethargy/stupor, coma

Internal Carotid Artery Strokes
- Contralateral hemiparesis
- Sensory perception deficit
- Hemianopsia, blurred vision, blindness
- Aphasia (dominant side)
- Headache
- Carotid bruit

Anterior Cerebral Artery Strokes
- Contralateral hemiparesis: leg more than arm
- Bladder incontinence
- Personality and behavioral changes
- Aphasia and amnesia
- Positive grasp and sucking reflex
- *Sensory perception* deficit (lower extremity)
- Memory impairment
- Ataxic gait

Vertebrobasilar Artery Strokes
- Headache and vertigo
- Possible coma
- Memory loss and confusion
- Flaccid paresis or paralysis (quadriparesis affecting all four extremities)
- Ataxia
- Vertigo
- Cranial nerve dysfunction (such as dysphagia from cranial nerve IX involvement)
- Visual deficits (one eye) or homonymous hemianopsia
- Sensory loss: numbness

not have disability or health insurance may worry about how their family will cope financially with the disruption in their lives. Early involvement of social services, the certified hospital chaplain, or psychological counseling may enhance coping skills.

Assess for emotional lability (uncontrollable emotional state), especially if the frontal lobe or right side of the brain has been affected. In such cases the patient often laughs and then cries unexpectedly for no apparent reason. Explain the cause of uncontrollable emotions to the family or significant others so that they do not feel responsible for these reactions.

Laboratory Assessment. Clinical history, physical assessment, and a National Institutes of Health Stroke Scale (NIHSS) score are usually enough to identify a stroke once it has occurred. No definitive laboratory tests confirm its diagnosis. Elevated hematocrit and hemoglobin levels are often associated with a severe or major stroke as the body attempts to compensate for lack of oxygen to the brain. An elevated white blood cell (WBC) count may indicate the presence of an infection or a response to physiologic stress or inflammation. Blood glucose and hemoglobin A1C levels are used to evaluate whether the client has diabetes and whether it is controlled.

In addition to other routine laboratory testing, the primary health care provider typically requests a prothrombin time (PT), an international normalized ratio (INR), and an activated partial thromboplastin time (aPTT) to establish baseline information before fibrinolytic or anticoagulation therapy may be started (Pagana et al., 2022).

Imaging Assessment. For definitive evaluation of a suspected stroke, a *computed tomography perfusion (CTP) scan* and/or *computed tomography angiography (CTA)* is used to assess the extent of ischemia of brain tissue. Cerebral aneurysms or AVM may also be identified. *Magnetic resonance angiography (MRA)* and multimodal techniques such as perfusion-weighted imaging enhance the sensitivity of the MRI to detect early changes in the brain, including confirming blood flow. *Ultrasonography* (carotid duplex scanning) may also be performed (see Chapter 35).

NCLEX Examination Challenge 38.1

Physiological Integrity

The nurse is caring for a client recently admitted with a left middle cerebral artery embolic stroke. Which of the following assessment findings would the nurse expect for this client? **Select all that apply.**
A. Left-sided hemiparesis
B. Right-sided tingling and numbness
C. Dysarthria
D. Ataxia
E. Vertigo

Analyze Cues and Prioritize Hypotheses: Analysis

Depending on stroke severity and/or response to immediate management, the priority collaborative problems for patients with a stroke may include:

1. Inadequate *perfusion* to the brain due to interruption of arterial blood flow and a possible increase in ICP
2. Decreased *mobility* and possible need for assistance to perform ADLs due to neuromuscular or impaired *cognition*
3. Aphasia and/or dysarthria due to decreased circulation in the brain (aphasia) or facial muscle weakness (dysarthria)
4. *Sensory perception* deficits due to altered neurologic reception and transmission

Generate Solutions and Take Actions: Planning and Implementation

Improving Cerebral Perfusion

Planning: Expected Outcomes. The patient with a stroke is expected to have improved cerebral *perfusion* to maintain adequate brain function and prevent further brain injury.

Interventions. Most strokes are treatable. Improvements in acute stroke management have helped to decrease deaths from stroke. Almost all large hospitals in the United States have designated stroke centers; however, community and rural acute care settings may not have access to a neurologist or other resources needed to manage an acute stroke. As a result, *teleneurology,* using two-way video health care technology, is a growing strategy to provide acute stroke consultation with a board-certified neurologist. Wilcock et al. (2021) performed a study examining hospitals that use teleneurology for stroke and found that they are more likely to give the fibrinolytic agent ("clot-busting drug") alteplase than hospitals without teleneurology. As a result, clinical outcomes are better for patients in hospitals that use teleneurology when compared with those hospitals that do not.

Interventions for patients experiencing strokes are determined primarily by the type and extent of the stroke. Nursing interventions are initially aimed at monitoring for neurologic changes or complications associated with stroke and its treatment. The two major treatment modalities for patients with acute ischemic stroke are IV fibrinolytic therapy and endovascular interventions. Regardless of the immediate management approach used, once the patient is stable, provide ongoing supportive care. Provide interventions to prevent and/or monitor for early signs of complications. Implement interventions to prevent patient falls. These health problems are discussed in appropriate chapters in this textbook.

Fibrinolytic Therapy. For selected patients with acute ischemic strokes, early intervention with IV fibrinolytic therapy ("clot-busting drug") is the standard of practice to improve blood flow to viable tissue around the infarction or through the brain. The success of fibrinolytic therapy for a stroke depends on the interval between the time that symptoms begin and treatment is available. IV (systemic) fibrinolytic therapy (also called *thrombolytic therapy*) for an acute ischemic stroke dissolves the cranial artery occlusion to reestablish blood flow and prevent cerebral infarction. *IV alteplase is the only drug approved at this time for the treatment of acute ischemic stroke.* The most important factor in determining whether to give alteplase is the time between symptom onset and time seen in the stroke center. Currently, the U.S. Food and Drug Administration (FDA) approves administration of alteplase within 3 hours of stroke onset. The American Stroke Association endorses extension of that time frame to 4.5 hours to administer this fibrinolytic for patients *unless* they fall into one or more of these categories (Powers et al., 2019):

- Age older than 80 years
- Anticoagulation regardless of international normalized ratio (INR)
- Imaging evidence of ischemic injury involving more than one-third of the brain tissue supplied by the middle cerebral artery
- Baseline National Institutes of Health Stroke Scale (NIHSS) score greater than 25
- History of both stroke and diabetes
- Evidence of active bleeding

Fibrinolytic therapy is explained to the patient and/or family member, and informed consent is obtained. The dosage of alteplase is based on the patient's actual weight at 0.9 mg/kg. The 2019 Clinical Practice Guidelines for management of patients with acute ischemic stroke recommend IV alteplase 0.9 mg/kg over 60 minutes with the initial 10% of that dose given as a bolus over the first minute. The newest recommendation for door-to-needle (DTN) time (ED admission to fibrinolytic therapy start) is 45 minutes (Powers et al., 2019).

Each hospital has strict protocols for mixing and administering the fibrinolytic drug and for monitoring the patient before and after fibrinolytic drug administration. In some cases, the patient's blood pressure may be too high to give the medication. In this instance, the patient receives a rapid-acting antihypertensive drug until the blood pressure is below 185/110 mm Hg (Powers et al., 2019). This level must be maintained during fibrinolytic therapy.

NURSING SAFETY PRIORITY
Drug Alert

In addition to frequent monitoring of vital signs, carefully observe for signs of intracerebral hemorrhage and other signs of bleeding during administration of fibrinolytic drug therapy. Additional best practice nursing interventions are listed in Box 38.4.

Endovascular Interventions. Endovascular procedures to improve **perfusion** include intraarterial thrombolysis using drug therapy, mechanical embolectomy (surgical blood clot [thrombosis] removal), and carotid stent placement. *Intraarterial thrombolysis* has the advantage of delivering the fibrinolytic agent directly into the thrombus within 6 hours of the stroke onset. It is particularly beneficial for some patients who have an occlusion of the middle cerebral artery or those who arrive in the ED after the window for IV alteplase. Patients having either fibrinolytic therapy and/or endovascular interventions are admitted to the critical care setting for intensive monitoring.

Carotid artery angioplasty with stenting is common to prevent or, in some cases, help manage an acute ischemic stroke. This

BOX 38.4 Best Practice for Patient Safety and Quality Care
Evidence-Based Nursing Interventions During and After IV Administration of Alteplase

- Admit the patient to a critical care or specialized stroke unit.
- Perform a double check of the drug. Use a programmable pump to deliver the initial dose over 60 minutes, with 10% of the dose given as a bolus over 1 minute. Do not manually push this drug.
- Perform neurologic assessments, including vital signs every 10 to 15 minutes during infusion and every 30 minutes after that for at least 6 hours; monitor hourly for 24 hours after treatment. Be consistent regarding the device used to obtain blood pressures because blood pressures can vary when switching from a manual to a noninvasive automatic to an intraarterial device.
- If systolic blood pressure is 185 mm Hg or greater or diastolic is 110 mm Hg or greater *prior to* alteplase or greater than 180/105 *after* alteplase during the first 24 hours, give antihypertensive drugs, such as labetalol, as prescribed (IV is recommended for faster response).
- To prevent bleeding, do not place invasive tubes, such as nasogastric (NG) tubes or indwelling urinary catheters, until the patient is stable (usually for 24 hours).
- Discontinue the infusion if the patient reports severe headache or has severe hypertension, bleeding, nausea, and/or vomiting; notify the primary health care provider immediately.
- Obtain a follow-up CT or MRI scan after fibrinolytic therapy and before starting antiplatelet or anticoagulant drugs.

interventional radiology procedure is usually done under moderate sedation. It may be performed by a cardiovascular surgeon or interventional radiologist. A technique using a distal/embolic protection device has made this procedure very safe. The device is placed beyond the stenosis through a catheter inserted into the femoral artery (groin) or radial artery (forearm). The device catches any clot debris that breaks off during the procedure. Placement of a carotid stent is performed to open a blockage in the carotid artery, typically at the division of the common carotid artery into the internal and external carotid arteries. Throughout the procedure, carefully assess the patient's neurologic and cardiovascular status.

NURSING SAFETY PRIORITY
Action Alert

Before discharge after carotid stent placement, teach the patient and family to report these symptoms to the primary health care provider immediately:
- Severe headache
- Change in LOC or **cognition** (e.g., drowsiness, new-onset confusion)
- Muscle weakness or motor dysfunction
- Severe neck pain
- Swelling at neck incisional site
- Hoarseness or dysphagia (due to nerve damage)

When the stroke is hemorrhagic and the cause is related to an AVM or cerebral aneurysm, the patient is evaluated for the optimal procedure to stop further bleeding. Some procedures can be used to prevent bleeding in an AVM or aneurysm that is discovered *before* symptom onset or SAH. Procedures occur in the interventional radiology suite or operating room.

Monitoring for Increased Intracranial Pressure. The patient is most at risk for increased ICP resulting from edema during the first 72 hours after onset of the stroke. Some patients may have worsening of their neurologic status starting within 24 to 48 hours after their endovascular procedure from increased ICP (Box 38.5).

Reassess patients with acute stroke and after endovascular treatment of stroke symptoms every 1 to 4 hours, depending on severity of the condition. Use the approved agency assessment strategy and documentation tools.

NURSING SAFETY PRIORITY
Critical Rescue

Be alert for symptoms of increased ICP in the stroke patient, and report any deterioration in the patient's neurologic status to the primary health care provider or Rapid Response Team immediately! *The first sign of increased ICP is a declining level of consciousness (LOC).*

Best practices for preventing or managing increasing ICP for patients experiencing a stroke include:
- Elevate the head of the bed per agency or primary health care provider protocol to improve **perfusion** pressure.
- Provide oxygen therapy to prevent hypoxia for patients with oxygen saturation of less than 95% or per agency or primary health care provider protocol or prescription.
- Maintain the head in a midline, neutral position to promote venous drainage from the brain.

BOX 38.5 Key Features

Increased Intracranial Pressure (ICP)

- Decreased level of consciousness (LOC) (earliest sign)
- Behavioral changes: restlessness, irritability, and confusion
- Headache
- Nausea and vomiting (may be projectile)
- Aphasia
- Change in speech pattern/dysarthria
- Change in sensorimotor status:
  - Pupillary changes: dilated and nonreactive pupils ("blown pupils") or constricted and nonreactive pupils (very late sign)
  - Cranial nerve dysfunction
  - Ataxia
- Seizures (usually within first 24 hours after stroke)
- Cushing triad (very late sign):
  - Severe hypertension
  - Widened pulse pressure
  - Bradycardia
- Abnormal posturing (very late sign) (see Chapter 35):
  - Decerebrate
  - Decorticate

- Avoid sudden and acute hip or neck flexion during positioning. Extreme hip flexion may increase intrathoracic pressure, leading to decreased cerebral venous outflow and elevated ICP. Extreme neck flexion also interferes with venous drainage from the brain and intracranial dynamics.
- Avoid the clustering of nursing procedures (e.g., giving a bath followed immediately by changing the bed linen). When multiple activities are clustered in a narrow time period, the effect on ICP can be a dramatic elevation.
- Hyperoxygenate the patient before and after suctioning to avoid transient hypoxemia and resultant ICP elevation from dilation of cerebral arteries.
- Provide airway management to prevent unnecessary suctioning and coughing that can increase ICP.
- Maintain a quiet environment for the patient experiencing a headache, which is common with cerebral hemorrhage or increased ICP.
- Keep the room lights low to accommodate any photophobia the patient may have.
- Closely monitor blood pressure, heart rhythm, oxygen saturation, blood glucose, and body temperature to prevent secondary brain injury and promote positive outcomes after stroke.

✚ NURSING SAFETY PRIORITY

Critical Rescue

For ischemic strokes, blood pressure is initially allowed to rise above 220 mm Hg systolic if the patient has not received IV alteplase or embolectomy. After IV alteplase or embolectomy, if the stroke patient's systolic BP is more than 180 mm Hg, notify the Rapid Response Team or primary health care provider immediately, and anticipate possible prescription of an IV antihypertensive medication. Monitor the patient's BP and mean arterial pressure (MAP) (normal MAP is 70 to 100 mm Hg; at least 60 mm Hg is necessary to perfuse major organs) every 5 minutes until the systolic BP is adequate to maintain brain **perfusion**. Avoid a sudden systolic BP drop to less than 120 mm Hg with drug administration, which may cause brain ischemia.

Ongoing Drug Therapy. Ongoing drug therapy depends on the type of stroke and the resulting neurologic dysfunction. In general, the purposes of drug therapy are to prevent further thrombotic or embolic episodes (with antithrombotics and anticoagulation) and to protect the neurons from hypoxia.

Antiplatelet drugs such as aspirin and clopidogrel are the standard of care for treatment following acute ischemic strokes and for preventing future strokes (Powers et al., 2019).

Sodium heparin and other anticoagulants, such as warfarin, a vitamin K antagonist (VKA), or non-VKA or direct oral anticoagulants (DOACs), are reserved for use in patients who have cardiopulmonary issues such as atrial fibrillation. *Anticoagulants are high-alert drugs that can cause bleeding, including intracerebral hemorrhage in the area of the ischemia.* A newer trend is to prescribe a DOAC rather than bridging heparinoids, such as low–molecular-weight heparin (LMWH) or unfractionated heparin, for patients with acute ischemic stroke. A study by Altavilla et al. (2019) showed a decrease in the incidence of bleeding and stroke recurrence by giving a DOAC instead of warfarin with bridging therapy.

An *initial* low dose of aspirin is safer and recommended within 24 to 48 hours after stroke onset (Green et al., 2021). Aspirin should not be given within 24 hours of fibrinolytic administration. Aspirin is an antiplatelet drug that prevents further clot formation by reducing platelet adhesiveness (clumping or "stickiness"). It can cause bruising, hemorrhage, and liver disease over a long-term period. Teach the patient to report any unusual bruising or bleeding to the primary health care provider or to call 911 if bleeding is severe or does not stop.

A calcium channel blocking drug that crosses the blood-brain barrier, such as nimodipine, may be given to treat or prevent cerebral vasospasm after a subarachnoid hemorrhage. Vasospasm, which usually occurs between 4 and 14 days after the stroke, slows blood flow to the area and causes ischemia. Nimodipine works by relaxing the smooth muscles of the vessel wall and reducing the incidence and severity of the spasm. In addition, this drug dilates collateral vessels to ischemic areas of the brain.

Stool softeners, analgesics for pain, and antianxiety drugs may also be prescribed as needed for symptom management. Stool softeners also prevent the Valsalva maneuver during defecation to prevent increased ICP.

Promoting Mobility and ADL Ability

Planning: Expected Outcomes. The patient with a stroke is expected to ambulate and provide self-care independently, with or without one or more assistive-adaptive devices.

Interventions. In collaboration with the rehabilitation therapists, assess the patient's functional ability for bed *mobility* skills, ambulation with or without assistance, and ADL ability, including feeding, bathing, and dressing. Patients who have had a stroke are at risk for aspiration due to impaired swallowing as a result of muscle weakness. *Therefore, the best practice for all suspected and diagnosed stroke patients is to maintain NPO status until their swallowing ability is assessed!* Follow agency guidelines for screening or use an evidence-based bedside swallowing screening tool to determine if dysphagia is present. Refer the patient to the speech-language pathologist (SLP) for a swallowing evaluation per stroke protocol as needed. If dysphagia is present, develop a collaborative plan of care to prevent aspiration and support nutrition. Collaborate with the registered dietitian nutritionist to ensure that nutritional needs are met. Monitor the patient's weight daily and serum prealbumin levels to detect any decrease from baseline.

Many patients who have an untreated stroke often have flaccid or spastic paralysis. It is not unusual for the patient to eventually have a flaccid arm and spastic leg on the affected side because the affected leg often regains function more quickly than the arm. Be sure to support the affected flaccid arm of the stroke patient, and teach assistive personnel (AP) to avoid pulling on it. Position the arm on a pillow while the patient is sitting to prevent it from hanging freely, which could cause shoulder subluxation. The physical therapist or occupational therapist provides a slinglike device to support the arm during ambulation. Chapter 7 describes interventions for rehabilitation, including improving *mobility* and promoting self-care.

Patients begin rehabilitation as soon as possible to regain function and prevent complications of immobility, such as pneumonia, atelectasis, and pressure injuries. Another major complication of impaired *mobility* is the development of venous thromboembolism (VTE), especially deep vein thrombosis (DVT), which can lead to a pulmonary embolism (PE). This risk is highest in older patients and in those with a severe stroke.

◎ CORE MEASURES
Venous Thromboembolism

> Per The Joint Commission's Core Measures for VTE, provide care to prevent this complication by applying intermittent sequential pneumatic (or compression) devices, changing the patient's position frequently, and ambulating the patient if possible. Report any indications of DVT to the primary health care provider and document in the patient's medical record. Chapter 30 discusses VTE in detail.

Promoting Effective Communication
Planning: Expected Outcomes. The patient with a stroke is expected to receive, interpret, and express spoken, written, and nonverbal messages, if possible. However, some patients may need to develop strategies for alternative methods of communication, such as pictures, images, or nonverbal language.

Interventions. Language or speech problems are usually the result of a stroke involving the dominant hemisphere. The left cerebral hemisphere is the speech center in most patients. Speech and language problems may be the result of aphasia or dysarthria. Aphasia is caused by cerebral hemisphere damage; dysarthria is the result of a loss of motor function to the tongue or the muscles of speech, causing facial weakness and slurred speech.

Aphasia can be classified in a number of ways. Most commonly, it is classified as expressive, receptive, or mixed. Expressive (Broca or motor) aphasia is the result of damage in the Broca area of the frontal lobe. It is a motor speech problem in which the patient generally understands what is said but cannot speak. The patient also has difficulty writing but may be able to read. Rote speech and automatic speech such as responses to a greeting are often intact. The patient is aware of the deficit and may become frustrated and angry.

Receptive (Wernicke or sensory) aphasia is caused by injury involving the Wernicke area in the temporoparietal area. The patient cannot understand the spoken or written word. Although perhaps able to talk, the language is often meaningless.

Usually, the patient has some degree of dysfunction in the areas of both expression and reception. This is known as *mixed* or *global aphasia*. Reading and writing ability are equally affected. Few patients have only expressive *or* receptive aphasia. In most cases, however, one type is dominant.

To help communicate with the patient with aphasia, use these guiding principles:

- Present one idea or thought in a sentence (e.g., "I am going to help you get into the chair).
- Use simple one-step commands rather than asking patients to do multiple tasks.
- Speak slowly but not loudly; use cues or gestures as needed.
- Avoid "yes" and "no" questions for patients with expressive aphasia.
- Use alternative forms of communication if needed, such as a computer, handheld mobile device, communication board, or flash cards (often with pictures).
- Do not rush the patient when speaking.

For specific communication strategies for the patient with aphasia or dysarthria, collaborate with the speech-language pathologist.

▓ INTERPROFESSIONAL COLLABORATION
Care of Patients With Aphasia

> For patients with moderate to severe aphasia or dysarthria, consult with the speech-language pathologist (SLP), who can complement your patient care with specialized knowledge of speech and language problems. The SLP may identify additional patient problems that could trigger the need for other team members to achieve positive outcomes for the patient who has experienced a stroke. According to the Interprofessional Education Collaborative Expert Panel's (2016) Competency of Roles and Responsibilities, using the unique and complementary abilities of other team members optimizes health and patient care (Slusser et al., 2019).

NCLEX Examination Challenge 38.2
Physiological Integrity

> A client was just admitted to the emergency department with a diagnosis of new-onset acute ischemic stroke. What drug would the nurse anticipate to treat the client at this time?
> A. Heparin
> B. Nimodipine
> C. Alteplase
> D. Aspirin

Managing Changes in Sensory Perception
Planning: Expected Outcomes. The major concern of patients with *sensory perception* deficits is to adapt to neurologic deficits. The patient with a stroke is expected to adapt to

sensory perception changes in vision, proprioception (body position sense), and/or peripheral sensation and to be free from injury.

Interventions. Patients with right hemisphere brain damage typically have difficulty with visual-perceptual or spatial-perceptual tasks. They often have problems with depth and distance perception and with discrimination of right from left or up from down. Because of these problems, patients can have difficulty with performing routine ADLs. Caregivers can help the patient adapt to these disabilities by using frequent verbal and tactile cues and by breaking down tasks into discrete steps. *Always approach the patient from the unaffected side, which should face the door of the room!*

Unilateral neglect (or inattention) occurs most commonly in patients who have had a right cerebral stroke. However, it can occur in any patient who experiences hemianopsia, in which the vision of one or both eyes is affected (Fig. 38.2). This problem places the patient at additional risk for injury, especially falls, because of an inability to recognize physical impairment on one side of the body or because of a lack of proprioception.

- Teach the patient to touch and use both sides of the body.
- When dressing, remind the patient to dress the affected side first.
- If homonymous hemianopsia is present, teach the patient to turn the head from side to side to expand the visual field because the same half of each eye is affected. This scanning technique is also useful when the patient is eating or ambulating.

Place objects within the patient's field of vision. A mirror may help visualize more of the environment. If the patient has diplopia, a patch may be placed over the affected eye and changed every 2 to 4 hours.

The patient with a left hemisphere lesion generally has memory deficits and may show significant changes in the ability to carry out simple tasks, such as eating and grooming. Help with ADLs, but encourage the patient to do as much as possible independently. To assist with memory problems, reorient the patient to the month, year, day of the week, and circumstances surrounding hospital admission. Establish a routine or schedule that is as structured, repetitious, and consistent as possible. Provide information in a simple, concise manner. Apraxia may be present. Typically, the patient with apraxia exhibits a slow, cautious, and hesitant behavioral style. The physical therapist helps the patient compensate for loss of positional sense.

Care Coordination and Transition Management

Eight core measures and quality indicators are associated with the care of stroke patients by the interprofessional health care team in acute care and in preparation for hospital discharge (TJC, 2021). Certification as a primary stroke center or a comprehensive stroke center is tied to consistent performance in achieving satisfactory core measures. The core measures may have additional implications in terms of reimbursement in the future.

⊚ **CORE MEASURES**

Interprofessional Care for Patients With Ischemic Stroke

The eight core measures for ischemic stroke care for all patients include:
- Venous thromboembolism (VTE) prophylaxis
- Discharge with antithrombotic therapy
- Discharge with anticoagulation therapy for atrial fibrillation/flutter
- Thrombolytic therapy as indicated
- Antithrombotic therapy reevaluated by end of hospital day 2
- Discharge on statin medication
- Stroke education provided and documented
- Assessment for rehabilitation

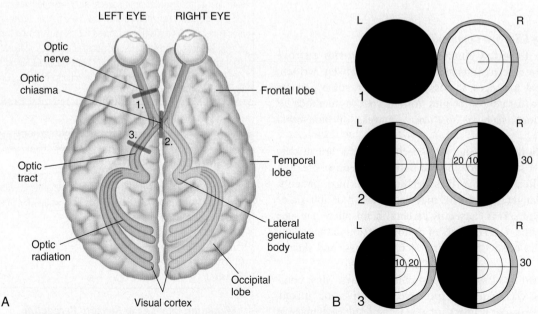

FIG. 38.2 (A) Site of lesions causing visual loss. *1,* Total blindness left eye. *2,* Bitemporal hemianopia. *3,* Left homonymous hemianopia. (B) Visual fields corresponding to the lesions shown at left. *1,* Total blindness left eye. *2,* Bitemporal hemianopia. *3,* Left homonymous hemianopia. (From Ball, J. W., Dains, J. E., Flynn, J. A., Solomon, B. S., & Stewart, R. W. [2023]. *Seidel's guide to physical examination* [10th ed.]. St. Louis: Elsevier.)

Nurses not only provide direct acute care to patients with stroke but also contribute to the peer review process to evaluate and monitor the care provided to patients with stroke who are planning transition from the hospital for continued care. According to the Centers for Medicare and Medicaid, stroke and preventable complications are in the top 10 causes of hospital readmission (https://www.cms.gov/medicare/medicare).

Many hospitals have developed transition-of-care systems to improve patient and family education, patient and family satisfaction, and 30-day hospital readmission rates. A classic systematic review of the literature performed by Oh et al. (2021) found that discharge education utilizing a teach-back method can reduce 30-day readmission by 45%. The concept of "hospital-at-home" is gaining popularity and can offer high-acuity care in the home with 24/7 telemedicine monitoring, as well as acute care provided by specialized nurses and health care providers. Improved clinical outcomes have been demonstrated during the first 30 postacute days to include: a decrease in hospital readmissions, a decrease in utilization of the ED, and a decrease in transfers to a skilled nursing facility. Technologic innovations in mobile health and telemedicine have offered new methods to extend care remotely to patients with stroke after hospital discharge; these methods include implantable loop monitors and follow-up virtual visits (Green et al., 2021).

The patient with a stroke may be discharged to home, a rehabilitation center, or a skilled nursing facility (SNF). Some patients have no significant neurologic dysfunction and are able to return home and live independently or with minimal support. Other patients are able to return home but require ongoing assistance with ADLs and supervision to prevent accidents or injury. The case manager (CM) coordinates speech-language, physical, and/or occupational therapy services to continue in the home or on an ambulatory care basis as needed. Patients admitted to an inpatient rehabilitation unit or facility or SNF require continued or more complex nursing care and extensive physical, occupational, recreational, speech-language, or cognitive therapy. The expected outcome for rehabilitation is to maximize the patient's abilities in all aspects of life. Chapter 7 discusses the role of nurses in the rehabilitation phase of care.

The three areas that should be included in patient and family education are disease prevention, disease-specific information, and self-management. The teaching plan may include lifestyle changes, drug therapy, ambulation and transfer skills, communication skills, safety precautions, nutritional management, activity levels, and self-management skills. Health teaching should focus on tasks that must be performed by the patient and the family after hospital discharge. Return demonstrations help to evaluate the family members' competency in tasks required for the patient's care (Fig. 38.3). Provide both written and verbal instruction in all of these areas. Home health services may be needed to provide ongoing care and education in the community. Specific teaching for stroke patients who are discharged to home is highlighted in Box 38.6.

As part of the discharge process, also inform the family about the signs and symptoms of depression and/or dementia that may occur within 3 months after a stroke. The strongest predictors of poststroke depression (PSD) are a history of depression,

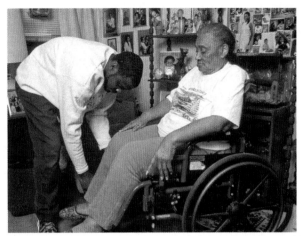

FIG. 38.3 Son adjusting his mother's wheelchair as part of caregiving responsibilities.

🏠 BOX 38.6 Home Health Care

Discharge Teaching for Home Care of Patients With Stroke

- Teach the patient and family about prescribed drugs to prevent another stroke and control hypertension. Instruct them about the name of each drug, the dosage, the timing of administration, how to take it, and possible side effects.
- Teach the patient how to climb stairs safely, if able; transfer from the bed to a chair; get into and out of a car; and use any aids for **mobility.**
- Provide important information regarding what to do in an emergency and where to call for nonemergency questions.
- Patients who have had a TIA or stroke are at risk for a new stroke. Teach family members to observe for and act on signs of a new stroke using the *FAST* mnemonic:
  - *Face* drooping
  - *Arm* weakness
  - *Speech* or language difficulty
  - *Time* to call 911

---

severe stroke, and poststroke physical or cognitive impairment. Patients may not exhibit typical signs of depression because of their cognitive, physical, and emotional impairments, including dementia. PSD is associated with increased morbidity and mortality, especially in older men.

Families may feel overwhelmed by the continuing demands placed on them. Family member caregivers are often uncertain about the progress of the patient and can become depressed the longer they provide care. Therefore, family members need to spend time away from the patient on a routine basis to continue to provide full-time care without sacrificing their own physical and emotional health. Refer the family to social services or other community resources for further support, counseling, and possible respite care.

Available resources include a variety of publications from the American Stroke Association (Stroke.org), including *Life after Stroke.* A good resource for stroke information and family support in Canada is the Heart and Stroke Foundation of Canada (www.heartandstroke.com). A website resource is *The Stroke Network,* which provides 24/7 online support for stroke survivors and caregivers of adult stroke patients (strokenet-work.org). Refer the patient and family members or significant others to local stroke support groups

For patients who require long-term symptom management or end-of-life care, refer the family to palliative care or hospice services. Chapter 8 provides a detailed description of end-of-life care and advance directives.

Evaluate Outcome: Evaluation

Evaluate the care of the patient with stroke based on the identified priority patient problems. The expected outcomes are that the patient:

- Has adequate cerebral **perfusion** to avoid long-term disability
- Maintains blood pressure and blood glucose within a safe, prescribed range
- Performs self-care and **mobility** activities independently, with or without assistive devices
- Learns to adapt to **sensory perception** changes, if present
- Communicates effectively or develops strategies for effective communication as needed
- Has adequate nutrition and avoids aspiration

✺ COGNITION CONCEPT EXEMPLAR: TRAUMATIC BRAIN INJURY

Traumatic brain injury (TBI) is damage to the brain from an external mechanical force and not caused by neurodegenerative or congenital conditions. TBI can lead to temporary and permanent impairment in **cognition, mobility, sensory perception,** and/or psychosocial function. As the term implies, patients who have any type of TBI experience trauma. The stress that follows a traumatic event affects each individual differently and can lead to long-lasting physical, mental, emotional, social, and spiritual distress. Nurses and other members of the interprofessional health team need to be aware of these effects and provide trauma-informed care as part of a patient-centered approach, described later under Interprofessional Collaborative Care.

Pathophysiology Review

Various terms are used to describe the brain injuries that occur when a mechanical force is applied either directly or indirectly to the brain. A force produced by a blow to the head is a *direct* injury, whereas a force applied to another body part with a rebound effect to the brain is an *indirect* injury. The brain responds to these forces by movement within the rigid cranial vault. It may also rebound or rotate on the brainstem, causing diffuse nerve axonal injury (shearing injuries). The brain may be contused (bruised) or lacerated (torn) as it moves over the inner surfaces of the cranium, which are irregularly shaped and sharp.

Movement or distortion within the cranial cavity is possible because of multiple factors. The first factor is how the brain is supported by cerebrospinal fluid (CSF) within the cranial cavity. When external force is applied to the head, the brain can be injured by the internal surfaces of the skull. The second factor is the consistency of brain tissue, which is very fragile, gel-like,

and prone to injury. Brain injury occurs both from initial forces on the cranium and brain and as a result of secondary injury related to mechanical pressure or cerebral edema.

The type of force and the mechanism of injury contribute to TBI. An *acceleration* injury is caused by an external force contacting the head, suddenly placing the head in motion. A *deceleration* injury occurs when the moving head is suddenly stopped or hits a stationary object (see Fig. 10.7). These forces may be sufficient to cause the cerebrum to rotate about the brainstem, resulting in shearing, straining, and distortion of the brain tissue, particularly of the axons in the brainstem and cerebellum. Small areas of hemorrhage (contusion, intracranial hemorrhage) may develop around the blood vessels that sustain the impact of these forces (stress), with destruction of adjacent brain tissue. Particularly affected are the basal nuclei and the hypothalamus, which are located deep in the brain.

Primary Brain Injury

Primary brain damage occurs at the time of injury and results from the physical stress (force) within the tissue caused by blunt or penetrating force. A primary brain injury may be categorized as focal or diffuse. A *focal* brain injury is confined to a specific area of the brain and causes localized damage that can often be detected with a CT scan or MRI. *Diffuse* injuries are characterized by damage throughout many areas of the brain. They begin at a microscopic level and are not initially detectable by CT scan. MRI has greater ability to detect microscopic damage, but these areas may not be imaged until necrosis occurs.

Primary brain injuries are also classified as either open or closed. An open traumatic brain injury occurs when the skull is fractured or when it is pierced by a penetrating object. The integrity of the brain and the dura is violated, and there is exposure to environmental contaminants. Damage may occur to the underlying vessels, dural sinuses, brain, and cranial nerves. In a closed traumatic brain injury, the integrity of the skull is intact, but damage to the brain tissue still occurs as a result of increased intracranial pressure or internal forces (Rogers, 2023).

TBI is further defined as mild, moderate, or severe (Table 38.3). Generally, the determination of severity of TBI is the result of the Glasgow Coma Scale (GCS) score immediately following resuscitation, the presence (or absence) of brain damage imaged by CT or MRI following the trauma, an estimation of the force of the trauma, and symptoms in the injured person.

One type of mild TBI is a concussion. A concussion is a traumatic injury to the brain caused by a blow to the head and may or may not result in some period of unconsciousness. Military personnel and people who participate in recreational or professional sports are especially at risk for concussions. Some patients report no immediate symptoms until later, which typically include impaired cognition (such as memory or thinking processes) and headache.

Secondary Brain Injury

Secondary injury to the brain includes any processes that occur *after* the initial injury and worsen or negatively influence patient outcomes. Secondary injuries result from physiologic, vascular,

TABLE 38.3	Differences Among Mild, Moderate, and Severe Traumatic Brain Injury	
Type of Traumatic Brain Injury	**Description**	**Symptoms**
Mild traumatic brain injury (mTBI)	Characterized by a blow to the head, transient confusion or feeling dazed or disoriented, and one or more of these conditions: (1) possible loss of consciousness for up to 30 minutes, (2) loss of memory for events immediately before or after the accident, and (3) focal neurologic deficit(s) that may or not be transient. Loss of consciousness does not have to occur for a person to be diagnosed with mTBI. No evidence of brain damage on a CT or MRI scan.	Includes a wide array of physical and cognitive problems that range from headache and dizziness to changes in behavior. Symptoms usually resolve within 72 hours. Symptoms may persist and last days, weeks, or months. Persistent symptoms following mTBI are also referred to as *postconcussion syndrome.*
Moderate	A moderate TBI is characterized by a period of loss of consciousness for 30 minutes to 6 hours and a Glasgow Coma Scale (GCS) score of 9 to 12. Often, but not always, focal or diffuse brain injury can be seen with a diagnostic CT or MRI scan. Posttraumatic *amnesia* (memory loss) may last up to 24 hours. May occur with either closed or open brain injury.	A short acute or critical care stay may be needed for close monitoring and to prevent secondary injury from brain edema, intracranial bleeding, or inadequate cerebral **perfusion.**
Severe	A severe TBI is defined by a GCS score of 3 to 8 and loss of consciousness for longer than 6 hours. Focal and diffuse damage to the brain, cerebrovascular vessels, and/or ventricles is common. Both open and closed head injuries can cause severe TBI, and injury can be focal or diffuse. CT and MRI scans can capture images of tissue damage quite early in the course of this illness.	Patients with severe TBI require management in critical care, including monitoring of hemodynamics, neurologic status, and possibly intracranial pressure (ICP). Patients with severe TBI are also at high risk for secondary brain injury from cerebral edema, hemorrhage, reduced **perfusion,** and the biomolecular cascade.

and biochemical events that are an extension of the primary injury.

The most common secondary injury from mild TBI (sometimes documented as mTBI), such as a concussion, is postconcussion syndrome. In this syndrome, the patient reports that headaches, impaired *cognition,* and dizziness continue to occur for at least 4 weeks after the initial brain injury. Other patients who have been diagnosed with concussions may experience only posttraumatic headaches or posttraumatic vertigo (a feeling of spinning or dizziness) for weeks to months after the initial injury. Additional symptoms of postconcussion syndrome that may occur include (Elliott et al., 2021):

- Irritability, depression, anxiety, and/or emotional lability
- Insomnia
- Difficulty concentrating or memory deficit (amnesia)
- Reduced alcohol tolerance

Some patients may not have been diagnosed as having a TBI because they are asymptomatic. However, later they may be diagnosed with chronic traumatic encephalopathy (CTE), an uncommon degenerative brain disease that occurs most often in military veterans, athletes, and others who experienced repetitive trauma to the brain. CTE can lead to dementia, depression, suicidal thinking, and substance use disorder. Although the disease is usually diagnosed by history and clinical presentation, it can only be confirmed at autopsy when the classic tau neurofibrillary tangles are evident (Rogers, 2023).

Another syndrome that can occur is second-impact syndrome (SIS). SIS is rare, and there is not an exact understanding of the pathophysiology. SIS occurs when the brain has not fully recovered from the initial TBI and sustains a second impact before recovery. The person will rapidly develop altered mental status and a loss of consciousness within seconds to minutes of the second hit, resulting in catastrophic neurologic injury (May et al., 2021). Most of these injuries occur in athletes. School nurses are in an ideal position to educate the public, coaches, parents, and athletes on the prevention of concussion and return-to-sports guidelines.

For patients with moderate or severe TBI, the most common secondary injuries result from hypotension and hypoxia, intracranial hypertension, and cerebral edema. Damage to the brain tissue occurs primarily because the delivery of oxygen and glucose to the brain is interrupted from cerebral edema and increasing pressure. Each of these problems is discussed in the following sections.

Hypotension and Hypoxia. Both hypotension, defined as a mean arterial pressure of less than 70 mm Hg, and hypoxemia, defined as a partial pressure of arterial oxygen (Pao_2) less than 80 mm Hg, restrict the flow of blood to vulnerable brain tissue. Hypotension may be related to shock (see Chapter 31) or other states of reduced **perfusion** to the brain, such as that caused by clot formation. Hypoxia can be caused by respiratory failure, asphyxiation, or loss of airway and impaired ventilation (see Chapter 26). These problems may occur as a direct result of moderate to severe brain injury or secondary to systemic injuries and comorbidities. Low blood flow and hypoxemia contribute to cerebral edema, creating a cycle of deteriorating **perfusion** and hypoxic damage. Patients with hypoxic damage related to moderate or severe brain injury face a poor prognosis and eventually experience impaired **cognition.**

Increased Intracranial Pressure. The cranial contents include brain tissue, blood, and cerebrospinal fluid (CSF). These components are encased in the relatively rigid skull. Within this space, there is little room for any of the components to expand or increase in volume. *A normal level of intracranial pressure (ICP) is 10 to 15 mm Hg.* Periodic increases in pressure occur with straining during defecation, coughing, or sneezing but do not harm the uninjured brain. A sustained ICP of greater than 20 mm Hg is considered detrimental to the brain because neurons begin to die.

As a result of brain injury, the increase in the volume of one component must be compensated for by a decrease in the volume of one of the other components. As a first response to an increase in the volume of any of these components, the CSF is shunted or displaced from the cranial compartment to the spinal subarachnoid space, or the rate of CSF absorption is increased. An additional response, if needed, is a decrease in cerebral blood volume by movement of cerebral venous blood into the sinuses or jugular veins. As long as the brain can compensate for the increase in volume and remain compliant, increases in ICP are minimal (Rogers, 2023).

Increased ICP is the leading cause of death from head trauma in patients who reach the hospital alive. It occurs when compliance no longer takes place and the brain cannot accommodate further volume changes. As ICP increases, cerebral *perfusion* decreases, leading to brain tissue ischemia and edema. If edema remains untreated, the brainstem may herniate downward through the foramen magnum or laterally from a unilateral lesion within one cerebral hemisphere, causing irreversible brain damage and possibly death (from brain herniation syndromes discussed later) (Rogers, 2023). Box 38.5 in the previous section on Stroke lists the common symptoms associates with increased ICP.

Hemorrhage. Hemorrhage, which causes a brain hematoma (collection of blood) or clot, may occur as part of the primary injury and begin at the moment of impact. It may also arise later from vessel damage as a secondary brain injury. Bleeding is caused by vascular damage from the shearing force of the trauma or direct physical damage from skull fractures or penetrating injury. *All hematomas are potentially life-threatening because they act as space-occupying lesions and are surrounded by edema.* Three major types of hemorrhage after TBI are epidural, subdural, and intracerebral hemorrhage. Subarachnoid hemorrhage may also occur.

An epidural hematoma results from arterial bleeding into the space between the dura and the inner skull (Fig. 38.4). It is often caused by a fracture of the temporal bone, which houses the middle meningeal artery. Patients with epidural hematomas have "lucid intervals" that last for minutes, during which time the patient is awake and talking. This follows a momentary unconsciousness that can occur within minutes of the injury (Rogers, 2023).

✚ NURSING SAFETY PRIORITY

Critical Rescue

After the initial interval, symptoms of neurologic impairment from hemorrhage can progress very quickly, with potentially life-threatening ICP elevation and irreversible structural damage to brain tissue. Monitor the patient suspected of epidural bleeding frequently (every 5 to 10 minutes) for changes in neurologic status. The patient can become quickly and increasingly symptomatic. *A loss of consciousness from an epidural hematoma is a neurosurgical emergency!* Notify the primary health care provider or Rapid Response Team immediately if these changes occur. Carefully document your assessments and identify any trends.

A subdural hematoma (SDH) results from venous bleeding into the space beneath the dura and above the arachnoid (see Fig. 38.4). It occurs most often from a tearing of the bridging veins within the cerebral hemispheres, from a laceration of brain tissue. *Bleeding from this injury occurs more slowly than from an epidural hematoma.* SDHs are subdivided into acute, subacute,

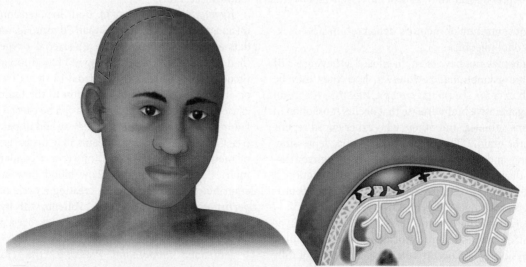

FIG. 38.4 Epidural hematoma (outside the dura mater of the brain), subdural hematoma (under the dura mater), and intracerebral hemorrhage (within the brain tissue).

and chronic. Acute SDH presents within 48 hours after impact; subacute SDH between 48 hours and 2 weeks, and chronic SDH from 2 weeks to several months after injury. SDHs have the highest mortality rate because they often are unrecognized until the patient presents with severe neurologic compromise.

The incidence of chronic SDHs (sometimes written as cSDH) nearly doubles when people are between 65 and 75 years of age and continues to increase in patients over 80 years old. Common causes of chronic SDHs in older adults include head trauma resulting from a fall and anticoagulant or antiplatelet therapy. Typical signs and symptoms include worsening headaches, paresis, acute confusion, and seizures. In some cases, patients may experience a decreased level of consciousness, including coma (Vacca & Argenti, 2018).

Traumatic intracerebral hemorrhage (ICH) is the accumulation of blood within the brain tissue caused by the tearing of small arteries and veins in the subcortical white matter (see Fig. 38.4). It often acts as a space-occupying lesion (e.g., a tumor) and may be potentially devastating, depending on its location. ICH may also produce significant brain edema and ICP elevations. A traumatic brainstem hemorrhage occurs as a result of a blow to the back of the head, fractures, or torsion injuries to the brainstem (vital sign center). *Brainstem injuries have a very poor prognosis.*

Brain Herniation Syndromes. In the presence of increased ICP, the brain tissue may shift and herniate downward. Of the several types of herniation syndromes (Fig. 38.5), *uncal herniation* is one of the most clinically significant because it is life-threatening. It is caused by a shift of one or both areas of the temporal lobe, known as the uncus. This shift creates pressure on the third cranial nerve (oculomotor). Late findings include dilated and nonreactive pupils, ptosis (eyelid drooping), and a rapidly deteriorating level of consciousness. *Central herniation* is caused by a downward shift of the brainstem and the diencephalon from a supratentorial lesion. It manifests clinically with Cheyne-Stokes respirations and pinpoint reactive pupils initially; then it may progress to nonreactive pupils and potential hemodynamic instability. *All herniation syndromes are potentially life-threatening, and the Rapid Response Team or primary health care provider must be notified immediately when they are suspected!*

Hydrocephalus. Hydrocephalus is an abnormal increase in CSF volume in the brain. It may be caused by impaired reabsorption of CSF at the arachnoid villi (from subarachnoid hemorrhage or meningitis), called a *communicating hydrocephalus*. It may also be caused by interference or blockage with CSF outflow from the ventricular system (from cerebral edema, tumor, or debris) (called a *noncommunicating hydrocephalus*). The ventricles may dilate from the relative increase in CSF volume. Ultimately, if not treated, additional CSF may lead to increased ICP.

Etiology and Genetic Risk

The most common causes of TBI in the United States are falls, intentional self-harm, motor vehicle crashes, and assaults. Falls among older adults are increasing as more baby boomers reach older adulthood. Firearm-related suicide is the most common cause of TBI-related deaths in the United States (CDC, 2021c). Alcohol and illicit drugs are significant contributing factors to the causes of TBI. Summer and spring months, evenings, nights, and weekends are associated with the greatest number of injuries. Young males are more likely than young females to have a TBI. Men tend to play more sports, enroll more often in military service, take more risks when driving, and consume larger amounts of alcohol than women. Falls are the most common cause of TBI in older adults and children.

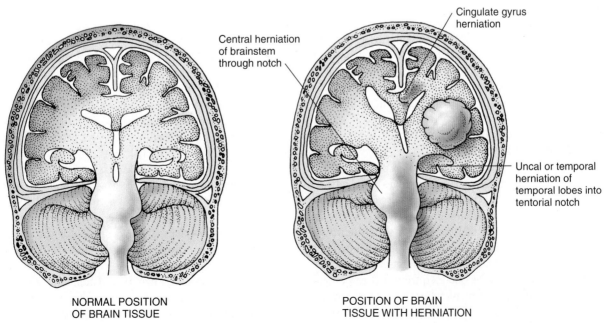

Central herniation of brainstem through notch

Cingulate gyrus herniation

Uncal or temporal herniation of temporal lobes into tentorial notch

NORMAL POSITION OF BRAIN TISSUE

POSITION OF BRAIN TISSUE WITH HERNIATION

FIG. 38.5 Herniation syndromes.

👤 PATIENT-CENTERED CARE: VETERAN HEALTH

Veterans and Traumatic Brain Injury

The United States is seeing increasing numbers of survivors of brain injury from wartime blast injuries. As a result, multiple types of TBI have become a major health problem among veterans of war and active military personnel. Be aware that most veterans who experienced a TBI also sustained other injuries, such as amputation and burns.

A number of veterans have mild TBI and postconcussion syndrome and can develop chronic traumatic encephalopathy (CTE). CTE is becoming more recognized as a TBI from repetitive brain injuries among active-duty military personnel and veterans.

Many veterans who have a TBI also experience posttraumatic stress disorder (PTSD), which affects their satisfaction with life. Symptoms such as headache pain, poor sleep quality, and dizziness can negatively impact their quality of life (Elliott et al., 2021). Nurses need to assess all active military members and veterans for indications of TBI and PTSD, and incorporate these needs into a patient-centered plan of care.

Incidence and Prevalence

Over 3 million people sustain a TBI in the United States every year; of these, more than 56,800 die (Williamson & Rajajee, 2023). The number of TBI-related emergency department visits, hospitalizations, and deaths has increased over the past several decades. In Canada, statistics are calculated for acquired brain injuries (ABIs), which include both traumatic *and* nontraumatic brain injuries, such as strokes.

Health Promotion and Maintenance

Nurses can educate the public on ways to decrease the incidence of TBI by using safe driving practices, such as wearing seat belts and never driving while impaired. . Teach people at risk about how alcohol and illicit drug use, including the use of marijuana, affect driving ability. Promote the use of helmets for skateboarding and bicycle and motorcycle riding. Teach gun safety to prevent unintentional injuries. Help prevent falls by providing a safe environment, especially for older adults. People need to be aware of environmental factors, such as inadequate lighting and loose rugs, that may increase the likelihood of falls. When possible, install safety equipment in bathtubs and showers. Evaluate balance and coordination as part of a fall prevention strategy inside the hospital and at home. Chapter 4 discusses fall prevention for older adults in detail.

Interprofessional Collaborative Care

Recognize Cues: Assessment

History. Obtaining an accurate history from a patient who has sustained a TBI may be difficult because of changes in the patient's *cognition.* The seriousness of the injury can cause amnesia (loss of memory). It is not unusual for the patient to experience amnesia for events before or after the injury. The patient with a moderate or severe brain injury may be unconscious or in a confused and combative state. If the patient cannot provide information, the history can be obtained from first responders or witnesses to the injury. Always ask when, where, and how the injury occurred. Did the patient lose consciousness; if so, for how long? Has there been a change in the level of consciousness (LOC)? If trauma is related to drug or alcohol consumption, it may be difficult to differentiate neurologic changes caused by head trauma from those produced by intoxication.

Determine whether the patient had fluctuating consciousness or seizure activity and whether there is a history of a seizure disorder. Obtain precise information about the circumstances of falls, particularly in the older patient. Recognize that many factors can contribute to death in older adults from TBI (see the Patient-Centered Care: Older Adult Health: Traumatic Brain Injury box).

👤 PATIENT-CENTERED CARE: OLDER ADULT HEALTH

Traumatic Brain Injury

- Brain injury is the fifth leading cause of death in older adults (CDC, 2021d).
- People who are 65 to 75 years old have the second highest incidence of brain injury of all age-groups (CDC, 2021d).
- Falls and motor vehicle crashes are the most common causes of brain injury (CDC, 2021d).
- Factors that contribute to high mortality are:
  - Falls causing subdural hematomas (closed head injuries), especially chronic subdural hematomas
  - Poorly tolerated systemic stress, which is increased by admission to a high-stimulus environment
  - Medical complications, such as hypotension, hypertension, and cardiac problems
  - Decreased protective mechanisms, which make patients susceptible to infections (especially pneumonia)
  - Decreased immunologic competence, which is further diminished by brain injury

Other pertinent information includes hand dominance, any diseases of or injuries to the eyes, and any allergies to drugs or food. Inquire about a history of alcohol or drug use because these substances may interfere with the neurologic baseline assessment. Consider whether the patient is a victim of violence if living in residential care or has a caregiver. *The Joint Commission and the Centers for Medicare and Medicaid Services require that all patients be screened for abuse and neglect when they are admitted to any type of health care facility.*

Physical Assessment/Signs and Symptoms. No two brain injuries are alike. The patient with a TBI may have a variety of signs and symptoms, depending on the severity of injury and the resulting increase in intracranial pressure (ICP) (see Box 38.5 under the Stroke section). Box 38.7 lists possible signs and symptoms of *mild* TBI (mTBI).

For any patient with a TBI, assess for signs of increased ICP, hypotension, hypoxemia (decreased blood level of oxygen), hypercarbia ($Paco_2$ greater than 40 to 45 mm Hg or increased partial pressure of carbon dioxide in arterial blood), or hypocarbia ($Paco_2$ less than 40 to 45 mm Hg or decreased partial pressure of carbon dioxide in arterial blood). *Hypercarbia* can cause cerebral vasodilation and contribute to elevated ICP. *Hypocarbia* is caused by hyperventilation and can lead to profound vasoconstriction with resulting ischemia. Carbon dioxide levels in an intubated patient can be determined with an end-tidal carbon dioxide ($ETco_2$) monitor, or capnography.

BOX 38.7   Key Features
Mild Traumatic Brain Injury

Physical Findings
- Appears dazed or stunned
- Loss of consciousness (if any) <30 minutes
- Headache
- Nausea
- Vomiting
- Balance or gait problems
- Dizziness
- Visual problems
- Fatigue
- Sensitivity to light
- Sensitivity to noise

Cognitive Findings
- Feeling mentally foggy
- Feeling slowed down
- Difficulty concentrating
- Difficulty remembering
- Amnesia about the events around the time of injury

Sleep Disturbances
- Drowsiness
- Sleeping less than usual
- Sleeping more than usual
- Trouble falling asleep

Emotional Changes
- Irritability
- Sadness
- Nervousness
- More "emotional"
- Depression

The early detection of changes in the patient's neurologic status enables the health care team to prevent or treat potentially life-threatening complications. *Be aware that subtle changes in blood pressure, consciousness, and pupillary reaction to light can be very informative about neurologic deterioration!*

Airway and Breathing Pattern Assessment. *The first priority is the assessment of the patient's ABCs—airway, breathing, and circulation!* Because TBI is occasionally associated with cervical spinal cord injuries, all patients with head trauma are treated as though they have cord injury until radiography proves otherwise. *Older adults are especially prone to cervical injuries at the first or second vertebral level, a life-threatening problem.* Assess for indicators of spinal cord injury, such as loss of **mobility** and **sensory perception,** tenderness along the spine, and abnormal head tilt.

✚ NURSING SAFETY PRIORITY
Critical Rescue

The upper cervical spinal nerves innervate the diaphragm to control breathing. Monitor all TBI patients for respiratory problems and diaphragmatic breathing, as well as for diminished or absent reflexes in the airway (cough and gag). Hypoxia and hypercapnia are best detected through arterial oxygen levels (partial pressure of arterial oxygen [Pao_2]), oxygen saturation (Spo_2), and end-tidal volume carbon dioxide measurement ($ETco_2$). Observe chest wall movement and listen to breath sounds. Provide respiratory support, including oxygen therapy and bed positioning. *Report any sign of respiratory problems immediately to the Rapid Response Team or primary health care provider!*

Injuries to the brainstem may cause a major life-threatening change in the patient's breathing pattern, such as Cheyne-Stokes respirations and/or apnea. In the unconscious patient, an artificial airway provides protection from aspiration and a route for oxygenation. Mechanical ventilation is often needed to support inadequate client respiratory effort.

Spine Assessment and Precautions. Patients with blunt trauma to the head or neck are typically transported from the scene of the injury to the hospital with a rigid cervical collar and a long spine board. *The expected outcome is to prevent new and secondary spine injury.* Spine precautions require placing the patient supine and aligning the spinal column in a neutral position so that there is no rotation, flexion, or extension. The long spine board is removed as soon as possible on arrival at the emergency department (ED) or ICU. The rigid cervical collar is maintained until definitive diagnostic studies to rule out cervical spine injury are completed.

Once the spine board is removed, spinal precautions are maintained until the primary health care provider indicates that it is safe to bend or rotate the cervical, thoracic, and lumbar spine. Spine precautions include:
- Bed rest
- No neck flexion with a pillow or roll
- No thoracic or lumbar flexion
- Manual control of the cervical spine anytime the rigid collar is removed
- Use of a "log-roll" procedure to reposition the patient

A hard, rigid cervical collar is used to maintain cervical spine ("C-spine") precautions and immobilization with a confirmed cervical injury. If the collar is ill-fitting or soiled, it may be changed according to hospital guidelines while a second qualified person maintains C-spine immobilization. Frequent assessment of the skin under the collar is important to monitor for skin breakdown.

Spine clearance is a clinical decision made by the primary health care provider, often in collaboration with the radiologist. Spine clearance includes determining the absence of acute bony, ligamentous, and neurologic abnormalities of the cervical spine based on history, physical examination, and/or negative radiologic studies.

Vital Signs Assessment. The mechanisms of autoregulation are often impaired as the result of a TBI. The more serious the injury, the more severe is the impact on *autoregulation* or the ability of cerebral vasculature to modify systemic pressure such that blood flow to the brain is sufficient. Monitor the patient's blood pressure and pulse frequently based on agency protocol and patient status. The patient may have hypotension or hypertension. Cushing triad, a classic but very late sign of increased ICP, consists of severe hypertension, a widened pulse pressure (increasing difference between systolic and diastolic values), and bradycardia. This triad of cardiovascular changes usually indicates imminent death.

Neurologic Assessment. Many hospitals use the Glasgow Coma Scale (GCS) to document neurologic status (see Chapter 35). A change of 2 points is considered clinically important; notify the primary health care provider of any deterioration of 2 points or more in GCS values.

The most important variable to assess with any brain injury is LOC! A decrease or change in LOC is typically the first sign of deterioration in neurologic status. A decrease in arousal, increased sleepiness, and increased restlessness or combativeness are all signs of declining neurologic status. Early indicators of a change in LOC include behavioral changes (e.g., restlessness, irritability) and disorientation, which are often subtle in nature. Report any of these signs and symptoms immediately to the primary health care provider or Rapid Response Team!

Use a bright light to assess pupillary size and reaction to light. Facial trauma may swell eyelids, making this assessment difficult. Consider whether drugs that affect pupillary dilation and constriction, such as anticholinergics or adrenergics, have been used recently.

✚ NURSING SAFETY PRIORITY

Critical Rescue

Check pupils of patients with TBI for size and reaction to light, particularly if the patient is unable to follow directions, to assess changes in level of consciousness. *Document any changes in pupil size, shape, and reactivity, and notify the Rapid Response Team or primary health care provider immediately because such changes could indicate an increase in ICP!*

Pupillary changes or eye signs differ depending on which areas of the brain are damaged. *Pinpoint and nonresponsive pupils are indicative of brainstem dysfunction at the level of the pons.* The *ovoid* pupil is regarded as the midstage between a normal-size and a dilated pupil. Asymmetric (uneven) pupils, loss of light reaction, or unilateral or bilateral dilated pupils are treated as herniation of the brain from increased ICP until proven differently. *Pupils that are fixed (nonreactive) and dilated are a poor prognostic sign. Patients with this problem are sometimes referred to as having "blown" pupils.* Pupillometers are utilized at some institutions to measure if a pupil is reactive in hard-to-assess patients (minimal reactivity, dark irises). Follow institution policy regarding the use of a pupillometer.

Check gross vision if the patient's condition permits. Have the patient read any printed material (e.g., your name tag) or count the number of fingers that you hold within the patient's visual field. Loss of vision is usually caused by either direct injury to the eye or injury to the occipital lobe.

Monitor for additional late signs of increased ICP. These manifestations include severe headache, nausea, vomiting (often projectile), and seizures. The primary health care provider may evaluate for papilledema (seen by ophthalmoscopic examination). Papilledema is edema and hyperemia (increased blood flow) of the optic disc. *It is always a sign of increased ICP.* Headache and seizures are a response to the injury and may or may not be associated with increased ICP. Always remember that the patient with a brain injury is at risk for potentially devastating ICP elevations during the first hours after the event and up to 3 to 4 days after injury, when cerebral edema can occur.

Assess for bilateral *motor* responses. The patient's motor loss or dysfunction usually appears contralateral (opposite side) to the site of the lesion, similar to that of a stroke. For example, a left-sided hemiparesis reflects an injury to the right cerebral hemisphere. Deterioration in *mobility* or the development of abnormal posturing or flaccidity is another indicator of progressive brain injury (see Chapter 35). These changes are the result of dysfunction within the pyramidal (motor) tracts of the spinal cord. Assess for brainstem or cerebellar injury, which may cause ataxia, decreased or increased muscle tone, and weakness. Remember that absence of motor function may also be an indicator of a spinal cord injury.

Carefully observe the patient's ears and nose for any signs of cerebrospinal fluid (CSF) leaks that result from a basilar skull fracture. Suspicious ear or nose fluid can be analyzed by the laboratory for glucose and electrolyte content. CSF placed on a white absorbent paper or linen can be distinguished from other fluids by the *"halo" sign,* a clear or yellowish ring surrounding a spot of blood. Although other body fluids can be used, a halo sign is most reliable when blood is in the center of the absorbent material because tears and saliva can also cause a clear ring in some conditions.

Palpate the patient's head gently to detect the presence of fractures or hematomas. Look for areas of ecchymosis (bruising), tender areas of the scalp, and lacerations. *Raccoon's eyes* are purplish discoloration around eyes that can follow fracture of the skull's base. When CT scans are used with head and brain injury, these fractures are often visualized before bruising appears.

Psychosocial Assessment. Patients with any level of TBI usually have varying degrees of psychosocial changes that may persist for a year or for a lifetime, depending on the severity of the injury and the person's response. Emotional lability and/or personality changes manifesting with temper outbursts, depression, risk-taking behavior, and denial of disability can occur. The patient may become talkative and develop a very outgoing personality. Memory, especially recent or short-term memory, is often affected. The patient may report difficulties in *cognition,* such as concentration or the ability to learn new information, and may have problems with insight and planning. Aggressive behavior, agitation, and sleep disorders may interfere with the ability to return to work or school. The ability to communicate and understand spoken and written language may be altered. Changes in *mobility* and *sensory perception* may require rehabilitation or the use of assistive devices. All these changes in health status may lead to difficulties within the family structure and with social and work-related interactions.

Imaging Assessment. The primary health care provider immediately requests a CT scan of the brain to identify the extent and scope of injury. This diagnostic test can identify the presence of an injury that requires surgical intervention, such as an epidural or subdural hematoma. An *MRI* may be done to detect subtle changes in brain tissue and show more specific detail of the brain injury. MRI is particularly useful in the diagnosis of diffuse axonal injury, but it is not recommended for patients with ICP-monitoring devices. Functional MRI, diffusion-weighted MRI, and MRI spectroscopy may be done to more specifically detect anoxic injury to the brain.

Analyze Cues and Prioritize Hypotheses: Analysis

The priority collaborative problems for patients with traumatic brain injury (TBI) vary greatly, depending on the severity of the event. The most common problems include:

1. Potential for decreased cerebral tissue *perfusion* due to primary event and/or secondary brain injury

2. Potential for decreased *cognition, sensory perception,* and/or *mobility* due to primary or secondary brain injury

3. Traumatic stress due to primary event and/or secondary injury

Generate Solutions and Take Actions: Planning and Implementation

Maintaining Cerebral Tissue Perfusion

Planning: Expected Outcomes. The expected outcome is that the patient will maintain adequate cerebral tissue *perfusion* with no evidence of secondary brain injury from cerebral edema and increased ICP.

Interventions. The patient with a *severe* TBI is admitted to the critical care unit or trauma center. Patients with *moderate* TBI are admitted to either the general nursing unit or the critical care unit, where they are closely observed for at least 24 hours. Those with *mild* TBI are usually sent home from the emergency department with instructions for home-based observation and primary health care provider follow-up. In some cases, the patient is hospitalized for 23-hour observation by staff. Cerebral *perfusion* is *not* typically affected by a mild TBI.

As with any critically injured patient, the priority for patients who have a moderate or severe TBI is to maintain a patent airway, breathing, and circulation! Specific nursing interventions for the patient with a TBI are directed toward preventing or detecting secondary brain injury or the conditions that contribute to secondary brain injury such as increased ICP, promoting fluid and electrolyte balance, and monitoring the effects of treatments and drug therapy. Providing health teaching and emotional support for the patient and family are vital parts of the plan of care.

If patients develop a subdural hematoma at any point after a TBI, a craniotomy is performed to evacuate the clot. Care of patients who undergo a craniotomy is discussed under Surgical Management in the Brain Tumor section.

Preventing and Detecting Secondary Brain Injury.
Take and record the patient's *vital signs* every 1 to 2 hours, or more often based on patient acuity. The primary health care provider may prescribe IV fluids or drug therapy to prevent severe hypertension or hypotension. Dysrhythmias and nonspecific ST-segment or T-wave changes may occur, possibly in response to stimulation of the autonomic nervous system or an increase in the level of circulating catecholamines (such as epinephrine) from the stress of trauma. *Document and report the presence of cardiac dysrhythmias, hypotension, and/or hypertension to the primary health care provider.* Obtain the target range for blood pressure and heart rate from the provider and monitor parameters.

The patient with a brain injury may develop a fever as a result of systemic trauma, blood in the cranium, a generalized inflammatory response to the injury, or from an infectious source. Fever from any cause is associated with higher morbidity and mortality rates. The occurrence of a neurogenic fever is rare, and all other sources of fever need to be ruled out. Maintenance of normothermia should be the goal and can be achieved by utilizing *targeted temperature monitoring (TTM).* TTM protocols allow the nurse to manage fever, evaluate effectiveness of

therapy, and manage any unwarranted side effects (e.g., shivering, electrolyte abnormalities). Shivering can be detrimental by increasing metabolic demand and may require the use of a paralytic agent and sedation. TTM can be implemented by using an invasive catheter placed by a health care provider or by the placement of an external cooling device to the body. Follow institutional guidelines on the management of TTM. The Brain Trauma Foundation and American College of Surgeons have developed TBI guidelines, and currently there is no evidence to support the use of prophylactic therapeutic hypothermia (<96.8°F [36°C]) in the management of TBI (Brain Trauma Foundation, 2022).

Arterial blood gas (ABG), oxygen saturation (SpO_2), and end-tidal carbon dioxide ($ETcO_2$) values are all used to evaluate respiratory status and guide mechanical ventilation therapy. Hyperventilation for the intubated patient during the first 24 hours after brain injury is usually avoided because it may produce ischemia by causing cerebral vasoconstriction. *Carbon dioxide is a very potent vasodilator that can contribute to increases in ICP.*

Prevent intermittent and sustained hypoxemia. Monitor peripheral oxygen saturation continuously in moderate to severe TBI. Hypoxemia damages brain tissue and contributes to cerebral vasodilation and increased ICP. Arterial oxygen levels (PaO_2) are maintained between 80 mm Hg and 100 mm Hg to prevent secondary injury. If available, hyperbaric oxygen therapy (HBOT) has been proposed as an adjunctive therapy; it uses high-dose oxygen to treat ischemia and hypoxia. HBOT is not FDA approved, but studies are being conducted worldwide to examine the feasibility and efficacy of using HBOT.

If the patient is intubated, provide 100% oxygen before and after each pass of the endotracheal suction catheter. Avoid overly aggressive hyperventilation with endotracheal suctioning because of the potential for hypocarbia. Cerebral ischemia caused by even transiently decreased oxygen and either high or low carbon dioxide levels contributes to secondary brain injury. Lidocaine given IV or endotracheally may be used to suppress the cough reflex; coughing increases ICP.

! NURSING SAFETY PRIORITY

Action Alert

Position the patient with TBI to avoid extreme flexion or extension of the neck and to maintain the head in the midline, neutral position. Log roll the patient during turning to avoid extreme hip flexion, and keep the head of the bed (HOB) elevated at least 30 degrees or as prescribed by the primary health care provider.

Generally, HOB elevation in patients with TBI is at 30 to 45 degrees to prevent aspiration. However, if increasing head elevation significantly lowers systemic blood pressure, the patient does not benefit from drainage of venous blood or CSF out of the skull from this position. If hypotension accompanies an elevated backrest position, the patient may be harmed. Avoid sudden vertical changes of the HOB in the older patient because the dura is tightly adhered to the skull and may pull away from the brain, leading to a subdural hematoma.

Patients with *severe* TBI often die. As the physiologic deterioration begins, keep in mind that the patient may be a potential organ donor. *Before* brain death is declared, contact the local organ-procurement organization. Determine whether the patient consented to be an organ donor. This information is typically on a driver's license or other state-issued card or advance directive. The patient's wishes should be followed unless the patient has a medical condition that prevents organ donation. The organ donor agency representative and/or primary health care provider discusses the possibility of organ procurement with the family. Some families may not agree with the patient's decision, which can cause an ethical dilemma. Many health care agencies have an ethics specialist or members of an ethics committee who can help with these situations.

Determining Brain Death. In 2010, the American Academy of Neurology guidelines for determining brain death were updated and remain the standard in the United States today. Four classic prerequisites must be met to establish a brain death diagnosis (Wijdicks et al., 2010):

- Coma of known cause as established by history, clinical examination, laboratory testing, and neuroimaging
- Normal or near-normal core body temperature [higher than 96.8°F (36°C)]
- Normal systolic blood pressure (higher than or equal to 100 mm Hg)
- At least one neurologic examination (many U.S. states and health care systems require two exams)

No consensus has been reached on who is qualified to perform head-to-toe brain-death neurologic examinations, but neurologists and critical care intensivists typically do them. Neuroimaging tests are not required to confirm brain death in most states or provinces, but are needed when a portion of the clinical exam or apnea test cannot be completed or uncertainty exists. It is important to note that there are different requirements between adults and children in determining brain death. Standard tests include four-vessel cerebral angiography and radionuclide cerebral perfusion scan; transcranial Doppler ultrasonography is gaining popularity and acceptance. Other tests that may be used are bedside electroencephalography (EEG), evoked potentials, cerebral computed tomography angiography (CTA), and/or magnetic cerebral angiography (Lewis & Kirschen, 2021).

Nurses need to be prepared to continue to provide intensive nursing care and to manage family grief reactions, including rejection of the diagnosis (Milliken & Uveges, 2020). Nursing is at the forefront to identify family conflict and guide ongoing communication among the health care team and family members. Early nursing interventions can include the engagement of pastoral care, a social worker, an ethics consultation, and palliative care.

Drug Therapy. *Mannitol*, an osmotic diuretic, is often used to treat cerebral edema by pulling water out of the extracellular space of the edematous brain tissue. It is most effective when given in boluses rather than as a continuous infusion. *Furosemide*, a loop diuretic, is often used as adjunctive therapy to reduce the incidence of rebound from mannitol. It also enhances the therapeutic action of mannitol, reduces edema and blood volume, decreases sodium uptake by the brain, and decreases the production of CSF at the choroid plexus.

Administer mannitol through a filter in the IV tubing or, if given by IV push, draw it up through a filtered needle to eliminate microscopic crystals. For the patient receiving either osmotic or loop diuretics, monitor for intake and output, severe dehydration, and indications of acute renal failure, weakness, edema, and changes in urine output. Serum electrolyte and osmolarity levels are measured every 6 hours. Mannitol is used to obtain a serum osmolarity of 310 to 320 mOsm/L, depending on primary health care provider preference and the desired outcome of therapy. Maintain strict measurement of output every hour. Check the patient's serum and urine osmolarity daily and sodium blood levels at regular intervals (Burchum & Rosenthal, 2022).

Hypertonic saline (HTS) is a hyperosmolar agent that can acutely reduce ICP and improve cerebral **perfusion** pressure, and works similarly to mannitol. The typical concentration used is 3% NaCl, but it can be as high as 23%. Nursing implications consist of continual neurologic assessments, monitoring of serial sodium concentrations and fluid status, and monitoring for pulmonary edema, especially if the patient has a history of cardiac or renal disease (Metheny & Moritz, 2021). Some organizations require an intensive care setting for close monitoring and a central line. The accompanying Evidence-Based Practice box summarizes a systematic review comparing the effect of mannitol when compared to hypertonic saline to reduce ICP.

📄 EVIDENCE-BASED PRACTICE

Is Hypertonic Saline or Mannitol the Best Treatment for Increased ICP?

DeNett, T., & Feltner, C. (2021). Hypertonic saline versus mannitol for the treatment of increased intracranial pressure in traumatic brain injury. *Journal of the American Association of Nurse Practitioners, 33*(4), 283–293. https://doi.org/10.1097/JXX.0000000000000340.

Increased intracranial pressure (ICP) occurring after traumatic brain injury (TBI) is associated with increased morbidity and mortality. If appropriate treatments are not initiated, brain herniation can occur and lead to death. A systematic review was completed to compare the efficacy of hypertonic saline (HTS) and mannitol in lowering ICP in patients with TBI. Four meta-analyses, three randomized controlled trials, and one retrospective cohort study met the inclusion criteria and were reviewed. The review found that HTS is an effective alternative to mannitol for increased ICP. Three of the studies suggested HTS may be superior to mannitol.

Level of Evidence: 1

The evidence in this paper was obtained in a systematic review using PubMed, Embase, CINAHL, and Web of Science.

Commentary: Implications for Practice and Research

Evidence demonstrates HTS to be as effective as mannitol for ICP reduction. Further research in a large multicenter clinical trial is needed to compare these two agents for superiority in the management of increased ICP. Providers should consider the properties of each agent, adverse effects, and potential benefits when selecting a hyperosmotic agent. Mannitol and HTS have similar effects on the treatment of ICP but can have serious side effects if monitored inappropriately. The nurse is in the position to monitor the infusion rate, frequency, and mode of administration of the selected hyperosmolar agent to obtain the best therapeutic effect, as well as to perform frequent patient assessments and recognize any side effects that require prompt evaluation.

Opioids such as fentanyl may be used with ventilated patients to decrease pain and control restlessness if the agitation is caused by pain. Fentanyl has fewer effects on blood pressure and heart rate than morphine and therefore may be a safer agent to manage pain for the patient with TBI. Propofol and midazolam (GABA-receptor agonists) provide sedation to decrease ICP but are not as effective for pain control. Most mechanically ventilated patients receive a combination of these drugs.

Maintaining or Managing Cognition, Sensory Perception, and Mobility

Planning: Expected Outcomes. The desired outcome is that the patient will not experience long-term decreased or altered *cognition, sensory perception,* and/or *mobility.* If alterations occur, the patient will receive rehabilitation services to achieve optimal functioning.

Interventions. An overwhelming majority of brain injury survivors have altered *cognition,* including decreased memory and impaired judgment. Cognitive impairments may interfere with the brain-injured patient's ability to function effectively in school, at work, and in personal life. *Cognitive rehabilitation* is a way of helping brain-injured patients regain function in areas that are essential for a return to independence and a reasonable quality of life.

If a large lesion of the parietal lobe is present, the patient may experience a loss of *sensory perception* for pain, temperature, touch, and proprioception, which prevents an appropriate response to environmental stimuli. A hazard-free environment is necessary to prevent injury (e.g., from burns if the patient's coffee is too hot). In collaboration with the rehabilitation therapist, integrate a sensory stimulation program into the comatose or stuporous patient's routine care activities. Sensory stimulation is done to facilitate a meaningful response to the environment. Present visual, auditory, or tactile stimuli one at a time, and explain the purpose and the type of stimulus presented. For example, show a picture of the patient's mother and say, "This is a picture of your mother." The picture is shown several times, and the same words are used to describe the picture. If auditory tapes or DVDs are used, they should be played no longer than 10 to 15 minutes. If the stimulus is presented for a longer period, it simply becomes "white noise" (meaningless background noise).

Some patients with TBI experience seizure activity as a result of primary or secondary brain injury. Be sure to initiate Seizure Precautions according to your agency's policy and procedure. Administer antiepileptic drugs (AEDs) to the patient as prescribed. Nursing care for patients experiencing seizures is described in Chapter 36.

Managing Traumatic Stress

Planning: Expected Outcomes. The desired outcome for the client who has a TBI is to develop strategies to cope with the traumatic event and receive appropriate care for adaptation and healing.

Interventions. The major role of the nurse and other members of the interprofessional health team is to recognize the effect of the trauma on the patient and utilize a trauma-informed approach to care. Trauma-informed care is an approach to health care involving understanding, acceptance, and support for victims of trauma through positive adaptation and healing. Effective nursing care requires an understanding of the patient's lived trauma experience. Demonstrating understanding may foster patient participation in care while helping patients meet their personal goals (Dowdell & Speck, 2022).

Trauma-informed care is built on six core principles, which nurses need to incorporate into their practice when caring for any patient who has experienced trauma (Dowdell & Speck, 2022):

- *Safety:* Patients who experience one or more traumatic events are often hypervigilant to environmental safety. Therefore, provide a safe space, including the environment, for the patient, without judgment regarding age, sexual orientation, gender identity, socioeconomic status, or social determinants of health. Be sure to ask patients how they want to be addressed.
- *Trustworthiness and transparency:* Transparency in communication helps to foster trust, which increases patients' participation in their care. Use clear, plain terminology, using knowledge of patients' health literacy, preferences, and values. Also consider the extent of their TBI and whether speech/language ability was affected.
- *Peer support:* Peer support for patients who survive trauma and their families usually includes other individuals who are trauma survivors. Assist patients and families to locate community resources for effective peer support to help them understand their experience and reaction to it.
- *Collaboration and mutual support:* Patients should be active partners in their care, including being supported about their health care decisions. For patients with a moderate to severe TBI, nurses need to be aware of the patients' goals and recognize that patients are experts on their lived trauma experience.
- *Empowerment:* This core principle is integral to all other principles in that patients should have a voice to make informed decisions about their care. Nurses and other health care staff should respect and support patients, even if they don't agree with their patients' decisions.
- *Culture and historical sensitivity:* Patients bring their life experiences, including a history of traumatic events, when they seek health care. Many patients who experienced one or more traumatic events have resulting emotional and mental health problems, including anxiety, depression, and insomnia. They may also employ harmful or unhealthy strategies, such as smoking, excess alcohol use, and overeating, to help cope with their stress. Be sure not to judge patients regarding their habits but help them develop more healthy behaviors by referring them to appropriate resources.

Care Coordination and Transition Management

The patient with a *mild* brain injury recovers at home after discharge from the emergency department (ED) or hospital (Box 38.8). Teach the patient who has sustained a *mild* brain injury that if signs and symptoms affecting physical, cognitive, or emotional functioning should occur, the patient should be referred to a health care provider trained in concussion management. Provide the patient and family with educational materials that will alert them to symptoms and management options.

The patient with a *moderate to severe* brain injury requires long-term case management and ongoing rehabilitation after hospitalization. Behavioral interventions are used by cognitive and brain injury rehabilitation specialists to help both the patient and family members develop adaptive strategies.

BOX 38.8 Patient and Family Education

Mild Traumatic Brain Injury

- For a headache, give acetaminophen every 4 hours as needed.
- Avoid giving the person sedatives, sleeping pills, or alcoholic beverages for at least 24 hours after TBI unless the primary health care provider instructs otherwise.
- Do not allow the person to engage in strenuous activity for at least 48 hours.
- Teach the caregiver to be aware that balance disturbances cause safety concerns and that the patient should provide for monitored or assisted movement.
- If any of these symptoms occur, take the person back to the emergency department or call 911 *immediately*:
  - Seizure
  - Severe, or worsening, headache
  - Persistent or severe nausea or vomiting
  - Blurred vision
  - Clear drainage from the ear or nose
  - Increasing weakness
  - Slurred speech
  - Progressive sleepiness
  - Unequal pupil size
- Keep follow-up appointments with the primary health care provider.

A number of specialized brain injury rehabilitation facilities are available in the United States and Canada. Some facilities offer noninvasive neuromodulation, which alters nerve activity through a targeted delivery of a stimulus to modulate abnormal neural pathway behavior caused by the injury (Bender Pape et al., 2020). Chapter 7 discusses interprofessional collaborative rehabilitative care in detail.

The major overall desired outcome for rehabilitation after brain injury is to maximize the patient's ability to return to the highest level of functioning. Activities such as occupational therapy, physical therapy, and speech-language therapy may continue in the home after discharge from the hospital or rehabilitation facility. Adaptation of the home environment to accommodate the patient safely may be needed. For example, smoke and fire alarms must function properly because the patient with a brain injury often loses the sense of smell. Home evaluations and referrals to outside agencies are completed before discharge. Be sure to refer the patient and family to the registered dietitian nutritionist for health teaching regarding healthy nutrition to prevent weight gain from decreased activity or stress eating. Many patients with TBI gain significant weight within a year of their injury, most likely because of inactivity.

Patients with personality and behavioral problems respond best to a structured and consistent environment. Instruct the family to develop a home routine that provides structure, repetition, and consistency. Remind the family about the importance of reinforcing positive behaviors rather than negative behaviors.

Most patients with *moderate to severe* TBI are discharged with varied long-term physical and cognitive disabilities. Changes in personality and behavior are very common. The patient and family must learn to cope with the patient's increased fatigue, irritability, temper outbursts, depression, loneliness, and memory problems. These patients often require constant supervision

at home, and families may feel socially isolated. Provide support and encouragement for the family and patient to help them get through each day.

Teach the family about the importance of regular respite care, either in a structured day-care respite program for the patient or through relief provided by a friend or neighbor. Family members, particularly the primary caregiver, may become depressed and have feelings of loneliness. In addition, they may feel angry with the patient because of the physical, financial, and emotional responsibilities that care has placed on them. To help the family cope with these problems, suggest that they join and actively participate in a local brain-injury support group.

Collaborate with the case manager to refer families and patients to local chapters of the Brain Injury Association of America (BIAA) (www.biausa.org) for information and support. The Brain Injury Association of Canada (www.braininjurycanada.ca) is available as a resource for patients in Canada. All of these organizations have a number of helpful publications on preventing and living with TBI. Other resources include religious, spiritual, and cultural leaders.

NCLEX Examination Challenge 38.3

Health Promotion and Maintenance

The nurse is teaching a client who recently experienced a mild traumatic brain injury about follow-up care at home. Which statement by the client indicates a need for further teaching?

A. "I can take acetaminophen every 4 hours as needed for headache."
B. "I should avoid taking any sedatives or alcohol for at least 24 hours."
C. "I should make an appointment for follow-up with my primary health care provider."
D. "I can go back to work as a construction worker as soon as I get home."

Evaluate Outcomes: Evaluation

Evaluate the care of the patient with TBI based on the identified priority problems. Expected outcomes are that the patient:

- Maintains cerebral tissue *perfusion*
- Learns to adapt to altered *mobility* and *sensory perception* changes, if any
- Has minimal alterations in *cognition* or understands how to compensate for *cognition* changes when necessary

BRAIN TUMORS

Brain tumors can arise anywhere within the brain structures and are named according to the cell or tissue where they originate; however, cerebral tumors are the most common. *Primary* tumors originate within the central nervous system (CNS) and rarely metastasize (spread) outside this area. *Secondary* brain tumors result from metastasis from other areas of the body, such as the lung, breast, kidney, skin, and GI tract.

Pathophysiology Review

Regardless of location, any tumor can expand and invade, infiltrate, compress, and displace normal brain tissue. Similar to the pathophysiologic changes that occur in patients with TBI, these changes can lead to cerebral edema or brain tissue inflammation, increased intracranial pressure (ICP), and neurologic deficits (focal or diffuse). In some cases, pituitary dysfunction can result. (See the Pathophysiology Review for TBI earlier in this chapter.)

Cerebral edema (vasogenic edema) results from changes in capillary endothelial tissue permeability that allows plasma to seep into the extracellular spaces. This leads to increased ICP and, depending on the location of the tumor, brain herniation syndromes. A variety of neurologic deficits result from edema, infiltration, distortion, and compression of surrounding brain tissue. The cerebral blood vessels may become compressed because of edema and increased ICP. This compression leads to ischemia (decreased blood flow) of the area supplied by the vessel. In addition, the tumor may enter the walls of the vessel, causing it to rupture and hemorrhage into the tumor bed or other brain tissue. Many patients who have brain tumors have headaches and seizures from interference with the brain's normal electrical activity.

Pituitary dysfunction may occur as the tumor compresses the pituitary gland and causes the syndrome of inappropriate antidiuretic hormone (SIADH) or arginine vasopressin deficiency (AVP-D) (central diabetes insipidus). These disorders result in severe fluid and electrolyte imbalances and can be life-threatening. (See Chapter 54 for a complete description of these disorders.)

Brain tumors are usually classified as benign, malignant, or metastatic. They may or may not be treated, depending on their location. Benign (noncancerous) tumors, such as meningiomas, can usually be removed and are generally associated with a positive outcome. Malignant or metastatic tumors, such as astrocytomas, require more aggressive intervention, including surgery, radiation, and/or chemotherapy.

A second classification system is based on location. Supratentorial tumors are located within the cerebral hemispheres above the tentorium (dural fold). Located beneath the tentorium is the infratentorial area (the area of the brainstem structures and cerebellum) where tumors may also occur (infratentorial tumors).

The exact cause of brain tumors is unknown. Several areas under investigation include genetic mutations and a variety of environmental factors. The use of cellular phones has been investigated as a cause of brain tumors, but findings are unconfirmed. Brain tumors account for a small percentage of all cancer deaths. Primary brain tumors are relatively uncommon, but many more patients have metastatic lesions. Malignant brain tumors are seen primarily in patients 40 to 70 years of age, and the survival rate is low compared with that of other cancers (Rogers, 2023).

Interprofessional Collaborative Care
Recognize Cues: Assessment
When possible, obtain a history from both the patient and family, including current signs and symptoms. A complete neurologic assessment is needed to establish baseline data and determine the nature and extent of neurologic deficits.

The signs and symptoms of brain tumors vary with the site of the tumor and are similar to those seen in patients with traumatic brain injury (TBI). In general, assess for these *common* symptoms of a brain tumor:

- Headaches that are usually more severe on awakening in the morning
- Nausea and vomiting
- Seizures (also called convulsions)
- Impaired *sensory perception,* such as facial numbness or tingling and visual changes
- Loss of balance or dizziness
- Weakness or paralysis in one part or one side of the body (hemiparesis or hemiplegia)
- Difficulty thinking, speaking, or articulating words
- Changes in *cognition,* mentation, or personality

Neurologic deficits result from the destruction, distortion, or compression of brain tissue. *Supratentorial (cerebral)* tumors usually result in paralysis, seizures, memory loss, cognitive impairment, language impairment, or vision problems. *Infratentorial* tumors produce ataxia, autonomic nervous system dysfunction, vomiting, drooling, hearing loss, and vision impairment. As the tumor grows, ICP increases, and the symptoms become progressively more severe.

Diagnosis is based on the history, neurologic assessment, clinical examination, and results of neurodiagnostic testing. Noninvasive diagnostic studies such as *CT* and *MRI scans* are conducted first. The CT scan can identify brain tissue abnormality, skull invasion, and bleeding quickly. Once an abnormality is found, an MRI The can identify more details about the tumor, including chemical composition, vascularity, extent of invasion, or whether a cellular wall is present. These details assist the neurosurgeon in deciding next steps—biopsy, complete or incomplete resection, or conservative management.

Take Actions: Interventions
Collaborative interventions depend on the type, size, and location of the tumor. For example, a small benign tumor may be monitored through CT and MRI scanning to assess its growth.

Nonsurgical Management. The desired outcomes of brain tumor management are to remove the tumor or decrease tumor size, improve quality of life, and improve survival time. The type of treatment selected depends on the tumor size and location, patient symptoms and general condition, and whether the tumor has recurred. In addition to traditional interventions, a number of experimental treatment modalities are being investigated. These include blood-brain barrier disruption, recombinant DNA, monoclonal antibodies, new chemotherapeutic drugs, and immunotherapy. Traditional *radiation therapy* may be used alone after surgery or in combination with chemotherapy and surgery. Chapter 18 discusses radiation treatment for patients with cancer.

Drug Therapy. The primary health care provider may prescribe a variety of drugs to treat the malignant or metastatic tumor, manage the patient's symptoms, and prevent complications. Chemotherapy may be given alone, in combination with radiation and surgery, and when tumors become larger. Although these drugs may control tumor growth or decrease tumor burden, the benefit does not last. Chemotherapy usually involves more than one agent that may be given orally, IV, intraarterially, and/or intrathecally through an Ommaya reservoir placed in a cranial ventricle. When given systemically, the drug must be lipid-soluble to cross the blood-brain barrier.

Commonly used oral drugs are lomustine, temozolomide (TMZ), procarbazine, and methotrexate. Vincristine may be given IV in combination with other drugs. Monitor for side effects of these drugs, which are similar to those of any chemotherapeutic drug. Chapter 18 describes general nursing implications for care of a patient receiving chemotherapy.

Direct drug delivery to the tumor is another treatment option. Disk-shaped drug wafers, such as carmustine, may be placed directly into the cavity created during surgical tumor removal (interstitial chemotherapy). This therapy is usually given for newly diagnosed high-grade malignant tumors, but recurrent tumors may also be treated with this method. Other drugs used are molecularly targeted. Examples include erlotinib, gefitinib, and bevacizumab (Burchum & Rosenthal, 2022).

Analgesics, such as codeine and acetaminophen, are given for headache. Dexamethasone is given to control cerebral edema. Levetiracetam or other antiepileptic drugs (AEDs) may be given to prevent seizure activity (see Chapter 36 for discussion of AEDs). Proton pump inhibitors may be administered to decrease gastric acid secretion and prevent the development of stress ulcers in high-risk patients.

Stereotactic Radiosurgery. Stereotactic radiosurgery (SRS) is an alternative to traditional surgery. Several techniques are used, including the modified linear accelerator (LINAC) using accelerated x-rays, a particle accelerator using beams of protons (cyclotron), and isotope seeds implanted in the tumor (brachytherapy). The Gamma Knife is a device that can be used in an SRS procedure, in which a single high dose of ionized radiation is used to focus multiple beams of gamma radiation produced by the radioisotope *cobalt-60* to destroy intracranial lesions selectively without damaging surrounding healthy tissue (Fig. 38.6). The Gamma Knife requires a frame to be attached to the skull to prevent any movement during the procedure. The procedure usually takes less than an hour to complete but may require general anesthesia and an overnight stay in the hospital.

Another system, called the *CyberKnife,* also uses the LINAC system to deliver high-energy x-ray photons, but is noninvasive and does not require a frame or general anesthesia. It can accommodate any form of patient movement (e.g., breathing, coughing) while delivering a precise, smaller treatment margin, allowing less exposure to healthy tissue. Patients can resume normal activity immediately after the treatment. Combining neurodiagnostic imaging tools, including MRI, CT, magnetic resonance angiography (MRA), and angiography, along with the Gamma Knife and CyberKnife, allows for precise localization of deep-seated or anatomically difficult lesions.

Both procedures are used primarily for brain tumors or arteriovenous malformations (AVMs) that are in a difficult location and therefore cannot be removed by craniotomy. These procedures may also be used with patients who decline conventional surgery, whose age and physical condition do not allow for general anesthesia, as an adjunct to radiation therapy, and for recurrent or residual AVMs or tumors after embolization or craniotomy.

Tumor Treating Fields. Tumor Treating Fields (TTFields) is a new technologic modality that delivers regional low-intensity, intermediate frequency-specific, alternating electric fields to a solid tumor. The therapy consists of placing transducers directly on the skin on opposite sides, directing alternating electric

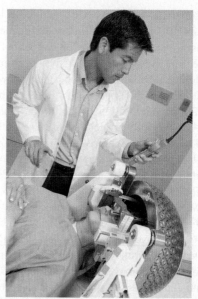

FIG. 38.6 A Gamma Knife treatment. The treatment beams are widely dispersed over the surface of the head to prevent damage to healthy brain tissue. The beams are intense only at the point of target. (© Getty Images. In Lampignano, J. P., & Kendrick, L. E. [2021]. *Bontrager's textbook of radiographic positioning and related anatomy* [10th ed.]. St. Louis: Elsevier.)

fields through the tumor and causing the cancer cells to slow or stop cell division, leading to death of the cancer cells and thus extending survival. The device is primarily used with patients diagnosed with glioblastoma multiforme (GBM).

GBM is a malignant primary tumor that arises from the astrocytes. This tumor represents only 1% of all primary tumors, but it grows rapidly and has no cure. The standard of care for GBM consists of surgical resection, chemotherapy, and radiation therapy. Overall survival is poor, with only 5% of patients surviving more than 5 years. In 2011, the FDA approved the use of TTFields in combination with the chemotherapeutic drug temozolomide (TMZ) for patients with recurrent GBM with a disease state refractory to surgical and radiation therapy.

Surgical Management. A craniotomy (surgical incision into the cranium to access the brain) may be performed to remove the tumor, improve symptoms related to the lesion, or decrease the tumor size (debulk). The challenge for the neurosurgeon is to remove the tumor as completely as possible without damaging normal tissue. Complete removal is possible with some benign tumors, which results in a "surgical cure." After surgery the patient is often admitted to the critical care unit or neurosurgical unit for frequent observation.

Preoperative Care. The patient having a craniotomy is typically very anxious about having the head opened and the brain exposed. Concerns are centered on the possibility of increased neurologic deficits after the surgery and the patient's self-image when part or all of the head is shaved. Provide reassurance that the surgeon will spare vital parts of the brain while removing or decreasing the size of the tumor. Teach the patient and family about what to expect immediately after surgery and throughout the recovery period. Some patients require short-term or long-term rehabilitation.

Other preoperative care is similar to that for any patient having surgery, as described in Chapter 9.

Operative Procedures. Surgery is performed under local or general anesthesia or sedation. Small tumors that are easily located may be removed by *minimally invasive surgery (MIS)*. For example, the transnasal approach using endoscopy can be performed for pituitary tumors. The patient has a short hospital stay and few complications after surgery. Stereotactic surgery using a rigid head frame can be done for tumors that are easily reached. This procedure requires only burr holes and local anesthesia because the brain has no sensory neurons for pain. Laser surgery can also be done.

For an *open traditional* craniotomy, the surgeon makes an incision along or behind the hairline after placing the patient's head in a skull fixation device. Several burr holes are drilled into the skull, and a saw is used to remove a piece of bone (bone flap) to expose the tumor area. The flap is stored carefully until the end of the procedure or for a later time. The tumor is located using imaging technology and removed or debulked (partially removed). After the tumor removal, the bone flap is replaced and held by small screws or bolts. A drain or monitoring device may be inserted. The surgeon creates a soft dressing "cap" over the top of the head to keep the surgical area clean and prevent the patient from touching the incision site.

Postoperative Care. The focus of postoperative care is to monitor the patient to detect changes in status and prevent or minimize complications, especially increased intracranial pressure (ICP).

! NURSING SAFETY PRIORITY

Action Alert

Assess neurologic and vital signs every 15 to 30 minutes for the first 4 to 6 hours after a craniotomy and then every hour. If the patient is stable for 24 hours, the frequency of these checks may be decreased to every 2 to 4 hours, depending on agency policy and the patient's condition. *Report immediately and document new neurologic deficits, particularly a decreased level of consciousness (LOC), motor weakness or paralysis, aphasia, decreased **sensory perception**, and sluggish pupil reaction to light!* Personality changes such as agitation, aggression, or passivity can also indicate worsening neurologic status.

Managing the Patient in the Immediate Postoperative Period. Periorbital edema and ecchymosis (bruising) around one or both eyes are not unusual and are treated with cold compresses to decrease swelling. Irrigate the affected eye(s) with warm saline solution or artificial tears to improve patient comfort. The patient in the critical care unit has routine cardiac monitoring because dysrhythmias may occur as a result of brain–autonomic nervous system–cardiac interactions or fluid and electrolyte imbalance.

Regardless of setting, ensure recording of the patient's intake and output for the first 24 hours. Anticipate fluid restriction to 1500 mL daily if there is pituitary involvement in either the tumor or surgical site and SIADH develops (see Chapter 54). Reposition the patient, being careful not to cause pressure on the operative site. Delegate or provide repositioning and deep

breathing every 2 hours. To prevent the development of venous thromboembolism (VTE), maintain intermittent sequential pneumatic devices until the patient ambulates.

For patients who have undergone *supratentorial* surgery, elevate the head of the bed 30 degrees or as tolerated to promote venous drainage from the head. *Position the patient to avoid extreme hip or neck flexion and maintain the head in a midline, neutral position to prevent increased ICP.* Turn the patient side to side or supine to prevent pressure injury and pneumonia.

Keep the patient with an *infratentorial* (brainstem) surgery flat or at 10 degrees, depending on the primary health care provider's prescription. Infratentorial approach is usually performed by a craniectomy (removal of pieces of bone), and the bone is not replaced, allowing space for any edema and preventing compression of the brainstem. Position the patient side-lying, alternating sides every 2 hours, for 24 to 48 hours or until ambulatory. This position prevents pressure on the neck-area incision site. It also prevents pressure on the internal tumor excision site from higher cerebral structures. Make sure that the patient remains on NPO status until awake and alert because edema around the medulla and lower cranial nerves may also cause vomiting and aspiration.

Check the head dressing every 1 to 2 hours for signs of drainage. Mark the area of drainage once during each shift for baseline comparison, although this practice varies by health care agency. A small or moderate amount of drainage is expected. Some patients may have a Hemovac or Jackson-Pratt drain in place for 24 to 72 hours after surgery. Measure the drainage every 8 hours, and record the amount and color. A typical amount of drainage is 30 to 50 mL every 8 hours. Follow the manufacturer's and neurosurgeon's instructions to maintain suction within the drain.

✚ NURSING SAFETY PRIORITY

Critical Rescue

After craniotomy, monitor the patient's dressing for excessive amounts of drainage. Report a saturated head dressing or drainage greater than 50 mL/8 hr immediately to the surgeon! *Monitor frequently for signs of increasing ICP!*

The usual laboratory studies monitored after surgery include complete blood count (CBC), serum electrolyte levels and osmolarity, and coagulation studies. Hormone and cortisol levels will be monitored with pituitary tumor surgery. The patient's hematocrit and hemoglobin concentration may be abnormally low from blood loss during surgery, diluted from large amounts of IV fluids given during surgery, or elevated if the blood was replaced. Hyponatremia (low serum sodium) may occur as a result of fluid volume overload, syndrome of inappropriate antidiuretic hormone (SIADH), or steroid administration.

Hypokalemia (low serum potassium) may cause cardiac irritability. Weakness, a change in LOC, and confusion are symptoms of hyponatremia and hypokalemia. Hypernatremia may be caused by meningitis, dehydration, or arginine vasopressin deficiency (AVP-D) (central diabetes insipidus). It manifests with muscle weakness, restlessness, extreme thirst, and dry mouth (see Chapter 54). Additional signs of dehydration such as decreased urinary output, thick lung secretions, and hypotension may be present. *Untreated hypernatremia can lead to seizure activity. DI should be considered if the patient voids large amounts of very dilute urine with an increasing serum osmolarity and electrolyte concentration.*

The patient may be mechanically ventilated for the first 24 to 48 hours after surgery to help manage the airway and maintain optimal oxygen levels. If the patient is awake or attempting to breathe at a rate other than that set on the ventilator, drugs such as propofol and fentanyl are given to treat pain and anxiety and promote rest and comfort. Suction the patient as needed. *Remember to hyperoxygenate the patient carefully before, during, and after suctioning!*

Drugs routinely given after surgery include antiepileptic drugs, histamine blockers or proton pump inhibitors for stress ulcer prevention, and glucocorticoids such as dexamethasone to reduce cerebral edema. Give acetaminophen for fever or mild pain. Antibiotics are typically prescribed to prevent infection during the immediate postoperative time or longer if a drain is present.

NCLEX Examination Challenge 38.4

Physiological Integrity

The nurse is caring for a client who returned from the PACU to the critical care unit following an open craniotomy to remove a frontal lobe malignant tumor. Which client finding would the nurse report to the surgeon or Rapid Response Team **immediately**?

A. Decline in level of consciousness
B. Report of headache
C. Drainage of 25 mL in 8 hours
D. Periorbital edema

Preventing and Managing Postoperative Complications. Postoperative complications are listed in Box 38.9. The major complications of *supratentorial* surgery are increased ICP from cerebral edema or hydrocephalus and hemorrhage.

Symptoms of *increased ICP* include severe headache, deteriorating LOC, restlessness, and irritability. Dilated pupils that are slow to react or nonreactive to light are late signs of increased ICP. Management of increased ICP is the same as that described under Interventions in the Traumatic Brain Injury section.

BOX 38.9 Postoperative Complications of Craniotomy

Early Postoperative Complications	Late Postoperative Complications
• Increased intracranial pressure (ICP)	• Wound infection
• Hematomas	• Meningitis
• Subdural hematoma	• Fluid and electrolyte imbalances
• Epidural hematoma	• Dehydration
• Subarachnoid hemorrhage	• Hyponatremia
• Hypovolemic shock	• Hypernatremia
• Hydrocephalus	• Seizures
• Respiratory complications	• Cerebrospinal fluid (CSF) leak
• Atelectasis	• Cerebral edema
• Hypoxia	
• Pneumonia	
• Neurogenic pulmonary edema	

Hydrocephalus (increased CSF in the brain) is caused by obstruction of the normal CSF pathway from edema, an expanding lesion such as a hematoma, or blood in the subarachnoid space. Rapidly progressive hydrocephalus produces the classic symptoms of increased ICP. Slowly progressive hydrocephalus manifests with headache, decreased LOC, irritability, blurred vision, and urinary incontinence. An intraventricular catheter may be placed to drain CSF during surgery or emergently after surgery for rapidly deteriorating neurologic function (ventriculostomy). If long-term treatment is required for chronic hydrocephalus, a surgical shunt is inserted to drain CSF to another area of the body. Additional information about shunts may be found in neuroscience nursing textbooks. Other complications listed in Box 38.9 are discussed in detail elsewhere in this chapter or this text.

Care Coordination and Transition Management

The patient with a brain tumor is managed at home if possible. Maintaining a reasonable quality of life is an important outcome for recovery and rehabilitation. Unless the patient has a significant degree of disability, no special preparation for home care is needed. Patients with hemiparesis need assistance to ensure that their home is accessible according to their method of *mobility* (e.g., cane, walker, or wheelchair). The environment should be made safe to prevent falls. For example, teach caregivers to remove scatter rugs and to place grab bars in the bathroom.

Information about the selection of rehabilitation or chronic care facility, if needed, can be obtained from the case manager (CM) or discharge planner. The selected facility should have experience in providing care for neurologically impaired patients. A psychologist should be available to provide input in the evaluation of the cognitive disabilities that the patient may have.

Seizures are a potential complication that can occur at any time for as long as 1 year or more after surgery. Provide the patient and family with information about seizure precautions and what to do if a seizure occurs. Teach the need for follow-up appointments to monitor for therapeutic levels of antiepileptic drugs (AEDs).

PATIENT-CENTERED CARE: CULTURE AND SPIRITUALITY

Malignant Brain Tumors

Be sure that the patient and family have access to resources for support. Discuss the ways in which they have coped with crises in the past, such as with the help of spiritual counselors or clergy. Provide hope and help them feel empowered to make the best decisions for their care and future. Listen to the patient's concerns, and offer ideas for other community resources, depending on the patient's specific needs. Psychological support is essential because of potential changes in self-esteem, potential decreases in ADL ability, and the prognosis for malignant brain tumors.

Refer the patient and the family or significant others to the American Brain Tumor Association (www.abta.org) or the National Brain Tumor Society (www.braintumor.org). The American Cancer Society (www.cancer.org) is also an appropriate community resource for patients with malignant tumors. In

Canada, the Brain Tumor Foundation of Canada (www.brain-tumour.ca) can be very useful for providing information and support to patients and their families who live there. Home care agencies are available to provide both the physical and rehabilitative care that the patient may need at home. Families should seek hospice services and palliative care if the patient has an untreatable or metastatic brain tumor and is terminally ill. (See Chapter 8 for additional information about end-of-life care.) Brain tumor support groups may also be a valuable asset to the patient and family.

GET READY FOR THE NEXT-GENERATION NCLEX® EXAMINATION!

Essential Nursing Care Points

Health Promotion/Disease Prevention

- The *Healthy People 2030* initiative recognizes the need for national attention to improve cardiovascular health and reduce deaths from heart disease and **stroke**. Specific objectives to help meet this goal include:
  - Increase the proportion of adult stroke survivors who participate in rehabilitation services.
  - Reduce stroke death (by controlling risk factors such as diabetes mellitus and high cholesterol).
- The CDC and other cardiovascular professional organizations recommend applying the ABCS of heart health *under medical supervision* to prevent strokes:
  - **A**spirin use when appropriate
  - **B**lood pressure control
  - **C**holesterol management
  - **S**moking cessation
- Blacks are twice as likely to smoke and have poorly controlled diabetes mellitus (DM) and hypertension when compared to Whites, making them more likely to die of stroke. Nurses need to identify specific determinants of health and educate people of color about the importance of managing DM and hypertension to prevent poor clinical outcomes.
- Nurses can educate the public on ways to decrease the incidence of **traumatic brain injury (TBI)** by using safe driving practices, such as wearing seat belts and never driving while impaired.
- Nurses should also educate individuals on the need to not drive or operate other riding devices when drinking alcohol or using drugs.
- Older adults need to take precautions to prevent falls, including creating a safe environment, to prevent TBI (see Chapter 4).

Chronic Disease Care

- Patients who are not candidates for emergency procedures that can resolve an evolving stroke usually have residual symptoms, such as aphasia, hemiplegia or hemiparesis, emotional lability, visual deficits, dysphagia, and incontinence.
- Residual symptoms of stroke depend on the extent and location of the injury.
- TBI can be mild, moderate, or severe. Mild TBI can result later in a chronic health problem called *postconcussion syndrome*.
- **Chronic traumatic encephalopathy (CTE)** is an uncommon degenerative brain disease that occurs most often in military veterans, athletes, and others who have experienced repetitive trauma to the brain.
- Residual symptoms of TBI depend on the extent and location of the injury.
- Veterans experience TBI (and often posttraumatic stress disorder [PTSD]) as a result of war blast injuries; be aware that other physical injuries often accompany the TBI, such as amputations and burns.

Regenerative or Restorative Care

- The priority for care of patients who experience a stroke or TBI is assessment of ABCs—*a*irway, *b*reathing, and *c*irculation—within the first 10 minutes after arriving to the emergency department (ED).
- Patients with residual stroke symptoms require an interprofessional care approach as part of the rehabilitation phase of care.
- The National Institutes of Health Stroke Scale (NIHSS) is a commonly used, valid, and reliable assessment tool that nurses complete as soon as possible after the patient arrives in the ED. This tool is used as one assessment to determine eligibility for IV fibrinolytics (Table 38.2).
- In addition to frequent monitoring of vital signs, carefully observe for signs of intracerebral hemorrhage and other signs of bleeding during administration of fibrinolytic drug therapy. Additional best practice nursing interventions are listed in Box 38.4.
- Endovascular procedures to improve *perfusion* include intraarterial thrombolysis using drug therapy, mechanical **embolectomy** (surgical blood clot [thrombosis] removal), and carotid stent placement.
- Nurses need to carefully monitor the patient's level of consciousness (LOC) following any neurologic cranial emergency, including stroke and TBI, because LOC decline is the first sign of increased intracranial pressure (ICP), a potentially life-threatening problem.
- Drug therapy using mannitol, hypertonic saline, and/or furosemide is used to decrease ICP when a patient has a major brain injury.
- Chemotherapy, stereotactic radiosurgery, and tumor treating fields are options to treat many brain tumors. In some cases, an open craniotomy is needed to remove or debulk the tumor.

Hospice/Palliative/Supportive Care

- For patients who require long-term symptom management or end-of-life stroke care, the nurse should refer the family to palliative care or hospice services. Chapter 8 provides a detailed description of end-of-life care and advance directives.
- Patients who have strokes or traumatic brain injury are often admitted to an inpatient rehabilitation unit or facility or skilled nursing facility and require continued or more complex nursing care and extensive physical, occupational, recreational, speech-language, or cognitive therapy. The expected outcome for rehabilitation is to maximize the patient's abilities in all aspects of life.
- Families should seek hospice services and palliative care if the patient has untreatable or metastatic brain tumor and is terminally ill.

Mastery Questions

1. The nurse is caring for a client receiving alteplase for an acute ischemic stroke. What is the **priority** nursing action for the client at this time?
   A. Position the client an upright sitting position.
   B. Monitor the client's heart rate frequently.
   C. Carefully observe for any indication of bleeding.
   D. Administer the drug based on the client's weight.

2. The nurse is preparing to administer mannitol for a client who sustained a severe traumatic brain injury this morning. Which of the following actions are appropriate for the nurse to take related to drug administration? **Select all that apply.**
   A. Document urinary output every 4 to 8 hours.
   B. Use a filtered needle if giving the drug via IV push.
   C. Monitor serum electrolyte levels daily.
   D. Monitor serum osmolality daily.
   E. Observe for symptoms of dehydration.

3. The nurse is observing a client with a mild traumatic brain injury for changes in level of consciousness (LOC). Which of the following client findings indicates an early change in LOC?
   A. Irritability
   B. Loss of reflexes
   C. Decorticate positioning
   D. Dizziness and vertigo

NGN Challenge 38.1

The nurse is caring for a 74-year-old diabetic client admitted to the ED.

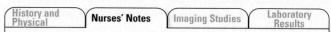

0655: Alert and oriented × 4; moves all extremities but states at home right arm felt weak and tingling. Now arm feels "more normal." PER-RLA; CNs intact. Lung sounds clear; S_1S_2 present. BS present × 4. Bilateral carotid bruits noted. T 99°F (37.2°C); HR 88 beats/min; RR 18 breaths/min; BP 168/92 mm Hg; Spo$_2$ 96% on RA. Long history of type 2 diabetes mellitus, hypertension, and alcohol use. 69-pack-year smoking history. Random nonfasting serum glucose = 231 mg/dL (12.8 mmol/L).

Complete the diagram by selecting from the choices below to specify what potential condition the client is likely experiencing, **2** nursing actions that are appropriate to take, and **2** parameters the nurse should monitor to assess the client's progress.

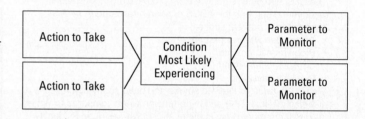

Actions to Take	Potential Conditions	Parameters to Monitor
Begin antiplatelet drug therapy	Traumatic brain injury	Platelet count
Administer supplemental oxygen therapy	Brain tumor	Serum glucose level
Anticipate potential carotid angioplasty with stenting	Acute ischemic stroke	Blood pressure
Give regular insulin per agency protocol	Transient ischemic attack	International Normalized Ratio
Change antihypertensive medication		Neurologic assessment

NGN Challenge 38.2

The nurse is caring for a 79-year-old client admitted to the neuroscience unit 2 days ago after falling at home and sustaining a head injury and fractured right humerus.

Vital Signs	Today	Yesterday	Admission Day
Temperature	99°F (37.2°C)	98.8°F (37.1°C)	98.8°F (37.1°C)
Heart rate	72 beats/min	70 beats/min	76 beats/min
Respiratory rate	20 breaths/min	18 breaths/min	18 breaths/min
Blood pressure	150/92 mm Hg	136/84 mm Hg	128/78 mm Hg
SpO2	95% on RA	96% on RA	96% on RA
Headache pain	5/10	5/10	4/10
GCS score	13	14	15

Tabs: History and Physical, Flow Sheet, Nurse's Notes, Laboratory Results

Complete the following sentence by selecting from the lists of options below.

The nurse analyzes the assessment findings and determines that the client most likely is experiencing **[1 Select]** as evidenced by **[2 Select]** and **[3 Select]** .

Options for 1	Options for 2	Options for 3
Epidural hematoma	Decreased SpO2	Decreased heart rate
Infection	Increased blood pressure	Increased headache pain
Increased intracranial pressure	Increased respiratory rate	Increased temperature
Stroke	A history of falling	Decreased GCS score

REFERENCES

Asterisk (*) indicates a classic or definitive work on this subject.

Altavilla, R., Caso, V., Bandini, F., Agnelli, G., Tsivgoulis, G., Yaghi, S., et al. (2019). Anticoagulation After Stroke in Patients with Atrial Fibrillation: To Bridge or Not With Low-Molecular-Weight Heparin? Stroke, 50(8), 2093–2100. https://doi.org/10.1161/STROKEAHA.118.022856.

Bender Pape, T., Herrold, A., Guernon, A., Aaronson, A., & Rosenow, J. (2020). Neuromodulatory interventions for traumatic brain injury. Journal of Head Trauma Rehabilitation, 35(6), 365–370. https://doi.org/10.1097/HTR.0000000000000643.

Brain Trauma Foundation. (2022). Management of severe traumatic brain injury. https://www.guidelinescentral.com/guideline/24234/#.

Burchum, J. L. R., & Rosenthal, L. D. (2022). Lehne's pharmacology for nursing care (11th ed.). St. Louis: Elsevier.

Camicia, M., Lutz, B., Summers, D., Klassman, L., & Vaughn, S. (2021). Nursing's role in successful stroke care transitions across the continuum: From acute care into the community. Stroke, 52(12), 794–805.

Centers for Disease Control and Prevention (CDC). (2021a). Stroke facts. www.cdc.gov/stroke/facts,htm.

Centers for Disease Control and Prevention (CDC). (2021b). Stroke signs & symptoms. https://www.cdc.gov/stroke/signs_symptoms.htmCenters for Disease Control and Prevention.

Centers for Disease Control and Prevention (CDC). (2021c). Heads Up. https://www.cdc.gov/headsup/index.html.

Centers for Disease Control and Prevention (CDC). (2021d). Traumatic brain injury: Get the facts. https://www.cdc.gov/traumatic-braininjury/get_the_facts.html.

DeNett, T., & Feltner, C. (2021). Hypertonic saline versus mannitol for the treatment of increased intracranial pressure in traumatic brain injury. Journal of the American Association of Nurse Practitioners, 33(4), 283–293. https://doi.org/10.1097/JXX.0000000000000340.

Dowdell, E. B., & Speck, P. M. (2022). Trauma-informed care in nursing practice. American Journal of Nursing, 122(4), 30–38.

Elliott, B., Chargualaf, K. A., & Patterson, B. (2021). Veteran-centered care in education and practice. New York, NY: Springer Publishing.

Green, T., McNair, N., Hinkle, J., Middleton, S., Miller, E., Perrin, S., et al. (2021). Care of the patient with acute ischemic stroke (Posthyperacute and Prehospital Discharge): Update to 2009 Comprehensive Nursing Care Scientific Statement. Stroke, 52, 00–00. https://doi.org/10.1161/STR.0000000000000357.

*Interprofessional Education Collaborative Expert Panel. (2016). Core competencies for interprofessional collaborative practice: Report of an expert panel (2nd ed.). Washington, D.C: Interprofessional Education Collaborative.

Lewis, A., & Kirschen, M. (2021). Brain Death/Death by Neurologic Criteria Determination. Neurocritical Care, 27(5), 1444–1464. https://doi.org/10.1212/CON.0000000000000987.

May, T., Foris, L., & Donnally, C., III. (2021). Second Impact Syndrome. [Updated 2021 Jul 6]. In: StatPearls [Internet]. Treasure Island (FL): StatPearls Publishing. Available from: https://www.ncbi.nlm.nih.gov/books/NBK448119/.

Metheny, N., & Moritz, M. (2021). Administration of 3% Sodium Chloride Via a Peripheral Vein. Journal of Infusion Nursing, 44(2), 94–102. https://doi.org/10.1097/NAN.0000000000000420Miller.

Milliken, A., & Uveges, M. (2020). Brain death: History, updates, and implications for nurses. American Journal of Nursing, 120(3), 32–38.

Office of Disease Prevention and Health Promotion. (n.d.). Heart disease and stroke. https://health.gov/healthypeople/objectives-and-data/browse-objectives/heart-disease-and-stroke.

Oh, E., Lee, H. J., Yang, Y. L., & Kim, Y. M. (2021). Effectiveness of discharge education with the teach-back method on 30-day readmission: A systematic review. Journal of Patient Safety, 17(4), 305–310. https://doi.org/10.1097/PTS.0000000000000596.

Pagana, K. D., Pagana, T. J., & Pagana, T. N. (2022). Mosby's manual of diagnostic and laboratory tests (7th ed.). St. Louis: Elsevier.

Powers, W.J., Rabinstein, A.A., Ackerson, T., Adeoye, O.M., Bambakidid, N.C., Becker, K., et al. (2019). American Heart Association/American Stroke Association Guideline: 2019 Update to the 2018 guidelines for the early management of patients with acute ischemic stroke—A guideline for healthcare professionals from the American Heart Association/American Stroke Association. Retrieved from https://www.ahajournals.org/doi/pdf/10.1161/STR.0000000000000211. https://strokeassociation.org/idc/groups/stroke-public/@wcm/@hcm/@sta/documents/downloadable/ucm_499252.pdf.

Rogers, J. L. (2023). *McCance and Huether's Pathophysiology: The biologic basis for disease in adults and children* (9th ed.). St. Louis: Mosby.

Slusser, M., Garcia, L. I., Reed, C.-R., & McGinnis, P. Q. (2019). *Foundations of interprofessional collaborative practice in health care*. St. Louis: Elsevier.

Smeltzer, S. C. (2021). Delivering quality healthcare for people with disability. Indianapolis. In *Sigma Theta Tau International Honor Society of Nursing*.

Stroke Awareness Foundation. (2021). *Stroke facts & statistics*. https://www.strokeinfo.org/stroke-facts-statistics/.

The Joint Commission. (2021). Stroke. https://www.jointcommission.org/measurement/measures/stroke/. http://www.jointcommission.org/specifications_manual_for_national_hospital_inpatient_quality_measures.aspx.

Towfighi, A., Benson, R. T., Tagge, R., Moy, C. S., Wright, C. B., & Ovbiagele, B. (2020). Inaugural health equity and actionable disparities in stroke: Understanding and problem-solving symposium. *Stroke, 51*(1), 3382–3391.

*Vacca, V. M., & Argenti, I. (2018). Chronic subdural hematoma: A common complexity. *Nursing, 48*(5), 25–31 2018.

Washington, H., Glaser, K., & Ifejika, N. (2021). Acute ischemic stroke. *American Journal of Nursing, 121*(9), 26–33. https://doi.org/10.1097/01.NAJ.0000790184.66496.1d.

Wells-Pittman, J., & Gullicksrud, A. (2020). Standardizing the frequency of neurologic assessment after acute stroke. *American Journal of Nursing, 120*(3), 48–54.

*Wijdicks, E. F., Varelas, P. N., Gronseth, G. S., Greer, D. M., et al. (2010). Evidence-based guideline update: Determining brain death in adults: Report of the quality standards subcommittee of the American Academy of Neurology. *Neurology, 74*(23), 1911–1918.

Wilcock, A., Schwamm, L., Zubizarreta, J., Zachrison, K., Uscher-Pines, L., Richard, J., et al. (2021). Reperfusion treatment and stroke outcomes in hospitals with telestroke capacity. *JAMA Neurology*, Mar 1;[e-pub]. https://doi.org/10.1001/jamaneurol.2021.0023.

Williamson, C., & Rajajee, V. (2023). Traumatic brain injury: Epidemiology, classification, and pathophysiology. *UpToDate*. Retrieved February 16, 2023, from https://www.uptodate.com/contents/traumatic-brain-injury-epidemiology-classification-and-pathophysiology.

Assessment and Concepts of Care for Patients With Eye and Vision Conditions

Cherie R. Rebar

http://evolve.elsevier.com/Iggy/

LEARNING OUTCOMES

1. Use knowledge of anatomy and physiology to perform a focused assessment related to visual *sensory perception.*
2. Teach evidence-based health promotion activities to help prevent visual problems and eye trauma.
3. Explain how genetic implications and physiologic aging affect visual *sensory perception.*
4. Plan collaborative care with the interprofessional team to promote *sensory perception* in patients with eye and vision problems.
5. Teach the patient and caregiver(s) about common drugs and other management strategies used for eye and vision problems.
6. Plan patient- and family-centered nursing interventions to decrease the psychosocial impact caused by living with eye and vision problems.
7. Apply knowledge of anatomy, physiology, and pathophysiology to provide evidence-based care for patients with eye and vision problems affecting *sensory perception.*
8. Analyze assessment and diagnostic findings to generate solutions and prioritize nursing care for patients with eye and vision problems.
9. Organize care coordination and transition management for patients with eye and vision problems.
10. Use clinical judgment to plan evidence-based nursing care to promote *sensory perception* and prevent complications in patients with eye and vision problems.
11. Incorporate factors that affect health equity into the plan of care for patients with eye and vision problems.

KEY TERMS

angle-closure glaucoma (ACG) A form of glaucoma that can have a sudden onset and is an emergency; characterized by a forward displacement of the iris, which presses against the cornea and closes the chamber angle, suddenly preventing outflow of aqueous humor. Also known as *primary angle-closure glaucoma (PACG), closed-angle glaucoma, narrow-angle glaucoma,* or *acute glaucoma.*

arcus senilis An opaque, bluish-white ring within the outer edge of the cornea.

cataract A lens opacity that distorts the image projected onto the retina.

enucleation Surgical removal of the entire eyeball.

glaucoma A condition in the eye that occurs with increased pressure and resulting hypoxia of photoreceptors and their synapsing nerve fibers.

hyperopia Farsightedness.

keratoconus Degeneration of the cornea.

keratoplasty Corneal transplant. The surgical removal of diseased corneal tissue and replacement with tissue from a human donor cornea.

macular degeneration Degeneration of the macula causing reduced central vision.

myopia Nearsightedness.

open-angle glaucoma (OAG) The most common form of glaucoma in the United States; characterized by increase in intraocular pressure due to reduced outflow of aqueous humor through the chamber angle. Also known as *primary open-angle glaucoma (POAG).*

photophobia Sensitivity to light.

presbyopia Age-related farsightedness.

retinal detachment The separation of the retina from the epithelium.

retinal hole A break in the retina, often caused by trauma or aging.

retinal tear A jagged and irregularly shaped break in the retina, which can result from traction on the retina.

secondary glaucoma Type of glaucoma that develops as a result of another health condition or trauma.

Vision is often thought of as most important sense. It helps people to assess surroundings; recognize danger; appreciate beauty; function as independently as possible; and work, play and interact with others. *Sensory perception* is the ability to perceive and interpret sensory input into one or more meaningful responses (see Chapter 3). Changes in the eye and vision can provide information about the patient's general health status and problems that might occur in self-care.

ANATOMY AND PHYSIOLOGY REVIEW

Visual *sensory perception* takes place when the eye and brain work together. Vision begins when light is changed into nerve impulses in the eye and the impulses are sent on to the brain to fully perceive images (Rogers, 2023). Systemic conditions and eye problems can change vision temporarily or permanently.

Structure

The eyeball, a round, ball-shaped organ, is located in the front part of the eye orbit. The orbit is the bony socket of the skull that surrounds and protects the eye along with the attached muscles, nerves, vessels, and tear-producing glands.

Layers of the Eyeball

The eye has three layers (Fig. 39.1). The external layer is the sclera (sometimes called the "white" of the eye) and the transparent cornea on the front of the eye.

The middle layer, or *uvea*, is heavily pigmented and consists of the choroid, the ciliary body, and the iris. The choroid, a dark brown membrane between the sclera and the retina, lines most of the sclera. It has many blood vessels that supply nutrients to the retina.

The ciliary body connects the choroid with the iris and secretes aqueous humor. The *iris* is the colored portion of the external eye; its center opening is the *pupil*. The muscles of the iris contract and relax to control pupil size and the amount of light entering the eye.

The innermost layer is the *retina*, a thin, delicate structure made up of sensory photoreceptors that begin the transmission of impulses to the optic nerve (Rogers, 2023). The retina contains blood vessels and two types of photoreceptors called *rods* and *cones*. The rods work at low light levels and provide peripheral vision. The cones are active at bright light levels and provide color and central vision.

The *optic fundus* is the area at the inside back of the eye that can be seen with an ophthalmoscope. This area contains the *optic disc*, a pinkish-orange or white depressed area where the nerve fibers that synapse with the photoreceptors join together to form the optic nerve and exit the eyeball. The optic disc contains only nerve fibers and no photoreceptor cells. To one side

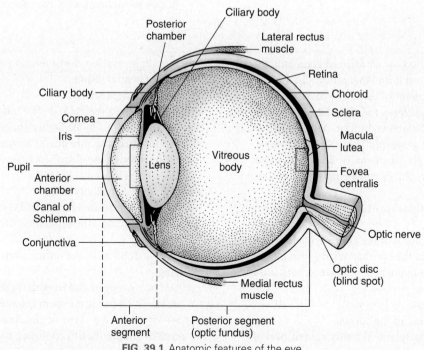

FIG. 39.1 Anatomic features of the eye.

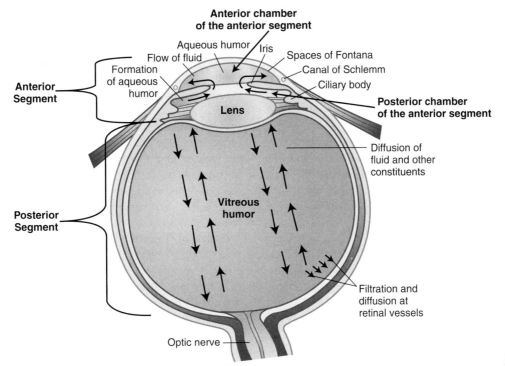

FIG. 39.2 Flow of aqueous humor.

of the optic disc is a small, yellowish pink area called the *macula lutea*. The center of the macula is the *fovea centralis*, where vision is most acute.

Refractive Structures and Media

Light waves pass through the cornea, aqueous humor, lens, and vitreous humor on the way to the retina. Each structure bends *(refracts)* the light waves to focus images on the retina. Together these structures are the eye's *refracting media.*

The *cornea* is the clear layer that forms the external bump on the front of the eye (see Fig. 39.1). The *aqueous humor* is a clear, watery fluid that fills the anterior and posterior chambers of the eye. This fluid is continually produced by the ciliary processes and passes from the posterior chamber, through the pupil, and into the anterior chamber. This fluid drains through the canal of Schlemm into the blood to maintain a balanced intraocular pressure (IOP), the pressure within the eye (Fig. 39.2).

The *lens* is a circular, convex structure that lies behind the iris and in front of the vitreous body. It is transparent and bends the light rays entering through the pupil to focus properly on the retina. The curve of the lens changes to focus on near or distant objects. A cataract is a lens opacity that distorts the image projected onto the retina.

The *vitreous body* is a clear, thick gel that fills the large vitreous chamber (the space between the lens and the retina). This gel transmits light and maintains eye shape.

The eye is a hollow organ and must be kept in the shape of a ball for vision to occur. To maintain this shape, the vitreous humor gel in the posterior segment and the aqueous humor in the anterior segment must be present in set amounts that apply pressure inside the eye to keep it inflated. This pressure is the *intraocular pressure (IOP).*

IOP has to be precisely accurate. If the pressure is too low, the eyeball is soft and collapses, preventing light from getting to the photoreceptors on the retina in the back of the eye. If the pressure becomes too high, the extra pressure compresses capillaries in the eye and nerve fibers. Pressure on retinal blood vessels prevents blood from flowing through them; therefore the photoreceptors and nerve fibers become hypoxic. Compression of the fine nerve fibers prevents intracellular fluid flow, which also reduces nourishment to the distal portions of these thin nerve fibers. Glaucoma occurs with increased pressure and resulting hypoxia of photoreceptors and their synapsing nerve fibers. Continued retinal hypoxia results in necrosis and death of photoreceptors, as well as permanent nerve fiber damage. Blindness occurs when photoreceptor and nerve fiber loss occur.

External Structures

The eyelids are thin, movable skinfolds that protect the eyes and keep the cornea moist. The *canthus* is the place where the two eyelids meet at the corner of the eye.

The *conjunctivae* are the mucous membranes of the eye. The palpebral conjunctiva is a thick membrane with many blood vessels that lines the undersurface of each eyelid. The thin, transparent bulbar conjunctiva covers the entire front of the eye.

A small *lacrimal gland,* which is located in the upper outer part of each orbit (Fig. 39.3), produces tears. Tears flow across the front of the eye, toward the nose, and into the inner canthus. They drain through the *punctum* (an opening at the nasal side of the lid edges) into the lacrimal duct and sac and then into the nose through the nasolacrimal duct.

Muscles, Nerves, and Blood Vessels

Six voluntary muscles rotate the eye and coordinate eye movements (Fig. 39.4 and Box 39.1). Coordinated eye movements ensure that both eyes receive an image at the same time so that only a single image is seen.

The muscles around the eye are innervated by cranial nerves (CNs) III (oculomotor), IV (trochlear), and VI (abducens). The *optic nerve* (CN II) is the nerve of sight, connecting the optic disc to the brain. The trigeminal nerve (CN V) stimulates the blink reflex when the cornea is touched. The facial nerve (CN VII) innervates the lacrimal glands and muscles for lid closure.

The ophthalmic artery brings oxygenated blood to the eye and the orbit. It branches to supply blood to the retina. The ciliary arteries supply the sclera, choroid, ciliary body, and iris. Outflow moves through several venous pathways that empty into the superior ophthalmic vein.

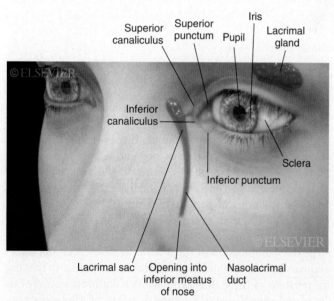

FIG. 39.3 Front view of the eye and adjacent structures. (From Elsevier Animation Gallery)

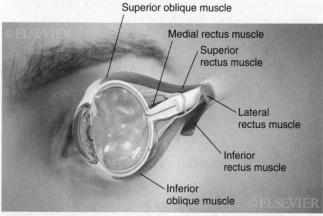

FIG. 39.4 Extraocular muscles. (From Elsevier Animation Gallery.)

Function

The four eye functions that provide clear images and vision are refraction, pupillary constriction, accommodation, and convergence.

Refraction bends light rays from the outside into the eye through curved surfaces and refractive media and finally to the retina. Each surface and medium bends (refracts) light differently to focus an image on the retina. *Emmetropia* is the perfect refraction of the eye in which light rays from a distant source are focused into a sharp image on the retina. Fig. 39.5 shows the normal refraction of light within the eye. Images fall on the retina inverted and reversed left to right. For example, an object in the lower nasal visual field strikes the upper outer area of the retina.

Errors of refraction are common. Hyperopia (farsightedness) occurs when the eye does not refract light enough. As a result, images converge behind the retina (see Fig. 39.5). In hyperopia, distant vision is normal, but near vision is poor. It is corrected with a convex lens in eyeglasses or contact lenses.

Myopia (nearsightedness) occurs when the eye overbends the light and images converge in front of the retina (see Fig. 39.5). Near vision is normal, but distance vision is poor. Myopia is corrected with a concave lens in eyeglasses or contact lenses.

Astigmatism is a refractive error caused by unevenly curved surfaces on or in the eye, especially the cornea. These uneven surfaces distort vision.

Pupillary constriction (miosis) and pupillary dilation (mydriasis) (Fig. 39.6) control the amount of light that enters the eye.

BOX 39.1 Functions of Ocular Muscles

Superior Rectus Muscle
- Together with the lateral rectus, this muscle moves the eye diagonally upward toward the side of the head.
- Together with the medial rectus, this muscle moves the eye diagonally upward toward the middle of the head.

Lateral Rectus Muscle
- Together with the medial rectus, this muscle holds the eye straight.
- Contracting alone, this muscle turns the eye toward the side of the head.

Medial Rectus Muscle
- Contracting alone, this muscle turns the eye toward the nose.

Inferior Rectus Muscle
- Together with the lateral rectus, this muscle moves the eye diagonally downward toward the side of the head.
- Together with the medial rectus, this muscle moves the eye diagonally downward toward the middle of the head.

Superior Oblique Muscle
- Contracting alone, this muscle pulls the eye downward.

Inferior Oblique Muscle
- Contracting alone, this muscle pulls the eye upward.

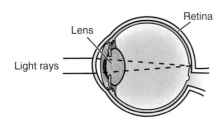

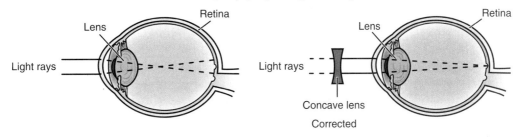

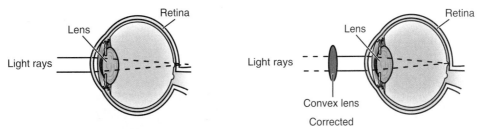

FIG. 39.5 Refraction and correction in emmetropia (A), myopia (B), and hyperopia (C). (From Banasik, J. [2022]. Pathophysiology [7th ed.]. St. Louis: Elsevier.)

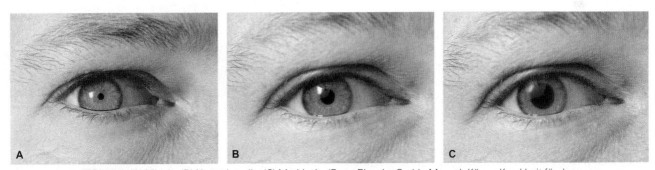

FIG. 39.6 (A) Miosis. (B) Normal pupils. (C) Mydriasis. (From Elsevier Gmbh, Mensch Körper Krankheit für den Rettungsdienst, 4. Auflage, 2022, Elsevier.)

If the level of light to one or both eyes is increased, both pupils constrict (become smaller). The amount of constriction depends on how much light is available and how well the retina can adapt to light changes. Certain drugs can alter pupillary constriction.

The process of maintaining a clear visual image when the gaze is shifted from a distant to a near object is known as *accommodation*. The healthy eye can adjust its focus by changing the curve of the lens.

Convergence is the ability to turn both eyes inward toward the nose at the same time. This action helps ensure that only a single image of close objects is seen.

Eye Changes Associated With Aging

Visual acuity decreases with age due to changes inside the eye (Touhy & Jett, 2023). Age-related changes of the nervous system and in the eye support structures also reduce visual function

PATIENT-CENTERED CARE: OLDER ADULT HEALTH

Changes in the Eye and Vision Related to Aging

Structure/Function	Change	Nursing Implications
Appearance	Eyes appear "sunken." Arcus senilis forms. Sclera yellows or appears blue.	Do not use eye appearance as an indicator of hydration status. Reassure that this change does not affect vision. Do not use sclera to assess for jaundice.
Cornea	Cornea flattens, which blurs vision and can cause or worsen astigmatism.	Encourage having annual eye examinations and wearing prescribed corrective lenses for best vision.
Ocular muscles	Muscle strength is reduced, making it more difficult to maintain an upward gaze or a focus on a single image.	Reassure that this is a normal finding and to refocus gaze frequently to maintain a single image.
Lens	Elasticity is lost, increasing the near point of vision (making the near point of best vision farther away). Lens hardens, compacts, and forms a cataract.	Encourage use of corrective lenses for reading. Emphasize the importance of annual eye examinations.
Iris and pupil	Decrease in ability to dilate results in small pupil size and poor adaptation to darkness.	Teach that good lighting is needed to avoid bumping into objects, tripping, and falling.
Color vision	Discrimination among greens, blues, and violets decreases.	Assess for any color-coded tools that are used for health purposes (e.g., does the patient use a color-coded medication dispenser? If so, it may be difficult to correctly distinguish colors that correspond with doses.)
Tears	Tear production is reduced, resulting in dry eyes, discomfort, and increased risk for corneal damage or eye infections.	Teach the proper use of lubricant eyedrops to reduce dryness. Teach to increase humidity in the home.

(see the Patient-Centered Care: Older Adult Health—Changes in the Eye and Vision Related to Aging box).

Structural changes occur with aging, including decreased eye muscle tone that reduces the ability to keep the gaze focused on a single object. The lower eyelid may relax and fall away from the eye *(ectropion)*, leading to dry eye signs and symptoms.

Arcus senilis, an opaque, bluish-white ring within the outer edge of the cornea, is caused by fat deposits (Fig. 39.7). This change does not affect vision.

Fatty deposits cause the sclera to develop a yellowish tinge. A bluish color may be seen as the sclera thins. With age, the iris has less ability to dilate, which leads to difficulty in adapting to dark environments. Older adults may benefit from additional light for reading and other "close-up" work and to avoid tripping over objects.

Functional changes also occur with aging. The lens yellows, hardens, shrinks, and loses elasticity, which reduces accommodation. The near point of vision (i.e., the closest distance at which the eye can see an object clearly) increases. Near objects, especially reading material, must be placed farther from the eye to be seen clearly (presbyopia). The far point (i.e., the farthest point at which an object can be distinguished) decreases. Together these changes narrow the visual field of an older adult.

General color perception decreases, especially for green, blue, and violet. More light is needed to stimulate the visual receptors. Intraocular pressure (IOP) is slightly higher in older adults.

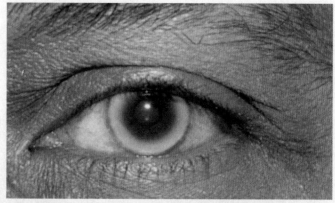

FIG. 39.7 Arcus senilis. (From Swartz, M. H. [2021]. *Textbook of physical diagnosis: History and examination* [8th ed]. St. Louis: Elsevier.)

Health Promotion/Disease Prevention

Impairment of vision impacts physical and psychological well-being and is identified as one of the top 10 disabilities in the United States (Centers for Disease Control and Prevention [CDC], 2022a). Many vision and eye problems can be avoided, and others can be corrected or managed if found early. Teach all adults about eye-protection methods, adequate nutrition that supports eye health, and the importance of regular eye examinations (See the Patient-Centered Care: Health Equity box.).

The risks for cataract formation and for cancer of the eye (ocular melanoma) increase with exposure to ultraviolet (UV)

PATIENT-CENTERED CARE: HEALTH EQUITY

Promoting Eye Health

Evidence shows that people with lower levels of education, food insecurity, financial concerns, and health care coverage through Medicaid are more likely to experience vision loss (CDC, 2022b). Advocate for all patients to gain timely access to eye examinations and eye health resources.

light. Teach adults to protect the eyes by using sunglasses that filter UV light whenever they are outdoors, at tanning salons, and when work involves UV exposure.

Vision can be affected by eye injury, which increases the risk for cataract formation and glaucoma. Teach adults to wear eye and head protection when working with particulate matter, fluid or blood spatter, high temperatures, or sparks. Protection should also be worn during participation in sports or any activity that increases the risk for the eye being hit by objects in motion. Teach adults to avoid rubbing the eyes to avoid trauma to outer eye surfaces.

Eye infections can lead to vision loss. Although the eye surface is not sterile, the sclera and cornea have no separate blood supply and therefore are at risk for infection. Teach adults to wash their hands before touching the eye or eyelid. Teach patients who use eyedrops about the proper technique to use these drugs and to not share eyedrops with others. If an eye has a discharge, teach the patient to use a separate eyedrop bottle for this eye and to wash the unaffected eye before washing the affected eye.

Other health problems, especially diabetes and hypertension, can seriously affect visual *sensory perception.* Teach patients with these conditions about the importance of controlling blood glucose levels and managing blood pressure to reduce the risk for vision loss. Annual evaluation by an eye care provider is needed to prevent eye complications and detect problems early. See Box 39.2 for specific recommendations about how often patients should be seen by an eye care provider for a general eye examination.

Eye care providers may recommend that adults older than 40 years have an eye examination annually that includes assessment of intraocular pressure and visual fields because the risk for both glaucoma and cataract formation increases with age.

! NURSING SAFETY PRIORITY

Action Alert

Teach adults to see a health care provider immediately when an eye injury occurs or an eye infection is suspected.

NCLEX Examination Challenge 39.1

Health Promotion and Maintenance

The nurse is caring for a healthy 54-year-old client presenting for an annual physical. The nurse would recommend that the client have an eye examination how frequently?

A. Once every year
B. Every 2 to 4 years
C. Every 3 to 5 years
D. Only when vision problems occur

BOX 39.2 Best Practice for Patient Safety and Quality Care

Basic Eye Examination Frequency

Age	Recommended Frequency
20–39 years, in good health with normal vision	Once in the 20s and once in the 30s unless there is an instance of visual impairment, infection, injury, eye pain, or diabetes **NOTE:** For people in this age category who wear contacts, annual examination is recommended.
20–39 years, Black	Every 2–4 years
20–39 years, White	Every 3–5 years
40–64 years, people of any race	Every 2–4 years
65 years and older, people of any race	Every 1–2 years
People with special risks (e.g., diabetes, eye surgery or trauma, glaucoma)	As recommended by the eye care provider (may be more frequent)

Adapted from American Academy of Ophthalmology. (2022). *Eye exam and vision testing basics.* <https://www.aao.org/eye-health/tips-prevention/eye-exams-101>; and PreventBlindness.org. (2022). *How often should I have an eye examination?* https://www.preventblindness.org/how-often-should-i-have-eye-exam.

RECOGNIZE CUES: ASSESSMENT

Patient History

General History

Collect information to determine whether problems with the eye or vision have an impact on ADLs or other daily functions.

Age is an important factor to consider when assessing visual *sensory perception* and eye structure. The incidence of glaucoma and cataract formation increases with aging. Presbyopia commonly begins in the 40s.

Sex assigned at birth may be important. Retinal detachments occur more often in men, and dry eye syndromes occur more often in women.

Occupation and leisure activities can affect eye health. Ask if the patient uses computers frequently because they may experience eyestrain. Machine operators are at risk for injury because of high speeds at which particles can be thrown at the eye. Chronic exposure to infrared or UV light may cause photophobia and cataract formation. Trauma to the face or head near the eye when playing sports such as baseball can damage external structures, the eye, the connections with the brain, or the area of the brain where vision is perceived. Teach all people to wear eye protection that is in keeping with their chosen occupation or sport.

Social habits such as smoking or vaping can be a significant risk factor for developing eye problems. Specifically, airborne formaldehyde can cause burning and watering of the eyes. Inquire about whether a patient smokes or vapes, and collect pertinent history regarding this practice.

BOX 39.3 Systemic Conditions and Common Drugs Affecting the Eye and Vision

Systemic Conditions and Disorders	Drugs
• Cardiac disease	• Adrenergic agonists
• COVID-19	• Adrenergic antagonists (beta blockers)
• Diabetes mellitus	• Antibiotics
• HIV-III (AIDS)	• Anticholinergics
• Hypertension	• Antihistamines[a]
• Lupus erythematosus	• Chemotherapy agents
• Multiple sclerosis	• Cholinergic agonists
• Pregnancy	• Corticosteroids[a]
• Sarcoidosis	• Decongestants[a]
• Thyroid problems	• Opioids
	• Oral contraceptives

[a] Prescription and over the counter.

Systemic health problems can affect vision. Check whether the patient has any condition listed in Box 39.3. Determine if the patient has, or recently had, conjunctivitis ("pink eye"), as this is one of the initial signs associated with COVID-19 (Gaur & Sarkar, 2022). Also ask if the patient is active duty military or is a veteran of the Armed Forces. These individuals may have experienced eye injury in the line of duty that needs to be further assessed. Ask about past accidents, injuries, surgeries (including laser surgeries), or head trauma that may have led to the present problem.

Drugs can also affect vision and the eye (see Box 39.3). Ask about the use of any prescription or over-the-counter drugs, especially decongestants and antihistamines, which cause eye dryness and may increase intraocular pressure. Document the name, strength, dose, and scheduling for all drugs the patient uses. Ocular effects from drugs include itching, foreign body sensation, redness, tearing, photophobia (sensitivity to light), and development of cataracts or glaucoma.

Nutrition History

Some eye problems are caused or worsened by vitamin deficiencies, so ask the patient about food choices. Vitamin A deficiency can cause eye dryness, keratomalacia, and blindness. Some nutrients and antioxidants, such as lutein, zeaxanthin, and beta carotene, help maintain retinal function (American

NCLEX Examination Challenge 39.2

Health Promotion and Maintenance

The nurse is caring for a client who wishes to take supplements to benefit their eye health. Which of the following supplements would the nurse discuss? **Select all that apply.**

A. Lutein
B. Zeaxanthin
C. Vitamin C
D. Magnesium
E. Saw palmetto

Optometric Association, 2023a; Mitra et al., 2021). A diet rich in fruits and red, orange, and dark green vegetables is important to eye health.

Family History and Genetic Risk

Ask about a family history of eye problems because some conditions have a familial tendency and some genetic problems lead to visual impairment.

Current Health Problems

Ask the patient about the onset of visual changes. Question whether the change occurred rapidly or slowly. Determine whether the signs and symptoms are present to the same degree in both eyes. If eye injury or trauma is involved, also ask:

• How long ago did the injury occur?
• What was the patient doing when it happened?
• If a foreign body was involved, what was its source?
• Was any first aid administered at the scene? If so, what kind, and what other actions were taken?

✚ NURSING SAFETY PRIORITY

Critical Rescue

Recognize that a sudden or persistent loss of visual *sensory perception* within the past 48 hours, eye trauma, a foreign body in the eye, or sudden ocular pain is an emergency. Respond by notifying the eye care provider immediately.

Physical Assessment

Inspection

Look for head tilting, squinting, or other actions that indicate that the patient is trying to attain clear vision. For example, patients with double vision may cock the head to the side to focus the two images into one, or they may close one eye to see clearly.

Assess for symmetry in the appearance of the eyes. Determine whether they are equally distant from the nose, are the same size, and have the same degree of prominence. Assess for their placement in the orbits and for symmetry of movement. *Exophthalmos (proptosis)* is protrusion of the eye. *Enophthalmos* is the sunken appearance of the eye.

Examine the eyebrows and eyelashes for hair distribution and determine the direction of the eyelashes. Eyelashes normally point outward and away from the eyelid. Assess the eyelids for *ptosis* (drooping), redness/hyperpigmentation, lesions, or swelling. The lids normally close completely, with the lid edges touching. When the eyes are open, the upper lid covers a small portion of the iris. The edge of the lower lid lies at the iris. No sclera should be visible between the eyelid and the iris.

Scleral and corneal assessment requires a penlight. Examine the sclera for color; it is usually white. In patients with light skin, a yellow color may indicate jaundice or systemic problems. In adults with dark skin, the normal sclera may appear yellow; and small, pigmented dots may be visible (Jarvis & Eckhart, 2024).

The cornea is best seen by directing a light at it from the side. It should be transparent, smooth, shiny, and bright. Any cloudy areas or specks may indicate injury.

Assess the blink reflex by bringing a hand quickly toward the patient's face. Tell the patient before you do this so they will be aware that you will be making a sudden movement with your hand. Use extreme caution when performing this maneuver, especially with confused patients. Patients with vision will blink.

Pupillary assessment involves examining each pupil separately and comparing the results. The pupils are usually round and of equal size, between 3 and 5 mm in diameter. About 20% of adults normally have a noticeable difference in the size of their pupils, which is known as anisocoria (Merck Manual, 2021). Pupil size varies in adults exposed to the same amount of light. Pupils are smaller in older adults, which reduces vision in low light conditions. Patients with myopia have larger pupils, whereas those with hyperopia have smaller pupils.

Observe pupils for response to light. Increasing light causes constriction, whereas decreasing light causes dilation. Constriction of both pupils is the normal response to direct light and to accommodation. Assess pupillary reaction to light by asking the patient to look straight ahead while you quickly bring the beam of a penlight in from the side and direct it at the right pupil. Constriction of the right pupil is a direct response to shining the penlight into that eye. Constriction of the left pupil when light is shined at the right pupil is known as a *consensual response*. Assess the responses for each eye. (You may see the abbreviation "PERRLA" in the electronic health record, which stands for **p**upils **e**qual, **r**ound, **r**eactive to **l**ight, and **a**ccommodation.)

Evaluate each pupil for speed of reaction. The pupil should immediately constrict when a light is directed at it (i.e., a *brisk* response). If the pupil takes more than 1 second to constrict, the response is *sluggish*. Pupils that fail to react are *nonreactive* or *fixed*. Compare the reactivity speed of right and left pupils and document any difference.

Assess for accommodation by asking the patient to focus on a distant object (which dilates the pupils), then place your finger about 3 inches (7–8 cm) from their nose and ask them to focus there (Jarvis & Eckhart, 2024). Pupils should constrict and there should be convergence of the axes of the eyes (Jarvis & Eckhart, 2024).

Vision Testing

Visual *sensory perception* is measured by first testing each eye separately and then testing both eyes together. Patients who wear corrective lenses are tested without and with their lenses. The eye care provider usually conducts this type of testing, which includes:

- Testing visual acuity to measure distance and near vision
- Using the *Snellen eye chart* to assess distance vision

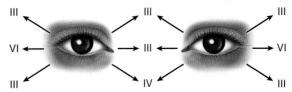

FIG. 39.8 Checking extraocular movements in the six cardinal positions indicates the functioning of cranial nerves III, IV, and VI. (From Silvestri, L. A., & Silvestri, A. E. [2023]. *Saunders comprehensive review for the NCLEX-RN® Examination* [9th ed.]. St. Louis: Elsevier.)

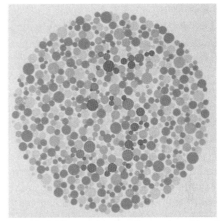

FIG. 39.9 An Ishihara color plate for testing color vision.

- Using the Rosenbaum Pocket Vision Screener or Jaeger card to assess near vision
- Testing for light perception
- Testing the visual field for degree of peripheral vision
- Assessing extraocular muscle function (Fig. 39.8) and eye alignment
- Assessing color vision via *Ishihara color plates* (Fig. 39.9)

Visual acuity in the United States is described in terms of what an average person can see on an eye chart from 20 feet away. For example, 20/20 vision means that the person can see at 20 feet what an average person can see from 20 feet away. Vision that is 20/40 means that the person can see at 20 feet what an average person can see at 40 feet. Only 35% of adults have 20/20 vision without correction, and about 75% of adults achieve 20/20 vision with correction (e.g., glasses, contacts, or surgery) (American Academy of Ophthalmology, 2022). In places outside of the United States, visual acuity is described in terms of what an average person can see on an eye chart that is 6 meters away; the goal is 6/6 vision (American Academy of Ophthalmology, 2022). A person is declared legally blind when the vision is 20/200 or less in the better eye, even with correction (American Academy of Ophthalmology, 2022).

Psychosocial Assessment

A patient with changes in visual *sensory perception* may be anxious about possible vision loss. Patients with severe visual defects may be unable to perform ADLs. Dependency from reduced vision can affect self-esteem. Ask patients how they feel about vision changes. Assess available family support, and the patient's coping techniques. Provide information about local resources and services as needed.

Diagnostic Assessment

Laboratory Assessment

Results of corneal cultures or conjunctival swabs and scrapings can help diagnose infections. If a culture is ordered, obtain a sample of the exudate from the conjunctiva or an ulcerated or inflamed area before antibiotics or topical anesthetics are instilled.

Imaging Assessment

CT is useful for assessing the eyes, the bony structures around the eyes, and the extraocular muscles. It can also detect tumors in the orbital space. A contrast agent is used unless trauma is suspected.

MRI is often used to examine the orbits and optic nerves and to evaluate ocular tumors. It cannot be used to evaluate injuries involving metal in the eyes. *Metal in the eye is an absolute contraindication for MRI.*

Radioisotope scanning is used to locate tumors and lesions. This test requires that the patient sign an informed consent form, and sedation may be used for those who are very anxious. A tracer dose of the radioactive isotope is given orally or by injection, and then the patient must lie still. The scanner measures the radioactivity emitted by the radioactive atoms concentrated in the area being studied. No special follow-up care is required.

Ultrasonography is used to examine the orbit and eye with high-frequency sound waves. This noninvasive test helps diagnose trauma, intraorbital tumors, proptosis, and choroidal or retinal detachments. It is also used to determine the length of the eye and any gross outline changes in the eye and the orbit in patients with cloudy corneas or lenses that reduce direct examination of the fundus.

Inform the patient that this test is painless. It is performed with the eyes closed or, when the eyes must remain open, with anesthetic eyedrops instilled first. The patient is usually positioned upright with the chin in the chin rest, although the test can be done with the patient lying back. The probe is touched against the patient's anesthetized cornea, and sound waves are bounced through the eye. The sound waves create a reflective pattern on a computer screen that can be examined for abnormalities. No special follow-up care is needed. Remind the patient not to rub or touch the eye until the anesthetic agent has worn off.

Other Diagnostic Assessment

Many tests are used to examine specific eye structures when patients have risks, signs and symptoms, or exposures. These tests are performed only by health care providers.

Slit-lamp examination magnifies the anterior eye structures (Fig. 39.10). The patient leans on a chin rest to stabilize the head. A narrow beam (slit) of light is aimed so that only a segment of the eye is brightly lit. The eye care provider can then locate the position of any abnormality in the cornea, lens, or anterior vitreous humor.

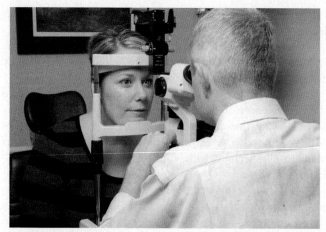

FIG. 39.10 Slit-lamp ocular examination. (From deWit, S. C., Stromberg, H. K., & Dallred, C. V. [2017]. *Medical-surgical nursing* [3rd ed.]. St. Louis: Elsevier.)

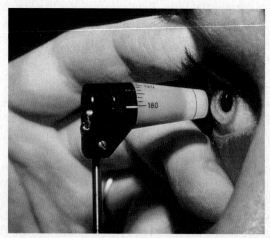

FIG. 39.11 Use of Goldmann applanation tonometer and a slit lamp to measure intraocular pressure. (From Friedman, N. J., Kaiser, P., & Pineda, R. [2021]. *The Massachusetts Eye and Ear Infirmary illustrated manual of ophthalmology* [5th ed.]. St. Louis: Elsevier.)

Corneal staining consists of placing fluorescein or other topical dye into the conjunctival sac, and then the eye is viewed through a blue filter. The procedure is noninvasive and is performed under aseptic conditions. The dye outlines corneal surface irregularities in a bright green color. This test is used to assess corneal trauma, problems caused by a contact lens, or the presence of foreign bodies, abrasions, ulcers, or other corneal disorders.

Tonometry measures intraocular pressure (IOP) with a tonometer, which applies pressure to the outside of the eye until it equals the pressure inside the eye. The thickness of the cornea affects how much pressure must be applied before indentation occurs. Tonometer readings are indicated for all patients older than 40 years of age. Adults with a family history of glaucoma should have their IOP measured once or twice a year. Normal readings range from 10 to 20 mm Hg (Gudgel, 2022). IOP varies throughout the day and typically peaks at certain times of the day. Always document the type and time of measurement.

The most common instrument used by eye care providers to measure IOP is the Goldmann applanation tonometer used with a slit lamp (Fig. 39.11). This method involves direct eye contact. Another instrument, the Tono-Pen XL (Fig. 39.12),

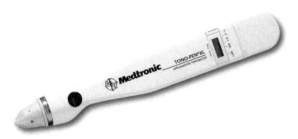

FIG. 39.12 The Tono-Pen XL. (Courtesy Medtronic Ophthalmics, Minneapolis, MN.)

BOX 39.4 Structures Assessed by Direct Ophthalmoscopy

Red Reflex
- Presence or absence

Optic Disc
- Color
- Margins (sharp or blurred)
- Cup size
- Presence of rings or crescents

Optic Blood Vessels
- Size
- Color
- Kinks or tangles
- Light reflection
- Narrowing
- Nicking at arteriovenous crossings

Fundus
- Color
- Tears or holes
- Lesions
- Bleeding

Macula
- Presence of blood vessels
- Color
- Lesions
- Bleeding

---

is designed for use by eye care providers in extended care or long-term care facilities or for other patients unable to be positioned behind a slit lamp. Evidence shows that the Goldmann tonometer remains the most reliable method of IOP assessment (Brusini et al., 2021).

Ophthalmoscopy allows viewing of the eye's external and interior structures with an *ophthalmoscope*. The health care provider positions the ophthalmoscope to see the patient's eye through the sight hole. A *red reflex* is usually seen in the pupil as a reflection of the light off of the retina. An absent red reflex in an adult may indicate a lens opacity or cloudiness of the vitreous. The provider can also examine the retina, optic disc, optic vessels, fundus, and macula with this tool. Box 39.4 lists the features that can be observed in each structure.

The use of an ophthalmoscope may raise anxiety in some patients. When working with a patient with confusion or a patient who does not speak the language used at the agency, use an interpreter service to ensure understanding and cooperation with the examination.

! NURSING SAFETY PRIORITY

Action Alert

Encourage caution when the health care provider is using an ophthalmoscope with a confused patient or one who does not understand the language spoken at the agency. This can serve to prevent accidental injury to the eye.

Fluorescein angiography, which is performed by a health care provider, provides a detailed image of eye circulation. Digital pictures are taken in rapid succession after the dye is given intravenously. This test helps to assess problems of retinal circulation (e.g., diabetic retinopathy, retinal hemorrhage, and macular degeneration) or to diagnose intraocular tumors.

Explain the procedure to the patient, check that the patient has signed the informed consent form, and instill mydriatic eyedrops (cause pupil dilation) 1 hour before the test. Teach that the dye may cause the skin to appear yellow for several hours after the test. The stain is eliminated through the urine, which may be green in appearance.

Encourage patients to drink fluids to help eliminate the dye. Remind them that any staining of the skin will disappear in a few hours. Instruct the patient to wear dark glasses and avoid direct sunlight until pupil dilation returns to normal because the bright light will cause eye discomfort.

Electroretinography (ERG) graphs the retina's response to light stimulation. This test is helpful in detecting and evaluating blood vessel changes from disease or drugs. The graph is obtained by placing an electrode on an anesthetized cornea. Lights at varying speeds and intensities are flashed, and the neural response is graphed. The measurement from the cornea is identical to the response that would be obtained if electrodes were placed directly on the retina.

Gonioscopy is a test performed when a high IOP is found and determines whether open-angle or closed-angle glaucoma is present. It uses a special lens that eliminates the corneal curve, is painless, and allows visualization of the angle where the iris meets the cornea.

Optical coherence tomography, ultrasonic imaging of the retina and optic nerve, creates a three-dimensional view of the back of the eye. It is often used in patients with ocular hypertension or who are at risk for glaucoma because of other health problems.

✷ SENSORY PERCEPTION CONCEPT EXEMPLAR: CATARACT

Pathophysiology Review

The lens is a transparent, elastic structure suspended behind the iris that focuses images onto the retina. A cataract is a lens opacity that distorts the image (Fig. 39.13). Cataracts develop usually in the patient's 50s as the lens thickens (Touhy & Jett, 2023). With time, as lens density increases and transparency is lost, visual **sensory perception** is greatly reduced. Both eyes may have cataracts, but the rate of progression is different in each eye.

Etiology and Genetic Risk

Cataracts may be present at birth or develop at any time although most people develop them later in life. They may be age related or caused by trauma or exposure to toxic agents. They also occur with other diseases and eye disorders (Box 39.5).

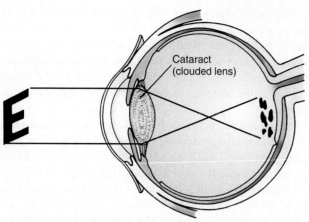

FIG. 39.13 Visual impairment produced by the presence of a cataract.

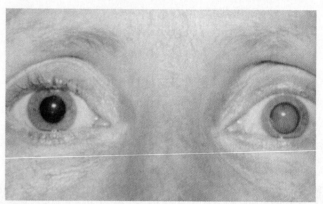

FIG. 39.14 Appearance of an eye with a mature cataract. (From Patton, K. T., & Thibodeau, G. A. [2016]. *Anatomy and physiology* [9th ed.]. St. Louis: Elsevier.)

BOX 39.5 Common Causes of Cataracts

Age
- Lens water loss and fiber compaction

Trauma
- Blunt injury to eye or head
- Penetrating eye injury
- Intraocular foreign bodies
- Radiation exposure, therapy

Toxin Exposure
- Corticosteroids
- Phenothiazine derivatives
- Miotic agents

Health Conditions
- Diabetes mellitus
- Hypoparathyroidism
- Down syndrome
- Chronic sunlight exposure

Complications
- Retinitis pigmentosa
- Glaucoma
- Retinal detachment

Incidence and Prevalence

The age-related cataract is the most common type. By age 75, more than half of all Americans have had a cataract (American Academy of Ophthalmology, 2023).

Health Promotion/Disease Prevention

Although most cases of cataracts in North America are age related, the onset of cataract formation occurs earlier with heavy sun exposure or exposure to other sources of ultraviolet (UV) light. Teach adults to reduce the risk for cataracts by wearing sunglasses that limit exposure to UV light whenever they are outdoors in the daytime. Cataracts also may result from direct eye injury. Urge adults to wear eye and head protection during sports, such as baseball, or any activity that increases the risk for the eye being hit. Individuals who smoke are at higher risk for development of cataracts versus nonsmokers (Boyd, 2022).

Interprofessional Collaborative Care

Care for the patient with cataracts occurs in the community, apart from the surgical procedure, which takes place in an ambulatory surgical setting.

Recognize Cues: Assessment

History. Age is important because cataracts are most prevalent in the older adult. Ask about these other predisposing factors:
- Recent or past trauma to the eye
- Exposure to radioactive materials, x-rays, or UV light
- Prolonged use of corticosteroids, chlorpromazine, or beta blockers
- Presence of intraocular disease (e.g., recurrent uveitis)
- Presence of systemic disease (e.g., diabetes mellitus, hypoparathyroidism, hypertension)
- Previous cataract, or family history of cataracts
- History of smoking, particularly if patient is a veteran, as studies show that cataract incidence is significantly higher among veterans who smoke compared with those who do not smoke (Brown et al., 2023)

Ask patients to describe their vision. For example, you might say, "Tell me what you can see well and what you have difficulty seeing."

Physical Assessment/Signs and Symptoms. Early signs and symptoms of cataracts include slightly blurred vision and decreased color perception. At first the patient may think that their glasses are smudged, or contacts are not fitting correctly. As lens cloudiness continues, blurred and/or double vision occurs, and the patient may have difficulty with ADLs. Patients commonly report increasing difficulty seeing at night, especially while driving. Without surgical intervention, visual impairment progresses to blindness. *No pain or eye redness is associated with age-related cataract formation.*

Unless a cataract has matured, it is not always visible to the naked eye on examination. Visual **sensory perception** is tested using an eye chart and brightness acuity testing. The health care provider will examine the lens with an ophthalmoscope and note any observed densities by size, shape, and location. A slit lamp can also be used to visualize the cornea, iris (and space between the cornea and iris), and lens. A retinal examination will also likely be performed to clearly see the back of the eye. As a cataract matures, the opacity makes it difficult to see the retina, and the red reflex may be absent. When this occurs, the pupil is bluish white (Fig. 39.14).

Psychosocial Assessment. Loss of vision is gradual, and the patient may not be aware of it until reading or driving is affected. The patient may have anxiety about loss of independence. Encourage the patient and family to express concerns about reduced vision.

Analyze Cues and Prioritize Hypotheses: Analysis

The priority collaborative problem for patients with cataracts is:
1. Impaired visual *sensory perception* due to cataracts

Generate Solutions and Take Actions: Planning and Implementation

The priority problem for the patient with cataracts is impaired visual *sensory perception,* which is a safety risk. Patients often live with reduced vision for years before the cataract is removed.

Improving Vision

Planning: Expected Outcomes. As long as patients do not have cognitive deficits, they are expected to recognize and report when ADLs cannot be performed safely and independently due to cataracts. At that time, surgery is indicated. For patients on Medicare, coverage is provided for (U.S. Department of Health and Human Services, 2023):

- A conventional intraocular lens (IOL) that is implanted during cataract surgery
- The cost of the facility, health care provider, and supplies needed to perform the surgery with implantation of the conventional IOL
- One pair of eyeglasses or contact lenses after each cataract surgery with IOL implantation

Interventions. Surgery is the only approach to treat cataracts and should be performed as soon as possible after vision is reduced and ADLs are affected. There are two main types of surgery to address cataracts: phacoemulsification (more common) and extracapsular cataract extraction (ECCE).

Preoperative Care. The eye care provider provides information about the procedure so that the patient can make informed decisions about treatment, and then obtains informed consent.

Preoperatively, assess how reduced vision affects ADLs. Teach that care before and after the procedure requires regular self-examination of the eye and possible instillation of different types of eyedrops several times daily for a prescribed period before surgery. In some cases, an ophthalmologist will not prescribe eyedrops before surgery, particularly in the case of *dropless cataract surgery* (Assil et al., 2020). Advise the patient to clarify with the ophthalmologist whether there is a need, or lack of need, to use them before the procedure. If patients are unable to instill the drops, help them make arrangements for this care.

For planning purposes, remind the patient that an adult will need to drive them home from the procedure following cataract surgery. Ask whether the patient takes any drugs that affect blood clotting, such as aspirin, warfarin, clopidogrel, and dabigatran. Communicate this information to the ophthalmologist because these drugs may need to be discontinued in select patients before cataract surgery.

Operative Procedures. The lens is often extracted by *phacoemulsification* (Fig. 39.15) (also called *phaco*). This procedure is usually done with local or topical anesthesia. A probe is inserted through the capsule, and high-frequency sound waves break the lens into small pieces, which are then removed by suction. The replacement intraocular lens (IOL), a small, clear, plastic lens, is placed inside the capsule to be positioned so that light rays are focused in the retina. Some patients have

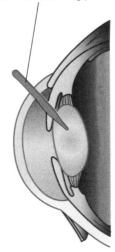

Sound wave and suctioning probe

Sound waves break up the lens, pieces are sucked out, and the capsule remains largely intact

FIG. 39.15 Cataract removal by phacoemulsification.

distant vision restored to 20/20 and may need glasses only for reading or close work. Some replacement lenses have multiple focal planes and may correct vision to the extent that glasses or contact lenses may not be needed.

In extracapsular cataract extraction (ECCE), which is often used for more advanced cataracts, the cataract is removed in one piece prior to the insertion of the replacement intraocular lens (IOL). Anesthesia around the eye is required to perform this procedure. Sutures are required to close the wound, resulting in a slower recovery compared with phacoemulsification.

Postoperative Care. Immediately after surgery, antibiotic and steroid ointments are instilled. The patient is usually discharged very soon following surgery, after stabilization and monitoring. Teach to wear dark glasses outdoors or in brightly lit environments until the pupil responds to light. Teach the patient and family members how to instill the prescribed eyedrops. Help them create a written schedule for the timing and the order of eyedrops administration. Remind the patient that vision in that eye will be blurred and to not drive or operate heavy machinery until the ointment is removed. Stress the importance of keeping all follow-up appointments.

Remind the patient that mild eye itching is normal, as is a "bloodshot" appearance. The eyelid may be slightly swollen; however, significant swelling or bruising is abnormal. Cool compresses may be beneficial. Discomfort at the site is controlled with acetaminophen or acetaminophen with oxycodone as prescribed. Aspirin is avoided because of its effects on blood clotting.

Pain early after surgery may indicate increased intraocular pressure (IOP) or hemorrhage. Instruct patients to contact the ophthalmologist if pain occurs with nausea or vomiting.

To prevent increases in IOP, teach the patient and family about activity restrictions. Activities that can cause a sudden rise in IOP are listed in Box 39.6.

Infection is a potential and serious complication. Teach the patient and family to observe for increasing eye redness, a decrease in vision, or an increase in tears and photophobia.

BOX 39.6   Activities That Increase Intraocular Pressure

- Bending from the waist
- Lifting objects weighing more than 10 lb (4.5 kg)
- Sneezing, coughing
- Blowing the nose
- Straining to have a bowel movement
- Vomiting
- Having sexual intercourse
- Keeping the head in a dependent position
- Wearing tight shirt collars or ties

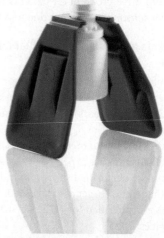

FIG. 39.16 Autosqueeze, a mechanism for self-administering eyedrops. (Courtesy Owen Mumford, Marietta, GA.)

Creamy white, dry, crusty drainage on the eyelids and lashes is normal. However, yellow or green drainage indicates infection and must be reported. Stress the importance of proper hand-washing to reduce the potential for infection.

Patients usually experience a dramatic improvement in vision within a day of surgery. Remind them that final best vision will not occur until 4 to 6 weeks after surgery.

! NURSING SAFETY PRIORITY

Action Alert

Instruct the patient who has had cataract surgery to immediately report any reduction of vision in the eye that just had the cataract removed.

Care Coordination and Transition Management

Patients are usually discharged within an hour or two following cataract surgery. Nursing interventions in that time frame focus on monitoring recovery and teaching. Some patients are pre-scribed to wear a light eye patch at night to prevent accidental rubbing. Instruct the patient to avoid getting water in the eye for 3 to 7 days after surgery.

Patients are prescribed eyedrops to use following surgery; remind them of the importance of adhering strictly to the pre-scribed administration times. If the patient has difficulty instill-ing eyedrops, a supportive neighbor, friend, or family member can be taught the procedure. Adaptive equipment that positions the bottle of eyedrops directly over the eye can also be pur-chased (Fig. 39.16).

Many patients are required to come back to the ophthalmol-ogist the day following cataract surgery for a follow-up appoint-ment. Ensure that patients have someone who can drive them to this appointment. Box 39.7 lists items to cover when assessing a patient who returns to the ophthalmologist the day following cataract surgery.

Although cataract surgery complications are not anticipated, teach the patient to immediately report any of these symptoms that occur:

- Sharp, sudden pain in the eye
- Bleeding or increased discharge from the eye
- Green or yellow, thick drainage from the eye
- Eyelid swelling

BOX 39.7   Assessing the Patient After Cataract Surgery

- Assess (after the ophthalmologist has removed any dressings):
  - Visual acuity in both eyes using a handheld eye chart
  - Visual fields of both eyes
  - Presence or absence of redness, tearing, and/or draining in the operative eye in comparison with the nonoperative eye
- Ask patients if they have:
  - Pain in or around the operative eye
  - Any changes in vision (decreased or improved) in the operative eye
  - Dark spots in their visual field
  - An increase in the number of floaters
  - Bright flashes of light in their visual field
- Remind the patient of:
  - Signs and symptoms of complications to report
  - Drug regimen information
  - Activity restrictions

- Reappearance of a bloodshot sclera after the initial appear-ance has cleared
- Decreased vision in the eye that had surgery
- Flashes of light or floating shapes seen in the eye

Remind the patient to continue to avoid activities that can increase IOP (see Box 39.6) and to follow any other activity restrictions. Cooking and light housekeeping are permitted, but vacuuming should be avoided for several weeks because of the forward flexion involved and the rapid opposing movements required.

Evaluate Outcomes: Evaluation

Evaluate the care of the patient with cataracts on the basis of improving visual ***sensory perception.*** The expected outcomes include that the patient will have improved visual ***sensory per-ception*** following surgery and recognize signs and symptoms of complications.

✳ SENSORY PERCEPTION CONCEPT EXEMPLAR: GLAUCOMA

Pathophysiology Review

Glaucoma is a group of eye disorders resulting in increased intraocular pressure (IOP). As described earlier in this chap-ter, the eye is a hollow organ. For proper eye function, the gel in the posterior segment (vitreous humor) and the fluid in the anterior segment (aqueous humor) must be present in set amounts that apply pressure inside the eye to keep it ball shaped.

In adults, the volume of the vitreous humor does not change. However, the aqueous humor is continuously made from blood plasma by the ciliary bodies located behind the iris and just in front of the lens (see Fig. 39.2). The fluid flows through the pupil into the bulging area in front of the iris. At the outer edges of the iris beneath the cornea, blood vessels collect fluid and return it to the blood. Usually about 1 mL of aqueous humor is always present, but it is continuously made and reabsorbed at a rate of about 5 mL daily.

A normal IOP requires a balance between production and outflow of aqueous humor (Rogers, 2023). If the IOP becomes too high, the extra pressure compresses retinal blood vessels and photoreceptors and their synapsing nerve fibers. This compression results in poorly oxygenated pho-toreceptors and nerve fibers. These sensitive nerve tissues become ischemic and die. When too many have died, vision is lost permanently. Tissue damage starts in the periphery and moves inward toward the fovea centralis. Untreated, glaucoma can lead to complete loss of visual *sensory per-ception.* Glaucoma is usually painless. The most common type progresses over time, and the patient may be unaware of gradual vision reduction.

There are various types of glaucoma (Box 39.8). The most common types are open-angle glaucoma and angle-closure glaucoma. Open-angle glaucoma (OAG), also known as *pri-mary open-angle glaucoma (POAG),* the most common form of glaucoma, usually affects both eyes and has no signs or symp-toms in the early stages. It develops slowly, with gradual loss of visual fields that may go unnoticed because central vision at first is unaffected.

BOX 39.8 Common Causes of Select Types of Glaucoma

Open-Angle Glaucoma
- Aging (over 40)
- Genetics
- Hypertension
- Increased intraocular pressure (IOP)

Angle-Closure Glaucoma
- Increased intraocular pressure (IOP) due to sudden blockage of aqueous humor drainage

Secondary Glaucoma
- Neovascular glaucoma (formation of new blood vessels on the iris (often occurs with diabetes)
- Steroid-induced glaucoma
- Trauma (known as *traumatic glaucoma*)
- Uveitis (known as *uveitic glaucoma*)

At times, patients may experience mild eye aching or head-aches. Late signs and symptoms occur after irreversible damage to optic nerve function and include seeing halos around lights, losing peripheral vision, and having decreased visual *sensory perception* that does not improve with eyeglasses. Outflow of aqueous humor through the chamber angle is reduced. Because the fluid cannot leave the eye at the same rate that it is produced, IOP gradually increases.

Angle-closure glaucoma (ACG), or *primary angle-closure glaucoma (PACG), closed-angle glaucoma, narrow-angle glau-coma,* or *acute glaucoma,* has a sudden onset and *is a medical emergency.* The problem is a forward displacement of the iris, which presses against the cornea and closes the chamber angle, suddenly preventing outflow of aqueous humor.

Secondary glaucoma arises as a result of another health con-dition or trauma. With secondary glaucoma, a known cause for the change in intraocular pressure is identifiable.

Etiology and Genetic Risk

Anyone can develop glaucoma. Some adults are at higher risk, such as adults older than 60 (especially Hispanic/Latino indi-viduals), African American people over 40 years of age, and those who have a family history of glaucoma (National Eye Institute, 2022).

Incidence and Prevalence

Glaucoma is a common cause of blindness in North America. It is usually age related, occurring in about 3 million adults in the United States (CDC, 2020a).

Health Promotion/Disease Prevention

There are no known ways to prevent glaucoma. The best preven-tion against damage that glaucoma can cause is for adults to have eye examinations with glaucoma checks done every 2 to 4 years before age 40, every 1 to 3 years between ages 40 and 54, every 1 to 2 years between ages 55 and 64, and every 6 to 12 months over the age of 65 (Glaucoma Research Foundation, 2022c).

Interprofessional Collaborative Care

Care for the patient with glaucoma generally takes place in the community setting. Members of the interprofessional team who collaborate most closely to care for this patient include the eye care provider and the nurse. For patients who experience psychosocial concerns related to decreased visual *sensory perception,* collaborate with the mental health provider (see the Interprofessional Collaboration: The Patient With Glaucoma box).

 INTERPROFESSIONAL COLLABORATION

The Patient With Glaucoma

The possibility or reality of vision loss can be distressing for patients. Numerous studies have identified a connection between glaucoma and the onset of anxiety and depression. More recent studies have begun to suggest that the anxiety and depression experienced by patients with glaucoma have an impact on the degree and progression of the disorder (Shin et al., 2021). Collaborate with a mental health professional when caring for patients who experience anxiety or depression related to changes in their sight.

You can support the patient at regular eye visits, and the mental health professional can provide ongoing counseling and support to the patient during this time of transition. According to the Interprofessional Education Collaborative (IPEC) Expert Panel's Competency of Roles and Responsibilities, using the unique and complementary abilities of other team members optimizes health and patient care (IPEC, 2016; Slusser et al., 2019).

Recognize Cues: Assessment

History. Ask about visual symptoms that have developed suddenly or over time. Symptoms of acute angle-closure glaucoma include a sudden visual loss, pain, conjunctival erythema, and corneal edema (Jacobs, 2022). In OAG, patients are often asymptomatic in the early stages. The visual fields first show a small loss of peripheral vision that gradually progresses to a larger loss.

Physical Assessment/Signs and Symptoms. Ophthalmoscopic examination shows cupping and atrophy of the optic disc. It becomes wider and deeper and turns white or gray. The sclera may appear reddened and the cornea foggy. Ophthalmoscopic examination performed by the health care provider reveals a shallow anterior chamber, a cloudy aqueous humor, and a moderately dilated, nonreactive pupil.

Diagnostic Assessment. An elevated intraocular pressure (IOP) is measured with tonometry. In open-angle glaucoma, the tonometry reading is often between 22 and 32 mm Hg (normal is 8–21 mm Hg [Gudgel, 2022]). In angle-closure glaucoma, the tonometry reading may be 30 mm Hg or higher. Visual field testing by perimetry is performed, as is visualization by gonioscopy to determine whether the angle is open or closed. Usually the optic nerve is imaged to determine to what degree nerve damage is present.

Analyze Cues and Prioritize Hypotheses: Analysis

The priority collaborative problems for patients with glaucoma include:

1. Impaired visual *sensory perception* due to glaucoma
2. Need for health teaching due to treatment regimen for glaucoma

Generate Solutions and Take Actions: Planning and Implementation

Supporting Visual Acuity via Health Teaching

Planning: Expected Outcomes. With proper intervention, the patient is expected to maintain optimum visual acuity as long as possible by adhering to the treatment regimen.

Interventions

Nonsurgical Management. Teach the patient that loss of visual *sensory perception* from glaucoma can be prevented by early detection, lifelong treatment, and close monitoring. Use of ophthalmic drugs that reduce ocular pressure can delay or prevent damage. Box 39.9 provides ways to help patients with reduced visual *sensory perception* to remain as independent as possible. Box 39.10 provides a list of interventions to care for the hospitalized patient or long-term care resident who has impaired vision due to glaucoma.

Drug therapy for glaucoma works to reduce IOP in several ways. Eyedrops can reduce the production of or increase the absorption of aqueous humor or constrict the pupil so that the ciliary muscle is contracted, allowing better circulation of the aqueous humor to the site of absorption. These drugs do not improve lost vision but prevent further damage by decreasing IOP. Close adherence to the prescribed dosage schedule is essential to receiving the maximum therapeutic effect of the eyedrops, so teach the patient to be dedicated in the regular timing of administration.

Prostaglandins, rho kinase inhibitors, nitric oxides, and miotic or cholinergic agents help drain fluid from the eye, which lowers eye pressure. Alpha-adrenergic agonists, beta blockers, and carbonic anhydrase inhibitors lower the amount of aqueous humor the eye makes. Systemic osmotic drugs such as IV mannitol may be given for angle-closure glaucoma to rapidly reduce IOP.

Remind patients that most eyedrops cause tearing, blurred vision, and a reddened sclera for a few minutes after instilling the drug. Some may also cause mild, but temporary, burning. Specific nursing implications related to drug therapy for glaucoma are listed in Table 39.1.

Vision rehabilitation is provided by specially trained therapists who teach ways of adaptive living for people with glaucoma and other forms of impaired vision (Glaucoma Research Foundation, 2022b). Certified vision rehabilitation therapists (CVRTs) can help the patient find adaptive ways to maximize their ability to read, use the computer, cook, work, and engage successfully in other ADLs (Duffy, 2021). Certified orientation and mobility specialists (COMSs or O&Ms) work with patients to develop skills to travel safely and independently, use Global Positioning System (GPS) navigation and public transportation, and use long canes (Duffy, 2021).

The priority teaching for the patient with glaucoma is about safety. Teach that the benefit of drug therapy occurs only when eye drops are used on the prescribed schedule; therefore patients must instill drops on time and not skip doses. Remind those who wear contact lenses to remove them before instilling eyedrops.

BOX 39.9 Patient and Family Education

Promoting Independent Living in Patients With Impaired Vision

Drug Therapy

- Assist with arranging for a neighbor, relative, friend, or home health nurse to visit weekly to organize the proper drugs for each day (if the patient is unable to do so).
- If the patient is to take drugs more than once each day, use a container of a different shape (with a lid) each time. For example, if the patient is to take drugs at 9 a.m., 3 p.m., and 9 p.m., the 9 a.m. drugs would be placed in a round container, the 3 p.m. drugs in a square container, and the 9 p.m. drugs in a triangular container.
- Place each day's drug containers in a separate box, with raised letters on the side of the box spelling out the day.
- Smartphone apps can be programmed with alarms to remind patients when to take medications (if they are unable to see an analog or digital clock).
- Some drug containers have alarms that can be set.

Communication

- Phones with large, raised block numbers are helpful. Those with black numbers on a white phone or white numbers on a black phone are most easily seen by a patient with low vision.
- Smartphones or apps that recognize vocal commands or have a programmable automatic dialing feature ("speed dial") are very helpful. Programmed numbers should include those for family, friends, neighbors, and 911.

Safety

- Leave furniture positioned the way the patient has it (due to familiarity).
- Eliminate rugs, as these increase the risk for falls.
- Appliance cords should be short and kept out of walkways.
- Unbreakable dishes, cups, and glasses are preferable to breakable ones.
- Cleansers and other toxic agents should be labeled with large, raised letters.

Food Preparation

- Meals on Wheels America is a service that many older adults appreciate. This service is local, bringing cooked, ready-to-eat meals. During meal delivery, a Meals on Wheels volunteer or staff member performs a basic safety check on the older adult and contacts emergency services or family if needed. The cost of the meal varies, depending on the patient's ability to pay. Some older adults do not have to pay anything to receive this valuable service.
- Many grocery stores and third-party apps offer delivery service. Customers can create a cart online or shop by phone. The store gathers the ordered food. They can have it ready for pickup, give it to a third party for delivery, or deliver it personally depending on services available in different areas. Costs vary; some stores charge for each delivery, whereas others are more affordable by offering an annual subscription fee.
- A microwave oven is a safer means of cooking than a standard stove. If the patient has and will use a microwave oven, others can prepare and label meals ahead of time and freeze them for later use. Also, many complete frozen dinners that comply with a variety of dietary restrictions are available to warm in the microwave.
- Friends or relatives may be able to help with food preparation. Often relatives do not know what to give an older adult for birthdays or other gift-giving occasions. One suggestion is a homemade prepackaged frozen dinner that the patient enjoys.

Personal Care

- Handgrips should be installed in bathrooms.
- The shower or tub floor should have a nonskid surface.
- Patients who shave should use an electric shaver rather than a razor.
- Have patients choose a hairstyle that they like and that is easy to care for; this promotes self-care. Home hair-care services are available in some areas.

Diversional Activity

- Some patients can read large-print books, newspapers, and magazines (available through local libraries and vision services).
- Most computers, smartphones, and tablets can adjust text size. This can enhance reading and communication.
- Many books, magazines, newspapers, and forms of entertainment are available by audiotape or by streaming.
- Card games, dominoes, and some board games are available in large, high-contrast print.

BOX 39.10 Best Practice for Patient Safety and Quality Care

Care of the Hospitalized Patient or Long-Term Care Resident With Reduced Vision

- Always knock or announce your entrance into the patient's room or area and introduce yourself; ensure that all members of the health care team also use this courtesy of announcement and introduction.
- Ensure that the patient's reduced vision is noted in the electronic health record, communicated to all staff, marked on the call board, and identified on the door of the person's room.
- Determine to what degree the patient can see, and provide opportunities for safe independence in as many ways as possible.
- Orient newly hospitalized patients to the environment, counting steps with them to the bathroom and reminding them to call for assistance.
- Help the patient place objects on the bedside table; do not move them without the person's permission.
- Remove all obstacles and clutter in walkways, especially to the bathroom.
- Ask the newly hospitalized patient what type of assistance is preferred for grooming, toileting, eating, and ambulating; communicate these preferences with staff.
- Describe food placement on a plate in terms of a clock face.
- Open milk cartons; open salt, pepper, and condiment packages; and remove lids from cups and bowls prior to meals.
- Unless the patient also has a hearing problem, use a normal tone of voice when speaking.
- When walking with the patient, offer your arm and walk a step ahead.

TABLE 39.1   Common Examples of Drug Therapy (Eyedrops)

Glaucoma

Drug Category	Selected Nursing Implications
Adrenergic Agonists	
Apraclonidine Brimonidine tartrate	Ask whether the patient is taking any antidepressants from the MAOI class. *These enzyme inhibitors increase blood pressure, as do the adrenergic agonists. When these agents are taken together, the patient may experience hypertensive crisis.* Teach the patient to wear dark glasses outdoors and to avoid too much sunlight exposure. *This type of drug can cause the eyes to become sensitive to light.* Teach the patient not to use the eyedrops with contact lenses in place and to wait 15 minutes after using the drug to put in contact lenses, if worn. *These drugs are absorbed by the contact lens, which can become discolored or cloudy.*
Beta-Adrenergic Blockers	
Betaxolol hydrochloride Carteolol Levobunolol Timolol	Ask whether the patient has moderate-to-severe asthma or COPD. *If these drugs are absorbed systemically, they constrict pulmonary smooth muscle and narrow airways.* Teach patients with diabetes to check their blood glucose levels more often when taking these drugs. *These drugs induce hypoglycemia and can mask the hypoglycemic symptoms.* Teach patients who also take oral beta blockers to check their pulse at least twice per day and to notify the primary health care and eye care providers if the pulse is consistently below 60 beats/min. *These drugs potentiate the effects of systemic beta blockers and can cause an unsafe decrease in heart rate and blood pressure.*
Carbonic Anhydrase Inhibitors	
Brinzolamide Dorzolamide	Ask whether the patient has an allergy to sulfonamide antibacterial drugs. *Drugs are similar to the sulfonamides; if a patient is allergic to the sulfonamides, an allergy is possible with these drugs.* Teach the patient to shake the drug before applying. *Drug separates on standing.* Teach the patient to not use the eyedrops with contact lenses in place and to wait 15 minutes after using the drug to put in the lenses. *These drugs are absorbed by the contact lens, which can become discolored or cloudy.*
Cholinergic Agonists	
Carbachol Echothiophate Pilocarpine	Teach to not administer more eyedrops than are prescribed and to report increased salivation or drooling to the primary health care and eye care providers. *These drugs are readily absorbed by conjunctival mucous membranes and can cause systemic side effects of headache, flushing, increased saliva, and sweating.* Teach to use good light when reading and to turn lights on in rooms. *The pupil of the eye will not open more to let in more light, and it may be harder to see objects in dim light. This can increase the risk for falls.*
Nitric Oxide	
Latanoprostene bunod	Teach to refrain from driving and using machinery while using this medication. *This drug can cause blurred vision.*
Prostaglandin Agonists	
Bimatoprost Latanoprost Tafluprost Travoprost	Teach to check the cornea for abrasions or trauma. *Drugs should not be used when the cornea is not intact.* Teach that eye color may darken, and eyelashes elongate, over time in the eye receiving one of these drugs. *Knowing the side effects in advance reassures the patient that their presence is expected and normal.* If only one eye is to be treated, teach *not* to place drops in the other eye to try to make the eye colors similar. *Using the drug in an eye with normal IOP can cause a lower-than-normal IOP, which reduces vision.* Caution that using more drops than prescribed can reduce drug effectiveness. *Drug action is based on blocking receptors, which can increase in number when the drug is overused.*
Rho Kinase Inhibitors	
Netarsudil	If the patient is dispensed a multiple-dose container, caution about cross-contamination. *Reports of bacterial keratitis have arisen when patients with other disorders (e.g., a concurrent corneal disorder) have accidentally contaminated the medication.*
Combination Drug	
Brimonidine tartrate and timolol maleate	Same as for each drug alone.

COPD, Chronic obstructive pulmonary disease; *MAOI,* monoamine oxidase inhibitor.

When more than one drop is prescribed, teach the patient to wait 5 to 10 minutes between drug instillations to prevent one drug from diluting another drug. Stress the need for good hand-washing, keeping the eyedrop container tip clean, and avoiding contact of the tip to any part of the eye. Explain potential interactions that may exist between medications and systemic effects that may occur when using these drugs. Also teach the technique of punctal occlusion (placing pressure on the corner of the eye near the nose) immediately after eyedrop instillation to prevent systemic absorption of the drug (Fig. 39.17).

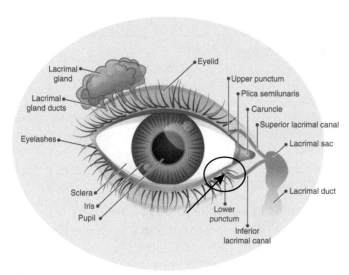

FIG. 39.17 Apply punctal occlusion in the circled area to prevent systemic absorption of eyedrops. (Used with permission from istockphoto.com, 2020, VectorMine.)

💊 NURSING SAFETY PRIORITY

Drug Alert

> Many eyedrops used for glaucoma therapy can be absorbed systemically and cause systemic problems. It is critical to teach punctal occlusion to patients using eyedrops for glaucoma therapy in order to minimize systemic absorption (see Fig. 39.17).

Surgical Management. Surgery can be performed when eyedrops for open-angle glaucoma are not effective at controlling IOP. A *laser trabeculoplasty* burns the trabecular meshwork, scarring it and causing the meshwork fibers to tighten. Tight fibers increase the size of the spaces between the fibers, improving outflow of aqueous humor and reducing IOP.

If glaucoma fails to respond to eyedrops and laser trabeculoplasty, an implanted shunt procedure (called *tube shunt surgery*) may be used. A small tube or filament is connected to a flat plate that is positioned on the outside of the eye in the eye orbit. The open part of the fine tube is placed into the front chamber of the eye. The fluid then drains through or around the tube into the area around the flat plate, where it collects and is reabsorbed into the bloodstream. Potential complications of glaucoma surgery include choroidal hemorrhage and choroidal detachment.

If laser *trabeculoplasty* and *tube shunt surgery* do not work, cyclophotocoagulation laser treatment may be done. This procedure causes the ciliary processes to shrink, which results in less production of aqueous humor and therefore lower IOP.

Laser peripheral iridotomy (LPI) is the first line of treatment for angle-closure glaucoma. A hole is created in the outer edge of the iris, which opens the angle in most patients; then the trabecular meshwork is exposed, and fluid can drain (Glaucoma Research Foundation, 2022a).

Care Coordination and Transition Management

Patients with glaucoma will need to instill eyedrops regularly as part of home care. If they are unable to instill or resistant to instilling their own eyedrops, teach the caregiver the proper technique or recommend adaptive equipment (see Fig. 39.16).

The patient will be seen as an outpatient every 1 to 3 months at the recommendation of the ophthalmologist, depending on how well controlled the IOP is. Teach the importance of good handwashing and keeping the tip of the eyedrop container clean. Remind the patient to instill eyedrops on time as recommended by the ophthalmologist and to not skip doses.

For the patient who had surgical management, teach the signs and symptoms of choroidal detachment and hemorrhage. These can occur during or after coughing, sneezing, straining at stools, or Valsalva maneuver. Serous detachment involves some degree of vision loss yet is usually painless. Hemorrhagic detachment involves an immediate loss of vision with sudden, excruciating, throbbing pain. Any vision loss, particularly when accompanied by pain, should be reported immediately to the eye care provider.

If needed, refer the patient to care services that can assist in the home. Support groups for individuals with vision impairment may also be helpful.

Evaluate Outcomes: Evaluation

Evaluate the care of the patient with glaucoma based on the identified priority patient problem. The primary expected outcome is that the patient will have optimum visual acuity as long as possible, as demonstrated by adherence to the treatment regimen.

CORNEAL DISORDERS

For a sharp retinal image, the cornea must be transparent and intact. Corneal problems may be caused by inflammation of the cornea (keratitis), degeneration of the cornea (keratoconus), or deposits in the cornea. All corneal problems reduce visual *sensory perception,* and some can lead to blindness.

CORNEAL ABRASION, ULCERATION, AND INFECTION

Pathophysiology Review

A *corneal abrasion* is a scrape or scratch injury of the cornea. This painful condition can be caused by a small foreign body, trauma, contact lens use, malnutrition, dry eye syndromes, and certain cancer therapies. The abrasion allows organisms to enter, leading to corneal infection. Bacterial, protozoal, and fungal infections can lead to *corneal ulceration,* a deeper injury. *This problem is an emergency* because the cornea has no separate blood supply, and infections that can permanently impair vision develop rapidly.

Interprofessional Collaborative Care

The patient with a corneal disorder has pain, reduced vision, photophobia, and eye secretions. Cloudy or purulent fluid may be present on the eyelids or lashes. Care for patients with a corneal disorder usually takes place in the community setting. Members of the interprofessional team who collaborate most closely to care for this patient include the eye care provider or family health care provider, and the nurse.

Recognize Cues: Assessment

Wear gloves when examining the eye. Anticipate the cornea to look hazy or cloudy with a patchy area of ulceration. When fluorescein stain is used, the patchy area appears green. Corneal scrapings (done by an eye care provider after anesthetizing the cornea with a topical agent) and microbial cultures are used to determine the causative organism. For culture, obtain swabs from the ulcer and its edges.

Take Actions: Interventions

Antiinfective therapy is started before the organism is identified because of the high risk for vision loss. A broad-spectrum antibiotic is prescribed first and may be changed when culture results are known. Steroids may be used with antibiotics to reduce the eye inflammation. Drugs can be given topically as eyedrops or injected subconjunctivally or intravenously. The nursing priorities are to begin the drug therapy, to ensure patient understanding of the drug therapy regimen, and to prevent infection spread.

Often the antiinfective therapy involves instilling eyedrops *every hour* for the first 24 hours. Teach the patient or family member how to instill the eyedrops correctly.

If the eye infection occurs only in one eye, teach the patient not to use the drug in the unaffected eye. Reinforce the importance of handwashing after touching the affected eye and before touching or doing anything to the healthy eye. If both eyes are infected, separate bottles of drugs are needed for each eye. Teach the patient to clearly label the bottles "right eye" and "left eye" and not to switch the drugs from eye to eye. Remind the patient not to wear contact lenses during the entire time that these drugs are being used because the eye is more vulnerable to infection or injury, and the drugs can cloud or damage the contact lenses.

> ### ! NURSING SAFETY PRIORITY
> #### Action Alert
>
> Teach the importance of applying eyedrops as often as prescribed, even at night, and to complete the entire course of antibiotic therapy. Treating the infection can save the vision in the infected eye. Remind the patient to make and keep all follow-up appointments.

Drug therapy may continue for weeks to ensure eradication of the infection. Teach patients to avoid using makeup around the eye until the infection has cleared. Instruct them to discard all open containers of contact lens solutions and bottles of eyedrops because these may be contaminated. Patients should not wear contact lenses for weeks to months until the infection is gone and the ulcer is healed.

> ### ◆ NURSING SAFETY PRIORITY
> #### Drug Alert
>
> Check the route of administration for ophthalmic drugs. Most are administered by the eye instillation route, not orally. Administering these drugs orally can cause systemic side effects and will not therapeutically treat the eye condition. Be sure to reinforce the correct route when teaching the patient.

KERATOCONUS

Pathophysiology Review

The cornea can permanently lose its shape, become scarred or cloudy, or become thinner, reducing useful visual *sensory perception.* Keratoconus, the degeneration of corneal tissue resulting in abnormal corneal shape, can occur with trauma or may be an inherited disorder (Fig. 39.18). Inadequately treated corneal infection and severe trauma can scar the cornea and lead to severe visual impairment that can be improved only through surgical interventions.

Interprofessional Collaborative Care

Keratoplasty (corneal transplant) is a surgical procedure to improve clarity for a permanent corneal disorder that obscures vision. The diseased corneal tissue is removed and replaced with tissue from a cornea donated by a human who has died.

Postoperative care involves comprehensive patient teaching. Local antibiotics are injected or instilled. Usually the eye is covered with a pressure patch and a protective shield until the patient returns to the ophthalmologist.

Teach the patient how to instill eyedrops. Instruct the patient to lie on the nonoperative side to reduce intraocular pressure (IOP). If a patch is to be used for more than a day, teach application processes. Instruct the patient to wear the shield at night for the first month after surgery and whenever around small children or pets in order to avoid injury. Instruct them *to avoid using* an ice pack on the eye.

Complications after surgery include bleeding, wound leakage, infection, and graft rejection. Teach patients to examine the eye (or have a family member or friend examine it) daily for the presence of infection or graft rejection. Graft rejection can occur and starts as inflammation in the cornea near the graft edge that moves toward the center. Vision is reduced, and the cornea becomes cloudy. Topical corticosteroids and other immunosuppressants are used to stop the rejection process. If rejection continues, the graft becomes opaque and blood vessels branch into the opaque tissue. Loss of vision, eye pain, redness in the eye, purulent drainage, an ongoing leak of clear fluid from the graft site (not tears) and light sensitivity need to be reported to the ophthalmologist right away.

The eye should be protected from any activity that can increase the pressure on, around, or inside the eye. Teach the

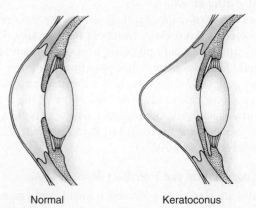

Normal   Keratoconus

FIG. 39.18 Profile of a normal cornea and one with keratoconus.

patient to avoid jogging, running, dancing, and any other activity that promotes rapid or jerky head motions for several weeks after surgery. Other activities that may raise IOP and should be avoided are listed in Box 39.6.

Eye donation is a common procedure and needed for corneal transplantation. The Eye Bank Association of America (EBAA, 2023) has published medical standards that detail donor eligibility and contraindications. If a deceased patient is a known eye donor, follow these recommended steps prior to donation:

- Raise the head of the bed 30 degrees.
- Instill prescribed antibiotic eyedrops.
- Close the eyes and apply a *small* ice pack.

RETINAL DISORDERS

MACULAR DEGENERATION

Pathophysiology Review

Macular degeneration, also known as *age-related macular degeneration* (AMD), is the deterioration of the macula (the area of central vision) and can be age related or exudative. It is the leading cause of blindness in individuals in the United States who are 65 years of age or older (CDC, 2020b). There are two types of AMD: *dry* and *wet*.

Dry AMD is the more common type of this condition. It is caused by a slow and gradual blockage of retinal capillaries by pigmented residue and photoreceptor waste products in the retina, allowing retinal cells in the macula to become ischemic and necrotic. Central vision declines, and patients describe mild blurring and distortion at first. Night vision is affected, and the ability to see clearly when reading is impaired. Eventually the patient loses all central vision.

Dry AMD progresses at a faster rate among smokers than among nonsmokers. Individuals with diabetes, hypertension, and high cholesterol are at risk for developing this condition. Other risk factors include being older than 55 years old, being White, smoking, and having a family history of AMD (National Eye Institute, 2021).

Wet (exudative) AMD progresses quickly. Patients experience a sudden decrease in vision after a detachment of pigment epithelium in the macula. Newly formed blood vessels, which have very thin walls, invade this injured area and cause fluid and blood to collect under the macula (like a blister), with scar formation and visual distortion. Wet (exudative) AMD can occur at any age, in only one eye or in both eyes. The patient with dry AMD can also develop wet (exudative) macular degeneration.

The risk for macular degeneration can be reduced by increasing long-term dietary intake of lutein, zeaxthin, vitamins C and E, and zinc (American Optometric Association, 2023b).

Interprofessional Collaborative Care

Recognize Cues: Assessment

An eye care provider will likely conduct indirect ophthalmoscopy to assess for gross macular changes, opacities, retinal concerns, and hemorrhage (Rebar & Rebar, 2019). IV fluorescein angiography may be performed by the eye care provider to locate leaking vessels, and the Amsler grid test may be conducted to demonstrate central visual field loss (Rebar & Rebar, 2019).

Take Actions: Interventions

Dry AMD has no cure. Management in the community setting is focused on slowing the progression of the vision loss and helping the patient maximize remaining vision and quality of life.

Central vision loss reduces the ability to read, write, recognize safety hazards, and drive. Suggest alternatives (e.g., large-print books, public transportation) and refer to community resources that provide adaptive equipment.

Management of patients with wet (exudative) AMD involves slowing the process and identifying further changes in visual perception. Fluid and blood may reabsorb in some patients. Laser therapy to seal the leaking blood vessels can limit the extent of the damage. Ocular injections with vascular endothelial growth factor inhibitors (VEGFIs), such as bevacizumab or ranibizumab, can improve vision in the patient with wet AMD. Aflibercept, a human recombinant fusion protein that functions as a VEGFI, and faricimab-svoa, a VEGFI and angiopoietin-2 (Ang-2) inhibitor, are other injectables used to treat wet AMD.

NCLEX Examination Challenge 39.4

Physiological Integrity

The nurse is caring for four outpatient clients being seen for an annual physical examination. Which client would the nurse identify as being at **highest** risk for development of dry age-related macular degeneration (AMD)?

A. 60-year-old client who recently began wearing glasses

B. 63-year-old client who has controlled hypertension

C. 67-year-old client with hypothyroidism

D. 69-year-old client with diabetes mellitus

RETINAL HOLES, TEARS, AND DETACHMENTS

Pathophysiology Review

A retinal hole is a break in the retina caused by trauma or that occurs with aging. A retinal tear is a jagged and irregularly shaped break in the retina, which can result from traction on the retina. A retinal detachment is the separation of the retina from the epithelium. Detachments are classified by the type and cause of their development.

One common cause of retinal holes, tears, and detachments is a *posterior vitreous detachment* (PVD). With aging, the vitreous gel often shrinks or thickens, causing it to pull away from the retina. The patient may experience small flashes of light seen as "shooting stars" or thin "lightning streaks" in one eye, most visible in a dark environment. These flashes of light may be accompanied by "floaters." In addition to aging, risk factors for PVD include extreme myopia, inflammation inside the eye, and cataract or eye laser surgery. When the PVD does not cause a retinal tear or detachment, no treatment is needed.

Interprofessional Collaborative Care
Recognize Cues: Assessment

The onset of a retinal detachment is usually sudden and painless. Patients may report suddenly seeing bright flashes of light (*photopsia*) or floating dark spots in the affected eye. During the initial phase of the detachment or if the detachment is partial, the patient may describe the sensation of a curtain being pulled over part of the visual field. The visual field loss corresponds to the area of detachment. Patients who report this type of concern to a telehealth triage nurse should be cautioned to have another individual drive them to their eye care provider of choice.

The eye care provider will perform an ophthalmoscopic examination. Detachments are seen as gray bulges or folds in the retina. Sometimes a hole or tear may be seen at the edge of the detachment.

Take Actions: Interventions

If a retinal hole or tear is discovered before it causes a detachment, the defect may be closed or sealed. Closure prevents fluid from collecting under the retina and reduces the risk for a detachment. Treatment involves creating a scar with *laser photocoagulation*—a procedure in which focused light beams seal tissue around the hole. *Cryopexy*, a procedure that involves a freezing probe, can be used to bind the retina and choroid together around the break.

Spontaneous reattachment of a totally detached retina is rare. Surgical repair—called *scleral buckling*—is needed to place the retina in contact with the underlying structures.

Preoperative Care. Most patients are anxious and fearful about the possible permanent loss of vision. Nursing priorities include providing information and support.

Instruct the patient to restrict activity and head movement before surgery to prevent further tearing or detachment. An eye patch is placed over the affected eye to reduce eye movement. Topical drugs are given before surgery to inhibit pupil constriction and accommodation.

Operative Procedures. Surgery is performed with the patient under general anesthesia. In scleral buckling, the ophthalmologist repairs wrinkles or folds in the retina and indents the eye surface to relieve the tugging pressure on the retina. The indentation or "buckling" is performed by placing a small piece of silicone against the outside of the sclera and holding it in place with an encircling band. This device keeps the retina in contact with the choroid for reattachment. Any fluid under the retina is drained.

Silicone oil or gas is placed inside the eye to promote retinal reattachment. These agents float up and against the retina to hold it in place until healing occurs.

Postoperative Care. After surgery an eye patch and shield are usually applied. Monitor the patient's vital signs, and check the eye patch and shield for drainage.

Activity after surgery varies. If oil or gas has been placed in the eye, teach the patient to keep the head in the position instructed by the ophthalmologist to promote reattachment.

Teach the patient to report sudden increase in pain or pain occurring with nausea to the ophthalmologist immediately. Remind the patient to avoid activities that increase intraocular pressure (IOP) (see Box 39.6).

Instruct the patient to avoid reading, writing, and work that requires close vision in the first week after surgery because these activities cause rapid eye movements and detachment. Teach the signs and symptoms of infection and detachment (sudden reduced visual acuity, eye pain, pupil that *does not constrict* in response to light) that must be reported to the ophthalmologist immediately.

REFRACTIVE ERRORS

Pathophysiology Review

The ability of the eye to focus images on the retina depends on the length of the eye from front to back and the refractive power of the lens system. Refraction is the bending of light rays. Problems in either eye length or refraction can result in refractive errors.

Myopia is nearsightedness, in which the eye overrefracts the light and the bent images fall in front of, not on, the retina. Hyperopia, also called *hypermetropia*, is farsightedness, in which refraction is too weak, causing images to be focused behind the retina. Presbyopia is the age-related problem in which the lens loses its elasticity and is less able to change shape to focus the eye for close work. As a result, images fall behind the retina. This problem usually begins in adults in their 40s. Astigmatism occurs when the curve of the cornea is uneven. Because light rays are not refracted equally in all directions, the image does not focus on the retina.

Interprofessional Collaborative Care
Recognize Cues: Assessment

Refractive errors are diagnosed through a refraction test. The patient is asked to view an eye chart while lenses of different strengths are systematically placed in front of the eye. With each lens strength, the patient is asked whether the lenses sharpen or worsen vision. The strength of the lens needed to focus the image on the retina is expressed in measurements called *diopters*.

Take Actions: Interventions

Nonsurgical Management. Refractive errors are corrected with eyeglasses or contact lenses that focus light rays on the retina (see Fig. 39.5). Hyperopic vision is corrected with a convex lens that moves the image forward. Myopic vision is corrected with a concave lens that moves the image back to the retina.

Surgical Management. Surgery can correct some refractive errors and enhance vision. The most common vision-enhancing surgery is laser in situ keratomileusis (LASIK). This procedure can correct nearsightedness, farsightedness, and astigmatism. The superficial layers of the cornea are lifted temporarily as a flap, and powerful laser pulses reshape the deeper corneal layers.

After reshaping is complete, the corneal flap is placed back into its original position.

Usually both eyes are treated at the same time, which is convenient for the patient, although this practice has risks. Many patients have improved vision within an hour after surgery, and complete healing takes up to 4 weeks. The outer corneal layer is not damaged, and pain is minimal.

Complications of LASIK are rare, yet include temporary or chronic dry eyes, halos around lights, double vision, light sensitivity, or vision loss. Risks for these complications are higher in patients with weak immune systems.

TRAUMA

Trauma to the eye or orbital area can result from almost any activity. Care varies, depending on the area of the eye affected, whether the globe of the eye has been penetrated, surrounding injuries, and the mechanism of trauma. If there is any type of object protruding from the area of injury, *do not attempt to remove it.* The provider of care will assess whether the object is holding other structures in place, and which mechanism of removal is appropriate.

FOREIGN BODIES

Eyelashes, dust, dirt, and airborne particles can come in contact with the conjunctiva or cornea and irritate or abrade the surface. The patient usually reports the feeling of something being in the eye and may have blurred vision. Pain occurs if the corneal surface is injured. Tearing and photophobia may be present.

Visual *sensory perception* is assessed before treatment. If nothing is seen on the cornea or conjunctiva, the eyelid is everted to examine the conjunctivae. The eye is examined with fluorescein, followed by irrigation with normal saline (0.9%) to gently remove the particles. Remember, if both eyes are affected, irrigate them simultaneously using separate personnel and equipment.

If an eye dressing or patch is applied after the foreign body is removed, tell the patient how long this must be left in place. Follow-up as directed by the eye care provider is needed to confirm that appropriate healing is taking place.

LACERATIONS

Lacerations are caused by sharp objects and projectiles. The injury occurs most commonly to the eyelids and cornea, although any part of the eye can be lacerated. The patient with a laceration should receive medical attention right away. *Corneal lacerations are an emergency because eye contents may prolapse through the laceration.* Symptoms include severe eye pain, photophobia, tearing, decreased vision, and inability to open the eyelid. If the laceration is the result of a penetrating injury, an object may be seen protruding from the eye.

Minor lacerations of the eyelid can be sutured in an emergency department, an urgent care center, or an eye care provider's office. A microscope is needed in the operating room if the patient has a laceration that involves the eyelid margin, affects the lacrimal system, involves a large area, or has jagged edges.

Antibiotics are given to reduce the risk for infection. Depending on the depth of the laceration, scarring may develop. If the scar alters vision, a corneal transplant may be needed later. If the eye contents have prolapsed through the laceration or if the injury is severe, enucleation (surgical eyeball removal) may be indicated.

PENETRATING INJURIES

A penetrating eye injury often leads to permanent loss of visual *sensory perception.* Glass, high-speed metal or wood particles, BB pellets, and bullets are common causes of penetrating injuries. The particles can enter the eye and lodge in or behind the eyeball. A wound may be visible. Depending on where the object enters and rests within the eye, vision may be affected. *Never remove an object protruding from the eye;* the health care provider will assess the immediate condition and determine how to proceed.

X-rays and CT scans of the orbit are usually performed. MRI is contraindicated because the procedure may move any metal-containing projectile and cause more injury.

Surgery is usually needed to remove the foreign object, and sometimes vitreal removal is needed. IV antibiotics are started before surgery, and a tetanus booster is given if necessary.

> **! NURSING SAFETY PRIORITY**
> *Action Alert*
>
> An object protruding from the eye is removed only by an eye care provider because it may be holding the eye structures in place. Improper removal can cause structures to prolapse out of the eye.

GET READY FOR THE NEXT-GENERATION NCLEX® EXAMINATION!

Essential Nursing Care Points

Health Promotion/Disease Prevention	Chronic Disease Care
• Teach ways to protect vision before loss or damage occurs. • Encourage patients to adhere to the recommended frequency for regular eye examinations based on their risk factors. • Orient newly hospitalized patients with impaired vision to their room, and remind them to call for help when ambulation is needed. • Ask about a family history of vision problems because some conditions have a genetic component.	• Regularly assess if assistive devices (e.g., glasses, contact lenses) are in good working order and serving the patient's current visual *sensory perception* needs. • Collaborate with the interprofessional team to increase independence and safety within the home environment and community for the patient with impaired vision. • Teach patients who use eyedrops to adhere strictly to the prescribed schedule.
Regenerative or Restorative Care	**Hospice/Palliative/Supportive Care**
• Teach patients who have had eye surgery to avoid activities that increase intraocular pressure (IOP). • Stress the importance of completing an antibiotic regimen for an eye infection or injury. • Never attempt to remove any object protruding from the eye.	• Encourage patients with vision loss to talk with an eye care specialist about the possibility of vision rehabilitation.

Mastery Questions

1. The telehealth nurse receives a call from a client who had surgery this morning to repair a retinal detachment. When the client reports pain in the affected eye with diminished visual acuity, which nursing response is appropriate?
   A. "Take acetaminophen to address the pain."
   B. "Contact your ophthalmologist right away."
   C. "This is a normal response to the type of surgery you had."
   D. "If the symptoms are still present in 24 hours, seek emergency care."

2. A client comes to the emergency department reporting the new sensation of something in the eye. Which of the following assessment data would the nurse anticipate that is consistent with a foreign body? **Select all that apply.**
   A. Pain
   B. Fever
   C. Tearing
   D. Photophobia
   E. Blurred vision

3. Which condition would the nurse anticipate when a client explains having slow, progressive visual disturbance over the past 2 years?
   A. Cataract
   B. Retinal hole
   C. Corneal abrasion
   D. Angle-closure glaucoma

NGN Challenge 39.1

The nurse is reviewing the health record of a client who is here for an eye examination.

- 64 years old
- Weight 130 lb (59 kg)
- Height 66 inches (167.6 cm)
- Medical history: Hypertension, type 2 diabetes
- Social history: Smokes 1 pack of cigarettes daily; denies alcohol or illicit substance use
- Family history: Hypertension, type 2 diabetes, glaucoma

NURSING FLOW SHEET

Date	Reason for Visit	Vision Acuity	Blood Pressure
6-17-2020	Annual eye exam; reports occasional dry eyes after working at the computer all day	20/20	130/86 mm Hg
6-26-2021	Annual eye exam; reports no changes in vision since last appointment	20/20	132/88 mm Hg
7-3-2022	Annual eye exam; reports noticing mild changes in vision stating, "Things are starting to look clouded over to me in my left eye. I must just be getting old."	20/60	150/98 mm Hg

Which of the following actions would the nurse plan to take at this time? **Select all that apply.**

- ○ Schedule client for cataract removal.
- ○ Prepare for scleral buckling procedure.
- ○ Teach about progressive nature of glaucoma.
- ○ Recognize these findings as a medical emergency.
- ○ Reassure that these findings are a normal part of aging.
- ○ Gather information to teach about eyedrop instillation.
- ○ Explain that drug therapy will halt the progression of eye changes.
- ○ Remind that accompanying symptoms such as eye redness will soon start.

NGN Challenge 39.2

The nurse reviews the notes for a 33-year-old client who has been brought by a coworker to the ophthalmologist.

History and Physical	Nurses' Notes	Imaging Studies	Laboratory Results

1111: Brought by car to emergency department by coworker. Reports being at work this morning in a meeting when suddenly they saw "shooting stars" in the left eye followed by the sensation of "someone closing a curtain" over the outer periphery of the eye. Denies pain. No other significant medical history is present. VS: T 98.2°F (36.8°C); HR 84 beats/min; RR 16 breaths/min; BP 124/92 mm Hg; SpO$_2$ 99% on RA.
Alert and oriented × 4; moves all extremities strongly and equally. PERRLA. Cranial nerves intact. Conjunctiva clear and sclera white bilaterally. Ophthalmologist in to see client.

Complete the diagram by selecting from the choices to specify what potential condition the client is likely experiencing, **2** nursing actions that are appropriate to take, and **2** parameters the nurse should monitor to assess the client's progress.

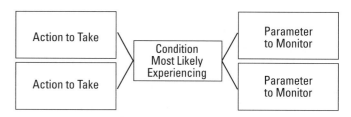

Actions to Take	Potential Conditions	Parameters to Monitor
Place in Trendelenburg position	Open angle glaucoma	Signs of infection in the eye
Recommend glasses to correct vision	Retinal tear	Drainage around the eye shield
Prepare for laser photocoagulation	Cataract	Formation of clouding over the eye
Place a patch over the unaffected eye	Myopia	Ability to see with newly prescribed glasses
Apply topical medication to inhibit pupil constriction and accommodation		Pupil that should begin to constrict to light

REFERENCES

American Academy of Ophthalmology. (2022). *What does 20/20 vision mean?* https://www.aao.org/eye-health/tips-prevention/what-does-20-20-vision-mean.

American Academy of Ophthalmology. (2023). *Eye health statistics.* Retrieved from https://www.aao.org/newsroom/eye-health-statistics#_edn1.

American Optometric Association. (2023). *Lutein & zeaxanthin.* https://www.aoa.org/patients-and-public/caring-for-your-vision/diet-and-nutrition/lutein.

American Optometric Association. (2023b). *Macular degeneration.* https://www.aoa.org/healthy-eyes/eye-and-vision-conditions/macular-degeneration?sso=y.

Assil, K., et al. (2020). Dropless cataract surgery: Modernizing perioperative medical therapy to improve outcomes and patient satisfaction. *Current Opinion in Ophthalmology, 31,* S1–S12. https://doi.org/10.1097/ICU.0000000000000708.

Boyd, K. (2022). Smoking and eye disease. *American Academy of Ophthalmology.* Retrieved from https://www.aao.org/eye-health/tips-prevention/smokers.

Brown, L., et al. (2023). Smoking and ocular morbidities in older adult veterans. *MedSurg Nursing, 32*(1), 51–56.

Brusini, P., Salvetat, M. L., & Zeppieri, M. (2021). How to measure intraocular pressure: An updated review of various tonometers. *Journal of Clinical Medicine, 10*(17), 3860. https://doi.org/10.3390/jcm10173860.

Centers for Disease Control and Prevention. (2020a). *Don't let glaucoma steal your sight!* Retrieved from https://www.cdc.gov/visionhealth/resources/features/glaucoma-awareness.html.

Centers for Disease Control and Prevention. (2020b). *Learn about age-related macular degeneration.* Retrieved from https://www.cdc.gov/visionhealth/resources/features/macular-degeneration.html.

Centers for Disease Control and Prevention. (2022a). *Fast facts of common eye disorders.* https://www.cdc.gov/visionhealth/basics/ced/fastfacts.htm.

Centers for Disease Control and Prevention. (2022b). *Vision health initiative: Social determinants of health, health equity, and vision loss.* https://www.cdc.gov/visionhealth/determinants/index.html.

Duffy, M. (2021). *Vision rehabilitation services.* VisionAware: American Printing House for the Blind. https://visionaware.org/everyday-living/essential-skills/vision-rehabilitation-services/.

Eye Bank Association of America (EBAA). (2023). *Medical standards/procedures manual.* http://restoresight.org/what-we-do/publications/medical-standards-procedures-manual/.

Gaur, A., & Sarkar, P. (2022). Eye: The hard-hit victim of COVID-19 Pandemic. *Journal of Ophthalmic & Vision Research, 17*(2), 290–295. https://doi.org/10.18502/jovr.v17i2.10805.

Glaucoma Research Foundation. (2022a). Laser iridotomy: Frequently asked questions. https://glaucoma.org/laser-iridotomy-frequently-asked-questions/.

Glaucoma Research Foundation. (2022b). *Vision rehabilitation therapies for living with glaucoma.* https://glaucoma.org/vision-rehabilitation-therapies-for-living-with-glaucoma/.

Glaucoma Research Foundation. (2022c). *What can I do to prevent glaucoma?* http://www.glaucoma.org/gleams/what-can-i-do-to-prevent-glaucoma.php.

Gudgel, D. (2022). *Eye pressure.* Retrieved from https://www.aao.org/eye-health/anatomy/eye-pressure.

Interprofessional Education Collaborative. (2016). *Core competencies for interprofessional collaborative practice: 2016 update.* Retrieved from https://nebula.wsimg.com/2f68a39520b-03336b41038c370497473?AccessKeyId=DC06780E69ED19E-2B3A5&disposition=0&alloworigin=1.

Jacobs, D. (2022). Open-angle glaucoma: Epidemiology, clinical presentation, and diagnosis. *UpToDate.* Retrieved May 18, 2023, from https://www.uptodate.com/contents/open-angle-glaucoma-epidemiology-clinical-presentation-and-diagnosis.

Jarvis, C., & Eckhardt, A. (2024). *Physical examination & health assessment* (9th ed.). St. Louis: Elsevier.

Merck Manual. (2021). *Professional version.* Anisocoria. Retrieved from https://www.merckmanuals.com/professional/eye-disorders/symptoms-of-ophthalmologic-disorders/anisocoria.

Mitra, S., Rauf, A., Tareq, A. M., Jahan, S., Emran, T. B., Shahriar, T. G., et al. (2021). Potential health benefits of carotenoid lutein: An updated review. *Food and Chemical Toxicology, 154*:112328.

National Eye Institute of the National Institutes of Health. (2021). *Age-related macular degeneration.* https://www.nei.nih.gov/learn-about-eye-health/eye-conditions-and-diseases/age-related-macular-degeneration.

National Eye Institute of the National Institutes of Health. (2022). *Glaucoma.* https://www.nei.nih.gov/learn-about-eye-health/eye-conditions-and-diseases/glaucoma.

Rebar, C., & Rebar, M. (2019). *L. Willis's Professional Guide to Pathophysiology* (4th ed.). Philadelphia, PA: Wolters Kluwer. Chapter 15: Sensory System.

Rogers, J. L. (2023). *McCance and Huether's Pathophysiology: The biologic basis for disease in adults and children* (9th ed.). St. Louis: Elsevier.

Shin, D. Y., Jung, K. I., Park, H. Y. L., et al. (2021). The effect of anxiety and depression on progression of glaucoma. *Scientific Reports, 11,* 1769. https://doi.org/10.1038/s41598-021-81512-0.

Slusser, M., et al. (2019). *Foundations of interprofessional collaborative practice* (1st ed.). St. Louis: Elsevier.

Touhy, T., & Jett, K. (2023). *Ebersole and Hess' Toward healthy aging* (11th ed.). St. Louis: Elsevier.

U.S. Department of Health and Human Services. (2023). *Medicare learning network Fact sheet: Medicare vision services.* https://www.cms.gov/outreach-and-education/medicare-learning-network-mln/mlnproducts/downloads/visionservices_factsheet_icn907165.pdf.

40

Assessment and Concepts of Care for Patients With Ear and Hearing Conditions

Cherie R. Rebar

http://evolve.elsevier.com/Iggy/

LEARNING OUTCOMES

1. Use knowledge of anatomy and physiology to perform a focused assessment related to auditory *sensory perception.*
2. Teach evidence-based health promotion activities to help prevent auditory problems and ear trauma.
3. Explain how genetic implications and physiologic aging affect auditory *sensory perception.*
4. Plan collaborative care with the interprofessional team to promote *sensory perception* in patients with ear and hearing problems.
5. Teach the patient and caregiver(s) about common drugs and other management strategies used for ear and hearing problems.
6. Plan patient- and family-centered nursing interventions to decrease the psychosocial impact caused by living with ear and hearing problems.
7. Apply knowledge of anatomy, physiology, and pathophysiology to provide evidence-based care for patients with ear and hearing problems affecting *sensory perception*.
8. Analyze assessment and diagnostic findings to generate solutions and prioritize nursing care for patients with ear and hearing problems.
9. Organize care coordination and transition management for patients with ear and hearing problems.
10. Use clinical judgment to plan evidence-based nursing care to promote *sensory perception* and prevent complications in patients with ear and hearing problems.
11. Incorporate factors that affect health equity into the plan of care for patients with ear and hearing problems.

KEY TERMS

cerumen The wax produced by glands within the external ear canal; helps protect and lubricate the ear canal.

conductive hearing loss Hearing loss that results from any physical obstruction of sound wave transmission (e.g., a foreign body in the external canal, a retracted or bulging tympanic membrane, or fused bony ossicles).

external otitis A painful irritation or infection of the skin of the external ear, with resulting allergic response or inflammation. When it occurs in patients who participate in water sports, external otitis is called *swimmer's ear.*

frequency The highness or lowness of tones (expressed in hertz). The greater the number of vibrations per second, the higher the frequency (pitch) of the sound; the lower the number of vibrations per second, the lower the pitch.

grommet A polyethylene tube that is surgically placed through the tympanic membrane to allow continuous drainage of middle ear fluids in the patient with otitis media.

intensity A quality of sound expressed in decibels (dB).

labyrinthectomy Surgical removal of the labyrinth.

mastoiditis An acute or chronic infection of the mastoid air cells caused by progressive otitis media.

Ménière disease Tinnitus, one-sided sensorineural hearing loss, and vertigo that is related to overproduction or decreased reabsorption of endolymphatic fluid, causing a distortion of the entire inner canal system.

mixed conductive-sensorineural hearing loss A profound hearing loss that results from a combination of both conductive and sensorineural types of hearing loss.

myringoplasty Simple surgical reconstruction of the eardrum.

myringotomy The surgical creation of a hole in the eardrum; performed to drain middle ear fluids and relieve pain in the patient with otitis media (middle ear infection).

nystagmus Involuntary eye movements.

ossiculoplasty Replacement of the ossicles within the middle ear.

otoscope An instrument used to examine the ear; consists of a light, a handle, a magnifying lens, and a pneumatic bulb for injecting air into the external canal to test eardrum mobility.

ototoxic Having a toxic effect on the inner ear structures.

presbycusis Sensorineural hearing loss, especially for high-pitched sounds; occurs as a result of aging.

sensorineural hearing loss Hearing loss that results from damage to the inner ear or auditory nerve (cranial nerve VIII).

swimmer's ear See *external otitis.*

threshold The lowest level of intensity at which pure tones and speech are heard by a patient about 50% of the time.

tinnitus A continuous ringing or noise perception in the ear.

vertigo A sense of whirling or turning in space.

Hearing is one of the five senses that allow *sensory perception.* It is used to assess surroundings, promote independence, warn of danger, appreciate music, and communicate with others. Hearing problems can evolve over long periods of time or occur suddenly. They can arise as a side effect of medications taken or a systemic health problem. These problems reduce the ability to fully communicate with the world and can lead to frustration, social isolation, and impaired functional ability.

ANATOMY AND PHYSIOLOGY REVIEW

Structure

The external ear, the middle ear, and the inner ear make up the ear's three divisions.

External Ear

The external ear develops in the embryo at the same time as the kidneys and urinary tract. Any adult with a defect of the external ear should also be examined for possible problems of the kidney and urinary systems.

The *pinna* is the part of the external ear that is composed of cartilage covered by skin and attached to the head at about a 10-degree angle at the level of the eyes. The external ear extends from the pinna through the external ear canal to the *tympanic membrane* (eardrum) (Fig. 40.1). It includes the *mastoid process,* which is the bony ridge located over the temporal bone behind the pinna. The ear canal is slightly **S** shaped and is lined with cerumen-producing glands, oil glands, and hair follicles. Cerumen (ear wax) helps protect and lubricate the ear canal.

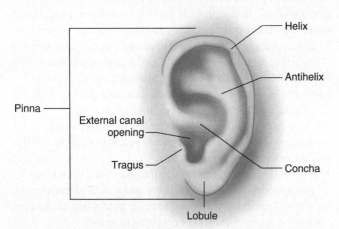

FIG. 40.1 Anatomic features of the external ear.

The distance from the opening of the ear canal to the eardrum in an adult is 1 to 1½ inches (2.5 to 3.75 cm).

Middle Ear

The eardrum separates the external ear and the middle ear. The middle ear consists of a compartment called the *epitympanum.* Located in the epitympanum are the top opening of the eustachian tube and three small bones known as the *bony ossicles,* which are the *malleus* (hammer), the *incus* (anvil), and the *stapes* (stirrup) (Fig. 40.2). The bony ossicles are joined loosely, thereby moving with vibrations created when sound waves hit the eardrum.

The eardrum is transparent, opaque, or pearly gray, and moves when air is injected into the external canal. The landmarks on the eardrum include the *annulus,* the *pars flaccida,* and the *pars tensa.* These correspond to the parts of the malleus that can be seen through the transparent eardrum. The eardrum is attached to the first bony ossicle, the malleus, at the umbo (Fig. 40.3). The umbo is seen through the eardrum membrane as a white dot and is one end of the long process of the malleus. The pars flaccida is that portion of the eardrum above the short process of the malleus. The pars tensa is that portion surrounding the long process of the malleus.

The middle ear is separated from the inner ear by the round window and the oval window. The eustachian tube begins at the floor of the middle ear and extends to the throat. The tube opening in the throat is surrounded by adenoid lymphatic tissue (Fig. 40.4). The eustachian tube allows the pressure on both sides of the eardrum to equalize. Secretions from the middle ear drain through the tube into the throat.

Inner Ear

The inner ear is on the other side of the oval window and contains the semicircular canals, the cochlea, the vestibule, and the distal end of the eighth cranial nerve (see Fig. 40.2). The *semicircular canals* are tubes made of cartilage and contain fluid and hair cells. These canals are connected to the sensory nerve fibers of the vestibular portion of the eighth cranial nerve. The fluid and hair cells within the canals help maintain the sense of balance.

The *cochlea,* the spiral organ of hearing, is divided into the scala tympani, the scala media, and the scala vestibuli. The scala media is filled with *endolymph,* and the scala tympani and scala vestibuli are filled with *perilymph.* These fluids protect the cochlea and the semicircular canals by allowing these structures to "float" in the fluids and be cushioned against abrupt head movements.

The *organ of Corti* is the receptor of hearing located on the membrane of the cochlea. The cochlear hair cells detect vibration from sound and stimulate the eighth cranial nerve.

The *vestibule* is a small, oval bony chamber between the semicircular canals and the cochlea. It contains the utricle and the saccule, organs that are important for balance.

Function

Auditory *sensory perception* occurs when sound is delivered through the air to the external ear canal. The sound waves strike the movable eardrum, creating vibrations. The eardrum is connected to the first bony ossicle, which allows the sound wave vibrations to be transferred from the eardrum to the malleus,

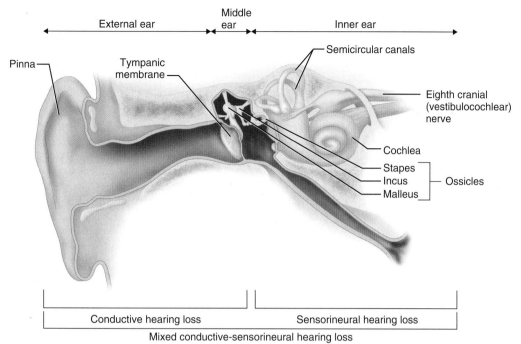

FIG. 40.2 Anatomic features of the middle and inner ear and areas involved in the three types of hearing loss.

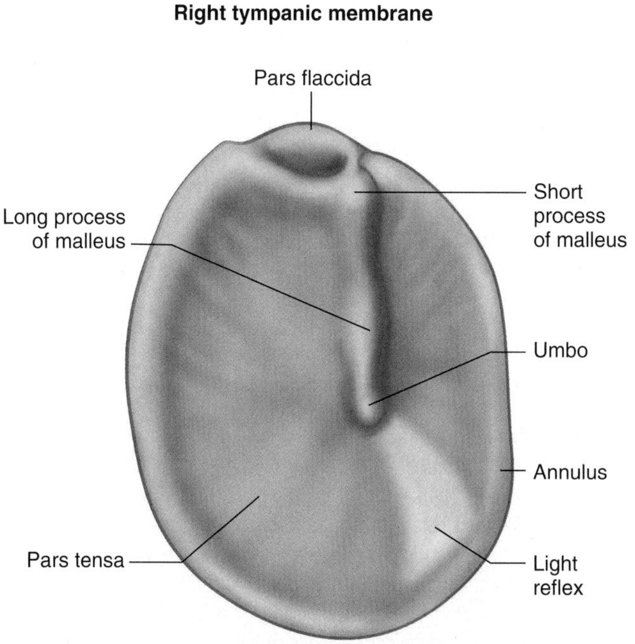

Right tympanic membrane

FIG. 40.3 Landmarks on the tympanic membrane.

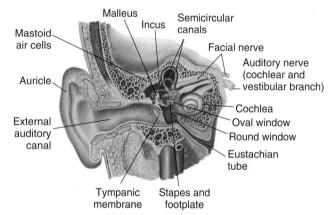

FIG. 40.4 Anatomic features and attached structures of the middle ear. (From Stewart, R.W., et. al. [2023]. *Seidel's Guide to physical examination: An interprofessional approach* [10th ed.]. St. Louis: Elsevier.)

the incus, and the stapes. From the stapes, the vibrations are transmitted to the cochlea. Receptors at the cochlea transduce (change) the vibrations into action potentials. The action potentials are conducted to the brain as nerve impulses by the cochlear portion of the eighth cranial (auditory) nerve. The nerve impulses are processed and interpreted as sound by the brain in the auditory cortex of the temporal lobe.

Ear and Hearing Changes Associated With Aging

All older adults should be screened for hearing acuity. Ear and hearing changes related to aging, and associated nursing adaptations and actions, are listed in the box titled Patient-Centered

Care: Older Adult Health: Age-Related Changes in the Ear and Hearing. Some of the ear changes do not cause harm; others affect the hearing ability of older adults.

✳ SENSORY PERCEPTION CONCEPT EXEMPLAR: HEARING LOSS

Pathophysiology Review

Loss of auditory *sensory perception* is common and may be conductive, sensorineural, or a combination of the two (see Fig. 40.2). Conductive hearing loss results from obstruction of sound wave transmission, such as a foreign body in the external canal, a retracted or bulging tympanic membrane, or fused bony ossicles. Tumors, scar tissue, and overgrowth of soft bony tissue *(otosclerosis)* on the ossicles from previous middle ear surgery also lead to conductive hearing loss.

👤 PATIENT-CENTERED CARE: OLDER ADULT HEALTH

Age-Related Changes in the Ear and Hearing

Ear or Hearing Change	Nursing Adaptations and Actions
Pinna becomes elongated because of loss of subcutaneous tissues and decreased elasticity.	Reassure the patient that this is normal. When positioning a patient on the side, do not "fold" the ear under the head.
Hair in the canal becomes coarser and longer, especially in men.	Reassure the patient that this is normal. More frequent ear irrigation may be needed to prevent cerumen attaching to hairs.
Cerumen is drier and becomes impacted more easily, reducing hearing function.	Request that the health care provider perform an assessment to determine whether the patient should self-irrigate the ears. If recommended, teach the patient (or caregiver, as necessary) to irrigate the ear canal as often as ordered by the primary health care provider.
Tympanic membrane loses elasticity and may appear dull and retracted.	Although this can indicate otitis media, do not use this as the only sign of this condition in older adults.
Hearing acuity decreases (in some people).	Tell the patient you will speak three words softly; then ask the patient to repeat them. You may have to repeat this test once or twice. If a deficit is assessed, refer the patient to a specialist to further assess hearing loss and recommend appropriate intervention. Do not assume that all older adults have a hearing loss!
The ability to hear high-frequency sounds is lost first. Older adults may have particular problems hearing the *f, s, sh,* and *pa* sounds.	Provide a quiet environment when speaking (close the door to the hallway), and face the patient. Avoid standing or sitting in front of bright lights or windows, which may interfere with the patient's ability to see your lips move. If the patient wears glasses, be sure that the patient is using them to enhance speech understanding. Speak slowly, clearly, and in a deeper voice while emphasizing beginning word sounds.

Data from Touhy, T., & Jett, K. (2022). *Ebersole and Hess' Gerontological nursing and healthy aging* (6th ed.). St. Louis: Elsevier; Touhy, T., & Jett, K. (2023). *Ebersole and Hess' Toward healthy aging* (11th ed.). St. Louis: Elsevier.

📄 EVIDENCE-BASED PRACTICE

The Effects of Providing Hearing Assistance in the Emergency Department

Dickson, V., et al. (2022). Providing hearing assistance to veterans in the emergency department: A qualitative study. *Journal of Emergency Nursing, 48*(3), 266-277.

Older adult veterans are at high risk for hearing loss due to exposure to combat-related noise exposure and age. More than 2 million veterans currently have severe hearing loss, which can dramatically affect the care they receive in busy emergency departments full of noise (Dickson et al., 2022). Effective communication among health care providers, nurses, and patients who are veterans is essential, yet hearing deficits in all older adults are often under-recognized and undertreated (Johns Hopkins Bloomberg School of Public Health, 2020).

With the desire to capture patient and provider perspectives about hearing issues experienced in the emergency department, this study was conducted to determine:
- Thoughts about hearing screenings in this setting
- Whether there are potential benefits of providing a hearing assistance device in this setting

Eleven participants—an appropriate sample for qualitative study purposes—took part in the study. All of the participants were older than 60, spoke English as their primary language, were likely to be discharged from the emergency department to home, and scored greater than or equal to 10 on the Hearing Handicap Inventory – Screen (Dickson et al., 2022). Following their use of an assistive hearing device during their emergency visit with the health care provider and nurse, they provided information about their experience.

Results indicated that the hearing screen and use of the assistive device were welcome and beneficial in improving the emergency department care experience (Dickson et al., 2022). Specific findings included the following:
1. Routine care does not support effective communication for veterans with hearing loss.
2. Screening for hearing loss in the emergency department was well-accepted for patients with non–life-threatening conditions.
3. Use of the hearing device made communication more effective and less tiresome for veterans and care providers.

Level of Evidence: VI
This research was designed as a qualitative study.

Commentary: Implications for Practice and Research
This study was conducted with the understanding that the average ED background noise level can make communication difficult for people with normal hearing. Therefore, people with a higher risk of hearing loss, such as veterans, could experience even more challenges with accurately hearing important care-related information (Dickson et al., 2022).

Facilitation of a brief hearing screening and voluntary use of a hearing assistive device can improve the care experience for veterans and clinicians. This improves the ability of veterans to understand their condition and associated needs, which means they can more actively participate in their own health care. This type of screening and the availability of a point-of-care accommodation in the form of a hearing assistive device could benefit patients with hearing loss in any care setting, not just the emergency department.

Any type of hearing loss can affect quality of life. It can also affect a patient's ability to understand information related to their health care. See the Evidence-Based Practice box.

Sensorineural hearing loss occurs when the inner ear or auditory nerve (cranial nerve VIII) is damaged. Prolonged exposure to loud noise damages the hair cells of the cochlea.

Many drugs are toxic to the inner ear structures, and their effects on hearing can be transient or permanent.

The differences in conductive and sensorineural hearing loss are listed in Table 40.1. Disorders that cause conductive hearing loss are often corrected with minimal or no permanent damage. Sensorineural hearing loss is often permanent.

TABLE 40.1 Comparison of Features of Conductive, Sensorineural, and Mixed Hearing Loss		
Conductive Hearing Loss	**Sensorineural Hearing Loss**	**Mixed Hearing Loss**
Causes Allergies Cerumen Eustachian tube dysfunction External otitis Fluid presence Foreign body Otitis media Perforation of the tympanic membrane	**Causes** Aging Auditory tumors Genetic hearing problems Head injury Health disorders (e.g., diabetes, Ménière disease, meningitis, stroke) Ototoxic drugs Prolonged noise exposure	**Causes** Combination of causes of conductive and sensorineural hearing loss (e.g., the patient has fluid in the ear, and the patient is exposed to prolonged noise in the personal work environment)
Assessment Findings Cerumen Hears better out of one ear Narrowing of ear canal Obstruction with a foreign body Otosclerosis Otitis externa Pain in the ear Report that one's own voice sounds strange Rupture of tympanic membrane Rinne test: bone conduction greater than air conduction in affected ear (will not hear fork at ear), and air conduction greater than bone conduction in unaffected ear Weber test: lateralization to affected ear	**Assessment Findings** Difficulty following conversations Dizziness Ear structures appear normal Hearing poorly in a loud environment Reports that speech of others is mumbled Tinnitus Rinne test: air conduction greater than bone conduction in most patients; some with severe loss may report bone conduction greater than air conduction if one ear functions better than the other Weber test: lateralization to unaffected or better-hearing ear	**Assessment Findings** Combination of any assessment findings associated with conductive and sensorineural hearing loss

Data from American Speech-Language-Hearing Association. (2023). Conductive hearing loss. https://www.asha.org/public/hearing/conductive-hearing-loss/; American Speech-Language-Hearing Association. (2023). Mixed hearing loss. https://www.asha.org/public/hearing/mixed-hearing-loss/ American Speech-Language-Hearing Association. (2023). Sensorineural hearing loss. https://www.asha.org/public/hearing/sensorineural-hearing-loss/; Weber, P. (2022). Evaluation of hearing loss in adults. *UpToDate*. Retrieved April 2, 2023, from https://www.uptodate.com/contents/evaluation-of-hearing-loss-in-adults.

Presbycusis is a sensorineural hearing loss that occurs with aging (Rogers, 2023). It is caused by degeneration of cochlear nerve cells, loss of elasticity of the basilar membrane, or a decreased blood supply to the inner ear. Higher intake of vitamin D and low-fat dietary patterns consisting of healthy fruits, vegetables, and meat are associated with reduced odds of development of hearing difficulties (Dawes et al., 2020).

Mixed conductive-sensorineural hearing loss includes a profound loss that results from a combination of these types of hearing loss. Mixed hearing loss involves damage to the inner and outer ear.

Etiology and Genetic Risk

Family history is important in determining genetic risk for hearing loss. Although most hearing loss resulting from a genetic mutation is noticed in childhood, some genetic problems can lead to progressive hearing loss in adults. For example, most people with Down syndrome who did not experience hearing loss as children will develop problems with hearing as they become young adults. Assess who in the family experienced hearing problems (and whether problems were present in one gender versus another), at what age the hearing loss was diagnosed, and whether both ears were affected.

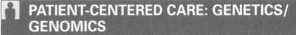

PATIENT-CENTERED CARE: GENETICS/GENOMICS

Genes and Hearing Loss

Mutations in several different genes are associated with hearing loss. One type of hearing loss among adults has a genetic basis with a mutation in gene *GJB2* (Online Mendelian Inheritance in Man [OMIM], 2023). This mutation causes poor production of the protein connexin 26, which has a role in the function of cochlear hair cells. Another vulnerability has been identified, substantiating a genetic predisposition for cisplatin-mediated sensorineural hearing loss (Tserga et al., 2019). Recognizing potential or actual genetic connections to hearing loss can help the nurse better collect a meaningful history that will influence care choices.

Incidence and Prevalence

Because hearing loss may be gradual and affect only some aspects of hearing, many adults are unaware that their hearing is impaired. The prevalence of adult hearing loss in the United States is estimated to be about 14% of the adult population between 20 and 69 years of age; this amount increases among people in their 70s and 80s (National Institute on Deafness and Other Communication Disorders, 2021).

Health Promotion/Disease Prevention

With proper care, hearing can be preserved to the greatest extent possible. Encourage patients to have simple hearing testing performed as part of their annual health assessment.

Teach adults to avoid using hairpins, ear candles, keys, cotton swabs, or toothpicks to clean the ear canal. These can scrape the skin of the canal, push cerumen up against the eardrum, and puncture the eardrum. If cerumen buildup is a problem, teach the patient to adhere only to the method of removal recommended by the primary health care provider.

Teach about the use of protective ear devices, such as over-the-ear headsets or foam ear inserts, when exposed to persistent loud noises. To prevent infections, suggest the use of earplugs when engaging in water sports and the use of an over-the-counter product such as Swim-EAR to help dry the ears after swimming.

! NURSING SAFETY PRIORITY

Action Alert

Teach patients the safe way to clean their ears, stressing that nothing smaller than their own fingertip should be inserted into the canal.

Interprofessional Collaborative Care

You will care for many patients with hearing loss. Often, they will not be seeking care for hearing issues, but for other health needs. Use the best practices strategies listed in Box 40.1 to communicate effectively with patients with hearing impairments.

Recognize Cues: Assessment

History. During the interview, sit in adequate light and face the patient to allow the patient to see you speak. The patient's posture and responses can provide information about hearing acuity. Tilting or turning the head to one side or leaning forward when listening to another person speak may indicate the presence of a hearing problem. Other indicators of hearing difficulty include asking the speaker to repeat statements or frequently saying "What?" or "Huh?" Assess whether the patient's responses match the question asked. For example, when you ask, "How old are you?" does the patient respond with an age or state something that may answer what the patient thought you said, such as "No, I am not cold."

Obtain data on age, demographics, personal and family history, socioeconomic status, occupational history, current health problems, and the use of remedies for ear problems. The patient's sex assigned at birth is important as some hearing disorders, such as otosclerosis, are more common in women.

Personal history includes past or current signs and symptoms of ear pain or discharge, vertigo (spinning sensation), tinnitus (ringing), decreased hearing, and difficulty understanding others when they talk. Ask about:

- Changes in hearing, when these began, and how fast (or slowly) they have progressed
- History of head or ear trauma or surgery

BOX 40.1   Best Practice for Patient Safety and Quality Care

Communicating With a Patient Who Is Hearing-Impaired

- Make sure that the room is well-lit and quiet.
- If available, offer the patient a hearing device, such as a personal digital amplifier.
- Get the patient's attention before you begin to speak.
- Position yourself directly in front of the patient. Be respectful of the patient's need for personal space.
- Ensure that you are not sitting or standing in front of a bright light or window, which can interfere with the patient's ability to see your lips move.
- If the patient indicates that one ear is better than the other, move closer to the better-hearing ear.
- Speak clearly and slowly; lowering your voice can be helpful to some patients.
- Do not shout (shouting often makes understanding more difficult).
- Keep hands and other objects away from your mouth when talking to the patient.
- Have the patient repeat your statements. Nodding of the head does not confirm that the patient understood.
- Rephrase sentences and repeat information to aid understanding.
- Use appropriate hand motions.
- Write messages on paper if the patient is able to read.
- Obtain the assistance of an interpreter if needed, and ensure that all members of the interprofessional team use this service.

- Number of past ear infections or perforations
- Presence of excessive cerumen
- Type and pattern of ear hygiene
- Drugs used (for any condition), as some are ototoxic (having a toxic effect on the inner ear structures), such as NSAIDs, certain antibiotics (e.g., aminoglycosides), diuretics, quinine-based medications, and certain cancer medications (American Tinnitus Association, 2022)
- Exposure to loud noise or music during occupational or social activities
- Air travel (especially in unpressurized aircraft)
- Health history of allergies, upper respiratory infections, COVID-19, cancer, hypothyroidism, atherosclerosis, human immunodeficiency virus (HIV) disease, or diabetes.

Physical Assessment: Signs and Symptoms. Techniques for assessment of patients with suspected loss of auditory *sensory perception* are found in Box 40.2. Remember to use Contact Precautions when assessing the ear because drainage may be present.

Tuning fork tests performed by the primary health care provider can help diagnose hearing loss. *Otoscopic examination,* performed by the primary health care provider with an otoscope, is used to assess the ear canal, eardrum, and middle ear structures that can be seen through the eardrum. Findings vary, depending on the cause of the hearing loss. The purpose of a brief otoscopic examination is to assess the patency of the external canal, identify lesions or excessive cerumen in the canal, and assess whether the tympanic membrane (eardrum) is intact or inflamed (Jarvis & Eckhardt, 2024).

BOX 40.2 Assessing the Patient With Suspected Hearing Loss

- Assess the ability to hear high-frequency consonants (*s, sh, f, th,* and *ch* sounds).
- Assess visible ear structures:
  - Position, size, and condition of the pinna; abnormalities include redness/hyperpigmentation, excessive warmth, crusting, scaling, nodules, and pain (Jarvis & Eckhardt, 2024).
  - Patency of the external canal; presence of cerumen or foreign bodies, edema, or inflammation
  - Mastoid process, which should be free from pain, redness/hyperpigmentation, and swelling
  - **NOTE:** The health care provider will assess the condition of the tympanic membrane for intactness and for the presence of edema, fluid, or inflammation.
- Assess functional ability, including:
  - Frequency of asking people to repeat statements
  - Withdrawal from social interactions or large groups
  - Shouting in conversation
  - Failing to respond when not looking in the direction of the sound
  - Answering questions incorrectly
- Assess hearing aids (if present) for cracks, debris, proper fit, and cleanliness.

Psychosocial Assessment. For patients with a loss of auditory *sensory perception,* communication can be challenging. They may isolate themselves because of difficulty in talking, listening, and interpreting what is said to them. Social and work isolation can lead to depression. Encourage patients to express their feelings and concerns about an actual or potential hearing loss.

NCLEX Examination Challenge 40.1

Psychosocial Integrity

Which statement by a client with progressive hearing loss would the nurse further assess as the **priority**?
A. "I think I may need a phone amplifier."
B. "It's getting harder for me to hear people in restaurants."
C. "It's easier for me to stay home than to go out and socialize."
D. "I would like to talk to the audiologist about getting better hearing aids."

Imaging Assessment. Imaging assessment can reveal some problems affecting hearing ability. Skull x-rays determine bony involvement in otitis media and the location of otosclerotic lesions. CT and MRI are used to determine soft-tissue involvement and the presence and location of tumors.

Other Diagnostic Assessments. Diagnostic assessments of hearing and balance can be useful in isolating the degree of hearing loss and, in some cases, the cause (Table 40.2).

Audiometry. Audiometry, performed by an audiologist, is the most reliable method of measuring the acuity of auditory *sensory perception.* Frequency is the highness or lowness of tones (expressed in hertz). The greater the number of vibrations

per second, the higher the frequency (pitch) of the sound. The fewer the vibrations per second, the lower the frequency.

Intensity of sound is expressed in decibels (dB). Threshold is the lowest level of intensity at which pure tones and speech are heard by a patient about 50% of the time. The lowest intensity at which a healthy ear can detect sound about 50% of the time is 0 dB. Conversational speech is around 60 dB, and a soft whisper is around 30 dB (Table 40.3). Sound at 110 dB is so intense (loud) that it can be painful for most people with normal hearing; this type of sound is akin to being near the speakers at a loud rock concert.

People with 20 to 40 dB of hearing loss may have mild difficulty hearing conversations in noisy settings (University of Iowa [UI], 2019). People with 41 to 55 dB of hearing loss have trouble hearing conversation even in quieter environments (UI, 2019). Those with 56 to 70 dB of hearing loss may not be able to hear a normal conversation, and if hearing loss is 71 to 90 dB, they can only hear if the speaker is right next to them (UI, 2019).

Analyze Cues and Prioritize Hypotheses: Analysis

The priority collaborative problems for the patient with any degree of hearing impairment include:
1. Decreased auditory *sensory perception* due to obstruction, *infection,* damage to the middle ear, or damage to the auditory nerve
2. Decreased communication due to difficulty hearing

Generate Solutions and Take Actions: Planning and Implementation

Increasing Hearing. Nursing care priorities focus on teaching the patient about the use of any prescribed drug therapy and appropriate assistive devices, helping the patient and caregivers to maintain or increase communication, and helping patients find community agency support.

Nonsurgical Management. Interventions include early detection of impaired auditory *sensory perception,* use of appropriate therapy, and use of assistive devices to augment the patient's usable hearing.

Early detection helps correct the problem causing the hearing loss. Assess for indications of hearing loss as covered in Box 40.2.

Drug therapy, if appropriate, is focused on correcting the underlying problem or reducing the side effects of problems occurring with hearing loss. Antibiotic therapy is used to manage external otitis and other ear infections. Teach patients the importance of taking the drug(s) exactly as prescribed. Caution patients not to stop the drug just because signs and symptoms have improved. By treating the *infection,* antibiotics reduce local edema and improve hearing. When *pain* is also present, analgesics are used. Many ear disorders induce vertigo and dizziness with nausea and vomiting. Antiemetic, antihistamine, and antivertiginous drugs can be prescribed to reduce these problems.

Assistive devices are useful for patients with permanent hearing loss. Amplifiers increase telephone volume, allowing the

TABLE 40.2   Diagnostic Studies and Associated Nursing Care

Test	Purpose	Associated Nursing Care
Audiometry	Used to test the ability to hear sounds. *Pure tone audiometry* is done in a soundproof area. The patient wears earphones and hears sounds directed to one ear at a time. The patient is to respond when a sound is heard. *Speech audiometry* is used to assess how loud speech must be before the patient can hear it well and how clearly the patient can understand and distinguish words that are spoken.	Describe test and confirm that no special preparation is needed. Clarify that pure tone audiometry takes about an hour, and speech audiometry takes about 10–15 minutes.
Auditory evoked potential (AEP)	Used to detect and estimate a patient's hearing level or degree of impairment. Can be used to help with the diagnosis of auditory disorders, multiple sclerosis, and neurologic disorders that affect balance.	Describe test, explaining that it is similar to an electroencephalogram (EEG). Other preparation is the same as that for BAEP.
Brainstem auditory evoked potential (BAEP) (also known as *auditory brainstem response*, or *ABR*)	Used to measure brain wave activity that happens when sounds are heard. Can be used to help with the diagnosis hearing loss and acoustic tumors.	Describe test and teach that electrodes will be placed on the scalp. Patients should wash their hair the night before the test and refrain from using lotions, moisturizers, or oils on the face. Small red spots may remain on the areas where the electrodes were placed, but these will resolve. Remind patients to wash their hair after the procedure to remove electrode gel.
Computerized dynamic posturography (CDP), also called *balance board testing* or *equilibrium platform testing*	Used to measure whether a patient can maintain steady balance as the platform the patient is standing on is manipulated. Can be used to identify problematic vestibular symptoms.	Describe test and confirm that no special preparation is needed. Teach that the patient will be placed into a safety harness to prevent falling. Explain that the platform the patient will stand on will move at different times, and the patient may be asked to maintain balance with the eyes shut during the test.
Electronystagmography (ENG)	Used to assess for central and peripheral disease of the vestibular system in the ear by detecting and recording nystagmus. Can be used to detect peripheral vestibular system disorders or to determine the site of a known lesion.	Describe test. Remind the patient to confirm with the health care provider which medications should be taken (or avoided) the day of the test, and to refrain from eating for at least 4 hours prior to testing. Explain that electrodes will be placed above and below the patient's eyes and that the patient may be instructed to look in different directions during the test. Teach that water and air may be introduced into the ear if the patient is undergoing caloric testing. Teach that dizziness and nausea may occur during the test and that another adult should be present to drive the patient home after testing.
Imaging assessment	CT (with or without contrast)—used to assess ear structures in great detail; can be used to assist with diagnosis of acoustic tumors. MRI—used to assess soft-tissue changes.	Describe test and teach to report claustrophobia prior to testing. A mild sedative may be prescribed. Open MRI is an option for those who need this test.
Laboratory tests	Used to assess whether an infection is present; microbial culture and antibiotic sensitivity can be performed for specific causative organism and the antibiotic that will best manage the infection.	Describe test. Confirm that no special preparation is needed and that blood work will be collected.
Tympanometry	Used to assess eardrum mobility, stiffness, or presence of puncture by changing air pressure in the external air canal.	Describe test and confirm that no special preparation is needed. Teach that there may be some discomfort while a probe is in the ear and that sounds heard during the procedure may be loud.

TABLE 40.3 **Decibel Intensity and Safe Exposure Time for Common Sounds**

Sound	Decibel Intensity (dB)	Typical Response
Threshold of hearing	0	Lowest level of intensity at which pure tones and speech are heard by a patient about 50% of the time
Watch ticking	20	No hearing damage/loss is usually experienced based on this exposure.
Soft whisper	30	No hearing damage/loss is usually experienced based on this exposure.
Average residence or office	40	No hearing damage/loss is usually experienced based on this exposure.
Conversational speech	60	No hearing damage/loss is usually experienced based on this exposure.
Washing machine or dishwasher	70	Noise may be annoying, but no hearing damage/loss is usually experienced based on this exposure.
City traffic (from inside a vehicle)	80	Noise may be annoying, but no hearing damage/loss is usually experienced based on this exposure.
Lawn mowers and leaf blowers	80–85	Hearing damage is possible after 2 hours of exposure.
Motorcycle	95	Hearing damage is possible after 50 minutes of exposure.
Loud entertainment venues (e.g., nightclubs, rock concerts)	105–110	Hearing loss is possible in less than 5 minutes of exposure.
Standing near sirens	120	Pain and ear injury
Standing near firecrackers	140–150	Pain and ear injury
Jet takeoff	150	Pain and ear injury

Data from Centers for Disease Control and Prevention. (2022). What noises cause hearing loss? https://www.cdc.gov/nceh/hearing_loss/what_noises_cause_hearing_loss.html.

caller to speak in a normal voice. Some phones also have a video display of words that are being spoken by the caller. Flashing lights activated by a ringing telephone or doorbell provide a visual alert. Video doorbell systems allow visualization of people outside. Some patients may have a service dog to alert them to sounds. Personal sound amplification products (PSAPs) offer solutions to situational activities that require a sound boost when a patient does not wish to have a hearing aid. These devices can help amplify sounds from a television or voices from people sitting at a table. Some devices are accessible via a headset or earpiece with Bluetooth capability, allowing patients to take calls or listen to music directly through their smartphones.

A hearing aid is a small electronic amplifier that assists patients with conductive hearing loss but is less effective for sensorineural hearing loss (Fig. 40.5). The styles vary by size, placement, and the degree to which they amplify sound. Most common hearing aids are small. Some are attached to the wearer's glasses and are visible to other people. Another type fits into the ear and is less noticeable. Newer devices fit completely in the canal with only a fine, clear filament visible. The cost of smaller hearing aids varies with size and quality. The audiologist will teach the patient how to wear and acclimate to the hearing aid that is selected.

Teach the patient how to care for the hearing aid (Box 40.3). Hearing aids are delicate devices that should be handled only by people who know how to care for them properly.

BOX 40.3 **Patient and Family Education**

Hearing Aid Care

- Keep the hearing aid dry.
- Clean the ear mold with mild soap and water while avoiding excessive wetting.
- Using a soft toothbrush or the brush that came with the device, clean debris from the hole in the middle of the part that goes into your ear.
- Turn off the hearing aid when not in use.
- Check and replace the battery frequently.
- Keep extra batteries on hand.
- Keep the hearing aid in a safe place.
- Avoid dropping the hearing aid or exposing it to temperature extremes.
- Avoid using hair spray, cosmetics, oils, or other hair and face products that might come into contact with the receiver.
- Check with your audiology provider to determine whether you can swim with your particular hearing aid(s). Some are water-resistant (and do not tolerate submersion); others are waterproof (and can be used while swimming).
- Adjust the volume to the lowest setting that allows you to hear to prevent feedback squeaking.
- If the hearing aid does not work:
  - Change the battery.
  - Check the connection between the ear mold and the receiver.
  - Check the on/off switch.
  - Clean the sound hole.
  - Adjust the volume.
  - Take the hearing aid to an authorized service center for repair.

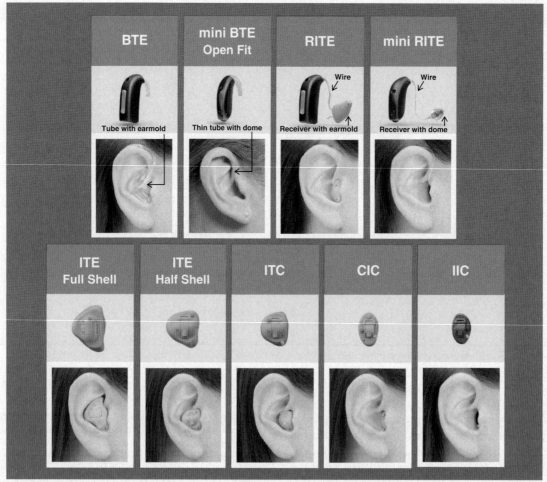

FIG. 40.5 Types of hearing aids. (From Oticon, Inc., Somerset, NJ. In Cifu, D.X., Lew, H.L., & Oh-Park, M. [2018]. *Geriatric rehabilitation.* Philadelphia: Elsevier.)

NCLEX Examination Challenge 40.2

Basic Care and Comfort

The nurse is caring for a client with progressive hearing loss. Which action would the nurse teach assistive personnel (AP) when delegating hearing aid care?

A. Clean the ear mold with alcohol to remove debris.
B. Store the cleaned devices in a dry, sealed container.
C. Immerse the hearing aid in warm water after cleaning it.
D. Take the hearing aid apart to assure that the inside is cleaned.

INTERPROFESSIONAL COLLABORATION

The Patient With Hearing Loss

The patient with hearing loss who needs hearing aids benefits from the services of an *audiologist.* Audiologists, members of the interprofessional team, are doctorally prepared individuals who can identify and manage problems with hearing or balance. They often see patients with conditions such as auditory nerve dysfunction, tinnitus, hearing loss, and auditory processing needs. They work with these patients on prevention of further hearing or balance problems and on ways of maximizing auditory ***sensory perception***.

According to the Interprofessional Education Collaborative (IPEC) Expert Panel's Competency of Roles and Responsibilities, using the unique and complementary abilities of other team members optimizes health and patient care (IPEC, 2016; Slusser et al., 2019).

Audiologists can also engage patients in audiologic rehabilitation, a process by which patients can relearn hearing skills that they have lost (American Speech-Language-Hearing Association, 2023). This process involves orientation to hearing aids, cochlear implants, and other hearing devices such as amplifiers, and instruction on how to use these to learn how to hear (or hear again).

For patients who do not need assistive devices but still have some degree of hearing loss, audiologic rehabilitation helps them learn skills to become better listeners. This type of rehabilitation can teach patients with any type of hearing loss how to use visual cues more effectively, and ways of improving and

enhancing communication (American Speech-Language-Hearing Association, 2023).

Cochlear implantation may help patients with sensorineural hearing loss. Although a superficial surgical procedure is needed to implant the device, the procedure does not enter the inner ear and thus is not considered a surgical correction for hearing impairment (Fig. 40.6). A small computer converts sound waves into electronic impulses. Electrodes are placed

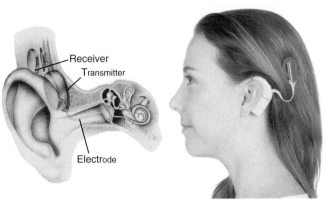

FIG. 40.6 Cochlear implant. (From Leonard, P.C. [2020]. *Quick and easy medical terminology* [9th ed.]. St. Louis: Elsevier.)

near the internal ear, with the computer attached to the external ear. The electronic impulses then directly stimulate nerve fibers.

Surgical Management. If nonsurgical management is ineffective, various surgical interventions are available for patients with specific disorders that have contributed to hearing loss.

Tympanoplasty. Tympanoplasty (Fig. 40.7) reconstructs the middle ear to improve conductive hearing loss. The procedures vary from simple reconstruction of the eardrum (myringoplasty) to replacement of the ossicles within the middle ear (ossiculoplasty).

Preoperative care. Teach the patient that systemic antibiotics may be given prior to the procedure to reduce the risk for **infection**. Remind patients to follow other measures to decrease the risks for infection, such as avoiding large crowds and people with upper respiratory infections, getting adequate rest, eating a balanced diet, and drinking adequate amounts of fluid.

Assure the patient that hearing loss immediately after surgery is normal because of canal packing and that hearing will improve when it is removed. Stress that forceful coughing increases middle ear pressure and must be avoided.

Operative procedures. Tympanoplasty can be done via a postaurical approach, endaural (through the ear canal) approach, or transcanal approach, or endoscopically (Fig. 40.8) (Brar et al., 2023). Surgery is performed only when the middle ear is free of infection. If an infection is present, the graft is more likely to become infected and not heal. Surgery of the eardrum and ossicles requires the use of a microscope and is a delicate procedure. Local anesthesia can be used, although general anesthesia is often used to prevent the patient from moving.

The surgeon can repair the eardrum with many materials, including tissue from a vein or muscle sheath. If the ossicles are damaged, more extensive surgery is needed for repair or replacement. The ossicles can be reached in several ways—through the ear canal, with an endaural incision, or by an incision behind the ear.

The surgeon removes diseased tissue and cleans the middle ear cavity. The patient's cartilage or bone, cadaver ossicles,

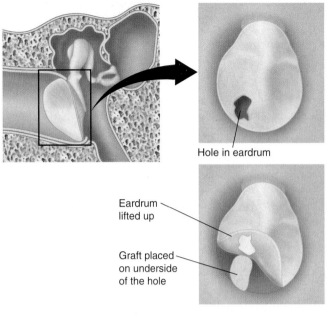

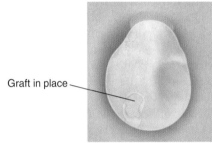

FIG. 40.7 Tympanoplasty.

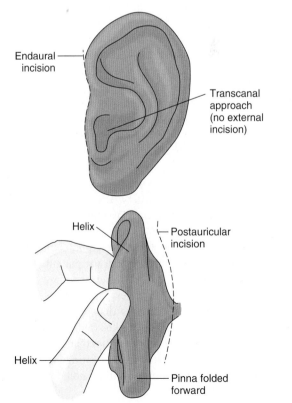

FIG. 40.8 Surgical approaches for repair of the ear and hearing structures.

stainless steel wire, or special polymers (Teflon) are used to repair or replace the ossicles.

Postoperative care. In an ossiculoplasty, a gelatin sponge soaked with ototopical antibiotic drops is packed in the ear canal; this will stay in place until the patient's follow-up visit (Young, 2022). If a skin incision is used, a dressing is placed over it. Keep the dressing clean and dry, using sterile technique for changes. Keep the patient flat, with the head turned to the side and the operative ear facing up for at least 12 hours after surgery. Give prescribed antibiotics to prevent *infection.*

Patients often report hearing improvement after removal of the canal packing. Until that time, communicate as with a patient who is hearing impaired, directing conversation to the unaffected ear. Instruct the patient in care and activity restrictions (Box 40.4), and teach that audiometry is usually performed 3 months after the procedure to assess hearing (Young, 2022).

Stapedectomy. A partial or complete stapedectomy with a prosthesis can correct some hearing loss, especially in patients with hearing loss related to otosclerosis. Although hearing usually improves after primary stapes surgery, some patients redevelop conductive hearing loss after surgery, and revision surgery is needed.

Preoperative care. To prevent *infection*, the patient must be free from external otitis at surgery. Teach the patient to follow measures that prevent middle ear or external ear infections, as noted in Box 40.5.

The surgeon will review the expected outcomes and possible complications of the surgery with the patient. The success rate of this procedure is high. However, there are always risks associated with this type of surgery, including complete and permanent hearing loss, dizziness that resolves the day after the procedure, development of tinnitus (although uncommon), and facial paralysis or taste abnormalities that arise due to nerve involvement. Remind the patient that hearing is initially worse after a stapedectomy, with improvement noted about 4 weeks after the procedure.

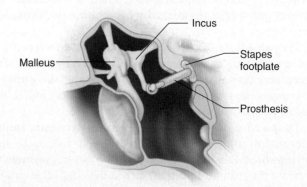

FIG. 40.9 Prosthesis used with stapedectomy. The stapes is removed, leaving the footplate. A metal or plastic prosthesis is connected to the incus and inserted through the hole to act as an artificial stapes.

Surgery is performed first on the ear with the greater hearing loss. If the surgery does not improve hearing, patients must decide to either attempt surgical correction of the other ear 6 months later or to continue to use an amplification device.

Operative procedures. A stapedectomy is usually performed through the external ear canal with the patient under local anesthesia. After removal of the affected ossicles, a piston-shaped prosthesis is connected between the incus and the footplate (Fig. 40.9). Because the prosthesis vibrates with sound as the stapes did, most patients have restoration of functional hearing.

Postoperative care. Remind the patient that improvement in hearing may not occur until 6 weeks after surgery. Drugs for *pain* help reduce discomfort, and antibiotics are used to prevent infection. Teach the patient about the precautions in Box 40.5.

The surgical procedure is performed in an area where cranial nerves VII, VIII, and X can be damaged by trauma or by swelling after surgery. *Assess for facial nerve damage or muscle weakness. Indications include an asymmetric appearance or drooping of features on the affected side of the face. Ask the patient about changes in taste or in facial perception of touch.* Vertigo, nausea, and vomiting can occur after surgery because of the nearness to inner ear structures.

Antivertiginous drugs (such as meclizine) and antiemetic drugs (such as ondansetron) may be prescribed. Prevent falls by assisting as needed. Instruct the patient to move slowly from a sitting to a standing position and to refrain from attempting to get out of bed or ambulate without assistance.

> ### ! NURSING SAFETY PRIORITY
> #### *Action Alert*
>
> Prevent injury by assisting the patient with ambulation during the first 1 to 2 days after stapedectomy. Keep top bed side rails up, and remind the patient to move the head slowly to avoid vertigo.

Totally Implanted Devices. Totally implanted devices, such as the Esteem®, can improve bilateral moderate to severe sensorineural hearing loss without any visible part (Envoy Medical, 2020). These devices have three totally implanted components: a sound processor, a sensor, and a driver. Vibrations of the eardrum and ossicles are picked up by the sensor and converted to electric signals that are processed by the sound processor. The processor is programmed to the patient's specific hearing pathology. The processor filters out some background noise and amplifies the desired sound signal. The signal is transferred to the computer, which then converts the processed signal into vibrations that are transmitted to the inner ear for auditory *sensory perception.*

The devices and the surgery may lead to possible complications, including temporary facial paralysis, changes in taste sensation, and ongoing or new-onset tinnitus. Unlike cochlear implants, the middle ear is entered, and it is considered a surgical procedure. Care before and after surgery is similar to that required with stapedectomy. The cost of the implant and procedure can be very high; currently this type of implantable device is not covered by Medicare or Medicaid, and only by select private insurers.

Maximizing Communication
Nonsurgical Management. Nursing priorities focus on facilitating communication and reducing anxiety. For communicating, use best practices that are listed in Box 40.1. Do not talk unnecessarily loudly to the patient because the sound may be projected at a higher frequency, making the patient less able to understand. Communicate by writing (if the patient is able to see, read, and write) or with pictures of familiar phrases and objects. Many television and streaming programs are now closed-captioned or subtitled.

Collaborate with members of the interprofessional team, such as the audiologist, who can help with maximizing hearing, which can improve communication. (See the Legal/Ethical Considerations box.)

Lip-reading and *sign language* can increase communication. Patients are taught special cues to look for when lip-reading and how to understand body language. However, the best lip-reader can still miss more than half of what is being said. Because even

> ### 🔍 LEGAL/ETHICAL CONSIDERATIONS
> #### Communication With Patients With Hearing Conditions
>
> Remember that you have a legal and ethical responsibility to make sure that you communicate effectively so that the patient receives the best care possible (National Association of the Deaf, 2023). Use all appropriate resources, based on the individual patient's abilities and needs, to ensure proper communication.

minimal lip-reading assists hearing, urge patients to wear their eyeglasses when talking with someone to see lip movement.

Sign languages, such as American Sign Language (ASL), combine speech with hand movements that signify letters, words, and phrases. These languages take time and effort to learn, and many people are unable to use them effectively.

Managing anxiety can increase the effectiveness of communication efforts. One source of anxiety is the possibility of permanent hearing loss. Provide accurate information about the likelihood of hearing returning. When the hearing impairment is likely to be permanent, reassure patients that communication and social interaction can be maintained with some practical modification.

Help patients use resources and communication to make social contact satisfying. Identify the patient's most satisfying activities and social interactions, and determine the effort necessary to continue them. The patient can alter activities to improve satisfaction. Instead of large gatherings, the patient might choose smaller groups. A meal at home with friends can substitute for dining out, or consider requesting a table in a quiet area of a restaurant.

Care Coordination and Transition Management

Patients with ear and hearing disorders rarely are hospitalized. Surgery, if needed, is often performed in an ambulatory surgery center. Follow-up hearing tests may be scheduled routinely or after surgical lesions are well healed, in about 12 weeks. To prevent *infection* after surgery, instruct patients to follow the information located in Box 40.5.

Provide written instructions to the patient and caregiver about how to take drugs and when to return for follow-up care, if needed. If eardrops are prescribed, teach proper instillation techniques, and obtain a return demonstration.

Teach patients with hearing aids how to effectively use and care for them. Remember that the costs associated with hearing devices can be extensive. Refer patients to appropriate agencies that specialize in working with patients with disorders affecting auditory *sensory perception.*

Evaluate Outcomes: Evaluation

Evaluate the care of the patient with hearing loss based on the identified priority patient problems. The expected outcomes include that the patient will:

- Maintain as much hearing as possible and/or use appropriate hearing compensation behaviors

- Successfully use a method (or methods) of communication that works best for the individual
- Successfully use assistive devices as needed

OTITIS MEDIA

Pathophysiology Review

The common forms of otitis media are acute otitis media, chronic otitis media, and serous otitis media. Each type affects the middle ear but has different causes and pathologic changes. If otitis progresses or is untreated, permanent conductive hearing loss may occur.

Acute otitis media and chronic otitis media are similar. An infecting agent in the middle ear causes inflammation of the mucosa, leading to swelling and irritation of the ossicles within the middle ear, followed by purulent inflammatory exudate. The acute form has a sudden onset and lasts 3 weeks or less. Chronic otitis media often follows repeated acute episodes, has a longer duration, and causes greater middle ear injury. It may be a result of the continuing presence of a biofilm in the middle ear. A *biofilm* is a community of bacteria working together to overcome host defense mechanisms to continue to survive and proliferate (see Chapter 21 for more information about biofilms). Therapy for complications associated with chronic otitis media usually involves surgical intervention.

The eustachian tube and mastoid, connected to the middle ear by a sheet of cells, are also affected by the **infection.** If the eardrum membrane perforates, the infection can thicken and scar the eardrum and middle ear if left untreated. Necrosis of the ossicles destroys middle ear structures and causes hearing loss.

Interprofessional Collaborative Care

Recognize Cues: Assessment

The patient with acute or chronic otitis media has ear **pain.** Acute otitis media causes more intense pain from increased pressure in the middle ear. Conductive hearing is reduced and distorted as sound-wave transmission is obstructed. The patient may notice tinnitus in the form of a low hum or a low-pitched sound. Headaches, malaise, fever, nausea, and vomiting can occur. As the pressure on the middle ear pushes against the inner ear, the patient may have dizziness.

Otoscopic examination is performed by the health care provider. Findings vary, depending on the stage of the condition. The eardrum is initially retracted, which allows landmarks of the ear to be seen clearly. At this early stage, the patient may have only vague ear discomfort. As the condition progresses, the eardrum's blood vessels dilate and appear red (Fig. 40.10). Later the eardrum becomes red, thickened, and bulging, with loss of landmarks. Decreased eardrum mobility is evident on inspection with a pneumatic otoscope. Pus may be seen behind the membrane.

With progression, the eardrum spontaneously perforates, and pus or blood drains from the ear (Fig. 40.11). The patient usually has a marked decrease in pain as the pressure on middle ear structures is relieved. Eardrum perforations often heal if the underlying problem is controlled. Simple central perforation does not interfere with hearing unless the ossicles are damaged or the perforation is large. Repeated perforations with extensive scarring cause hearing loss.

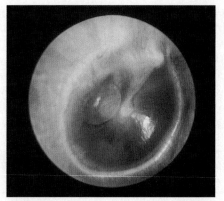

FIG. 40.10 Otoscopic view of otitis media.

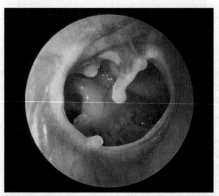

FIG. 40.11 Otoscopic view of a perforated tympanic membrane.

Take Actions: Interventions

Nonsurgical Management. Bed rest limits head movements, which can decrease **pain.** Application of very mild heat may help reduce pain. Systemic antibiotic therapy is needed to address the **infection.** Teach patients to complete the antibiotic therapy as prescribed and to not stop taking the drug even when they begin to feel better. Analgesics such as ibuprofen and acetaminophen can be used to relieve pain and reduce fever. For severe pain, opioid analgesics may be prescribed. Antihistamines and decongestants can also be prescribed to decrease fluid in the middle ear.

Surgical Management. If **pain** persists after antibiotic therapy and the eardrum continues to bulge, a myringotomy (surgical opening of the eardrum) may be performed. This procedure drains middle ear fluids and immediately relieves pain.

The procedure requires only a small surgical incision, which is often performed in an office or clinic under local anesthesia, yet can also be done in a surgical suite under general anesthesia. The incision heals rapidly. For relief of pressure caused by serous otitis media and for patients who have repeated episodes of otitis media, a small grommet (polyethylene tube) may be surgically placed through the eardrum to allow continuous drainage of middle ear fluids (Fig. 40.12).

Priority care after surgery includes teaching the patient to keep the external ear and canal clean and dry while the incision is healing. Hair-washing and showering should be avoided for several days so that water and chemicals are not introduced into

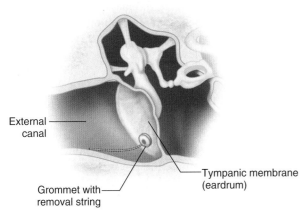

External canal

Grommet with removal string

Tympanic membrane (eardrum)

FIG. 40.12 Grommet through the tympanic membrane. A small grommet is placed through the tympanic membrane away from the margins, which allows prolonged drainage of fluids from the middle ear.

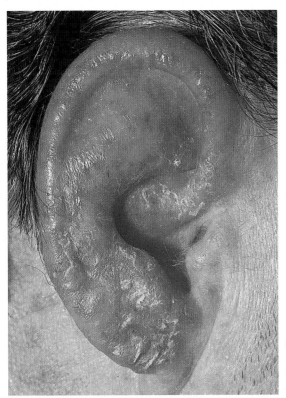

FIG. 40.13 External otitis. (From Habif, T.P. [2016]. *Clinical dermatology* [6th ed.]. Philadelphia: Elsevier.)

the ear. Other instructions after surgery are listed in Box 40.4 earlier in this chapter.

EXTERNAL OTITIS

Pathophysiology Review

External otitis (Fig. 40.13) is a painful condition caused when irritating or infective agents come into contact with the skin of the external ear. The result is an allergic response or inflammation with or without **infection.** Affected skin becomes red, swollen, and tender to touch or movement. Swelling of the ear canal can lead to temporary hearing loss from obstruction. Allergic external otitis is often caused by contact with cosmetics, hair

sprays, earphones, earrings, or hearing aids. The most common infectious organisms are *Pseudomonas aeruginosa, Proteus vulgaris, Staphylococcus aureus,* and *Escherichia coli* (Kesser, 2022).

External otitis occurs more often in hot, humid environments, especially in the summer, and is known as swimmer's ear because it often occurs in people involved in water sports. Patients who have traumatized their external ear canal with sharp or small objects (e.g., hairpins, cotton-tipped applicators) or with headphones also are more susceptible to external otitis. Others at risk include people with general allergies, psoriasis, eczema, and seborrheic dermatitis (Kesser, 2022).

Necrotizing or *malignant otitis* is the most virulent form of external otitis. This extremely rare condition occurs most often in older adults with diabetes or in patients with human immunodeficiency virus (HIV) (Grandis, 2023). Organisms spread beyond the external ear canal into the ear and skull. In progressive cases, osteomyelitis of the base of the skull and the temporomandibular joint develop (Grandis, 2023). Although rare, death from complications such as meningitis or brain abscess is possible.

Interprofessional Collaborative Care
Recognize Cues: Assessment

Signs and symptoms of external otitis range from mild itching to **pain** with movement of the pinna or tragus, particularly when upward pressure is applied to the external canal. Patients report feeling as if the ear is plugged and hearing is reduced. The temporary hearing loss can be severe when inflammation obstructs the canal and prevents sounds from reaching the eardrum.

Take Actions: Interventions

Treatment focuses on reducing inflammation, edema, and **pain.** Cleaning is the first step, as cerumen, desquamated skin, and other purulent material must be removed from the ear canal (Goguen & Durand, 2023). The primary health care provider will conduct the cleaning through an otoscope. Once the ear canal is clean, eardrops will be much more effective.

Nursing priorities include enhancing comfort measures, such as applying heat to the ear for 20 minutes three times a day. This can be accomplished by using washcloths warmed with water and placed inside a plastic bag. This method of treatment can be applied after a dry washcloth is laid over the affected ear to keep the plastic bag from compromising tissue integrity. A heating pad placed on the lowest setting can also be used. Teach the patient that minimizing head movements reduces pain.

Topical antibiotic and steroid therapies are generally prescribed to decrease inflammation and pain. Watch the patient or caregiver administer the eardrops to make sure that proper technique is used. Oral or IV antibiotics are used in severe cases, especially when **infection** spreads to surrounding tissue or when area lymph nodes are enlarged.

Analgesics, including opioids, may be needed for **pain** relief during the initial days of treatment. Ibuprofen or acetaminophen can relieve less severe pain. Teach the patient to place a cotton ball coated with petroleum jelly into the ear when showering. The patient must be taught to avoid water sports, ear buds, and hearing aids for at least 7 to 10 days. People who swim should be taught to wear earplugs when swimming. Finally, teach the patient to use preventive measures for minimizing ear canal moisture, trauma, or exposure to materials that lead to local irritation or contact dermatitis.

CERUMEN OR FOREIGN BODIES

Pathophysiology Review

Cerumen (earwax) is the most common cause of an impacted ear canal. Foreign bodies, such as small vegetables, beads, pencil erasers, and insects, can also be impacting. Although uncomfortable, cerumen or foreign bodies are rarely emergencies and can be removed carefully by a health care professional. Cerumen impaction in older adults is common, and removal often improves hearing in older adults.

Interprofessional Collaborative Care

Recognize Cues: Assessment

Patients may report a sensation of fullness in the ear, with or without hearing loss, and may have ear *pain,* itching, dizziness, or bleeding from the ear. Cerumen or a foreign body may be visible with direct inspection.

Take Actions: Interventions

When the occluding material is cerumen, management options include watchful waiting, manual removal, or the use of ceruminolytic agents followed by manual removal or irrigation.

If the cerumen is thick and dry or cannot be removed easily, the primary health care provider may recommend use of a ceruminolytic product such as Debrox. This helps to soften the wax before removal by the provider. Another approach is manual removal by the health care provider. Irrigation, performed by the nurse, is another effective way to remove cerumen. Caution patients to avoid self-treatment without consultation with the primary health care provider.

If an insect is suspected as a foreign body in the ear, it is killed before removal unless it can be coaxed out by a flashlight. A topical anesthetic can be placed in the ear canal for pain relief. Warm mineral oil, olive oil, or baby oil can be instilled into the ear to suffocate the insect, which is then removed by the primary health care provider with ear forceps. If a foreign body cannot be removed in the outpatient setting, surgical removal under general anesthetic may be required.

! NURSING SAFETY PRIORITY

Action Alert

Do not irrigate the ear of a patient with an eardrum perforation or otitis media because this may spread the *infection* to the inner ear. Also, do not irrigate the ear when the foreign object is vegetable matter because this material expands when wet, making the impaction worse. An experienced health care professional performs removal of vegetable matter.

MASTOIDITIS

Pathophysiology Review

The lining of the middle ear is continuous with the lining of the mastoid air cells, which are embedded in the temporal bone.

Mastoiditis is an *infection* of the mastoid air cells caused by progressive otitis media. It is a rare condition in adults; however, it can occur as a complication of acute or chronic otitis media. If not managed appropriately, it can lead to brain abscess, meningitis, and death.

Interprofessional Collaborative Care

Recognize Cues: Assessment

The signs and symptoms of mastoiditis include redness/hyperpigmentation, *pain*, and swelling behind the ear. The pinna usually is edematous, and the auricle is displaced posteriorly or downward (Lustig & Limb, 2023). Patients may have low-grade fever, malaise, and ear drainage. CT should be performed if mastoiditis is suspected. If intracranial complications are anticipated, an MRI will be ordered instead of a CT scan (Lustig & Limb, 2023).

Take Actions: Interventions

Interventions focus on stopping the *infection* before it spreads to other structures. IV antibiotics are used but do not easily penetrate the infected bony structure of the mastoid. Cultures of the ear drainage determine which antibiotics should be most effective. Surgical removal of the infected tissue is needed if the infection does not respond to antibiotic therapy within a few days. Mastoidectomy with myringotomy is a common treatment. All infected tissue must be removed so that the infection does not spread to other structures. If cholesteatoma—a keratinized, desquamated epithelial collection in the middle ear or mastoid—is present, a tympanomastoidectomy is performed (Lustig & Limb, 2023).

TINNITUS

Tinnitus (continuous ringing or noise perception in the ear) is a common ear problem that can occur in one or both ears. Diagnostic testing cannot confirm tinnitus; however, testing is performed to assess hearing and rule out other disorders. A Tinnitus and Hearing Survey, Tinnitus Screener, or Tinnitus Handicap Inventory: Screening Version tool can be used to help determine whether intervention for tinnitus is warranted (U.S. Department of Veterans Affairs, 2022).

Signs and symptoms range from mild ringing, which can go unnoticed during the day, to a loud roaring in the ear, which can seriously interfere with thinking and attention span. Factors that contribute to tinnitus include age, sclerosis of the ossicles, Ménière disease, certain drugs (aspirin, NSAIDs, high-ceiling diuretics, quinine, aminoglycoside antibiotics), exposure to loud noise, and other inner ear problems. Research indicates that there may be a link between a new onset of tinnitus and COVID-19 infection (Bento & Campos, 2022), so always query patients with a recent onset of symptoms about whether they have a history of this virus.

The problem and its management vary with the underlying cause. Behavioral therapies such as tinnitus retraining therapy, biofeedback, and cognitive behavioral therapy are effective for some patients (Dinces, 2021). Select medications that have been used with varying degrees of success include intratympanic dexamethasone and low doses of carbamazepine (Dinces, 2021). Therapy is also focused on ways to mask tinnitus with ambient background noise, sound machines, fans, or music set on low volumes (Dinces, 2021). Refer patients with tinnitus to local and online support groups as needed, and to the American Tinnitus Association.

 PATIENT-CENTERED CARE: VETERAN HEALTH

Noise Exposure in Veterans

Veterans who have served are often exposed to noise, particularly if they have been around gunfire, detonation of weapons, explosives, or aircraft. Tinnitus is the top compensated service-connected disability and affects over 2.7 million veterans (U.S. Department of Veterans Affairs, 2023). Nurses must remember to assess patients for veteran status and inquire about occupational exposure (Elliott, 2019). Provide a quiet and private environment for care, be mindful of coexisting conditions that the veteran may have, and communicate with a multimodal approach, using visual handouts and demonstrations (Elliott, 2019).

MÉNIÈRE DISEASE

Pathophysiology Review

Ménière disease is a condition that includes a classic trio of symptoms—episodic vertigo, tinnitus, and hearing loss (Moskowitz & Dinces, 2022). Symptoms usually occur in adults between the ages of 20 and 40 years (Moskowitz & Dinces, 2022). Episodes, also called "attacks," can last several days, although some patients always report ongoing symptoms of varying intensity. Patients can be almost totally incapacitated during an attack, and recovery can take hours to days. Although most patients have a window of forewarning when an attack is beginning, others experience Tumarkin otolithic crises, known as *sudden drop attacks*, in which the patient falls to the ground with no warning (Wu et al., 2019).

The pathophysiology leading to this condition is not fully understood. However, it is known that Ménière disease is progressive, leading to an excess of endolymphatic fluid that builds up within the inner ear, causing distortion and distention of portions of the labyrinth system (Moskowitz & Dinces, 2022). This distortion decreases hearing by dilating the cochlear duct, causes vertigo because of damage to the vestibular system, and stimulates tinnitus. At first, hearing loss is reversible, but repeated damage to the cochlea from increased fluid pressure can lead to permanent hearing loss.

Interprofessional Collaborative Care

Recognize Cues: Assessment

Signs and symptoms include vertigo, hearing loss, and tinnitus. Vertigo is often accompanied by nausea, vomiting, headache, and nystagmus. Blood pressure, pulse, and respirations may be elevated. Hearing loss occurs first with the low-frequency tones; in some patients, it progresses to include all levels and eventually becomes permanent. Patients may describe the tinnitus as having variable pitch and intensity, which may fluctuate or remain continuous.

Take Actions: Interventions

Nonpharmacologic treatment for Ménière disease includes diet and lifestyle adjustments, as some patients with this condition are sensitive to triggers such as high salt intake, certain foods, other illnesses, stress, and fatigue (Vestibular Disorders Association, 2022). Teach patients how to modify their diet accordingly, if foods seem to be a trigger. It is also important to teach the client to avoid activities that place them at risk of experiencing vertigo, such as standing on chairs or ladders. Patients with sudden drop attacks should not drive, and may be subject to having a driver's license suspended for safety purposes (Wu et al., 2019).

Teach patients to move the head slowly to prevent worsening of the vertigo. Institute and teach fall precautions to all patients with Ménière disease. Vestibular rehabilitation therapy (VRT) uses exercise activities to improve balance, which can be helpful.

Pharmacologic treatment is used to reduce symptoms. Diuretics can be prescribed to decrease endolymph volume, which reduces vertigo, hearing loss, tinnitus, and aural fullness. Gentamicin is sometimes prescribed to control vertigo (Vestibular Disorders Association, 2022). Promethazine can be given for nausea and vomiting. For patients who do not respond to pharmacologic intervention, intratympanic gentamicin may be recommended to destroy vestibular tissue, or intratympanic steroids can be used (Vestibular Disorders Association, 2022).

When drug therapy is ineffective in controlling symptoms or attacks, other procedures may be considered. Decompression or shunting of the endolymphatic sac has been shown to have favorable outcomes in controlling vertigo. Finally, labyrinthectomy can be done in extreme cases in which the patient already has significant hearing loss or continuous disabling vertigo. This surgical procedure destroys the bony and membranous labyrinth by removal of the neuroepithelium, resulting in total hearing loss on the operative side.

NCLEX Examination Challenge 40.3
Physiological Integrity

Which of the following client statements regarding Ménière disease demonstrates to the nurse an understanding of this condition? **Select all that apply.**
A. "I am not going to drive when I have an attack."
B. "Surgery is going to be required to fix this problem."
C. "If I begin to feel dizzy, I will sit or lie down immediately."
D. "When I drink a lot of caffeine, the vertigo seems to be worse."
E. "This problem may come and go over the course of my lifetime."

VESTIBULAR SCHWANNOMA/ACOUSTIC NEUROMA

A vestibular schwannoma, also known as an *acoustic neuroma*, is a benign tumor of the vestibulocochlear nerve (cranial nerve VIII)

PATIENT-CENTERED CARE: HEALTH EQUITY

Social Determinants of Health and Vestibular Schwannoma Management

Social determinants of health (SDOH) influence the care of patients. The Area Deprivation Index (ADI) is a tool that reveals general socioeconomic conditions in an area; these data can influence care. Evidence shows that a higher ADI score is associated with a higher vestibular schwannoma tumor grade, often requiring radiation (Ellsperman et al., 2023). Advocate for all patients to be assessed quickly when symptoms of vestibular schwannoma are present.

that often damages other structures as it grows. Depending on the size and exact location of the tumor, damage to hearing, facial movements, and sensation can occur. A vestibular schwannoma can cause neurologic signs and symptoms as the tumor enlarges in the brain.

Signs and symptoms begin with tinnitus and progress to gradual sensorineural hearing loss. Later, patients have constant mild to moderate vertigo. As the tumor enlarges, nearby cranial nerves are damaged. Without treatment, brainstem compression, cerebellar tonsil herniation, hydrocephalus, or death can occur (Park et al., 2023).

The tumor is diagnosed with an MRI. If the patient cannot tolerate an MRI, a high-resolution CT with and without contrast can be used (Park et al., 2023). Treatment involves surgery, radiation, or watchful observation. If surgery is performed, risks include hearing loss, facial weakness, persistent headaches, and/or vestibular disturbances (Park et al., 2023). Because these tumors grow very slowly, even patients who have had surgery need prolonged follow-up.

GET READY FOR THE NEXT-GENERATION NCLEX® EXAMINATION!

Essential Nursing Care Points

Health Promotion/Disease Prevention	Chronic Disease Care
• Assess whether there is a family history of hearing problems, as some genetic problems can lead to progressive hearing loss in adults. • Ensure that all members of the interprofessional team use a medical interpreter as needed for the patient with a hearing impairment. • Teach ways to protect hearing before loss or damage occurs. • Regularly evaluate drugs that are taken to determine whether they carry a risk for ototoxicity.	• Teach patients with progressive and chronic hearing loss about supportive and financial resources that can be of assistance. • Regularly assess whether assistive devices (e.g., hearing aids) are in good working order and serving the patient's current auditory *sensory perception* needs.
Regenerative or Restorative Care	**Hospice/Palliative/Supportive Care**
• Protect the patient with vertigo or dizziness from tinnitus or injury by teaching the patient to sit or lie down immediately at the onset of symptoms. • Teach patients with tinnitus or who have undergone ear surgery to move the head slowly to prevent dizziness or vertigo.	• Encourage patients with hearing loss to talk with an audiologist about audiologic rehabilitation.

Mastery Questions

1. The nurse is caring for a client who is deaf. Which communication method would the nurse use when beginning to perform care?
   A. Ask the client to read lips.
   B. Talk to the family member.
   C. Enunciate words when speaking.
   D. Use a board for pictures and writing.

2. The nurse is teaching older adults at a community health fair. Which of the following hearing changes associated with aging would the nurse discuss? **Select all that apply.**
   A. Hair in the ear thickens and accumulates.
   B. Hearing acuity changes in all older adults.
   C. Cerumen dries and becomes more easily impacted.
   D. The ability to hear high-frequency pitches diminishes first.
   E. Sounds such as *f, s, sh,* and *pa* become more difficult to discern.

NGN Challenge 40.1

The nurse reviews the Nurses' Notes for a 79-year-old client seeing the primary health care provider today for a 6-month follow-up appointment.

Health History	**Nurses' Notes**	Vital Signs	Laboratory Results

March 23
Height: 62 in (157.5 cm); weight: 134 lb (60.8 kg). Vital signs: T 98.8°F (37.1°C); HR 62 beats/min; RR 16 breaths/min; BP 124/86 mm Hg. SpO₂ 97% on RA.
Here for regular 6-month follow-up. History of hypertension and hypercholesterolemia controlled by medication. Client reports getting consistent readings of 120s over 80s when she takes her blood pressure at home. No reports of swelling, shortness of breath, chest pain, or pressure. States that her only new concern is noticing that she must have people repeat what they are saying more frequently than normal. States it isn't tremendously bothersome at this time. Health care provider conducted full examination with no concerning findings. Amlodipine and simvastatin refilled. Will return for follow-up in 6 months.

October 1
Height: 62 in (157.5 cm); weight: 136 lb (61.7 kg). Vital signs: T 98.6°F (37°C); HR 66 beats/min; RR 16 breaths/min; BP 126/82 mm Hg. SpO₂ 98% on RA.
Here for regular 6-month follow-up. History of hypertension and hypercholesterolemia controlled by medication. Client reports getting consistent readings of 120s over 80s when she takes her blood pressure at home. No reports of swelling, shortness of breath, chest pain, or pressure. Admits to slight ongoing sinus tenderness over the past 3 days, with onset of nasal congestion. Reports that she feels "like someone has their hands over my ears." Reports coughing up green mucus. Denies dizziness. Also states that she has noted a decline in hearing since March and that her family is now telling her she needs hearing aids. She says that even with the television turned up loud, it is hard to understand what is being said, and that speaking on a telephone sounds "muffled." Health care provider to see patient.

Complete the diagram by selecting from the choices below to specify what potential condition the client is likely experiencing, **2** nursing actions that are appropriate to take, and **2** parameters the nurse should monitor to assess the client's progress.

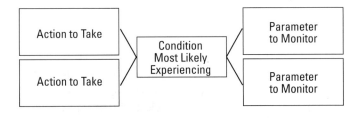

Actions to Take	Potential Conditions	Parameters to Monitor
Refer to audiologist	Otitis externa	Body temperature
Teach about dietary triggers	Progressive hearing loss	Ongoing dizziness
Schedule myringotomy	Mastoiditis	Ability to hear
Ensure that CT is performed	Ménière disease	Efficacy of new hearing aids
Explore client's feelings about hearing		Results of CT scan

NGN Challenge 40.2

The nurse is reviewing the nursing flow sheet for a 46-year-old client admitted last night with dizziness, nausea, and vomiting. The electronic health record indicates that the client was at home yesterday morning and had a sudden spinning sensation. When it didn't resolve, her spouse brought her to the ED in the early evening. She was admitted for observation and given meclizine.

Highlight client findings on the Nursing Flow Sheet at 0210 and documentation for 0210 that are of **immediate** concern to the nurse.

Time	March 10 1712 (ED)	March 10 2202 (Admission)	March 11 0210
Temperature	98.8°F (37.17°C)	98.6°F (37°C)	98.6°F (37°C)
Heart rate	80 beats/min	74 beats/min	60 beats/min
Respiratory rate/SpO₂	20 breaths/min; 98%	18 breaths/min; 98%	14 breaths/min; 97%
Blood pressure	120/70 mm Hg	118/72 mm Hg	100/64 mm Hg

2202: Alert and oriented × 4; CN check normal; PERRLA; equal movement and grasp all 4 extremities. Reports earlier severe vertigo. Still with moderate vertigo. Headache 5/10. CT scan ordered by emergency health care provider for tomorrow morning.

0210: Drowsy but can be awakened; oriented × 3, not sure of day but oriented to person, place, and situation. Words are slightly slurred. Reports feeling very sleepy and mouth is very dry. Headache 3/10. Reports moderate vertigo with dry mouth. She says she has a new ringing in her ears.

REFERENCES

American Speech-Language-Hearing Association. (2023). *Adult audiologic (hearing) rehabilitation.* https://www.asha.org/public/hearing/adult-audiologic-rehabilitation/.

American Tinnitus Association. (2022). *Causes.* https://www.ata.org/understanding-facts/causes.

Bento, R. F., & Campos, T. V. (2022). Hearing loss, tinnitus, and dizziness and their relation with Covid-19: What is the current evidence? *International Archives of Otorhinolaryngology, 26,* 1–2.

Brar, S., Watters, C., & Winters, R. (2023). Tympanoplasty. [Updated 2023 Jan 3]. In: *StatPearls* [Internet]. Treasure Island, FL: StatPearls Publishing; 2023 Jan-. Available from: https://www.ncbi.nlm.nih.gov/books/NBK565863/

Dawes, P., et al. (2020). Relationship between diet, tinnitus, and hearing difficulties. *Ear and Hearing, 41*(2), 289–299.

Dickson, V., et al. (2022). Providing hearing assistance to veterans in the emergency department: A qualitative study. *Journal of Emergency Nursing, 48*(3), 266–277.

Dinces, E. (2021). Treatment of tinnitus. *UpToDate.* Retrieved May 17, 2023, from https://www.uptodate.com/contents/treatment-of-tinnitus.

Elliott, B. (2019). Tinnitus and hearing impairment in the veteran population. *MedSurg Matters!, 38*(3), 8–10.

Ellsperman, S., Bellile, E., Fryatt, R., Hoi, K., Wang, J., Fayson, S., Banakis Hartl, R. & Stucken, E. (2023). The impact of social determinants of health on vestibular schwannoma management: A single institution review. *Otology & Neurotology, 44* (5), 507–512. doi: 10.1097/MAO.0000000000003883.

Envoy Medical. (2020). *Esteem.* http://esteemhearing.com/.

Goguen, L., & Durand, M. (2023). External otitis: Treatment. *UpTo-Date*. Retrieved May 17, 2023, from https://www.uptodate.com/contents/external-otitis-treatment.

Grandis, J. (2023). Malignant (necrotizing) external otitis. *UpToDate*. Retrieved May 17, 2023, from https://www.uptodate.com/contents/malignant-necrotizing-external-otitis.

Interprofessional Education Collaborative. (2022). *Core competencies for interprofessional collaborative practice: 2016 update.* Retrieved May 17, 2023, from https://ipec.memberclicks.net/assets/2016-Update.pdf.

Jarvis, C., & Eckhardt, A. (2024). *Physical examination & health assessment* (8th ed.). St. Louis: Elsevier.

Johns Hopkins Bloomberg School of Public Health. (2020). *Hearing loss prevalence in the U.S.: Increased, undiagnosed, undertreated.* https://www.jhucochlearcenter.org/sites/default/files/2020-12/Fact%20Sheet%20-%20Hearing%20Loss%20Prevalence%20(Cochlear%20Center%20for%20Hearing%20and%20Public%20Health)v1.pdf.

Kesser, B. (2022). *External otitis (acute). Merck manual: Professional version.* Retrieved from: https://www.merckmanuals.com/professional/ear,-nose,-and-throat-disorders/external-ear-disorders/external-otitis-acute.

Lustig, L., & Limb, C. (2023). Chronic otitis media, cholesteatoma, and mastoiditis in adults. *UpToDate.* Retrieved May 17, 2023, from https://www.uptodate.com/contents/chronic-otitis-media-and-cholesteatoma-in-adults.

Moskowitz, H., & Dinces, E. (2022). Meniere disease: Evaluation, diagnosis and management. *UpToDate.* Retrieved May 17, 2023, from https://www.uptodate.com/contents/meniere-disease-evaluation-diagnosis-and-management.

National Association of the Deaf. (2023). *Hospitals and other health care facilities.* Retrieved from https://www.nad.org/resources/health-care-and-mental-health-services/health-care-providers/hospitals-and-other-health-care-facilities/.

National Institute on Deafness and Other Communication Disorders (NIDCD). (2021). *Quick statistics about hearing.* http://www.nidcd.nih.gov/health/statistics/Pages/quick.aspx.

Online Mendelian Inheritance in Man (OMIM). (2023). *Gap junction proteins, beta-2.* GJB2. www.omim.org/entry/121011.

Park, J. K., Vernick, D. M., & Ramakrishna, N. (2023). Vestibular schwannoma (acoustic neuroma). *UpToDate.* Retrieved June 19, 2023, from https://www.uptodate.com/contents/vestibular-schwannoma-acoustic-neuroma.

Rogers, J. L. (2023). *McCance and Huether's Pathophysiology: The biologic basis for disease in adults and children* (9th ed.). St. Louis: Elsevier.

Slusser, M., Garcia, L., Reed, C., & McGinnis, P. (2019). *Foundations of interprofessional collaborative practice in health care.* St. Louis: Elsevier.

Touhy, T., & Jett, K. (2022). *Ebersole and Hess' gerontological nursing healthy aging* (6th ed.). St. Louis: Elsevier.

Tserga, E., Nandwani, T., Edvall, N. K., et al. (2019). The genetic vulnerability to cisplatin ototoxicity: A systematic review. *Scientific Reports, 9,* 3455. https://doi.org/10.1038/s41598-019-40138-z.

University of Iowa [UI]. (2019). *Iowa head and neck protocols: How to read an audiogram.* https://medicine.uiowa.edu/iowaprotocols/how-read-audiogram.

U.S. Department of Veterans Affairs. (2022). *Tinnitus questionnaires, surveys and interviews.* https://www.ncrar.research.va.gov/ClinicianResources/TinnitusQuestionnaires.asp.

U.S. Department of Veterans Affairs. (2023). *Veterans benefits administration annual benefits report: Fiscal year 2022.* https://www.benefits.va.gov/REPORTS/abr/docs/2022-abr.pdf#.

Vestibular Disorders Association. (2022). *Ménière disease.* https://vestibular.org/article/diagnosis-treatment/types-of-vestibular-disorders/menieres-disease/.

Wu, V., et al. (2019). Approach to Ménière disease management. *Canadian Family Physician, 65*(7), 463–467.

Young, A., & Ng, M. (2022). Ossiculoplasty. [Updated 2022 Apr 17]. In *StatPearls [Internet].* Treasure Island (FL): StatPearls Publishing. 2022 Jan-. Available from: https://www.ncbi.nlm.nih.gov/books/NBK563162/.

41

Assessment of the Musculoskeletal System

Donna D. Ignatavicius

http://evolve.elsevier.com/Iggy/

LEARNING OUTCOMES

1. Use knowledge of anatomy and physiology to perform a focused assessment of the musculoskeletal system.
2. Teach evidence-based health promotion activities to help prevent musculoskeletal health conditions or trauma.
3. Demonstrate clinical judgment to interpret assessment findings in a patient with a musculoskeletal health condition.
4. Identify factors that affect health equity for patients with musculoskeletal health conditions.
5. Explain how genetic implications and physiologic aging of the musculoskeletal system affect *mobility.*
6. Interpret assessment findings for patients with a suspected or actual musculoskeletal condition.
7. Plan evidence-based care and support for patients undergoing diagnostic testing of the musculoskeletal system.

KEY TERMS

arthralgias Joint aches and discomfort.

arthritis Joint inflammation.

arthroscopy A diagnostic or surgical procedure in which a fiberoptic tube is inserted into a joint for direct visualization of the ligaments, menisci, and articular surfaces of the joint.

bone scan A radionuclide test in which radioactive material is injected for viewing the entire skeleton.

bursitis Inflammation of bursae, which are small sacs lined with synovial membrane located at joints and bony prominences to prevent friction between bone and structures next to bone.

dermatomyositis Polymyositis that occurs with a purplish skin rash.

effusion Fluid accumulation, such as in a joint.

fascia Dense fibrous tissue that surrounds skeletal muscle, which contains the muscle's blood, lymph, and nerve supply.

gout A genetically linked arthritis caused by an inborn error of purine metabolism.

kyphosis Outward curvature of the thoracic spine causing a "humped back."

lordosis An inward abnormal curvature of the lumbar spine.

muscle atrophy Skeletal muscle deterioration that results when muscles are not regularly exercised and they deteriorate from disuse.

muscular dystrophy A group of genetically linked diseases that cause chronic skeletal muscle weakness and organ dysfunction due to smooth muscle involvement.

myopathy A problem in muscle tissue often resulting in weakness.

neuropathy A problem in nerve tissue often resulting in weakness and decreased *sensory perception.*

neurovascular assessment (also called a *circ check*) An assessment that includes palpation of pulses in the extremities below the level of injury and assessment of sensation, movement, color, temperature, and pain in the injured part.

osteoblasts Bone-forming cells.

osteoclasts Bone-destroying cells.

osteomalacia Softening of bone in adults due to inadequate vitamin D.

osteopenia Decreased bone density (bone loss) that occurs as one ages.

osteoporosis A chronic disease of cellular regulation in which bone loss causes significant decreased density and possible fracture.

Paget disease A chronic metabolic disorder that causes bone to become fragile and misshapen.

physical disability A limitation in mobility or activity that can affect one or more ADLs, such as walking, transferring, bathing, toileting, or dressing; the limitation often requires the use of special equipment such as a cane or wheelchair.

polymyositis An uncommon chronic rheumatic disease that is characterized by inflammation of multiple muscles.

scoliosis An abnormal lateral curvature of the spine.

synovial joints Body joints that are lined with synovium, a membrane that secretes synovial fluid for lubrication and shock absorption.

✵ PRIORITY AND INTERRELATED CONCEPTS

The priority concept for this chapter is:
- *Mobility*

The interrelated concepts for this chapter are:
- *Sensory Perception*
- *Pain*

The musculoskeletal system is the second largest body system. It includes the bones, joints, and skeletal muscles, as well as the supporting structures needed to move them. *Mobility* is a basic human need that is essential for performing ADLs. When a patient cannot move to perform ADLs or other daily routines, self-esteem and a sense of self-worth can be diminished. Chapter 3 briefly reviews the concept of mobility.

Disease, surgery, and trauma can affect one or more parts of the musculoskeletal system, often leading to decreased mobility. When *mobility* is impaired for a long time, other body systems are affected. For example, prolonged immobility can lead to skin breakdown, constipation, joint contractures, and venous thromboembolism. If nerves are damaged by trauma or disease, patients may also have both impaired *sensory perception* and *pain*. (See Chapter 3 for a review of these health concepts.)

ANATOMY AND PHYSIOLOGY REVIEW

As the term implies, the musculoskeletal system consists of a skeletal and muscular system.

Skeletal System

The skeletal system consists of 206 bones and multiple joints. The growth and development of these structures occur during childhood and adolescence and are not discussed in this text. Common physical skeletal differences among selected racial/ethnic groups are listed in Table 41.1.

Bones

Types and Structure. Bone can be classified in two ways: by *shape* and by structure. For example, *long bones,* such as the femur, are cylindric with rounded ends and often bear weight. *Short bones,* such as the phalanges, are small and bear little or no weight.

The second way bone is classified is by *structure* or composition. As shown in Fig. 41.1, the outer layer of bone, or cortex, is composed of dense, compact bone tissue. The inner layer, in the medulla, contains spongy, cancellous tissue (Rogers, 2023). Almost every bone has both tissue types but in varying quantities.

The structural unit of the cortical compact bone is the haversian system, which is detailed in Fig. 41.1. The haversian system is a complex canal network containing microscopic blood vessels that supply nutrients and oxygen to bone and lacunae, which are small cavities that house osteocytes (bone cells).

The softer cancellous tissue contains large spaces, or trabeculae, which are filled with red and yellow marrow. Hematopoiesis

TABLE 41.1	Musculoskeletal Differences in Selected Ethnic Groups
Racial or Ethnic Group	**Typical Musculoskeletal Differences**
Black	Greater bone density than Whites, Asian/Pacific Islanders, and Hispanics
	Accounts for decreased incidence of osteoporosis
Amish	Greater incidence of dwarfism than in other populations
Chinese American	Bones shorter and smaller with less bone density
	Increased incidence of osteoporosis
Egyptian American	Shorter in stature than Whites and Blacks
Filipino/Vietnamese	Short in stature; adult height about 5 feet
Irish American	Taller and broader than other Whites
	Less bone density than Blacks

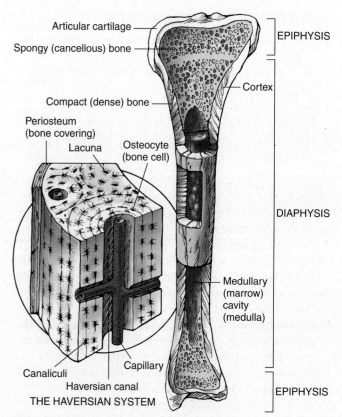

FIG. 41.1 Structure of a typical long bone. The cortex, or outer layer, is composed of dense, compact tissue. The microscopic structure of this compact cortical tissue is the haversian system.

(production of blood cells) occurs in the red marrow. The yellow marrow contains fat cells, which can be dislodged and enter the bloodstream to cause *fat embolism syndrome (FES),* a life-threatening complication. In the deepest layer of the periosteum are osteogenic cells, which later differentiate into osteoblasts (bone-forming cells) and osteoclasts (bone-destroying cells) (Rogers, 2023).

Bone is a very vascular tissue. Each bone has a main nutrient artery, which enters near the middle of the shaft and branches into ascending and descending vessels. These vessels supply the cortex, the marrow, and the haversian system. Very few nerve fibers are connected to bone. Sympathetic nerve fibers control dilation of blood vessels. Sensory nerve fibers transmit pain signals experienced by patients who have primary lesions of the bone, such as bone tumors.

Function. The skeletal system:
- Provides a framework for the body and allows the body to be weight bearing, or upright
- Supports the surrounding tissues (e.g., muscle and tendons)
- Assists in movement through muscle attachment and joint formation
- Protects vital organs, such as the heart and lungs
- Manufactures blood cells in red bone marrow
- Provides storage for mineral salts (e.g., calcium and phosphorus)

Bone is a very dynamic tissue. It undergoes a continuous process of formation and resorption, or destruction, at equal rates until the age of 35 years. In later years, bone resorption increases, decreasing bone mass and predisposing patients to injury, especially older women.

Bone accounts for about 99% of the *calcium* in the body and 90% of the *phosphorus*. In healthy adults, the serum concentrations of calcium and phosphorus maintain an inverse relationship. As calcium levels rise, phosphorus levels decrease. When serum levels are altered, calcitonin and parathyroid hormone (PTH) work to maintain equilibrium. If the calcium in the blood is decreased, the bone, which stores calcium, releases calcium into the bloodstream in response to PTH stimulation. Chapter 13 describes these electrolytes in more detail.

Calcitonin is produced by the thyroid gland and *decreases* the serum calcium concentration if it is increased above its normal level. Calcitonin inhibits bone resorption and increases renal excretion of calcium and phosphorus as needed to maintain balance in the body.

Vitamin D and its metabolites are produced in the body and transported in the blood to promote the absorption of calcium and phosphorus from the small intestine. They also seem to enhance PTH activity to release calcium from the bone. A decrease in the body's vitamin D level can result in osteomalacia (softening of bone) in the adult (Rogers, 2023).

When serum calcium levels are lowered, *parathyroid hormone* (PTH, or parathormone) secretion increases and stimulates bone to promote osteoclastic activity and *release* calcium to the blood. PTH reduces the renal excretion of calcium and facilitates its absorption from the intestine. If serum calcium levels increase, PTH secretion diminishes to preserve the bone calcium supply. This process is an example of the feedback loop system of the endocrine system.

Adrenal glucocorticoids regulate protein metabolism, either increasing or decreasing catabolism to reduce or intensify the organic matrix of bone. They also aid in regulating intestinal calcium and phosphorus absorption.

Estrogens stimulate osteoblastic activity and inhibit PTH. When estrogen levels decline at menopause, women are susceptible to low serum calcium levels with increased bone loss (osteoporosis). *Androgens,* such as testosterone in men, promote anabolism (body tissue building) and increase bone mass.

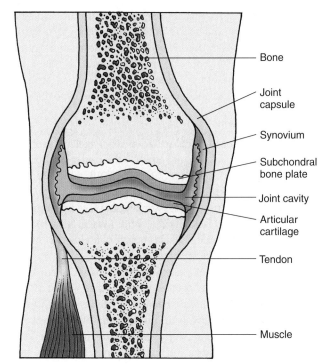

FIG. 41.2 Structure of a synovial joint. Synovium lines the joint capsule but does not extend into the articular cartilage.

Thyroxine (T_4) is one of the principal hormones secreted by the thyroid gland. Its primary function is to increase the rate of protein synthesis in all types of tissue, including bone. *Insulin* works together with growth hormone to build and maintain healthy bone tissue. More information about these hormones can be found in the endocrine health problem chapters of this text.

Joints. A *joint* is a space in which two or more bones come together. The major function of a joint is to provide movement and flexibility in the body.

There are three types of joints in the body:
- Synarthrodial, or completely immovable, joints (e.g., in the cranium)
- Amphiarthrodial, or slightly movable, joints (e.g., in the pelvis)
- Diarthrodial (synovial), or freely movable, joints (e.g., the elbow and knee)

Although any of these joints can be affected by disease or injury, the synovial joints are most commonly involved, as discussed in Chapter 43. The diarthrodial, or synovial, joint is the most common type of joint in the body. Synovial joints are the only type lined with synovium, a membrane that secretes synovial fluid for lubrication and shock absorption. As shown in Fig. 41.2, the synovium lines the internal portion of the joint capsule but does not normally extend onto the surface of the cartilage at the spongy bone ends. Articular cartilage consists of a collagen fiber matrix impregnated with a complex ground substance. Patients with arthritis (joint inflammation) often have synovitis (synovial inflammation) and breakdown of the cartilage. Bursae, small sacs lined with synovial membrane, are located at joints and bony prominences to prevent friction between bone and structures next to bone. These structures can also become inflamed, causing painful bursitis.

Synovial joints are described by their anatomic structures. For example, *ball-and-socket* joints (shoulder, hip) permit movement in any direction. *Hinge* joints (elbow) allow motion in one plane—flexion and extension. The knee is often classified as a hinge joint, but it rotates slightly, as well as flexes and extends. It is best described as a *condylar* type of synovial joint.

Muscular System

In contrast to smooth and cardiac muscle, skeletal muscle is striated voluntary muscle controlled by the central and peripheral nervous systems. The junction of a peripheral motor nerve and the muscle cells that it supplies is sometimes referred to as a *motor end plate*. Muscle fibers are held in place by connective tissue in bundles, or fasciculi. The entire muscle is surrounded by dense fibrous tissue, or fascia, which contains the muscle's blood, lymph, and nerve supply.

The main function of skeletal muscle is movement of the body and its parts. When bones, joints, and supporting structures are adversely affected by injury or disease, the adjacent muscle tissue is often involved, limiting **mobility.** During the aging process, muscle fibers decrease in size and number, even in well-conditioned adults. Muscle atrophy results when muscles are not regularly exercised, and they deteriorate from disuse or aging.

Supporting structures for the muscular system are very susceptible to injury. They include tendons (bands of tough, fibrous tissue that attach muscles to bones) and ligaments, which attach bones to other bones at joints.

Musculoskeletal Changes Associated With Aging

Osteopenia, or decreased bone density (bone loss), occurs as one ages. Many older adults, especially thin White women, have *severe* osteopenia, a disease called osteoporosis. This condition can cause kyphosis (outward curvature of the thoracic spine causing a "humped back") and gait changes, which predispose the person to fractures (Jarvis & Eckhardt, 2024). Chapter 42 discusses this health problem in detail.

Synovial joint cartilage can become less elastic and compressible as a person ages. As a result of these cartilage changes and continued use of joints, the joint cartilage becomes damaged, leading to osteoarthritis (OA). Genetic defects in cartilage may also contribute to joint disease. The most common joints affected are the weight-bearing joints of the hip, knee, and cervical and lumbar spine, but joints in the shoulder and upper extremity, feet, and hands also can be affected. Refer to Chapter 43 for a complete discussion of OA.

In older adults, musculoskeletal changes can cause decreased coordination, loss of muscle strength, gait changes, and a risk for falls with injury. (See Chapter 4 for a discussion on fall prevention.) The box titled Patient-Centered Care: Older Adult Health: Changes in the Musculoskeletal System Related to Aging lists the major anatomic and physiologic changes and related nursing interventions to ensure patient safety (Touhy & Jett, 2022).

Health Promotion/Disease Prevention

Many health problems of the musculoskeletal system can be prevented through health promotion strategies and avoidance

PATIENT-CENTERED CARE: OLDER ADULT HEALTH

Changes in the Musculoskeletal System Related to Aging

Physiologic Change	Nursing Interventions	Rationales
Decreased bone density	Teach safety tips to prevent falls (see Chapter 4).	Porous bones are more likely to fracture.
	Reinforce need to exercise, especially weight-bearing exercise.	Exercise slows bone loss.
Increased bone prominences	Prevent pressure on bone prominences.	There is less soft tissue to prevent skin breakdown.
Kyphosis and widened gait, shift in the center of gravity, which could cause imbalance and falls	Teach proper body mechanics; instruct the patient to sit in supportive chairs with arms. Assess need for ambulatory device, such as cane or walker; ensure use of supportive shoes.	Correction of posture problems can help prevent further deformity; the patient should have support to ensure improved balance, such as ambulatory devices.
Joint cartilage degeneration (osteoarthritis [OA]) (see Chapter 43)	Provide moist heat, such as a shower or warm, moist compresses or heating pad.	Moist heat increases blood flow to the area and promotes **mobility**.
Decreased range of motion (ROM)	Assess the patient's ability to perform ADLs and **mobility**.	The patient may need assistance with ADLs and ambulation.
Muscle atrophy, decreased strength	Teach isometric and isotonic exercises.	Exercises increase muscle strength.
Slowed movement	Do not rush the person; be patient.	The patient may become frustrated if hurried or sustain a fall.

of risky lifestyle behaviors to prevent injury and disease. For example, women may slow the process of bone loss by taking vitamin D and calcium supplements and increasing these nutrients in their diet. Weight-bearing activities, such as walking and strengthening exercises, can reduce risk factors for osteoporosis and maintain muscle strength (Rogers, 2023).

Accidents, lifestyle, and substance abuse can contribute to the occurrence of musculoskeletal injury. Young men are at the greatest risk for traumatic injury related to motor vehicle or scooter crashes, and should use these devices safely and avoid substance use. Young and middle-aged adults tend to engage more than other groups in high-impact sports, such as excessive jogging or running. These activities can cause musculoskeletal injury to soft tissues and bone.

Older adults are at the greatest risk for falls that result in fractures and soft tissue injury. Teach older adults and their families or caregivers to prevent falls by implementing the evidence-based strategies that are described in Chapter 4.

Tobacco smoking also has negative effects on the musculoskeletal system and can slow bone healing. The nicotine in tobacco is the primary cause of these effects (Niu & Lim, 2020).

Excessive alcohol intake can decrease vitamins and nutrients that the person needs for bone and muscle tissue growth. Teach individuals who use these substances about the potential effects on their bone health. For all patients, develop a patient-centered health promotion plan to help promote bone health and prevent musculoskeletal injury. Additional health promotion/disease prevention strategies can be found in other chapters of this unit related to specific conditions of the musculoskeletal system.

RECOGNIZE CUES: ASSESSMENT

Patient History

In the assessment of a patient with an actual or potential musculoskeletal condition, a detailed and accurate history is helpful in identifying priority problems and nursing interventions. The history reveals information about the patient that can direct the physical assessment.

Mobility limitation is the major cause of physical disability, requiring many individuals to use ambulatory aids such as canes and walkers or wheelchairs, especially for middle-aged and older adults. Patients who are physically disabled may also have difficulty with one or more functional activities, such as bathing, toileting, and dressing (Smeltzer, 2021).

PATIENT-CENTERED CARE: HEALTH EQUITY

Physical Disability and Social Determinants of Health

Physical disability occurs most commonly in older adults from Hispanic, American Indian/Alaska Native, and other racial groups when compared to Whites (Smeltzer, 2021). Social determinants of health, such as being at poverty level, having low levels of education, and being unemployed or underemployed when compared with Whites, are likely responsible for these differences (Smeltzer, 2021).

When taking a personal health history, question the patient about any traumatic injuries and sports activities, no matter when they occurred. An injury to the lumbar spine 30 years ago may have caused a patient's current low back pain and possible disability. A motor vehicle crash or sports injury can cause osteoarthritis years after the event. Ask patients whether they are following a pain management plan, including the use of substances such as cannabis (marijuana).

Previous or current illness or disease may affect musculoskeletal status. For example, a patient with diabetes who is treated for a foot ulcer is at high risk for acute or chronic osteomyelitis (bone infection). In addition, diabetes slows the healing process. Ask the patient about any previous hospitalizations and illnesses or complications. Inquire about the

ability to perform ADLs independently or if assistive-adaptive devices are used.

Current lifestyle also contributes to musculoskeletal health. When assessing a patient with a possible musculoskeletal alteration, inquire about occupation or work life. A person's occupation can cause or contribute to an injury. For instance, fractures are common in patients whose jobs require manual labor, such as housekeepers, mechanics, and industrial workers. Certain occupations, such as computer-related jobs, may predispose a person to carpal tunnel syndrome (entrapment of the median nerve in the wrist) or neck pain.

Ask about allergies, particularly allergy to dairy products, and previous and current use of drugs (prescribed, over-the-counter, and illicit). Allergy to dairy products could lead to decreased calcium intake. Some drugs, such as steroids, can negatively affect calcium metabolism and promote bone loss. Inquire about herbs, vitamin and mineral supplements, or biologic compounds that may be used for arthritis and other musculoskeletal conditions, such as glucosamine and chondroitin. These integrative therapies are commonly used by patients with various types of arthritis and arthralgias (joint aches and discomfort).

Nutrition History

A brief review of the patient's nutrition history helps determine any risks for inadequate nutrient intake. For example, most people, especially women, do not get enough calcium in their diets. Determine whether the patient has had a significant weight gain or loss and whether the weight change was expected.

Ask the patient to recall a typical day of food intake to help identify deficiencies and excesses in the diet. Lactose intolerance is a common problem that can cause inadequate calcium intake. People who cannot afford to buy food, or who have food insecurity, are especially at risk for undernutrition.

Inadequate protein or insufficient vitamin C or D in the diet slows bone and tissue healing. Obesity places excess stress and strain on bones and joints, with resulting trauma to joint cartilage. In addition, obesity inhibits *mobility* in patients with musculoskeletal conditions, which predisposes them to complications such as respiratory and circulatory problems. People with eating disorders such as anorexia nervosa and bulimia nervosa are also at risk for osteoporosis related to decreased intake of calcium and vitamin D.

Family History and Genetic Risk

Obtaining a family history helps to identify disorders that have a familial or genetic tendency. For example, osteoporosis and gout (a genetically linked arthritis caused by an inborn error of purine metabolism) often occur in several generations of a family. Positive family history of these types of disorders can increase risks to the patient. Chapters 42 and 43 provide a more complete description of musculoskeletal conditions that have strong genetic links.

Current Health Problems

The most common reports of people with a musculoskeletal condition are *pain* and/or weakness, either of which can impair *mobility.* Collect data pertinent to the patient's presenting health problem:

- Date and time of onset
- Factors that cause or exacerbate (worsen) the problem
- Course of the problem (e.g., intermittent or continuous)
- Signs and symptoms (as expressed by the patient) and the pattern of their occurrence
- Measures that improve signs and symptoms (e.g., heat, ice)

Assessment of pain can present many challenges. *Pain* can be related to bone, muscle, or joint problems. It may be described as acute or chronic, depending on the onset and duration. Pain with movement could indicate a fracture and/or muscle or joint injury. Assess the intensity by using a pain scale and asking the patient to rate the level of pain being experienced. Quality of pain may be described as dull, burning, aching, or stabbing. Determine the location of pain and areas to which it radiates. With any assessment, it is always best if patients describe the pain in their own words and point to its location, if possible. Chapter 6 describes acute and persistent pain in detail.

Weakness may be related to individual muscles or muscle groups. Determine whether weakness occurs in proximal or distal muscles or muscle groups. Proximal weakness (near the trunk of the body) may indicate myopathy (a problem in muscle tissue). Distal weakness and impaired *sensory perception* (especially in lower extremities) may indicate neuropathy (a problem in nerve tissue). Muscle weakness in the lower extremities may increase the risk for falls and injury. Weakness in the upper extremities may interfere with *mobility* and functional ability.

Assessment of the Musculoskeletal System

Although bones, joints, and muscles are usually assessed during a head-to-toe approach, each subsystem is described separately for emphasis and understanding. For physical assessment of the musculoskeletal system, use inspection, palpation, and range of motion (ROM). A focused assessment is described in this chapter. More specific assessment techniques are discussed in the musculoskeletal problem chapters in this unit.

Observe the patient's posture, gait, and general *mobility* for gross deformities and disability. Note unusual findings and coordinate with the physical or occupational therapist for an in-depth physical assessment, if needed.

Posture includes the person's body build and alignment when standing and walking. Assess the curvature of the spine and the length, shape, and symmetry of extremities. Fig. 41.3 illustrates several common spinal deformities. *Lordosis* (an inward

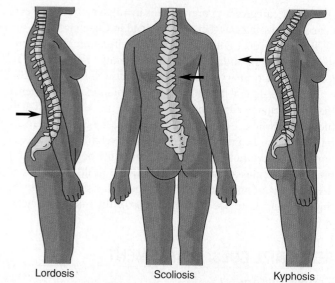

Lordosis   Scoliosis   Kyphosis

FIG. 41.3 Common spinal deformities.

abnormal curvature of the lumbar spine) is a common finding in adults who have abdominal obesity. Scoliosis (an abnormal lateral curvature of the spine) is common in children and young adults (Jarvis & Eckhardt, 2024).

Many patients with lower extremity musculoskeletal conditions eventually have a problem with *gait.* The rehabilitation therapist usually evaluates the patient's balance, steadiness, and ease and length of stride. Any limp or other asymmetric leg movement or deformity should be noted.

If the extremities are affected by a musculoskeletal condition, assess arms or legs at the same time for side-to-side comparisons. For example, inspect and palpate both arms and shoulders for deformity, poor alignment, tenderness or pain, and *mobility.* A shoulder injury may prevent the patient from combing hair with the affected arm, but severe arthritis may inhibit movement in both arms. Assess the elbows and wrists in a similar way.

Because the hand has multiple joints in a single digit, assessment of hand function is perhaps the most critical part of the examination. If the hands are affected, inspect and palpate the metacarpophalangeal (MCP), proximal interphalangeal (PIP), and distal interphalangeal (DIP) joints (Fig. 41.4). The same digits are compared on the right and left hands. Determine the range of motion (ROM) for each joint by observing active movement. If movement is not possible, evaluate passive motion. For a quick and easy assessment of ROM, ask the patient to make a fist and then appose each finger to the thumb. If the patient can perform these maneuvers, ROM of the hand is not seriously restricted.

During the skeletal assessment, note the size, shape, tone, and strength of major skeletal muscles. Ask the patient to demonstrate muscle strength. Apply resistance by holding the extremity and asking the patient to move against resistance. As an option, place your hands on the upper arms and ask the patient to try to raise the arms. Although movement against resistance is not easily quantified, several scales used by therapists are available for grading the patient's strength.

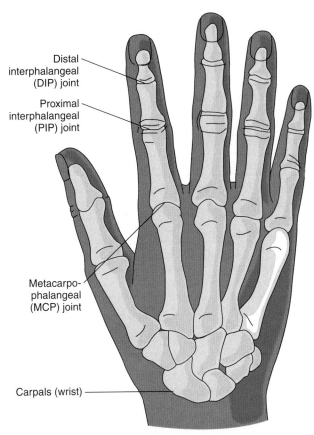

Distal interphalangeal (DIP) joint

Proximal interphalangeal (PIP) joint

Metacarpo-phalangeal (MCP) joint

Carpals (wrist)

FIG. 41.4 Small joints of the hand.

Mobility and Functional Assessment

In collaboration with the physical or occupational therapist, assess the patient's need for ambulatory devices, such as canes and walkers, during transfer from bed to chair and while walking. Observe the patient's ability to perform ADLs, such as dressing and bathing. *Pain*, deformity, and/or impaired *sensory perception* may limit physical *mobility* and function. Coordinate with the rehabilitation therapists to assess the patient's functional status, if needed. A discussion of functional assessment is found in Chapter 7.

Assess major bones, joints, and muscles by inspection, palpation, and determination of ROM. Pay special attention to areas that are affected or may be affected, according to the patient's history, physical disability, or current problem.

As long as the patient can function to meet personal needs, an assessment of ROM is not needed. Observe the client's skin for color, elasticity, and lesions that may relate to musculoskeletal dysfunction. For instance, redness/hyperpigmentation or warmth may indicate an inflammatory process and/or pressure injury to skin.

Evaluation of the hip joint relies primarily on determination of its degree of *mobility* because the joint is deep and difficult to inspect or palpate. *The patient with hip joint pain usually experiences it in the groin or has pain that radiates to the knee or lower back.* The knee is readily accessible for physical assessment, particularly when the patient is sitting and the knee is flexed. Fluid accumulation, or effusion, is easily detected in the knee joint. Limitations in movement with accompanying pain are common findings. The knees may be poorly aligned, as in genu

valgum ("knock-knee") or genu varum ("bowlegged") deformities (Jarvis & Eckhardt, 2024).

The ankles and feet are often neglected in the physical assessment. However, they contain multiple bones and joints that can be affected by disease and injury. Observe and gently palpate ankles and feet if are affected by musculoskeletal conditions.

Neurovascular Assessment

While completing a physical assessment of the musculoskeletal system, perform an assessment of peripheral vascular and nerve integrity if the patient has a current injury. Beginning with the injured side, always compare one extremity with the other.

> **! NURSING SAFETY PRIORITY**
> *Action Alert*
>
> Perform a complete neurovascular assessment (also called a *circ check*), which includes palpation of pulses in the extremities below the level of injury and assessment of sensation, movement, color, temperature, capillary refill, and pain in the injured part. If pulses are not palpable, use a Doppler to find pulses in the extremities. This assessment is described in detail in Chapter 44.

Psychosocial Assessment

The data from the history and physical assessment provide clues for anticipating psychosocial problems. For instance, prolonged absence from employment or permanent physical disability may cause job or career loss. Further stress may be experienced if chronic *pain* continues and the patient cannot cope with numerous stressors. Assess for anxiety and depression, which are common when patients have chronic pain. Deformities resulting from musculoskeletal disease or injury, such as an amputation, can affect a person's body image and self-concept. Help patients identify support systems and coping mechanisms that may be useful if they have long-term musculoskeletal health conditions. Encourage them to verbalize feelings related to loss and body image changes. Refer patients and families for psychological or spiritual counseling if needed and if it is culturally appropriate. Additional information about psychosocial assessment may be found under specific discussions of musculoskeletal conditions in this unit.

Diagnostic Assessment
Laboratory Assessment

The common laboratory tests used in assessing patients with musculoskeletal disorders are outlined in Table 41.2 (Pagana & Pagana, 2022). There is no special patient preparation or follow-up care for any of these tests. Teach the patient about the purpose of the test and the procedure that can be expected. Additional tests performed for patients with connective tissue diseases, such as rheumatoid arthritis, are described in Chapter 43.

Disorders of bone and the parathyroid gland are often reflected in an alteration of the serum calcium or phosphorus level. Therefore, these electrolytes, especially calcium, are monitored. A decrease in serum calcium could indicate bone density loss.

Alkaline phosphatase (ALP) is an enzyme normally present in blood. The concentration of ALP increases with bone or liver damage. In metabolic bone disease and bone cancer, the enzyme concentration rises in proportion to the osteoblastic activity,

TABLE 41.2   Laboratory Profile

Musculoskeletal Assessment

Test	Normal Range for Adults	Significance of Abnormal Findings
Serum calcium	9.0–10.5 mg/dL (2.10–2.50 mmol/L) *Older adults:* decreased	*Hypercalcemia* (increased calcium) • Metastatic cancers of the bone • Paget disease • Bone fractures in healing stage *Hypocalcemia* (decreased calcium) • Osteoporosis • Osteomalacia
Serum phosphorus (phosphate)	3.0–4.5 mg/dL (0.97–1.45 mmol/L) *Older adults:* decreased	*Hyperphosphatemia* (increased phosphorus) • Bone fractures in healing stage • Bone tumors *Hypophosphatemia* (decreased phosphorus) • Osteomalacia
Alkaline phosphatase (ALP)	30–120 units/L (40–160 IU/L) *Older adults:* slightly increased	*Elevations* may indicate: • Metastatic cancers of the bone or liver • Paget disease (a chronic metabolic disorder that causes bone to become fragile and misshapen) • Osteomalacia
Serum muscle enzymes Creatine kinase (CK-MM)	Total CK: *Men:* 55–170 units/L (20–215 IU/L) *Women:* 30–135 units/L (20–160 IU/L) CK-MM: 96%–100%	*Elevations* may indicate: • Muscle trauma • Muscular dystrophy (a group of genetically linked diseases that cause chronic skeletal muscle weakness and organ dysfunction due to smooth muscle involvement) • Effects of electromyography
Lactate dehydrogenase (LDH)	Total LDH: 100–190 units/L (45–90 IU/L) *Older adults:* slightly increased LDH_1: 17%–27% LDH_2: 27%–37% LDH_3: 18%–25% LDH_4: 3%–8% LDH_5: 0%–5%	*Elevations* may indicate: • Skeletal muscle necrosis (cell death) • Extensive cancer • Muscular dystrophy
Aspartate aminotransferase (AST)	0-35 units/L 97–40 IU/L *Older adults:* slightly increased	*Elevations* may indicate: • Skeletal muscle trauma • Muscular dystrophy
Aldolase (ALD)	3.0–8.2 units/dL (less than 8 U/L)	*Elevations* may indicate: • Polymyositis (an uncommon chronic rheumatic disease that is characterized by inflammation of multiple muscles) or dermatomyositis (polymyositis that occurs with a purplish skin rash) • Muscular dystrophy

which indicates bone formation. The level of ALP is normally slightly increased in older adults (Pagana & Pagana, 2022).

The major *muscle enzymes* affected in skeletal muscle disease or injuries are:

• Creatine kinase (CK-MM)
• Lactate dehydrogenase (LDH)
• Aspartate aminotransferase (AST)
• Aldolase (ALD)

As a result of damage, the muscle tissue releases additional amounts of these enzymes, which increases serum levels.

Imaging Assessment

Radiography. The skeleton is very visible on *standard x-rays.* Anteroposterior and lateral projections are the initial screening views used most often. Bone density, alignment, swelling, and intactness can be seen on x-ray. The conditions of joints can be determined, including the size of the joint space, the smoothness of articular cartilage, and synovial swelling. Soft-tissue involvement may be evident but not clearly differentiated.

Computed tomography (CT) is very useful for detecting musculoskeletal conditions, particularly those of the vertebral column and joints. The scanned images can be used to create additional images from other angles or to create three-dimensional images and view complex structures from any position. The nurse or radiology technologist should ask the patient about iodine-based contrast allergies if contrast will be used. Otherwise, there is no pre- or postprocedural care required.

Magnetic Resonance Imaging. *Magnetic resonance imaging (MRI),* with or without the use of contrast media, is commonly used to diagnose musculoskeletal disorders. It is more accurate than CT for many spinal and knee problems. MRI is most appropriate for joints and soft tissue, such as muscles, tendons, and ligaments.

Magnetic resonance arthrography (MRA) combines arthrography (contrast medium injection into a joint) and MRI. It is particularly useful for diagnosing problems of the shoulder and the type and degree of rotator cuff tears. The patient's shoulder is typically injected with contrast medium under fluoroscopy. Then the patient is taken for an MRI, where the shoulder is examined.

Ultrasonography. Sound waves produce an image of the tissue in ultrasonography. An ultrasound procedure may be used to view:

- Soft-tissue disorders, such as masses and fluid accumulation
- Traumatic joint injuries
- Osteomyelitis (bone infection)
- Surgical hardware placement

A jellylike substance applied to the skin over the site to be examined promotes the movement of a metal probe. No special preparation or posttest care is necessary. A quantitative ultrasound (QUS) may be done for determining fractures or bone density. Bone-density testing is discussed in Chapter 43.

Bone Scan. The bone scan is a radionuclide test in which radioactive material (nucleotide) is injected for viewing the entire skeleton. It is occasionally used to detect bone tumors, arthritis, osteomyelitis (bone infection), osteoporosis, vertebral compression fractures, and unexplained bone *pain.*

Because bone takes up the nucleotide slowly, the nuclear medicine physician or technician administers the isotope 4 to 6 hours before scanning. Other tests that require contrast media or other isotopes cannot be given during this time.

Depending on the tissue to be examined, the patient is taken to the nuclear medicine department 4 to 6 hours after injection. The procedure takes 30 to 60 minutes, during which time the patient must lie still for accurate test results to be achieved. The scan may be repeated at 24, 48, and/or 72 hours.

No special care is required after the test. The radioisotope is excreted in stool and urine, but no precautions are taken in handling the excreta. Remind the patient to push fluids to facilitate urinary excretion.

Other Diagnostic Assessments

Biopsies. In a bone biopsy, the physician extracts a specimen of the bone tissue for microscopic examination. This invasive test may confirm the presence of infection or neoplasm, but it is not commonly done today. One of two techniques may be used to retrieve the specimen: needle (closed) biopsy or incisional (open) biopsy.

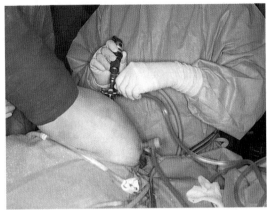

FIG. 41.5 An arthroscope is used in the diagnosis of pathologic changes in the joints. This patient is undergoing arthroscopy of the shoulder.

Muscle biopsy may be performed to confirm a diagnosis of atrophy (as in muscular dystrophy) or inflammation (as in polymyositis). The procedures and care for patients undergoing muscle biopsy are the same as those for patients undergoing bone biopsy.

Arthroscopy. Arthroscopy may be used as a diagnostic test or a surgical procedure. An arthroscope is a fiberoptic tube inserted into a joint for direct visualization of the ligaments, menisci, and articular surfaces of the joint. The knee and shoulder are most commonly evaluated. In addition, synovial biopsy and surgery to repair traumatic injury can be done through the arthroscope as an ambulatory care or same-day surgical procedure.

Patient Preparation. Arthroscopy is performed on an ambulatory care basis as same-day surgery. The patient must have *mobility* in the joint being examined. Those who cannot move the joint or who have an infected joint are not candidates for the procedure.

If the procedure is done for surgical repair, the patient may have a physical therapy consultation before arthroscopy to learn the exercises that are necessary after the test. ROM exercises are also taught but may not be allowed immediately after arthroscopic surgery. The nurse in the surgeon's office or at the surgical center can teach these exercises or reinforce the information provided by the physical therapist. The nurse also reinforces the explanation of the procedure and posttest care and ensures that the patient has signed an informed consent form.

Procedure. The patient is usually given local, light general, or epidural anesthesia, depending on the purpose of the procedure. As shown in Fig. 41.5, the arthroscope is inserted through a small incision shorter than ¼ inch (0.6 cm). Multiple incisions may be required to allow inspection at a variety of angles. After the procedure, a dressing may be applied, depending on the amount of manipulation during the test or surgery.

! NURSING SAFETY PRIORITY

Action Alert

After a bone biopsy, watch for bleeding from the puncture or incision site and for tenderness, redness/hyperpigmentation, or warmth that could indicate infection. Mild analgesics may be used.

! NURSING SAFETY PRIORITY

Action Alert

The priority for care after arthroscopy is to assess the neurovascular status of the patient's affected limb per agency or surgeon protocol. Monitor and document distal pulses, warmth, color, capillary refill, *pain,* movement, and sensation of the affected extremity.

Follow-up Care. The immediate care after arthroscopy is the same for patients having the procedure for diagnostic purposes as it is for those having it for surgical intervention.

Encourage the patient to perform exercises as taught before the procedure, if appropriate. For the mild discomfort experienced after a diagnostic arthroscopy, the primary health care provider prescribes a mild analgesic, such as acetaminophen. If postoperative, the patient may have short-term activity restrictions, depending on the musculoskeletal problem. Ice is often used for 24 hours, and the extremity should be elevated for 12 to 24 hours. When arthroscopic surgery is performed, the primary health care provider usually prescribes a short-term opioid-analgesic combination, such as oxycodone and acetaminophen.

Although complications are not common, monitor and teach the patient to observe for:

- Swelling
- Severe joint or limb *pain*
- Thrombophlebitis
- Infection

Teach the patient to immediately contact the primary health care provider if these conditions are observed. Otherwise, the health care provider usually sees the patient about 1 week after the procedure to check for complications.

NCLEX Examination Challenge 41.2
Physiological Integrity

A client who had arthroscopic surgery for knee ligament repair reports increased swelling and pain two days after the procedure. What action would be the **best** for the nurse to recommend for the client at this time?
A. Apply ice four times a day.
B. Elevate the leg on two pillows.
C. Notify your surgeon immediately.
D. Continue taking analgesia as directed.

GET READY FOR THE NEXT-GENERATION NCLEX® EXAMINATION!

Essential Assessment Points

- Bone is a very dynamic, vascular tissue that undergoes a continuous process of formation and resorption (destruction).
- Three of the most common physiologic changes of aging that affect the musculoskeletal system include a decrease in bone density (osteopenia), degeneration of joint cartilage, and muscle atrophy.
- To promote bone health, individuals should consume adequate calcium to help prevent bone loss and should avoid risky behaviors that could cause musculoskeletal injury.
- Physical disability caused by limitations in *mobility* occurs most commonly in people of color when compared with Whites; this health inequity is most likely related to social determinants of health.
- The most common symptoms reported by clients with musculoskeletal conditions are *pain* and weakness.
- Assessment of the musculoskeletal system should include a comparison of extremities, mobility, and functional assessment, if needed.
- Clients with physical disability or musculoskeletal health conditions often experience anxiety, depression, and/or body image issues.
- Laboratory tests to help determine the presence of musculoskeletal conditions are listed in Table 41.2.
- Imaging tests and arthroscopy can aid in visualizing musculoskeletal health conditions.
- Teach clients having an arthroscopy for diagnosis or surgery to report severe or increased pain and swelling to their surgeon immediately.

Mastery Questions

1. The nurse is assessing an older adult admitted to an assisted-living facility. Which of the following musculoskeletal changes of aging would the nurse expect? **Select all that apply.**
   A. Scoliosis
   B. Kyphosis
   C. Osteoarthritis
   D. Muscle atrophy
   E. Slowed movement
   F. Joint contractures

2. The nurse is reviewing serum laboratory test results for a client who sustained a fractured femur several weeks ago. Which finding would the nurse expect for this client?
   A. Decreased aldolase
   B. Increased calcium
   C. Decreased phosphorous
   D. Increased alkaline phosphatase

REFERENCES

Jarvis, C., & Eckhardt, A. (2024). *Physical examination & health assessment* (9th ed.). St. Louis: Elsevier.

Niu, S., & Lim, F. (2020). The effects of smoking on bone health and healing. *American Journal of Nursing, 120*(7), 40–45.

Pagana, K. D., & Pagana, T. J. (2022). *Mosby's manual of diagnostic and laboratory tests* (7th ed.). St. Louis: Elsevier.

Rogers, J. L. (2023). *McCance and Huether's Pathophysiology: The biologic basis for disease in adults and children* (9th ed.). St. Louis: Elsevier.

Smeltzer, S. C. (2021). *Delivering quality healthcare for people with disability.* Indianapolis: Sigma Theta Tau International Honor Society of Nursing.

Touhy, T. T. & Jett, K. (2022). *Ebersole and Hess' Gerontological nursing and healthy aging* (6th ed.). St. Louis: Elsevier.

42

Concepts of Care for Patients With Musculoskeletal Conditions

Donna D. Ignatavicius

http://evolve.elsevier.com/Iggy/

LEARNING OUTCOMES

1. Plan collaborative care with the interprofessional team to promote *mobility* in patients with osteoporosis.
2. Teach adults how to decrease the risk for osteoporosis.
3. Teach the patient and caregiver(s) about common drugs and other management strategies used for osteoporosis.
4. Plan patient- and family-centered nursing interventions to decrease the psychosocial impact caused by living with bone cancer.
5. Apply knowledge of anatomy, physiology, and pathophysiology to provide evidence-based care for patients with osteoporosis affecting *cellular regulation.*
6. Analyze assessment and diagnostic findings to generate solutions and prioritize nursing care for patients with musculoskeletal conditions.
7. Organize care coordination and transition management for patients with bone cancer.
8. Use clinical judgment to plan evidence-based nursing care to promote mobility and prevent complications in patients with musculoskeletal conditions.
9. Incorporate factors that affect health equity into the plan of care for patients with osteoporosis.

KEY TERMS

bone mineral density (BMD) The amount of mineral in bone that determines bone strength; peaks between 25 and 30 years of age.

bunionectomy Surgical removal of the first metatarsal bony overgrowth and bursa with realignment to manage pain.

dual x-ray absorptiometry (DXA) A noninvasive radiographic scan to assess bone mineral density.

Dupuytren contracture (or deformity) A slowly progressive thickening of the palmar fascia, resulting in flexion contracture of the fourth (ring) and fifth (little) fingers of the hand.

fragility fracture A fracture caused by osteoporosis.

ganglion A round, benign cyst often found on a wrist or foot joint or tendon.

hallux valgus deformity A common foot problem in which the great toe drifts laterally at the first metatarsophalangeal (MTP) joint.

kyphosis Outward curvature of the thoracic spine causing a "humpback."

osteomalacia Loss of bone related to lack of vitamin D, which causes bone softening.

osteomyelitis Infection in bone caused by bacteria (most often), viruses, parasites, or fungi; the infection may be acute or chronic.

osteonecrosis (also known as avascular necrosis) Bone death secondary to lack of or disruption in blood supply to the affected bone, usually from trauma or chronic steroid therapy.

osteopenia Loss of bone mass.

osteoporosis A chronic disease of cellular regulation in which bone loss causes significant decreased density and possible fracture.

Paget disease A chronic, slowly progressive skeletal metabolic bone disorder that causes rapid bone destruction and reformation, causing bone pain, arthritis, fractures, and deformities.

plantar fasciitis An inflammation of the plantar fascia, which is located in the area of the arch of the foot, causing pain.

PRIORITY AND INTERRELATED CONCEPTS

The priority concepts for this chapter are:
- *Mobility*
- *Infection*
- *Cellular Regulation*

The *Cellular Regulation* concept exemplar for this chapter is Osteoporosis.

The interrelated concept for this chapter is:
- *Pain*

Musculoskeletal conditions include diseases of *cellular regulation* (e.g., osteoporosis and cancer), bone tumors, bone *infection*, and a variety of deformities and syndromes. Older adults are at the greatest risk for most of these problems, although *primary* bone cancer is most often found in adolescents and young adults.

Almost all musculoskeletal health problems result in decreased *mobility* and acute or persistent (chronic) *pain.* These concepts are reviewed in Chapter 3. This chapter focuses on selected adult musculoskeletal conditions not covered in Chapter 43 on arthritis and Chapter 44 on musculoskeletal trauma. Musculoskeletal conditions that are seen most often in children, such as scoliosis and progressive muscular dystrophies, are not included in this chapter because they are included in pediatric textbooks.

CELLULAR REGULATION CONCEPT EXEMPLAR: OSTEOPOROSIS

Pathophysiology Review

Osteoporosis is a chronic disease of *cellular regulation* in which bone loss causes significant decreased density and possible fracture. It is often referred to as a *silent disease* because the first sign of osteoporosis in most people is diagnosed after a fracture. For this reason, osteoporosis is often underdiagnosed and undertreated in multiple populations (Cochran et al., 2022).

According to *Healthy People 2030* (2023) data, 50% of all postmenopausal women will have a fragility fracture (fracture caused by osteoporosis; sometimes referred to as a "bone attack") in their lifetime. Twenty-five percent of men over 50 years of age will also have an osteoporosis-related fracture. Any fracture places individuals with bone loss at a very high risk for future fractures. This risk is especially high for women of color and Asian/Pacific Islander women when compared with White women as discussed later in this chapter (Crandall et al., 2021).

Osteoporosis is a major global health problem. In less affluent or famine countries, many people have both osteoporosis *and* osteomalacia as a result of dietary deficiencies. Osteomalacia is loss of bone related to lack of vitamin D, which causes bone softening. Vitamin D is needed for calcium absorption in the small intestine. As a result of vitamin D deficiency, normal bone building is disrupted, and calcification does not occur to harden the bone. Table 42.1 compares these two bone diseases.

Bone is a living, changing tissue that is constantly undergoing changes in a process referred to as *bone remodeling,* a type of *cellular regulation.* Osteoporosis and osteopenia (loss of bone mass) occur when osteoclastic (bone resorption) activity is greater than osteoblastic (bone-building) activity. The result is a decreased bone mineral density (BMD). BMD is the amount of mineral that determines bone strength; it peaks between 25 and 30 years of age. Before and during the peak years, osteoclastic activity and osteoblastic activity work at the same rate. After the peak years, osteoclastic activity exceeds bone-building activity, and bone density decreases. BMD decreases most rapidly in postmenopausal women as serum estrogen levels diminish. Although estrogen does not build bone, it helps prevent bone loss. *Trabecular,* or *cancellous* (spongy), bone is lost first, followed by loss of *cortical* (compact) bone. The hip, wrist, and spinal column have the highest amount of cancellous bone and are therefore the most likely to fracture first.

Standards for the diagnosis of osteoporosis are based on BMD testing that provides a T-score for the patient. A T-score represents the number of standard deviations above or below (designated with a minus sign) the average BMD for young, healthy adults. The T-score in a healthy 30-year-old adult is 0. Osteopenia is present when the T-score is at −1 and above −2.5. Osteoporosis is diagnosed in a person who has a T-score at or lower than −2.5 (Cochran et al., 2022). Severe or established osteoporosis is defined as the presence of osteoporosis plus one or more fractures.

Osteoporosis can be classified as generalized or regional. *Generalized* osteoporosis involves many structures in the skeleton and is further divided into two categories: primary and secondary. *Primary* osteoporosis is more common and occurs in postmenopausal women and in men in their seventh or eighth decade of life. *Secondary* osteoporosis may result from other medical conditions, such as hyperparathyroidism; long-term drug therapy, such as with corticosteroids; or prolonged decreased *mobility,* such as that seen with spinal cord injury. Treatment of the secondary type is directed toward the cause of the osteoporosis when possible.

TABLE 42.1	Differential Features of Osteoporosis and Osteomalacia	
Characteristic	**Osteoporosis**	**Osteomalacia**
Definition	Decreased bone mass caused by multiple factors	Bone softening caused by lack of calcification
Primary etiology	Lack of calcium and estrogen or testosterone	Lack of vitamin D
Radiographic findings	Osteopenia (bone loss), fractures	Fractures
Calcium level	Low or normal	Low or normal
Phosphate level	Normal	Low or normal
Parathyroid hormone	Normal	High or normal
Alkaline phosphatase	Normal	High

Regional (localized) osteoporosis, an example of secondary disease, can occur when a limb is immobilized related to a fracture, injury, or paralysis. Decreased **mobility** for longer than 8 to 12 weeks can result in this type of osteoporosis. Bone loss also occurs when people spend prolonged time in a gravity-free or weightless environment (e.g., astronauts).

Etiology and Genetic Risk

Primary osteoporosis is caused by a combination of genetic, lifestyle, and environmental factors. Box 42.1 lists the major potentially modifiable and nonmodifiable risk factors that can contribute to the development of this disease (Cochran et al., 2022).

PATIENT-CENTERED CARE: GENETICS/GENOMICS

Genetic Factors Associated With Osteoporosis

The genetic and immune factors that cause osteoporosis are very complex. Strong evidence demonstrates that genetics is a significant factor. Many genetic changes have been identified as possible causative factors, but there is no agreement about which ones are most important or constant in all patients. For example, changes in the vitamin D₃ receptor *(VDR)* gene and calcitonin receptor *(CTR)* gene have been found in some patients with the disease. Receptors are essential for the uptake and use of these substances by the cells (Rogers, 2023).

The bone morphogenetic protein 2 *(BMP-2)* gene has a key role in bone formation and maintenance. Some osteoporotic patients who had fractures have changes in their *BMP-2* gene. Alterations in the growth hormone 1 *(GH-1)* gene have been discovered in petite Asian-American women who are highly predisposed to bone loss (Rogers, 2023).

Hormones, tumor necrosis factor (TNF), interleukins, and other substances in the body help control osteoclasts in a very complex pathway. The identification of the importance of the cytokine receptor activator of nuclear factor kappa-B ligand (RANKL), its receptor RANK, and its decoy receptor osteoprotegerin (OPG) has helped researchers understand more about the activity of osteoclasts in metabolic bone disease. Disruptions in the RANKL, RANK, and OPG system can lead to increased osteoclast activity in which bone is rapidly broken down (Rogers, 2023). Knowledge of these physiologic changes has contributed to the development of new drugs to manage osteoporosis (see the Drug Therapy section later in this chapter).

PATIENT-CENTERED CARE: GENDER HEALTH

Gender Differences in Osteoporosis

Primary osteoporosis most often occurs in women after menopause or after removal of both ovaries as a result of decreased estrogen levels. Obese women can store estrogen in their tissues for use as necessary to maintain a normal level of serum calcium better than thinner women and are therefore less likely to develop osteoporosis and resulting fractures.

Men over 50 years of age also develop osteoporosis as they age because their testosterone levels decrease. Testosterone is the major sex hormone that builds bone tissue. Older men are often underdiagnosed and undertreated and should be screened for osteopenia and osteoporosis.

The relationship of osteoporosis to nutrition is well established. For example, excessive caffeine in the diet can cause calcium loss in the urine. A diet lacking enough calcium and vitamin D stimulates the parathyroid gland to produce parathyroid hormone (PTH). PTH triggers the release of calcium from the bony matrix. Activated vitamin D is needed for calcium uptake in the body. Malabsorption of nutrients in the small intestine also contributes to low serum calcium levels. Institutionalized or homebound patients who are not exposed to sunlight may be at a higher risk because they do not receive adequate vitamin D for the metabolism of calcium (Cochran et al., 2022).

Calcium loss occurs at a more rapid rate when phosphorus intake is high. (Chapter 13 describes the usual relationship between calcium and phosphorus in the body.) People who drink large amounts of carbonated beverages each day (over 40 ounces [1200 mL]) are at high risk for calcium loss and subsequent osteoporosis, regardless of age or gender.

Protein deficiency may also affect **cellular regulation.** Because 50% of serum calcium is protein bound, protein is needed to use calcium. However, excessive protein intake may increase calcium loss in the urine. For example, people who are on high-protein, low-carbohydrate diets, such as the Atkins diet, may consume too much protein to replace other foods that are not allowed.

Incidence and Prevalence

Osteoporosis or osteopenia is a health problem for more than 54 million Americans (Noel et al., 2021). According to *Healthy People 2030,* 1 in 10 people over 50 years of age in the United States have osteoporosis.

PATIENT-CENTERED CARE: HEALTH EQUITY

Issues in Diagnosis and Treatment of Osteoporosis

Body build, weight, and race/ethnicity seem to influence who gets the disease. Osteoporosis occurs most often in older, lean-built White women, particularly those who do not exercise regularly. However, dark-skinned individuals are at risk for decreased vitamin D, which is needed for adequate calcium absorption in the small intestines. Dietary preferences or intolerances, sun avoidance, or the inability to afford high-nutrient food may influence anyone's rate of bone loss. For example, many non-Hispanic Blacks often have lactose intolerance and cannot drink regular milk or eat other dairy-based foods. As an alternative, lactose-free milk, almond milk, or soy milk provides calcium, although these types of milk may be cost-prohibitive.

For a number of years, researchers have described health inequities between White, and non-Hispanic Black, Asian/Pacific Islander, and Hispanic groups. These minority groups receive less screening and treatment for bone loss, including after experiencing a fracture, when compared with White individuals. The reasons for those differences for *some* individuals in these groups likely include social determinants of health such as (Noel et al., 2021):
- Lack of access to health care for minority groups
- Lower educational level
- Lower socioeconomic status

Nurses need to teach members of minority groups about how to promote bone health and the need for screening for bone loss.

 PATIENT-CENTERED CARE: VETERAN HEALTH

Osteopenia and Osteoporosis

Another group in which bone loss may be underdiagnosed is the veteran population. Although postmenopausal women are at the highest risk, male and female veterans often have osteopenia or osteoporosis, which may be diagnosed after a low-trauma fracture (Elliott et al., 2021). All veterans should be screened for bone mineral density and treated aggressively to prevent future potentially debilitating fragility fractures.

Health Promotion/Disease Prevention

The *Healthy People 2030* initiative recognizes the need for national attention to the prevention of osteoporosis and fragility fractures.

♥ **MEETING *HEALTHY PEOPLE 2030* OBJECTIVES**

Osteoporosis

To prevent fractures and disabilities related to osteoporosis, these objectives have been outlined:
- Reduce the proportion of adults with osteoporosis.
- Increase the proportion of older adults who get screened for osteoporosis.
- Reduce hip fractures among older adults.
- Increase the proportion of older adults who get treatment for osteoporosis after a fracture.

Osteoporosis prevention begins with education for young women who need to be aware of appropriate health and lifestyle practices that can prevent this potentially disabling disease. Nurses can play a vital role in patient education for women of any age to prevent and manage osteoporosis.

The focus of evidence-based osteoporosis prevention at any age is to decrease modifiable risk factors to promote patient safety. For example, teach patients who do not include enough dietary calcium examples of best foods to eat, such as dairy products and dark green leafy vegetables. Teach them to read food labels for sources of calcium content. Recognize that individuals who are experiencing food insecurity may not be able to purchase these expensive foods. Explain the importance of sun exposure (but not so much as to get sunburned) and adequate vitamin D in the diet (Cochran et al., 2022).

Teach people at high risk for bone loss the importance of smoking cessation (if needed), weight loss (if needed), and avoidance of excessive alcohol use to promote bone health. Teach them to limit the number of carbonated beverages consumed each day. Remind patients who have sedentary lifestyles about the importance of exercise and which types of exercise build bone tissue. Weight-bearing exercises, such as regularly scheduled walking, are preferred. Teach people at high risk to avoid activities that cause jarring, such as horseback riding and jogging, to prevent potential vertebral compression fractures.

Remind all postmenopausal women and men over 50 years of age to request bone loss screening from their primary health care provider. For older adults over 65 years old, Medicare pays for bone mineral testing (described later in this section) every 2 years. Although their risk is less than that of Whites, be sure to teach people of color and those of Asian descent to have bone loss screening by no later than 50 years of age.

🛡 **NURSE WELL-BEING REMINDER!**

Remember: Be sure to increase calcium and vitamin D in your diet, get regular exercise, and, to the extent possible, follow a healthy lifestyle to help prevent osteopenia or osteoporosis. If you are postmenopausal or a male over 50 years of age, seek screening for bone mineral density. If you have experienced either a high- or a low-trauma fracture, be aware that you are at high risk for future fractures and should seek postfracture treatment and monitoring.

Interprofessional Collaborative Care

Recognize Cues: Assessment

History. A complete health history with assessment of risk factors is important in the prevention, early detection, and treatment of osteoporosis. Patients who have risk factors for osteoporosis are at increased risk for fractures when falls occur. In some cases the fracture occurs before the fall. Include a fall risk assessment in the health history, especially for older adults. Assess for evidence-based fall risk factors as described in Chapter 4.

Physical Assessment/Signs and Symptoms. When performing a musculoskeletal assessment, inspect the vertebral column. The classic "dowager's hump," or kyphosis (outward curvature of the thoracic spine causing a "humpback") is often present (Fig. 42.1). Older patients may state that they have gotten shorter, perhaps as

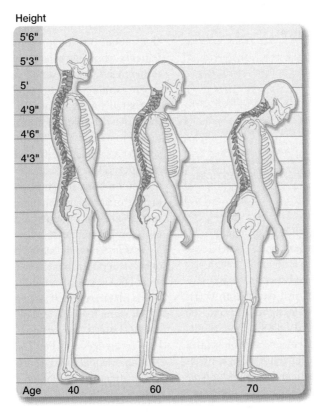

FIG. 42.1 Normal spine at age 40 years and osteoporotic changes at ages 60 and 70 years. These changes can cause a loss of as much as 6 inches in height and can result in the so-called *dowager's hump (far right)* in the upper thoracic vertebrae.

much as 2 to 3 inches (5–7.5 cm), within the previous 20 years. Take or delegate the taking of height and weight measurements and compare with previous measurements if they are available (Jarvis & Eckhardt, 2024).

 NATIONAL PATIENT SAFETY GOALS

Fall Prevention

The Joint Commission's National Patient Safety Goals (NPSGs) specify the need to reduce risk for harm to patients resulting from falls. Hospitals and long-term care facilities have risk management programs to assess for the risk for falls. For patients at high risk, communicate this information to other members of the health care team using colored armbands, posted signs, or other easy-to-recognize methods. Chapter 4 discusses fall prevention in health care agencies and at home in more detail.

The patient may have back pain, which often occurs after lifting, bending, or stooping. The pain may be sharp and acute or persistent (chronic). *Pain* is worse with activity and is often reduced by rest. Back pain accompanied by tenderness and voluntary restriction of spinal movement suggests one or more compression vertebral fractures (i.e., one of the most common and painful types of osteoporotic or fragility fracture). *Mobility* restriction and spinal deformity may result in constipation, abdominal distention, reflux esophagitis, and respiratory compromise in severe cases. The most likely area for spinal fracture is between T8 and L3, the most movable part of the vertebral column.

Fractures are also common in the distal end of the radius (wrist) and the upper third of the femur (hip). Ask the patient to locate all areas that are painful, and observe for signs and symptoms of fractures such as swelling and malalignment. Signs and symptoms of fractures are discussed in Chapter 44.

Psychosocial Assessment. Women associate osteoporosis with menopause, getting older, and becoming less independent. The disease can result in decreased *mobility,* deformity, and disability that can affect the patient's well-being and life satisfaction. Quality of life may be further affected by persistent (chronic) *pain,* insomnia, depression, and fear of falling (Touhy & Jett, 2022).

Assess the patient's concept of body image, especially if the patient is severely kyphotic. For example, the patient may have difficulty finding clothes that fit properly. Social interactions may be avoided because of a change in appearance or the physical limitations of being unable to sit in chairs in restaurants, movie theaters, and other places. Changes in sexuality may occur as a result of poor self-esteem or the discomfort caused by positioning during intercourse.

Because osteoporosis poses a risk for fractures, teach the patient to be very cautious about activities. The threat of fracture can create anxiety and fear and result in further limitation of social or physical activities. Assess for these feelings to assist in treatment decisions and health teaching. For example, the patient may not exercise as prescribed for fear that a fracture will occur.

NCLEX Examination Challenge 42.1

Health Promotion and Maintenance

The nurse is providing health teaching to a postmenopausal client about osteoporosis prevention and screening. Which statement by the client indicates a **need for further teaching**?

A. "I'm planning to have my DXA scan next week because I should get one every year."

B. "I signed up for a virtual smoking cessation program with my partner so we can quit together."

C. "I joined a group of coworkers who take a walk at lunchtime every day."

D. "I'll try to eat more foods high in calcium like dairy products and green leafy vegetables."

Laboratory Assessment. Serum calcium and vitamin D_3 levels should be routinely monitored (at least once a year) for all women and for men older than 50 years who are at a high risk for the disease. Serum calcium should be between 9.0 and 10.5 mg/dL (2.10 and 2.50 mmol/L). Total 25-hydroxyvitamin D (D_2 plus D_3) levels should be between 25 and 80 ng/mL (75 and 200 nmol/L) (Pagana et al., 2022; Pagana et al., 2019). These results can help determine the need for supplements and preventive measures to slow bone loss. No definitive laboratory tests confirm a diagnosis of primary osteoporosis, although a number of *bone turnover markers* can provide information about bone resorption and formation activity. Although not commonly tested for, these markers are sensitive to bone changes and can be used to monitor effectiveness of treatment for osteoporosis or to detect bone changes early in the disease process. Examples of these markers are osteocalcin and bone-specific alkaline phosphatase (BSAP).

Imaging Assessment. Conventional x-rays of the spine and long bones show decreased bone density, but only after a large amount of bone loss has occurred. Fractures can also be seen on x-rays. According to the Bone Health and Osteoporosis Foundation (BHOF) (formerly the National Osteoporosis Foundation), all postmenopausal women and men age 50 and older should be evaluated for osteoporosis risk to determine the need for BMD testing and/or vertebral imaging.

The most commonly used screening and diagnostic radiographic test for measuring bone mineral density (BMD) is dual x-ray absorptiometry (DXA). The spine and hip are most often assessed when a central DXA (cDXA) scan is performed. If spinal deformity is present, the wrist may also be assessed. Many primary health care providers recommend that women in their 40s have a baseline screening DXA scan so later bone changes can be detected and compared. DXA is a noninvasive, painless scan that emits less radiation than a chest x-ray. It is the most common test currently used but has limitations. First, BMD alone explains only part of the bone change and provides no information on cellular activity. Second, there are variations among different DXA systems. In addition, DXA may not be as useful for very tall or very obese patients.

Tell patients that their height is measured before a DXA scan. The patient stays dressed but is asked to remove any metallic objects such as belt buckles, coins, keys, or jewelry that might interfere with the test. The results are displayed on a computer graph, and a T-score is calculated. No special follow-up care

for the test is required. However, the patient needs to discuss the results with the primary health care provider for any decisions about possible preventive or management interventions. Patients who have osteopenia or osteoporosis usually have follow-up DXA scans every 2 years.

For some patients, *CT-based absorptiometry* (qualitative computed tomography [QCT]) may be performed. This test measures the volume of bone density and strength of the vertebral spine and hip. The peripheral QCT (pQCT) scan measures the same at the forearm or tibia. High-resolution pQCT (HR-pQCT) of the radius and tibia provides additional information on bone structure and architecture. These tests are predictive of spine and/or hip fractures in women; however, they require greater amounts of radiation when compared with the more traditional DXA.

Vertebral imaging can be performed using lateral spine x-rays or lateral vertebral fracture assessment, which is available as part of most DXA systems. According to the clinical guidelines outlined by the BHOF, vertebral imaging is indicated for these groups:

- All women age 70 and older and all men age 80 and older if BMD is less than or equal to a T-score of 1.0
- Women ages 65 to 69 and men ages 70 to 79 if BMD is less than or equal to a T-score of 1.5
- Postmenopausal women and men age 50 and older with certain risk factors, such as significant height loss, history of low-trauma fracture, or being on long-term corticosteroids

The most promising imaging test for diagnosing bone disease is the use of *MRI* to assess bone marrow composition. MRI does not involve radiation and can be used to view bone in ways that other techniques cannot. To determine the presence of osteoporosis, quantitative MRI procedures provide information about yellow bone marrow content, diffusion, and perfusion to the bone. *Perfusion* to osteoporotic bone is lower than to bone of normal bone density. Fat marrow content, sometimes referred to as *bone marrow adipose tissue (BMAT),* is higher in patients with bone loss compared with those with normal BMD (Xiaojuan & Schwartz, 2020). These tests are more reliable and offer more information about bone change than BMD measurements alone but are very expensive and not widely used yet.

Several imaging tests are available for community-based screening because these devices are more portable. However, they lack the preciseness and reliability of the previously discussed imaging procedures. Examples include peripheral DXA (pDXA) and peripheral quantitative ultrasound densitometry (pQUS). The *pDXA scan* assesses BMD of the heel, forearm, or finger. It is often used for large-scale screening purposes. *pQUS* is an effective and low-cost screening tool that can detect osteoporosis and predict risk for hip fracture. The heel, tibia, and patella are most commonly tested. This procedure requires no special preparation, is quick, and has no radiation exposure or specific follow-up care (Pagana et al., 2022). Both tests are commonly used for screening at community health fairs, skilled nursing facilities (SNFs), and women's health centers.

Analyze Cues and Prioritize Hypotheses: Analysis

The priority problem for patients with osteoporosis or osteopenia is *potential for fractures due to weak, porous bone tissue.*

Generate Solutions and Take Actions: Planning and Implementation

Planning: Expected Outcomes. The expected outcome is that the patient will avoid fractures by preventing falls, managing risk factors, and adhering to preventive or treatment measures for bone loss.

Interventions. The patient is predisposed to fractures, so nutrition therapy, lifestyle changes, and drug therapy are used to slow bone resorption and form new bone tissue. Self-management education (SME) can help prevent osteoporosis or slow the progress.

Nutrition Therapy. The nutritional considerations for the treatment of a patient with a diagnosis of osteoporosis are the same as those for preventing the disease. Teach patients about the need for adequate amounts of calcium and vitamin D for bone remodeling. Instruct them to avoid excessive alcohol and caffeine consumption. People who are lactose intolerant can choose a variety of soy and rice products that are fortified with calcium and vitamin D. In addition, calcium and vitamin D are added to many fruit juices, bread, and cereal products. Be sure to evaluate whether individuals can afford to purchase these expensive foods and beverages before nutritional health teaching.

A variety of nutrients are needed to maintain bone health. *The promotion of a single nutrient will not prevent or treat osteoporosis.* Help the patient develop a nutrition plan that is most beneficial in maintaining bone health; the plan should emphasize fruits and vegetables, low-fat dairy and protein sources, increased fiber, and moderation in alcohol and caffeine (Cochran et al., 2022).

Lifestyle Changes. Exercise is important in the prevention and management of osteoporosis. It also plays a vital role in *pain* management, cardiovascular function, and an improved sense of well-being.

In collaboration with the primary health care provider, the physical therapist may prescribe exercises for strengthening the abdominal and back muscles for those at risk for vertebral fractures. These exercises improve posture and support for the spine. Abdominal muscle tightening, deep breathing, and pectoral stretching are stressed to increase lung capacity. Exercises for the extremity muscles include muscle-tightening, resistive, and range-of-motion (ROM) exercises to improve *mobility.* Muscle strengthening also helps to prevent falls and promote balance. Swimming and yoga provide overall muscle exercise. Assess the individual's ability to afford or participate in these exercises. Evaluate the individual's housing arrangement, food security status, and financial ability before considering health teaching.

In addition to exercises for muscle strengthening, a general weight-bearing exercise program should be implemented. Teach patients that walking for 30 minutes three to five times a week is the single most effective exercise for osteoporosis prevention. Remind them to avoid any activity that would cause jarring of the body, such as jogging and horseback riding. These activities can cause compression fractures of the vertebral column.

In addition to nutrition and exercise, other lifestyle changes may be needed. Teach the patient to avoid tobacco in any form, especially active or passive cigarette smoking (Cochran et al., 2022). Remind women not to consume more than one alcoholic drink per day (5 ounces each); instruct men not to have more than two alcoholic drinks per day.

Drug Therapy. Evidence shows that drug therapy should be used for postmenopausal women and men age 50 and older when the BMD T-score for the hip or lumbar spine is below or equal to −2.5 with no other risk factors, or when the T-score is below −1.5 with risk factors or previous fracture. Anyone age 50 or older who had a hip or vertebral fracture should also be treated (Cochran et al., 2022). The primary health care provider may prescribe a bisphosphonate, estrogen agonist/antagonist (formerly called *selective estrogen receptor modulator* [SERM]), parathyroid hormone (PTH), RANKL inhibitor, sclerostin inhibitor, or a combination of several drugs to treat or prevent osteoporosis (Table 42.2).

Bisphosphonates are the most common drugs used for osteopenia. Bisphosphonates are considered antiresorptive drugs because they slow bone resorption by binding with crystal elements in bone, especially spongy, cancellous bone tissue. Some of the drugs in this classification are also approved for Paget disease and hypercalcemia caused by cancer. Paget disease is a chronic, slowly progressive skeletal metabolic bone disorder that causes rapid bone destruction and reformation, causing bone pain, arthritis, fractures, and deformities.

> ### 💊 NURSING SAFETY PRIORITY
> #### *Drug Alert*
>
> Two of the most recent additions to the bisphosphonates are IV zoledronic acid and IV pamidronate. For management of osteoporosis, zoledronic acid is needed only once a year, and pamidronate is given every 3 to 6 months. Both drugs are associated with transient influenza-type symptoms, especially after the first dose. Less commonly, both drugs have been linked to a complication called jaw osteonecrosis (also known as *avascular necrosis,* or *bone death*), in which infection and necrosis of the mandible or maxilla occur (Burchum & Rosenthal, 2022). The incidence of this serious problem is low, but it can be a complication of this infusion therapy.
>
> To promote safety, teach patients to take oral bisphosphonates early in the morning with 8 ounces of water and wait 30 to 60 minutes in an upright position before eating. If chest discomfort (a symptom of esophageal irritation) occurs, instruct patients to discontinue the drug and contact their health care provider. Patients with poor renal function, hypocalcemia, or gastroesophageal reflux disease (GERD) should not take bisphosphonates. *Teach patients to have an oral assessment and preventive dentistry before beginning any bisphosphonate therapy.* To promote safety, instruct them to inform any dentist who is planning invasive treatment, such as a tooth extraction or implant, that they are taking a bisphosphonate drug.
>
> Teach patients that they should not take bisphosphonates continuously as lifelong management owing to long-term adverse effects such as esophageal cancer, atrial fibrillation, jaw osteonecrosis, and severe musculoskeletal pain. The decision to continue the drug after 2 years is made based on follow-up DXA scan results. If bone loss is maintained or bone density increases, the bisphosphonate is discontinued. If bone loss continues to occur, the drug can be continued for up to 5 years (Burchum & Rosenthal, 2022).

A newer drug class is *RANK ligand (receptor activator of nuclear factor kappa-B ligand) inhibitors,* such as denosumab. This drug is given subcutaneously twice a year by a health care professional. RANKL inhibitors work to prevent bone loss by inhibiting osteoclastic-mediated bone resorption.

TABLE 42.2   Common Examples of Drug Therapy

Osteopenia and Osteoporosis

Drug Category	Selected Nursing Implications
Calcium (With Vitamin D)	
Calcium and vitamin D$_3$ may be taken separately or in combination.	Take a third of the daily dose at bedtime *because no weight-bearing activity to build bone occurs while sleeping.*
	Encourage increased fluids, unless medically contraindicated, *to help prevent urinary calculi (stones).*
	Teach patient to take the drugs with 6–8 ounces of water *to help dissolve them.*
	Assess for a history of urinary stones before giving calcium.
	Monitor calcium level *to determine drug effectiveness.*
	Observe for signs of hypercalcemia, such as calcium deposits under the skin, cardiac dysrhythmias, changes in skeletal muscle tone, and urinary stones, *which may indicate calcium excess.*
	Teach patients to check with their primary health care providers about recommended doses to take.
Bisphosphonates	
Common examples of bisphosphonates:	Teach patients to take drug on an empty stomach first thing in the morning with a full glass of water *to help prevent esophagitis, esophageal ulcers, and gastric ulcers.*
• Alendronate	
• Ibandronate	Remind patients to take drug 30 minutes before food, drink, and other drugs *to prevent interactions.*
• Risedronate	Instruct the patient to remain upright, sitting or standing, for 30 minutes after taking the drug *to help prevent esophagitis (esophageal inflammation).*
• Pamidronate (IV)	
• Zoledronic acid (IV)	Instruct the patient to have a dental examination before starting the drug *because it can cause jaw and maxillary osteonecrosis, particularly if oral hygiene is poor.*
	Do not give the drug to patients who are sensitive to aspirin *because bronchoconstriction may occur.*
	For IV drug, infuse over 15–30 minutes *to prevent rare complications such as atrial fibrillation.*
	For IV drugs, check the patient's serum creatinine before and after administering the medication *because it can cause renal insufficiency or acute kidney injury.*
Estrogen Agonists/Antagonists	
Example of estrogen agonists/antagonists:	Teach the patient the signs and symptoms of venous thromboembolism (VTE), especially in the first 4 months of therapy, *because these drugs can cause VTE.*
• Raloxifene	Monitor liver function tests (LFTs) in collaboration with the primary health care provider *because the drug can increase LFT values.*
RANKL Inhibitors	
Common examples of RANKL inhibitors:	Teach patients to report new musculoskeletal pain, especially in the back, and skin reactions, not just at the injection site.
• Denosumab	Teach patients to report signs and symptoms of infection, *a common adverse effect.*
	Monitor levels of calcium, magnesium, and phosphorus *because the drug can cause severe hypocalcemia;* patients with impaired renal function are especially at risk.
	Instruct the patient to have a dental examination before starting the drug *because it can cause jaw and maxillary osteonecrosis, particularly if oral hygiene is poor.*

One of the newest drugs for osteoporosis is a monoclonal antibody called *romosozumab*, the first drug in a class of sclerostin inhibitors. This drug incorporates antiresorptive and anabolic (bone-building) properties by blocking actions of sclerostin, an inhibitor of bone formation. Patients who have had a stroke or myocardial infarction in the past 12 months should not take this drug (Cochran et al., 2022). Romosozumab is given only to women who can no longer become pregnant and should be avoided in any patient who has hypocalcemia (Burchum & Rosenthal, 2022).

Teriparatide and abaloparatide are *parathyroid hormone–related protein drugs* that build bone and should not be used long-term. These drugs are available as daily subcutaneous injections and are indicated for patients who have had a previous fracture or who have multiple risk factors. For the best clinical outcome, postmenopausal women who have a T-score of less than –2.5 should take romosozumab for 1 year *or* teriparatide/abaloparatide for 2 years followed by an antiresorptive drug such as a bisphosphonate (Cochran et al., 2022).

Care Coordination and Transition Management

Home Care Management. Patients with osteoporosis are usually managed at home unless they have major fragility fractures. Some patients do not know that they have osteoporosis until they experience a fall and have one or more fractures.

Remind patients to have follow-up DXA scans as prescribed to determine the effectiveness of drug therapy. For example, some patients maintain or gain bone mass and can discontinue their prescribed drug as directed by their primary health care provider. After discontinuation of medication, follow-up scans determine whether drug therapy needs to be restarted or another drug prescribed. This process helps to reduce the potential adverse effects that are associated with certain drug classifications.

Part of your responsibility is to collaborate with members of the interprofessional health care team to ensure that the patient's home is safe and hazard free to help prevent falling. In some cases, home modifications may be needed, such as ramps instead of stairs or handrails near toilets and bathtubs and showers. Teach patients to prevent clutter in the home for clear pathways, avoid slippery floors, wear rubber-soled shoes, and avoid scatter rugs. Chapter 4 describes fall prevention in detail.

Self-Management Education. Teach patients about lifestyle practices that can help prevent additional bone loss. For example, to help prevent vitamin D deficiency, daily sun exposure (at least 5 minutes each day) is the most important source of vitamin D. If vitamin D levels remain low, teach patients to increase calcium and vitamin D sources in the diet.

Some people are lactose intolerant or do not use dairy products because of vegan diets. However, many products are available for people who avoid dairy products. Soy and rice milk, tofu, and soy products are substitutes, but they are expensive. Teach patients to choose products that are fortified with vitamin D.

If patients are on drug therapy for osteopenia or osteoporosis, teach them to adhere to the medication regimen and take the prescribed drug(s) as instructed. Lack of adherence to long-term therapy for osteoporosis and bone health promotion practices is a major problem that results in increased fractures, hospital stays, and health care costs.

Health Care Resources. Refer patients to the Bone Health and Osteoporosis Foundation (www.bhop.org) in the United States for information regarding the disease and its treatment. The Osteoporosis Society of Canada (www.osteoporosis.ca) has similar services. Large health care systems often have osteoporosis specialty clinics and support groups for patients with osteoporosis.

Evaluate Outcomes: Evaluation

Evaluate the care of the patient with osteoporosis or at risk for osteoporosis based on the identified priority patient problem. Expected outcomes are that the patient:

- Continues to follow up with DXA screenings as recommended to assess ongoing bone health
- Makes necessary changes in lifestyle to help prevent further bone loss
- Does not experience a fragility fracture due to bone loss

OSTEOMYELITIS

Pathophysiology Review

Infection in bony tissue can be a severe and difficult-to-treat problem. Osteomyelitis (bone infection) can result in chronic recurrence, loss of function, persistent (chronic) ***pain,*** amputation, or even death due to sepsis.

Bacteria (most common), viruses, parasites, or fungi can cause osteomyelitis. Invasion by one or more pathogenic microorganisms stimulates the inflammatory response in bone tissue. The inflammation produces an increased vascular leak and edema, often involving the surrounding soft tissues. Once inflammation is established, the vessels in the area become thrombosed and release exudate (pus) into bony tissue. Ischemia of bone tissue follows and results in necrotic bone. This area of necrotic bone separates from surrounding bone tissue, and *sequestrum* is formed. The presence of sequestrum prevents bone healing and causes superimposed infection, often in the form of bone abscess that can lead to chronic osteomyelitis (Rogers, 2023). As shown in Fig. 42.2, the cycle repeats

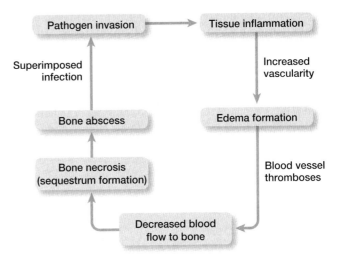

FIG. 42.2 Infection cycle of osteomyelitis.

itself as the new infection leads to further inflammation, vessel thromboses, and necrosis. Because bone is a dynamic tissue and attempts to heal itself, osteoblasts often lay new bone tissue over the infected tissue, making it difficult for drug therapy to penetrate into the infected bone.

Osteomyelitis may be categorized as *exogenous,* in which infectious organisms enter from outside the body as in an open fracture or after surgery, or *endogenous (hematogenous),* in which organisms are carried by the bloodstream from other areas of infection in the body. A third category is *contiguous,* in which bone infection results from skin infection of adjacent tissues. Osteomyelitis can be further divided into two major types: acute and chronic (Rogers, 2023).

Each type of bone infection has its own causative factors. Pathogenic microbes favor bone that has a rich blood supply and a marrow cavity. *Acute hematogenous infection* results from bacteremia, underlying disease, or nonpenetrating trauma. Urinary tract infections, particularly in older men, tend to spread to the lower vertebrae. Long-term IV catheters can be primary sources of infection. Patients undergoing long-term hemodialysis and IV drug users are also at risk for osteomyelitis. *Salmonella* infections of the GI tract may spread to bone. Patients with sickle cell disease and other hemoglobinopathies often have multiple episodes of salmonellosis, which can cause bone infection (Rogers, 2023).

Poor dental hygiene and periodontal (gum) infection can be causative factors in *contiguous* osteomyelitis in facial bones. Minimal nonpenetrating trauma can cause hemorrhages or small-vessel occlusions, leading to bone necrosis. Regardless of the source of infection, many infections are caused by *Staphylococcus aureus.* Treatment of infection may be complicated further by the presence of *methicillin-resistant Staphylococcus aureus* (MRSA) or other multidrug-resistant organisms (MDROs), which are very common in hospitalized and other institutionalized patients as discussed in Chapter 19. The most common causes of MRSA in patients with musculoskeletal health problems are postoperative surgical site infections (SSIs) and infections from surgically implanted devices, such as an open reduction, internal fixation device.

The most common cause of contiguous spread in older adults is found in those who have slow-healing foot ulcers. Multiple organisms tend to be responsible for the resulting osteomyelitis (Rogers, 2023).

Penetrating trauma leads to acute osteomyelitis by direct inoculation. A soft tissue *infection* may be present as well. Animal bites, puncture wounds, skin ulcerations, and bone surgery can result in osteomyelitis. The most common offending organism is *Pseudomonas aeruginosa*, but other gram-negative bacteria may be found.

If bone *infection* is misdiagnosed or inadequately treated, *chronic osteomyelitis* may develop, especially in older adults who have foot ulcers. Inadequate care management results when the treatment period is too short or when the treatment is delayed or inappropriate. About half of cases of chronic osteomyelitis are caused by gram-negative bacteria, especially in older adults (Rogers, 2023).

Interprofessional Collaborative Care
Recognize Cues: Assessment
Bone *pain,* with or without other signs and symptoms, is a common concern of patients with osteomyelitis. The pain is often described as a constant, localized, pulsating sensation that worsens with movement. Perform a complete pain assessment as described in Chapter 6.

The patient with acute osteomyelitis has fever, usually with temperature higher than 101°F (38.3°C). Older adults may not have an extreme temperature elevation because of a lower core body temperature and compromised immune system that occur with normal aging. The area around the infected bone swells and is tender when palpated. Erythema (redness)/hyperpigmentation and heat may also be present. Fever, swelling, and erythema/hyperpigmentation are less common in those with chronic osteomyelitis (Box 42.2). When vascular compromise is severe, patients may not experience *pain* because of nerve damage from lack of adequate perfusion.

When vascular insufficiency is suspected, assess circulation in the distal extremities. Ulcerations may be present on the feet or hands, indicating inadequate healing ability as a result of impaired *perfusion.*

The patient with osteomyelitis often has an elevated white blood cell (leukocyte) count, which may be double the normal value. The erythrocyte sedimentation rate (ESR) may be normal early in the course of the disease but may rise as the condition progresses. It may remain elevated for as long as 3 months after drug therapy is discontinued and can be used to monitor the effectiveness of treatment.

If bacteremia (bacteria in the bloodstream that could lead to septic shock) is present, a blood culture identifies the offending organisms to determine which antibiotics should be used in treatment. Both aerobic and anaerobic blood cultures are performed before drug therapy begins. Further diagnostic testing using a variety of radionuclide scans or MRI may be performed to assess the extent of the infection and perfusion in the affected area.

Take Actions: Interventions
If a wound is present, surgical débridement is performed to remove as much of the necrotic and infected tissue as possible. A local antimicrobial is applied into the wound bed. Then the primary health care provider typically prescribes at least 6 weeks of IV antimicrobial therapy based on the wound culture and sensitivity results. This therapy is often followed by oral antimicrobial therapy for 4 to 8 weeks. In the presence of copious wound drainage, follow Contact Precautions to prevent the spread of the offending organism to other patients and health care personnel. Teach patients, visitors, and staff members how to use these precautions. (See Chapter 19 for a discussion of Contact Precautions.)

More than one antimicrobial agent may be needed to combat multiple types of organisms. The nurse gives the drugs at specifically prescribed times so therapeutic serum levels are achieved. Observe for the actions, side effects, and toxicity of these drugs. Teach family members or other caregivers in the home setting how to administer drug therapy if they are continued after hospital discharge or are used only at home. Some patients may need to be admitted to a skilled nursing facility (SNF) for IV drug therapy. For patients with MRSA infection, IV vancomycin, IV daptomycin, or linezolid (IV or oral) may be used. Oral linezolid allows older patients to remain at home or in an assisted-living facility rather than being admitted to an SNF (Burchum & Rosenthal, 2022).

The optimal drug regimen for patients with *chronic* osteomyelitis is not well established. Prolonged therapy for more than 3 months is typically needed to eliminate the *infection.* Patients are usually cared for in the home or skilled care setting with long-term vascular access catheters, such as a peripherally inserted central catheter (PICC). After discontinuation of IV drugs, oral therapy may be needed. Patients and families must understand the complications of inadequate treatment or failure to follow up with their primary health care provider.

Drugs are also needed to manage *pain.* Patients often experience acute and persistent (chronic) pain and must receive a regimen of drug therapy for control. Chapter 6 describes pharmacologic and nonpharmacologic interventions for both acute and persistent (chronic) pain.

A treatment to increase tissue perfusion for patients with chronic, unremitting osteomyelitis is the use of a hyperbaric chamber or portable device to administer hyperbaric oxygen (HBO) therapy. These devices are usually available in large tertiary care centers and may not be accessible to all patients who might benefit from them. With HBO therapy, the affected area

---

BOX 42.2 Key Features
Acute Versus Chronic Osteomyelitis

Acute Osteomyelitis
- Fever; temperature usually above 101°F (38.3°C)
- Swelling around the affected area
- Possible erythema/hyperpigmentation and heat in the affected area
- Tenderness of the affected area
- Bone pain that is constant, localized, and pulsating; worsens with movement

Chronic Osteomyelitis
- Foot ulcer(s) or bone surgery (most commonly)
- Sinus tract formation
- Localized *pain*
- Drainage from the affected area (usually due to bone abscess)

is exposed daily to a high concentration of oxygen that diffuses into the tissues to promote healing. In conjunction with high-dose drug therapy and surgical débridement, HBO has proven very useful in treating a number of anaerobic infections. Other wound-management therapies are described in Chapter 21.

BONE TUMORS

Pathophysiology Review

Bone tumors may be classified as benign (noncancerous) or malignant (cancerous). *Benign* bone tumors are often asymptomatic and may be discovered on routine x-ray examination or as the cause of pathologic fractures. The cause of benign bone tumors is not known. Tumors may arise from several types of tissue. The most common benign bone tumor is the *osteochondroma*. Although its onset is usually in childhood, the tumor grows until skeletal maturity and may not be diagnosed until adulthood. The tumor may be a single growth or multiple growths and can occur in any bone. The femur and the tibia are most often involved (Rogers, 2023).

Malignant (cancerous) bone tumors may be primary (those that begin in bone) or secondary (those that originate in other tissues and metastasize [spread] to bone). *Primary tumors* occur most often in people between 10 and 30 years of age and make up a small percentage of bone cancers. As with other forms of cancer, the exact cause of bone cancer is unknown, but genetic and environmental factors are likely causes. *Metastatic lesions* most often occur in the older age-group and account for most bone cancers in adults (Rogers, 2023).

Osteosarcoma, or osteogenic sarcoma, is the most common type of *primary* malignant bone tumor. More than 50% of cases occur in the distal femur, followed in decreasing order of occurrence by the proximal tibia and humerus. The tumor is relatively large, causing acute *pain* and swelling. The involved area is usually warm because the blood flow to the site increases. The center of the tumor is sclerotic from increased osteoblastic activity. The periphery is soft, extending through the bone cortex in the classic sunburst appearance associated with the neoplasm (which is visible on x-ray). Osteosarcoma typically metastasizes (spreads), which results in death.

Although *Ewing sarcoma* is not as common as other tumors, it is the most malignant (Rogers, 2023). Like other primary tumors, it causes *pain* and swelling. In addition, systemic signs and symptoms, particularly low-grade fever, leukocytosis, and anemia, are common. The pelvis and the lower extremity are most often affected. Pelvic involvement is a poor prognostic sign. It often extends into soft tissue. Death results from metastasis to the lungs and other bones. Although the tumor can be seen in patients of any age, it usually occurs in children and young adults in their 20s.

Primary tumors of the prostate, breast, kidney, thyroid, and lung are called *bone-seeking* cancers because they spread to the bone more often than other primary tumors. The vertebrae, pelvis, femur, and ribs are the bone sites commonly affected. Simply stated, primary tumor cells, or seeds, are carried to bone through the bloodstream. *Fragility fractures caused by metastatic bone are a major concern in patient care management.*

Interprofessional Collaborative Care

Recognize Cues: Assessment

Assess for *pain*, the most common symptom of most bone tumors. Pain can range from mild to severe. It can be caused by direct tumor invasion into soft tissue, compressed peripheral nerves, or a resulting pathologic or fragility fracture. Severe, unrelenting pain is the primary concern for patients who have metastatic bone disease, particularly when the patient moves. Perform a complete pain assessment of the patient as a baseline to plan care as described in Chapter 6.

When the tumor affects the lower extremities or the small bones of the hands and feet, local swelling may be detected as the tumor enlarges. In some cases, muscle atrophy or muscle spasm may be present. Marked disability and impaired *mobility* may occur in those with advanced metastatic bone disease.

Patients with malignant bone tumors may be young adults whose productive lives are just beginning. They need strong support systems to help cope with the diagnosis and its treatment. Family, significant others, and health care professionals are major components of the needed support. Determine which systems or resources are available.

Patients often experience a loss of control over their lives when a diagnosis of cancer is made. As a result, they become anxious and fearful about the outcome of their illness. Coping with the diagnosis becomes a challenge. As patients progress through the grieving process, there may be initial denial. Identify the anxiety level and assess the stage or stages of the grieving process. Explore any maladaptive behavior, indicating ineffective coping mechanisms. Chapter 18 further describes the psychosocial assessment of patients with cancer.

Routine x-rays are used to find bone tumors and bone metastasis. CT and MRI are useful for complex anatomic areas, such as the spinal column and sacrum. These tests are particularly helpful in evaluating the extent of soft tissue involvement. Metastatic lesions may increase or decrease bone density, depending on the amount of osteoblastic and osteoclastic activity.

In some cases a needle bone biopsy may be performed, usually under fluoroscopy to guide the surgeon. Needle biopsy is an ambulatory care procedure with rare complications. After biopsy, the cancer is staged for size and degree of spread. One popular method is the TNM system, based on tumor size and number (T), the presence of cancer cells in lymph nodes (N), and metastasis (spread) to distant sites (M) (see Chapter 18 for further discussion).

The patient with a *malignant* bone tumor typically shows elevated serum alkaline phosphatase (ALP) levels, indicating the body's attempt to form new bone by increasing osteoblastic activity. The patient with Ewing sarcoma or metastatic bone cancer often has anemia and leukocytosis (increased white blood cells). The progression of Ewing sarcoma may be evaluated by elevated serum lactate dehydrogenase (LDH) levels.

In some patients with bone metastasis from the breast, kidney, or lung, the serum calcium level is elevated. Massive bone destruction stimulates release of the mineral into the bloodstream. In patients with Ewing sarcoma and bone metastasis, the erythrocyte sedimentation rate (ESR) may be elevated because of secondary tissue inflammation (Pagana et al., 2022).

Take Actions: Interventions

Because *pain* is often due to direct primary tumor invasion, treatment is aimed at reducing the size of or removing the tumor. *Benign* or small primary malignant bone tumors are usually completely removed for a potential cure. The expected outcome of treating *metastatic* bone tumors is palliative rather than curative. Palliative therapies may prevent further bone destruction and improve patient function. A combination of nonsurgical and surgical management is used for bone cancer. Collaborate with members of the interprofessional health care team to plan high-quality care to achieve positive patient outcomes. The following discussion focuses on interventions for patients with malignant bone tumors or metastatic bone cancer.

Nonsurgical Management. In addition to analgesics for local *pain* relief, chemotherapy and radiation therapy are often given to shrink the malignant tumor. For patients with painful metastatic spinal involvement, bracing and short-term immobilization may be appropriate.

The primary health care provider may prescribe *chemotherapy* to be given alone or in combination with radiation or surgery. Certain proliferating tumors, such as Ewing sarcoma, are sensitive to cytotoxic drugs. Others, such as chondrosarcomas, are often totally drug resistant. Chemotherapy seems to work best for small primary or metastatic tumors, and may be administered before or after surgery. In most cases the primary health care provider prescribes a combination of agents. The drugs selected are determined in part by the primary source of the cancer in metastatic disease. For example, when metastasis occurs from breast cancer, estrogen and progesterone blockers may be used. Chapter 18 describes the general nursing care of patients who receive chemotherapy. *Remember that all chemotherapeutic agents are categorized as high-alert medications* (Institute for Safe Medication Practices, 2022).

Other drugs are given for specific metastatic cancers, depending on the location of the primary site. For example, biologic agents, such as cytokines, are given to stimulate the immune system to recognize and destroy cancer cells, especially in patients with renal cancer. Zoledronic acid and pamidronate are two IV bisphosphonates that are approved for bone metastasis from the breast, lung, and prostate (Burchum & Rosenthal, 2022). These drugs help protect bones and prevent fractures. Although rare, inform patients that osteonecrosis of the jaw may also occur, especially in those who have invasive dental procedures. Monitor associated laboratory tests, such as serum creatinine and electrolytes, because these drugs can be toxic to the kidneys and cause acute kidney injury (AKI). Bisphosphonates are described earlier in the Osteoporosis section and in Table 42.2.

Denosumab is a RANKL inhibitor that is also approved for metastatic bone disease (Burchum & Rosenthal, 2022). The drug binds to a protein that is essential for the formation, function, and survival of osteoclasts. By preventing the protein from activating its receptor, the drug decreases bone loss and increases bone mass and strength.

Radiation therapy, either brachytherapy or external radiation, is used for selected types of malignant tumors. For patients with Ewing sarcoma and early osteosarcoma, radiation may be the treatment of choice in reducing tumor size and thus pain.

For patients with metastatic disease, radiation is given primarily for palliation. The therapy is directed toward the painful sites to provide a better quality of life. One or more treatments are given, depending on the extent of disease. With precise planning, radiation therapy can be used with minimal complications. The general nursing care for patients receiving radiation therapy is described in Chapter 18.

Interventional radiologists can perform several noninvasive procedures to help relieve *pain* in the patient with metastasis to the spinal column. For example, *microwave ablation (MWA)* can be done under moderate sedation or general anesthesia to kill the targeted tissue with heat by using microwaves. Most patients have pain relief or control after this ambulatory care procedure.

Surgical Management. Primary malignant bone tumors are usually reduced or removed with surgery, and surgery may be combined with radiation or chemotherapy. In addition to the nature, progression, and extent of the tumor, the patient's age and general health state are considered. As for any patient preparing for cancer surgery, the patient with bone cancer needs psychological support from the nurse and other members of the health care team.

Wide or radical resection procedures are used for patients with bone sarcomas to salvage the affected limb. Wide excision is removal of the lesion surrounded by an intact cuff of normal tissue and leads to cure of low-grade tumors only. A radical resection includes removal of the lesion, the entire muscle, bone, and other tissues directly involved. It is the procedure used for high-grade tumors.

In some cases, an allograft may be implanted with internal fixation for patients who do not have metastases. This is a common procedure for sarcomas of the proximal femur. Allograft procedures for the knee are also performed, particularly in young adults. Preoperative chemotherapy is given to enhance the likelihood of success. Allografts with adjacent tendons and ligaments are harvested from cadavers and can be frozen or freeze-dried for a prolonged period. The graft is fixed with a series of bolts, screws, or plates.

The surgical incision for a limb salvage procedure is often extensive. A pressure dressing with wound suction is typically maintained for several days. The patient who has undergone a limb salvage procedure has some degree of impaired physical *mobility* and a self-care deficit. The nature and extent of the alterations depend on the location and extent of the surgery.

After upper extremity surgery, the patient can engage in active-assistive exercises by using the opposite hand to help achieve motions such as forward flexion and abduction of the shoulder. Continuous passive motion (CPM) using a CPM machine may be initiated as early as the first postoperative day for either upper extremity or lower extremity procedures.

After lower extremity surgery, the emphasis is on strengthening the quadriceps muscles by using passive and active motion when possible. Maintaining muscle tone is an important prerequisite to weight bearing, which progresses from toe touch or partial weight bearing to full weight bearing by 2 to 3 months after surgery. Coordinate the patient's plan of care for ambulation and muscle strengthening with the physical therapist.

The patient who has had a bone graft may have a cast or other supportive device for several months. Weight bearing is prohibited until there is evidence that the graft is incorporated into the adjacent bone tissue.

During the recovery phase, the patient may also need assistance with ADLs, particularly if the surgery involves the upper extremity. Assist if needed, but at the same time encourage the patient to do as much as possible unaided. Some patients need assistive-adaptive devices for a short period while they are healing. Coordinate the patient's plan of care for promoting independence in ADLs with the occupational therapist.

Care Coordination and Transition Management

After medical treatment for any type of primary bone tumor, the patient is usually managed at home with follow-up care. When home support is not available, the patient may be admitted to a long-term care facility for extended or hospice care. Coordinate the patient's transition and continuity of care with the case manager and other interprofessional health team members, depending on the patient's needs.

In collaboration with the occupational therapist, evaluate the patient's home environment for structural barriers that may hinder *mobility*. The patient may be discharged with a cast, a walker, crutches, or a wheelchair. Assess support system for availability of assistance if needed.

Accessibility to eating and toileting facilities is essential to promote ADL independence. Because the patient with metastatic disease is susceptible to pathologic fractures, potential hazards that may contribute to falls or injury should be removed.

For the patient receiving intermittent chemotherapy or radiation on an ambulatory care basis, emphasize the importance of keeping appointments. Review the expected side and toxic effects of the drugs with the patient and family. Teach how to treat less serious side effects and when to contact the primary health care provider. If the drugs are administered at home via long-term IV catheter, explain and demonstrate the care involved with daily dressing changes and potential catheter complications. Chapter 15 describes the health teaching required for a patient receiving infusion therapy at home.

If patients have undergone surgery, they have a wound and the potential for impaired *mobility*. Teach the patient, family, and/or significant others how to care for the wound. Help the patient learn how to perform ADLs and mobility activities independently for self-management. Coordinate with the occupational therapist to assist in ADL teaching and provide or recommend assistive and adaptive devices, if necessary. The physical therapist can teach the proper use of any needed ambulatory aids, such as a walker or cane, and routine exercises.

Pain management can be a major challenge, particularly for the patient with metastatic bone disease. Discuss the various options for persistent pain relief, including relaxation and music therapy. Emphasize the importance of techniques that worked during hospitalization. See Chapter 6 for cancer pain assessment and management.

The patient with bone cancer may fear that the malignancy will return. Acknowledge this fear but reinforce confidence in the health care team and medical treatment chosen. Mutually establish realistic outcomes regarding returning to work and participating in recreational activities. Encourage the patient to resume a functional lifestyle, but caution that it should be gradual. Certain activities, such as participating in sports, may be prohibited.

Help the patient with advanced metastatic bone disease prepare for death. Palliative and hospice care at home is often needed for these patients. The nurse and other support personnel assist the patient through the stages of death and dying. Identify resources that can help the patient write a will, visit with distant family members, or do whatever is needed for a peaceful death.

PATIENT-CENTERED CARE: CULTURE AND SPIRITUALITY

Medical Aid in Dying

Patients who have metastatic bone cancer are usually older adults who have severe, unrelenting *pain.* Some patients may request medical aid in dying to prevent further pain and suffering and to experience a more peaceful or "good" death. Although nurses cannot directly assist a patient in dying, they can provide health teaching, support, and palliative care. Ten states, the District of Columbia, and nine countries currently have legalized medical aid in dying. Some nurses and other health care professionals may not agree with a patient's request to hasten death using a barbiturate. However, they are obligated to provide information to patients and families to help them make informed patient-centered decisions (Roy, 2022). Chapter 8 describes end-of-life care in detail.

In addition to family and significant others, cancer support groups are helpful to the patient with bone cancer. Some organizations, such as *I Can Cope,* provide information and emotional support. Others, such as *CanSurmount,* are geared more toward patient and family education. The American Cancer Society (www.cancer.org) and the Canadian Cancer Society (www.cancer.ca) can also provide education and resources for patients and families.

COMMON DISORDERS OF THE HAND

Specific localized health problems affecting the hand or part of the hand may affect the musculoskeletal system. Two of these problems are discussed here. Dupuytren contracture or deformity is a slowly progressive thickening of the palmar fascia, resulting in flexion contracture of the fourth (ring) and fifth (little) fingers of the hand (Fig. 42.3). The third or middle finger is occasionally affected. Although Dupuytren contracture is a common problem,

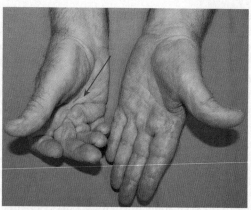

FIG. 42.3 Dupuytren disease with coalescence of scar tissue affecting multiple adjacent digits resulting in flexion contractures at the MCP and PIP joints. (From Chung, KC. [2022]. *Operative techniques in hand and wrist surgery* [4th ed.]. St. Louis: Elsevier.)

the cause is unknown. It usually occurs in older White men, tends to occur in families, is most common in people with diabetes, and can be bilateral (Rogers, 2023). Symptoms include:

- Inability to grasp objects
- Inability to lay hand flat on table
- Development of hard "cords" (buildup of collagen)

When hand function becomes impaired, treatment is needed. A noninvasive treatment was recently approved that does not require surgery for repair. The patient receives an injection of clostridial collagenase (Xiaflex) into the cord, which breaks down the diseased collagen. The next day the patient's affected finger is straightened under local anesthesia. This typically successful treatment does not require follow-up occupational therapy and is not painful.

In some cases surgery is performed. A partial or selective fasciectomy (cutting of fascia) is performed to release the contracture. After removal of the surgical dressing, a splint may be used and occupational therapy is ordered for at least 6 weeks. Nursing care is similar to that for the patient with carpal tunnel repair (see Chapter 44).

A **ganglion** is a round, benign cyst, often found on a wrist or foot joint or tendon. The synovium surrounding the tendon degenerates, allowing the tendon sheath tissue to become weak and distended. Ganglia are painless on palpation, but they can cause joint discomfort after prolonged joint use or minor trauma or strain. The lesion can rapidly disappear and then recur. Ganglia are most likely to develop in people between 15 and 50 years of age. With local or regional anesthesia in a primary health care provider's office or clinic, the fluid within the cyst can be aspirated through a small needle. A cortisone injection may follow. If the cyst is very large, it is removed using a small incision. Teach patients to avoid strenuous activity for 48 hours after surgery and report any signs of inflammation to their primary health care provider.

COMMON DISORDERS OF THE FOOT

The **hallux valgus deformity** is a common foot problem in which the great toe drifts laterally at the first metatarsophalangeal

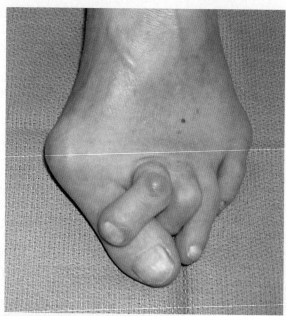

FIG. 42.4 Crossover toe deformity in a patient with hallux valgus. (From Miller M. D., et al. [2020]. *Essential orthopaedics* [2nd ed.]. St. Louis: Elsevier.)

(MTP) joint (Fig. 42.4). The first metatarsal head becomes enlarged, resulting in a *bunion*. As the deviation worsens, the bony enlargement causes pain, particularly when shoes are worn. Women are affected more often than men. Hallux valgus often occurs as a result of poorly fitted shoes, in particular those with narrow toes and high heels. Other causes include osteoarthritis, rheumatoid arthritis, foot and ankle surgery, and family history.

For some patients who are of advanced age or are not surgical candidates, custom-made shoes can be made to fit the deformed feet and provide comfort and support. A plaster mold is made to conform to each foot; shoes can be made from these molds. Teach the patient to consult with a podiatrist or foot clinic to be evaluated for custom shoes.

Surgery is the treatment of choice for hallux valgus correction. The traditional surgical procedure, a simple **bunionectomy**, involves removal of the bony overgrowth and bursa and realignment to manage *pain*. When other toe deformities accompany the condition or if the bony overgrowth is large, several *osteotomies*, or bone resections, may be performed. Fusions may also be performed. Screws or wires are often inserted to stabilize the bones in the great toe and first metatarsal during the healing process. If both feet are affected, one foot is usually treated at a time. Surgery usually is performed as a same-day procedure. *Be sure to assess neurovascular status and pain control before allowing the patient to be discharged.* Teach the patient to avoid full weight bearing until cleared by the surgeon and to wear an orthopedic boot at all times while awake. The healing time after surgery may be 12 weeks or longer because the feet receive less blood flow than other parts of the body as a result of their distance from the heart. Some patients experience a return of the deformity in later years.

The newer minimally invasive surgical procedure, or lapiplasty, involves several small incisions; this procedure usually improves stabilization and prevents return of the deformity. The patient wears an orthopedic boot or shoe for about 2 to 6 weeks and is able to bear weight 2 or 3 days after surgery.

NCLEX Examination Challenge 42.3

Physiological Integrity

The nurse is assessing a middle-aged client immediately after a traditional (open) right bunionectomy. Which client finding would the nurse report to the surgeon?

A. Right pedal pulse 2+
B. Swelling in right great toe
C. 5/10 pain in right great toe
D. Right toe capillary refill more than 5 seconds

Plantar fasciitis is an inflammation of the plantar fascia, which is located in the area of the arch of the foot. It is often seen in middle-age and older adults, as well as in athletes, especially runners. Obesity is also a contributing factor. Patients report severe *pain* in the arch of the foot, especially when getting out of bed. The pain is worsened with weight bearing. Although most patients have unilateral plantar fasciitis, the problem can affect both feet (Rogers, 2023).

Most patients respond to conservative management, which includes rest, ice, stretching exercises, strapping of the foot to maintain the arch, shoes with good support, and orthotics. NSAIDs or steroids may be needed to control *pain* and inflammation. If conservative measures are unsuccessful, endoscopic surgery to remove the inflamed tissue may be required. Teach the patient about the importance of adhering to the treatment plan and to follow the physical therapist's instruction regarding exercise.

GET READY FOR THE NEXT-GENERATION NCLEX® EXAMINATION!

Essential Nursing Care Points

Health Promotion/Disease Prevention

- The *Healthy People 2030* initiative recognizes the need for national attention to the prevention of osteoporosis and fragility fractures.
- Osteoporosis prevention begins with education for young women who need to be aware of appropriate health and lifestyle practices that can prevent this potentially disabling disease, such as smoking cessation (if needed), regular exercise, and increased calcium and vitamin D intake.
- Nurses need to teach postmenopausal women and men over 50 years of age to have bone mineral density (BMD) screening by dual x-ray absorptiometry (DXA) to detect osteopenia (bone loss) or osteoporosis (severe loss of bone mass).

Chronic Disease Care

- Osteoporosis is a chronic disease of *cellular regulation* in which bone loss causes significant decreased density and possible fracture.
- The patient who has osteoporosis is predisposed to fractures, so nutrition therapy, lifestyle changes, and drug therapy are used to slow bone resorption and form new bone tissue.
- The primary health care provider may prescribe bisphosphonates, estrogen agonist/antagonists (formerly called *selective estrogen receptor modulators* [SERMs]), parathyroid hormone (PTH), RANKL inhibitor, sclerostin inhibitor, or a combination of several drugs to treat or prevent osteoporosis (see Table 42.2).
- Osteomyelitis (bone infection) can result in chronic recurrence, loss of function, persistent (chronic) *pain,* amputation, or even death due to sepsis.
- Patients who have *chronic* osteomyelitis usually require more than 3 months of IV and/or oral antimicrobial therapy at home or in a health care facility; nurses need to teach family or other caregivers how to administer the drug through a peripherally inserted central catheter (PICC line).

Regenerative or Restorative Care

- The patient with acute osteomyelitis has fever, usually with temperature higher than 101°F (38.3°C).
- The primary health care provider typically prescribes at least 6 weeks of IV antimicrobial therapy based on the wound culture and sensitivity results; this therapy is usually followed by oral antimicrobial therapy for 4 to 8 weeks.
- Primary bone tumors are typically treated with a combination of chemotherapy, radiation therapy, and surgery to remove the tumor, if possible.
- A noninvasive treatment for Dupuytren contracture is an injection of clostridial collagenase (Xiaflex) into the "cord," which breaks down the diseased collagen; this treatment does not require follow-up occupational therapy and is not painful.
- The nurse provides health teaching for patients having minimally invasive surgery to correct a hallux valgus deformity to include weight-bearing and activity restrictions.

Hospice/Palliative/Supportive Care

- Palliative and hospice care at home is often needed for patients who have metastatic bone cancer.
- Some patients with metastatic bone cancer may request medical aid in dying to prevent further pain and suffering and to experience a more peaceful or "good" death rather than severe pain and suffering.
- Although nurses cannot directly assist a patient in dying, they can provide health teaching, support, and palliative care.

Mastery Questions

1. The nurse is planning teaching for an older client who is at risk for osteoporosis. Which of the following **modifiable** client risk factors would the nurse consider as part of the teaching plan? **Select all that apply.**
   A. Older age
   B. Corticosteroids for lung disease
   C. Lack of regular exercise
   D. Parental history of osteoporosis
   E. Postmenopause
   F. Food insecurity

2. The nurse is planning care for a client who had an osteosarcoma surgically removed from the left lower leg. What is the nurse's **priority** for immediate postoperative care?
   A. Monitor for symptoms of wound infection.
   B. Assess for symptoms of venous thromboembolism.
   C. Evaluate neurovascular status in the left foot.
   D. Observe for surgical site bleeding.

NGN Challenge 42.1

42.1.1

The nurse is caring for a 55-year-old client transferred from the urgent care center to the acute medical unit.

Highlight the findings that would require **immediate** follow-up.

History and Physical	Nurses' Notes	Vital Signs	Laboratory Results

1100: Admitted to unit for diabetic ulcer on the right ankle that had been healing. Client followed by primary health care provider for type 1 diabetes mellitus that has been uncontrolled for several years. Provider's office closed on weekend and client concerned that drainage from wound was becoming more copious and foul smelling. H/O hypertension and hypercholesterolemia, but both controlled by drug therapy. Works remotely at a computer every day. States it is difficult to exercise on a regular basis or eat healthy. FSBG: 216 mg/dL (12 mmol/L); height: 68 in (173 cm); weight: 169 lb (76.7 kg). VS: T 100.6°F (38.2°C); HR 88 beats/min; RR 22 breaths/min; BP 122/74 mm Hg; SpO$_2$ 96% on RA. IV line started in left forearm with 0.9% NS at 100 mL/hr.

42.1.2

The nurse is caring for a 55-year-old client transferred from the urgent care center to the acute medical unit.

History and Physical	Nurses' Notes	Vital Signs	Laboratory Results

1100: Admitted to unit for diabetic ulcer on the right ankle that had been healing. Client followed by primary health care provider for type 1 diabetes mellitus that has been uncontrolled for several years. Provider's office closed on weekend and client concerned that drainage from wound was becoming more copious and foul smelling. H/O hypertension and hypercholesterolemia, but both controlled by drug therapy. Works remotely at a computer every day. States it is difficult to exercise on a regular basis or eat healthy. FSBG: 216 mg/dL (12 mmol/L); height: 68 in (173 cm); weight: 169 lb (76.7 kg). VS: T 100.6°F (38.2°C); HR 88 beats/min; RR 22 breaths/min; BP 122/74 mm Hg; SpO$_2$ 96% on RA. IV line started in left forearm with 0.9% NS at 100 mL/hr.

1220: Returned from Radiology for right ankle x-ray. Wound culture and sensitivity sent to lab. Blood drawn for culture, BMP, and CBC. Full-thickness right ankle ulcer 3 cm × 2.25 cm; draining large amount of yellowish, foul drainage. Gauze dressing applied. States right ankle pain is 6/10, especially when ambulating to BR.

Complete the following sentence by selecting from the lists of options below.

The client is at high risk for **[1] [Select]** as evidenced by **[2] [Select]** and **[3] [Select]**.

Options for 1	Options for 2	Options for 3
Osteoporosis	Tachypnea	Draining full-thickness wound
Diabetic ketoacidosis	Tachycardia	Hyperglycemia
Osteomyelitis	Fever	Uncontrolled diabetes mellitus
Septic shock	High blood pressure	Obesity

42.1.3

The nurse is caring for a 55-year-old client transferred from the urgent care center to the acute medical unit.

History and Physical	**Nurses' Notes**	Vital Signs	Laboratory Results

1100: Admitted to unit for diabetic ulcer on the right ankle that had been healing. Client followed by primary health care provider for type 1 diabetes mellitus that has been uncontrolled for several years. Provider's office closed on weekend and client concerned that drainage from wound was becoming more copious and foul smelling. H/O hypertension and hypercholesterolemia, but both controlled by drug therapy. Works remotely at a computer every day. States it is difficult to exercise on a regular basis or eat healthy. FSBG: 216 mg/dL (12 mmol/L); height: 68 in (173 cm); weight: 169 lb (76.7 kg). VS: T 100.6°F (38.2°C); HR 88 beats/min; RR 22 breaths/min; BP 122/74 mm Hg; Spo$_2$ 96% on RA. IV line started in left forearm with 0.9% NS at 100 mL/hr.

1220: Returned from Radiology for right ankle x-ray. Wound culture and sensitivity sent to lab. Blood drawn for culture, BMP, and CBC. Full-thickness right ankle ulcer 3 cm × 2.25 cm; draining large amount of yellowish, foul drainage. Gauze dressing applied. States right ankle pain is 6/10, especially when ambulating to BR.

Complete the following sentence by selecting from the list of word choices below.

The *priority* for the client at this time is to manage **[Word Choice]** to prevent **[Word Choice]**.

Word Choices
Sepsis
Blood glucose
Wound infection
Diabetic ketoacidosis
Right foot gangrene

42.1.4

The nurse is caring for a 55-year-old client transferred from the urgent care center to the acute medical unit.

History and Physical	**Nurses' Notes**	Vital Signs	Laboratory Results

1100: Admitted to unit for diabetic ulcer on the right ankle that had been healing. Client followed by primary health care provider for type 1 diabetes mellitus that has been uncontrolled for several years. Provider's office closed on weekend and client concerned that drainage from wound was becoming more copious and foul smelling. H/O hypertension and hypercholesterolemia, but both controlled by drug therapy. Works remotely at a computer every day. States it is difficult to exercise on a regular basis or eat healthy. FSBG: 216 mg/dL (12 mmol/L); height: 68 in (173 cm); weight: 169 lb (76.7 kg). VS: T 100.6°F (38.2°C); HR 88 beats/min; RR 22 breaths/min; BP 122/74 mm Hg; Spo$_2$ 96% on RA. IV line started in left forearm with 0.9% NS at 100 mL/hr.

1220: Returned from Radiology for right ankle x-ray. Wound culture and sensitivity sent to lab. Blood drawn for culture, BMP, and CBC. Full-thickness right ankle ulcer 3 cm × 2.25 cm; draining large amount of yellowish, foul drainage. Gauze dressing applied. States right ankle pain is 6/10, especially when ambulating to BR.

Based on the client's findings, select 4 nursing interventions that would be appropriate to meet the client's priority need.

- ○ Administer sliding scale insulin per protocol.
- ○ Begin IV broad-spectrum antibiotic therapy.
- ○ Initiate supplemental oxygen via nasal cannula.
- ○ Prepare the client for possible surgical wound débridement.
- ○ Apply an orthopedic boot to the right leg.
- ○ Elevate the client's right leg at all times.
- ○ Monitor FSBG 4 times a day before meals.

42.1.5

The nurse is caring for a 55-year-old client admitted yesterday with uncontrolled type 1 diabetes mellitus and infected right ankle diabetic ulcer. The client had a surgical wound débridement and has been diagnosed with right ankle acute osteomyelitis. Preliminary wound culture results indicate methicillin-resistant *Staphylococcus aureus* (MRSA) infection.

Which of the following nursing interventions would the nurse undertake at this time? **Select all that apply.**

- ○ Place client on contact precautions.
- ○ Draw daily fasting blood glucose (FBS).
- ○ Begin continuous IV insulin drip.
- ○ Change IV antibiotic to vancomycin.
- ○ Administer acetaminophen every 4 hours.
- ○ Perform neurovascular assessment every 4 hours.

42.1.6

A 55-year-old client who was hospitalized for an infected right ankle diabetic ulcer was discharged 4 weeks ago to continue IV vancomycin at home via a peripherally inserted central catheter (PICC) line. The home health nurse visits the home to evaluate the client's progress and compares assessment data from the client's previous hospitalization with current assessment findings.

For each client finding, indicate if the client has improved or not improved.

Previous Client Finding	Current Client Finding	Improved	Not Improved
Right ankle ulcer 3 cm × 2.25 cm; draining large amount of yellowish, foul drainage	Right ankle ulcer 2.8 cm × 2 cm; minimal tannish drainage without odor		
Temperature on admission: 100.6°F (38.2°C)	Current temperature: 98°F (36.7°C)		
FSBG: 216 mg/dL (12 mmol/L)	FSBG: 110 mg/dL (6.1 mmol/L)		
PICC line in place for antibiotic therapy	No redness at insertion site		
No report of feeling depressed	States feeling depressed		

REFERENCES

Burchum, J. L. R., & Rosenthal, L. D. (2022). *Lehne's pharmacology for nursing care* (11th ed.). St. Louis: Elsevier.

Cochran, T., Iyer, T. K., & Batur, P. (2022). Osteoporosis management. *Journal of Women's Health, 31*(2), 154–157.

Crandall, C. J., Hunt, R. P., LaCroix, A. Z., Robbins, J. A., Wactawski-Wende, J., Johnson, K. C., et al. (2021). *After the initial fracture in postmenopausal women, were do subsequent fractures occur?*. https://doi.org/10.1016/j.eclinm.2021.100826.eCollection2021May.

Elliott, B., Chargualaf, K. A., & Patterson, B. (2021). *Veteran-centered care in education and practice*. New York City, NY: Springer Publishing.

Healthy People 2030. (2023). Osteoporosis. https://health.gov/healthy-people/objectives-and-data/browse-objectives/osteoporosis.

Institute for Safe Medication Practices. (2022). *ISMPs list of high-alert medications*. www.ismp.org/Tools/highalertmedications.pdf.

Jarvis, C., & Eckhardt, A. (2024). *Physical examination & health assessment* (8th ed.). St. Louis: Elsevier.

Noel, S. E., Santos, M. P., & Wright, N. C. (2021). Racial and ethnic disparities in bone health and outcomes in the United States. *Journal of Bone and Mineral Research*. https://doi.org/10.1012/jbmr.4417.

Pagana, K. D., Pagana, T. J., & Pagana, T. N. (2022). *Mosby's manual of diagnostic and laboratory tests* (7th ed.). St. Louis: Elsevier.

Pagana, K. D., Pagana, T. J., & Pike-MacDonald, S. A. (2019). *Mosby's Canadian manual of diagnostic and laboratory tests* (2nd ed.). Toronto, ON: Elsevier.

Rogers, J. L. (2023). *McCance and Huether's Pathophysiology: The biologic basis for disease in adults and children* (9th ed.). St. Louis: Elsevier.

Roy, K. (2022). Medical aid in dying: What every nurse needs to know. *American Journal of Nursing, 122*(3), 30–37.

Touhy, T. A., & Jett, K. F. (2022). *Ebersole and Hess' gerontological nursing and healthy aging* (6th ed.). St. Louis: Elsevier.

Xiaojuan, L., & Schwartz, A. V. (2020). MRI assessment of bone marrow composition in osteoporosis. *Current Osteoporosis Reports, 18*, 57–66.

43

Concepts of Care for Patients With Arthritis and Total Joint Arthroplasty

Donna D. Ignatavicius

http://evolve.elsevier.com/Iggy/

LEARNING OUTCOMES

1. Plan collaborative care with the interprofessional team to promote *mobility* in patients with arthritis.
2. Teach adults how to decrease the risk for osteoarthritis.
3. Teach the patient and caregiver(s) about common drugs affecting *immunity* and other management strategies used for rheumatoid arthritis.
4. Plan patient- and family-centered nursing interventions to decrease the psychosocial impact caused by living with arthritis.
5. Apply knowledge of anatomy, physiology, and pathophysiology to provide evidence-based care for patients with arthritis.
6. Analyze assessment and diagnostic findings to generate solutions and prioritize nursing care for patients who have arthritis.
7. Organize care coordination and transition management for patients having total joint arthroplasty.
8. Use clinical judgment to plan evidence-based nursing care to decrease *pain* and *inflammation* in patients with arthritis.
9. Incorporate factors that affect health equity into the plan of care for patients with arthritis.

KEY TERMS

arthritis Inflammation of one or more joints.

arthrocentesis An invasive diagnostic procedure performed at the bedside or in a primary health care provider's office to aspirate a sample of synovial fluid for analysis and to relieve pressure caused by excess fluid.

crepitus A grating sound caused by loosened bone and cartilage in a synovial joint.

exacerbations Flare-ups of disease (that typically alternate with disease remissions).

gout The body's inflammatory response to large amounts of uric acid (a result of purine metabolism) in the blood (hyperuricemia) and other body fluids.

joint coach A family care partner who can help the patient having a total joint arthroplasty through the perioperative period and assist with discharge needs.

joint effusion The presence of excess joint fluid, especially common in the knee.

mobility technician A specially trained nursing assistant whose primary responsibility is to ambulate hospitalized patients.

orthopedic patient navigator A nurse who coordinates care as the single point of contact for a patient who has orthopedic surgery.

osteoarthritis The progressive deterioration and loss of articular (joint) cartilage and bone in one or more joints.

osteonecrosis Bone death secondary to lack of or disruption in blood supply to the affected bone, usually from trauma or chronic steroid therapy.

osteophytes Bone spurs caused by irregular bony overgrowth.

paresthesias Burning and tingling sensations, especially in the extremities.

peripheral nerve block (PNB) A single injection or continuous infusion by a portable pump (e.g., continuous femoral nerve blockade, or CFNB) to provide regional/local anesthesia during and/or after surgery.

primary arthroplasty First-time joint arthroplasty.

quadriceps-setting exercises ("quad sets") Postoperative exercises designed to decrease the risk of deep vein thrombosis by straightening the legs and pushing the back of the knees into the bed.

regenerative therapies Minimally invasive treatment modalities, such as stem cell therapy and platelet-rich plasma, that are used to repair joint cartilage.

revision arthroplasty An arthroplasty done to replace an implant that has loosened or failed.

rheumatoid arthritis A chronic, progressive, systemic inflammatory autoimmune disease process that affects primarily the synovial joints.

Sjögren syndrome A condition in which the patient has dry eyes (keratoconjunctivitis sicca [KCS], or the sicca syndrome), dry mouth (xerostomia), and dry vagina (in some cases). This health problem may occur as a separate condition or be associated with late-stage rheumatoid arthritis or other autoimmune arthritis-related disease.

subcutaneous nodules Soft, round, movable nodules that often occur along the ulnar side of the arm in patients with advanced rheumatoid arthritis.

KEY TERMS—cont'd

subluxation Partial joint dislocation.

synovitis Inflammation of joint synovium.

total joint arthroplasty (TJA) The surgical creation of a functional (synovial) joint using implants, also sometimes called a *total joint replacement (TJR).*

vasculitis Inflammation of blood vessel walls that can decrease arterial blood flow.

 PRIORITY AND INTERRELATED CONCEPTS

The priority concepts for this chapter are:
- *Mobility*
- *Immunity*

The *Mobility* concept exemplar for this chapter is Osteoarthritis.
The *Immunity* concept exemplar for this chapter is Rheumatoid Arthritis.

The interrelated concepts for this chapter are:
- *Pain*
- *Inflammation*

Arthritis means *inflammation* of one or more joints. However, in clinical practice arthritis is categorized as either noninflammatory or inflammatory. Although there are many types of arthritis and diseases in which arthritis occurs as a symptom, the two most common types, osteoarthritis and rheumatoid arthritis, are the focus of this chapter.

The major exemplar for the concept of *mobility* is osteoarthritis (OA), a noninflammatory, localized disorder. The major exemplar for *immunity* is rheumatoid arthritis (RA), a systemic, autoimmune inflammatory disorder. Both of these health problems can cause joint *pain* and stiffness. These priority concepts are reviewed briefly in Chapter 3. Other autoimmune disorders causing arthritis are discussed elsewhere in this text.

✳ MOBILITY CONCEPT EXEMPLAR: OSTEOARTHRITIS

Osteoarthritis is the most common arthritis and a major cause of impaired *mobility,* persistent *pain,* and disability among adults in the United States and the world.

Pathophysiology Review

Osteoarthritis (OA) is the progressive deterioration and loss of articular (joint) cartilage, bone, and other connective tissues in one or more joints. As people age or experience joint injury, proteoglycans and water can decrease in the joint. The production of synovial fluid, which provides joint lubrication and nutrition, also declines because of the decreased synthesis of hyaluronic acid and less body fluid in older adults compared with younger adults (Rogers, 2023). Although OA occurs more often in the older population, some older adults do not develop the disease.

In patients of any age with OA, enzymes such as stromelysin break down the articular matrix. In early disease the cartilage changes from its normal bluish-white, translucent color to an opaque and yellowish-brown appearance. As cartilage and the bone beneath the cartilage begin to erode, the joint space narrows and osteophytes (bone spurs caused by irregular bony overgrowth) form (Fig. 43.1). As the disease progresses, fissures, calcifications, and ulcerations develop and the cartilage thins. Inflammatory cytokines (enzymes) such as interleukin-1 (IL-1) may enhance this deterioration. The body's normal repair process cannot overcome the rapid process of degeneration (Rogers, 2023). Secondary joint *inflammation* can occur when joint involvement is severe. Joint inflammation, also called synovitis, is evident when the joint is red, warm, painful, and swollen.

Eventually the cartilage disintegrates, and pieces of bone and cartilage "float" in the diseased joint, causing crepitus, a grating sound caused by the loosened bone and cartilage in a synovial joint. The resulting joint *pain* and stiffness can lead to decreased *mobility* and muscle atrophy. Muscle tissue helps support joints, particularly those that bear weight (e.g., hips, knees).

Etiology and Genetic Risk

The cause of OA is a combination of many factors. For patients with *primary* OA, aging and genetic factors are major contributors. Weight-bearing joints (hips and knees), the vertebral column, and the hands are most commonly affected, probably because they are used most often or bear the mechanical stress of body weight and many years of use.

Secondary OA occurs less often than primary disease and can result from joint injury and obesity at younger ages. Injury to the joints from excessive use, trauma, or other joint disease (e.g., rheumatoid arthritis) predisposes a person to OA. Heavy manual occupations (e.g., carpet laying, construction, farming) cause high-intensity or repetitive stress to the joints. The risk for hip and knee OA is increased in professional and amateur athletes, especially football players, runners, and gymnasts. Fractures or other joint tissue injuries can lead to OA years after the trauma. Certain metabolic diseases (e.g., diabetes mellitus, Paget disease of the bone) and blood disorders (e.g., hemophilia, sickle cell disease) can also cause arthritis.

OA occurs in people who are obese much more commonly than in those who are not obese (Arthritis Foundation, 2023). Weight-bearing joints such as hips and knees are most often affected in obese individuals.

Incidence and Prevalence

The prevalence of OA varies among different populations but is a universal problem. Most people older than 60 years have joint changes that can be seen on x-ray examination, although not all of these adults actually develop the disease. According to the

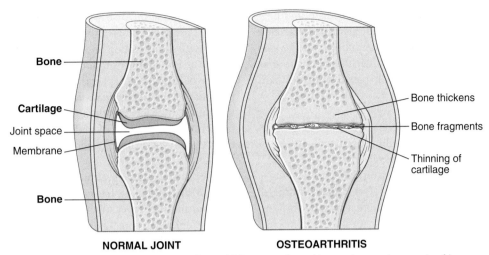

FIG. 43.1 In osteoarthritis *(right)*, the joint bone thickens, cartilage thins, and some fragments of bone may develop. Compare this evidence of disease with a normal joint *(left)*. (From Chabner, D. E. [2023]. *Medical terminology: A short course* [9th ed.]. St. Louis: Elsevier.)

Arthritis Foundation (2023) estimates, over 33 million people in the United States have symptomatic OA, and the disease is the fifth most common cause of disability worldwide.

PATIENT-CENTERED CARE: GENDER HEALTH

Osteoarthritis in Women

More men than women younger than 55 years old have OA caused by athletic or traumatic injuries. After age 55 women have the disease more often than men. Although the cause for this difference is not known, contributing factors may include increased obesity in women after having children and broader hips in women than men (Arthritis Foundation, 2023). Be sure to assess all patients in the hospital or community-based setting, particularly those who are older and obese, for signs and symptoms of OA.

PATIENT-CENTERED CARE: VETERAN HEALTH

Osteoarthritis in the Military and Veteran Population

Almost all OA that occurs among the military population is the result of combat injury. OA occurs twice as often among members of the military who are younger than 40 years of age compared with the general population (Arthritis Foundation, 2023). Osteoarthritis among the military and veteran population is associated with comorbidities related to cardiovascular health, including obesity, diabetes mellitus, and hypertension. While obesity and diseases associated with obesity contribute to OA development, veterans who have mental health issues such as posttraumatic stress disorder, depression, and anxiety are also at higher risk for OA when compared to the general population (Elliott et al., 2021). Possible factors that may explain this relationship include the likelihood that veterans with mental health disorders may not exercise regularly or may gain weight due to lack of energy or motivation. Assess all active military and veteran patients for reports of joint pain, previous traumatic events, and comorbidities, including both physical and mental health disorders, to ensure appropriate management.

BOX 43.1 MEETING *HEALTHY PEOPLE 2030* OBJECTIVES

Osteoarthritis

To better manage osteoarthritis and promote quality of life:
- Reduce the proportion of adults with arthritis causing moderate or severe joint pain.
- Reduce the proportion of adults whose arthritis limits their work.
- Reduce the proportion of adults whose arthritis limits their activities.
- Increase the proportion of adults with arthritis who get counseling for physical activity.

Health Promotion/Disease Prevention

The *Healthy People 2030* (2022) initiative recognizes the need for national attention to help reduce and better manage arthritis (Box 43.1).

Based on these objectives and the risk factors for OA, teach adults to:
- Maintain proper nutrition to prevent obesity, or participate in an evidence-based weight-reduction program if needed.
- Take care to avoid injuries, especially those that can occur from professional or amateur sports.
- Avoid participating in risky behaviors that could cause trauma and subsequent arthritis.
- Take adequate work breaks to rest joints in jobs where repetitive motion or joint stress is common.
- Stay active and maintain a healthy lifestyle, including regular physical activity and exercise, if possible.

Interprofessional Collaborative Care
Recognize Cues: Assessment

History. Patients with OA usually seek medical attention for their joint pain in ambulatory care settings. However, you will also care for those who have OA as a secondary diagnosis in acute and chronic care facilities. Ask the patient about the course of the disease. Collect information specifically related to OA, such as the nature and location of joint pain and how much pain and suffering the patient is experiencing. *Remember that older patients may underreport pain, resulting in inadequate management.* Use a 0-to-10 scale or other assessment tool as appropriate to assess pain intensity. Chapter 6 discusses pain assessment in detail.

Other questions to ask include:

- If joint stiffness has occurred, where and for how long?
- When and where has any joint swelling occurred?
- How much discomfort are you having?
- How much is your *pain* disrupting your daily life?
- What do you do to control the discomfort, *pain,* or stiffness?
- Do you have any loss of *mobility* or difficulty in performing ADLs?

Because this disease occurs more often in older women, age and gender are important factors for the nursing history. Ask patients about their occupation, nature of work, history of injury (including falls), weight history, and current or previous involvement in sports or the military. A history of obesity is significant, even for those currently within the ideal range for body weight. Document any family history of arthritis. Determine whether the patient has a current or previous medical condition that may cause joint symptoms.

Physical Assessment/Signs and Symptoms. In the early stage of the disease the signs and symptoms of OA may appear similar to those of rheumatoid arthritis (RA) (discussed later in this chapter) or other types of arthritis. The distinction between OA and RA becomes more evident as the disease progresses. Table 43.1 compares the major characteristics of both diseases and their common drug therapies. Some patients have both types of arthritis or an additional type, such as gout.

The typical patient with OA is a middle-age or older woman who reports *persistent (chronic) joint **pain** and stiffness.* Early in the course of the disease, these symptoms are reduced after rest or sleep and worsen after extended activity. Later, they may occur with slight motion or even when at rest. Because cartilage has no nerve supply, the *pain* is caused by joint and soft-tissue involvement and spasms of the surrounding muscles, or secondary joint *inflammation*. During the joint examination the patient may have tenderness on palpation or when putting the joint through range of motion. Some patients with hip OA report groin pain that is referred to the thigh, back, knee, or buttock.

Crepitus (a coarse grating sound caused by loosened bone and cartilage) may be felt or heard as the joint goes through range of motion, especially the knee joint. One or more joints may be affected. The patient may also report joint stiffness that usually lasts *less than* 30 minutes after a period of inactivity (Rogers, 2023).

On inspection, knee joints affected by osteoarthritis are often enlarged because of bony hypertrophy (overgrowth). The enlarged knee feels hard on palpation. Joint effusions (excess joint fluid) are common when the knees are inflamed. The presence of *inflammation* indicates a secondary synovitis.

About half of patients with hand involvement have *Heberden nodes* (bony nodules at the distal interphalangeal [DIP] joints) and *Bouchard nodes* (bony nodules at the proximal interphalangeal [PIP] joints) (Fig. 43.2). Although OA is *not* typically a bilateral, symmetric disease, these large bony nodes appear on both hands, especially in women. The nodes may be painful and red. Some patients experience *pain* when developing nodes or when nodes are palpated. These deformities tend to be familial and are often a cosmetic concern to patients.

Observe any *atrophy of skeletal muscle* from disuse. The vicious cycle of the disease discourages the movement of painful joints, which may result in contractures, muscle atrophy, and further *pain*. *Loss of function* or decreased *mobility* may result,

TABLE 43.1	**Differential Features of Rheumatoid Arthritis and Osteoarthritis**	
Characteristic	**Rheumatoid Arthritis**	**Osteoarthritis**
Typical onset (age)	35–45 yr	Older than 60 yr
Gender affected	Female (2–3:1)	Female (2:1)
Risk factors or cause	Autoimmune (genetic basis) Emotional stress (triggers exacerbation) Environmental factors	Aging Genetic factor (possible) Obesity Trauma Occupation
Disease process	Inflammatory	Likely degenerative with secondary *inflammation*
Disease pattern	Bilateral, symmetric, multiple joints Usually affects upper extremities first Distal interphalangeal joints of hands spared Systemic	May be unilateral, single joint Affects weight-bearing joints and hands, spine Metacarpophalangeal joints spared Nonsystemic
Laboratory findings	Elevated rheumatoid factor, antinuclear antibody, and ESR	Normal or slightly elevated ESR
Common drug therapy	NSAIDs (short-term use) Methotrexate Biological response modifiers	NSAIDs (short-term use) Acetaminophen Other analgesics

ESR, Erythrocyte sedimentation rate.

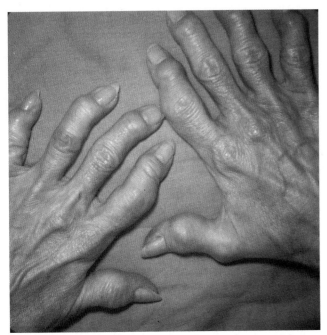

FIG. 43.2 Osteoarthritic hands with Heberden (distal interphalangeal) and Bouchard (proximal interphalangeal) nodes on multiple fingers and thumbs. Note angular changes at distal joints as a result of loss of joint cartilage and instability. (From Beaty, J. H., & Azar, F. M. [2021]. *Campbell's operative orthopaedics* [14th ed.]. St. Louis: Elsevier.)

depending on which joints are involved. Hip or knee pain may cause the patient to limp and restrict walking distance.

OA can affect the spine, especially the lumbar region at the L3–4 level or the cervical region at C4–6 (neck). Compression of spinal nerve roots may occur as a result of vertebral facet bone spurs. The patient typically reports radiating pain, stiffness, and muscle spasms in one or both extremities (Rogers, 2023).

Severe *pain* and deformity often interfere with ambulation and self-care. In addition to performing a musculoskeletal assessment, collaborate with the physical and occupational therapists to assess functional ability. Assess the patient's *mobility* and ability to perform ADLs. Chapter 7 describes functional assessment in detail.

Psychosocial Assessment. OA is a chronic condition that may cause changes in lifestyle and physical disability. An inability to care for oneself in advanced disease can result in role changes and other losses. Persistent *pain* interferes with quality of life, including sexuality. Patients may not have the energy for sexual intercourse or may find positioning uncomfortable.

Patients with continuous *pain* from arthritis may develop depression or anxiety. The patient may also have a role change in the family, workplace, or both. To identify changes that have been or need to be made, ask about the patient's roles before the disease developed. Identify coping strategies to help live with the disease. Ask the patient about expectations regarding treatment for OA.

In addition to role changes, joint deformities and bony nodules often alter body image and self-esteem. Observe the patient's response to body changes. Does the patient ignore them or seem overly occupied with them? Ask patients directly how they perceive their body image. Document your assessment findings in the interprofessional health record per agency policy.

Laboratory Assessment. The primary health care provider uses the history and physical examination to make the diagnosis of OA. The results of routine laboratory tests are usually normal but can be helpful in screening for associated conditions. The erythrocyte sedimentation rate (ESR) and high-sensitivity C-reactive protein (hsCRP) may be slightly elevated when secondary synovitis occurs. The ESR also tends to rise with age and infection.

Imaging Assessment. Routine x-rays are useful in determining structural joint changes. Specialized views are obtained when the disease cannot be visualized on standard x-ray film but is suspected. Magnetic resonance imaging (MRI) may be used to determine vertebral or knee involvement.

Analyze Cues and Prioritize Hypotheses: Analysis

The priority collaborative problems for patients with osteoarthritis (OA) include:

1. Persistent *pain* due to joint swelling, cartilage deterioration, and/or secondary joint *inflammation*
2. Potential for decreased *mobility* due to joint *pain* and muscle atrophy

Generate Solutions and Take Actions: Planning and Implementation

In 2019 the Osteoarthritis Research Society International (OARSI) committee updated its evidence-based expert consensus guidelines for patients with knee, hip, and polyarticular OA (Bannuru et al., 2019). The Arthritis Foundation supports the OARSI recommendations and advocates for a self-management program for all patients who have osteoarthritis. These guidelines have major implications for nursing care as described in the following section.

Managing Persistent Pain

Planning: Expected Outcomes. The patient with OA is expected to have a *pain* level that is acceptable to the patient (e.g., at a 2–3 or less on a pain intensity scale of 0 to 10).

Interventions. No drug therapy can influence the course and progression of OA. Optimal management of patients with OA requires a multimodal approach (combination of therapies) to manage persistent *pain*. Perform a pain assessment before and after implementing interventions (see Chapter 6).

Nonsurgical Management. Management of persistent joint *pain* can be challenging for both the patient and the health care professional. Drug therapy and a variety of nonpharmacologic therapies are used to manage the patient with OA. Chapter 6 elaborates on interventions for persistent noncancer pain.

Drug therapy. The purpose of drug therapy is to reduce *pain* and *inflammation* caused by cartilage destruction, muscle spasm, and/or synovitis. The American Pain Society, Arthritis Foundation, American Geriatrics Society, and OARSI committee recommend regular *acetaminophen* or *NSAIDs* as the primary drugs of choice (Bannuru, et al., 2019).

NURSING SAFETY PRIORITY

Drug Alert

> The standard ceiling dose of acetaminophen is 4000 mg each day. However, patients may be at risk for liver damage if they take more than 3000 mg daily, have alcoholism, or have liver disease. *Older adults are particularly at risk because of normal changes of aging such as slowed excretion of drug metabolites.* Remind patients to read the labels of over-the-counter (OTC) or prescription drugs that could contain acetaminophen before taking them. Teach them that their liver enzyme levels may be monitored while taking this drug (Burchum & Rosenthal, 2022).

Diclofenac 1% topical gel, a topical NSAID, is recommended for relief of mild to moderate *pain* for knee OA (Bannuru et al., 2019). Teach patients to apply the drug according to directions, including using the dosing card that is packaged with the drug. Remind patients to avoid heat application to any area where the gel is applied and not to take any other NSAID while using the drug. Instruct them to expect it will take at least 2 weeks before diclofenac gel is effective for joint pain reduction or relief (Burchum & Rosenthal, 2022).

If acetaminophen or topical agents do not relieve discomfort, oral *NSAIDs* may be prescribed. These traditional drugs supported by OARSI guidelines include oral COX-2 nonselective and selective NSAIDs. Patients who have a history of cardiovascular events such as stroke or myocardial infarction should not take oral NSAIDs (Bannuru et al., 2019).

Before beginning oral NSAID therapy, baseline laboratory information is obtained, including a complete blood count (CBC) and complete metabolic panel (CMP). Celecoxib, a COX-2 inhibitor, is the preferred drug choice unless the patient has hypertension, kidney disease, or cardiovascular history.

 NURSING SAFETY PRIORITY

Drug Alert

> All of the COX–2 inhibiting drugs are thought to cause cardiovascular disease, such as myocardial infarction and hypertension, due to vasoconstriction and increased platelet aggregation (clumping). All NSAIDs can cause GI side effects, bleeding, and acute kidney injury if used long-term (Burchum & Rosenthal, 2022). Therefore, they are prescribed at the lowest effective dose. Remind patients to take celecoxib with food to decrease GI distress. Teach your patient about potential adverse effects and the need to report them to the primary health care provider. Examples include having dark, tarry stools; shortness of breath; edema; frequent dyspepsia; hematemesis (bloody vomitus); and changes in urinary output.

Other agents that are recommended for the knee joint are intraarticular corticosteroid and hyaluronic acid (HA) injections to help manage pain (Bannuru et al., 2019). Corticosteroid injections help to decrease joint inflammation, which can reduce pain. Hyaluronic acid is a very viscous solution that provides lubrication within the joint to improve mobility and provide pain relief. Several types of HA preparations are available. Be sure to remind patients to tell their provider if they have egg or poultry allergies because they may not be candidates for this treatment (Burchum & Rosenthal, 2022). Both corticosteroid and HA injections may be administered once or several times over months.

Nonpharmacologic interventions. In addition to drug therapy, a number of evidence-based nonpharmacologic measures are recommended for patients with OA, including rest balanced with exercise, joint positioning, heat or cold applications, weight control, and ambulatory (gait) aids (Bannuru et al., 2019). In combination with a weight-management program, if needed, a structured exercise program is highly recommended for patients who have hip and polyarticular OA. Aquatic exercises are recommended for patients who have knee OA. Collaborate with the physical therapist (PT) to plan a program for structured exercises to support affected joints.

Teach the patient to *position joints in their functional position.* For example, when in a supine position (recumbent), the patient should use a small pillow under the head or neck but avoid the use of other pillows. The use of large pillows under the knees or head may result in flexion contractures. Remind patients to use proper posture when standing and sitting to reduce undue strain on the vertebral column. Teach the patient to wear supportive shoes; foot insoles may help relieve pressure on painful metatarsal joints (Gourdine, 2019).

Many patients apply *heat* or *cold* for temporary relief of *pain.* Heat may help decrease the muscle tension around the tender joint and thereby decrease pain and stiffness. Suggest hot showers and baths, hot packs or compresses, and moist heating pads. *Regardless of treatment, teach patients to check that the heat source is not too heavy or so hot that it causes burns.* A temperature just above body temperature is adequate to promote comfort.

If needed, collaborate with the PT to provide special heat treatments, such as paraffin dips, diathermy (using electrical current), and ultrasonography (using sound waves). A 15- to 20-minute application is usually sufficient to temporarily reduce pain, spasm, and stiffness. Cold packs or gels that feel hot and cold at the same time may also be used.

Cold therapy has limited use for most patients in promoting comfort. Cold works by numbing nerve endings and decreasing secondary joint *inflammation,* if present.

Gradual *weight loss* for obese patients may lessen the stress on weight-bearing joints, decrease *pain,* and perhaps slow joint degeneration. If needed, collaborate with the registered dietitian nutritionist or other weight-management professional to provide more in-depth teaching and meal planning or to make referrals to community resources for weight reduction.

Minimally invasive regenerative therapies, such as stem cell therapy and platelet-rich plasma (PRP), are being used for knee OA to delay or substitute for surgery. PRP has shown very effective results in treating knee OA because it is rich in growth factor, which stimulates regeneration of knee cartilage, reduces pain, and improves joint function (Mogoi et al., 2019).

Complementary and integrative health. Some patients with OA report that a variety of integrative therapies are useful. However, the evidence supporting their effectiveness is inconsistent and inconclusive. Determine whether the patient is using integrative therapies and, if so, which therapies to assess for drug-herb interactions or other potentially adverse events.

Topical *capsaicin* products are safe over-the-counter (OTC) drugs. They work by blocking or modifying substance P and other neurotransmitters for *pain.* Tell the patient using capsaicin to expect a burning sensation for a short time after applying it. Recommend the use of plastic gloves for application. To prevent burning of eyes or other body areas, wash hands immediately after applying the substance.

Dietary supplements may complement traditional drug therapies. Glucosamine and chondroitin are widely used and are reported to be the most effective nonprescription supplements taken that may reduce pain and improve functional ability. Glucosamine may decrease *inflammation,* and chondroitin may play a role in strengthening cartilage. However, the evidence to support their use is inconsistent and is not included in the most recent OARSI evidence-based guidelines (Bannuru et al., 2019; Arthritis Foundation, 2023).

Medical marijuana (cannabis). Medical marijuana (cannabis) has been used for many years to assist in pain management. Patients with osteoarthritis pain have reported the effectiveness of cannabinoids, and there is a growing body of scientific evidence that supports these reports. Both plant-based and man-made cannabinoids may be effective for pain control (Clark, 2021).

PATIENT-CENTERED CARE: HEALTH EQUITY

Pain Management for Osteoarthritis

Persistent pain from osteoarthritis is reported to be more severe and disabling among older African Americans when compared to Whites, making them likely to experience decreased mobility, function, and quality of life (Booker & Herr, 2021). Older African Americans are less likely to receive prescription pain medication or surgery, and are more likely to use integrative therapies to manage pain. Social determinants of health, such as decreased access to health care, social isolation, and financial constraints, contribute to this health inequity. Research demonstrates that older African Americans also lack adequate knowledge about osteoarthritis self-management (Booker & Herr, 2021). Nurses need to advocate for all older adults to ensure that they are aware of how to manage their osteoarthritis pain and access available health resources, including surgical options.

Surgical Management. Surgery may be indicated when conservative measures and/or drug therapy no longer provide *pain* control, when *mobility* becomes so restricted that patients cannot participate in activities, and when the desired quality of life cannot be maintained. The most common surgical procedure for OA is total joint arthroplasty (TJA) (surgical creation of a functional [synovial] joint using implants), also known as *total joint replacement (TJR).* Almost any synovial joint of the body can be replaced with a prosthetic system that consists of at least two implants—one for each joint surface. The hip and knee are most often replaced, but shoulder and ankle arthroplasties are becoming increasingly common as a result of advances in technology. TJAs are expected to increase as the older adult population grows over the next 20 years.

TJA is a procedure used most often to manage the pain of OA and improve *mobility,* although other conditions causing cartilage and bone destruction may require the surgery. These disorders include rheumatoid arthritis (RA), congenital anomalies, trauma, and osteonecrosis. Osteonecrosis is bone death secondary to lack of or disruption in blood supply to the affected bone, usually from trauma or chronic steroid therapy. The affected bone site is most commonly the femoral or humeral head, distal femur, or proximal tibia.

The *contraindications* for TJA are active infection anywhere in the body and rapidly progressive *inflammation.* An active infection elsewhere in the body or from the joint being replaced can result in an infected TJA and subsequent prosthetic failure. Severe medical problems, such as uncontrolled diabetes or hypertension, put the patient at risk for major postoperative complications. Therefore, these problems should be stabilized before surgery. Patients who smoke should plan to enroll in a smoking-cessation program and stop smoking prior to surgery to help prevent cardiovascular complications of surgery.

Some patients may be assigned to an orthopedic patient navigator, a nurse who coordinates care as the single point of contact for a patient who has orthopedic surgery. This nurse provides support for the patient and family, both inside and outside the hospital. Specific responsibilities of an orthopedic patient navigator include (Teng et al., 2021):

- Provide orthopedic nursing expertise based on current evidence
- Provide services throughout the continuum of care
- Act as patient advocate and educator
- Collect, trend, and analyze data to improve clinical outcomes.

Total hip arthroplasty. The number of total hip arthroplasty (THA) procedures (also known as *total hip replacement [THR]*) has steadily increased over the past 40 years. If the patient has a joint replacement for the first time, it is referred to as primary arthroplasty. If the implant loosens or fails for any reason, revision arthroplasty may be performed to replace the previous one. Availability of improved joint implant materials and better custom design features allow longer life of a THA. Although adult patients of any age can undergo THA, the procedure is performed most often in those older than 60 years. *The special needs and normal physiologic changes of older adults often complicate the perioperative period and may result in additional postoperative complications.*

PREOPERATIVE CARE. As with any surgery, preoperative care begins with assessing the patient's level of understanding about the surgery and the patient's ability to participate in the postoperative plan of care. Identifying a joint coach (family care partner) can help the patient through the perioperative period and assist with discharge needs. Many hospitals have a Joint Academy or Joint Camp in which members of the interprofessional health care team provide educational classes prior to surgery. Jones et al. (2022) conducted a retrospective study, which demonstrated that these classes impacted postoperative outcomes (see the Evidence-Based Practice box).

The surgeon explains the procedure and postoperative expectations (including possible complications) during the office visit, but this patient education may have occurred weeks or months before the scheduled elective surgery. Information may be provided in a notebook, pamphlet, DVD, video, or online so that the patient can review it at home and share with the joint coach and other family members. This review is particularly useful to patients with inadequate reading skills or poor memory.

 ## PATIENT-CENTERED CARE: CULTURE AND SPIRITUALITY

Health Literacy

Written materials or other media provided in the language appropriate for the patient's reading level and culture are essential. If an interpreter is needed to be sure that the information is understood, one needs to be provided for the patient at each appointment, while in the hospital, and when discharged to home or inpatient rehabilitation services.

 ## EVIDENCE-BASED PRACTICE

What is the Impact of Preoperative Total Joint Arthroplasty Education on Outcomes?

Jones, E. D., Davidson, C. J., & Cline, T. W. (2022). The effect of preoperative education prior to hip or knee arthroplasty on immediate postoperative outcomes. *Orthopaedic Nursing, 41*(1), 4–12.

The researchers conducted a retrospective chart review of 707 patients over 50 years of age who had either a total hip or total knee arthroplasty to determine immediate postoperative outcomes related to ambulation and mobility. When compared to patients who did not participate in preoperative education, patients who participated in preoperative classes facilitated by physical therapy had the following clinical outcomes:

- Significantly shorter hospital length of stay (representing a savings of almost $1000 per patient)
- Greater mobility, as demonstrated by achieving more degrees of hip or knee flexion and ambulating longer distances

Level of Evidence: 3
This study compared two groups of patients—one group who participated in classes and one group that did not. Therefore, it is a quasiexperimental study.

Commentary: Implications for Practice and Research
Although this study measured mobility outcomes related to classes offered by physical therapists, nurses are in the unique role of reinforcing exercises and ambulation for patients hospitalized for total hip or knee arthroplasties. Interprofessional health team communication is needed to ensure the plan of care to achieve optimal clinical outcomes. Additional research is needed to study patients in multiple Joint Replacement Centers to validate findings.

Preoperative rehabilitation, or "prehab," is essential to prevent functional decline after surgery and provide a quicker functional recovery. As part of prehab, the patient and joint coach learn postoperative exercises, transfer and positioning techniques, and ambulation with a walker or crutches, depending on the patient's age and stability. Other best practices for preoperative patient and family education are summarized in Box 43.2.

In addition, patients preparing for elective orthopedic surgery may be screened for their risk of postoperative *delirium.* Jones and Taylor (2019) described a quality improvement initiative for identifying delirium risk to anticipate the need for safety sitters to prevent patient falls. Delirium is discussed in Chapters 3 and 4, and in mental health textbooks.

For patients not at risk for delirium, *Enhanced Recovery After Surgery (ERAS) programs,* also called "fast track," "accelerated track," or "rapid recovery" programs, are common in Total Joint Replacement Centers to improve patient outcomes, such as a shortened hospital length of stay (LOS), improved patient experiences, and enhanced functional outcomes. Patients who participate in this type of program also have fewer hospital readmissions.

In addition to usual preoperative laboratory tests and x-rays, the surgeon may ask the patient with RA to undergo a cervical spine x-ray if having general anesthesia. Those with RA often have cervical spine disease that can lead to subluxation (partial joint dislocation) during intubation. A CT scan and/or MRI may be done to assess the operative joint and surrounding soft tissues, especially if the patient is undergoing a robotic-assisted THA.

Ask patients to check with their surgeon about which drugs they can take the morning of surgery with a small amount of water, including antihypertensives, thyroid hormone supplements, and antidiabetic agents. Some drugs, such as NSAIDs and anticoagulants/antiplatelets, are discontinued 5 to 10 days before surgery to prevent surgical bleeding. See Chapter 9 for additional general preoperative care interventions and teaching.

OPERATIVE PROCEDURES. Similar to other orthopedic surgeries, the patient receives an *IV antibiotic,* usually a cephalosporin such as cefazolin or cefuroxime, within an hour before the initial surgical incision per the Surgical Care Improvement Project (SCIP) Core Measures to help prevent infection. If the patient has a beta-lactam allergy, vancomycin or clindamycin is administered 2 hours before the initial incision (Bodden & Coppola, 2018).

Several different types of anesthesia are used for THA surgeries and are administered by an anesthesiologist or nurse anesthetist. These options include general anesthesia, neuraxial (spinal or epidural) anesthesia, regional nerve blocks, or a combination of these agents. Patients receiving neuraxial or regional anesthetics may also be given IV moderate sedation to keep them unaware of their environment during the procedure. The benefit of a regional block is that the patient may receive extended *pain* relief, often up to 24 hours after surgery. Chapter 9 describes complications and nursing implications associated with varying types of anesthesia.

BOX 43.2 Patient and Family Education

Preoperative Care and Education for Patients Having a Total Hip Arthroplasty

Topic Area	Health Teaching
Nutrition Assessment	Stress the need for preoperative assessment for clinical malnutrition, which is associated with prolonged postoperative rehabilitation and surgical complications.
	Collaborate with the registered dietitian nutritionist for nutritional assessment.
Pain Assessment and Management	Assess for use of opioids for persistent pain before surgery.
	Teach the patient and joint coach about multimodal pain management options.
Venous Thromboembolism (VTE) Prevention	Teach the need for anticoagulant drug therapy, which should start within 24 hours after surgery and continue for at least 14 days after surgery.
	For patients taking anticoagulants or antiplatelet drugs before surgery, plan for interruption of these drugs for 5 to 10 days before surgery.
	Teach the need for frequent mobilization after surgery; early mobility also helps to prevent constipation.
	Teach the need for compression stockings and/or sequential compression devices during the hospital stay.
Infection Prevention	Teach the patient to expect to receive an IV antibiotic before surgery and possibly up to 24 hours after surgery.
	Teach the importance of screening for nares (nose) colonization of *Staphylococcus aureus* 2–4 weeks before surgery.
	Teach the need to use nasal mupirocin ointment twice a day for 1 week (or longer, depending on the nasal culture) before surgery.
	Teach the need to bathe with chlorhexidine gluconate (CHG) solution or wipes for at least the night before and the morning of surgery (a longer period of time may be needed, depending on agency or surgeon protocol).
	Teach the patient to sleep on clean linens and not to use lotions or powders after the CHG baths; remind the patient to avoid sleeping with pets in the bed.

For most patients, *tranexamic acid (TXA)* is used to reduce blood loss during the THA surgical procedure. TXA is an antifibrinolytic agent that improves postoperative hemoglobin and hematocrit and decreases the need for blood transfusions. Preventing hypothermia is another important goal during THA surgery because it is associated with increased blood loss, increased risk for infection, and increased risk for a cardiac event. Patients with a low body mass index (BMI) are at the highest risk for hypothermia (Bodden & Coppola, 2018).

Some patients are candidates for *minimally invasive surgery (MIS)*, using a small incision (usually 4 inches [10.16 cm] instead of 6 to 12 inches [15.24 to 30.48 cm] for traditional surgery) with special instruments, cameras, and computers to reduce muscle cutting and stretching. This newer technique cannot be used for patients who are obese or those with osteoporosis. It is done only for primary THAs, not for revision surgeries. Like those of any MIS, the benefits of minimally invasive THA are decreased soft tissue damage, blood loss, and postoperative *pain.* Patients usually have a shorter hospital stay and quicker recovery. They are generally satisfied with the cosmetic appearance of the incision because there is less scarring. Postoperative complications are less common in patients who undergo minimally invasive ("mini") hip arthroplasty compared with those having the traditional technique.

Hip resurfacing is an alternative to total hip replacement surgery. This procedure is most often performed for younger patients or for those with early-stage cartilage loss of the weight-bearing surface of the femoral head. Instead of completely removing the femoral head and inserting the stem into the femoral canal, the surgeon removes the cartilage from the surface and an artificial cap is placed over the existing natural femoral head.

Two components are used in the THA—the acetabular implant and the femoral implant (Fig. 43.3). A noncemented prosthesis is commonly used for younger patients. Bone surfaces are smoothed as they are prepared to receive the artificial implants. The noncemented components are press-fitted into the prepared bone. The acetabular cup may be placed using computer- or robotic-assisted guidance. For cemented prostheses, polymethyl methacrylate (an acrylic fixating substance) is typically used. It often contains an antibiotic to reduce the risk of infection. The hybrid surgical technique usually involves a cemented femoral component and a noncemented acetabular component. A closed wound drainage system is not commonly used today for a THA because it can contribute to increased blood loss and cause hematoma formation (Bodden & Coppola, 2018). A surgical pressure dressing is applied before the patient is discharged to the postanesthesia care unit (PACU).

Considerations of a noncemented prosthesis include protection of weight-bearing status to allow bone to grow into the prosthesis and decreased problems with loosening of the prosthesis. With a cemented prosthesis, cement can fracture or deteriorate over time, leading to loosening of the prosthesis. These problems cause *pain* and can lead to the need for a revision arthroplasty. In revision arthroplasty the old prosthesis is removed and new implants are placed. Bone graft may be added if bone loss is significant. Outcomes from revision arthroplasty may not be as positive as with primary arthroplasty, particularly for obese patients.

Three surgical approaches are commonly used to perform a THA. Nursing care and patient education differ slightly depending on which approach is used. Be sure to confirm the surgeon's

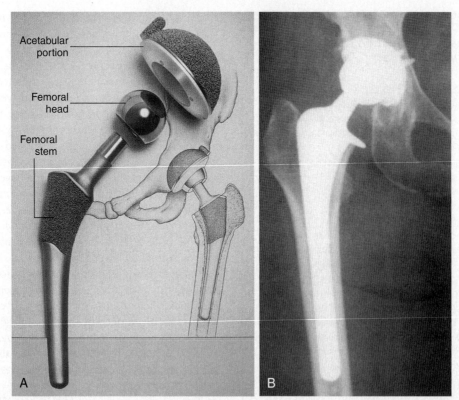

Acetabular portion

Femoral head

Femoral stem

A

B

FIG. 43.3 (A) Acetabular and femoral components of a total hip arthroplasty. (B) Radiograph showing a hip after placement of a cementless Harris-Galante implant. The bone grows into the porous metal to stabilize it to the skeleton. (From Chabner, D. E. [2021]. *The language of medicine* [12th ed.]. St. Louis: Elsevier.)

surgical method for each patient. For the *anterior approach,* the hip joint can be exposed without detaching surrounding muscles. Therefore, this approach has the least likely chance of postoperative hip dislocation and may have the quickest postoperative recovery.

Both of the other surgical methods, *direct lateral* and *posterolateral approaches,* require detaching and/or cutting into large skeletal muscles, which can cause severe postoperative **pain** and a high risk for hip dislocation. The posterolateral approach has the highest risk for dislocation and is therefore seldom used.

POSTOPERATIVE CARE. The typical hospital stay for the patient having a traditional THA is 3 days unless the patient participates in an ERAS program. Some younger patients stay in the hospital only overnight. The goal for rapid recovery programs is for the patients to have same-day THA surgery.

In addition to providing the routine postoperative care discussed in Chapter 9, assess for and help prevent possible postoperative complications. One of the most common complications after a THA is hip dislocation. Other complications include venous thromboembolism, infection, and complications of decreased **mobility.**

PREVENTING HIP DISLOCATION. As described earlier, the risk for hip dislocation depends on the operative approach used by the surgeon.

⚠ NURSING SAFETY PRIORITY

Action Alert

Teach patients to maintain correct positioning of the hip joint and leg at all times. After returning from the postanesthesia care unit (PACU), place the patient in a supine position with the head slightly elevated. One or two regular bed pillows are used in most cases to remind patients to keep their legs abducted if they had one of the two lateral surgical approaches. *If an abduction device with straps is used to prevent dislocation, be sure to loosen the straps every 2 hours and check the patient's skin for irritation or breakdown.* Place and support the affected leg in neutral rotation. The procedure for postoperative turning is not universal and is specified by agency policy or surgeon preference. Turning the patient to the operative side provides "splinting" of the operative hip but may be too painful for some patients. If the patient is turned to the nonoperative side, the operative leg needs to be fully supported with pillows to prevent slipping of the leg into an adducted position that can lead to dislocation. Teach the patient and family about precautions to prevent hip dislocation.

Older adults may have difficulty understanding health teaching because they often become acutely confused after a THA as a result of surgery, anesthesia, and/or unfamiliar environments. The Patient-Centered Care: Older Adult Health box highlights special nursing care of older adults in the postoperative period.

PATIENT-CENTERED CARE: OLDER ADULT HEALTH

Special Postoperative Care of the Older Adult With a Total Hip Arthroplasty

When caring for older adults, be sure to incorporate these postoperative evidence-based nursing actions:

- For patients who had a *posterolateral or direct lateral surgical approach*, use an abduction pillow or splint (rather than bed pillows) to keep their legs apart and prevent adduction, especially if the patient is very restless or has an altered mental state. Hip adduction can cause the surgical hip to become partially or completely dislocated.
- Keep the patient's heels off the bed to prevent pressure injuries.
- Do not rely on fever as a sign of infection; older patients often have infection without fever. Be alert to decreasing mental status and/or elevated white blood cell count as indicators of infection.
- When assisting the patient out of bed, move slowly to prevent orthostatic (postural) hypotension. Allow the patient to sit on the side of the bed for a brief period of time before standing; have the patient stand for a brief period before beginning ambulation.
- Encourage the patient to deep breathe and cough and to use the incentive spirometer every 2 hours to prevent atelectasis and pneumonia.
- On the surgical day, get the patient out of bed to a recliner chair to prevent complications of decreased **mobility.**
- Anticipate the patient's need for pain medication, especially if unable to verbalize the need for **pain** control. For patients on a multimodal pain protocol, assess the need to medicate for breakthrough pain (see Chapter 6).
- Expect a temporary change in mental state immediately after surgery as a result of the anesthetic and unfamiliar sensory stimuli. Reorient the patient frequently.

Observe the patient carefully for signs and symptoms of hip dislocation, including reports of sudden intense **pain** or sudden agitation for the patient who is unable to communicate, affected leg rotation, and/or leg shortening. If the surgical hip becomes dislocated, the surgeon may be able to manipulate and relocate it after the patient receives moderate sedation. If the hip does not reduce into position, the patient may have surgical reduction in the operating room (OR).

! NURSING SAFETY PRIORITY

Action Alert

As with other musculoskeletal surgery, *monitor neurovascular assessments* frequently for a possible compromise in circulation to the affected distal extremity following a THA. Check and document color, temperature, distal pulses, capillary refill, movement, and sensation. The procedure for performing a thorough lower-extremity neurovascular assessment is described in detail in Chapter 41. Remember to compare the operative leg with the nonoperative leg. These assessments are performed at the same time the vital signs are checked. Report any changes in neurovascular assessment to the surgeon, and carefully monitor for changes. Early detection of changes in neurovascular status can prevent permanent tissue damage.

PREVENTING POSTOPERATIVE COMPLICATIONS. The most potentially life-threatening and commonly occurring complication after THA is venous thromboembolism (VTE), which includes deep vein thrombosis (DVT) and pulmonary embolism (PE). *Older patients are especially at increased risk for VTE because of age and decreased circulation before surgery. Obese patients, patients who currently smoke, and those with a history of VTE are also at high risk for thrombi.*

Preventive evidence-based postoperative interventions include a combination of **p**harmacology, **a**mbulation, and **c**ompression (PAC) (Tubog, 2019). *Anticoagulants* such as subcutaneous low-molecular-weight heparin (LMWH) or factor Xa inhibitors are effective drugs in preventing VTE in patients having a THA. Patients are usually on anticoagulants for 10 days to several weeks after surgery, depending on surgeon preference and the patient's response and risk factors.

The use of subcutaneous LMWH, such as enoxaparin and dalteparin, is common for patients with total hip or knee arthroplasty. As an alternative to LMWH, subcutaneous fondaparinux, a factor Xa–inhibiting agent, may be prescribed for some patients undergoing these surgeries. Newer Xa inhibitors, rivaroxaban and apixaban, may be given orally to patients who undergo THA. You do not need to monitor the prothrombin time or international normalized ratio (INR) for patients receiving these drugs because they do not affect coagulation values. However, for other older anticoagulants such as warfarin, patients are at risk for bleeding due to impaired clotting. A complete discussion of nursing care associated with patients taking anticoagulants is found in Chapter 30.

Early *ambulation* and exercise also help prevent VTE. Be sure that the patient ambulates at least three times a day. Teach the patient about leg exercises, which should begin in the immediate postoperative period and continue through the rehabilitation period. These exercises include plantar flexion and dorsiflexion (heel pumping), circumduction (circles) of the feet, gluteal and quadriceps muscle setting, and straight-leg raises (SLRs). Teach the patient to perform gluteal exercises by pushing the heels into the bed and to achieve quadriceps-setting exercises ("quad sets") by straightening the legs and pushing the back of the knees into the bed. In addition to preventing clots, these exercises improve muscle tone, which helps restore the function of the extremity.

Intermittent pneumatic *compression* devices, also called bilateral sequential compression devices (SCDs), are important in preventing VTE by increasing venous blood flow during periods of inactivity. However, clients often report that these devices are hot and bulky to wear, which affects their willingness to use them. Some surgeons prescribe antiembolism stockings, which are less effective but are more widely accepted by clients.

Monitor the surgical incision and vital signs carefully—every 4 hours for the first 24 hours and every 8 to 12 hours thereafter, following facility and surgeon protocols. Observe for signs of infection, such as an elevated temperature, increased redness/hyperpigmentation around the incision, and excessive or foul-smelling drainage from the incision. These signs and symptoms may be seen as early as 2 to 3 days after surgery. *An older patient may not have a fever with infection but instead may experience an altered mental state, especially delirium.* If you suspect this problem, obtain a sample of any drainage for culture and sensitivity to determine the causative organisms and the antibiotics that may be needed for treatment.

MANAGING POSTOPERATIVE PAIN. Although hip arthroplasty is performed to relieve joint *pain,* patients experience varying levels of pain related to the surgical procedure. Pain control protocols vary, depending on the region of the country, anesthesiologist/nurse anesthetist, and surgeon. Many patients equate pain control with opioids (Morland, 2019). However, in view of the opioid crisis, a *multimodal pain management* approach is best practice for patients having a major joint arthroplasty.

Immediate pain control may be achieved by short-term patient-controlled analgesia (PCA), or IV push, typically with morphine or hydromorphone. Pizzi et al. (2020) demonstrated that oral patient-controlled analgesia with oxycodone is effective in managing pain for patients having total joint arthroplasty. Nonopioid drugs are used as part of the multimodal analgesic approach because they act at different pain receptor sites. Examples of these drugs include (Bodden & Coppola, 2018; Goode et al., 2019):

- Continuous peripheral nerve block (e.g., bupivacaine, ropivacaine)
- NSAIDs (e.g., ketorolac, celecoxib)
- NMDA receptor antagonists (e.g., ketamine)
- Gabapentinoids (e.g., gabapentin, pregabalin)

Chapter 6 contains information on the nursing care associated with these pain medications.

Nonpharmacologic methods for acute and chronic pain control, such as cryotherapy and music therapy, can also be used to decrease the amount of drug therapy used. Chapter 6 describes these methods in detail.

PROMOTING POSTOPERATIVE MOBILITY AND ACTIVITY. Depending on the time of day that the surgery is performed, the patient with a THA gets out of bed with assistance the night of surgery to prevent problems related to decreased *mobility* (e.g., VTE, pneumonia), especially in older adults.

! NURSING SAFETY PRIORITY

Action Alert

Be sure to assist with the patient's first time getting out of bed to prevent falls and observe for dizziness. When getting the patient out of bed, put a gait belt on and then stand on the same side of the bed as the affected leg. After the patient sits on the side of the bed, remind the patient to stand on the unaffected leg and pivot to the chair with guidance. *To avoid injury, do not lift the patient!*

A recent approach to ensure early ambulation of patients who have total joint replacements is the use of a **mobility technician**, a specially trained nursing assistant whose primary responsibility is to ambulate hospitalized patients (Lisevick et al., 2020). Some patients have late-day surgeries, when physical therapy departments are closed, preventing ambulation on the same surgical day. Mobility technicians ambulate patients on the surgical day and continue regularly scheduled ambulation during the entire hospital stay.

The surgeon, type of prosthesis, and surgical procedure determine the amount of weight bearing that can be applied to the affected leg. A patient with a cemented implant is usually allowed immediate weight bearing as tolerated (WBAT). Typically, only minimal weight bearing is initially permitted for patients with noncemented prostheses. When x-ray evidence of bony ingrowth can be seen, the patient can progress to partial weight bearing (PWB) and then to full weight bearing (FWB) over a period of weeks.

In collaboration with the physical therapist (PT), teach the patient how to follow weight-bearing restrictions. Most patients use a walker, but younger adults may use crutches. They are usually advanced to a single cane or crutch if they can walk without a severe limp 4 to 6 weeks after surgery. When the limp disappears, they no longer need an ambulatory/assistive device and may be permitted to sit in chairs of normal height, use regular toilets, and drive a car. The timing to resume driving may be slightly longer in a patient who has had surgery on the right hip because of patient safety concerns.

NCLEX Examination Challenge 43.2

Safe and Effective Environment

The nurse plans care for a client who underwent an anterior total hip arthroplasty this morning. What is the **priority** action that the nurse would include?

A. Administer continuous peripheral nerve block per agency protocol.
B. Keep the operative leg adducted for the first 2 days after surgery.
C. Assist the client to get out of bed and ambulate this evening.
D. Monitor for dislocation of the operative hip while in bed.

PROMOTING POSTOPERATIVE SELF-MANAGEMENT. With the increase in ERAS programs that emphasize a structured approach and rapid recovery, the length of stay in the acute care hospital is typically less than 3 days if there are no postoperative complications. Patients experiencing postoperative complications often stay longer. Keep in mind that Medicare patients need a 3-day qualifying hospital stay to receive rehabilitation in a skilled inpatient unit. Discharge from the acute care facility may be to the home, a rehabilitation unit, a transitional care unit, or a skilled unit or long-term care facility for continued rehabilitation before discharge to home. The interprofessional team provides written instructions for posthospital care and reviews them with patients and their joint coaches. Be sure to provide a copy of these instructions for the patient.

Acute rehabilitation usually takes several weeks, depending on the patient's age and progress and the type of prosthesis used. However, it usually takes 6 weeks or longer for complete recovery. Patients who are discharged to their homes often are able to attend physical therapy sessions in an office or ambulatory care setting. Others have no means or cannot use community resources and need physical therapy in the home, depending on their health insurance coverage. *Collaborate with the case manager to determine which option is best for your patient.* Box 43.3 outlines the most important health teaching for you to provide to the patient being discharged after a THA.

HOSPITAL READMISSION AFTER THA. The most common complications of THA surgery that cause readmission to the hospital include thromboembolic problems, such as DVT and

BOX 43.3 Patient and Family Education

Care of Patients With Total Hip Arthroplasty After Hospital Discharge

Hip Precautions

- Do not sit or stand for prolonged periods.
- Do not cross your legs beyond the midline of your body.
- For *posterolateral or direct lateral surgical approach* patients: Do not bend your hips more than 90 degrees.
- For *anterior surgical approach* patients: Do not hyperextend your operative leg behind you.
- Do not twist your body when standing.
- Use the prescribed ambulatory aid such as a walker when walking.
- Use assistive/adaptive devices as needed (e.g., sock aids, shoehorns, dressing sticks, extenders [also see Chapter 7]).
- Do not put more weight on your affected leg than allowed and instructed.
- Call 911 if you experience any signs or symptoms of hip dislocation, including sudden difficulty bearing weight on the surgical leg, leg shortening or rotation, or a feeling that the hip has "popped" with immediate intense **pain.**
- Resume sexual intercourse as usual on the advice of your surgeon.

Pain Management

- Report increased hip or anterior thigh pain to the surgeon immediately.
- Take oral analgesics as prescribed and only as needed.
- Do not overexert yourself; take frequent rests.
- Use ice or cryotherapy as needed with operative hip to decrease or prevent swelling and minimize pain.

Incisional Care

- Follow the instructions provided regarding dressing changes, if needed. Some surgeons use specialty clear dressings that do not need to be changed. No dressing may be needed if a skin sealant was used.
- Inspect your hip incision every day for redness/hyperpigmentation, heat, or drainage; if any of these are present, call your surgeon immediately.
- Do not bathe the incision or apply anything directly to the incision unless instructed to do so. Shower according to the surgeon's instructions.

Other Care

- Continue walking and performing the leg exercises as you learned them in the hospital. Do not increase the amount of activity unless instructed to do so by the therapist or surgeon.
- Do not cross your legs; this will help prevent blood clots.
- Report pain, redness/hyperpigmentation, or swelling in your legs to your surgeon immediately.
- Call 911 for acute chest pain or shortness of breath (could indicate pulmonary embolus).
- Follow the bleeding precautions learned in the hospital to prevent bleeding; avoid using a straight razor, avoid injuries, and report bleeding or excessive bruising to your surgeon immediately.
- Be sure to follow up with outpatient physical therapy for your exercise and ambulation program to build strength, **mobility,** and endurance (if discharged to home).
- Follow up with visits to the surgeon's office as instructed.

stroke; surgical site infection (SSI); and systemic infections, including pneumonia and sepsis. Men of advanced age and those with comorbidities, such as heart failure and diabetes, are at the highest risk for hospital readmission after a THA (Bodden & Coppola, 2018).

Total knee arthroplasty. As the population ages, more adults are undergoing total knee arthroplasty (TKA, also known as *total knee replacement [TKR]*). The increased demand for TKA in the United States is due to osteoarthritis and obesity, which is a contributing factor to OA in weight-bearing joints. Osteoarthritis is discussed earlier in this chapter. Patients who have rheumatoid arthritis or posttraumatic arthritis caused by a physical injury may also need a TKA (Mori & Ribsam, 2018). Similar to the THA, patients who experience a failed primary TKA may undergo revision arthroplasty.

TKAs are most often performed as unilateral procedures, meaning that *one* knee is replaced during surgery. However, a growing number of patients choose to have *both* knees done at one time or within 3 to 6 months of each other. Having both knees replaced at one time is referred to as simultaneous bilateral total knee arthroplasty (BTKA). Simultaneous BTKA is sometimes done for patients who have moderate to severe arthritis in both knees.

With careful patient selection and the use of evidence-based practices, some patients may have a unilateral TKA in an ambulatory surgery center (ASC) instead of in a hospital with an inpatient stay. Research demonstrates that patients who have same-day surgery for a knee replacement have a low postoperative complication rate, high patient satisfaction rate, and minimal postdischarge health care utilization (Mascioli et al., 2021).

Partial knee replacements are used for patients with minimal cartilage loss in specified areas of the involved knee and are typically done more often in younger patients. Minimally invasive surgery (MIS) is also an option for either partial or total knee arthroplasty for this population. Severe bone loss, obesity, and previous knee surgeries are contraindications for this type of surgery. Patients who have MIS procedures have less **pain** and blood loss and greater range of motion to promote a faster postoperative recovery.

PREOPERATIVE CARE. TKA is performed when joint **pain** can no longer be managed by conservative measures. When limited **mobility** severely prevents patients from participating in work or activities they enjoy, this procedure can restore a high quality of life. The preoperative care and teaching for patients undergoing a TKA are similar to that for THA (see Evidence-Based Practice box in the THA section earlier in this chapter). However, precautions for positioning are not the same because joint dislocation is not a common complication. Differences in patient and family teaching depend on the procedure used by the orthopedic surgeon and established best practices.

The use of Enhanced Recovery After Surgery (ERAS) programs for many types of surgery has improved outcomes for patients having a TKA. As part of this program, patients have a screening to determine their *nutritional status*, including identifying those who are malnourished and/or obese. Obesity is linked to health problems, such as heart disease, diabetes, hypertension, and stroke, and can impair bone and wound healing. Obese patients who have a TKA typically have a longer length of stay in the hospital and are more likely than other patients to be transferred to a skilled nursing facility for rehabilitation. Therefore, the surgeon may request that the patient lose 20 lb or more before surgery to promote improved postoperative recovery.

Patients who have had bariatric surgery may have chronic anemia and bone loss due to insufficient nutrients. Bone health is a concern for adults of any age who have a history of bariatric surgery. Chapter 52 discusses obesity and bariatric surgery in detail.

Planning for postdischarge *transitions of care* begins before surgery, including identifying a joint coach (family care partner) who plays an active role in patient care through the perioperative care. *Preoperative rehabilitation* ("prehab") is important to enhance functional ability and provide a quicker postoperative recovery. All patients are given verbal and either written or video preoperative instructions, which include the activity protocol to follow after surgery. The PT and OT provide information about transfers, ambulation, postoperative exercises, and ADL assistance. Patients should practice walking with walkers or crutches to prepare them for ambulation after TKA. Teach patients about the possible need for assistive/adaptive devices to assist with ADLs, including an elevated toilet seat, safety handrails, and dressing devices such as a long-handled shoehorn. Some third-party payers may cover these devices, depending on the patient's condition and age. Teach the patient and family how and where this equipment can be obtained to have it available after surgery. Case managers or social workers may arrange for needed items to be delivered to the patient's room before discharge.

A *pain management* assessment and plan before surgery are essential to promote a satisfactory postoperative patient experience. Patients with persistent preoperative pain may have mental health problems, such as anxiety, depression, and/or substance use disorder. Some patients have been treated with long-term analgesics, including opioids, for many years before surgery. These factors place patients having major joint arthroplasty at high risk for severe postoperative pain that can be challenging to manage (Jackman, 2019).

Best practices for postoperative management of persistent pain patients include to (Jackman, 2019):
- Identify at-risk patients preoperatively.
- Establish trust and discuss the postoperative pain management plan.
- Perform a comprehensive preoperative and postoperative assessment of pain and reassessment.
- Use multimodal and alternative pain management modalities.
- Consult the pain management team if needed and available.
- Manage mental health/psychological disorders that may be present.
- Plan continuing pain management for and after discharge.

Teach patients that they will need to shower with a chlorhexidine gluconate (CHG) body wash or use CHG wipes the night before and the morning of surgery to decrease bacteria on the skin that could cause infection. Remind them to wear clean nightwear, sleep on clean linen, and avoid having pets in their bed. All patients having a TKA should be treated for at least a week with nasal mupirocin ointment to prevent surgical site infection from *Staphylococcus aureus* (Mori & Ribsam, 2018).

Ask patients to check with their surgeon about which drugs they can take the morning of surgery with a small amount of water, including antihypertensives, thyroid hormone supplements, and antidiabetic agents. Some drugs, such as NSAIDs and anticoagulants/antiplatelets, are discontinued 5 to 10 days before surgery to prevent surgical bleeding. See Chapter 9 for additional general preoperative care interventions and teaching.

OPERATIVE PROCEDURES. As with the hip, the knee can be replaced with the patient under a variety of anesthetic agents, including general or neuraxial (epidural or spinal) anesthesia. One of the more recent advances in postoperative pain management for TKA is the use of a **peripheral nerve block (PNB)**, most commonly a femoral nerve block (FNB) using a local anesthetic. An IV moderate sedation agent is used in addition to the neuraxial or PNB drug. PNB may be either a single injection or continuous infusion by a portable pump (e.g., continuous femoral nerve blockade, or CFNB). In addition, other local medications may be injected into the knee or surrounding tissues to assist in the reduction of severe pain that usually occurs after knee surgery and to minimize perioperative bleeding. Sasse et al. (2020) reported that adding a ketorolac periarticular injection decreased pain and improved postoperative mobility for patients having a TKA.

An antibiotic, usually an IV cephalosporin (cefazolin or cefuroxime), is given within 60 minutes before the surgical incision and proximal tourniquet inflation per the SCIP Core Measures to aid in the prevention of infection. If giving a fluoroquinolone or vancomycin, the infusion should begin 2 hours (120 minutes) before the incision and tourniquet inflation (Mori & Ribsam, 2018). In the *traditional surgery,* the surgeon makes a central longitudinal incision about 6 to 8 inches (15.24 to 20.32 cm) long. Osteotomies of the femoral and tibial condyles and of the posterior patella are performed, and the surfaces are prepared for the prosthesis. The femoral prosthesis is often noncemented (using a press-fit) with the tibial component being cemented.

Total knee arthroplasties require multiple bone incisions and extensive soft tissue involvement, which can result in significant blood loss. Interventions that may reduce blood loss include:
- Tourniquet use during surgery
- Fibrin sealants
- Tranexamic acid (TXA), an antifibrinolytic agent

While these interventions may be effective, most of them also have disadvantages. For example, using an operative tourniquet can increase postoperative pain. The strongest evidence supports TXA use during surgery for blood loss reduction (Mori & Ribsam, 2018). This drug improves postoperative hemoglobin and hematocrit and decreases the need for blood transfusions. The surgeon also applies a compression (pressure) dressing from the toes to the thigh to decrease edema and bleeding.

Minimally invasive TKA may be performed using a shorter incision and special instruments to spare muscle and other soft tissue. Computer-guided or robotic equipment may be used to ensure accurate positioning of the knee implants.

POSTOPERATIVE CARE. Provide the usual postoperative care needed for any patient who has surgery (see Chapter 9). Specific nursing care of the patient with a TKA is similar to that for the patient with a total hip arthroplasty, as described in the previous section.

✚ NURSING SAFETY PRIORITY

Critical Rescue

If the patient has a continuous femoral nerve blockade (CFNB), perform and document neurovascular assessment every 2 to 4 hours, or according to hospital protocol. Be sure that patients can perform dorsiflexion and plantar flexion motions of the affected foot without pain in the lower leg. In addition, monitor these patients for signs and symptoms that indicate absorption of the local anesthetic into the patient's system, including:

- Metallic taste
- Tinnitus
- Nervousness
- Slurred speech
- Bradycardia
- Hypotension
- Decreased respirations
- Seizures

Document and report these new-onset signs and symptoms to the surgeon, anesthesiologist/nurse anesthetist, or Rapid Response Team immediately, and carefully continue to monitor the patient for any changes.

Since joint dislocation is rare after TKA, there are no special positioning precautions required to prevent adduction. Maintain the operative leg in a neutral position, avoiding both internal and external rotation. Do not place a pillow under the replaced knee or hyperextend the knee.

MANAGING POSTOPERATIVE PAIN. In the immediate postoperative period, the surgeon prescribes some form of cryotherapy (cold application) to decrease swelling, hematoma formation, and ***pain*** at the surgical site. The affected knee is typically very swollen and discolored for a number of weeks after surgery. These problems are more common with this type of surgery than with hip surgery. Several types of cryotherapy are used, including ice/gel pack compression and circulating cold water cryotherapy devices.

In general, ***pain*** control measures for patients with TKA are similar to those with total hip arthroplasty. Many patients report high ratings on the pain intensity scale and require analgesic medications longer than patients with THA, particularly if they have had bilateral knee surgery. Similar to best practices for managing pain in patients having a THA, a multimodal analgesic approach including a variety of opioid and nonopioid drugs is used (see earlier discussion in this chapter). For some younger patients, IV acetaminophen may be effective in managing TKA pain.

Nonpharmacologic pain modalities are becoming an integral part of the comprehensive pain management plan. For example, music therapy is an effective strategy for many postoperative patients having a TKA to reduce pain.

PREVENTING POSTOPERATIVE COMPLICATIONS. Some complications that affect patients with THA may also affect those having

unilateral or bilateral TKA, such as venous thromboembolism (VTE) and infection. Complications generally depend on the overall health of the patient.

Average-risk patients begin anticoagulant therapy within 24 hours after surgery and continue for at least 14 days. Common drugs used include fondaparinux, apixaban, dabigatran, rivaroxaban, low-dose unfractionated heparin, and low-molecular-weight heparin. Mechanical VTE prevention includes pneumatic or sequential compression devices and/or compression stockings that are applied before surgery and worn during the hospital stay.

A recent integrative literature review to determine evidence-based nursing practices to prevent complications for patients with bilateral TKA found a lack of clinical practice guidelines for both nursing and surgeon care (Pietsch et al., 2018). Assessments and interventions associated with impaired clotting and infection are described in the Postoperative Care section of the discussion of Total Hip Arthroplasty.

PROMOTING POSTOPERATIVE SELF-MANAGEMENT. The desired outcome for discharge from the acute hospital unit is that the patient can walk with crutches or a walker and has adequate flexion in the operative knee for ambulation, including walking up and down stairs. Patients are able to bear weight as tolerated unless the prosthesis is not cemented. Patients may be discharged to their homes or to an acute rehabilitation unit, transitional care unit, or skilled unit in a long-term care facility for therapy after 1 to 3 days in acute care. Patients participating in Enhanced Recovery After Surgery (ERAS) programs have a shorter hospital length of stay and fewer complications or readmissions.

For some patients, home care services may provide physical therapy and nursing care for 1 to 2 weeks followed by outpatient therapy. *Collaborate with the case manager to determine which option is best for your patient.* During the home rehabilitation phase, the use of a stationary bicycle or continuous passive motion (CPM) machine may help gain flexion (Fig. 43.4). These patients typically return to work and other usual activities in 6 weeks, depending on their age, type of surgery, and other health status factors. Total recovery from a TKA surgery takes 6 weeks or longer, especially for those older than 75 years.

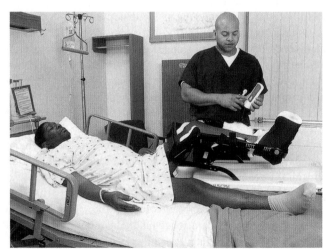

FIG. 43.4 A continuous passive motion (CPM) machine in use.

HOSPITAL READMISSION AFTER TKA. The primary causes of readmission after a TKA are infection and VTE. Women who have a longer postoperative hospital stay and are discharged to an inpatient rehabilitation facility or skilled nursing facility are at the greatest risk for these complications (Causey-Upton et al., 2019).

NCLEX Examination Challenge 43.3

Health Promotion and Maintenance

The nurse is assessing a client with a history of severe bilateral knee osteoarthritis in preparation for possible total knee arthroplasty. Which client risk factor would be of **most concern** for the client considering surgery?

A. Obesity
B. Diabetes mellitus
C. Over 65 years of age
D. Severe osteoarthritis

Other joint arthroplasties. The shoulder and other upper-extremity joints do not bear weight and therefore tend to have less arthritis and subsequent pain. Preoperative teaching for patients having any of these surgeries depends on the surgeon's technique and postoperative protocols.

Total shoulder arthroplasty (TSA) has gained increasing popularity as newer prostheses and technology have been developed. This procedure usually decreases arthritic or traumatic pain, and increases the patient's ability to perform ADLs. Because the shoulder joint is complex and has many articulations (joint surfaces), subluxation or complete dislocation is a potential complication. Usually the glenohumeral joint, created by the glenoid cavity of the shoulder blade (scapula) and the head of the humerus, is replaced because it moves the most and is therefore most affected by arthritis. A cemented or noncemented hemiarthroplasty (replacement of part of the joint), typically the humeral component, may be performed as an alternative to TSA.

After surgery the patient may be placed in an abduction immobilizer or pillow device to protect the joint from excessive motion until rehabilitation therapy begins. *Do not remove these devices unless instructed to do so by the surgeon.*

In addition to the potential for dislocation, postoperative complications are similar to those for other total joint replacements and include infection and neurovascular compromise. *As for any other total joint arthroplasty, perform frequent neurovascular assessments at least every 4 to 8 hours.* The procedure for performing a thorough upper-extremity neurovascular assessment is described in detail in Chapter 41. Document and report any significant changes to the surgeon immediately. The hospital stay for TSA is shorter than for a total hip or knee replacement and may be performed as a same-day procedure. Rehabilitation with an OT generally takes several months.

Improving Mobility

Planning: Expected Outcomes. The patient with osteoarthritis (OA) is expected to maintain or improve a level of *mobility* and activity that allows independent function with or without an assistive ambulatory device.

BOX 43.4 **Patient and Family Education**
Exercises for Patients With Osteoarthritis

- Follow the exercise instructions that have been prescribed specifically for you. There are no universal exercises; your exercises have been specifically tailored to your needs.
- Do your exercises on both "good" and "bad" days. Consistency is important.
- Respect pain. Reduce the number of repetitions when the inflammation is severe and you have more pain.
- Use active rather than active-assist or passive exercise whenever possible.
- Do not substitute your normal activities or household tasks for the prescribed exercises.
- Avoid resistive exercises when your joints are severely inflamed.

Interventions. Management of the patient with OA often requires an interprofessional health team effort. If needed, consult and collaborate with the physical therapist (PT) and occupational therapist (OT) to meet the outcome of independent function and *mobility.* Major interventions include therapeutic exercise and the promotion of ADLs and ambulation by teaching about health and the use of assistive devices.

Aquatic activities may be therapeutic, such as swimming to enhance chest and arm muscles and reduce knee OA pain. Aerobic exercises (e.g., walking, biking, swimming, aerobic dance) are also recommended. Exercises may be prescribed by rehabilitation therapists for the patient with OA, but you will need to reinforce their techniques and principles. The ideal time for exercise is immediately after the application of heat. To prevent further joint damage, teach patients to carefully follow the instructions for exercise outlined in Box 43.4.

Collaborate with the PT to evaluate the patient's need for ambulatory aids, such as canes or walkers. Although some patients do not like to use these aids or may forget how to use them, they can help prevent further joint deterioration and pain. Collaborate with the OT, if needed, to provide suggestions and devices for assistance for ADLs. Chapter 7 discusses rehabilitation therapies in more detail.

Care Coordination and Transition Management

Be aware that most patients older than 60 years will have some degree of arthritis and possibly persistent *pain* that needs to be managed. The patient with OA is not usually hospitalized for the disease itself but may be admitted for surgical management or other health issue.

Arthritis is one of the most common physical disabilities that patients experience. Many patients with physical disability have mobility and/or self-care limitations. Others may have difficulty with one or more instrumental activities of daily living (IADLs), such as preparing meals or housekeeping. These patients may be admitted to the hospital or other facility for other unrelated health problems such as cardiac events or cancer surgeries. Many patients report that their disability is ignored by health care professionals who may not know how to address the effects of their disability. Be sure to incorporate the presence of any physical disability into the plan of care for all patients in any setting as highlighted in Box 43.5 (Smeltzer, 2021).

BOX 43.5   Best Practice for Patient Safety and Quality Care

Planning Care for Patients Who Have Physical Disability Caused by Arthritis

- Assess the patient's mobility and ADL and IADL function, and incorporate those abilities into the plan of care.
- If needed, refer the patient to appropriate rehabilitation therapists (PT and/ or OT) for evaluation of mobility and/or ADL function.
- If the patient is able to ambulate with or without a walker or other gait aid, continue to ambulate the patient daily, if possible, in any inpatient setting.
- Assess the patient's coping skills in living with a physical disability; refer the patient to appropriate inpatient or community resources as needed to improve coping and quality of life.
- Determine whether the patient is aware of or has obtained preventive health screenings and practices healthy lifestyle habits, if the patient's living situation supports those activities.
- Assess any social determinants of health that affect the ability of the patient to have access to health care; incorporate these factors into the patient's plan of care by providing community resources and referrals.

BOX 43.6   Home Health Care

Evidence-Based Instructions for Joint Protection

Teach patients with arthritis to:

- Use large joints instead of small ones; for example, place your purse strap over your shoulder instead of grasping the purse with your hand.
- Do not turn a doorknob clockwise. Turn it counterclockwise to avoid twisting your arm and promoting ulnar deviation (especially for patients who also have rheumatoid arthritis).
- Use two hands instead of one to hold objects.
- Sit in a chair that has a high, straight back.
- When getting out of bed, do not push off with your fingers; use the entire palm of both hands.
- Do not bend at your waist; instead, bend your knees while keeping your back straight.
- Use long-handled devices, such as a hairbrush with an extended handle.
- Use assistive/adaptive devices, such as Velcro closures and built-up utensil handles to protect your joints.
- Do not use pillows in bed except a small one under your head.
- Avoid twisting or wringing your hands; use a device or rubber grip to open jars or bottles.

Home Care Management. If weight-bearing joints are severely involved, the patient may have difficulty going up or down stairs. Making arrangements to live on one floor with accessibility to all rooms is often the best solution. A home care nurse or case manager may collaborate with a rehabilitation therapist to assess the need for structural alterations to the home to accommodate ambulatory aids and enable the patient to perform ADLs. For example, a seat and handrails may need to be installed in the shower. If the patient has undergone a total hip or knee arthroplasty, an elevated toilet seat is necessary for several weeks after surgery to prevent excessive hip flexion. Throw rugs and other environmental hazards should be removed to prevent tripping and falls.

Self-Management Education. Self-management education (SME) is an effective, psychosocially focused, nonpharmacologic intervention. Learning how to protect joints is the most important part of patient and family education. Preventing further damage to joints slows the progression of OA and minimizes ***pain.*** Explain the general principles of joint protection and give practical examples as outlined in Box 43.6.

As with other diseases in which drugs and nutrition therapy are used, teach the patient and family the drug therapy protocol, desired effects and potential side effects, and toxic effects. Emphasize the importance of reducing weight and eating a well-balanced diet to promote tissue healing.

Many patients with arthritis look for a cure after becoming frustrated and desperate about the course of the disease and treatment. Better control of arthritis is possible, but cure is not yet available. Unfortunately, tabloids, books, media, and the Internet often report "curative" remedies. People spend billions of dollars each year on quackery, including liniments, special diets, and magnets. More hazardous substances such as snake oil and industrial cleaners are also advertised as remedies. Refer the patient to the Arthritis Foundation for up-to-date information about these "cures." The practice of wearing a copper bracelet will not cure arthritis, but it will not cause harm.

However, if the patient is using a potentially harmful substance or method, reinforce the need to avoid the unproven remedy and explain why it should not be used. Respect the patient's preferences, values, and beliefs for using benign remedies that do not cause harm.

With most types of arthritis, patients must live with a persistent, unpredictable, and painful disorder. Their roles, self-esteem, and body image may be affected by these diseases. Body image is usually not as devastating in OA as in the inflammatory arthritic diseases such as RA. The psychosocial component associated with having arthritis is discussed in more detail later in this chapter in the Rheumatoid Arthritis section.

Health Care Resources. The patient who has undergone surgery may need help from community resources. After an arthroplasty, the patient may need assistance with ***mobility.*** The patient may be discharged to home or an inpatient rehabilitation unit. Collaborate with the case manager and surgeon to determine the best placement. If the patient is discharged to home, home care nurses may be approved for third-party payment for several visits, depending on the presence of any existing systemic diseases. A home care aide may visit the home to help with hygiene-related needs, and a PT may work with ambulatory and ***mobility*** skills. For older patients, a family member, significant other, or other caregiver should be in the home for at least the first few weeks when the patient needs the most assistance. Emphasize the need for patient safety, especially interventions to prevent falls, as described in Chapter 4.

Provide written instructions about the required care, regardless of whether the patient goes home or to another inpatient facility. *As required by The Joint Commission's National Patient Safety Goals (NPSGs) and other health care accrediting organizations, hand-off communication with the new care provider is essential for seamless continuity of care and care coordination.*

The Arthritis Foundation (www.arthritis.org) is an important community resource for all patients with all types of arthritis.

This organization provides information to laypeople and health care professionals and refers patients and their families to other resources as needed. Local support groups can help them cope with these diseases.

Evaluate Outcomes: Evaluation

Evaluate the care of the patient with OA on the basis of the identified priority problems. The expected outcomes are that the patient:

- Achieves pain control to a pain intensity level of 2 to 3 on a scale of 0 to 10 or at a level that is acceptable to the patient
- Does not experience complications associated with total joint arthroplasty (if performed)
- Moves and functions in own environment independently with or without assistive devices

✴ IMMUNITY CONCEPT EXEMPLAR: RHEUMATOID ARTHRITIS

Pathophysiology Review

Rheumatoid arthritis (RA) is a chronic, progressive, systemic inflammatory autoimmune disease process that affects primarily the synovial joints. *Systemic* means that this disease can affect any or all parts of the body while affecting many joints.

In patients with RA, transformed autoantibodies (rheumatoid factors [RFs]) that attack healthy tissue, especially synovium, are formed, causing *inflammation.* The disease then begins to involve the articular cartilage, joint capsule, and surrounding ligaments and tendons. *Immunity* and inflammatory factors cause cartilage damage in patients with RA (Rogers, 2023):

- CD4 helper T cells and other immune cells in synovial fluid promote cytokine release, especially interleukin-1 (IL-1) and tumor necrosis factor–alpha (TNFA), which attack cartilage.
- Neutrophils and other inflammatory cells in the joint are activated and break down the cartilage.
- Immune complexes deposit in synovium, and osteoclasts are activated.
- B and T lymphocytes of the immune system are stimulated and increase the inflammatory response. (Also see Chapter 16 for a complete discussion of the inflammatory response.)

The synovium then thickens and becomes hyperemic, fluid accumulates in the joint space, and a pannus forms. The pannus is vascular granulation tissue composed of inflammatory cells; it erodes articular cartilage and eventually destroys bone. As a result, in late disease, fibrous adhesions, bony ankyloses (abnormal fusion of bones in the joint), and calcifications occur. Bone loses density, and secondary osteoporosis exists.

Permanent joint changes may be avoided if RA is diagnosed early. Early and aggressive treatment to suppress synovitis may lead to a remission. RA is a disease characterized by natural remissions and exacerbations (flare-ups). Interprofessional health care team management helps control the disease to decrease the intensity and number of exacerbations. Preventing flares helps prevent joint erosion and permanent joint damage.

Because RA is a systemic disease, areas of the body besides the synovial joints can be affected. Inflammatory responses similar to those occurring in synovial tissue may occur in any organ or body system in which connective tissue is prevalent. If blood vessel *inflammation* (vasculitis) occurs, the organ supplied by that vessel can be affected, leading to eventual failure of the organ or system in late disease.

Etiology and Genetic Risk

The etiology of RA remains unclear, but research suggests a *combination of environmental and genetic factors.* Some researchers also suspect that female reproductive hormones influence the development of RA because it affects women more often than men—usually young to middle-age women. Others suspect that infectious organisms may play a role, particularly the Epstein-Barr virus (Rogers, 2023). Physical and emotional stressors have been linked to exacerbations of the disorder and may be contributing factors or "triggers" to its development.

👤 PATIENT-CENTERED CARE: GENETICS/GENOMICS

Rheumatoid Arthritis and Immunity

Research has shown that there is a strong association between RA and several human leukocyte antigen (HLA)–*DR* alleles. The cause of this association is not clear, but most HLA diseases are autoimmune (Rogers, 2023). *DR* alleles, especially *DR4* and *DRB1*, are the primary genetic factors contributing to the development of RA. *DR4* is associated with more severe forms of the disease. Other contributing factors are being researched.

Incidence and Prevalence

RA affects over 1.5 million people, and Whites have the disease more often than other groups. Women are two to three times more likely to have RA compared with men (Rogers, 2023). The cause for these trends is not known.

👤 PATIENT-CENTERED CARE: HEALTH EQUITY

Health Disparities in Rheumatoid Arthritis

Research data over a 13-year period from 2005 to 2018 demonstrate that when compared to other groups, African Americans have a higher prevalence of rheumatoid arthritis, particularly those who have an educational level of less than high school and a low family income. The impact of these social determinants of health needs further research, but the stress of poverty may contribute to the risk for developing the disease (Xu & Wu, 2021). Assess patients for these factors and incorporate into their plan of care.

Interprofessional Collaborative Care
Recognize Cues: Assessment

The onset of rheumatoid arthritis (RA) may be acute and severe or slow and progressive; patients may have vague symptoms that last for several months before diagnosis. The onset of the disease is more common in the winter months than in the warmer months. The signs and symptoms of RA can be categorized as early or late disease and as joint (articular) or systemic (extraarticular), as briefly summarized in Box 43.7.

BOX 43.7   **Key Features**

The Patient With Rheumatoid Arthritis

Common Early Signs and Symptoms (Early Disease)	Common Late Signs and Symptoms (Advanced Disease)
Joint • Inflammation **Systemic** • Low-grade fever • Fatigue • Weakness • Anorexia • Paresthesias	**Joint** • Deformities (e.g., swan neck or ulnar deviation) • Moderate-to-severe **pain** and morning stiffness **Systemic** • Osteoporosis • Severe fatigue • Anemia • Weight loss • Muscle atrophy • Subcutaneous nodules • Peripheral neuropathy • Vasculitis • Pericarditis • Fibrotic lung disease • Sjögren syndrome • Kidney disease

Physical Assessment/Signs and Symptoms. In the *early* stage of RA the patient typically reports joint *inflammation,* generalized weakness, and fatigue. Anorexia, weight loss of about 2 to 3 lb (1 kg), and persistent low-grade fever are common. In patients with early disease, the upper-extremity joints are involved initially—often the proximal interphalangeal (PIP) and metacarpophalangeal (MCP) joints of the hands. These joints may be slightly reddened, warm, stiff, swollen, and tender or painful, particularly on palpation (caused by synovitis). The typical pattern of joint involvement in RA is bilateral and symmetric (e.g., both wrists). The number of joints involved usually increases as the disease progresses.

The presence of only *one* hot, swollen, painful joint (out of proportion to the other joints) may mean that the joint is infected. *Refer the patient to the primary health care provider (generally the rheumatologist) immediately if this is the case.* Single hot, swollen joints are considered infected until proven otherwise and require immediate long-term antibiotic treatment.

As the disease advances, the joints become progressively inflamed and very painful. The patient usually has frequent morning stiffness, which can last for several hours after awakening. On palpation the joints feel soft and look puffy because of synovitis and effusions. The fingers often appear spindlelike. Note any muscle atrophy (which can result from disuse secondary to joint pain) and a decreased range of motion in the affected joints.

Most or all synovial joints are eventually affected. The temporomandibular joint (TMJ) may be involved in severe disease, but such involvement is uncommon. When the TMJ is affected, the patient may have pain when chewing or opening the mouth.

When the spinal column is involved, the cervical joints are most likely to be affected. During clinical examination, gently palpate the posterior cervical spine and identify it as cervical pain, tenderness, or loss of motion.

✚ NURSING SAFETY PRIORITY

Critical Rescue

Cervical RA may result in subluxation, especially of the first and second vertebrae. This complication may be life-threatening because branches of the phrenic nerve that supply the diaphragm are restricted and respiratory function may be compromised. The patient is also in danger of becoming quadriparetic (weak in all extremities) or quadriplegic (paralyzed in all extremities). If cervical pain (may radiate down one arm) or loss of range of motion is present in the cervical spine, keep the neck straight in a neutral position to prevent permanent damage to the spinal cord or spinal nerves. *Notify the Rapid Response Team and primary health care provider immediately about these neurologic changes!*

Joint deformity occurs as a late articular manifestation, and secondary osteoporosis can cause bone fractures. Observe common deformities, especially in the hands and feet (Fig. 43.5). Extensive wrist involvement can result in carpal tunnel syndrome (see Chapter 44 for assessment and management of carpal tunnel syndrome).

Gently palpate the tissues around the joints to elicit pain or tenderness associated with other rheumatoid complications, unless the patient is having severe joint **pain.** For example, Baker cysts (enlarged popliteal bursae behind the knee) may occur and cause tissue compression and pain. Tendon rupture is also possible, particularly rupture of the Achilles tendon.

Numerous extraarticular signs and symptoms are associated with advanced disease. Assess the patient to ascertain systemic involvement. In addition to increased joint swelling and tenderness, *moderate to severe weight loss, fever,* and *extreme fatigue* are common in late disease exacerbations, often called *flare-ups.* Some patients have the characteristic soft, round, movable subcutaneous nodules, which usually appear on the ulnar surface of the arm, on the fingers, or along the Achilles tendon. These nodules can disappear and reappear at any time and are associated with severe, destructive disease. Rheumatoid nodules are usually not a problem themselves; however, they occasionally open and become infected and may interfere with ADLs. Accidentally bumping the nodules may cause discomfort. Occasionally nodules occur in the lungs.

Inflammation of the blood vessels results in vasculitis, particularly of small to medium-size vessels. When arterial involvement occurs, major organs can become ischemic and malfunction. Assess for ischemic skin lesions that appear in groups as small, brownish spots, most commonly around the nail bed. Monitor the number of lesions, note their location each day, and report vascular changes to the health care provider. Increased lesions indicate increased vasculitis, and a decreased number indicates decreased vasculitis. Also carefully assess any larger lesions that appear on the lower extremities. These lesions can lead to ulcerations, which heal slowly as a result of decreased circulation. Peripheral neuropathy associated with decreased

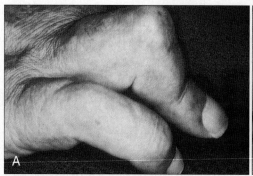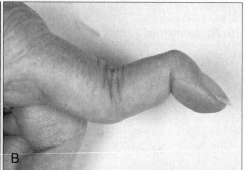

FIG. 43.5 Common joint deformities seen in rheumatoid arthritis. (A) Boutonniere deformity. (B) Swan neck deformity. (From Hochberg, M. C., Gravallese, E. M., Silman, A. J., et al. [2019]. *Rheumatology* [7th ed.]. Philadelphia: Elsevier.)

circulation can cause footdrop and paresthesias (burning and tingling sensations), usually in older adults.

Respiratory complications may manifest as *pleurisy, pneumonitis, diffuse interstitial fibrosis,* and *pulmonary hypertension.* Cardiac complications include *pericarditis* and *myocarditis.* These health problems are discussed elsewhere in this text. Assess for eye involvement, which typically manifests as *iritis* and *scleritis.* If either of these complications is present, the sclera of one or both eyes is reddened and the pupils have an irregular shape. Visual disturbances may occur.

Several syndromes are seen in patients with advanced RA. The most common is Sjögren syndrome, which includes a triad of:

- Dry eyes (keratoconjunctivitis sicca [KCS], or the sicca syndrome)
- Dry mouth (xerostomia)
- Dry vagina (in some cases)

Note the patient's report of dry mouth or dry eyes. Some patients state that their eyes feel "gritty," as if sand is in their eyes. Inspect the mouth for dry, sticky membranes and the eyes for redness/hyperpigmentation and lack of tearing.

Psychosocial Assessment. Rheumatoid arthritis (RA) and other inflammatory types of arthritis are chronic diseases that can be disabling if not well controlled. Fear of becoming dependent, uncertainty about the disease process, altered body image, devaluation of self, frustration, and depression are common psychosocial problems. Physical limitations and persistent **pain** may limit the patient's **mobility.** These limitations can result in role changes in the family and society. For example, the person may be unable to cook for the family or be an active sexual partner. In addition, extreme fatigue often causes patients to desire an early bedtime and napping, and may result in a reluctance to socialize.

Body changes caused by joint changes and drug therapy (if used) may also cause poor self-esteem and body image. Because many societies value people with physically fit, attractive bodies, the patient with RA may be embarrassed to be seen in public places. The patient may grieve or experience degrees of depression. The patient may have feelings of helplessness caused by a loss of control over a disease that can "consume" the body. Fortunately, newer drugs have improved the treatment of RA and provide the patient with hope and better disease control. Only a small percentage of patients with RA become wheelchair dependent.

Living with a chronic disease and its associated **pain** is difficult for the patient and family. Chronic suffering and pain affect quality of life. Assess the patient's emotional and mental status in relation to the disease and its problems. Evaluate the patient's support systems and resources. Patients who are knowledgeable about their disease and treatment options feel emotionally stronger to cope with their disease and better able to discuss treatment options with their primary health care provider.

Laboratory Assessment. Laboratory tests help support a diagnosis of RA, but no single test or group of tests can confirm it. The test for *rheumatoid factor (RF)* measures the presence of unusual antibodies of the immunoglobulins G (IgG) and M (IgM) types that develop in a number of connective tissue diseases. Many patients with RA have a positive titer (greater than 1:80), *especially in older adults* (Pagana et al., 2022). However, the presence of RF is not diagnostic for RA.

One of the newest laboratory tests, used to detect the level of *anti–cyclic citrullinated peptide (anti-CCP),* is very specific and sensitive in detecting early RA. The presence of anti-CCP is also a marker for aggressive and erosive late-stage disease.

The *antinuclear antibody (ANA)* test measures the titer of a group of antibodies that destroy the nuclei of cells and cause tissue death in patients with autoimmune disease. The fluorescent method is sometimes referred to as *FANA.* If this test result is positive (a value higher than 1:40), various subtypes of this antibody are identified and measured.

An elevated *erythrocyte sedimentation rate (ESR),* or "sed rate," (greater than 20 mm/hr) can confirm **inflammation** or infection anywhere in the body. An elevated ESR helps support a diagnosis of an unspecified inflammatory disease. The test is most useful to monitor the course of a disease, especially for inflammatory autoimmune diseases. In general the more severe the disease gets, the higher the ESR rises; as the disease improves or goes into remission, the ESR level decreases.

Measurement of the *high-sensitivity C-reactive protein,* or *hsCRP,* is another useful test to measure **inflammation** and may be done with or instead of the ESR. As the name implies, it is more sensitive to inflammatory changes than the ESR. It is also very useful for detecting infection anywhere in the body.

The presence of most chronic diseases usually causes mild to moderate anemia, which contributes to the patient's fatigue. Therefore, monitor the patient's complete blood count (CBC) for a low hemoglobin, hematocrit, and red blood cell (RBC) count. An increase in white blood cell (WBC) count is consistent with an inflammatory response. A decrease in the WBC count may indicate Felty syndrome, a pulmonary complication associated with late RA (Rogers, 2023). Thrombocytosis (increased platelets) can also occur in patients with late RA. Additional laboratory tests may be performed, depending on the body systems and organs that may be affected by the disease. For example, if heart involvement is suspected, the primary health care provider may request cardiac enzyme testing.

Other Diagnostic Assessment. A standard x-ray is used to visualize the joint changes and deformities typical of RA. A CT scan may help determine the presence and degree of cervical spine involvement.

An arthrocentesis is an invasive diagnostic procedure that may be used for patients with joint swelling caused by excess synovial fluid (effusion). It may be performed at the bedside or in a health care provider's office or clinic. After administering a local anesthetic, the provider inserts a large-gauge needle into the joint (usually the knee) to aspirate a sample of synovial fluid and to relieve pressure caused by excess fluid. The fluid is analyzed for inflammatory cells and immune complexes, including RF. Fluid from patients with RA typically reveals increased WBCs, cloudiness, and volume.

Teach the patient to use ice and to rest the affected joint for 24 hours after arthrocentesis. Often the primary health care provider will recommend acetaminophen as needed for discomfort. If increased pain or swelling occurs, teach the patient or family to notify the primary health care provider immediately.

MRI may be performed to assess spinal column disease or other joint involvement. Because RA can affect multiple body systems, tests to diagnose specific systemic manifestations are performed as needed. For example, nerve conduction studies help confirm peripheral neuropathy. Pulmonary function tests help determine the presence of lung involvement.

NCLEX Examination Challenge 43.4
Physiological Integrity

The nurse is caring for a client who has severe advanced rheumatoid arthritis who is admitted to the Urgent Care Center for upper respiratory symptoms, including a nagging cough. Which of the following assessment findings would the nurse expect that are related to the client's arthritis? **Select all that apply.**

A. Low-grade fever
B. Hand joint deformities
C. Report of severe fatigue
D. Inflamed wrist and ankle joints
E. Morning stiffness

Analyze Cues and Prioritize Hypotheses: Analysis

The priority collaborative problems for patients with rheumatoid arthritis (RA) include:

1. Chronic *inflammation* and persistent *pain* due to systemic autoimmune disease process

2. Potential for decreased *mobility* due to joint deformity, muscle atrophy, and fatigue
3. Potential for decreased self-esteem image due to joint deformity

Generate Solutions and Take Actions: Planning and Implementation

Patients who have RA are managed in the community under the supervision of a qualified primary health care provider. The expected outcome for management is that the disease goes into remission and its progression slows to decrease *pain,* prevent joint destruction, and increase *mobility.* When patients with RA are admitted to the inpatient acute care or long-term care facility, it is usually for health problems other than for complications of arthritis. Whether the patient is in a facility or community, be sure to plan interventions to manage persistent *pain* and *inflammation*, as well as the potential for decreased *mobility* and decreased self-esteem.

Managing Chronic Inflammation and Pain

Planning: Expected Outcomes. The patient with RA is expected to have a *pain* level that is acceptable to the patient (e.g., at a 2–3 on a pain intensity scale of 0 to 10). A major focus of pain management is drug therapy to modify or prevent the progression of the disease, thereby decreasing joint and systemic *inflammation.*

Interventions. As in other types of arthritis, the interprofessional health care team manages *pain* by using a combination of pharmacologic and nonpharmacologic measures. Total joint arthroplasty (TJA) may be indicated when other measures fail to relieve pain. TJA is discussed in the Osteoarthritis section of this chapter.

Drug Therapy. Some drugs prescribed for RA have antiinflammatory and/or analgesic actions. For example, NSAIDs are sometimes used for early RA to help decrease *pain* and *inflammation.* The choice of which one to prescribe depends on the patient's needs and tolerance and the scientific evidence supporting the drug therapy. To decrease GI problems, the NSAID may be given with an H_2-blocking agent such as famotidine. If there is no clinical change after 6 to 8 weeks, the primary health care provider may discontinue the current NSAID and try another one or change to a different drug class.

Other drugs affect *immunity* through immunosuppression, thus modifying the progress of the disease to reduce *pain* and inflammation. Initially most patients are managed with *disease-modifying antirheumatic drugs (DMARDs).* As the name implies, these drugs are given to slow the progression of the disease. For best results, they should be started early in the disease process.

First-line disease-modifying antirheumatic drugs. Methotrexate *(MTX),* an immunosuppressive medication, in a low once-a-week dose is the mainstay of therapy for RA because it is effective and relatively inexpensive. It is a slow-acting drug, taking 4 to 6 weeks to begin to control joint *inflammation* (Burchum & Rosenthal, 2022). Observe for desired therapeutic drug effects, such as a decrease in joint *pain* and swelling.

Monitor patients for potential adverse effects, such as decreases in WBCs or platelets (as a result of bone marrow suppression) or elevations in liver enzymes or serum creatinine.

NURSING SAFETY PRIORITY
Drug Alert

Patients taking MTX are at risk for infection caused by impaired or decreased drug-induced *immunity.* Teach them to avoid crowds and people who are ill. Remind patients to avoid alcoholic beverages while taking MTX to prevent liver toxicity. Teach them to observe and report other side and toxic effects, which include mouth sores and acute dyspnea from pneumonitis. Although not commonly occurring, lymph node tumor (lymphoma) and pneumonitis (lung *inflammation*) have been associated in those who have RA and are taking MTX. Folic acid, one of the B vitamins, is often given to those who are taking MTX to help decrease some of the drug's side effects (Burchum & Rosenthal, 2022).

NURSING SAFETY PRIORITY
Drug Alert

The most serious adverse effect of hydroxychloroquine is retinal damage. Teach patients to report blurred vision or headache. Remind them to have an eye examination before taking the drug and then every 6 months afterward to detect changes in the cornea, lens, or retina. If this rare complication occurs, the primary health care provider discontinues the drug (Burchum & Rosenthal, 2022).

Pregnancy is not recommended while taking methotrexate because birth defects are possible. *Strict birth control is recommended for childbearing women who are in need of MTX to control their RA.* If pregnancy is ever desired, instruct the patient to consult the rheumatologist and an obstetric/gynecologic (OB/GYN) health care provider. Generally, the primary health care provider discontinues the drug at least 3 months before planned pregnancy. MTX may be restarted after birth if the patient does not breast-feed (Burchum & Rosenthal, 2022).

Another DMARD sometimes used for RA is *hydroxychloroquine.* This drug slows the progression of mild rheumatoid disease before it worsens. It is an antimalarial drug that helps suppress the immune response to decrease joint and muscle *pain.* Patients generally tolerate hydroxychloroquine quite well. In a few cases mild stomach discomfort, light-headedness, or headache has been reported. The drug should not be used for patients who have known cardiac disease or dysrhythmias (Burchum & Rosenthal, 2022).

Biological response modifiers. As a group, *biological response modifiers (BRMs),* sometimes called *biologics,* are one of the newest and most effective classes of DMARDs and include interleukins, tumor necrosis factor (TNF) inhibitors, and monoclonal antibodies (Table 43.2). Any one of the BRMs may be tried. If one drug is not effective, the primary health care provider prescribes another drug in the same class. All these drugs are expensive, and insurance companies may not completely pay for their use.

Teach patients receiving any one of the BRMs that they are at a high risk for developing impaired *immunity* and subsequent infection. Instruct them to stay away from people with infections and to avoid large crowds if possible. Remind patients with multiple sclerosis (MS), tuberculosis (TB), or a positive TB test that they should not receive BRMs because they make patients susceptible to flare-ups of these diseases. Determine whether the patient has had a recent negative purified protein derivative (PPD) test for TB. If not, a PPD skin test is typically administered and the selected BRM is not started until a negative test result is confirmed (Burchum & Rosenthal, 2022). Collaborate with the primary health care provider to ensure that this process is complete. Most of these drugs are given parenterally and require health teaching for self-administration.

Other drugs. The newest classification of DMARDs is the *Janus kinase (JAK)-inhibiting drugs,* often called *JAK inhibitors.* Like other BRMs, these drugs have been approved for

TABLE 43.2 Common Examples of Drug Therapy
Disease-Modifying Antirheumatic Drugs

Drug Category	Selected Nursing Implications
Tumor Necrosis Factor (TNF) Inhibitor Examples of TNF inhibitors: • Etanercept • Infliximab • Golimumab	• For etanercept, teach patient to report injection site reaction, *which may indicate a local allergic response and cause pain.* • Teach patients to report signs and symptoms of infection.
Interleukin (IL)-6 Receptor Antagonist Examples of IL-6 receptor antagonists: • Anakinra • Tocilizumab	• Monitor the WBC count of patients receiving any of these drugs, *which can cause a marked decrease, making patients susceptible to infection.* • Monitor liver enzymes *because drugs can cause liver dysfunction.*
Janus Kinase (JAK) Inhibitor Examples of JAK inhibitors: • Tofacitinib • Baricitinib • Upadacitinib	• Be aware that tofacitinib has a black box warning about the increased risk of cardiac events, cancer, and blood clots when taking this drug. • Teach patients to report signs and symptoms of infection.

other types of arthritis and autoimmune disorders (see Table 43.2).

A few drugs may be given in combination with or instead of the previously described drugs. It is not unusual for a patient to be taking several disease-modifying drugs, such as methotrexate, a BRM, and an adjunct medication. Each drug works differently to relieve symptoms and slow the progression of the disease. For example, sulfasalazine, a sulfa drug, may be given in combination with other drugs to reduce inflammation and pain. Be aware that this drug should not be used for patients who have a sulfa allergy. Common side effects of sulfasalazine include nausea, vomiting, and skin rash (Burchum & Rosenthal, 2022).

Glucocorticoids (steroids)—usually prednisone—may be given for their fast-acting antiinflammatory and immunosuppressive effects. Prednisone may be given in high dose for short duration (pulse therapy) or as a low chronic dose. Moderate-dose short-term tapering bridge therapy may be used when inflammation is symptomatic and other RA medications are insufficient or have not yet had an effect.

Chronic steroid therapy can result in numerous complications, such as:

- Diabetes mellitus
- Impaired or decreased *immunity*
- Fluid and electrolyte imbalances
- Hypertension
- Osteoporosis
- Glaucoma

Some drug effects are dose related, whereas others are not. Observe the patient for complications associated with chronic steroid therapy, and report them to the primary health care provider. For example, if blood pressure becomes elevated or significant laboratory values change, notify the primary health care provider.

Patients with RA may experience one or a few joints that have more *pain* and *inflammation* than the others. Cortisone injections in single joints may be used to temporarily relieve local *pain* and *inflammation*. Have the patient ice and rest the joint for 24 hours after the procedure. Oral analgesics are also sometimes needed during that time.

Nonpharmacologic Interventions. Adequate rest, proper positioning, and ice and heat applications are important in pain management. If acute *inflammation* is present, ice packs may be applied to "hot" joints for pain relief until the inflammation lessens. The ice pack should not be too heavy. At home the patient can use a small bag of frozen peas or corn as an ice pack.

Heated paraffin (wax) dips may help increase comfort of arthritic hands. Finger and hand exercises are often done more easily after paraffin treatment. To relieve morning stiffness or the pain of late-stage disease, recommend a hot shower rather than a sponge bath or a tub bath. It is often difficult for the patient with RA to get into and out of a bathtub, although special hydraulic lifts, tub chairs, and walk-in bathtubs are available to facilitate bathing. Safety (grab) bars and nonskid tread in the tub or shower floor are important safety features

to discuss with all patients. Some older adults prefer using shower chairs and a walk-in shower that does not have a ledge that could cause falls.

Hot packs applied directly to involved joints may be beneficial if they are not too heavy. Most physical therapy departments have machines that keep hot packs ready for when they are needed. Teach patients to use the microwave or stovetop heating instructions to warm heat packs at home. Remind them to follow the instructions given with each heating device used.

Plasmapheresis (sometimes called *plasma exchange*) is an in-hospital procedure prescribed by a primary health care provider in which the patient's plasma is treated to remove the antibodies causing the disease. Although not commonly done, this procedure may be combined with steroid pulse therapy for patients with severe, life-threatening disease.

Complementary and Integrative Health. Some patients may have **pain** relief from hypnosis, acupuncture, imagery, music therapy, or other techniques. Stress management is also popular as a pain relief intervention. Chapter 6 discusses these therapies in more detail.

Adequate nutrition is an important part of the management of RA. Obesity should be avoided or treated if present. The inflammatory state may place a greater burden on the metabolism of some essential nutrients. This catabolic state may be related to increased cytokine production, specifically tumor necrosis factor.

According to the Arthritis Foundation (2023), no one food causes or cures arthritis; however, healthy nutrition in general is important. Refer patients to the Arthritis Foundation's publications regarding diet and arthritis. Teach patients to take any herbal or nutrition supplement under the supervision of a qualified health care provider to prevent adverse events and drug-food or drug-drug interactions.

Other integrative therapies are safe and have been scientifically proven to be effective to help control RA **pain** for most people. Examples include mind-body therapies, such as relaxation techniques, imagery, and spiritual practices. For information about these techniques, see Chapter 6.

Promoting Mobility

Planning: Expected Outcomes. Patients with RA often have decreased *mobility* related to multiple joint deformities and muscle atrophy. Fatigue and generalized weakness also contribute to decreased mobility. The expected outcome is that the patient will be able to independently perform ADLs with or without ambulatory and assistive devices.

Interventions. Although the physical appearance of a patient with severe RA may create the image that ADL independence is not possible, a number of alternative and creative methods can be used to perform these activities. *Do not perform these activities for the patient unless asked. Those with RA do not want to be dependent.* For example, hand deformities often prevent a patient from opening packages of food such as a box of crackers; however, the patient may prefer to use the teeth to open the crackers rather than depend on someone else.

In the hospital or long-term care facility, a patient may not eat because of the barriers of heavy plate covers, milk cartons, small packages of condiments, and heavy containers. Styrofoam or paper cups may bend and collapse as the patient attempts to hold them. A china or heavy plastic cup with handles may be easier to manipulate. Collaborate with the registered dietitian nutritionist to help with access to food and total independence in eating.

INTERPROFESSIONAL COLLABORATION

Care of Patients With Rheumatoid Arthritis

Even though many patients with severe or late-stage rheumatoid arthritis (RA) often adapt to their pain and deformity, they may still need assistance with ADLs. For example, when fine motor activities (e.g., squeezing a tube of toothpaste) become impossible, patients often use larger joints or body surfaces that can substitute for smaller ones. Devices such as long-handled brushes can help patients brush their hair; dressing sticks can assist with putting on pants. Consult with OT to help patients learn to function as independently as possible. According to the Interprofessional Education Collaborative (IPEC) Expert Panel's Competency of Roles and Responsibilities, using the unique and complementary abilities of health care team members can optimize clinical outcomes (IPEC, 2016; Slusser et al., 2019).

Additional nursing interventions depend in part on identifying the factors contributing to fatigue. For example, persistent **pain,** sleep disturbances, and weakness are associated with increased fatigue. Anemia may also be a contributing factor and may be treated with iron (if an iron deficiency anemia is present), folic acid, or vitamin supplements prescribed by the primary health care provider. Chronic normochromic or chronic hypochromic anemia often occurs in most chronic systemic diseases. Assess for drug-related blood loss such as that caused by NSAIDs by checking the stool for gross or occult blood. *Older white women are the most likely to experience GI bleeding as a result of taking these medications* (Burchum & Rosenthal, 2022).

If fatigue and decreased **mobility** result from muscle atrophy, the primary health care provider prescribes an aggressive physical therapy program to strengthen muscles and prevent further atrophy. Patients also experience increased fatigue when **pain** prevents them from getting adequate rest and sleep. Measures to facilitate sleep include promoting a quiet environment, giving warm beverages, and administering hypnotics or relaxants as prescribed if necessary.

In addition to identifying and managing specific reasons for fatigue, determine the patient's usual daily activities and teach principles of *energy conservation.* Box 43.8 provides specific suggestions for conserving energy and thus increasing activity tolerance and **mobility.**

Enhancing Self-Esteem

Planning: Expected Outcome. The patient with RA often has multiple joints that are inflamed or deformed, causing a potential for decreased self-esteem. Therefore,

---

BOX 43.8   Patient and Family Education
Energy Conservation for the Patient With Arthritis

- Balance activity with rest. Take one or two naps each day.
- Pace yourself; do not plan too much for one day.
- Set priorities. Determine which activities are most important and do them first.
- Delegate responsibilities and tasks to your family and friends.
- Plan ahead to prevent last-minute rushing and stress.
- Learn your own activity tolerance and do not exceed it.

the expected outcome is that the patient will verbalize a positive perception of self as a result of interprofessional interventions.

Interventions. Body image and self-esteem may be affected by the disease process. Determine the patient's perception of these changes and the impact of the reactions of family and significant others. The most important intervention is to communicate acceptance of the patient. When a trusting relationship is established, encourage the patient to express personal feelings.

As a reaction to body changes and joint deformity and the presence of a chronic, painful disease, some patients display behaviors indicative of loss. They may use coping strategies that range from denial or fear to anger or depression. In an attempt to regain control over the effects of the disease process, they may appear to be "manipulative and demanding" and sometimes may be referred to as having an "arthritis personality." *This personality, which represents a negative label, is a myth; avoid using these terms.* Patients are trying to cope with the effects of their illness and should be treated with patience and understanding. Continually assess and accept these behaviors, but remain realistic in discussing goals to improve self-esteem and body image. Emphasize their strengths and help them identify previously successful coping strategies. If needed, consult with mental health professionals or religious/spiritual leaders to help patients cope with this potentially debilitating chronic disease.

Care Coordination and Transition Management

Patients with rheumatoid arthritis (RA) are usually managed at home, but in some cases they may be institutionalized in a long-term care facility if they become restricted to bed or a wheelchair. Some patients may be transferred to a rehabilitation facility for several weeks to help develop strategies, techniques, and skills for independent living at home. Chapter 7 discusses the rehabilitation process in detail. Keep in mind that patients with RA can become physically disabled. Box 43.5 provides considerations for caring for patients who are physical disabled by arthritis in any health setting.

Home Care Management. The amount of home care preparation depends on the severity of the disease. Structural changes may be necessary if there are deficits in performing ADLs or **mobility.** Doors must be wide enough to accommodate

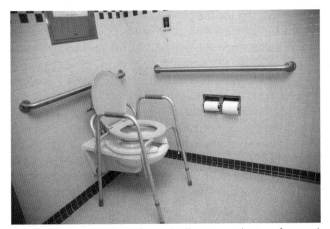

FIG. 43.6 Handrails and an elevated toilet seat make transfers easier and safer for the patient.

a wheelchair or walker if one is used. Ramps are needed to prevent the patient in a wheelchair from becoming homebound. If the person cannot use stairs, access to facilities for all ADLs on one floor is needed. Handrails should be available in the bathroom and halls.

To promote continued homemaking functions, countertops and appliances may require structural changes. The patient may also require handrails and elevated chairs and toilet seats, which facilitate safe transfers (Fig. 43.6). *These devices are especially important for older adults with arthritis.*

Self-Management Education. Self-management education (SME) is a vital role for nurses in collaborative management of arthritis. Many people have signs and symptoms of joint *inflammation* but do not seek medical attention. Teach them to seek professional health care to reduce *pain* and prevent disability.

Teach patients to discuss any questions with their primary health care provider before trying any over-the-counter or home remedies. Some remedies may be harmful. Check with the Arthritis Foundation for the latest information on arthritis myths and quackery (www.arthritis.org).

Provide information to the patient and family about drug therapy, joint protection, energy conservation, rest, and exercise as summarized in the boxes presented earlier in the RA section.

Assess the patient's coping strategies. The patient with RA often reports being on an "emotional roller coaster" from coping with a chronic illness every day. Control over one's life is an important human need. The patient with an unpredictable chronic disease may lose this control, and this lowers self-esteem. Health care providers must allow the patient to make decisions about care. Families and significant others must also include the patient in decision making. Although the patient's behavior may be perceived as demanding or manipulative, self-esteem cannot be improved without this important aspect of interpersonal relationships.

Increased dependency also affects a sense of control and self-esteem. Some people ignore their health needs and portray

a tough image for others by insisting that they need no assistance. Emphasize to the patient and family that asking for help may be the best decision at times to prevent further joint damage and disease progression.

RA may also affect work and social roles. The patient may have physical difficulty doing tasks that require lifting, climbing, grasp, or gross motor or fine motor activities. The severity of RA disease may cause difficulty with the total number of hours worked. Some people with RA can do their jobs well without problem; others may have varying degrees of difficulty. Those who can no longer do their jobs may need to discuss the possibility of a lighter workload with their employers; others may need to file for disability with their company and the U.S. Social Security Administration.

Health Care Resources. The need for health care resources for the patient with RA is often similar to that for the patient with osteoarthritis. A home care nurse or aide, physical therapist, or occupational therapist may be needed during severe exacerbations or as the disease progresses. In collaboration with the case manager, identify these resources, and make sure that they are available as needed. The Arthritis Foundation is an excellent source of information and support.

Arthritis support groups and self-help courses provide the education and support that patients, families, and friends need. Refer the patient to a psychological counselor or religious or spiritual leader for emotional support and guidance during times of crisis or as needed. Identify and recommend other support systems within the family and community when necessary.

Patients who have severe advanced RA often develop depression, anxiety, excessive stress, and a poor quality of life as a result of pain and deformity. Many patients also have anorexia and dyspnea, which could be best managed by palliative care providers. Refer patients and their families to a local palliative care program for symptom management to improve quality of life.

Evaluate Outcomes: Evaluation

Evaluate the care of the patient with RA on the basis of the identified priority problems. The expected outcomes are that the patient:

- Achieves *pain* control to a pain intensity level of 2 to 3 or less on a scale of 0 to 10 or at a level that is acceptable to the patient
- Moves and functions in own environment independently with or without assistive devices
- Verbalizes increased self-esteem and positive perception of self

GOUT

Primary gout is the most common inflammatory disease that can cause arthritis and systemic complications, such as kidney disease, if not treated. However, most patients seek treatment for painful arthritis, which can prevent further symptoms and control disease progression.

Pathophysiology Review

Gout is the body's inflammatory response to a large amount of uric acid (a result of purine metabolism) in the blood (hyperuricemia) and other body fluids. Purine is a by-product of certain proteins. When the concentration of serum uric acid is above 6.8 mg/dL, it deposits as urate crystals in connective tissues, including the synovial fluid of joints. If hyperuricemia is not treated, over time the patient can develop gouty arthritis and possibly urate deposits under the skin called *tophi*. Factors that contribute to the development of gout include gender and age (usually men over 50 years of age), genetic predisposition, chronic alcohol consumption, obesity, and diuretic therapy, especially thiazides (Rogers, 2023). Secondary gout occurs more commonly in women as a result of thiazide therapy.

Interprofessional Collaborative Care

Recognize Cues: Assessment

The symptoms of gout and gouty arthritis depend on the phase of disease progression (Rogers, 2023).

- Phase 1. Asymptomatic hyperuricemia: The patient has an elevated uric acid level but no arthritic or kidney symptoms. Some patients never progress beyond this phase of the disease.
- Phase 2. Acute gouty arthritis: In this phase of the disease, the patient has an acute "attack" in one single joint, often the metatarsal joint of the great toe. The patient reports severe or excruciating pain in the inflamed joint. Pain and inflammation may last from several hours to several days and then may resolve without treatment. These episodes may occur over months to years, especially when triggered by alcohol, high protein intake, or certain drugs. After having multiple gouty attacks, the patient is considered to have chronic gout.
- Phase 3. Tophaceous arthritis. Over many years without adequate management, the patient may experience the development of tophi, kidney stones, and kidney disease. Due to the effectiveness of currently used drugs, few patients today progress to this phase of gout.

Take Actions: Interventions

The goal of treatment for patients diagnosed with gout is to maintain their serum uric acid level to less than 6 mg/dL. Drug therapy is the major treatment modality used to meet this goal.

Drug therapy for the patient who is diagnosed with gout depends on the phase of the disease. The diagnosis of gout is often made when the patient has the first acute arthritic episode, or *acute* gouty arthritis. If the patient seeks medical treatment, the drugs of choice for an acute gout episode are either an NSAID, steroid, or colchicine. *Colchicine* works by inhibiting the migration of leukocytes to the inflamed joint to decrease inflammation. However, it does not affect uric acid level or prevent additional attacks. Teach the patient that GI distress may occur, including diarrhea, abdominal pain, nausea, and vomiting. Remind the patient to take the drug with food to help minimize these potential side effects (Burchum & Rosenthal, 2022).

To decrease a patient's uric acid level, the patient may be prescribed a *uricosuric drug* such as probenecid to excrete excess uric acid via the kidneys. Probenecid can be safely administered with colchicine.

For chronic gout, some patients take a uric acid biosynthesis inhibitor, also known as a xanthine oxidase inhibitor, such as allopurinol or febuxostat. These drugs work to reduce the production of uric acid in the body. Although febuxostat is the newest in this drug class, it has a greater risk for patients to experience an adverse cardiovascular event (Burchum & Rosenthal, 2022).

When none of these drugs work to manage a patient's severe chronic gout, pegloticase may be prescribed. This drug is administered every two weeks by intravenous infusion under medical supervision. Each dose should be infused slowly over no less than two hours (Burchum & Rosenthal, 2022).

To help prevent a gouty arthritic attack or flare-up, teach patients the importance of avoiding or limiting substances that can trigger an attack, including:

- Red meat such as ground beef
- Organ meats such as liver
- Shellfish such as shrimp
- Alcohol, especially beer

In addition, review the patient's drug profile to identify any medications that could cause a gouty arthritic attack, such as a thiazide diuretic. If the patient is obese, collaborate with the registered dietitian nutritionist for a referral to a community weight-loss program.

GET READY FOR THE NEXT-GENERATION NCLEX® EXAMINATION!

Essential Nursing Care Points

Health Promotion/Disease Prevention

- The *Healthy People 2030* initiative recognizes the need for national attention to help reduce and better manage arthritis, including the need to reduce the number of adults who have moderate or severe pain that limits their work and other activities.
- Nurses need to teach patients to maintain proper nutrition to prevent obesity, a risk factor for both osteoarthritis and gout.
- Nurses need to teach patients who have gout to avoid or limit red or organ meats, shellfish, and alcohol.
- Practicing joint protection and energy conservation techniques are essential as part of managing rheumatoid arthritis.

Chronic Disease Care

- Chronic arthritis is a major cause of physical disability in adult patients, especially among older adults.
- **Osteoarthritis (OA)** is the progressive deterioration and loss of articular cartilage, bone, and other connective tissues in one or more joints.
- The priority problem for patients who have OA is persistent joint *pain,* which can limit *mobility* and the ability to perform ADLs independently.
- The primary health care provider typically prescribes acetaminophen or topical agents such as diclofenac 1% gel to relieve local joint pain in one or more synovial joints; NSAIDs may be used if these first-line drugs are ineffective at reducing pain.
- **Rheumatoid arthritis (RA)** is a chronic, progressive, systemic inflammatory autoimmune disease that affects primarily synovial joints.
- Disease-modifying antirheumatic drugs (DMARDs) are the mainstay of drug therapy for RA because they slow the progression of the disease process; methotrexate is the first-line drug used because it is very effective.
- Biological response modifiers are immunomodulating drugs used alone or in combination with other drugs to slow the RA disease process (see Table 43.2).
- **Gout** is the body's inflammatory response to a large amount of uric acid (a result of purine metabolism) in the blood (hyperuricemia) and other body fluids.

Regenerative or Restorative Care

- **Total joint arthroplasty** is a surgical procedure used most often to manage pain of OA and improve *mobility*.
- Formal preoperative teaching using an interprofessional approach results in optimal postoperative patient outcomes.
- For patients not at risk for delirium, Enhanced Recovery After Surgery (ERAS) programs improve postoperative outcomes for patients having a total hip arthroplasty (THA) or total knee arthroplasty (TKA).
- For patients who undergo a posterolateral or direct lateral surgical approach for THA, nurses need to ensure that patients keep their legs apart, using several pillows or a special abduction pillow or splint.
- Neurovascular status should be carefully monitored in the operative leg for patients who undergo a THA or TKA.
- The most potentially life-threatening postoperative complication of a THA or TKA is venous thromboembolism (VTE); evidence-based postoperative interventions to help prevent VTE include pharmacology (anticoagulants), early ambulation, and compression with stockings or devices.
- Patients who undergo a THA or TKA require 6 weeks or more of rehabilitative therapy.

Hospice/Palliative/Supportive Care

- Patients who have severe advanced RA often develop depression, anxiety, excessive stress, and a poor quality of life as a result of and deformity.
- Patients who have total hip or knee arthroplasty require acute rehabilitation after hospital discharge in either an inpatient or community setting. Some patients may qualify for home rehabilitation therapy.
- Refer patients who have advanced RA disease and their families to a local palliative care program for symptom management to improve quality of life.

Mastery Questions

1. The nurse is assessing a client who was recently diagnosed with osteoarthritis in multiple joints. Which of the following assessment findings would the nurse expect this client might have? **Select all that apply.**
   A. Subcutaneous nodules
   B. Hot, swollen joints
   C. Knee effusions
   D. Joint pain
   E. Anemia

2. The nurse is teaching a client who has moderate pain due to rheumatoid arthritis. Which statement by the client indicates a **need for further teaching** about how to protect affected joints?
   A. "I should use large joints instead of smaller ones whenever possible."
   B. "I plan to use those rubber grips to help me open jars or bottles."
   C. "I need to get some long-handled devices to help me dress and brush my hair."
   D. "I will use my recliner more so that I can put my feet up to decrease joint swelling."

3. The nurse is teaching a client who is starting on etanercept for rheumatoid arthritis. Which statement would the nurse **include** in the teaching?
   A. "Be sure to take this drug with food to prevent GI distress such as nausea and vomiting."
   B. "You will be monitored carefully because this drug can cause an adverse cardiac event."
   C. "Be sure to report any symptoms of possible infection to your primary health care provider."
   D. "You will need to have your liver enzymes monitored frequently to detect any damage."

NGN Challenge 43.1

The nurse reviews recent vital signs and lab results for a 72-year-old client who has been receiving infliximab for rheumatoid arthritis for the past 2 years.

History and Physical	Vital Signs	Nurses' Notes	Laboratory Results
Today	**0400**	**1200**	**2000**
Temperature	99.8°F (37.7°C)	100.4°F (38°C)	100.8°F (38.2°C)
Heart Rate	84 beats/min	87 beats/min	90 beats/min
Respiratory Rate	16 breaths/min	18 breaths/min	20 breaths/min
Blood Pressure	128/72 mm Hg	124/70 mm Hg	116/64 mm Hg
SpO_2 (RA)	96%	97%	95%

History and Physical	Laboratory Results	Nurses' Notes	Vital Signs	
Laboratory Test	**Results 2 Days Ago**	**Results Yesterday**	**Results Today**	**Reference Range**
White Blood Cell (WBC) Count	10,500/mm^3 (10.5 × 10^9/L)	12,000/mm^3 (12 × 10^9/L)	14,700/mm^3 (14.7 × 10^9/L)	5000–10,000/mm^3 (5.0–10.0 × 10^9/L)
Blood Urea Nitrogen (BUN)	22 mg/dL (7.86 mmol/L)	28 mg/dL (10 mmol/L)	31 mg/dL (11.07 mmol/L)	10–20 mg/dL (2.9–8.2 mmol/L)
Potassium (K)	4.8 mEq/L (4.8 mmol/L)	4.9 mEq/L (4.9 mmol/L)	4.9 mEq/L (4.9 mmol/L)	3.5–5.0 mEq/L (3.5–5.0 mmol/L)
Sodium (Na)	146 mEq/L (146 mmol/L)	148 mEq/L (148 mmol/L)	150 mEq/L (150 mmol/L)	136–145 mEq/L (136–145 mmol/L)

Complete the following sentence by selecting from the lists of options below.

The client's *priority* condition is most likely **1 [Select]** as evidenced by the client's **2 [Select]** and **3 [Select]**.

Options for 1	Options for 2	Options for 3
Hypotension	Low SpO_2	Fever
Acute kidney injury	Elevated BUN	Tachycardia
Infection	Elevated sodium	Tachypneic
Dehydration	Elevated WBC count	Low blood pressure

NGN Challenge 43.2

The nurse is caring for a 65-year-old client who had a left total knee arthroplasty 2 days ago.

History and Physical	Nurses' Notes	Imaging Studies	Laboratory Results

0615: States was ambulating in hallway with walker at 0430 because of sharp pain in operative leg that started last evening and made the client awaken early this morning. Posterior left calf reddened and slightly swollen; tender and warm when lightly touched. Pedal pulses present and equal. Cap refill <3 sec in both feet. Client in bed at present with left leg elevated on two pillows; instructed to stay in bed until surgeon visit in the next hour. Saline lock remains in place in left forearm. Current VS: T 99.2°F (37.3°C), HR 82 beats/min, RR 18 breaths/min, BP 120/66 mm Hg.

Complete the diagram by selecting from the choices below to specify which potential condition the client is most likely experiencing, **2** nursing actions that are appropriate to take, and **2** parameters the nurse should monitor to assess the client's progress.

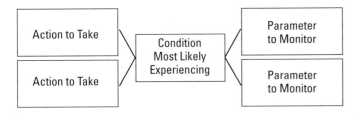

Actions to Take	Potential Conditions	Parameters to Monitor
Compare measurements of both leg calves	Infection	Presence of chest pain
Obtain blood cultures per agency protocol	Deep vein thrombosis	Pedal pulses
Prepare to administer continuous heparin infusion or other direct-acting anticoagulant	Compartment syndrome	Dyspnea or increased respiratory effort
Request order for antibiotic therapy	Peripheral vascular disease	Hemoglobin and hematocrit levels
Draw blood for CBC and coagulation studies		Level of consciousness

REFERENCES

Asterisk (*) indicates a classic or definitive work on this subject.

Arthritis Foundation. (2023). *Osteoarthritis.* https://www.arthritis.org/disease/osteoarthritis.

Bannuru, R. R., Osani, M. C., Vaysbrot, E. E., Arden, N. K., Bennell, K., Bierma-Zeinstra, S. M. A., et al. (2019). OARSI guidelines for the non-surgical management of knee, hip, and Polyarticular osteoarthritis. *Osteoarthritis and Cartilage, 27*(11), 1578–1589.

*Bodden, J., & Coppola, C. (2018). *Best practice guideline: Total hip replacement (arthroplasty).* Chicago, IL: SmithBucklin (for the National Association of Orthopaedic Nursing).

Booker, S., & Herr, K. (2021). Voices of African American older adults on the implications of social and health-related policies for osteoarthritis pain care. *Pain Management Nursing, 22*(1), 50–57.

Burchum, J. L. R., & Rosenthal, L. D. (2022). *Lehne's pharmacology for nursing care* (10th ed.). St. Louis: Elsevier.

Causey-Upton, R., Howell, D. M., Kitzman, P. H., Custer, M. G., & Dressler, E. V. (2019). Factors influencing discharge readiness after total knee replacement. *Orthopaedic Nursing, 38*(1), 6–14.

Clark, C. S. (2021). *Cannabis: A handbook for nurses.* Philadelphia, PA: Wolters Kluwer Health.

Elliott, B., Chargualaf, K. A., & Patterson, B. (2021). *Veteran-centered care in education and practice.* New York, NY: Springer Publishing.

Goode, V. M., Morgan, B., Muckler, V. C., Cary, M. P., Jr., Zbed, C. E., & Zychowicz, M. (2019). Multimodal pain management for major joint replacement surgery. *Orthopaedic Nursing, 38*(2), 150–156.

Gourdine, J. (2019). Review of nonsurgical treatment guidelines for lower extremity osteoarthritis. *Orthopaedic Nursing, 38*(5), 303–308.

Healthy People 2030. (2022). Arthritis https://health.gov/healthypeople/objectives-and-data/browse-objectives/arthritis.

*Interprofessional Education Collaborative. (2016). *Core competencies for interprofessional collaborative practice: 2016 update.* Washington, DC: Interprofessional Education Collaborative.

Jackman, C. (2019). Perioperative pain management for the chronic pain patient with long-term opioid use. *Orthopaedic Nursing, 38*(2), 159–163.

Jones, E. D., Davidson, L. J., & Cline, T. W. (2022). The effect of preoperative education prior to hip or knee arthroplasty on immediate postoperative outcomes. *Orthopaedic Nursing, 41*(1), 4–12.

Jones, L., & Taylor, T. (2019). Identifying acute delirium on acute care units. *Medsurg Nursing, 28*, 172–175 181.

Lisevick, A. B., Kelly, S., Cremins, M. S., Vellansky, S. S., McCann, G. P., LeBlanc, K., et al. (2020). Mobility technicians: A viable solution to early ambulation of total joint replacement patients. *Orthopaedic Nursing, 39*(5), 333–337.

Mascioli, A. A., Shaw, M., Boykin, S., Mahedevan, P., Wilder, J. H., Bell, J. W., et al. (2021). Total knee arthroplasty in freestanding ambulatory surgery centers: 5-year retrospective chart review of 90-day postsurgical outcomes and health care utilization. *Journal of the American Academy of Orthopaedic Surgeons, 29*(23), e1184–e1192.

Mogoi, V., Elder, B., Hayes, K., & Huhman, D. (2019). Effectiveness of platelet-rich plasma in management of knee osteoarthritis in a rural clinic. *Orthopaedic Nursing, 38*(3), 193–198.

*Mori, C., & Ribsam, V. (2018). *Best practice guideline: Total knee replacement (arthroplasty)*. SmithBucklin (for the National Association of Orthopaedic Nursing).

Morland, R. (2019). Evolution of the national opioid crisis. *Nursing, 39*(5), 51–56.

Pagana, K. D., Pagana, T. J., & Pagana, T. N. (2022). *Mosby's manual of diagnostic and laboratory tests* (7th ed.). St.Louis: Elsevier.

Pietsch, T., David, J., & Vergara, F. (2018). Integrative review for patients with bilateral total knee arthroplasty: A call for nursing practice guidelines. *Orthopaedic Nursing, 37*(4), 237–243.

Pizzi, L. J., Bates, M., Chelly, J. E., & Goodrich, C. J. (2020). A prospective randomized trial of an oral patient-controlled analgesia device versus usual care following total hip arthroplasty. *Orthopaedic Nursing, 39*(1), 37–46.

Rogers, J. L. (2023). *Pathophysiology: The biologic basis for disease in adults and children* (9th ed.). St. Louis: Elsevier.

Sasse, L., Laessig-Stary, B., & Abitz, T. (2020). Periarticular ketorolac improves outcomes for patients with joint replacements. *Orthopaedic Nursing, 39*(1), 47–50.

Slusser, M. M., Garcia, L. I., Reed, C.-R., & McGinnis, P. Q. (2019). *Foundations of interprofessional collaborative practice in health care*. St. Louis: Elsevier.

Smeltzer, S. C. (2021). Delivering quality healthcare for people with disability. Indianapolis. In *Sigma Theta Tau International Honor Society of Nursing*.

Teng, L. J., Goldsmith, L. J., Sawhney, M., & Jussaume, L. (2021). Hip and knee replacement patients' experiences with an orthopedic patient navigator: A qualitative study. *Orthopaedic Nursing, 40*(5), 292–298.

Tubog, T. D. (2019). Combined intermittent pneumatic leg compression and pharmacological prophylaxis for prevention of venous thromboembolism. *Orthopaedic Nursing, 38*(4), 270–272.

Xu, Y., & Wu, Q. (2021). Prevalence trend and disparities in rheumatoid arthritis among US adults, 2005-2018. *Journal of Clinical Medicine, 10*, 3289. https://doi.org/10.3390/jcm10153289.

44

Concepts of Care for Patients With Musculoskeletal Trauma

Donna D. Ignatavicius

http://evolve.elsevier.com/Iggy/

LEARNING OUTCOMES

1. Plan collaborative care with the interprofessional team to promote *mobility, perfusion*, and *tissue integrity* in patients with lower extremity amputations.
2. Teach adults how to decrease the risk for musculoskeletal trauma.
3. Teach the patient and caregiver(s) about common drugs and other management strategies used for amputations affecting *sensory perception.*
4. Plan patient- and family-centered nursing interventions to decrease the psychosocial impact caused by musculoskeletal injury.
5. Apply knowledge of anatomy, physiology, and pathophysiology to provide evidence-based care for patients with fractures.
6. Analyze assessment and diagnostic findings to generate solutions and prioritize nursing care for patients who have amputations.
7. Organize care coordination and transition management for patients having surgery to manage musculoskeletal trauma.
8. Use clinical judgment to plan evidence-based nursing care to promote *mobility* and decrease *pain* in patients with fractures.
9. Incorporate factors that affect health equity into the plan of care for patients planning amputation.

KEY TERMS

acute compartment syndrome (ACS) A serious but uncommon limb-threatening condition in which increased pressure within one or more compartments (that contain muscle, blood vessels, and nerves) reduces circulation to the lower leg or forearm.

amputation The removal of a part of the body.

ankle-brachial index A measure of blood flow in the lower extremities. It is calculated by dividing ankle systolic pressure by brachial systolic pressure. A normal ABI is 0.9 or higher.

avascular necrosis (also known as *osteonecrosis*) The death of bone tissue.

bone reduction Realignment of the bone ends for proper healing that is accomplished by a *closed* (nonsurgical) method or an *open* (surgical) procedure.

carpal tunnel syndrome (CTS) A common condition in which the median nerve in the wrist becomes compressed, causing pain and numbness.

cast A rigid device (synthetic or, less commonly, plaster) that immobilizes the affected body part while allowing other body parts to move.

closed (simple) fracture A fracture that does not extend through the skin (no visible wound).

complex regional pain syndrome (CRPS) A poorly understood dysfunction of the central and peripheral nervous systems that leads to severe, persistent pain.

ergonomics The study of how equipment and furniture can be arranged so that people can do work or other activities more efficiently and comfortably without injury.

external fixation A surgical procedure in which pins or wires are inserted through the skin and affected bone and then connected to a rigid external frame outside the body to immobilize the fracture during healing.

fascia iliaca compartment block (FICB) A regional anesthetic technique to manage pain for patients who have a fractured hip. The anesthetic agent (such as levobupivacaine) blocks the femoral, lateral cutaneous, and obturator nerves while avoiding the risk of injury to the femoral artery and vein.

fasciotomy A procedure for acute compartment syndrome in which the surgeon cuts through fascia to relieve pressure and tension on vital blood vessels and nerves.

fat embolism syndrome (FES) A serious but uncommon complication of fractures in which fat globules are released from the yellow bone marrow into the bloodstream within 12 to 48 hours after injury. These globules clog small blood vessels that supply vital organs, most commonly the lungs, and impair organ perfusion.

fracture A break or disruption in the continuity of a bone that often affects mobility and causes pain.

fragility fracture A fracture caused by osteoporosis or other disease that weakens bone.

internal fixation A surgical procedure in which metal pins, screws, rods, plates, or prostheses are inserted inside the body to immobilize a fracture during healing.

neuroma A sensitive tumor consisting of damaged nerve cells that forms most often in patients with amputations of an upper extremity but that can occur anywhere.

open (compound) fracture A fracture that extends through the skin, causing a visible wound.

opioid-induced constipation (OIC) Constipation that can result from taking opioids for a long period of time.

phantom limb pain (PLP) A persistent altered sensory perception in the amputated body part that is unpleasant or painful.

repetitive stress injury (RSI) A fast-growing occupational injury that occurs in people whose jobs require repetitive hand activities, such as pinching or grasping during wrist flexion; carpal tunnel syndrome (CTS) is the most common RSI.

subcutaneous emphysema The appearance of bubbles under the skin because of air trapping.

traction The application of a pulling force to a part of the body to provide bone alignment or relief of muscle spasm.

vertebroplasty Minimally invasive techniques in which bone cement is injected through the skin (percutaneously) directly into a vertebral fracture site to provide stability and immediate pain relief.

✳ PRIORITY AND INTERRELATED CONCEPTS

The priority concepts for this chapter are:
- *Mobility*
- *Perfusion*

The *Mobility* concept exemplar for this chapter is Fracture.
The *Perfusion* concept exemplar for this chapter is Amputation.

The interrelated concepts for this chapter are:
- *Pain*
- *Tissue Integrity*
- *Sensory Perception*

Musculoskeletal trauma accounts for about two-thirds of all injuries and is one of the primary causes of disability in the United States. It includes health problems that range from simple muscle strain to multiple bone fractures with severe soft tissue damage. This chapter focuses on the most common types of musculoskeletal trauma that nurses are likely to encounter in practice.

Fractures and other musculoskeletal trauma limit a patient's *mobility* in varying degrees, depending on the severity and extent of the injury. These injuries can also result in severe acute and/or persistent *pain* and altered *sensory perception.* Amputations result in impaired *tissue integrity* and are often performed because of inadequate arterial *perfusion* caused by chronic disease. These health concepts are reviewed in Chapter 3 of this text. In some cases, bleeding from traumatic injuries can lead to hemorrhage and hypovolemic shock, described elsewhere in this text.

Musculoskeletal injury often results in stress-related disorders such as posttraumatic stress disorder (PTSD) and acute stress disorder (Breazeale et al., 2022). In addition, common postinjury symptoms include anxiety, sleep disturbances, and depression. When caring for patients who experience musculoskeletal trauma, be sure to assess for risk factors, symptoms,

and behaviors associated with these psychosocial disorders. Common risk factors include (Breazeale et al., 2022):
- Female
- Older age
- High-intensity acute pain
- High injury severity

If you suspect patients are at risk for or have symptoms consistent with any of these problems, refer them to qualified mental health care providers for prompt management. Refer to your mental health textbook for related nursing interventions for patients with these disorders.

✳ MOBILITY CONCEPT EXEMPLAR: FRACTURE

A fracture is a break or disruption in the continuity of a bone that often affects *mobility* and causes *pain*. It can occur anywhere in the body and at any age.

Pathophysiology Review

All fractures have the same basic pathophysiologic mechanism and require similar patient-centered, interprofessional collaborative care, regardless of fracture type or location.

Classification of Fractures

A fracture can be classified by the extent of the break:
- *Complete fracture.* The break is across the entire width of the bone in such a way that the bone is divided into two distinct sections. If bone alignment is altered or disrupted, the fracture is also referred to as a *displaced* fracture. The ends of bone sections of a displaced fracture are more likely to damage surrounding nerves, blood vessels, and other soft tissues.
- *Incomplete fracture.* The fracture does not divide the bone into two portions because the break is through only part of the bone. This type of fracture is not typically displaced.

A fracture can also be described by the extent of associated soft tissue damage: **open** (or **compound**) or **closed** (or **simple**) (Fig. 44.1). The skin surface over the broken bone is disrupted

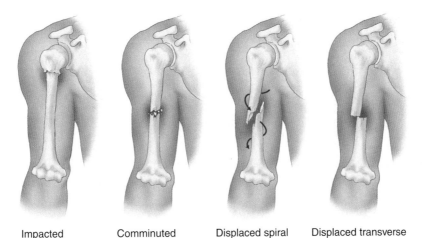

Impacted   Comminuted   Displaced spiral   Displaced transverse

FIG. 44.1 Common types of fractures. The spiral and transverse fractures are also displaced. The ends of broken bones in displaced fractures often pierce the surrounding skin, resulting in open fractures; however, these two examples are closed fractures. (From Leonard, P. C. [2022]. *Building a medical vocabulary: With Spanish translations* [11th ed.]. St. Louis: Elsevier.)

in a *compound* fracture, which causes an external wound. These fractures are often graded to define the extent of tissue damage. A *simple* fracture does not extend through the skin and therefore has no visible wound.

In addition to being identified by type, fractures are described by their cause. A *fragility fracture* (also known as a *pathologic* or *spontaneous fracture*) occurs after minimal trauma to a bone that has been weakened by disease. For example, a patient with bone cancer or osteoporosis can easily have a fragility fracture (see Chapter 42 for a discussion of these disorders). A *fatigue (stress) fracture* results from excessive strain and stress on the bone. This problem is commonly seen in recreational and professional athletes. *Compression fractures* are produced by a loading force applied to the long axis of cancellous bone. They commonly occur in the vertebrae of older patients with osteoporosis and are extremely painful.

Stages of Bone Healing

When a bone is fractured, the body immediately begins the healing process to repair the injury and restore the body's equilibrium. Fractures heal in five stages that are a continuous process and not single stages.

- In stage 1, within 24 to 72 hours after the injury, a hematoma forms at the site of the fracture because bone is extremely vascular.
- Stage 2 occurs in 3 days to 2 weeks, when granulation tissue begins to invade the hematoma. This then prompts the formation of fibrocartilage, providing the foundation for bone healing.
- Stage 3 of bone healing occurs as a result of vascular and cellular proliferation. The fracture site is surrounded by new vascular tissue known as a *callus* (within 3 to 6 weeks). *Callus* formation is the beginning of a nonbony union.
- As healing continues in stage 4, the callus is gradually resorbed and transformed into bone. This stage usually takes 3 to 8 weeks.
- During the fifth and final stage of healing, consolidation and remodeling of bone continue to meet mechanical demands.

This process may start as early as 4 to 6 weeks after fracture and can continue for up to 1 year, depending on the severity of the injury and the age and health of the patient. Fig. 44.2 summarizes the stages of bone healing.

In young, healthy adult bone, healing takes about 4 to 6 weeks. In the older person who has reduced bone mass, healing time is lengthened. Complete healing may take 3 months or longer in people who are older than 70 years. Other factors, such as the severity of the trauma, the type of bone injured, how the fracture is managed, and/or the presence of infection or **avascular necrosis (AVN)**, also called *osteonecrosis,* can also impact healing.

PATIENT-CENTERED CARE: OLDER ADULT HEALTH

The Effect of Age on Bone Healing

Bone healing is often affected by the aging process. Bone formation and strength rely on adequate nutrition. Calcium, phosphorus, vitamin D, and protein are necessary for the production of new bone (see Chapter 42). For women, the loss of estrogen after menopause decreases the body's ability to form new bone tissue. Chronic diseases can also affect the rate at which bone heals. For instance, peripheral vascular diseases, such as arteriosclerosis, reduce arterial circulation to bone. Thus the bone receives less oxygen and fewer nutrients, both of which are needed for healing and repair.

Complications of Fractures

Regardless of the type or location of the fracture, several limb- and life-threatening acute and chronic complications can result from the injury. Signs and symptoms of beginning complications must be treated early to prevent serious consequences. In some cases, careful monitoring and assessment by the nurse can prevent these complications from occurring or worsening.

Acute Complications of Fractures. Common acute complications of fractures include venous thromboembolism (VTE) and bone or soft tissue infection. *Venous thromboembolism (VTE)* includes deep vein thrombosis (DVT) and its major

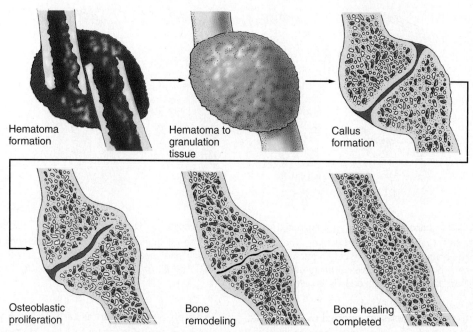

FIG. 44.2 Stages of bone healing.

complication, pulmonary embolism (PE). It is the most common complication of lower extremity surgery or trauma and the most often fatal complication of musculoskeletal surgery. Chapter 30 discusses VTE, including prevention and management, in detail.

Whenever there is trauma to tissues, the body's defense system is disrupted. Wound infections are the most common type of infection resulting from orthopedic trauma. They range from superficial skin infections to deep wound abscesses. Infection can also be caused by implanted hardware used to repair a fracture surgically, such as screws, pins, plates, or rods. Clostridia infections can result in gas gangrene or tetanus and can prevent the bone from healing properly.

Bone infection, or osteomyelitis, is most common with open fractures in which *tissue integrity* is altered and after surgical repair of a fracture (see Chapter 42 for discussion of osteomyelitis). For patients experiencing this type of trauma, the risk for health care agency–acquired infections is increased. These infections are common, and many result from multidrug-resistant organisms, such as methicillin-resistant *Staphylococcus aureus* (MRSA). Reducing MRSA infection is a primary desired outcome for all health care agencies. Chapter 19 discusses prevention and management of infection in detail.

Several complications of fractures are rare but are potentially limb- or life-threatening, including acute compartment syndrome and fat embolism syndrome. Acute compartment syndrome (ACS) is a serious limb-threatening condition in which increased pressure within one or more compartments (that contain muscle, blood vessels, and nerves) reduces circulation to the lower leg or forearm.

The pathophysiologic changes of increased compartment pressure are sometimes referred to as the *ischemia-edema cycle*. Capillaries within the muscle dilate, which raises capillary (arterial) and venous pressure. Capillaries become more permeable because of the release of histamine by the ischemic muscle tissue, and venous drainage decreases. As a result, plasma proteins leak into the interstitial fluid space and edema occurs. Edema increases pressure on nerve endings and causes severe pain. The pain experienced is greater than expected for the nature of the injury. ***Perfusion*** to the area is reduced, and further ischemia results. ***Sensory perception*** deficits or paresthesia generally appears before changes in vascular or motor signs. The color of the tissue pales/becomes ashen, and pulses begin to weaken but rarely disappear. The affected area is usually palpably tense, and acute severe ***pain*** occurs with passive motion of the extremity. If the condition is not treated, cyanosis, tingling, numbness, paresis, and necrosis can occur. Box 44.1 summarizes the sequence of pathophysiologic events in compartment syndrome and the associated clinical assessment findings.

The pressure to the compartment can be from an external or internal source, but fracture is present in most cases of ACS. Tight, bulky dressings and casts are examples of *external* pressure causes. Blood or fluid accumulation in the compartment is a common source of *internal* pressure. ACS is not limited to patients with musculoskeletal problems. It can also occur in those with severe burns, extensive insect bites or snakebites, or massive infiltration of IV fluids. In these situations, edema increases internal pressure in one or more compartments. Patients with ACS may need a surgical procedure known as a fasciotomy. In this procedure, the surgeon cuts through the fascia to relieve pressure and tension on vital blood vessels and nerves. The wound remains open and requires care to begin to heal from the inside out. The surgeon usually closes the wound with a skin graft in several days. Wound care is described in Chapter 21 and in basic nursing fundamentals textbooks.

Long-term problems resulting from compartment syndrome include infection, persistent motor weakness in the affected

BOX 44.1   Key Features
Acute Compartment Syndrome

Physiologic Change	Clinical Findings
Increased compartment pressure	No change
Increased capillary permeability	Edema
Release of histamine	Increased edema
Increased blood flow to area	Pulses present Pink tissue
Pressure on nerve endings	Acute pain
Increased tissue pressure	Referred pain to compartment(s)
Decreased tissue perfusion	Increased edema
Decreased oxygen to tissues	Pallor/ash gray appearance
Increased production of lactic acid	Unequal pulses Flexed posture
Anaerobic metabolism	Cyanosis
Vasodilation	Increased edema
Increased blood flow	Tense muscle swelling
Increased tissue pressure	Tingling Numbness
Increased edema	Paresthesia
Muscle ischemia	Severe pain unrelieved by drugs
Tissue necrosis	Paresis/paralysis

TABLE 44.1   Fat Embolism Versus Blood Clot (Pulmonary) Embolism

Fat Embolism	Blood Clot Embolism
Definition	
Obstruction of the pulmonary (or other organ) vascular bed by fat globules	Obstruction of the pulmonary artery by a blood clot or clots
Origin	
Most from fractures of the long bones; occurs usually within 48 hr of injury	Most from deep vein thrombosis in the legs or pelvis; can occur anytime
Assessment Findings	
Altered mental status (earliest sign)	Same as for fat embolism, except no petechiae
Increased respirations, pulse, temperature	
Chest pain	
Dyspnea	
Crackles	
Decreased Sao₂	
Petechiae (not present in all patients)	
Mild thrombocytopenia	
Treatment	
Bed rest	Preventive measures (e.g., leg exercises, antiembolism stockings, SCDs)
Gentle handling	
Oxygen	Bed rest
Hydration (IV fluids)	Oxygen
Possibly steroid therapy	Possibly mechanical ventilation
Fracture immobilization	Anticoagulants
	Thrombolytics
	Possible surgery: pulmonary embolectomy, vena cava umbrella

Sao₂, Arterial oxygen saturation; *SCD*, sequential compression device.

extremity, contracture, and myoglobinuric renal failure. In extreme cases, amputation becomes necessary.

Fat embolism syndrome (FES) is another serious complication of fractures in which fat globules are released from the yellow bone marrow into the bloodstream within 12 to 48 hours after an injury. These globules clog small blood vessels that supply vital organs, most commonly the lungs, and impair organ *perfusion*. FES usually results from fractures or fracture repair but may also occur, although less often, in patients experiencing pancreatitis, osteomyelitis, blunt trauma, or sickle cell disease.

The earliest signs and symptoms of FES are a low arterial oxygen level (hypoxemia), dyspnea, and tachypnea (increased respirations). Headache, lethargy, agitation, confusion, decreased level of consciousness, seizures, and vision changes may follow. Nonpalpable, red-brown petechiae—a macular, measleslike rash—may appear over the neck, upper arms, and/or chest. This rash is a classic manifestation but is usually the last sign to develop (Rogers, 2023).

Abnormal laboratory findings include:

- Decreased Pao₂ level (often below 60 mm Hg)
- Increased erythrocyte sedimentation rate (ESR)
- Decreased serum calcium levels
- Decreased red blood cell and platelet counts
- Increased serum level of lipids

These changes in blood values are poorly understood, but they aid in diagnosis of the condition.

The chest x-ray often shows bilateral infiltrates but may be normal. The chest CT often reveals a patchy distribution of opacities. An MRI of the brain can show evidence of neurologic deficits from hypoxemia. FES can result in respiratory failure or death, often from pulmonary edema. When the lungs are affected, the complication may be misdiagnosed as a pulmonary embolism from a blood clot (Table 44.1).

Chronic Complications of Fractures. Avascular necrosis, delayed bone healing, and chronic regional pain syndrome are later chronic complications of musculoskeletal trauma. Blood supply to the bone may be disrupted, causing decreased *perfusion* and death of bone tissue, or avascular necrosis. This problem is most often a complication of hip fractures or any fracture in which there is displacement of bone. Surgical repair of fractures also can cause necrosis because the hardware can interfere with circulation. Patients on long-term corticosteroid therapy, such as prednisone, are also at high risk for ischemic necrosis.

Delayed union is a fracture that has not healed within 6 months of injury. Some fractures never achieve union; that is, they never completely heal (*nonunion*). Others heal incorrectly (*malunion*). These problems are most common in patients with tibial fractures, fractures that involve many treatment techniques (e.g., cast, traction), and pathologic fractures. Union may also be delayed or not achieved in the older patient due to poor bone health. If bone does not heal, the patient typically has persistent *pain* and decreased *mobility* from deformity.

Complex regional pain syndrome (CRPS), formerly called *reflex sympathetic dystrophy (RSD)*, is a poorly understood dysfunction of the central and peripheral nervous systems that leads to severe, persistent *pain* and other symptoms. Genetic factors may play a role in the development of this devastating complication. CRPS most often results from fractures or other traumatic musculoskeletal injury and commonly occurs in the feet and hands (Thurlow & Gray, 2018). In some cases, specific nerve injuries are present, but in others no injury can be identified. To facilitate soft tissue healing and *prevent* CRPS, the physical therapist asks the patient to frequently apply a variety of objects with varying surface types directly to the skin to desensitize it. These objects can be rough, smooth, hard, soft, sharp (but not enough to damage the skin), or dull.

When CRPS is present, a triad of signs and symptoms is present, including (Thurlow & Gray, 2018):

- Abnormalities of the autonomic nervous system (changes in color, temperature, and sensitivity of skin over the affected area, excessive sweating, edema)
- Motor symptoms (paresis, muscle spasms, loss of function)
- Altered *sensory perception* symptoms (intense burning pain that becomes intractable [unrelenting])

In addition to physical chronic complications of fractures, many patients develop postinjury chronic stress disorders, including PTSD. As mentioned earlier, many patients also experience anxiety, sleep disturbances, and depression.

Etiology and Genetic Risk

The primary cause of a fracture is trauma from a motor vehicle crash or fall, especially in older adults. The trauma may be a direct blow to the bone or an indirect force from muscle contractions or pulling forces on the bone. Sports, vigorous exercise, and malnutrition are contributing factors. Bone diseases, such as osteoporosis, increase the risk for a fracture in older adults (see Chapter 42). Genetic factors that increase risk for fracture are discussed with these specific health problems throughout this text.

Incidence and Prevalence

The incidence of fractures depends on the location of the injury. Rib fractures are the most common type in the adult population. Femoral shaft fractures occur most often in young and middle-age adults.

PATIENT-CENTERED CARE: OLDER ADULT HEALTH

Fractures and Aging

The incidence of proximal femur (hip) fractures is highest in older adults. Humeral fractures are also common in older adults; the older the person, usually the more proximal is the fracture. Wrist (Colles) fractures are typically seen in middle and late adulthood and usually result from a fall. These fractures are sometimes referred to as *FOSH fractures* (fall out-stretched hand). Middle-age and older adults, especially women, have a higher incidence of osteoporosis, which increases the risk for fragility fractures.

PATIENT-CENTERED CARE: VETERAN HEALTH

Musculoskeletal Trauma in Active Military and Veteran Population

The primary type of injury experienced by individuals in military training and service is musculoskeletal trauma, most often strains, sprains, and stress fractures in lower extremities. Injuries of the lower back in the lumbar spinal region are also common, most likely caused by carrying heavy equipment and supplies. Chronic inflammation and pain from these injuries lead to high rates of physical disability in this group (Elliott et al., 2021). When caring for patients who are serving or who have served in the military, assess whether they experienced a physical injury and if they have residual symptoms that affect their function or quality of life.

Health Promotion/Disease Prevention

Airbags have decreased the number of severe injuries and deaths, but they have *increased* the number of leg and ankle fractures, especially in older adults. Focus health teaching on risks for musculoskeletal injury, including:

- Osteoporosis screening and self-management education (see Chapter 42)
- Fall prevention (see Chapter 4)
- Home safety assessment and modification, if needed
- Dangers of substance use and driving
- Preventing overuse injuries for recreational and professional athletes
- Helmet use when riding bicycles, motorcycles, and other small motorized vehicles/devices

Remind individuals that if they smoke, they are more likely to have a fracture, experience severe pain from a musculoskeletal injury or surgery, and have a slower bone and tissue healing time than those who do not smoke. Therefore, refer patients to a well-respected smoking-cessation program.

Interprofessional Collaborative Care
Recognize Cues: Assessment

History. The patient with a new fracture typically reports moderate to severe *pain.* Delay the detailed interview for a nursing history until the patient is more comfortable; then ask about the cause of the fracture. Certain types of force (e.g., incisional, crush, acceleration, or deceleration), shearing, and friction lead to most musculoskeletal injuries. As a result, several body systems are often affected.

Incisional injuries, as from a knife wound, and *crush* injuries cause hemorrhage and decreased *perfusion* to major organs. *Acceleration or deceleration* injuries cause direct trauma to the spleen, brain, and kidneys when these organs are moved from their fixed locations in the body. *Shearing and friction* damage *tissue integrity* and cause a high level of wound contamination.

Asking about the events leading to the injury helps identify which forces were experienced and therefore which body systems or parts of the body to assess. For example, a forward fall often results in a Colles fracture of the wrist because people try to catch themselves with an outstretched hand. Knowing the mechanism of injury also helps determine whether other types of injury, such as head or spinal cord injury, might be present.

Obtain a substance use history regardless of the patient's age. For example, a young adult may have had an excessive amount of alcohol and/or drugs, which contributed to a motor vehicle crash or a fall at the work site. Many older adults also consume alcohol and an assortment of prescribed and over-the-counter drugs, which can cause dizziness and loss of balance. *Assess adults of all ages about opioid use for persistent pain before the fracture. This information is essential for developing a pain management plan for the patient.*

Ask about the patient's occupation and recreational activities. Some occupations are more hazardous than others. For instance, construction work is potentially more physically dangerous than office work. Certain hobbies and recreational activities, such as skiing, are also extremely hazardous. Contact sports, such as football and ice hockey, often result in musculoskeletal injuries, including fractures. Other activities do not have such an obvious potential for injury but can cause fractures nonetheless. For instance, daily jogging or running can lead to fatigue (stress) fractures.

Physical Assessment/Signs and Symptoms. The patient with a fracture often has trauma to other body systems. Therefore assess all major body systems *first* for life-threatening cues, especially when patients have head, chest, and/or abdominal trauma. Some fractures can cause internal organ damage, resulting in hemorrhage. When a pelvic fracture is suspected, assess vital signs, skin color, and level of consciousness for indications of possible hypovolemic shock from internal blood loss. Remember that if there is one pelvic fracture, there is usually another fracture in the pelvis, even if it is small or hairline. Check the urine for blood, which indicates possible damage to the urinary system, often the bladder. If the patient cannot void, suspect that the bladder or urethra has been damaged. Complete assessment of organ function is described elsewhere in this text.

Patients with severe or multiple fractures of the arms, legs, or pelvis have severe acute **pain.** Vertebral compression fractures are also extremely painful. Patients *with a fractured hip may have groin pain or pain referred to the back of the knee or lower back. Pain* is usually caused by muscle spasm and edema that result from the fracture.

! NURSING SAFETY PRIORITY
Action Alert

Patients with one or more fractured ribs have severe pain when they take deep breaths. Monitor respiratory status, which may be severely compromised from pain or pneumothorax (air in the pleural cavity). Assess the patient's *pain* level, and manage pain *before* continuing the physical assessment.

For fractures of the shoulder and upper arm, the physical assessment is best performed with the patient in a sitting or standing position, if possible, so that shoulder drooping or other abnormal positioning can be seen. Support the affected arm and flex the elbow to promote comfort during the assessment. For more distal areas of the arm, perform the assessment with the patient in a supine position so that the extremity can be elevated to reduce swelling.

Place the patient in a supine position for assessment of the legs and pelvis. A patient with an impacted hip fracture may be able to walk for a short time after injury, although this is not recommended.

When inspecting the site of a possible fracture, look for a change in bone alignment. The bone may appear deformed, a limb may be internally or externally rotated, and/or one or more bones may also be dislocated (out of their joint capsules). Observe for extremity shortening or a change in bone shape.

If the skin is intact (closed fracture), the area over the fracture may be ecchymotic (bruised) from bleeding into the underlying soft tissues. Subcutaneous emphysema, the appearance of bubbles under the skin because of air trapping, may be present but is usually seen later.

! NURSING SAFETY PRIORITY
Action Alert

Swelling at the fracture site is rapid and can result in marked neurovascular compromise as a result of decreased arterial **perfusion.** *Gently perform a thorough neurovascular assessment and compare extremities.* Assess skin color and temperature, **sensory perception, mobility, pain,** and pulses distal to the fracture site. If the fracture involves an extremity and the patient is not in severe pain, check the nails for capillary refill by applying pressure to the nail and observing for the speed of blood return (usually less than 3 seconds). If nails are brittle or thick, assess the skin next to the nail. Checking for capillary refill is not as reliable as other indicators of **perfusion.**

Box 44.2 describes the procedure for a neurovascular assessment, which evaluates **c**irculation, **m**ovement, and **s**ensation (CMS) function.

Psychosocial Assessment. The psychosocial status of a patient with a fracture depends on the extent of the injury, possible complications, coping ability, and availability of support systems. Hospitalization is not required for a single, uncomplicated fracture, and the patient returns to usual daily activities within a few days. Examples include a single fracture of a bone in the finger, wrist, foot, or toe.

In contrast, a patient suffering severe or multiple traumas may be hospitalized for weeks to months and may undergo many surgical procedures, treatments, and prolonged rehabilitation. These disruptions in lifestyle can create a high level of stress, anxiety, and/or depression. Long-term psychosocial problems commonly occur in these patients.

⚇ PATIENT-CENTERED CARE: CULTURE AND SPIRITUALITY
Long-Term Recovery From Musculoskeletal Trauma

For patients experiencing long-term recovery from fractures and other trauma, stress, anxiety, and depression can affect relationships between the patient and family members or friends. Assess patients' feelings, and ask how they coped with previously experienced stressful events. Body image and sexuality may be altered by deformity, treatment modalities for fracture repair, or long-term immobilization. Establish a trusting relationship and determine the patient's spiritual beliefs and practices. Assess the availability of love and support systems, such as family, friends, church or temple, or community groups, who can help patients during the acute and rehabilitation phases when multiple or severe fractures occur.

BOX 44.2 Best Practice for Patient Safety and Quality Care

Assessment of Neurovascular Status in Patients With Musculoskeletal Injury

Assessment Method	Normal Findings
Skin Color Inspect the area distal to the injury.	No change in pigmentation compared with other parts of the body.
Skin Temperature Palpate the area distal to the injury (the dorsum of the hands is most sensitive to temperature).	The skin is warm.
Movement Ask the patient to move the affected area or the area distal to the injury (active motion).	The patient can move without discomfort.
Move the area distal to the injury (passive motion).	No difference in comfort compared with active movement.
Sensation Ask the patient if numbness or tingling is present (paresthesia).	No numbness or tingling.
Palpate with a paper clip (especially the web space between the first and second toes or the web space between the thumb and forefinger).	No difference in sensation in the affected and unaffected extremities. (Loss of sensation in these areas indicates peroneal nerve or median nerve damage.)
Pulses Palpate the pulses distal to the injury.	Pulses are strong and easily palpated; no difference in the affected and unaffected extremities.
Capillary Refill (Least Reliable) Press the nail beds distal to the injury until blanching occurs (or the skin near the nail if nails are thick and brittle).	Blood returns (return to usual color) within 3 sec (5 sec for older patients).
Pain Ask the patient about the location, nature, and frequency of the pain.	Pain is usually localized and is often described as stabbing or throbbing. (Pain out of proportion to the injury and unrelieved by analgesics might indicate compartment syndrome.)

Active patients of any age or those who are older and live alone may become depressed during the healing process, especially if experiencing persistent *pain* that can decrease energy levels. Patients who were previously active and otherwise healthy often feel vulnerable and can become very anxious when they are not able to return to their usual level of activity. Provide hope that appropriate pain management will improve their comfort level and restore energy to return to their usual life habits. Some patients may benefit from counseling or psychotherapy services to help them with symptoms of stress, depression, and/or anxiety.

Laboratory Assessment. No special laboratory tests are available for assessment of fractures. Hemoglobin and hematocrit levels may often be low because of bleeding caused by the injury. If extensive soft tissue damage is present, the erythrocyte sedimentation rate (ESR) may be elevated, which indicates the expected inflammatory response. If this value and the white blood cell (WBC) count increase during fracture healing, the patient may have a bone or soft tissue infection. During the healing stages, serum calcium and phosphorus levels may increase as the affected bone releases these elements into the blood.

Imaging Assessment. The primary health care provider requests standard *x-rays* to confirm a diagnosis of fracture, which often reveals bone disruption, malalignment, or deformity. If the x-ray does not show a fracture but the patient is symptomatic, the x-ray is usually repeated with additional views.

The *CT* scan is useful in detecting fractures of complex structures, such as the hip and pelvis. It also identifies compression fractures of the spine. *MRI* is useful in determining the amount of soft tissue damage that may have occurred with the fracture.

Analyze Cues and Prioritize Hypotheses: Analysis

The priority collaborative problems for patients with fractures include:

1. Acute *pain* due to fractured bone(s), soft tissue damage, muscle spasm, and edema
2. Decreased *mobility* due to *pain,* muscle spasm, and soft tissue damage
3. Potential for neurovascular compromise due to impaired tissue *perfusion*

Generate Solutions and Take Actions: Planning and Implementation

Managing Acute Pain

Planning: Expected Outcomes. The patient with a fracture is expected to state adequate *pain* control is achieved (a 2 to 3 on a pain scale of 0 to 10) after fracture reduction and immobilization.

Interventions. A fracture can happen anywhere and may be accompanied by multiple injuries to vital organs or major vessels (e.g., thoracic aorta dissection or tear). Interprofessional collaborative care depends on the severity and extent of the injury and the number of fractures the patient has.

Emergency Care: Fracture. For any patient who experiences trauma in the community, first call 911 and assess for **a**irway, **b**reathing, and **c**irculation (ABCs, or primary survey). Then provide lifesaving care if needed before being concerned about the fracture or other injury. If cardiopulmonary resuscitation (CPR) is needed, ensure circulation first, followed by airway and breathing (Box 44.3).

After a head-to-toe assessment (secondary survey) and patient stabilization by the prehospital team, pain is often managed with short-term IV opioids such as fentanyl, hydromorphone, or morphine sulfate. Depending on the severity of the injury, other drugs to decrease opioid use, such as NSAIDs and regional nerve blocks, are also administered. Cardiac monitoring for patients who are older than 50 years is established before

BOX 44.3   Best Practice for Patient Safety and Quality Care

Emergency Care of the Patient With an Extremity Fracture

- Assess the patient's **a**irway, **b**reathing, and **c**irculation (ABCs); establish any ABC that is affected by the injury.
- Perform a quick head-to-toe assessment.
- Remove the patient's clothing (cut if necessary) to inspect the affected area while supporting the area above and below the injury. Do not remove shoes unless the foot or ankle is injured because this can cause increased trauma.
- Apply direct pressure on the area if there is bleeding and pressure over the proximal artery nearest the fracture.
- Remove jewelry on the affected extremity in case of swelling.
- Keep the patient warm and in a supine position.
- Check the neurovascular status of the area distal to the fracture, including temperature, color, sensation, movement, and capillary refill. Compare affected and unaffected limbs.
- Immobilize the extremity by splinting; include joints above and below the fracture site. Recheck circulation after splinting.
- Cover any open areas with a dressing (preferably sterile).

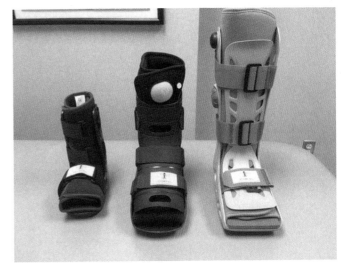

FIG. 44.3 Walking boots of various sizes and types. (From Porter, D. A., & Schon, L. C. [2021]. *Baxter's The foot and ankle in sport* [3rd ed.]. St. Louis: Elsevier.)

drug administration. In the emergency department (ED) or urgent care center, fracture management begins with reduction and immobilization of the fracture while attending to continued *pain* assessment and management.

Nonsurgical Management. Bone reduction, or realignment of the bone ends for proper healing, may be accomplished by a closed method or an open (surgical) procedure. Nonsurgical management includes closed reduction and immobilization with a bandage, splint, boot, or cast. In some cases, dislocated bones are also reduced, such as when the distal tibia and fibula are dislocated with a fractured ankle.

The primary health care provider selects the treatment method based on the type, location, and extent of the fracture. These interventions prevent further injury and reduce *pain.*

For each modality, the primary nursing concern is assessment and prevention of neurovascular dysfunction or compromise. Assess and document the patient's neurovascular status every hour for the first 24 hours and every 1 to 4 hours thereafter, depending on the injury and agency/primary health care provider protocol. Elevate the fractured extremity higher than the heart, and apply ice for the first 24 to 48 hours as needed to reduce edema.

Closed reduction and immobilization. *Closed* reduction is the most common nonsurgical method for managing a simple fracture. While applying a manual pull, or traction, on the bone, the primary health care provider moves the bone ends so that they realign. Moderate sedation is used during this procedure for patient comfort. The nurse monitors the patient's oxygen saturation (and possibly end-tidal carbon dioxide [$ETCO_2$] level) to ensure adequate rate and depth of respirations during the procedure. *If the $ETCO_2$ becomes too low (below 30 mm Hg) and the respiratory rate falls to 10 breaths/min, rub the patient's sternum and encourage breathing.* An x-ray confirms that the bone ends are approximated (aligned) before the bone is immobilized, and a splint or other device is applied to keep the bone in alignment.

Splints and orthopedic boots/shoes. For certain areas of the body, such as the scapula (shoulder) and clavicle (collarbone), a commercial immobilizer may be used to keep the bone in place during healing. Because upper extremity bones do not bear weight, splints may be sufficient to keep bone fragments in place for a closed fracture. Thermoplastic, a durable, flexible material for splinting, allows custom fitting to the patient's body part. Splints for lower extremities are also custom fitted using flexible materials and held in place with elastic bandages. When possible, splints are preferred over casts to prevent the complications that can occur with casting. Splints also allow room for extremity swelling without causing decreased arterial *perfusion.*

For foot or toe fractures, orthopedic shoes may be used to support the injured area during healing. For ankles or the lower part of the leg, padded orthopedic boots supported by multiple Velcro straps to hold the boot in place may be used (Fig. 44.3). These devices are especially useful when the patient is allowed to bear weight on the affected leg.

Casts. For more complex fractures or fractures of the lower extremity, the primary health care provider or orthopedic technician may apply a cast to hold bone fragments in place after reduction. A cast is a rigid device that immobilizes the affected body part while allowing other body parts to move. It also allows early *mobility* and reduces *pain.* Although its most common use is for fractures, a cast may be applied for correction of deformities (e.g., clubfoot) or for prevention of deformities (e.g., those seen in some patients with rheumatoid arthritis).

Fiberglass, a waterproof synthetic casting material, is used most often for fracture immobilization (Fig. 44.4). Fiberglass can dry and become rigid within minutes and decreases the risk for impaired *tissue integrity.* *Plaster* was the traditional material used for casts but is used much less often today. When first applied, a plaster cast feels hot because an immediate chemical reaction occurs; it soon becomes damp and cool. This type of cast takes at least 24 hours to dry, depending on the size and location of the cast. A wet cast feels cold, smells musty, and is grayish. The cast is dry when it feels hard and firm, is odorless, and has a shiny white appearance.

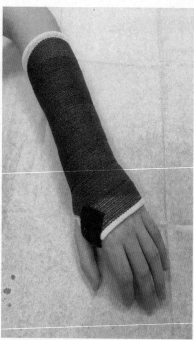

FIG. 44.4 Synthetic fiberglass cast used to immobilize the wrist. (From Bevers, M. S. A. M., et al. [2020]. The feasibility of high-resolution peripheral quantitative computed tomography [HR-pQCT] in patients with suspected scaphoid fractures. *Journal of Clinical Densitometry, 23*[3], 432–442.)

If *tissue integrity* under the cast is impaired, the primary health care provider, orthopedic technician, or specially educated nurse cuts a window in the cast so that the wound can be observed and cared for. The piece of cast removed to make the window must be retained and replaced after wound care to prevent localized edema in the area. This is most important when a window is cut from a cast on an extremity. Tape or elastic bandage wrap may be used to keep the "window" in place. A window is also an access for taking pulses, removing wound drains, or preventing abdominal distention when the patient is in a body or spica cast.

If the cast is too tight, it may be cut with a cast cutter to relieve pressure or allow tissue swelling. The primary health care provider may choose to bivalve the cast (i.e., cut it lengthwise into two equal pieces). Either half of the cast can be removed for inspection or for provision of care. The two halves are then held in place by an elastic bandage wrap. Before the cast is cut, inform the patient that the cast cutter will not injure the skin but that warmth might be felt during the procedure.

When a patient has an *arm cast,* teach the patient to elevate the arm above the heart to reduce swelling. The hand should be higher than the heart. Ice may be prescribed for the first 24 to 48 hours. When the patient is walking or standing, the arm is supported with a sling placed around the neck to alleviate fatigue caused by the weight of the cast. The sling should distribute the weight over a large area of the shoulders and trunk, not just the neck. Some primary health care providers prefer that the patient not use a sling after the first few days in an arm cast, particularly a short-arm cast. This encourages normal movement of the mobile joints and enhances bone healing. For many wrist fractures, a splint is used to immobilize the area instead of a cast to accommodate for edema formation.

A *leg cast* allows **mobility** and requires the patient to use ambulatory aids such as crutches or a walker. A cast shoe, sandal, or boot that attaches to the foot or a rubber walking pad attached to the sole of the cast assists in ambulation (if weight bearing is allowed) and helps prevent damage to the cast. Teach the patient to elevate the affected leg on several pillows to reduce swelling and to apply ice for the first 24 hours or as prescribed.

Before the cast is applied, explain its purpose and the procedure for its application. With a *plaster* cast, warn the patient about the heat that will be felt immediately after the wet cast is applied. *Do not cover a new plaster cast.* Allow for air-drying, and handle the cast with the palms of the hand to prevent damage.

> ! **NURSING SAFETY PRIORITY**
>
> *Action Alert*
>
> Check to ensure that any type of cast is not too tight, and frequently monitor and document neurovascular status—usually every hour for the first 24 hours after application if the patient is hospitalized. You should be able to insert a finger between the cast and the skin. Teach the patient to apply ice for the first 24 to 36 hours to reduce swelling and inflammation.

Inspect the cast at least once every 8 to 12 hours for drainage, alignment, and fit. Plaster casts act like sponges and absorb drainage, whereas synthetic casts act like a wick pulling drainage away from the drainage site. Document the presence of any drainage on the cast. However, the evidence is unclear on whether drainage should be circled on the cast because it may increase anxiety and is not a reliable indicator of drainage amount. *Immediately report to the primary health care provider any sudden increases in the amount of drainage or change in the integrity of the cast.* After swelling decreases, it is not uncommon for the cast to become too loose and need replacement. If the patient is not admitted to the hospital, provide instructions regarding cast care.

During hospitalization, assess for other complications resulting from casting that can be serious and life-threatening, such as infection, circulation impairment, and peripheral nerve damage. If the patient returns home after cast application, teach how to monitor for these complications and when to notify the primary health care provider.

Infection can result from impaired *tissue integrity* under the cast (pressure necrosis). If pressure necrosis occurs, the patient typically reports a very painful "hot spot" under the cast, and the cast may feel warmer in the affected area. Teach the patient or family to smell the area for mustiness or an unpleasant odor that would indicate infected material. If the infection progresses, a fever may develop. Teach the patient to never put anything down inside the cast, such as a hanger or pencil, to scratch an itch because this action can cause significant skin damage.

Circulation impairment causing decreased **perfusion** and *peripheral nerve damage* can result from tightness of the cast. Teach the patient to assess for circulation at least daily, checking for numbness, increased **pain,** and the ability to move the area distal to the extremity. Remind patients to wiggle their toes and move them up and down.

The patient with a cast may be immobilized for a prolonged period, depending on the extent of the fracture and the type of cast. In this case, assess for complications of decreased **mobility,** such as skin breakdown, pneumonia, atelectasis, venous thromboembolism, and constipation.

Because of prolonged immobilization, a joint may become contracted, usually in a fixed state of flexion. Osteoarthritis and osteoporosis may develop from lack of weight bearing. Muscle can also atrophy from lack of exercise during prolonged immobilization of the affected body part, usually an extremity.

NCLEX Examination Challenge 44.1
Safe and Effective Care Environment

The nurse is assessing a client who sustained a right displaced closed ankle fracture as a result of falling. What would be the nurse's **priority** assessment related to the fracture?

A. Observing for bleeding at the fracture site
B. Monitoring neurovascular status
C. Assessing lower extremity alignment
D. Observing for bruising around the fracture site

Traction. Traction is the application of a pulling force to a part of the body to provide bone reduction or as a last resort to decrease muscle spasm (thus reducing *pain*). A patient in traction is often hospitalized, but in some cases home care is possible even for skeletal traction.

Although not frequently used today, the two major types of traction are skin and skeletal traction. *Skin traction* involves the use of a Velcro boot (Buck traction) (Fig. 44.5), belt, or halter, which is usually secured around the affected leg. The primary purpose of skin traction is to decrease painful muscle spasms that accompany hip and proximal femur fractures. A weight is used as a pulling force, which is limited to 5 to 10 lb (2.3 to 4.5 kg) to prevent injury to the skin.

In *skeletal traction,* screws are surgically inserted directly into bone (e.g., femoral condyles for distal femur fractures). These allow the use of longer traction time and heavier weights, usually 15 to 30 lb (6.8 to 13.6 kg). Skeletal traction aids in bone realignment but impairs the patient's *mobility*. Use pressure-reduction measures and monitor for indications of impaired *tissue integrity*. Pin site care is also an important part of nursing management to prevent infection. Keep pin sites clean and document the nature of any drainage. Follow the agency's or primary health care provider's protocol for pin care.

⚠ NURSING SAFETY PRIORITY
Action Alert

When patients are in traction, weights are not removed without a primary health care provider's order. They should not be lifted manually or allowed to rest on the floor. Weights should be freely hanging at all times. Teach this important point to assistive personnel on the unit, to other personnel such as those in the radiology department, and to visitors. Inspect the skin at least every 8 hours for signs of irritation or inflammation. When possible, remove the belt or boot that is used for skin traction every 8 hours to inspect under the device. Assess neurovascular status of the affected body part per agency or primary health care provider protocol to detect impaired *perfusion* and *tissue integrity*. The patient's circulation is typically monitored every hour for the first 24 hours after traction is applied and every 4 hours thereafter.

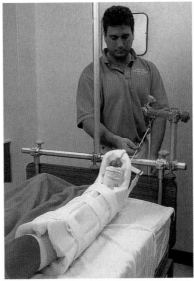

FIG. 44.5 Skin traction with a hook-and-loop fastener (Velcro) boot may occasionally be used for hip fractures. (Courtesy Smith & Nephew, Inc., Orthopaedics Divisions, Memphis, TN.)

Drug therapy. After fracture treatment, the patient often has *pain* for a prolonged time during the healing process. The primary health care provider commonly prescribes opioid and nonopioid analgesics, NSAIDs, and possibly muscle relaxants.

For patients with severe *pain*, opioid and nonopioid drugs are alternated or given together to manage pain both centrally in the brain and peripherally at the site of injury. For severe or multiple fractures, short-term patient-controlled analgesia (PCA) with morphine, fentanyl, or hydromorphone is used. Oxycodone and oxycodone with acetaminophen or hydrocodone with acetaminophen are common oral opioid drugs that can be very effective for most patients with fracture pain. NSAIDs and other drugs are given to decrease associated tissue inflammation; however, they can slow bone healing.

For patients who have less severe injury, the analgesic may be given on an as-needed basis. Collaborate with the patient regarding the best times for the strong analgesics to be given (e.g., before a complex dressing change, after physical therapy sessions, or at bedtime). Assess the effectiveness of the analgesic and its side effects. Constipation is a common side effect of opioid therapy, especially for older adults. Assess for frequency of bowel movements and administer stool softeners or laxatives as needed for opioid-induced constipation (OIC). Encourage fluids, high-fiber foods, and activity as tolerated. Be aware that other drugs, such as anticholinergics, calcium channel blockers, antidepressants, and diuretics, may cause medication-induced constipation (MIC) (Burchum & Rosenthal, 2022).

Physical therapy. Collaborate with the physical therapist (PT) to assist with pain control and edema reduction by using ice/heat packs, electrical muscle stimulation ("e-stim"), and special treatments such as dexamethasone iontophoresis. Iontophoresis is a method for absorbing dexamethasone, a synthetic steroid, through the skin near the painful area to decrease inflammation and edema. A small device delivers a minute amount of electricity via electrodes that are placed on the skin. The patient may describe the sensation as a pinch or slight sting. The electrical current increases the ability of the skin to absorb the drug from a topical patch into the affected soft tissue.

When acute *pain* is not adequately controlled, some patients experience a chronic, intense burning pain and edema that are associated with complex regional pain syndrome (CRPS). This syndrome often results from fractures and other musculoskeletal trauma as described earlier in this chapter.

Surgical Management. For some types of fractures, closed reduction is not sufficient. Surgical intervention may be needed to realign the bone to enhance the healing process.

Preoperative care. Teach the patient and family what to expect during and after the surgery. The preoperative care for a patient undergoing orthopedic surgery is similar to that for anyone having surgery with general or epidural anesthesia. Some patients may also receive a regional nerve blockade, which promotes comfort immediately after surgery. (See Chapter 9 for a thorough discussion of general preoperative nursing care.)

Operative procedures. Open reduction with internal fixation (ORIF) is one of the most common methods of reducing and immobilizing a fracture. External fixation with closed reduction is used when patients have soft tissue injury (open fracture). Although nurses do not determine which surgical technique is used, understanding the procedures helps in planning patient teaching and care.

Because ORIF permits early *mobility,* it is often the preferred surgical method. *Open* reduction allows the surgeon to directly view the fracture site. Internal fixation uses metal pins, screws, rods, plates, or prostheses inside the body to immobilize a fracture during healing. The surgeon makes one or more incisions to gain access to the broken bone(s) and implants one or more devices into bone tissue after each fracture is reduced. A cast, boot, or splint may be placed to maintain immobilization during the healing process, depending on the body part affected.

After the bone achieves union, the metal hardware may be removed, depending on the location and type of fracture. Hardware is removed most frequently in ankle fractures, depending on the severity of the injury. If the metal implants are not bothersome, they may remain in place. Examples of internal fixation devices for fractured hips are discussed later in this chapter.

An alternative modality for the management of fractures is the external fixation apparatus, as shown in Fig. 44.6. External fixation is a surgical procedure in which pins or wires are inserted through the skin and affected bone and then connected to a rigid external frame outside the body to stabilize the fracture during healing. The system may be used for upper or lower extremity fractures or for fractures of the pelvis, especially for open fractures when wound management is needed. After a fixator is removed, the patient may be placed in a cast, boot, or splint until healing is complete or may undergo internal fixation.

External fixation has several advantages over other surgical techniques:
- There is minimal blood loss compared with internal fixation.
- The device allows early ambulation and exercise of the affected body part while relieving pain.

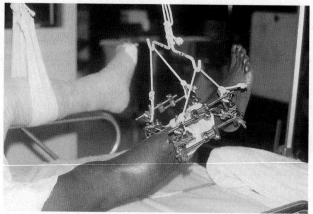

FIG. 44.6 Example of an external fixation device on the right leg. The left leg is in a splint. (From Rogers, J.L. [2023]. *McCance & Huether's Pathophysiology: The biologic basis for disease in adults and children* [9th ed.]. St. Louis: Elsevier.)

- The device maintains alignment in closed fractures that will not maintain position in a cast and stabilizes comminuted fractures that require bone grafting.

A disadvantage of external fixation is an increased risk for pin site *infection.* Pin site infections can lead to osteomyelitis, which is serious and difficult to treat (see Chapter 42).

Postoperative care. The postoperative care for a patient undergoing ORIF or external fixation is similar to that provided for any patient undergoing surgery (see Chapter 9). Because bone is a vascular, dynamic body tissue, the patient is at risk for complications specific to fractures and musculoskeletal surgery. IV ketorolac is often given in the postanesthesia care unit (PACU) or soon after discharge to the postsurgical area to reduce inflammation and *pain.* Aggressive pain management starts as soon as possible after surgery to prevent the development of persistent pain and promote early *mobility.* Patients who had a regional nerve blockade typically have little or no pain immediately after surgery for about 18 to 24 hours. However, when the anesthetic begins to wear off, be sure that the patient is medicated to prevent severe pain. Use nonpharmacologic measures for pain management, such as imagery, distraction, music therapy, and other measures that the patient prefers and are allowed by agency policy to promote comfort.

Additional information about postoperative care may be found later in this chapter in sections that discuss fractures to specific sites. Depending on the fractures that are repaired, some ORIF procedures are performed as same-day surgeries. Patients stay in the hospital up to 23 hours after surgery.

For patients with an *external fixator,* assess the pin sites every 8 to 12 hours for drainage, color, odor, and severe redness/hyperpigmentation, which indicate inflammation and possible *infection.* In the first 48 to 72 hours, *clear* fluid drainage or weeping is expected, which creates crusting around the pins. Although no standardized method or evidence-based protocol for pin site care has been established, recommendations have been made based on current evidence. A systematic review of pin site care found that pin site crusts should not be removed because they protect the patient from infection (Georgiades, 2018).

The patient with an external fixator may have a disturbed body image. The frame may be large and bulky, and the affected area may have massive tissue damage with dressings. Be sensitive to this possibility in planning care. Teach about alterations to clothing that may be required while the fixator is in place.

Procedures for Nonunion. Some management techniques are not successful because the bone does not heal. Several additional options are available to the primary health care provider to promote bone union, such as electrical bone stimulation, bone grafting, and ultrasound fracture treatment.

For selected patients, *electrical bone stimulation* may be successful. This procedure is based on research showing that bone has electrical properties that are used in healing. The exact mechanism of action is unknown. A noninvasive, external system delivers a small continuous electrical charge directed toward the nonhealed bone. There are no known risks with this system, although patients with pacemakers cannot use this device on an arm. Implanted direct-current stimulators are placed directly in the fracture site and have no external apparatus. Both systems require several months of treatment.

Another method of treating nonunion is *bone grafting*. In most cases, chips of bone are taken from the iliac crest or other site and are packed or wired between the bone ends to facilitate union. Allografts from cadavers may also be used. These grafts are frozen or freeze-dried and stored under sterile conditions in a bone bank.

Bone banking from living donors is becoming increasingly popular. If qualified, patients undergoing total hip arthroplasty may donate their femoral heads to the bank for later use as bone grafts for others. Careful screening ensures that the bone is healthy and that the donor has no communicable disease. The bone cannot be donated without written consent.

One of the newest modalities for fracture healing is *low-intensity pulsed ultrasound*. Used for slow-healing fractures or for new fractures as an alternative to surgery, ultrasound treatment has had excellent results. The patient applies the treatment for about 20 minutes each day. It has no contraindications or adverse effects.

Increasing Mobility

Planning: Expected Outcomes. The patient with a fracture is expected to increase physical ***mobility*** and be free of complications associated with immobility. Fracture patients are also expected to move purposefully in their own environment independently with or without an ambulatory device unless restricted by traction or other modality.

Interventions. The interventions necessary for this patient problem can be grouped into two types: those that help increase and promote ***mobility*** and those that prevent complications of decreased ***mobility***. Interventions to prevent complications of decreased mobility are briefly summarized in Chapter 3. Additional information may be found in nursing fundamentals textbooks.

Many patients with musculoskeletal trauma, including fractures, are referred by their primary health care provider for rehabilitation therapy with a physical therapist (PT) (usually for lower extremity injuries) and/or occupational therapist (OT) (usually for upper extremity injuries). The timing for this referral depends on the nature, severity, and treatment modality of the fracture(s) or other musculoskeletal trauma.

For example, some patients who have an ORIF for an ankle fracture begin therapy when the incisional staples or wound closure strips are removed and an orthopedic boot is fitted. Based on the initial evaluation, the PT performs gentle manipulative exercises to increase range of motion. The therapist may also begin to help the patient with *laterality,* a concept to help the brain identify the injured foot from the uninjured foot. Computer programs and mirror-box therapy can help reprogram the brain as part of *cognitive retraining.* In mirror-box therapy for an injured foot, the patient covers the affected foot while looking at and moving the uninjured foot in front of the mirror. The brain often perceives the foot in the mirror as the injured foot.

Stimulation by touch also helps the brain acknowledge the injured foot. The PT teaches the patient to frequently touch the injured area and use various materials and objects against the skin to desensitize it. These interventions improve **mobility** and decrease the risk for complex regional pain syndrome, discussed earlier in this chapter.

The success of rehabilitation is affected by the patient's motivation and willingness to perform prescribed exercises and activities between PT visits. For example, rehabilitation for ankle surgery may take several months, depending on the severity of the injury and the age and general health of the patient.

When weight bearing begins for lower extremity fractures about 6 weeks after surgery, the PT teaches the patient how to begin with toe-touch or partial weight bearing using crutches or a walker. Muscle-strengthening exercises of the affected leg help with ambulation because atrophy can begin shortly after injury.

The use of crutches, knee-walker scooter, or a walker increases **mobility** and assists in ambulation. The patient may progress to a cane after the bone heals. *Crutches* are the most commonly used ambulatory aid for many types of lower extremity musculoskeletal trauma (e.g., fractures, sprains, amputations). In most agencies, the physical therapist or emergency department/ambulatory care nurse fits the patient for crutches and teaches how to ambulate with them. Reinforce those instructions, and evaluate whether the patient is using the crutches correctly.

Walking with crutches or a knee-walker scooter requires strong arm muscles, balance, and coordination. For this reason, these ambulatory aids are not often used for older adults; traditional walkers and canes are preferred. Crutches can cause upper extremity bursitis or axillary nerve damage if they are fitted or used incorrectly. For that reason, the top of each crutch is padded. To prevent pressure on the axillary nerve, there should be two to three finger-breadths between the axilla and the top of the crutch when the crutch tip is at least 6 inches (15 cm) diagonally in front of the foot. The crutch is adjusted so that the elbow is flexed no more than 30 degrees when the palm is on the handle (Fig. 44.7). The distal tips of each crutch are rubber to prevent slipping.

There are several types of gaits for walking with crutches. The most common one for musculoskeletal injury is the three-point gait, which allows little weight bearing on the affected leg. The types of crutch-walking gaits are discussed in fundamentals of nursing books.

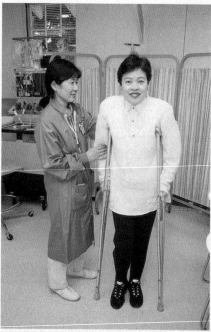

FIG. 44.7 Assisting the patient with crutch walking. Note how the therapist guards the patient and how the patient's elbows are at no more than 30 degrees of flexion.

A *walker* is most often used by the older patient who needs additional support for balance. The physical therapist assesses the strength of the upper extremities and the unaffected leg. Strength is improved with prescribed exercises as needed.

A *cane* is sometimes used if the patient needs only minimal support for an affected leg. The straight cane offers the least support. A hemi-cane or quad-cane provides a broader base for the cane and therefore more support. The cane is placed on the *unaffected* side and should create no more than 30 degrees of flexion of the elbow. The top of the cane should be parallel to the greater trochanter of the femur or stylus of the wrist. To ambulate, teach the patient to step forward with the cane and affected side at the same time for support. Then move the unaffected leg forward. Chapter 7 and fundamentals textbooks describe how to use these ambulatory devices in more detail.

Preventing and Monitoring for Neurovascular Compromise

Planning: Expected Outcomes. The patient with a fracture is expected to have no compromise in neurovascular status as evidenced by adequate **perfusion** (circulation), **mobility** (movement), and **sensory perception** (sensation) (CMS). If severe compromise occurs, the patient is expected to have early and prompt emergency treatment to prevent severe tissue damage.

Interventions. Perform neurovascular (NV) assessments (also known as "*circ checks*" or *CMS assessments*) frequently before and after fracture treatment. Patients who have extremity casts, splints with elastic bandage wraps, and open reduction with internal fixation (ORIF) or external fixation are especially at risk for NV compromise. If **perfusion** to the distal extremity is impaired, the patient reports increased **pain**, impaired **mobility**, and decreased **sensory perception.** If these symptoms are allowed to progress, patients are at risk for acute compartment syndrome (ACS), as described earlier in this chapter.

In some cases, compartment pressure may be monitored on a onetime basis with a handheld device with a digital display, or pressure can be monitored continuously. Monitoring is recommended for comatose or unresponsive high-risk patients with multiple trauma and fractures.

Care Coordination and Transition Management

The patient with an *uncomplicated* fracture is usually discharged to home from the emergency department or urgent care center. Older adults with hip or other fractures or patients with multiple traumas are hospitalized and then transferred to home, a rehabilitation setting, or a long-term care facility for rehabilitation. Collaborate with the case manager or the discharge planner in the hospital to ensure patient-centered care coordination. Be sure to communicate the plan of care clearly to the health care agency receiving the patient using the SBAR (situation, background, assessment, recommendation) communication method or other agency-specific system.

Home Care Management. If the patient is discharged to home, the nurse, rehabilitation therapist, or case manager (CM) may assess the home environment for structural barriers to **mobility** such as stairs. Be sure that the patient has easy access to the bathroom. Ask about small pets, scatter rugs, waxed floors, and walkway areas that could increase the risk for falls. If patients need to use a wheelchair or other ambulatory aids, make sure that they can use them safely and that there is room in the house to ambulate with these devices. The physical therapist may teach the patient how to use stairs, but older adults or those using crutches may experience difficulty performing this task. Depending on the age and condition of the patient, a home health care nurse may make one or two visits to check that the home is safe and that the patient and family are able to follow the interprofessional plan of care.

Self-Management Education. The patient with a fracture may be discharged from the hospital, emergency department, office, or clinic with a bandage, splint, boot, or cast. Provide verbal and written instructions on the care of these devices.

The patient may also need to continue wound care at home. Instruct the patient and family about how to assess and dress the wound to promote healing and prevent **infection.** Teach them how to recognize complications and when and where to seek professional health care if complications occur. Additional educational needs depend on the type of fracture and fracture repair.

Encourage patients and their families to ensure adequate foods high in protein and calcium that are needed for bone and tissue healing. For patients with lower extremity fractures, less weight bearing on long bones can cause anemia. The red bone marrow needs weight bearing to simulate red blood cell production. Encourage foods high in iron content. Teach the patient to take a daily iron-added multivitamin (take with food to prevent possible nausea) and a stool softener with a stimulant to prevent opioid-induced constipation.

Teach patients about the need for follow-up visits to the primary health care provider to assess bone healing and determine when casts or other devices can be discontinued. Box 44.4 describes care of the affected extremity after removal of the cast.

NCLEX Examination Challenge 44.2

Physiological Integrity

The nurse is teaching the client who had a right closed tibial fracture repair how to walk with a cane after cast removal. Which statement by the client indicates understanding about the health teaching?

A. "I should use the cane only when I feel I need support for my right leg."
B. "I should step forward with the cane and my left leg when I walk."
C. "I should use the cane on my left side for support when I walk."
D. "I should stay in bed for a few days while my leg continues to heal.

Health Care Resources. Arrange for follow-up care at home if needed. If there is severe bone and tissue damage, be realistic and help the patient and family understand the long-term nature of the recovery period. Multiple treatment techniques and surgical procedures required for complications can be mentally and emotionally draining for the patient and family.

An older or incapacitated patient may need assistance with ADLs, which can be provided by home care aides if family or other caregivers are unavailable. In collaboration with the case manager, anticipate the patient's needs and arrange for these services.

Evaluate Outcomes: Evaluation

Evaluate the care of the patient with one or more fractures based on the identified priority patient problems. The expected outcomes include that the patient:

🏠 BOX 44.4 Home Health Care

Care of the Extremity After Cast Removal

Teach patients to:
- Remove scaly, dead skin carefully by soaking; do not scrub.
- Move the extremity carefully. Expect smaller circumference, discomfort, weakness, and decreased range of motion.
- Support the extremity with pillows or your orthotic device until strength and movement return.
- Exercise slowly as instructed by your physical therapist.
- Wear support stockings or elastic bandages to prevent swelling (for lower extremity).

- States that adequate *pain* control (a 2 to 3 on a 0 to 10 pain scale) is achieved to accomplish ADLs
- Ambulates independently with or without an assistive device (if not restricted by traction or other device)
- Is free of physiologic consequences of decreased *mobility*
- Has adequate blood flow to maintain tissue *perfusion* and function
- Is free of fracture complications

LOWER EXTREMITY FRACTURES

Hip Fracture

Hip fracture is the most common musculoskeletal injury in older adults and one of the most frequently seen injuries in any health care setting or community. It has a high mortality rate as a result of multiple complications related to surgery, depression, and decreased *mobility.* Over half of older adults experiencing a hip fracture are unable to live independently, and many die within the first year. Fortunately, the incidence of hip fractures is decreasing, most likely owing to early management of bone loss and a decrease in the number of people who smoke. Smoking contributes to bone loss (Rosenberg, 2020).

Pathophysiology Review

Hip fractures include those involving the upper third of the femur and are classified as *intracapsular* (within the joint capsule) or *extracapsular* (outside the joint capsule). These types are further divided according to fracture location (Fig. 44.8).

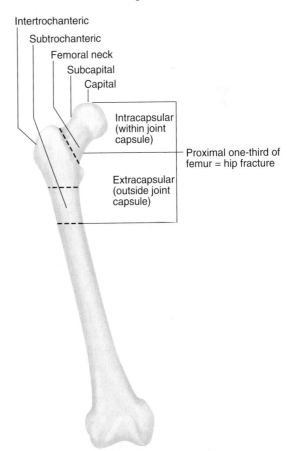

FIG. 44.8 Types of hip fractures.

In the area of the femoral neck, disruption of the blood supply to the head of the femur is a concern, which can result in ischemic or avascular necrosis (AVN) of the femoral head. AVN causes death and necrosis of bone tissue and results in pain and decreased *mobility.* This problem is most likely in patients with displaced fractures.

Osteoporosis is the biggest risk factor for hip fractures (see Chapter 42). This disease weakens the upper femur (hip), which causes it to break and lead to a fall. In some cases, a fall causes the fracture of the weakened hip, often referred to as a fragility fracture. The number of people with hip fracture is expected to increase as the population ages, and the associated health care costs will be tremendous (Conley et al., 2020).

👤 PATIENT-CENTERED CARE: OLDER ADULT HEALTH

Fragility Hip Fractures

Teach older adults about the risk factors for fragility hip fractures, including physiologic aging changes, disease processes, drug therapy, and environmental hazards. Physiologic changes include sensory changes such as diminished visual acuity and hearing; changes in gait, balance, and muscle strength; and joint stiffness. Disease processes such as osteoporosis, foot disorders, bony metastases, and changes in cardiac function increase the risk for fracture. These diseases are discussed elsewhere in this textbook. Drugs, such as diuretics, antihypertensives, antidepressants, sedatives, opioids, and alcohol, are factors that increase the risks for falling in older adults. Use of three or more of these drugs at the same time drastically increases the risk for falls. Throw rugs, loose carpeting, floor clutter, inadequate lighting, uneven walking surfaces or steps, and pets are environmental hazards that also cause falls.

The older adult with hip fracture usually reports groin pain or pain behind the knee on the affected side. In some cases, the patient has pain in the lower back or no pain at all. However, the patient is unable to stand without pain. X-ray or other imaging assessment confirms the diagnosis.

Interprofessional Collaborative Care

The expected outcome of interprofessional collaborative care is to relieve pain by reducing and immobilizing the hip fracture. Almost all patients have surgery to meet this outcome. Keep in mind that some older adults are high-risk surgical patients because of physiologic changes of aging and multiple comorbidities.

Preoperative Care. Patients usually receive IV morphine or hydromorphone after admission to the emergency department and may receive morphine or hydromorphone PCA or epidural analgesia after surgery. However, an integrative review of 38 research articles by Wennberg et al. (2018) found that first responders and emergency department staff do not adequately assess or manage pain among older adults who experience hip fracture. The authors recommended that nurses and other health professionals should continuously assess and better manage pain, which could improve cognition and patient satisfaction.

A major desired outcome for older adults experiencing a hip fracture is to achieve effective preoperative and postoperative

pain management while avoiding adverse drug effects. A preoperative alternative to opioid administration is fascia iliaca compartment block (FICB), a regional anesthetic technique using levobupivacaine or other drug to block femoral, lateral cutaneous, and obturator nerves. This procedure avoids the risk of injury to the femoral artery and vein. The benefits of FICB include effective pain relief without opioids and minimal cost (Williams et al., 2019).

Some older adults who experience a hip fracture may be placed temporarily in skin traction in an attempt to reduce pain from muscle spasms. However, a recent systematic review demonstrated that skin traction is ineffective in preoperative pain management (Sammut et al., 2021).

Postoperative Care. The treatment of choice is surgical repair by ORIF, when possible, to reduce pain and allow the older patient to be out of bed and ambulatory. Depending on the exact location of the fracture, an ORIF may include an intramedullary rod, pins, prostheses (for femoral head or femoral neck fractures, also known as a *hemiarthroplasty*), or a compression screw. Figs. 44.9 and 44.10 illustrate examples of these devices. Epidural, spinal, and/or general anesthesia is used. Occasionally a patient will be so debilitated that surgery cannot be done. In these rare cases, nonsurgical options include pain management and bed rest to allow natural fracture healing.

Before and after a hip repair, older adults frequently experience acute confusion (delirium) (see Chapter 3). They may pull at tubes or the surgical dressing or attempt to climb out of bed, possibly falling and causing self-injury. Other patients stay awake all night and sleep during the day. Keep in mind that some patients have a quiet delirium. Monitor the patient frequently to prevent falls. Use evidence-based fall prevention strategies, and ask the family or other visitors to let staff know if the patient is attempting to get out of bed. Chapter 4 describes fall prevention strategies and delirium management in detail.

Best practices for care of patients with fragility hip fractures can be summarized by reviewing the 12 internationally accepted nursing quality indicators (MacDonald et al., 2018).

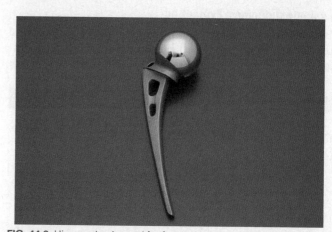

FIG. 44.9 Hip prosthesis used for femoral head or neck fractures (hemiarthroplasty). (Courtesy Smith & Nephew, Inc., Orthopaedics Divisions, Memphis, TN.)

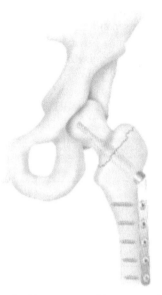

FIG. 44.10 Compression hip screw used for open reduction with internal fixation (ORIF) of the hip.

These indicators and associated postoperative nursing care are outlined in Box 44.5.

! NURSING SAFETY PRIORITY

Action Alert

Patients who have a *hemiarthroplasty* for fractured hip repair are at risk for hip dislocation or subluxation. Be sure to prevent hip adduction and rotation to keep the operative leg in proper alignment. Regular pillows or abduction devices can be used for patients who are confused or restless. If straps are used to hold the device in place, make sure that they are not too tight, and check the skin every 2 hours for signs of pressure. Perform neurovascular assessments to ensure that the device is not interfering with arterial circulation or peripheral nerve conduction.

Many patients recover fully from hip fracture repair and regain their functional ability. They are typically discharged to their home, rehabilitation unit or center, or a skilled nursing facility for physical and occupational therapy. However, some patients are not able to return to their prefracture ADL and *mobility* level. Family caregivers often have unexpected responsibilities caring for patients during their recovery. Hip fracture resource centers can be very useful in providing caregiver support. For some patients, palliative or end-of-life care may be needed.

Other Fractures of the Lower Extremity

Other fractures of the lower extremity may or may not require hospitalization. However, if the patient has severe or multiple fractures, especially with soft tissue damage, hospital admission is usually required. Patients who have surgery to repair their injury may also be hospitalized. Coordinate care with the physical and occupational therapists regarding transfers, positioning, and ambulation. Collaborate with the case manager regarding placement after discharge. Most patients go home unless there is no support system or additional rehabilitation is needed. Health teaching and ensuring continuity of care are essential.

BOX 44.5 Best Practice for Patient Safety and Quality Care

Quality Indicators for Postoperative Nursing Care of Older Adults With Hip Fractures

Nursing Quality Indicator	Nursing Care Best Practice
Timing of Surgery	Ensure that the patient has surgery within 24–48 hours of the fracture, depending on the patient's condition.
Early and Frequent Mobility	Assist the patient to get out of the bed to stand, walk, or sit on the side of the bed on the day of surgery. Walk the patient 1–2 times a day on the first postoperative day.
Malnutrition Prevention	Conduct a nutritional screening on admission. Provide a diet as tolerated with daily oral nutritional supplements postoperatively.
Catheter-Associated Urinary Tract Infection (CAUTI) Prevention	Avoid the use of an indwelling urinary catheter, if possible. If a urinary catheter must be used, the catheter should be removed within 24 hours, if possible.
Pain Management	Use a multimodal pain management approach based on frequent pain assessments. Use geriatric drug dosing and regional nerve blocks if feasible.
Delirium	Complete cognitive screening on admission. Screen the patient each day for delirium.
Pneumonia Prevention	Keep the head of the patient's bed elevated to at least 30 degrees. Perform dysphagia screening and provide frequent mouth care.
Constipation Prevention	Assess daily for bowel movement. Implement an evidence-based bowel protocol, including preventive stool softeners and laxatives.
Venous Thromboembolism (VTE) Prevention	Implement an evidence-based VTE prevention protocol.
Pressure Injury Prevention	Perform a valid pressure injury risk assessment on admission. Perform daily skin assessments. Follow an evidence-based pressure injury prevention protocol/plan of care, including the need to keep the patient's heels off the bed to prevent breakdown.
Care Transitions/Preparing for Home	Provide patient self-management health teaching. Teach the need to follow up with the primary health care provider 4–6 weeks after discharge.
Bone Health	Teach the patient the need to follow up on personal bone health to prevent future fractures.

Fractures of the *lower two-thirds of the femur* usually result from trauma, often from a motor vehicle crash. A femur fracture is seldom immobilized by casting because the powerful muscles of the thigh become spastic, which causes displacement of bone ends and significant pain. Extensive hemorrhage can occur with femur fracture.

Surgical treatment is ORIF with plates, nails, rods, or a compression screw. In a few cases in which extensive bone fragmentation or severe tissue trauma is found, external fixation may be used. Healing time for a femur fracture may be 6 months or longer. Skeletal traction, followed by a full-leg brace or cast, may be used in nonsurgical treatment.

Trauma to the lower leg most often causes fractures of both the *tibia* and the *fibula,* particularly the lower third, and is often referred to as a *tib-fib* fracture. The major treatment techniques are closed reduction with casting, internal fixation, and external fixation. If closed reduction is used, the patient may wear a cast for 6 to 10 weeks. Because of poor **perfusion** to parts of the tibia and fibula, delayed union is not unusual with this type of fracture. Internal fixation with nails or a plate and screws, followed by a long-leg cast for 4 to 6 weeks, is another option. Since the fibula is a non–weight-bearing bone, occasionally no fixation is required. When the fractures cause extensive skin and soft tissue damage, the initial treatment may be external fixation, often for 6 to 10 weeks, usually followed by application of a cast until the fracture is completely healed. The patient is typically non–weight bearing and uses ambulatory aids such as crutches.

Ankle fractures are described by their anatomic place of injury. For example, a bimalleolar (Pott) fracture involves the medial malleolus of the tibia and the lateral malleolus of the fibula. The small talus that makes up the rest of the ankle joint may also be broken. An ORIF is usually performed using two incisions: one on the medial (inside) aspect of the ankle and one on the lateral (outer) side. Several screws or nails are placed into the tibia, and a compression plate with multiple screws keeps the fibula in alignment. Weight bearing is restricted until the bone heals.

Treatment of fractures of the foot or phalanges (toes) is similar to that of other fractures. Phalangeal fractures may be more painful but are not as serious as most other types of fractures. Crutches are used for ambulation if weight bearing is restricted, but many patients can ambulate while wearing an orthopedic shoe or boot while the bone heals.

FRACTURES OF THE CHEST AND PELVIS

Chest trauma may cause fractures of the ribs or sternum. The major concern with rib and sternal fractures is the potential for puncture of the lungs, heart, or arteries by bone fragments or ends. *Assess airway, breathing, and circulation status **first** for any patient having chest trauma!* Fractures of the lower ribs may damage underlying organs, such as the liver, spleen, or kidneys. These fractures tend to heal on their own, without surgical intervention. Patients are often uncomfortable during the healing process and require analgesia. They also have a high risk for pneumonia because of shallow breathing caused by **pain** on inspiration. Encourage them to breathe normally if possible, and ensure that their pain is well managed.

Because the pelvis is very vascular and is close to major organs and blood vessels, associated internal damage is the major focus in fracture management. After head injuries, pelvic fractures are the second most common cause of death from trauma. In young adults, pelvic fractures typically result from motor vehicle crashes or falls from buildings. Falls are the most common cause in older adults. The major concern related to pelvic injury is venous oozing or arterial bleeding. Loss of blood volume leads to hypovolemic shock.

> ### ❗ NURSING SAFETY PRIORITY
> #### *Action Alert*
>
> Assess for internal abdominal trauma by checking for blood in the urine and stool and by monitoring the abdomen for the development of rigidity or swelling. The trauma team may use CT scanning or ultrasound for assessment of hemorrhage. Ultrasound is noninvasive, rapid, reliable, and cost-effective, and it can be done at the bedside.

There are many classification systems for pelvic fractures. A system that is particularly useful divides fractures of the pelvis into two broad categories: non–weight-bearing fractures and weight-bearing fractures.

When a *non–weight-bearing* part of the pelvis is fractured, such as one of the pubic rami or the iliac crest, treatment can be as minimal as bed rest on a firm mattress or bed board. This type of fracture can be quite painful, and the patient may need stool softeners to facilitate bowel movements because of hesitancy to move. Well-stabilized fractures usually heal in 2 months.

A *weight-bearing* fracture (such as multiple fractures of the pelvic ring, creating instability, or a fractured acetabulum) necessitates external fixation or ORIF or both. Progression to weight bearing depends on the stability of the fracture after fixation. Some patients can fully bear weight within days of surgery, whereas others managed with traction may be unable to bear weight for as long as 12 weeks. For complex pelvic fractures with extensive soft tissue damage, external fixation may be required.

COMPRESSION FRACTURES OF THE SPINE

Most vertebral fractures are caused by osteoporosis or metastatic bone cancer. Compression fractures result when trabecular or cancellous bone within the vertebra becomes weakened and causes the vertebral body to collapse. The patient has *severe pain* (especially when moving), deformity (kyphosis), and possible neurologic compromise. As discussed in the Osteoporosis section of Chapter 42, the patient's quality of life is reduced by the impact of this problem.

Nonsurgical management includes bed rest, analgesics, nerve blocks, and physical therapy to maintain muscle strength. Vertebral compression fractures (VCFs) that remain painful and impair **mobility** may be treated with vertebroplasty or kyphoplasty. These procedures are minimally invasive techniques in which bone cement is injected through the skin (percutaneously) directly into the fracture site to provide stability and immediate pain relief. In addition to vertebroplasty, radiologists and orthopedic surgeons may do a kyphoplasty (using a balloon) or the preferred vertebral augmentation (using a different cavity-creating device) to partially reexpand a compressed vertebral body.

Minimally invasive procedures can be done in an operating or interventional radiology suite by a surgeon or interventional radiologist. They can be done with moderate sedation or general anesthesia. IV ketorolac may be given before the procedure to reduce inflammation. Large-bore needles are placed into the fracture site using fluoroscopy or CT guidance. Then the deflated balloon is inserted through the needles and inflated in the fracture site, and the cement is injected.

Patients may have the procedures in an ambulatory care setting and return home after 2 to 4 hours or be admitted to the hospital for an overnight stay. Box 44.6 outlines the preprocedure and postprocedure care for percutaneous interventions for vertebral compression fractures.

Before discharge, teach the patient to report any signs or symptoms of infection from puncture sites. Remind the patient to avoid a soaking bath for 1 week, use analgesics as needed, resume activity slowly, and contact the primary health care provider for questions or concerns. Surgery generally reduces preoperative pain significantly.

BOX 44.6 Best Practice for Patient Safety and Quality Care

Nursing Care for Patients Having Vertebroplasty or Kyphoplasty

Provide *preprocedure care*, including:

- Check the patient's coagulation laboratory test results; platelet count should be more than 100,000/mm³ (100 × 10⁹/L).
- Make sure that all anticoagulant drugs were discontinued as requested by the surgeon or interventional radiologist.
- Assess and document the patient's neurologic status, especially extremity movement and sensation.
- Assess the patient's pain level.
- Assess the patient's ability to lie prone for at least 1 hour.
- Establish an IV line in a size suitable for surgery, and take vital signs.

Provide *postprocedure care*, including:

- Place the patient in a flat supine position for 1 to 2 hours or as requested by the surgeon or interventional radiologist.
- Monitor and record vital signs and frequent neurologic assessments; report any change immediately to the physician.
- Apply an ice pack to the puncture site if needed to relieve pain.
- Assess the patient's pain level, and compare it with the preoperative level; give mild analgesic as needed.
- Monitor for complications, such as bleeding at the puncture site or shortness of breath; report these findings immediately if they occur.
- Assist the patient with ambulation.

Before discharge, teach the patient and family the following:

- Avoid driving or operating machinery for the first 24 hours because of drugs used during the procedure.
- Monitor the puncture site for signs of infection, such as redness/hyperpigmentation, pain, swelling, or drainage.
- Keep the dressing dry, and remove it the next day.
- Begin usual activities, including walking, the next day, and slowly increase the activity level over the next few days.

✴ PERFUSION CONCEPT EXEMPLAR: AMPUTATION

An **amputation** is the removal of a part of the body. Advances in microvascular surgical procedures for limb salvage, better use of antibiotic therapy, and improved surgical techniques for traumatic injury and bone cancer have reduced the number of elective amputations. The psychosocial aspects of the procedure are as devastating as the physical impairments that result. The loss is complete and permanent and causes a change in body image and self-esteem. Collaborate with members of the interprofessional team, including prosthetists, rehabilitation therapists, psychologists, case managers, and physiatrists (rehabilitation physicians), when providing care to the patient who undergoes an amputation.

Pathophysiology Review

Amputations may be elective or traumatic. Most amputations are *elective* and are related to complications of peripheral arterial disease (PAD) that result in decreased **perfusion** (ischemia) to distal areas of the lower extremity. *Traumatic* amputations most often result from accidents or war.

Levels of Amputation

Elective lower extremity (LE) amputations are performed much more frequently than upper extremity amputations. Several types of LE amputations may be performed.

The loss of any or all of the small toes presents a minor disability. Loss of the great toe is significant because it affects balance, gait, and "push-off" ability during walking. Midfoot amputations and the Syme amputation are common procedures for peripheral vascular disease. In the Syme amputation, most of the foot is removed, but the ankle remains. The advantage of this surgery over traditional amputations below the knee is that weight bearing can occur without the use of a prosthesis and with reduced pain.

An intense effort is made to preserve knee joints with below-the-knee amputation (BKA). When the cause for the amputation extends beyond the knee, above-knee or higher amputations are performed. Hip disarticulation, or removal of the hip joint, and hemipelvectomy (removal of half of the pelvis with the leg) are more common in younger patients than in older ones who cannot easily handle the cumbersome prostheses required for ambulation. The higher the level of amputation, the more energy is required for **mobility**. These higher-level procedures are sometimes done for cancer of the bone, osteomyelitis, or trauma as a last resort.

An amputation of any part of the upper extremity is generally more incapacitating than one of the legs. The arms and hands are necessary for ADLs such as feeding, bathing, dressing, and driving a car. In the upper extremity, as much length as possible is saved to maintain function. Early replacement with a prosthetic device is vital for the patient with this type of amputation.

Complications of Amputation

The most common complications of amputations are:

- Hemorrhage leading to hypovolemic shock
- Infection

- Phantom limb *pain*
- Neuroma
- Flexion contractures

When a person loses part or all of an extremity either by surgery or by trauma, major blood vessels are severed, which causes *hemorrhage*. If the bleeding is uncontrolled, the patient is at risk for hypovolemic shock and possibly death.

As with any surgical procedure or trauma, infection can occur in the wound or the bone (osteomyelitis). The older adult who is malnourished and confused is at the greatest risk because excreta may soil the wound or the patient may remove the dressing and pick at the incision. Preventing infection is a major emphasis in hospitals and other health care settings.

Persistent *pain* is a frequent complication of amputation. This sensation is felt in the amputated part immediately after surgery and usually diminishes over time. When it persists and is unpleasant or painful, it is referred to as **phantom limb pain (PLP)**. PLP is more common in patients who had chronic limb pain before surgery and less common in those who have traumatic amputations. The patient reports pain in the removed body part shortly after surgery, usually after an above-the-knee amputation (AKA). The *pain* is often described as intense burning, crushing, or cramping. Some patients report that the removed part is in a distorted, uncomfortable position. They experience numbness and tingling, referred to as *phantom limb sensation,* and pain. Others state that the most distal area of the removed part feels as if it is retracted into the residual limb end. For most patients, the pain is triggered by touching the residual limb or by temperature or barometric pressure changes, concurrent illness, fatigue, anxiety, or stress. Routine activities such as urination can trigger the pain. If *pain* is long-standing, especially if it existed before the amputation, any stimulus can cause it, including touching any part of the body.

Neuroma, a sensitive tumor consisting of damaged nerve cells, forms most often in amputations of the upper extremity but can occur anywhere. The patient may or may not have pain. It is diagnosed by sonography and can be treated either surgically or nonsurgically. Surgery to remove the neuroma may be performed, but it often regrows and is more painful than before the surgery. Nonsurgical modalities include peripheral nerve blocks, steroid injections, and cognitive therapies such as hypnosis.

Flexion contractures of the hip or knee are most frequently seen in patients with amputations of the lower extremity. This complication must be avoided so that the patient can ambulate with a prosthetic device. Proper positioning and active range-of-motion exercises in the early postoperative period help prevent this complication.

Etiology and Genetic Risk

Diabetes mellitus is typically the underlying cause of peripheral arterial disease (PAD), which leads to lower extremity amputation for many patients. Amputation should be considered only after other interventions have failed to restore circulation to the lower extremity, sometimes referred to as *limb salvage procedures* (e.g., percutaneous transluminal angioplasty [PTA]). These procedures are discussed elsewhere in this text.

Trauma to a limb is the second leading cause of amputation and is the primary cause of *upper extremity* amputation. For example, an individual may clean lawn mower blades without disconnecting the machine. A motor vehicle crash or industrial machine accident may also cause an amputation.

Incidence/Prevalence

Over 2 million people live with amputations in the United States. People of color are most likely to have limb loss due to diabetes mellitus and PAD (Amputee Coalition, 2021).

PATIENT-CENTERED CARE: HEALTH EQUITY

Elective Lower Extremity Amputations

Research on the incidence of elective lower extremity amputations demonstrates the following health equity issues (Amputee Coalition, 2021; Fanaroff et al., 2021):
- Black individuals are less likely than Whites to undergo limb salvage procedures. Therefore, Black individuals, especially men, are twice as likely to have a lower extremity amputation due to diabetes mellitus as a result of peripheral arterial disease (PAD).
- Hispanics are 30% more likely than Whites to have a major lower extremity amputation related to diabetic foot infection. Indigenous people are 70% more likely than insured nonindigenous people to have a lower extremity amputation.

Studies have shown that social determinants of health, especially low household income and lack of health care access, are largely responsible for these health inequities (Fanaroff et al., 2021). Assess all patients who have diabetes mellitus and PAD to determine their access to health care and health insurance status. Teach patients how to manage their disease, and identify community resources that can help them with self-management as needed.

PATIENT-CENTERED CARE: VETERAN HEALTH

Traumatic Amputations

The number of traumatic amputations has increased during recent wars as a result of hidden land mines (IEDs), bombs, and motor vehicle crashes (e.g., in Iraq and Afghanistan). Multiple limbs or parts of limbs are amputated as a result of these events. Thousands of veterans experience trauma to multiple limbs and must adjust to major changes in their lifestyles. Many veterans have multiple amputations that affect **mobility** and ADL function. Additionally, many veteran amputees have comorbid physical and mental health problems, including traumatic brain injury (TBI) and posttraumatic stress disorder (PTSD) (Elliott et al., 2021).

Health Promotion/Disease Prevention

Typical patients undergoing elective amputation are middle-age or older people of color who have diabetes and a lengthy history of smoking. Many of these patients have not cared for their feet properly due to lack of knowledge, which results in a nonhealing, infected foot ulcer and possibly gangrene. Therefore, adherence to the disease management plan may help prevent the need for later amputation. Lifestyle habits such as maintaining a healthy weight, regular exercise, and avoiding smoking can help prevent or manage chronic diseases such as diabetes and poor blood circulation.

The second largest group of patients who undergo amputations consists of young men involved in motorcycle or other vehicular crashes, who are injured by industrial equipment, or who have been in combat or accidents in war. These individuals may experience either a traumatic amputation or undergo a surgical amputation because of a severe crushing injury and massive soft tissue damage. Teach young people the importance of taking safety precautions to prevent injury at work and to avoid speeding or driving while drinking alcohol.

Interprofessional Collaborative Care
Recognize Cues: Assessment

Physical Assessment/Signs and Symptoms. Monitor neurovascular status in the affected extremity that will be electively amputated. When the patient has peripheral vascular disease, check the circulation in both legs. Assess skin color, temperature, sensation, and pulses in both affected and unaffected extremities. Capillary refill can be difficult to determine in the older adult related to thickened and opaque nails. In this situation, the skin near the nail bed can be used. Capillary refill is a less reliable cue than other indicators. Observe and document any discoloration of the skin, edema, ulcerations, presence of necrosis, and hair distribution on the lower extremities.

Psychosocial Assessment. People react differently to the loss of a body part. Be aware that an amputation of only a portion of one finger, especially the thumb, can be traumatic to the patient. The thumb is needed for hand activities. Therefore, the loss must not be underestimated. Patients undergoing amputation face a complete, permanent loss. Evaluate their psychological preparation for a planned amputation, and expect them to go through the grieving process. Adjusting to a traumatic, unexpected amputation is often more difficult than accepting a planned one.

Attempt to determine the patient's willingness and motivation to withstand prolonged rehabilitation after the amputation. Asking questions about how the patient has dealt with previous life crises can provide clues. Adjustment to the amputation and rehabilitation is less difficult if the patient is willing and has the resources to make needed changes.

PATIENT-CENTERED CARE: VETERAN HEALTH

Psychological Impact of Amputations

The young military servicemember may be bitter, hostile, or depressed if experiencing one or more traumatic amputations while being deployed. Active military members are often medically discharged due to their physical and emotional limitations. However, this practice is beginning to change as advances in reconstruction improve (Elliott et al., 2021). Older veterans typically have elective amputations as a result of peripheral arterial disease.

The patient with one or more amputations experiences an altered self-concept. The physical alterations affect body image and self-esteem. For example, a young veteran may think that an intimate relationship with a partner is no longer possible or desirable. An older adult may feel a loss of independence. Assess the patient's feelings about self to identify areas in which emotional support is needed. Consult with the certified hospital chaplain, other spiritual leader, or hospital social worker if the patient is hospitalized. Counseling resources are also available in the community and through the Department of Veterans Affairs health system in the United States.

PATIENT-CENTERED CARE: CULTURE AND SPIRITUALITY

Family Response to Amputation

In addition to assessing the patient's psychosocial status, assess the family's reaction to the surgery or trauma. The family's response usually correlates directly with the patient's progress during recovery and rehabilitation and the patient's values and beliefs. Rehabilitation for patients who experience multiple limb traumas, including amputation, can be as long as 9 to 15 months (Elliott et al., 2021). Expect the family to grieve for the loss, and allow them time to adjust to the change. Establish a trusting relationship, and reassure the patient and family that you are available to listen to their concerns and needs.

Assess the patient's and family's coping abilities, and help them identify personal strengths and weaknesses. Assess the patient's religious, spiritual, and cultural beliefs. Some groups (e.g., Jewish) require that the amputated body part be stored for later burial with the rest of the body or buried immediately. Other cultural customs and rituals may apply, depending on the group with which the patient associates.

Diagnostic Assessment. The surgeon determines which tests are performed to assess for viability of the limb based on blood flow. A number of noninvasive techniques are available for this evaluation. For complete accuracy, the surgeon does not rely on any single test.

One procedure is measurement of segmental limb blood pressures, which can also be used by the nurse at the bedside. In this test, an ankle-brachial index (ABI) is calculated by dividing ankle systolic pressure by brachial systolic pressure. A normal ABI is 0.9 or higher.

Blood flow in an extremity can also be assessed by other noninvasive tests, including *Doppler* ultrasonography or laser Doppler flowmetry and transcutaneous oxygen pressure ($TcPO_2$). The ultrasonography and laser Doppler measure the speed of blood flow in the limb. The $TcPO_2$ measures oxygen pressure to indicate blood flow in the limb and has proven reliable for predicting healing.

Analyze Cues and Prioritize Hypotheses: Analysis

The collaborative problems for patients with amputations include:
1. Potential for decreased tissue *perfusion* in residual limb due to soft tissue damage, edema, and/or bleeding
2. Acute and/or persistent *pain* due to soft tissue damage, muscle spasm, and edema
3. Decreased *mobility* due to pain, muscle spasm, soft tissue damage, and/or lack of balance due to a missing body part
4. Decreased self-esteem due to one or more ADL deficits, disturbed self-concept and body image, and/or lack of support systems

Generate Solutions and Take Actions: Planning and Implementation
Monitoring for Decreased Tissue Perfusion

Planning: Expected Outcomes. The patient with one or more amputations is expected to have adequate peripheral *perfusion* to the residual (surgical) limb(s) as evidenced by warm, usual-color skin.

Interventions. A *traumatic* amputation requires rapid emergency care to possibly save the severed body part for reattachment to promote **perfusion** and prevent hemorrhage. If the severed body part(s) is mutilated or crushed, it cannot be used.

Emergency Care: Traumatic vs. Elective Amputation. For a person who has a *traumatic amputation* in the community, first call 911. Assess the patient for airway or breathing problems. Examine the amputation site and apply direct pressure with layers of dry gauze or other cloth, using clean gloves if available. Many nurses carry gloves and first-aid kits for this type of emergency. Elevate the extremity above the patient's heart to decrease the bleeding. Do not remove the dressing to prevent dislodging the clot.

The fingers are the most likely part to be amputated and replanted. The current recommendation for prehospital care is to wrap the completely severed finger in dry sterile gauze (if available) or a clean cloth. Put the finger in a watertight, sealed plastic bag. *Place the bag in ice water, never directly on ice, at 1 part ice and 3 parts water.* Avoid contact between the finger and the water to prevent tissue damage. Do not remove any semi-detached parts of the digit. Be sure that the part goes with the patient to the hospital.

For patients with a *planned (elective) surgical amputation,* the nurse's primary focus is to monitor for signs indicating that there is sufficient tissue **perfusion** and no hemorrhage. The skin flap at the end of the residual (remaining) limb should be pink in a light-skinned person and not discolored (lighter or darker than other usual skin pigmentation) in a dark-skinned patient. The area should be warm but not hot. Assess the closest proximal pulse for presence and strength and compare it with that in the other extremity. However, if the patient has bilateral vascular disease, comparison of limbs may not be an accurate way of measuring blood flow. Use a Doppler device to determine if the affected side is being perfused. Monitor vital signs per agency protocol.

✚ NURSING SAFETY PRIORITY
Critical Rescue

If the patient has decreased tissue **perfusion**, notify the surgeon or Rapid Response Team immediately to communicate your assessment findings! If the patient's blood pressure drops and the pulse increases, suspect covert (hidden) bleeding. To check for the presence of overt (obvious) bleeding, be sure to lift the residual limb and feel under the pressure dressing for dampness or drainage. If bleeding occurs, apply direct pressure and notify the Rapid Response Team or primary health care provider immediately. Continue to monitor the patient until help arrives.

Managing Acute and/or Persistent Pain

Planning: Expected Outcomes. The patient with an amputation is expected to state that adequate **pain** control is achieved after appropriate management.

Interventions. All patients experience **pain** as a result of either a traumatic or surgical (elective) amputation. Some patients also report pain in the missing body part (phantom limb pain [PLP]). Be sure to determine which type the patient has.

❗ NURSING SAFETY PRIORITY
Action Alert

If the patient reports PLP, recognize that the **pain** is real and should be managed promptly and completely! It is *not* therapeutic to remind the patient that the limb cannot be hurting because it is missing. To prevent increased pain, handle the residual limb carefully when assessing the site or changing the dressing.

Opioid analgesics are not as effective for PLP as they are for residual limb pain. IV infusions of calcitonin during the week after amputation can reduce PLP. The primary health care provider prescribes other drugs on the basis of the type of PLP the patient experiences. For instance, beta-blocking agents such as propranolol are used for constant, dull, burning pain. Antiepileptic drugs such as pregabalin and gabapentin may be used for knifelike or sharp burning (neuropathic) pain. Antispasmodics such as baclofen may be prescribed for muscle spasms or cramping. Some patients improve with antidepressant drugs as adjuvant therapy.

Other pain management modalities are described in Chapter 6. Incorporate them into the plan of care if agreeable with the patient by collaborating with specialists who are trained to perform them. For example, physical therapists often use massage, heat, transcutaneous electrical nerve stimulation (TENS), mirror therapy, and ultrasound therapy for pain control. Yildirim & Sen (2020) found that mirror therapy, in which the patient regularly practices exercises with the affected and unaffected extremity in front of a mirror, helps to decrease phantom limb pain.

Consult with the certified hospital chaplain or social worker to provide emotional support based on the patient's preferences and beliefs. A psychologist may be needed to provide diagnostic assessment and/or psychotherapy.

Promoting Mobility

Planning: Expected Outcomes. The patient with an amputation is expected to have adequate **mobility** and be free of complications associated with decreased mobility.

Interventions. Collaborate with the physical and/or occupational therapists to begin exercises as soon as possible after surgery. If the amputation is planned, the therapist may work with the patient before surgery to start muscle-strengthening exercises and evaluate the need for ambulatory aids, such as crutches. If the patient can practice with these devices before surgery, learning how to ambulate after surgery is much easier.

For patients with above- or below-the-knee amputations, teach range-of-motion (ROM) exercises for prevention of flexion contractures, particularly of the hip and knee. A trapeze and an overhead frame aid in strengthening the arms and allow the patient to move independently in bed. Teach the patient how to perform ROM exercises. Be sure to turn the patient every 2 hours or teach the patient how to turn independently. Move the patient slowly to prevent muscle spasms.

A firm mattress is essential for preventing contractures with a leg amputation. Assist the patient into a prone position every 3 to 4 hours for 20- to 30-minute periods if tolerated and not contraindicated. This position may be uncomfortable initially, but it helps prevent hip flexion contractures. Instruct the patient to pull the residual limb close to the other leg and contract the

INTERPROFESSIONAL COLLABORATION

Care of Patients Who Have an Amputation

Interprofessional collaborative care depends on the type and location of the amputation. For example, an above-the-knee amputation (AKA) has the potential for more postoperative complications than does a partial foot amputation. Regardless of where the amputation occurs, collaborate with the rehabilitation therapists to improve ambulation and/or enable the patient to be independent in ADLs. For many amputations, prostheses can be used to substitute for the missing body part. According to the Interprofessional Education Collaborative (IPEC) Expert Panel's Competency of Roles and Responsibilities, using the unique and complementary abilities of other team members optimizes health and patient care (Slusser et al., 2019).

gluteal muscles of the buttocks for muscle strengthening. After staples are removed, the physical therapist may begin resistive exercises, which should also be done at home.

For above- and below-the-knee amputations, teach the patient how to push the residual limb down toward the bed while supporting it on a soft pillow at first. Then instruct the patient to continue this activity using a firmer pillow and then progress to a harder surface. This activity helps prepare the residual limb for prosthesis and reduces the incidence of phantom limb *pain* and sensation.

Elevation of a lower-leg residual limb on a pillow while the patient is in a supine position is controversial. Some practitioners advocate avoiding this practice at all times because it promotes hip or knee flexion contracture. Others allow elevation for the first 24 to 48 hours to reduce swelling and subsequent *pain.* Inspect the residual limb daily to ensure that it lies completely flat on the bed.

Before an elective amputation, the patient often sees a certified prosthetist-orthotist (CPO) so that planning can begin for the postoperative period. Arrangements for replacing an arm part are especially important for the patient to achieve self-management. Some patients are fitted with a temporary prosthesis at the time of surgery. Others, particularly older patients with vascular disease, are fitted after the residual limb has healed.

The patient being fitted for a leg prosthesis should bring a sturdy pair of shoes to the fitting. The prosthesis will be adjusted to that heel height.

Several devices help shape and shrink the residual limb in preparation for the prosthesis. Rigid, removable dressings are preferred because they decrease edema, protect and shape the limb, and allow easy access to the wound for inspection. An air splint, a plastic inflatable device, is sometimes used for this purpose. One of its disadvantages is air leakage and loss of compression. Wrapping with elastic bandages can also be effective in reducing edema, shrinking the limb, and holding the wound dressing in place.

For wrapping to be effective, reapply the bandages every 4 to 6 hours or more often if they become loose. Figure-eight wrapping prevents restriction of blood flow. Decrease the tightness of the bandages while wrapping in a distal-to-proximal direction. After wrapping, anchor the bandages to the highest joint, such as above the knee for below-the-knee amputations.

The design of and materials for prostheses have improved dramatically over the past 20 years. Computer-assisted design and computer-assisted manufacturing (CAD-CAM) is used for a custom fit. One of the most important developments in lower extremity prosthetics is the ankle-foot prosthesis, such as the Flex-Foot for more active amputees.

Another innovation for patients who have extensive or high amputation is a surgical procedure designed to improve client function and *mobility.* During *osseointegration reconstruction*, the surgeon anchors an implant (usually metal) to the residual bone of the amputation which is then attached to a prosthesis using a transcutaneous connector. This procedure has been improved since its initial introduction over 30 years ago.

Promoting Self-Esteem

Planning: Expected Outcomes. The patient with an amputation is expected to adapt to the amputation to achieve a positive self-esteem and have an active and productive life.

Interventions. The patient often experiences feelings of inadequacy as a result of losing a body part, especially an older adult who was in poor health before surgery. If patients are unable to adapt psychologically to the amputation, they may have difficulty adapting to a possible lifestyle change. If possible, arrange for the patient to meet with a rehabilitated, active amputee who is about the same age as the patient.

The use of the word *stump* in referring to the remaining portion of the limb (residual limb) continues to be controversial. Patients have reported feeling as if they were part of a tree when the term is used. However, some rehabilitation specialists who routinely work with amputees believe the term is appropriate because it forces the patient to realize what has happened and promotes adjustment to the amputation. *Assess the patient to determine which term is preferred.*

Assess the patient's verbal and nonverbal references to the affected area. Some patients behave euphorically (extremely happy) and seem to accept the loss. *Do not jump to the conclusion that acceptance has occurred.* Ask patients to describe their feelings about changes in body image and self-esteem. Patients may verbalize acceptance but refuse to look at the area during a dressing change. This inconsistent behavior is not unusual and should be documented and shared with other health care team members.

With advancements in prostheses and surgical techniques, many patients can return to their jobs and other activities. Professional athletes who use prostheses are often quite successful in sports. Patients with amputations ski, hike, golf, bowl, and participate in other physically demanding activities. Many amputees participate actively in organized and recreational sports.

If a job or career change is necessary, collaborate with a social worker or vocational rehabilitation specialist to evaluate the patient's skills. A supportive family or significant other is important for the adjustment to this change. The patient may also think that an intimate relationship is no longer possible because of physical changes. Discuss sexuality issues with patients and their partners as needed. Professional assistance from a sex therapist, intimacy coach, or psychologist may be needed.

Help the patient and family set realistic desired outcomes, and take one day at a time. Help them recognize personal strengths. If the desired outcomes are unrealistic, frustration and disappointment may decrease motivation during rehabilitation. Basic principles of rehabilitation are discussed in Chapter 7.

NCLEX Examination Challenge 44.3

Psychosocial Integrity

The nurse is interviewing a client who is planning to have an elective below-the-knee amputation for a nonhealing diabetic ulcer and gangrene. The client expresses feeling sad and useless without both legs. What would be the nurse's **best** response?

A. "You're only going to lose part of one leg, so you still will have both legs."

B. "Would you like to talk with our social worker or certified hospital chaplain?"

C. "Why don't you wait and see how you feel after surgery tomorrow?"

D. "Can you tell me more about your feelings of sadness and uselessness?"

Care Coordination and Transition Management

The patient is discharged directly to home or to a skilled facility or rehabilitation facility, depending on the extent of the amputation. When rehabilitation is not feasible, as in the older adult with dementia or other debilitating impairment, the patient may be discharged to a long-term care facility. Coordinate this transfer with the case manager or discharge planner to ensure continuity of care.

Home Care Management. At home, the patient with a leg amputation needs to have enough room to use a wheelchair if the prosthesis is not yet available. The patient must be able to use toileting facilities and have access to areas necessary for self-management, such as the kitchen. Structural home modifications may be needed before the patient goes home.

Self-Management Education. After the sutures or staples are removed, the patient begins residual limb care. A home care nurse may be needed to teach the patient or family how to care for the limb and the prosthesis if it is available (Box 44.7).

The limb should be rewrapped several times a day with an elastic bandage applied in a figure-eight manner. For many patients, a shrinker stocking or sock is easier to apply. After the limb is

healed, it is cleaned each day with the rest of the body during bathing with soap and water. Teach the patient and/or family to inspect it every day for signs of inflammation or skin breakdown.

> **! NURSING SAFETY PRIORITY**
>
> **Action Alert**
>
> Collaborate with the prosthetist to teach the patient about care of the prosthesis to ensure its reliability and proper function. These devices are custom-made, taking into account the patient's level of amputation, lifestyle, and occupation. Proper teaching regarding correct cleansing of the socket and inserts, wearing of the correct liners, and assessment of footwear is essential before discharge, as is the setup of a schedule of follow-up care. This information may need to be reviewed by the home care nurse.

Health Care Resources. A patient who seems to adjust to the amputation during hospitalization may realize that it is difficult to cope with the loss after discharge from the hospital. Teach the patient and family about available resources and support from organizations such as the Amputee Coalition of America (ACA) (www.amputee-coalition.org) and the Amputation Foundation (www.amputationfoundation.org).

> **👤 PATIENT-CENTERED CARE: VETERAN HEALTH**
>
> **Services and Resources**
>
> Teach patients who are veterans about the many resources that can help them adjust to one or more amputations. In addition to specialty clinics and other services offered by the Department of Veterans Affairs in the United States, many other community and military services exist to help veterans adapt their lifestyle and remain active. Many of these services also assist families of veterans who have been injured (Table 44.2).

Evaluate Outcomes: Evaluation

Evaluate the care of the patient with one or more amputations based on the identified priority patient problems. The expected outcomes include that the patient:

- Have adequate *perfusion* to the residual limb
- State that *pain* is controlled to between a 2 and 3 or as acceptable to the patient on a 0-to-10 pain intensity assessment scale

> **🏠 BOX 44.7   Home Health Care**
>
> **The Patient With a Lower Extremity Amputation in the Home**
>
> Assess the residual limb for:
> - Adequate circulation
> - Infection
> - Healing
> - Flexion contracture
> - Dressing/elastic wrap
>
> Assess the patient's ability to perform ADLs in the home.
> - Evaluate the patient's ability to use ambulatory aids and care for the prosthetic device (if available).
> - Assess the patient's pain level (intensity and quality).
> - Assess the patient's nutritional status.
> - Assess the patient's ability to cope with body image change.

TABLE 44.2   Examples of Military and Community Resources for Veterans With Amputations in the United States

Resource	Website Address
Hope for the Warriors™	www.hopeforthewarriors.org
Military OneSource	www.militaryonesource.com
Veterans Affairs	www.va.gov
Amputee Coalition of America	www.amputee-coalition.org
Wounded Warrior Project	www.woundedwarriorproject.org
American Amputee Foundation	www.americanamputee.org
Amputee Coalition of Canada	www.amputeecoalitioncanada.org

- Perform *mobility* skills independently and not experience complications of decreased mobility
- Have a positive self-esteem and lifestyle adaptation to live a productive, high-quality life

CARPAL TUNNEL SYNDROME

Pathophysiology Review

Carpal tunnel syndrome (CTS) is a common condition in which the median nerve in the wrist becomes compressed, causing pain and numbness. The carpal tunnel is a rigid canal that lies between the carpal bones and a fibrous tissue sheet. A group of tendons surrounds the synovium and shares space with the median nerve in the carpal tunnel. When the synovium becomes swollen or thickened, this nerve is compressed (Rogers, 2023).

The median nerve supplies motor, sensory, and autonomic function for the first three fingers of the hand and the palmar aspect of the fourth (ring) finger. Because the median nerve is close to other structures, wrist flexion causes nerve impingement, and extension causes increased pressure in the lower portion of the carpal tunnel.

CTS is the most common type of repetitive stress injury (RSI). RSIs are the fastest-growing type of occupational injury. People whose jobs require repetitive hand activities, such as pinching or grasping during wrist flexion (e.g., factory workers, computer operators, jackhammer operators), are predisposed to CTS. In more recent years, young adults have an increased incidence of CTS due to texting and other cell phone use. It can also result from overuse in sports activities such as golf, tennis, or racquetball.

CTS usually presents as a chronic problem. Acute cases are rare. Excessive hand exercise, edema or hemorrhage into the carpal tunnel, or thrombosis of the median artery can lead to acute CTS. Patients with hand burns or a Colles fracture of the wrist are particularly at risk for this problem. In most cases, the cause may not result in nerve deficit for years.

CTS is also a common complication of certain metabolic and connective tissue diseases. For example, synovitis (inflammation of the synovium) occurs in patients with rheumatoid arthritis (RA). The hypertrophied synovium compresses the median nerve. In other chronic disorders such as diabetes mellitus, inadequate blood supply can cause median nerve neuropathy or dysfunction, resulting in CTS.

 PATIENT-CENTERED CARE: GENDER HEALTH

Carpal Tunnel Syndrome in Women

Women, especially those older than 50 years, are much more likely than men to experience CTS, probably due to the higher prevalence of diseases such as RA in women (Rogers, 2023). The problem usually affects the dominant hand but can occur in both hands simultaneously.

Health Promotion/Disease Prevention

Most businesses recognize the hazards of repetitive motion as a primary cause of occupational injury and disability. Both men and women in the labor force are experiencing increasing numbers of RSIs. Occupational health nurses have played an important role in ergonomics and in the development of ergonomically designed furniture and various aids to decrease CTS and other musculoskeletal injuries. Ergonomics is the study of how equipment and furniture can be arranged so that people can do work or other activities more efficiently and comfortably without injury.

U.S. federal and state legislation has been passed to ensure that all businesses, including health care organizations (HCOs), provide *ergonomically appropriate workstations* for their employees (Occupational Safety and Health Administration [OSHA]). The Joint Commission also requires that hospitals and other HCOs provide a safe work environment for all staff. In Canada, each province requires the work setting to have joint health and safety committees in which employees are actively involved in setting safety standards (Canadian Centre for Occupational Health and Safety). Box 44.8 lists best practices for preventing CTS in the health care setting.

Interprofessional Collaborative Care

Recognize Cues: Assessment

A diagnosis is often made based on the patient's history and report of hand pain and numbness and without further assessment. Patients typically report a "pins and needles" sensation in the first three fingers and nocturnal burning pain that is relieved by activity upon waking. Strenuous hand activity can exacerbate the pain and numbness (Rogers, 2023).

The primary health care provider performs several tests for abnormal sensory findings. The Phalen wrist test, sometimes called the *Phalen maneuver*, produces paresthesia in the median nerve distribution (palmar side of the thumb, index and middle fingers, and half of the ring finger) within 60 seconds as a result of increased internal carpal pressure. The patient is asked to relax the wrist into flexion or to place the back of the hands together and flex both wrists at the same time. The Phalen test is positive in most patients with CTS (Jarvis & Eckhardt, 2024).

BOX 44.8 Best Practice for Patient Safety and Quality Care

Health Promotion Activities to Prevent Carpal Tunnel Syndrome

- Become familiar with federal and state laws regarding workplace requirements to prevent repetitive stress injuries such as carpal tunnel syndrome (CTS).
- When using equipment or computer workstations that can contribute to developing CTS, assess that they are ergonomically appropriate, including:
  - Specially designed wrist rest devices
  - Geometrically designed computer keyboards
  - Chair height that allows good posture
- Take regular short breaks away from activities that cause repetitive stress, such as working at computers and using cell phones and other handheld devices.
- Stretch fingers and wrists frequently during work hours.
- Stay as relaxed as possible when using equipment that causes repetitive stress.

In addition to inspecting for muscle atrophy and task performance, observe the wrist for swelling. Gently palpate the area and note any unusual findings. Autonomic changes may be evidenced by skin discoloration, nail changes (e.g., brittleness), and increased or decreased hand sweating.

Take Actions: Interventions

The primary health care provider uses conservative measures before surgical intervention. However, CTS can recur with either type of treatment. Management depends on the patient, but established best practices have not been determined.

Nonsurgical Management. Aggressive drug therapy and immobilization of the wrist are the major components of nonsurgical management. Teach the patient the importance of these modalities in the hope of preventing surgical intervention.

NSAIDs are the most commonly prescribed drugs for the relief of *pain* and inflammation, if present, but they do not slow the progression of CTS (Blevins, 2020). In addition to or instead of systemic medications, the primary health care provider may inject corticosteroids directly into the carpal tunnel. If the patient responds to the injection, several additional weekly or monthly injections are given. Teach the patient to take NSAIDs with or after meals to reduce gastric irritation.

A splint or hand brace may be used to immobilize the wrist during the day, during the night, or both. Many patients experience temporary relief with these devices. The occupational therapist places the wrist in the neutral position or in slight extension.

Some patients report fewer symptoms after beginning yoga or another exercise routine. Wrist-stretching exercises may be recommended, including wrist extension and flexion stretches (Blevins, 2020).

Surgical Management. The nurse in the surgeon's office or ambulatory surgical or hand center reinforces the teaching provided by the surgeon regarding the nature of the carpal tunnel release (CTR) surgery. Postoperative care is reviewed so that the patient knows what to expect. Chapter 9 describes general preoperative care in detail.

During surgery, the transverse carpal ligament is resected to relieve pressure on the median nerve. One of three procedures may be used: endoscopic CTR, mini-open CTR, and ultrasound-guided CTR. There is no evidence that one type of procedure is more effective than the other; it is basically surgeon preference and expertise.

The most common surgery is the endoscopic carpal tunnel release (ECTR). In this procedure, the surgeon makes a very small incision (less than ½ inch [1.2 cm]) through which the endoscope is inserted. The surgeon then uses special instruments to free the trapped median nerve. Although ECTR is less invasive and costs less than the open procedure, the patient may have a longer period of postoperative pain and numbness compared with recovery from open carpal tunnel release (OCTR). Surgical treatment seems to be more effective than conservative measures over the long term.

After surgery, monitor vital signs and check the dressing carefully for drainage and tightness. If ECTR has been performed, the dressing is very small. The surgeon may require

that the patient's affected hand and arm be elevated above heart level for several days to reduce postoperative swelling. Check the neurovascular status of the fingers every hour during the immediate postoperative period, and encourage the patient to move them frequently. Offer pain medication and assure the patient that a prescription for analgesics will be provided before discharge. Discomfort should not last more than 24 to 72 hours (Blevins, 2020).

Hand movements, including lifting heavy objects, may be restricted for 4 to 6 weeks after surgery. The patient can expect weakness for weeks or perhaps months. Teach the patient to report any changes in neurovascular status, including increased pain, bleeding, or infection, to the surgeon's office immediately.

Remind the patient and family that the surgical procedure might not be a cure. For example, synovitis may recur with rheumatoid arthritis and may recompress the median nerve. Multiple surgeries and other treatments are common with CTS.

The patient may need help with self-management activities during recovery. Ensure that assistance in the home is available before discharge; this is usually provided by the family or significant others. Major surgical complications are rare after CTS surgery.

KNEE INJURIES

In addition to the bone and muscle problems already discussed, trauma can cause cartilage, ligament, and tendon injury. Many musculoskeletal injuries are the result of playing sports (professional and recreational) or doing other strenuous physical activities. The popularity of all-terrain vehicles (ATVs) and skateboarding has increased injuries in younger patients. Sports injuries have become so common that large metropolitan hospitals have sports medicine clinics and physicians who specialize in this field.

The principles of injury to one part of the body are similar to those of other sports injuries and accidents. For example, a tendon rupture in a knee is cared for in the same manner as a tendon rupture in the wrist. Box 44.9 lists general emergency measures for sports-related injuries.

BOX 44.9 Best Practice for Patient Safety and Quality Care

Emergency Care of Patients With Sports-Related Injuries

- Do not move the victim until spinal cord injury is ascertained (see Chapter 37 for assessment of spinal cord injury).
- Use RICE:
  - **Rest** the injured part; immobilize the joint above and below the injury by applying a splint if needed.
  - Apply **ice** intermittently for the first 24 to 48 hours (heat may be used thereafter).
  - Use **compression** for the first 24 to 48 hours (e.g., elastic wrap).
  - **Elevate** the affected limb to decrease swelling.
- Always assume that the area is fractured until x-ray studies are done.
- Assess neurovascular status in the area distal to the injury.

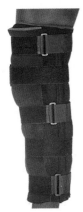

FIG. 44.11 Knee immobilizer. (From Ostendorf, W. R., Perry, A. G., & Potter, P. A. [2020]. *Nursing interventions & clinical skills* [7th ed.]. St. Louis: Elsevier.)

Because the knee is most often injured, it is discussed as a typical example of musculoskeletal trauma. Trauma to the knee results in *internal derangement*, a broad term for disturbances of an injured knee joint. When surgery is required to resolve the problem, most surgeons prefer to perform the procedure through an arthroscope when possible. A description of arthroscopy is presented in Chapter 41. Postoperative care for knee surgeries generally includes analgesics, physical therapy, and bracing or splinting, often using a knee immobilizer (Fig. 44.11). All patients require frequent neurovascular monitoring. Rehabilitation services may be needed after repair of severe knee injuries. Table 44.3 lists examples of common knee injuries and their interprofessional management.

ROTATOR CUFF INJURIES

The musculotendinous, or rotator, cuff of the shoulder functions to stabilize the head of the humerus in the glenoid cavity during shoulder abduction. Young adults usually sustain a tear of the cuff by substantial trauma, such as may occur during a fall, while throwing a ball, or with heavy lifting. Older adults tend to have small tears related to aging, repetitive motions, or falls, and the tears are initially painless. Later, pain typically begins to limit arm motion and the patient seeks medical attention.

The patient with a torn rotator cuff has shoulder *pain* and cannot easily abduct the arm at the shoulder. When the arm is abducted, the patient usually drops it because abduction cannot be maintained (drop arm test). Pain is more intense at night and with overhead activities. Partial-thickness tears are more painful than full-thickness tears, but full-thickness tears result in more weakness and loss of function. Muscle atrophy is commonly seen, and *mobility* is reduced (Rogers, 2023). Diagnosis is confirmed with x-rays, MRI, ultrasonography, and/or CT scans.

The primary health care provider usually treats the patient with partial-thickness tears conservatively with NSAIDs, intermittent steroid injections, physical therapy, and activity limitations while the tear heals. Physical therapy treatments may include ultrasound, electrical stimulation, ice, and heat.

For patients who do not respond to conservative treatment in 3 to 6 months or for those who have a complete (full-thickness) tear, the surgeon repairs the cuff using mini-open or arthroscopic procedures. An interscalene nerve block may be used to extend analgesia for an open repair. If a peripheral nerve block is used, remind the patient that the arm will feel numb and cannot be moved for up to 20 or more hours after surgery. Observe, report, and document complications of respiratory distress and neurovascular compromise.

After surgery, the affected arm is usually immobilized for several weeks. Pendulum exercises are started on the third or fourth postoperative day and progress to active exercises in about 2 weeks. Patients then begin rehabilitation in the ambulatory-care occupational therapy department. Teach them that they may not have full function for several months.

NCLEX Examination Challenge 44.4

Physiological Integrity

The nurse is assessing a client who injured the left knee while playing football with friends. Which of the following nursing actions are appropriate for this acute injury? **Select all that apply.**

A. Elevate the affected leg to decrease swelling.
B. Apply warm compresses on the affected knee.
C. Recommend that the client get an x-ray.
D. Apply an elastic sleeve or wrap on the affected knee.
E. Rest as much as possible so that the knee can heal.

TABLE 44.3 Examples of Acute Soft Tissue Musculoskeletal Injuries

Acute Injury/Description	Management
Sprain: excessive stretching of a ligament	Immobilization, RICE, possible surgery if severe
Strain: excessive stretching of a muscle or tendon	Heat/cold, activity limitations, NSAIDs, muscle relaxants, possible tendon repair
Ligament tear (such as anterior cruciate ligament in knee): damage to ligament most often caused by sports or vehicular crash	RICE, surgery if does not heal or is severe (usually arthroscopic)
Meniscus tear: damage to knee cartilage caused by sports or other trauma	RICE, bracing, splinting, NSAIDs, surgery (usually arthroscopic)
Tendon rupture (such as the Achilles tendon in heel): often caused by sports or wearing high-heeled shoes; in some cases can occur after taking fluoroquinolones such as ciprofloxacin (Cipro)	RICE, NSAIDs, orthotic devices, ultrasound, surgery if severe or does not heal
Patellofemoral pain syndrome (PFPS): knee pain caused by overuse of the knee joint; also called *runner's knee*	Rest, splinting, bracing, NSAIDs, possibly surgery as last resort
Joint dislocation: displacement of a bone from its usual position in a synovial joint	Manual joint relocation; possible surgery

GET READY FOR THE NEXT-GENERATION NCLEX® EXAMINATION!

Essential Nursing Care Points

Health Promotion/Disease Prevention

- To prevent fragility fractures, the nurse should teach patients at risk to have regular screening for osteopenia and osteoporosis and to implement measures to prevent falls.
- Nurses need to teach patients to avoid risky physical activities that could result in one or more fractures or amputations.
- Nurses should teach patients who have diabetes and/or peripheral arterial disease (PAD) to self-manage their disease and engage in a healthy lifestyle (if resources are available to meet that goal) to help prevent elective amputation.
- To reduce the risk of carpal tunnel syndrome and other work-related injuries, individuals should have ergonomically designed equipment or workstations available to reduce injury, take regular short breaks from tasks that cause repetitive stress, and frequently stretch fingers and wrists.

Chronic Disease Care

- Patients who experience amputation often have **phantom limb pain (PLP)**, which is usually described as a persistent *pain* perceived in the removed body part.
- PLP should be managed appropriately and completely using a variety of long-term drug therapy, including beta-blocking agents such as propranolol, antiepileptic drugs such as gabapentin, and antispasmodics such as baclofen.
- **Complex regional pain syndrome (CRPS)** is a chronic complication associated with fractures in which the client has severe, persistent *pain*, autonomic symptoms such as edema and coolness, and loss of function of the fracture area.

Regenerative or Restorative Care

- Common complications of fractures or fracture repair include infection and venous thromboembolism (VTE).
- Less common but potentially limb- or life-threatening complications of fractures include **acute compartment syndrome (ACS)** and **fat embolism syndrome (FES)**. Table 44.1 differentiates VTE and FES.
- Patients with ACS may need a surgical procedure known as a **fasciotomy**.
- The patient who has a fracture often has trauma to other parts of the body. Therefore, nurses should assess all major body systems *first* for life-threatening complications, such as head, chest, or abdominal injury.
- The primary management for any fracture is reduction and immobilization; casts, splints, or surgery may be used. Traction is used less often as part of fracture management.
- Nurses should monitor for infection surrounding pin sites for external fixation or skeletal traction, making sure not to remove crusting that can occur around the pins.
- Traumatic amputations are common among active military service members and individuals who engage in risky behaviors; elective amputations are common among individuals who have diabetes mellitus and peripheral arterial disease, particularly in those who are unable to self-manage their diseases or do not know how to do so.
- Table 44.2 lists examples of military and community resources for veterans who have undergone amputations.
- Table 44.3 lists common soft tissue musculoskeletal injuries and briefly describes their management.

Hospice/Palliative/Supportive Care

- After hip fracture repair, some patients are unable to return to their prefracture ADLs and *mobility* level. Family caregivers often have unexpected responsibilities caring for patients during their recovery. For some patients, palliative or end-of-life care may be useful.
- Patients who experience major fractures and amputations often require extensive rehabilitation to improve ADL ability and mobility.
- Rehabilitation after multiple traumatic amputations often takes 9 to 15 months.
- Patients who have soft tissue injuries of the knee or upper extremity often require rehabilitation to return to baseline ADL ability and mobility.

Mastery Questions

1. A client who had an elective left above-the-knee amputation 2 days ago reports severe pain of 9 on a 0-to-10 pain intensity scale in the left foot. What would be the nurse's **most appropriate** action at this time?
   A. Administer the analgesic medication that is ordered for pain.
   B. Remind the client that the left foot was removed as part of the amputation.
   C. Assess circulation and massage the left residual limb.
   D. Provide a mirror for the client to help visualize the loss of the lower leg.

2. The nurse is planning care for a client who has a new compound fracture of the left wrist. For what complication would the nurse determine the client is **most** at risk?
   A. Fat embolism syndrome (FES)
   B. Venous thromboembolism (VTE)
   C. Acute compartment syndrome (ACS)
   D. Infection

3. The nurse is assessing a client who sustained a right tibia-fibula closed fracture with a large amount of soft tissue injury. For which of the following **common** complications would the nurse carefully monitor? **Select all that apply.**

A. Infection
B. Delayed union
C. Acute compartment syndrome (ACS)
D. Fat embolism syndrome (FES)
E. Bone malunion

NGN Challenge 44.1
44.1.1

The nurse is caring for a 39-year-old client who was admitted yesterday afternoon to the orthopedic unit.

History and Physical	Nurses' Notes	Vital Signs	Laboratory Results

1430: Returned from PACU following reduction of tib-fib fractures with external fixation. Very drowsy but arousable; oriented × 3. IV of 0.9% NS infusing at 100 mL/hr in right forearm. PCA continuous basal morphine for pain to be D/C'd tomorrow a.m. States that pain is 3/10 in left leg and 2/10 in left arm, using a 0-to-10 pain intensity scale. VS: T 97.8°F (36.6°C); HR 75 beats/min & regular; RR 18 breaths/min; BP 116/66 mm Hg; Spo$_2$ 100% on 2 L/min O$_2$ via NC. D/C when fully awake. Both feet cool; pedal pulses equal at 2+; left foot cap refill <3 sec; no swelling in left foot. Fixator in place and left leg elevated on pillow. Left lower leg swollen; wound covered with sterile gauze to be changed every 8 hours per protocol. Left full arm cast in place. Left hand slightly swollen and cooler than right hand; able to move all fingers; cap refill <3 sec.

1710: Drowsy at times but easily awakened; oriented × 3. IV of 0.9% NS infusing at 100 mL/hr in right forearm. Spo$_2$ 95% on room air. Has not voided since transfer from PACU. States that pain in surgical leg has increased to 5/10. Occasional use of PCA; encouraged to use PCA more often. No pain in left arm. Left hand slightly swollen; able to move all fingers; cap refill <3 sec. Both feet cool; pedal pulse in (R) leg 2+, 1+ in (L) leg; left foot cap refill <3 sec. Fixator in place and left leg elevated on pillow.

Select the 2 client findings that would be of **immediate** concern to the nurse.
○ Drowsy but easily awakened
○ Both feet cool
○ Spo$_2$ 95% on room air
○ Pain increased from 3 to 5 in surgical leg
○ Left hand slightly swollen
○ Has not voided since transfer from PACU
○ Left pedal pulse decreased from 2+ to 1+

44.1.2

The nurse is caring for a 39-year-old client who was admitted yesterday afternoon to the orthopedic unit.

History and Physical	Nurses' Notes	Vital Signs	Laboratory Results

1430: Returned from PACU following reduction of tib-fib fractures with external fixation. Very drowsy but arousable; oriented × 3. IV of 0.9% NS infusing at 100 mL/hr in right forearm. PCA continuous basal morphine for pain to be D/C'd tomorrow a.m. States that pain is 3/10 in left leg and 2/10 in left arm. VS: T 97.8°F (36.6°C); HR 75 beats/min & regular; RR 18 breaths/min; BP 116/66 mm Hg; Spo$_2$ 100% on 2 L/min O$_2$ via NC. D/C when fully awake. Both feet cool; pedal pulses equal at 2+; left foot cap refill <3 sec; no swelling in left foot. Fixator in place and left leg elevated on pillow. Left lower leg swollen; wound covered with sterile gauze to be changed every 8 hours per protocol. Left hand slightly swollen and cooler than right hand; able to move all fingers; cap refill <3 sec.

1710: Drowsy at times but easily awakened; oriented × 3. IV of 0.9% NS infusing at 100 mL/hr in right forearm. Spo$_2$ 95% on room air. Has not voided since transfer from PACU. States that pain in surgical leg has increased to 5/10. Occasional use of PCA; encouraged to use PCA more often. No pain in left arm. Left hand slightly swollen and cooler than right hand; able to move all fingers; cap refill <3 sec. Both feet cool; pedal pulse in (R) leg 2+, 1+ in (L) leg; left foot cap refill <3 sec. Fixator in place and left leg elevated on pillow.

Complete the following sentence by selecting from the lists of options below.

The client is at risk for **1 [Select]** as evidenced by **2 [Select]**.

Options for 1 (Client Condition)	Options for 2 (Client Finding)
Urinary retention	Left pedal pulse decreased from 2+ to 1+
Complex regional pain syndrome	Both feet are cool
Neurovascular compromise	Pain increased from 3 to 5 in the surgical leg
Peripheral arterial disease	Not voiding since transfer from the PACU

44.1.3

The nurse is caring for a 39-year-old client in the orthopedic unit following a tib-fib fracture external fixation yesterday.

History and Physical	**Nurses' Notes**	Vital Signs	Laboratory Results

0550: Alert & oriented × 3. IV converted to saline lock due to client voiding × 3 during the night. No report of pain in left arm; arm cast intact and no hand swelling. Able to move all fingers; cap refill <3 sec. States that left lower leg continues to be painful even when using PCA as instructed. Currently reports a 7/10 pain with a "pins and needles" sensation in the left foot. (L) pedal pulse absent; (R) pedal pulse 2+. Left foot cooler than right foot; (L) cap refill at 5 sec; (R) cap refill <3 sec. Left lower leg continues to be swollen; no redness or drainage from pin sites. Surgeon notified about latest assessment and will make rounds within the hour.

Complete the following sentence by selecting from the list of word choices below.

The nurse would determine that the *priority* for the client's care is to manage early symptoms associated with **[Word Choice]**.

Word Choices
Wound infection
Complex regional pain syndrome
Acute arterial occlusion
Acute compartment syndrome

44.1.4

The nurse is caring for a 39-year-old client in the orthopedic unit following a tib-fib fracture external fixation yesterday.

History and Physical	**Nurses' Notes**	Vital Signs	Laboratory Results

0550: Alert & oriented × 3. IV converted to saline lock due to client voiding × 3 during the night. No report of pain in left arm; arm cast intact and no hand swelling. Able to move all fingers; cap refill <3 sec. States that left lower leg continues to be painful even when using PCA as instructed. Currently reports a 7/10 pain with a "pins and needles" sensation in the left foot. (L) pedal pulse absent; (R) pedal pulse 2+. Left foot cooler than right foot; (L) cap refill at 5 sec; (R) cap refill <3 sec. Left lower leg continues to be swollen; no redness or drainage from pin sites. Surgeon notified about latest assessment and will make rounds within the hour.

The nurse anticipates orders from the surgeon based on the client's most recent findings Select whether the following anticipated orders are indicated or not indicated for the client at this time.

Potential Orders	**Indicated**	**Not Indicated**
Start IV infusion of 0.9% NS		
Insert an indwelling urinary catheter		
Prepare client for surgery		
Apply ice to left leg four times a day		
Type and crossmatch for 2 units packed RBCs		
Notify Radiology to schedule left leg arteriography		

44.1.5

The nurse is caring for a 39-year-old client in the orthopedic unit following a tib-fib fracture external fixation yesterday.

History and Physical	**Nurses' Notes**	Vital Signs	Laboratory Results

0550: Alert & oriented × 3. IV converted to saline lock due to client voiding × 3 during the night. No report of pain in left arm; arm cast intact and no hand swelling. Able to move all fingers; cap refill <3 sec. States that left lower leg continues to be painful even when using PCA as instructed. Currently reports a 7/10 pain with a "pins and needles" sensation in the left foot. (L) pedal pulse absent; (R) pedal pulse 2+. Left foot cooler than right foot; (L) cap refill at 5 sec; (R) cap refill <3 sec. Left lower leg continues to be swollen; no redness or drainage from pin sites. Surgeon notified about latest assessment and will make rounds within the hour.
0710: Surgeon examined client and scheduled a fasciotomy to relieve compartmental pressure.
1525: Returned from PACU after left lower leg fasciotomy. VS: T 97.8°F (36.6°C); HR 78 beats/min & regular; RR 16 breaths/min; BP 110/62 mm Hg; Spo₂ 96% on room air. Both feet warm; pedal pulses both 2+. Bulky dressing covering lower leg fasciotomy incision. Reports pain in left leg and foot as 3/10.

Which of the following postoperative actions would the nurse take at this time? **Select all that apply.**

○ Perform fixator pin care every 12 hours per protocol
○ Inspect fixator pin sites for redness or drainage
○ Perform lower extremity circulation checks every 4 hours
○ Provide wound care to skin graft site
○ Use sterile moist dressing for fasciotomy site

44.1.6

The client visits the surgeon for the first follow-up appointment since being discharged from the hospital. The nurse assesses the client before the examination by the surgeon and compares current findings with the below Nurses' Notes documented in the hospital.

History and Physical	**Nurses' Notes**	Vital Signs	Laboratory Results

0550: Alert & oriented × 3. IV converted to saline lock due to client voiding × 3 during the night. No report of pain in left arm; arm cast intact and no hand swelling. Able to move all fingers; cap refill <3 sec. States that left lower leg continues to be painful even when using PCA as instructed. Currently reports a 7/10 pain with a "pins and needles" sensation in the left foot. (L) pedal pulse absent; (R) pedal pulse 2+. Left foot cooler than right foot; (L) cap refill at 5 sec; (R) cap refill <3 sec. Left lower leg continues to be swollen; no redness or drainage from pin sites. Surgeon notified about latest assessment and will make rounds within the hour.

0710: Surgeon examined client and scheduled a fasciotomy to relieve compartment pressure.

1525: Returned from PACU after left lower leg fasciotomy. VS: T 97.8°F (36.6°C); HR 78 beats/min & regular; RR 16 breaths/min; BP 110/62 mm Hg; SpO_2 96% on RA. Both feet warm; pedal pulses both 2+. Bulky dressing covering lower leg fasciotomy incision. Reports pain in left leg and foot as 3/10.

For each current client finding, indicate if the client's condition has improved or worsened.

Current Client Findings	Improved	Worsened
Pain in left lower leg 1/10		
Ambulating independently with crutches		
Redness and purulent drainage around two pin sites		
Fasciotomy skin graft approximated and healing		

REFERENCES

Amputee Coalition. (2021). *Race and ethnicity disparities in limb loss.* https://www.amputee-coalition.org/resources/race-ethnic-disparity-limb-loss/.

Blevins, S. (2020). Carpal tunnel syndrome. *MEDSURG Nursing,* 29(1), 53–55.

Breazeale, S., Barrett, S., Holland, W., & Webb, M. (2022). Pain and mental health symptoms after traumatic orthopedic injury. *AJN,* 122(9), 26–36.

Burchum, J., & Rosenthal, L. (2022). *Lehne's pharmacology for nursing care* (11th ed.). St. Louis: Elsevier.

Conley, R. B., Adib, G., Adler, R. A., Akesson, K. E., Alexander, I. M., & Amenta, K. C. (2020). Secondary fracture prevention: Consensus clinical recommendations from a multistakeholder coalition. *Orthopaedic Nursing,* 39(3), 145–161.

Elliott, B., Chargualaf, K. A., & Patterson, B. (2021). *Veteran-centered care in education and practice.* New York, NY: Springer Publishing.

Fanaroff, A. C., Yang, L., Nathan, A. S., Khatana, S. A. M., Julien, H., Wang, T. Y., et al. (2021). Geographic and socioeconomic disparities in major lower extremity amputation rates in metropolitan areas. *Journal of the American Heart Association.* https://doi.org/10.1161/JAHA.121.021456.

*Georgiades, D. S. (2018). A systematic integrative review of pin site crusts. *Orthopaedic Nursing,* 37(1), 36–42.

Jarvis, C., & Eckhardt, A. L. (2024). *Physical examination & health assessment* (9th ed.). St. Louis: Elsevier.

*MacDonald, V., Maher, A. B., Mainz, H., Meehan, A. J., Brent, L., Hommel, A., et al. (2018). Developing and testing an international audit of quality indicators for older adults with fragility fractures. *Orthopaedic Nursing,* 37(2), 115–121.

Rogers, J. L. (2023). *McCance and Huether's Pathophysiology: The biologic basis for disease in adults and children* (9th ed.). St. Louis: Elsevier.

Rosenberg, K. (2020). Incidence of hip fractures is decreasing. *American Journal of Nursing,* 120(12), 69.

Sammut, R., Attard, M., Mangion, D., & Trapani, J. (2021). The effectiveness of skin traction in reducing pain in adults with a hip fracture: A systematic review. *International Journal of Orthopaedic and Trauma Nursing,* 43. https://doi.org/10.1016/j.ijotn.2021.100880.

Slusser, M. M., Garcia, L. I., Reed, C.-R., & McGinnis, P. Q. (2019). *Foundations of interprofessional collaborative practice in health care.* St. Louis: Elsevier.

*Thurlow, G., & Gray, B. (2018). Complex regional pain syndrome. *International Journal of Orthopaedic and Trauma Nursing,* 40, 44–47.

*Wennberg, P., Andersson, H., & Sundstrom, B. W. (2018). Patients with suspected hip fractures in the chain of emergency care: An integrative review of the literature. *International Journal of Orthopaedic and Trauma Nursing,* 29, 16–31.

Williams, M. G., Jeffery, Z., Corner, H. W., Charity, J., Quantick, M., & Sartin, N. (2019). A robust approach to implementing fascia iliaca compartment nerve blocks in hip fracture patients. *Orthopaedic Nursing,* 37(3), 185–189.

Yildirim, M., & Sen, S. (2020). Mirror therapy in the management of phantom limb pain. *AJN,* 120(3), 41–46.

45

Assessment of the Gastrointestinal System

Charity Lynn Hacker

http://evolve.elsevier.com/Iggy/

LEARNING OUTCOMES

1. Use knowledge of anatomy and physiology to perform a focused assessment of the GI system.
2. Teach evidence-based health promotion activities to help prevent GI health problems or trauma.
3. Identify factors that affect health equity for patients with GI health problems.
4. Explain how genetic implications and physiologic aging of the GI system affects *nutrition* and *elimination*.
5. Interpret assessment findings for patients with a suspected or actual GI problem.
6. Plan evidence-based care and support for patients undergoing diagnostic testing of the GI system.

KEY TERMS

amylase An enzyme that converts starch and glycogen into simple sugars; found most commonly in saliva and pancreatic fluids.

borborygmus Rumbling or gurgling sounds in the stomach and intestines related to food, fluid, or gas movement. Also known as *borborygmi*.

bruit An audible swishing sound produced when the volume of blood or the diameter of the blood vessel changes.

colonoscopy An endoscopic examination of the entire large bowel.

digestion The mechanical and chemical process in which complex foodstuffs are broken down into simpler forms that can be used by the body.

dyspepsia An epigastric burning sensation, often referred to as "heartburn."

endoscope A tube that allows viewing and manipulation of internal body areas.

endoscopic retrograde cholangiopancreatography (ERCP) A procedure in which the bile ducts, pancreatic duct, and gallbladder are visualized through endoscopy.

endoscopy The direct visualization of the GI tract by means of a flexible fiberoptic endoscope.

enteroscopy Visualization of the small intestine.

esophageal stricture Narrowing of the esophageal opening.

esophagogastroduodenoscopy (EGD) The visual examination of the esophagus, stomach, and duodenum by means of a fiberoptic endoscope.

flatulence Gas in the lower GI tract.

guaiac-based fecal occult blood test (gFOBT) A diagnostic test that measures the presence of blood in the stool from GI bleeding—a common finding associated with colorectal cancer.

lipase An enzyme secreted by the pancreas that facilitates the breakdown of triglycerides into fatty acids.

NPO (nothing by mouth) No eating, drinking (including water), or smoking.

PQRST A mnemonic (memory device) that may help in the assessment of abdominal pain. The letters represent these areas *P*, precipitating or palliative (What brings it on? What makes it better or worse?); *Q*, quality or quantity (How does it look, feel, or sound?); *R*, region or radiation (Where is it? Does it spread anywhere?); *S*, severity scale (How bad is it [on a scale of 0–10]? Is it getting better, worse, or staying the same?); *T*, timing (What are the onset, duration, and frequency?).

reflux Reverse or backward flow.

sigmoidoscopy An endoscopic examination of the rectum and sigmoid colon using a flexible scope.

steatorrhea Fatty stools.

virtual colonoscopy Three-dimensional images of the colon and rectum created by use of an abdominal and pelvic CT scan.

The mouth, esophagus, stomach, small and large intestines, and rectum make up the *alimentary canal,* also known as the *gastrointestinal (GI) tract.* The GI system is formed when the salivary glands, liver, gallbladder, and pancreas secrete substances into this tract (Fig. 45.1). The main functions of the GI tract, with the aid of organs such as the pancreas and the liver, are the digestion of food to adequately meet the body's **nutrition** needs, and the **elimination** of waste resulting from digestion. The GI tract is susceptible to numerous health problems, including structural or mechanical alterations, impaired motility, infection, inflammation or autoimmune disease, and cancer.

ANATOMY AND PHYSIOLOGY REVIEW

Structure

The lumen, or inner wall, of the GI tract consists of four layers: mucosa, submucosa, muscularis, and serosa (Fig. 45.2). The *mucosa,* the innermost layer, includes a thin layer of smooth muscle and specialized exocrine gland cells. It is surrounded by the *submucosa,* which is made up of connective tissue. The *submucosa* layer is surrounded by the muscularis. The *muscularis* is composed of both circular and longitudinal smooth muscles that work to keep contents moving through the tract. The outermost layer, the *serosa,* is composed of connective tissue. Although the GI tract is continuous from the mouth to the anus, it is divided into specialized regions. The mouth, pharynx, esophagus, stomach, and small and large intestines each perform a specific function. In addition, the secretions of the salivary, gastric, and intestinal glands; liver; and pancreas empty into the GI tract to aid digestion.

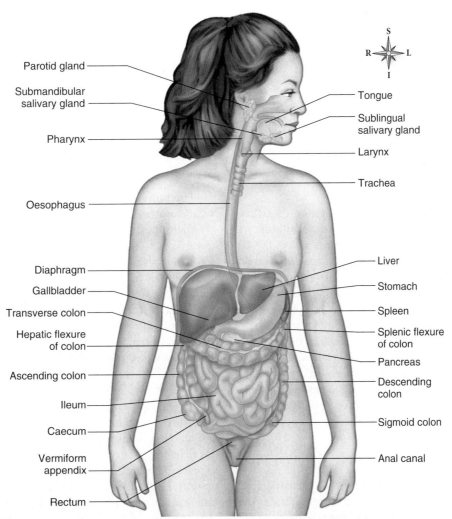

FIG. 45.1 The GI system (GI tract) can be thought of as a tube (with necessary structures) extending from the mouth to the anus for a 25-foot length. The structure of this tube *(shown enlarged)* is basically the same throughout its length. (From Patton, K. T., & Thibodeau, G. A. [2022]. *Anatomy and physiology* [11th ed.]. St. Louis: Elsevier.)

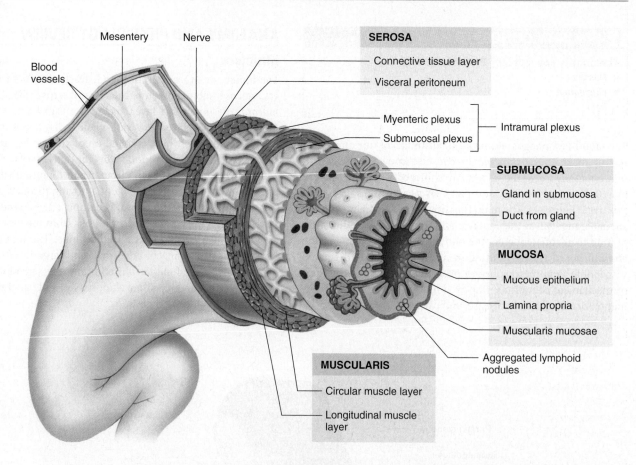

FIG. 45.2 Wall of the GI tract. (From Patton, K. T., & Thibodeau, G. A. [2022]. *Anatomy and physiology* [11th ed.]. St. Louis: Elsevier.)

Function

The functions of the GI tract include secretion, digestion, absorption, motility, and *elimination.* Food and fluids are ingested, swallowed, and propelled along the lumen of the GI tract to the anus for elimination. The smooth muscles contract to move food from the mouth to the anus. Before food can be absorbed, it must be broken down to a liquid called *chyme.* Digestion is the mechanical and chemical process through which complex foodstuffs are broken down into simpler forms that can be used by the body. During digestion, the stomach secretes hydrochloric acid, the liver secretes bile, and digestive enzymes are released from accessory organs, aiding in food breakdown. After the digestive process is complete, *absorption* takes place as the nutrients produced by digestion are moved from the GI tract into the body's circulatory system for use.

Oral Cavity

The oral cavity (mouth) includes the buccal mucosa, lips, tongue, hard palate, soft palate, teeth, and salivary glands. The buccal mucosa is the mucous membrane lining the inside of the mouth. The tongue is involved in speech, taste, and *mastication* (chewing). Small projections called *papillae* cover the tongue and provide a roughened surface, permitting the movement of

food in the mouth during chewing. The hard palate and the soft palate together form the roof of the mouth.

Adults have 32 permanent teeth: 16 each in upper and lower arches. The different types of teeth function to prepare food for digestion by cutting, tearing, crushing, or grinding the food. Swallowing begins after food is taken into the mouth and chewed. Saliva is secreted in response to the presence of food in the mouth and begins to soften the food. Saliva contains a specific mixture of products, including salivary amylase and salivary lipase, that break down carbohydrates and lipids, respectively (Ogobuiro et al., 2022).

Esophagus

The *esophagus* is a muscular canal that extends from the pharynx (throat) to the stomach and passes through the center of the diaphragm. Its primary function is to move food and fluids from the pharynx to the stomach. At the upper end of the esophagus is a sphincter referred to as the *upper esophageal sphincter (UES).* When at rest, the UES is closed to prevent the movement of air into the esophagus during respiration. The portion of the esophagus just above the gastroesophageal (GE) junction is referred to as the *lower esophageal sphincter (LES).* When at rest, the LES is normally closed to prevent reflux of gastric contents into the esophagus. If the

LES does not work properly, gastroesophageal reflux disease (GERD) can develop.

Stomach

The *stomach* is located in the midline and left upper quadrant (LUQ) of the abdomen and has three functional regions: the fundus, body, and antrum. Anatomically, the *cardia* is the narrow portion of the stomach that is below the gastroesophageal (GE) junction. The *fundus* is the area nearest to the cardia. The main area of the stomach is referred to as the *body* or *corpus*. The *antrum* (pylorus) is the distal (lower) portion of the stomach and is separated from the duodenum by the pyloric sphincter. Both ends of the stomach are guarded by sphincters (cardiac [LES] and pyloric), which aid in the transport of food through the GI tract and prevent backflow.

Smooth muscle cells that line the stomach are responsible for gastric motility. The stomach is also richly innervated with intrinsic and extrinsic nerves. Parietal cells lining the wall of the stomach secrete hydrochloric acid, whereas chief cells secrete pepsinogen (a precursor to pepsin, a digestive enzyme). Parietal cells also produce intrinsic factor, a substance that aids in the absorption of vitamin B_{12}. Absence of intrinsic factor causes pernicious anemia.

After ingestion of food, the stomach functions as a food reservoir where the digestive process begins, using mechanical movements and chemical secretions. The stomach mixes or churns the food, breaking apart the large food molecules and mixing them with gastric secretions to form chyme, which then empties into the duodenum. The *intestinal phase* begins as the chyme passes from the stomach into the duodenum, causing distention. The upper small intestine produces several hormones and enzymes—including secretin and cholecystokinin, which inhibit further acid production and decrease gastric motility—that facilitate the functions of the GI tract (Ogobuiro et al., 2022).

Pancreas

The *pancreas* is a long and flat, pear-shaped organ that lies behind the stomach and extends horizontally from the duodenal C-loop to the spleen. The pancreas is divided into portions known as the head, the body, and the tail (Fig. 45.3).

Two major cellular bodies (exocrine and endocrine) within the pancreas have separate functions. The exocrine part consists of cells that secrete enzymes needed for digestion of carbohydrates, fats, and proteins (proteases, amylase, and lipase). The endocrine part of the pancreas is made up of the *islets of Langerhans,* with alpha cells producing glucagon and beta cells producing insulin, as well as delta and pancreatic peptide cells. The hormones produced are essential in the regulation of metabolism.

Liver and Gallbladder

The liver is the largest organ in the body (other than skin) and is located mainly in the right upper quadrant (RUQ) of the abdomen. The right and left hepatic ducts transport bile from the liver. It receives its blood supply from the hepatic artery and portal vein, resulting in about 1200 mL of blood flow through the liver every minute.

The liver performs more than 400 functions in three major categories: storage, protection, and metabolism. It produces bile, which facilitates the digestion of fats and lipids. It stores many minerals and vitamins, such as iron; copper; fat-soluble vitamins A, D, and E; and water-soluble vitamin B_{12} (Kalra et al., 2022).

The protective function of the liver involves phagocytic *Kupffer cells,* which are part of the body's reticuloendothelial system. They engulf harmful bacteria and anemic red blood cells. The liver also detoxifies potentially harmful compounds (e.g., drugs, chemicals, alcohol). Therefore the risk for drug toxicity increases with aging because of decreased liver function.

The liver functions in the metabolism of proteins that are vital for survival. It breaks down amino acids to remove ammonia, which is then converted to urea and is excreted via the

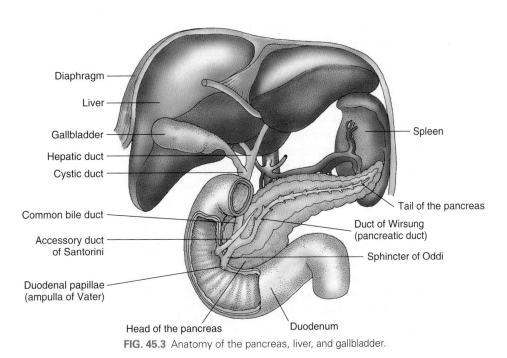

FIG. 45.3 Anatomy of the pancreas, liver, and gallbladder.

kidneys as urine (Barmore et al., 2022). It synthesizes several plasma proteins, including albumin, prothrombin, and fibrinogen. The liver's role in carbohydrate metabolism involves storing and releasing glycogen as the body's energy requirements change. The organ also synthesizes, breaks down, and temporarily stores fatty acids and triglycerides.

The liver forms and continually secretes bile, which is essential for the breakdown of fat. The secretion of bile increases in response to gastrin, secretin, and cholecystokinin. Bile is secreted into small ducts that empty into the common bile duct (CBD) and into the duodenum at the *sphincter of Oddi.* However, if the sphincter is closed, the bile goes to the gallbladder for storage.

The *gallbladder* is a pear-shaped, bulbous sac that is located underneath the liver. It is drained by the cystic duct, which joins with the hepatic duct from the liver to form the CBD. The gallbladder collects, concentrates, and stores the bile that has come from the liver. It releases the bile into the duodenum via the CBD when fat is present.

Small Intestine

The small intestine is the longest and most convoluted portion of the digestive tract, measuring an average of 9 to 16 feet (3–5 m) in length in an adult. It is composed of three different regions: the duodenum, jejunum, and ileum. The *duodenum* is the first 8 to 10 inches (20–25 cm) of the small intestine and is attached to the distal end of the pylorus. The common bile duct and pancreatic duct join to form the ampulla of Vater, emptying into the duodenum at the duodenal papilla. This papillary opening is surrounded by muscle known as the *sphincter of Oddi.* The 8-foot (2.5-m) portion of the small intestine that follows the sphincter of Oddi is the *jejunum.* The last 10 feet (3 m) of the small intestine is called the *ileum.* The ileocecal valve separates the entrance of the ileum from the cecum of the large intestine.

The inner surface of the small intestine has a velvety appearance because of numerous mucous membrane fingerlike projections. These projections are called *intestinal villi.* In addition to the intestinal villi, the small intestine has circular folds of mucosa and submucosa, which increase the surface area for digestion and absorption.

The small intestine has three main *functions:* movement (mixing and peristalsis), digestion, and absorption. Because the intestinal villi increase the surface area of the small intestine, it is the major organ of absorption of the digestive system. The small intestine mixes and transports the chyme to combine with many digestive enzymes. It takes an average of 3 to 6 hours for the contents to be passed by peristalsis through the small intestine. Intestinal enzymes aid the body in the digestion of proteins, carbohydrates, and lipids.

Large Intestine

The large intestine extends about 5 to 6 feet in length from the ileocecal valve to the anus and is lined with columnar epithelium that has absorptive and mucous cells. It begins with the *cecum,* a dilated, pouchlike structure that is inferior to the ileocecal opening. At the base of the cecum is the vermiform appendix, which recent theories have tied to the maintenance of intestinal immunity (Hodge et al., 2022). The large intestine then extends upward from the cecum as the colon. The colon consists of four divisions: ascending colon, transverse colon, descending colon, and sigmoid colon. The sigmoid colon empties into the rectum.

Beyond the sigmoid colon, the large intestine bends downward to form the rectum. The last 1 to 1½ inches (3–4 cm) of the large intestine are called the *anal canal,* which opens to the exterior of the body through the anus. The internal and external sphincter muscles surround the anal canal and control defecation.

The large intestine's *functions* are movement, absorption, and *elimination.* Movement in the large intestine consists mainly of segmental contractions, such as those in the small intestine, to allow enough time for the absorption of water and electrolytes. In addition, peristaltic contractions are triggered by colonic distention to move the contents toward the rectum, where the material is stored until the urge to defecate occurs. Absorption of water and some electrolytes occurs in the large intestine to reduce the fluid volume of the chyme. This process creates a more solid material, the feces, for *elimination.*

GI Changes Associated With Aging

As people age, and especially after 65 years of age, physiologic changes occur in the GI system. Common digestive and *elimination* changes can affect *nutrition.* The Patient-Centered Care: Older Adult Health—GI System Changes Associated With Aging box lists common GI changes in older adults.

👤 PATIENT-CENTERED CARE: OLDER ADULT HEALTH

GI System Changes Associated With Aging

Physiologic Change	Disorders Related to Change
Atrophy of the gastric mucosa leads to decreased hydrochloric acid levels (hypochlorhydria).	Decreased absorption of iron and vitamin B_{12} and proliferation of bacteria. Atrophic gastritis occurs as a consequence of bacterial overgrowth.
Peristalsis decreases, and nerve impulses are dulled.	Decreased sensation to defecate can result in postponement of bowel movements, which leads to constipation and impaction.
Distention and dilation of pancreatic ducts change. Calcification of pancreatic vessels occurs with a decrease in lipase production.	Decreased lipase level results in decreased fat absorption and digestion. Steatorrhea (fatty stool) occurs because of decreased fat digestion.
A decrease in the number and size of hepatic cells leads to decreased liver weight and mass. This change and an increase in fibrous tissue lead to decreased protein synthesis and changes in liver enzymes. Enzyme activity and cholesterol synthesis are diminished.	Decreased enzyme activity depresses drug metabolism, which leads to accumulation of drugs—possibly to toxic levels.
Intestinal microbiota abnormalities occur during the aging process (Flint & Tadi, 2023).	Dysfunctional microbial activity contributes to anorexia and subsequent undernutrition.

RECOGNIZE CUES: ASSESSMENT

Patient History

General History

The purpose of the health history is to determine the events related to the current health problem (Box 45.1). Ask questions about changes in appetite, weight, and stool. Determine the patient's experience with *pain,* if that is a concern.

Collect data about the patient's age, gender, and culture. This information can be helpful in assessing who is likely to have particular GI system disorders. For instance, older adults are more at risk for stomach cancer than are younger adults. Younger adults are at higher risk for inflammatory bowel disease (IBD). The exact reasons for these differences continue to be studied. Colon cancer, once a disease that primarily affected older adults, is increasing in prevalence in adults under 50 years old (Lotfollahzadeh et al., 2022).

NCLEX Examination Challenge 45.1

Health Promotion and Maintenance

Which of the following GI findings in the older adult would the nurse associate with aging? **Select all that apply.**

A. Increased lipase levels
B. More frequent bowel movements
C. Elevated bacterial growth
D. Retention of drug products
E. Enhanced fat absorption

Finally, ask whether the patient has traveled outside of the country recently or has been camping near lakes and streams in any location. This information may provide clues about the cause of symptoms such as diarrhea.

Nutrition History

A *nutrition* history is important when assessing GI system function. Many conditions arise because of alterations in intake and absorption of nutrients. The purpose of a nutrition assessment is to gather information about how well the patient's needs are being met. Inquire about any special diet and whether there are any known food allergies. Ask the patient to describe the usual foods that are eaten daily and the times at which meals are taken.

Ask if there is a personal or family history of lactose intolerance. Some individuals have lactose intolerance for much of their lives, and others develop it as they get older (Fawley, 2021). Estimates project that about 50% of U.S. adults have acquired lactose intolerance over their lifetime, with prevalence being higher in African American, Asian, Hispanic, Native American, and Jewish individuals (Fawley, 2021).

Health problems can also affect *nutrition;* therefore explore changes that have occurred in eating habits because of illness.

BOX 45.1   Best Practice for Patient Safety and Quality Care

Questions for GI Health History

- What is your typical daily food intake?
- What medications are you taking? (Obtain name, dose, and frequency)
- Do you take any vitamins, minerals, or herbal supplements? If so, what are they?
- How is your appetite? Has there been a recent change?
- Have you lost or gained weight recently? If so, was the weight loss or gain intentional?
- Are you on a special diet? If so, what kind, and for what purpose?
- Do you have difficulty chewing or swallowing?
- Do you wear dentures? If so, how well do they fit?
- Do you experience indigestion or "heartburn"? If so, how often? What seems to cause it? What helps it?
- Have you had GI disorders or surgeries in the past? If so, what are they and when did they occur?
- Is there a family history of GI health problems?
- Do you smoke (or vape), or have you ever smoked (vaped) in the past?
- Do you chew or have you ever chewed tobacco?
- Do you drink alcoholic beverages? If so, what kind, how much, and how many each week?
- Do you have pain, diarrhea, constipation, or gas? Do any specific foods accompany the problem?
- Have you traveled out of the country recently? If so, where and when?
- What is your usual bowel *elimination* pattern? Frequency? Character?
- Do you use laxatives to produce a bowel movement? If so, how frequently?
- Do you have any pain or bleeding associated with bowel movements?
- Have you experienced changes in your usual bowel pattern or stool?
- Have you ever had an endoscopy or a colonoscopy? If so, which one, and when?

Assess for anorexia, changes in taste, and any difficulty or *pain* with swallowing (dysphagia) that could be associated with esophageal disorders. Recognize that one of the symptoms associated with COVID-19 is loss of taste, which sometimes resolves and sometimes persists. Also ask if abdominal *pain* or discomfort occurs with eating and whether the patient has experienced nausea, vomiting, or dyspepsia (an epigastric burning sensation, often referred to as "heartburn"). Unknown food allergies may be a cause of these symptoms. Inquire about unintentional weight loss because some GI cancers may present in this manner. Assess for alcohol and caffeine consumption because both substances are associated with many GI disorders, such as gastritis and peptic ulcer disease.

The patient's socioeconomic status may have a profound impact on *nutrition.* People who have limited budgets, such as some older adults or the unemployed, may not be able to purchase foods required for a balanced diet. They may substitute less expensive and less effective over-the-counter (OTC) medications or herbs for prescription drugs. People who live in "food deserts" (i.e., places with little access to fresh fruits and vegetables [U.S. Department of Agriculture, 2022] and other healthy foods) may also be affected by lack of *nutrition.* Necessary medical care may be delayed, and patients may not seek health care until conditions are well advanced.

PATIENT-CENTERED CARE: CULTURE AND SPIRITUALITY

Cultural and Spiritual Nutrition Observances

Cultural and spiritual observations are important to understand when obtaining a complete **nutrition** history. Ask about preferred foods, and determine if these may contribute to GI symptoms the patient reports. For example, spices or hot peppers used in cooking can aggravate or precipitate indigestion. Note spiritual observations such as fasting or abstinence, and whether these may have an impact on the patient's nutrition health or symptoms that are occurring.

Family History and Genetic Risk

Ask about a family history of GI disorders. Some GI health problems have a genetic predisposition. For example, familial adenomatous polyposis (FAP) is an inherited autosomal dominant disorder that predisposes the patient to colon cancer (Centers for Disease Control and Prevention [CDC], 2023a). Pertinent genetic risks are discussed with the GI problems in later chapters.

Current Health Problems

Because GI signs and symptoms are often vague and difficult for the patient to describe, it is important to obtain a chronologic account of the current problem, symptoms, and any treatments taken. If a patient has kept a diary of dates, symptoms, and treatments used, this can be helpful to establish patterns. Ask about the location, quality, quantity, and timing of each symptom (onset, duration), and factors that may aggravate or alleviate it (see Box 45.1).

Changes in bowel habits are common assessment findings. Obtain this information from the patient:
- Pattern of bowel movements
- Color and consistency of the feces
- Occurrence(s) of diarrhea or constipation
- Actions taken to relieve diarrhea or constipation, and whether they were successful
- Presence of frank blood or tarry stools
- Presence of abdominal distention or gas
- Weight gain or loss that has been unintentional

Assess the patient's:
- Normal weight
- Weight gain or loss
- Timing of significant weight gain or loss
- Changes in appetite or oral intake

Pain is a common concern of patients with GI tract disorders. Abdominal pain is often vague and difficult to evaluate. The mnemonic **PQRST** may be helpful in conducting a pain assessment (Jarvis & Eckhardt, 2024):

P: Precipitating or palliative factors
- What were you doing when the pain started?
- What caused it?
- What makes it better or worse?
- What seems to trigger it (e.g., stress, position, certain activities)?

Q: Quality or quantity
- Describe the feeling (e.g., sharp, dull, stabbing, burning, crushing, throbbing, nauseating, shooting, twisting, or stretching).

R: Region or radiation
- Where is the pain located?
- Does it radiate? (Where?)
- Does it feel as if it travels or moves around?
- Did it start elsewhere and is now localized to one spot?

S: Severity scale
- How severe is the pain on a scale of 0 to 10, with 0 being no pain and 10 being the worst pain ever?
- Does it interfere with activities?
- How bad is it at its worst?
- Does it force you to sit down, lie down, slow down?
- How long does an episode last?

T: Timing
- When or at what time did the pain start?
- How long did it last?
- How often does it occur (e.g., hourly, daily, weekly, monthly)?
- Is it sudden or gradual?
- What were you doing when you first experienced it?
- When do you usually experience it (e.g., daytime, night, early morning)?
- Are you ever awakened by it?
- Does it lead to anything else?
- Is it accompanied by other signs and symptoms?
- Does it ever occur before, during, or after meals?
- Does it occur seasonally?

Skin changes may result from GI tract disorders such as liver and biliary system obstruction. Ask whether these clinical signs and symptoms have occurred in the past or are currently present:
- Skin discolorations or rashes
- Itching
- Jaundice
- Increased bruising or tendency to bleed

Physical Assessment/Signs and Symptoms

Physical assessment involves a comprehensive examination of the patient's **nutrition** status, mouth, and abdomen. Nutrition assessment is discussed in detail in Chapter 52. Oral assessment is described in Chapter 46.

In preparation for assessment of the abdomen, ask the patient to empty the bladder and then to lie in a supine position with knees bent, keeping the arms at the sides to prevent tensing of the abdominal muscles.

The abdomen is assessed by using the four techniques of examination in a specific order. Nurse generalists perform inspection, auscultation, and light palpation. Health care providers perform inspection, auscultation, deep palpation, and percussion. These sequences are preferred so that palpation and percussion do not increase intestinal activity and bowel sounds. If appendicitis or an abdominal aneurysm is suspected, palpation is not done. Avoid auscultating or palpating any pulsating abdominal mass; this can be a life-threatening abdominal aortic aneurysm. Report this finding to the health care provider immediately.

Inspection

The abdominal examination usually begins with inspection of the patient's right side and proceeds in a systematic fashion (Fig. 45.4):

- Right upper quadrant (RUQ)
- Left upper quadrant (LUQ)
- Left lower quadrant (LLQ)
- Right lower quadrant (RLQ)

Table 45.1 lists the organs that lie in each of these areas.

If areas of **pain** or discomfort are noted from the history, they are cautiously assessed last in the examination sequence. This sequence should prevent the patient from tensing abdominal muscles because of the pain, which can make the examination difficult.

Inspect the skin and note any of these findings:

- Overall asymmetry of the abdomen
- Discoloration or scarring
- Abdominal distention
- Bulging flanks
- Taut, glistening skin
- Skin folds
- Subcutaneous fat noted
- Location, size, and description of any pressure injuries

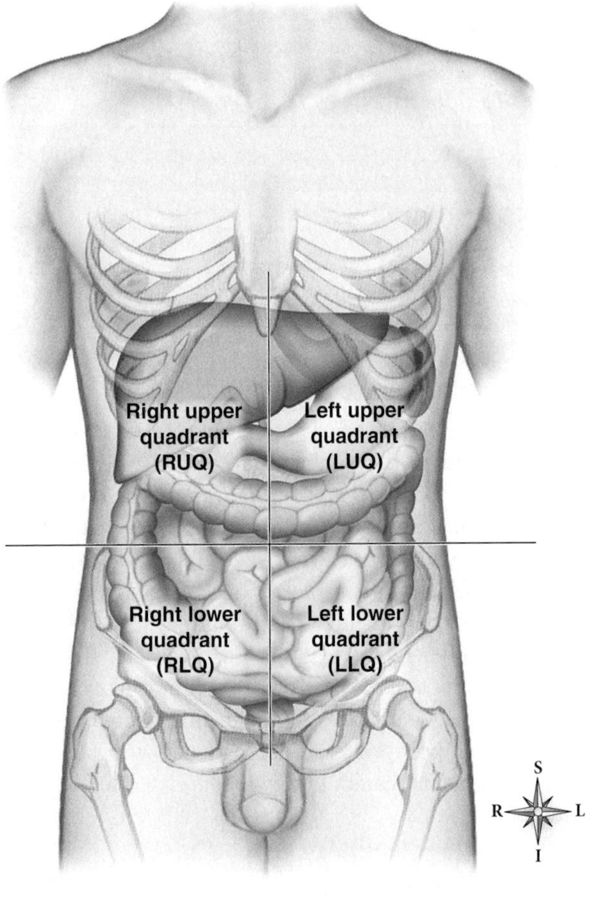

Observe the contour and symmetry of the abdomen, which can be rounded, flat, concave, or distended. It is best determined when standing at the side of the bed or treatment table and looking down on the abdomen. View the abdomen at eye level from the side. Asymmetry of the abdomen can indicate problems affecting the underlying body structures (see Table 45.1). Note the shape and position of the umbilicus for any deviations.

! NURSING SAFETY PRIORITY
Action Alert

> Peristaltic movements are rarely seen unless the patient is thin and has increased peristalsis. If these movements are observed, note the quadrant of origin and the direction of peristaltic flow. Report this finding to the health care provider because it may indicate an intestinal obstruction.

Finally, observe abdominal movements, including the normal rising and falling with inspiration and expiration, and note any distress during movement. Occasionally pulsations may be visible, particularly in the area of the abdominal aorta.

! NURSING SAFETY PRIORITY
Action Alert

> If a bulging, pulsating mass is present during inspection of the abdomen, *do not touch* the area with hands or a stethoscope because the patient may have an abdominal aortic aneurysm, a life-threatening problem. Notify the health care provider of this finding immediately!

Auscultation

Bowel sounds are created as air and fluid move through the GI tract. They are normally heard as relatively high-pitched, irregular gurgles with a normal frequency range of 5 to 30 per minute (Jarvis & Eckhardt, 2024). They are characterized as normal, hypoactive, or hyperactive. They are diminished or absent after abdominal surgery or in the patient with peritonitis or paralytic ileus. The most reliable method for assessing the return of peristalsis after abdominal surgery is to ask if flatus has been passed within the past 8 hours or a stool has been produced within the past 12 to 24 hours.

Increased high-pitched bowel sounds, especially loud, gurgling sounds, result from increased motility of the bowel (**borborygmus**). These sounds are usually heard in the patient with diarrhea or gastroenteritis or are heard above a complete intestinal obstruction.

Auscultation of the abdomen is performed with the diaphragm of the stethoscope because bowel sounds are usually high pitched. Place the stethoscope lightly on the abdominal wall, beginning in the RLQ in the area of the ileocecal valve, where bowel sounds are normally present (Jarvis & Eckhardt, 2024). Proceed with listening to other quadrants.

FIG. 45.4 Topographic division of the abdomen into quadrants. (From Patton, K. T., & Thibodeau, G. A. [2022]. *Anatomy and physiology* [11th ed.]. St. Louis: Elsevier.)

TABLE 45.1 Location of Body Structures in Each Abdominal Quadrant and Midline

Right Upper Quadrant (RUQ)	Left Upper Quadrant (LUQ)
• Most of the liver	• Left lobe of the liver
• Gallbladder	• Stomach
• Duodenum	• Spleen
• Head of the pancreas	• Body and tail of the pancreas
• Hepatic flexure of the colon	• Splenic flexure of the colon
• Part of the ascending and transverse colon	• Part of the transverse and descending colon

Midline
- • Abdominal aorta
- • Uterus (if enlarged)
- • Bladder (if distended)

Right Lower Quadrant (RLQ)	Left Lower Quadrant (LLQ)
• Cecum	• Part of the descending colon
• Appendix	• Sigmoid colon
• Right ureter	• Left ureter
• Right ovary and fallopian tube	• Left ovary and fallopian tube
• Right spermatic cord	• Left spermatic cord

During auscultation, also listen for vascular sounds or **bruits** ("swooshing" sounds) over the abdominal aorta, the renal arteries, and the iliac arteries. A bruit heard over the aorta usually indicates the presence of an aneurysm. *If this sound is heard, do not percuss or palpate the abdomen. Notify the health care provider immediately of your findings!*

Palpation

The purpose of palpation is to determine the size and location of abdominal organs and to assess for the presence of masses or tenderness. Palpation of the abdomen consists of two types: light and deep. Nurse generalists perform light palpation. The technique of *light palpation* is used to detect large masses and areas of tenderness. Place the first four fingers of the palpating hand close together and then place them lightly on the abdomen and proceed smoothly and systematically from quadrant to quadrant. Depress the abdomen to a depth of ½ to 1 inch (1.25–2.5 cm). Proceed with a rotational movement of the palpating hand. Note any areas of tenderness or guarding because these areas will be examined last and cautiously during deep palpation. While performing light palpation, note signs of rigidity, which, unlike voluntary guarding, is a sign of peritoneal inflammation. Only health care providers, such as physicians, physician associates, and advance practice nurses, should perform deep palpation. Deep palpation is used to further determine the size and shape of abdominal organs and masses.

Percussion

Percussion may be done by the health care provider to determine the size of solid organs; to detect the presence of masses, fluid, and air; and to estimate the size of the liver and spleen. The percussion notes heard in the abdomen are termed *tympanic* (the high-pitched, loud, musical sound of an air-filled intestine) or *dull* (the medium-pitched, softer, thudlike sound over a solid organ, such as the liver).

The liver and spleen can be percussed. An enlarged liver is called *hepatomegaly*. Dullness heard in the left anterior axillary line indicates enlargement of the spleen (*splenomegaly*). Mild to moderate splenomegaly can be detected by percussion before the spleen becomes palpable.

NCLEX Examination Challenge 45.2
Physiological Integrity

While performing an abdominal assessment on a client, the nurse notes rigidity over the left upper quadrant. Which GI disorder would the nurse anticipate?
A. Gastroenteritis
B. Peritoneal inflammation
C. Intestinal obstruction
D. Paralytic ileus

Psychosocial Assessment

Psychosocial assessment focuses on how the GI health problem affects the patient's life and lifestyle. Remember that patients are often reluctant to discuss **elimination** problems, which may be very personal and embarrassing. The interview focus is on whether usual daily activities have been interrupted or disturbed.

Ask about recent stressful events, as stress has been associated with the development or exacerbation (flare-up) of irritable bowel syndrome (IBS) and other GI disorders. If patients are diagnosed with cancer, it is likely that they will experience the stages of the grieving process. Patients may be depressed, angry, or in denial. Appropriately refer patients who need ongoing support to a mental health professional.

Diagnostic Assessment
Laboratory Assessment

To make an accurate assessment of the many possible causes of GI system abnormalities, laboratory testing of blood, urine, and stool specimens may be performed.

Serum Tests. A *complete blood count (CBC)* aids in the diagnosis of anemia and infection. It also detects changes in the blood's formed elements. In adults, GI bleeding is the most frequent cause of anemia. It is associated with GI cancer, peptic ulcer disease, diverticulitis, and inflammatory bowel disease.

Prothrombin time (PT) is useful in evaluating levels of clotting factors. PT measures the rate at which prothrombin is converted to thrombin, a process that depends on vitamin K–associated clotting factors. Hepatocellular liver disease leads to a prolonged PT secondary to impaired synthesis of clotting proteins (National Library of Medicine, 2022).

Many electrolytes are altered in GI tract dysfunction. For example, calcium is absorbed in the GI tract and may be measured to detect malabsorption. Excessive vomiting or diarrhea causes sodium or potassium depletion, thus requiring replacement.

Assays of serum enzymes are important in the evaluation of liver damage. Aspartate aminotransferase (AST) and alanine aminotransferase (ALT) are two enzymes found in the liver and other organs. These enzymes are elevated in most liver disorders, but their levels are highest in conditions that cause necrosis, such as hepatitis and cirrhosis.

Elevations in serum amylase and lipase may indicate acute pancreatitis, a serious inflammation of the pancreas characterized by a sudden onset of abdominal pain, nausea, and vomiting. In this disease, serum amylase levels begin to elevate within 24 hours of onset and remain elevated for up to 5 days. Serum amylase and lipase are not elevated when extensive pancreatic necrosis is present because there are few pancreatic cells manufacturing the enzymes.

Bilirubin, the primary pigment in bile, is normally conjugated and excreted by the liver and biliary system. It is measured as total serum bilirubin, conjugated (direct) bilirubin, and unconjugated (indirect) bilirubin. These measurements are important in the evaluation of jaundice and liver and biliary tract functioning. Elevations in direct and indirect bilirubin levels and/or gamma-glutamyl transferase (GGT) can indicate impaired excretion.

The serum level of ammonia may also be measured to evaluate hepatic function. Ammonia is normally used to rebuild amino acids or is converted to urea for excretion. Elevated levels are seen in conditions that cause hepatocellular injury, such as cirrhosis, hepatitis, and hepatic encephalopathy (National Library of Medicine, 2021).

Two primary oncofetal antigens—cancer antigen (CA) 19-9 and carcinoembryonic antigen (CEA)—are evaluated to monitor the efficacy of cancer therapy and assess for the recurrence of cancer in the GI tract. These antigens may also be increased in benign GI conditions. Table 45.2 lists blood tests commonly used to diagnose and then monitor GI disorders.

Urine Tests. Amylase can be detected in the urine. In acute pancreatitis, renal clearance of amylase is increased. Amylase levels in the urine remain elevated 5 to 7 days after onset of disease processes, even after serum levels return to normal within 1 to 2 days (Pagana et al., 2022). This becomes an important finding in patients who are symptomatic for several days or longer.

Urine *urobilinogen* is a form of bilirubin that is converted by the intestinal flora and excreted in the urine. Its measurement is useful in the evaluation of hepatic and biliary obstruction, because the presence of bilirubin in the urine often occurs before jaundice is seen.

Stool Tests. The American Cancer Society (ACS) recommends regular screening to detect colorectal cancer early when it can most effectively be treated (ACS, 2020). Options include an annual high-sensitivity fecal immunochemical test (FIT), an annual guaiac-based fecal occult blood test (gFOBT) (such as the Hemoccult II Sensa), or a multitargeted stool DNA (mt-sDNA) test performed every 3 years (ACS, 2020). These tests use a take-home, multisample method rather than having the test done during a digital rectal examination.

PATIENT-CENTERED CARE: HEALTH EQUITY

Colorectal Cancer Incidence

Black, American Indian, and Alaska Native people are disproportionately affected by the incidence of colorectal cancer (Siegel et al., 2023). Advocate for regular screening for all patients so that colon cancer can be detected in its earliest stages and successfully treated.

The traditionally used gFOBT (e.g., Hemoccult II Sensa) requires an active component of guaiac and is therefore more likely than the FIT (e.g., OC-Sensor) to yield false-positive results. In addition, patients having the guaiac-based test must avoid NSAIDs for 7 days prior to and during the collection period, as well as red meat and vitamin C more than 250 mg/day for 3 days prior to and during the test period (CliaWaived, 2020). Patient adherence is likely to be higher with the FIT method because drugs and food do not interfere with the test results.

As an alternative to the gFOBT or FIT, a multitargeted stool DNA test (mt-sDNA) can be completed every 3 years (ACS, 2020). Available only by prescription, this type of at-home diagnostic kit (such as Cologuard) is shipped directly to the patient after the health care provider has ordered the testing. Although less specific in detection than a colonoscopy, this type of testing can be encouraging to patients who may be fearful of undergoing a traditional colonoscopy or have concerns about financial coverage.

The cost of at-home colorectal cancer screening tests is covered by Medicare and Medicare Advantage (U.S. Centers for Medicare and Medicaid Services, n.d.a, n.d.b). It also is covered, based on the Affordable Care Act, by most private insurances. Medicare reports that there is no out-of-pocket cost for the client for the mt-sDNA test or fecal occult testing if screening guidelines are met and the health care provider orders the tests (U.S. Centers for Medicare and Medicaid Services, n.d.b).

Once received in the mail, the tests are easy to complete. The patient does not have to undergo any special preparation, such as the bowel cleansing that is required prior to a traditional colonoscopy. The patient collects one stool sample and returns it via a prepaid postage container. Although false-negative or false-positive

TABLE 45.2 **Laboratory Profile**

GI Assessment

Test (Serum)	Normal Range for Adults	Select Potential Significances of Variance From Normal
Alanine aminotransferase (ALT)	4–36 units/L (4–36 SI units/L) **NOTE:** Values may be slightly higher in older adults, men, and African American people.	*Increased* levels: • Hepatitis (significant elevation) • Cirrhosis (moderate elevation) • Pancreatitis (mild elevation)
Albumin	3.5–5.0 g/dL (35–50 g/L)	*Increased* levels: • Dehydration *Decreased* values: • Liver disease • Undernutrition
Alkaline phosphatase	30–120 units/L (0.5–2.0 μkat/L) **NOTE:** Values may be slightly higher in older adults.	*Increased* levels: • Cirrhosis • Intrahepatic or extrahepatic biliary obstruction • Liver tumor *Decreased* levels: • Hypophosphatemia • Undernutrition
Ammonia	10–80 mg/dL (6–47 μmol/L)	*Increased* levels: • Hepatic disease such as cirrhosis • Portal hypertension • GI bleeding with mild liver disease • GI obstruction with mild liver disease • Hepatic encephalopathy and hepatic coma
Amylase	60–120 Somogyi units/dL (30–220 units/L) **NOTE:** Values may be slightly higher in older adults.	*Increased* levels: • Cholecystitis • GI disease (e.g., perforated peptic ulcer, perforated or necrotic bowel) • Pancreatitis, acute or chronic
Aspartate aminotransferase (AST)	0–35 units/L (0–0.58 μkat/L) **NOTE:** Values may be slightly higher in older adults and lower in females.	*Increased* levels: • Cirrhosis • Hepatic metastasis • Hepatitis • Liver injury, drug induced *Decreased* levels: • Renal dialysis, chronic • Renal disease, acute
Bilirubin (total)	0.3–1.0 mg/dL (5.1–17 μmol/L) **Critical value:** **Adult >12 mg/dL**	*Increased* levels: • Cirrhosis • Hemolysis • Hepatitis
Bilirubin, conjugated (direct)	0.1–0.3 mg/dL (1.7–5.1 μmol/L)	*Increased* levels: • Biliary obstruction • Gallstones • Liver metastasis
Bilirubin, unconjugated (indirect)	0.2–0.8 mg/dL (3.4–12.0 μmol/L)	*Increased* levels: • Cirrhosis • Hemolysis • Hepatitis
Calcium (total)	9.0–10.5 mg/dL (2.25–2.62 mmol/L) **NOTE:** Values may be slightly lower in older adults. **Critical values:** **<6 or >13 mg/dL (<1.5 or >3.25 mmol/L)**	*Increased* levels: • Hyperparathyroidism • Metastasis to the bone *Decreased* levels: • Hypoalbuminemia • Hypoparathyroidism • Malabsorption • Pancreatitis

TABLE 45.2 Laboratory Profile—cont'd

GI Assessment

Test (Serum)	Normal Range for Adults	Select Potential Significances of Variance From Normal
Cancer antigen (CA) (CA 19-9)	0–37 units/mL	*Increased* levels: • Cancer of the pancreas, stomach, colon, gallbladder • Gallstones • Pancreatitis, acute
Carcinoembryonic antigen (CEA)	<5 ng/mL (5 mcg/L)	*Increased* levels: • Cancer (GI, breast, lung, pancreatic, hepatobiliary) • Cirrhosis • Crohn's disease • Inflammation associated with colitis, cholecystitis, pancreatitis, diverticulitis • Peptic ulcer
Cholesterol	<200 mg/dL Canadian: 3.5–5.2 mmol/L	*Increased* levels: • Pancreatitis • Biliary obstruction *Decreased* levels: • Liver cell damage
Lipase	0–160 units/L (0–160 units/L)	*Increased* levels: • Biliary disease • Bowel obstruction • Pancreatitis, acute or chronic • Peptic ulcer disease
Potassium	3.5–5.0 mEq/L (3.5–5.0 mmol/L) **Critical values: <3 or >6.1 mEq/L**	*Increased* levels: • Hyperkalemia • Hemolysis • Renal failure, acute or chronic *Decreased* levels: • Ascites • Diarrhea • Gastric suctioning
D-Xylose absorption	20–57 mg/dL (60-min plasma) 30–58 mg/dL (120-min plasma)	*Decreased* levels: • Malabsorption • Short-bowel syndrome

Data from Pagana, K., Pagana, T., & Pagana, T. (2022). *Mosby's manual of diagnostic and laboratory tests* (7th ed.). St. Louis: Elsevier.

results are possible, home-based screening tests are a cost-effective tool for identifying colorectal cancer. All positive results must be followed up by a colonoscopy for further investigation.

Encourage patients to talk openly with their health care provider to determine if a home-based screening test is appropriate. People who have a personal or family history of colon cancer, who have a condition that places them at risk (such as inflammatory bowel disease or Crohn's disease) (CDC, 2023a), or who have had previous positive results from another type of colon cancer screening test should be taught that a traditional colonoscopy is preferred over an at-home test. Emphasize the need to promptly follow up with the health care provider after the test to discuss results and possible subsequent actions that need to be taken.

Stool samples may also be collected to test for *ova and parasites* to aid in the diagnosis of parasitic infection. They may also be tested for *fecal fats* when steatorrhea (fatty stools) or malabsorption is suspected. Fat is normally absorbed in the small intestine in the presence of biliary and pancreatic secretions; in malabsorption, fat is abnormally excreted in the stool. Stool samples can also be tested to detect the presence of infectious agents, such as *Clostridium difficile*, a common cause of diarrhea in older adults and patients on prolonged antibiotic therapy.

Imaging Assessment

Radiographic examinations and similar diagnostic procedures are useful in detecting structural and functional disorders of the GI system. Provide information about preparation for the examination, provide an explanation of the procedure, and teach the required postprocedure care.

A *plain film of the abdomen* may be the first x-ray study that the health care provider requests when diagnosing a GI problem. This film can reveal masses, tumors, and strictures or obstructions. Patterns of bowel gas appear light on the abdominal film and can be useful in detecting an obstruction (ileus). No preparation is required except to wear a hospital gown and remove any jewelry or belts, which may interfere with the film.

When abdominal *pain* is severe or bowel perforation is suspected, an *acute abdomen series* may be requested. This procedure consists of a chest x-ray, a supine abdomen film, and an upright abdomen film. The chest x-ray may reveal a hiatal hernia, and an upright abdomen film may show air in the peritoneum from a bowel perforation. Although x-rays are helpful, diagnostic ultrasound and CTs are used more often (Patterson et al., 2022).

The American Cancer Society screening guidelines include the following imaging procedures as options to determine the presence of colorectal cancer and polyps in adults older than 45 years (ACS, 2020):

- Flexible sigmoidoscopy (FSIG) every 5 years, *or*
- CT colonography (virtual colonoscopy) every 5 years, *or*
- Colonoscopy every 10 years

CT, also referred to as a *CT scan,* provides a noninvasive cross-sectional x-ray view that can detect tissue densities and abnormalities in the abdomen, including the liver, pancreas, spleen, and biliary tract. It may be performed with or without contrast medium. If contrast medium is ordered, ask about any previous reactions to contrast medium and identify all severe allergies to medications. The patient is to remain on **nothing by mouth (NPO)** status for at least 4 hours before the test if a contrast medium is to be used. IV access is required for injection of the contrast medium. Advise the patient that a warm and flushed feeling, or a metallic taste, may be experienced on injection. The patient who has claustrophobia may require a mild sedative to tolerate the study. The radiologic technician instructs the patient to lie still and to hold the breath when asked, as a series of images are taken. The test takes about 10 minutes without contrast, or about 30 minutes with contrast.

Like other parts of the body, the abdomen and its organs may also be evaluated with *MRI,* such as *magnetic resonance cholangiopancreatography (MRCP).* Because of the use of powerful magnets, the patient will be asked about the presence of any medical implants, and precautions are taken to ensure that the patient meets requirements for this type of testing. Although this type of imaging takes longer than a CT scan, it does not expose patients to radiation.

Other Diagnostic Assessment

Endoscopy. Endoscopy is direct visualization of the GI tract using a flexible fiberoptic endoscope, a tube that allows viewing and manipulation of internal body areas. It is commonly ordered to evaluate bleeding; ulceration; inflammation; tumors; and cancer of the esophagus, stomach, biliary system, or bowel. Specimens for biopsy and cell studies (e.g., *Helicobacter pylori*) can be obtained through the endoscope. There are several types of endoscopic examinations, and the patient must sign an informed consent form before having any of these invasive studies performed.

Esophagogastroduodenoscopy. Esophagogastroduodenoscopy (EGD) is a visual examination of the esophagus, stomach, and duodenum by means of a fiberoptic endoscope. If GI bleeding is found during an EGD, the health care provider can use clips, thermocoagulation, injection therapy, or a topical hemostatic agent (U.S. Centers for Medicare and Medicaid Services, 2019). If the patient has an esophageal stricture, a narrowing of the esophageal opening, it can be dilated during EGD. Gastric lesions can be visualized using this procedure, and suspicion for celiac disease can be affirmed.

Usually patients are asked to avoid anticoagulants, aspirin, or other NSAIDs for several days to a week before EGD unless it is absolutely necessary. The patient can take regularly prescribed medications the morning of the test unless otherwise instructed by the health care provider. Patients with diabetes should consult their primary health care provider for special instructions. Teach the patient to remain NPO for 6 to 8 hours before the procedure. If the patient has dentures, they are removed. Explain that a flexible tube will be passed down the esophagus while the patient is under moderate sedation. Midazolam, fentanyl, or propofol is commonly used for sedation (Cohen, 2022). *These drugs can depress the rate and depth of the patient's respirations.* Atropine may be administered to dry secretions. A local anesthetic is sprayed to inactivate the gag reflex and facilitate passage of the tube. Explain that this anesthetic will depress the gag reflex and that swallowing will be difficult.

After the drugs are given, the patient is placed in a position with the head of the bed elevated. A bite block is inserted to prevent biting down on the endoscope and to protect the teeth. The health care provider passes the tube through the mouth and into the esophagus (Fig. 45.5). The procedure takes about 15 to 30 minutes.

During the test, the endoscopy nurse monitors the patient's respirations for rate and depth. Oxygenation adequacy is

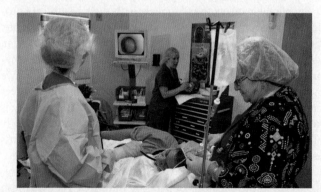

FIG. 45.5 Esophagogastroduodenoscopy allows visualization of the esophagus, the stomach, and the duodenum. If the esophagus is the focus of the examination, the procedure is called *esophagoscopy.* If the stomach is the focus, the procedure is called *gastroscopy.*

measured via an oxygen analyzer such as a pulse oximeter. Ventilation is measured via capnography, capnometry, or mass spectroscopy (American Society of Anesthesiologists, 2020). Shallow respirations decrease the amount of carbon dioxide that the patient exhales. *If the patient's respiratory rate is below 10 breaths/min or the exhaled carbon dioxide level falls below 20%, the nurse typically uses a stimulus such as a sternal rub to encourage deeper and faster respirations.*

After the test, check vital signs frequently (usually every 15–30 minutes) until the sedation begins to wear off. The side rails of the bed are raised during this time. Keep the patient NPO until the gag reflex returns (usually in 30–60 minutes). IV fluids that were started before the procedure can be discontinued when the patient is able to tolerate oral fluids without nausea or vomiting.

> ### ❗ NURSING SAFETY PRIORITY
> #### Action Alert
>
> *The priority for care to promote patient safety after esophagogastroduodenoscopy is to prevent aspiration.* Do not offer fluids or food by mouth until you are sure that the gag reflex is intact! Monitor for signs of perforation, such as **pain,** bleeding, or fever.

Because EGD is most often performed as an ambulatory care procedure requiring moderate sedation, be sure that patients have someone to drive them home. Remind the patient to not drive for at least 12 to 18 hours after the procedure because of sedation. Explain that a hoarse voice or sore throat may persist for several days after the test. Throat lozenges can be used to relieve throat discomfort.

Endoscopic Retrograde Cholangiopancreatography. Endoscopic retrograde cholangiopancreatography (ERCP) includes visual and radiographic examination of the liver, gallbladder, bile ducts, and pancreas to identify the cause and location of obstruction. It is commonly used today for therapeutic purposes rather than for diagnosis. After a cannula is inserted into the common bile duct, a radiopaque dye is instilled, and several x-ray images are obtained. The health care provider may perform a papillotomy (a small incision in the sphincter around the ampulla of Vater) to remove gallstones. If a biliary duct stricture is found, plastic or metal stents may be inserted to keep the ducts open. Biopsy samples of tissue are also frequently taken during this test.

The patient prepares for this test in the same manner as for an EGD. Perform medication reconciliation to determine if the patient is taking anticoagulants, NSAIDs, antiplatelet drugs, or antihyperglycemic agents. The health care provider will determine whether drugs are safe to take and whether any will need to be stopped before the test.

The patient must be NPO for 6 to 8 hours before the test. Be sure that dentures are removed prior to the test. Ask about prior exposure to x-ray contrast media and any sensitivities or allergies. IV access is required to administer drugs that cause moderate sedation. Ask the patient about any implantable medical devices, such as a cardiac pacemaker. Modern pacemakers generally are not affected by electrocautery; however, it is recommended that implantable defibrillators be deactivated, if possible, when electrocautery is used (Tringali et al., 2022).

The endoscopic procedure and nursing care for a patient having an ERCP are similar to those for the EGD procedure, except that the endoscope is advanced farther into the duodenum and into the biliary tract. Once the cannula is in the common duct, contrast medium is injected, and x-rays are taken to view the biliary tract. A tilt table assists in distributing the contrast medium to all areas to be assessed. The patient is placed in a left lateral position for viewing the common bile duct. Once the cannula is placed, the patient is moved to the prone position. After examination of the biliary tree, the cannula is directed into the pancreatic duct for examination. The ERCP lasts from 30 minutes to 2 hours, depending on the treatment that may be done.

After the test, assess vital signs frequently, usually every 15 minutes, until the patient is stable. To prevent aspiration, check to ensure that the gag reflex has returned before offering fluids or food. Discontinue IV fluids that were started before the procedure when the patient is able to tolerate oral fluids without nausea or vomiting.

> ### ❗ NURSING SAFETY PRIORITY
> #### Action Alert
>
> After endoscopic retrograde cholangiopancreatography (ERCP), teach about the importance of monitoring for unexpected yet severe postprocedure complications, including cholecystitis, pancreatitis, infection, bleeding, perforation, and biloma (Johns Hopkins Medicine, 2023). The patient has severe **pain** if any of these complications occur. Fever is present in sepsis. These problems do not occur immediately after the procedure; they may take several hours to 2 days to develop.

Colicky abdominal **pain** and flatulence can result from air instilled during the procedure. Instruct the patient to report abdominal pain, fever, nausea, or vomiting that fails to resolve after returning home. Be sure that patients have someone to drive them home if the test was done on an ambulatory care basis. Remind the patient to not drive for at least 12 to 18 hours after the procedure because of sedation.

Small Bowel Capsule Endoscopy. Small bowel endoscopy, or enteroscopy, provides a view of the small intestine. Video capsule endoscopy (VCE) is a procedure that uses a small-bowel enteroscopy device to visualize the entire small bowel (Hanscom et al., 2021), including the distal ileum. These devices are used to evaluate and locate the source of GI bleeding. Before the development of the VCE capsule endoscopes, viewing the small intestine was inadequate. The capsule battery lasts around 10 hours, so it is not used to view the colon.

Prepare the patient by explaining the procedure, the purpose, and what to expect during the testing. The patient must not eat or drink, including water, for 12 hours before the test and be NPO for the first 2 hours of the testing. The patient may drink clear liquids after 2 hours and have a light lunch after 4 hours (American Society for Gastrointestinal Endoscopy, 2020).

At the time of the procedure, the patient's abdomen is marked for the location of the sensors, and the sensors are applied. The patient wears an abdominal belt that houses a data recorder to capture the transmitted images. After the capsule is swallowed with a glass of water, the patient may return to normal activity, but should try to avoid vigorous activity and remain calm for the remainder of the study. At the end of the procedure, the patient returns the capsule equipment to the facility for downloading to a central computer. The procedure lasts about 8 hours or until the capsule is passed from the body.

Because the capsule endoscope is a single-use device that moves through the GI tract by peristalsis and is excreted naturally, explain to the patient that the capsule will be seen in the stool and is discarded after **elimination.** No other follow-up is necessary. The patient should report to the health care provider any signs or symptoms of GI obstruction, fever, chest pain, or difficulty breathing or if the capsule is not passed within 2 weeks.

Colonoscopy. Colonoscopy is an endoscopic examination of the entire large bowel. Be sure to fully assess all patients who may need a colonoscopy. The American Cancer Society recommends that beginning at age 45 years all healthy men and women should have a colonoscopy every 10 years or choose another equally effective recommended screening option (ACS, 2020). Evidence currently shows that younger adults with obesity are developing colon cancer, possibly due to chronic low-level inflammation that leads to cancer over a period of time (CDC, 2022). Those at high risk for cancer (e.g., family history) or those who had polyps removed should have the test more often.

The health care provider can obtain tissue biopsy specimens or remove polyps through the colonoscope during this procedure. A colonoscopy can also evaluate the cause of chronic diarrhea or locate the source of GI bleeding. Topical hemostatic agents or other methods may be used to manage the bleeding.

Patient Preparation. Patients who have their first colonoscopy are often very anxious. Provide information about the procedure, level of sedation, and possibility of **pain** (Lee, 2022). Reassure them that pain will be controlled with medication as needed.

Remind patients to avoid aspirin, anticoagulants, and antiplatelet drugs for several days before the procedure. Patients with diabetes should check with their primary health care provider about drug therapy requirements on the day of the test because they are NPO.

The health care provider will prescribe the specific method of preparation of the bowel, which begins the night before the procedure. Drinkable solutions can be chilled to improve taste. Teach the patient to partake of a clear liquid diet the day before the scheduled colonoscopy. An electrolyte replacement drink or other sports drinks will be recommended by the health care provider to replace electrolytes that are lost during bowel preparation. Teach to avoid red, orange, or purple (grape) beverages or gelatin. The patient should be NPO for several hours before the procedure, based on the health care provider's instructions.

Watery diarrhea usually begins in about an hour after starting the bowel preparation process. In some cases the patient may also require laxatives, suppositories (e.g., bisacodyl), or one or more small-volume cleansing enemas (e.g., Fleet).

The failure to achieve adequate bowel preparation prior to this procedure can lead to decreased visualization of adenoma or unsuccessful colonoscopy. Patient education and the type of bowel preparation solution are critical to a successful procedure (Lee, 2022).

Procedure. IV access is necessary for the administration of moderate sedation. The health care provider prescribes drugs to aid in relaxation, usually IV midazolam, fentanyl, or propofol (Lee & Salzman, 2021). Alternative therapies, such as using music, can improve the person's experience with a colonoscopy, although it is not a substitute for sedation or pain medication.

Initially the patient is placed on the left side with the knees drawn up while the endoscope is placed into the rectum and moved to the cecum. Air or carbon dioxide may be instilled for better visualization. Research indicates that the use of carbon dioxide is associated with decreased patient **pain** and distention (Lee & Salzman, 2021). The entire procedure lasts about 30 to 60 minutes. Atropine sulfate is kept available in case of bradycardia resulting from vasovagal response.

During the test, monitor the patient's respirations for rate and depth, and the oxygen saturation level via pulse oximetry. Shallow respirations decrease the amount of carbon dioxide that the patient exhales. If the patient's respiratory rate is below 10 breaths/min or the exhaled carbon dioxide level falls below 20%, use a stimulus such as a sternal rub to encourage deeper and faster respirations.

Follow-up Care. Check vital signs every 15 minutes until the patient is stable. Maintain NPO status and keep the side rails up until the patient is fully alert. Ask the patient to lie on the left side to promote comfort and encourage passing flatus. Observe for signs of perforation (severe **pain**) and hemorrhage, such as a rapid drop in blood pressure. Reassure the patient that a feeling of fullness, cramping, and passage of flatus is expected for several hours after the test. Fluids are permitted after the patient passes flatus to indicate that peristalsis has returned. Discontinue IV fluids that were started before the procedure when the patient can tolerate oral fluids without nausea or vomiting.

If a polypectomy or tissue biopsy was performed, there may be a small amount of blood in the first stool after the colonoscopy. Complications of colonoscopy are not common. *Report excessive bleeding or severe **pain** to the health care provider immediately* (Box 45.2).

As with other endoscopic procedures, the patient will need someone to provide transportation home if the procedure was done in an ambulatory care setting. Remind the patient to avoid driving and making important or legal decisions for the rest of the day after the procedure because of the effects of sedation.

Virtual Colonoscopy. A noninvasive imaging procedure to obtain multidimensional views of the entire colon is the *CT colonography,* known as virtual colonoscopy (Fig. 45.6). The bowel preparation and dietary restrictions are similar to those for traditional colonoscopy. However, if a polyp is detected during a virtual colonoscopy or if bleeding is found, the patient must have a follow-up invasive colonoscopy for treatment. Therefore the advantage of the traditional colonoscopy is that both diagnostic testing and minor surgical procedures can be done at the same time.

BOX 45.2   Best Practice for Patient Safety and Quality Care

Care of the Patient After a Colonoscopy

- Do not allow the patient to take anything by mouth until sedation wears off
- Take vital signs every 15 to 30 minutes until the patient is alert.
- Keep patient in left lateral position to promote passing of flatus.
- Keep the top side rails up until the patient is alert.
- Assess for rectal bleeding or severe pain.
- Remind the patient that fullness and mild abdominal cramping are expected for several hours.
- Assess for signs and symptoms of bowel perforation, including severe abdominal pain and guarding. Fever may occur later.
- Assess for signs and symptoms of hypovolemic shock, including dizziness, light-headedness, decreased blood pressure, tachycardia, pallor/ash gray skin, and altered mental status (this may be the first sign in older adults).
- If the procedure is performed in an ambulatory care setting, arrange for another person to drive the patient home.
- Teach the patient to refrain from driving, making legal decisions, or carrying out other work that requires focus for the rest of the day.

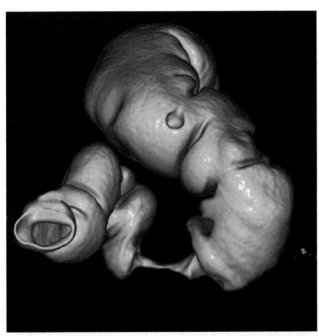

FIG. 45.6 Virtual colonoscopy. (From Bushong, S. C. [2021]. *CT colonography [virtual colonoscopy]: Radiologic science for technologists: Physics, biology, and protection* [12th ed.]. St. Louis: Elsevier.)

Sigmoidoscopy. Proctosigmoidoscopy, referred to as a sigmoidoscopy, is an endoscopic examination of the rectum and sigmoid colon using a flexible scope. This procedures screens for colon cancer, investigates the source of GI bleeding, and can be used to diagnose or monitor inflammatory bowel disease. If sigmoidoscopy is used as an alternative to colonoscopy for colorectal cancer screening, it is recommended that screening begin at 45 years of age and be done every 5 years thereafter (ACS, 2020). Patients at high risk for cancer may require more frequent screening.

As with similar tests, the health care provider will determine which medicines, such as NSAIDs and anticoagulants, should be discontinued prior to the procedure. Teach the patient to consume a clear liquid diet for a period of time determined by the health care provider before the test. A laxative may be prescribed for the night before the test. A cleansing enema or sodium biphosphate (Fleet) enema is usually required the morning of the procedure.

The patient is placed on the left side in the knee-chest position. Moderate sedation is not required. The endoscope is lubricated and inserted into the anus to the required depth for viewing. Tissue biopsy may be performed during this procedure, but the patient cannot feel it. The examination usually lasts between 5 and 15 minutes.

Inform the patient that mild gas ***pain*** and flatulence may be experienced from air instilled into the rectum during the examination. If a biopsy specimen was obtained, a small amount of bleeding may be observed. Instruct the patient that excessive bleeding should be reported immediately to the health care provider.

PATIENT-CENTERED CARE: HEALTH EQUITY

Health Literacy

Personal health literacy—the degree to which people can find, understand, and use information and services to make health-related decisions—varies dramatically among people (CDC, 2023b). This can affect how well they adhere to preprocedure and postprocedure expectations. Lack of adherence can result in omitting important screening or evaluative opportunities. Assess all people to determine if they fully understand testing procedures and requirements by having them explain the test, preparation, and follow-up in their own words (Smith et al., 2021). If there is misunderstanding, provide gentle clarification until understanding is achieved.

Ultrasonography. Ultrasonography is a technique in which high-frequency, inaudible vibratory sound waves are passed through the body via a transducer. The echoes created by the sound waves are then recorded and converted into images for analysis. Ultrasonography is commonly used to view soft tissues, such as the liver, spleen, pancreas, and biliary system. The advantages of this test are that it is painless, is noninvasive, requires no radiation, and requires no specific preparation.

The patient may be fasting, depending on the abdominal organs to be examined. Explain that it will be necessary to lie still during the study.

The patient is usually placed in a supine position. The technician applies insulating gel to the end of the transducer and on the area of the abdomen under study. This gel allows airtight contact of the transducer with the skin. The technician moves the transducer back and forth over the skin until the desired images are obtained. The study takes about 15 to 30 minutes. No follow-up care is necessary.

Endoscopic Ultrasonography. Endoscopic ultrasonography (EUS) provides images of the GI wall and high-resolution images of the digestive organs. The ultrasonography is performed through the endoscope. This procedure is useful in diagnosing the presence of lymph node tumors; mucosal tumors; and tumors of the pancreas, stomach, and rectum. The patient preparation and follow-up care are similar to those for both endoscopy and ultrasonography.

Liver-Spleen Scan. A liver-spleen scan uses IV injection of a radioactive material that is taken up primarily by the liver and secondarily by the spleen. The scan evaluates the liver and spleen for tumors or abscesses, organ size and location, and blood flow.

Teach the patient about the need to lie still during the scanning. Provide assurance that the injection has only small amounts of radioactivity and is not dangerous. Ask female patients of childbearing age if they may be pregnant or are currently breast-feeding. The radionuclide can be found in breast milk, and radiation from x-rays or scans should be avoided in pregnancy.

A radioactive injection is given through an IV line, and a wait of about 15 minutes is necessary for uptake. The patient is placed in many different positions while the scanning takes place. Tell the patient that the radionuclide is eliminated from the body through the urine in 24 hours. Careful handwashing after toileting decreases the exposure to any radiation present in the urine.

GET READY FOR THE NEXT-GENERATION NCLEX® EXAMINATION!

Essential Assessment Points

- Differentiate GI changes associated with aging from abnormal findings.
- Remind patients to have someone available to drive them home after an endoscopic procedure because of the effects of moderate sedation.
- Check for the return of the gag reflex after an endoscopic procedure before offering fluids or food; aspiration may occur if the gag reflex is not intact.
- Use effective communication when teaching patients and caregivers what to expect during tests and procedures associated with GI assessment.
- Teach to carefully follow instructions for bowel preparation before diagnostic testing; the bowel must be clear to visualize the colon.
- Use inspection, auscultation, and light palpation to assess the GI system; the health care provider will perform percussion.
- Do not palpate or auscultate any abdominal pulsating mass because it could be a life-threatening aortic aneurysm.
- Identify and report complications of GI testing to the health care provider.
- Interpret laboratory results related to GI assessment and report abnormal findings to the health care provider.
- Monitor vital signs, and assess for bleeding, fever, and pain following an endoscopic procedure.

Mastery Questions

1. Immediately following an esophagogastroduodenoscopy (EGD), which of the following interventions would the nurse implement to promote client safety? **Select all that apply.**
   A. Remind the client to drive themselves safely home.
   B. Do not allow any food or drink until the gag reflex returns.
   C. Check vital signs hourly until sedation wears off.
   D. Discontinue IV fluids upon completion of the procedure.
   E. Ensure only one side rail is up throughout recovery.

2. Which of the following statements would the nurse include when educating a client who is scheduled to have a video capsule endoscopy (VCE)? **Select all that apply.**
   A. "You will wear an abdominal belt with a data recorder throughout the test."
   B. "The capsule is a single-use item and will be discarded on elimination."
   C. "Contact your health care provider if the capsule is not passed within 3 days."
   D. "No drink or food should be consumed in the 12 hours prior to the testing."
   E. "There are no restrictions you have to observe before and during the testing period."

REFERENCES

American Cancer Society (ACS). (2020). *American Cancer Society Guideline for Colorectal Cancer Screening.* https://www.cancer.org/cancer/colon-rectal-cancer/detection-diagnosis-staging/acs-recommendations.html.

American Gastroenterological Association. (2020). *The fact about GI health disparities.* https://gastro.org/news/the-facts-about-gi-health-disparities/.

American Society for Gastrointestinal Endoscopy. (2020). *Understanding capsule endoscopy.* www.asge.org/home/for-patients/patient-information/understanding-capsule-endoscopy.

American Society of Anesthesiologists (ASA). (2020). *Standards for Basic Anesthetic Monitoring.* https://www.asahq.org/standards-and-guidelines/standards-for-basic-anesthetic-monitoring.

Barmore, W., Azad, F., & Stone, W. (2022). Physiology, Urea Cycle. [Updated 2022 May 15]. In *StatPearls [Internet].* Treasure Island (FL): StatPearls Publishing. 2022 Jan-. Available from: https://www.ncbi.nlm.nih.gov/books/NBK513323/.

Centers for Disease Control and Prevention (CDC). (2022). *Obesity and Cancer.* https://www.cdc.gov/cancer/obesity/index.htm.

Centers for Disease Control and Prevention (CDC). (2023a). *What are the Risk Factors for Colorectal Cancer?* https://www.cdc.gov/cancer/colorectal/basic_info/risk_factors.htm.

Centers for Disease Control and Prevention. (2023b). *What is health literacy?* https://www.cdc.gov/healthliteracy/learn/index.html.

CliaWaived. (2020). *Hemoccult II sensitive (fecal occult blood) tests.* https://cliawaived.com/hemoccult-ii-sensa-fecal-occult-blood-tests.html.

Cohen, J. (2022). Gastrointestinal endoscopy in adults: Procedural sedation administered by endoscopists. *UpToDate.* Retrieved May 7, 2023, from https://www.uptodate.com/contents/gastrointestinal-endoscopy-in-adults-procedural-sedation-administered-by-endoscopists.

Fawley, R. (2021). Lactose intolerance. *American College of Gastroenterology.* https://gi.org/topics/lactose-intolerance-in-children/.

Flint, B., & Tadi, P. (2023). Physiology, Aging. [Updated 2023 Jan 4]. In *StatPearls* [Internet]. Treasure Island (FL): StatPearls Publishing; 2023 Jan-. Available from: https://www.ncbi.nlm.nih.gov/books/NBK556106/.

Hanscom, M., Stead, C., Feldman, H., Marya, N. B., & Cave, D. (2021). Video capsule endoscopy and device-assisted enteroscopy. *Digestive Diseases and Sciences,* 1–14. Advance online publication. https://doi.org/10.1007/s10620-021-07085-0.

Hodge, B., Kashyap, S., & Khorasani-Zadeh, A. (2022). Anatomy, Abdomen and Pelvis, Appendix. [Updated 2022 Aug 8]. In *StatPearls* [Internet]. Treasure Island, FL: StatPearls Publishing; 2023 Jan-. Available from: https://www.ncbi.nlm.nih.gov/books/NBK459205/.

Jarvis, C., & Eckhardt, A. (2024). *Physical examination & health assessment* (8th ed.). St. Louis: Elsevier.

Johns Hopkins Medicine. (2023). In *Endoscopic retrograde cholangiopancreatography (ERCP).* https://www.hopkinsmedicine.org/health/treatment-tests-and-therapies/endoscopic-retrograde-cholangiopancreatography-ercp.

Kalra, A., Yetiskul, E., Wehrle, C., & Tuma, F. (2022). Physiology, Liver. [Updated 2022 May 8]. In *StatPearls [Internet]*. Treasure Island (FL): StatPearls Publishing. 2022 Jan-. Available from: https://www.ncbi.nlm.nih.gov/books/NBK535438/.

Lee, L. (2022). Patient education: Colonoscopy (Beyond the basics). *UpToDate.* Retrieved May 7, 2023, from https://www.uptodate.com/contents/colonoscopy-beyond-the-basics.

Lee, L., & Salzman, J. (2021). Overview of colonoscopy in adults. *UpToDate.* Retrieved May 6, 2023, from https://www.uptodate.com/contents/overview-of-colonoscopy-in-adults.

Lotfollahzadeh, S., Recio-Boiles, A., & Cagir, B. (2022). Colon cancer. [Updated 2022 Dec 3]. In *StatPearls* [Internet]. Treasure Island, FL: StatPearls Publishing; 2023 Jan-. Available from: https://www.ncbi.nlm.nih.gov/books/NBK470380/.

National Library of Medicine. (2021). *Ammonia levels.* https://medlineplus.gov/lab-tests/ammonia-levels/.

National Library of Medicine. (2022). *Prothrombin Time Test and INR (PT/INR).* https://medlineplus.gov/lab-tests/prothrombin-time-test-and-inr-ptinr/.

Ogobuiro, I., Gonzales, J., & Tuma, F. (2022). Physiology, Gastrointestinal. [Updated 2022 Apr 21]. In *StatPearls [Internet]*. Treasure Island (FL): StatPearls Publishing. 2022 Jan-. Available from: https://www.ncbi.nlm.nih.gov/books/NBK537103/.

Pagana, K. D., Pagana, T. J., & Pagana, T. N. (2022). *Mosby's manual of diagnostic and laboratory tests* (7th ed.). St. Louis: Elsevier.

Patterson, J., Kashyap, S., & Dominique, E. (2022). Acute abdomen. [Updated 2022 Jul 11]. In *StatPearls [Internet]*. Treasure Island (FL): StatPearls Publishing. 2022 Jan-. Available from: https://www.ncbi.nlm.nih.gov/books/NBK459328/.

Siegel, R., et al. (2023). Colorectal cancer statistics, 2023. *CA: A Cancer Journal for Clinicians, 73,* 233–254.

Smith, G., Lai, V., & Poon, S. (2021). Building the case for health literacy in gastroenterology. *Gastrointestinal Nursing, 19*(7). https://doi.org/10.12968/gasn.2021.19.7.26.

Tringali, A., Loperfido, S., & Costamagna, G. (2022). Uncommon complications of endoscopic retrograde cholangiopancreatography (ERCP). *UpToDate.* Retrieved May 7, 2023, from https://www.uptodate.com/contents/uncommon-complications-of-endoscopic-retrograde-cholangiopancreatography-ercp.

U.S. Centers for Medicare and Medicaid Services. (n.d.a). Fecal occult blood test. https://www.medicare.gov/coverage/fecal-occult-blood-tests

U.S. Centers for Medicare and Medicaid Services. (n.d.b). Multi-target Stool DNA Test. https://www.medicare.gov/coverage/multi-target-stool-dna-tests

U.S. Centers for Medicare and Medicaid Services. (2019). *Diagnostic and Therapeutic Esophagogastroduodenoscopy.* https://www.cms.gov/medicare-coverage-database/view/lcd.aspx?LCDId=33583&articleId=57063&Cntrctr=All&UpdatePeriod=458.

U.S. Department of Agriculture. (2022). *Food access research atlas.* https://www.ers.usda.gov/data-products/food-access-research-atlas/documentation/.

46

Concepts of Care for Patients With Oral Cavity and Esophageal Conditions

Charity Lynn Hacker

http://evolve.elsevier.com/Iggy/

LEARNING OUTCOMES

1. Plan collaborative care with the interprofessional team to promote **tissue integrity** and **nutrition** in patients with oral cavity and esophageal problems.
2. Teach adults how to decrease the risk for oral cavity and esophageal problems.
3. Teach the patient and caregiver(s) about common drugs and other management strategies used for oral cavity and esophageal problems.
4. Plan patient- and family-centered nursing interventions to decrease the psychosocial impact caused by living with oral cavity and esophageal problems.
5. Apply knowledge of anatomy, physiology, and pathophysiology to provide evidence-based care for patients with oral cavity and esophageal problems affecting **tissue integrity** and **nutrition**.
6. Analyze assessment and diagnostic findings to generate solutions and prioritize nursing care for patients with oral cavity and esophageal problems.
7. Organize care coordination and transition management for patients with oral cavity and esophageal problems.
8. Use clinical judgment to plan evidence-based nursing care to promote **tissue integrity** and **nutrition** and prevent complications in patients with oral cavity and esophageal problems.
9. Incorporate factors that affect health equity into the plan of care for patients with oral cavity and esophageal problems.

KEY TERMS

aphthous stomatitis Noninfectious stomatitis.

Barrett's epithelium Columnar epithelium (instead of the normal squamous cell epithelium) that develops in the lower esophagus during the process of healing from gastroesophageal reflux disease. It is considered premalignant and is associated with an increased risk of cancer in patients with prolonged disease.

candidiasis An infection caused by the fungus *Candida albicans.*

dysphagia Difficulty swallowing.

erythroplakia A velvety red mucosal lesion, most often occurring in the oral cavity.

esophageal stricture Narrowing of the esophageal opening.

esophagogastroduodenoscopy (EGD) The visual examination of the esophagus, stomach, and duodenum by means of a fiberoptic endoscope.

gastroesophageal reflux (GER) Condition that occurs as a result of backward flow of stomach contents into the esophagus.

gastroesophageal reflux disease (GERD) An upper gastrointestinal disease caused by the backward flow (reflux) of gastrointestinal contents into the esophagus.

hiatal hernia A condition, also called a *diaphragmatic hernia*, that involves the protrusion of the stomach through the esophageal hiatus of the diaphragm into the chest.

leukoplakia White, patchy lesions on a mucous membrane.

minimally invasive esophagectomy (MIE) A laparoscopic surgical procedure to remove part of the esophagus; may be performed in patients with early-stage cancer.

reflux esophagitis Damage to the esophageal mucosa, often with erosion and ulceration, in patients with gastroesophageal reflux disease.

regurgitation Backward flow of stomach contents into the esophagus.

sialadenitis Inflammation of a salivary gland.

stomatitis Inflammation of the oral mucosa; characterized by painful single or multiple ulcerations that impair the protective lining of the mouth. The ulcerations are commonly referred to as "canker sores."

upper endoscopy See *esophagogastroduodenoscopy.*

volvulus Obstruction of the bowel caused by twisting of the bowel.

xerostomia Very dry mouth caused by a severe reduction in saliva flow.

A HEALTHY ORAL CAVITY

Inside the mouth, teeth tear, grind, and crush food into small particles to promote swallowing, beginning the process of digestion. Saliva enzymes begin carbohydrate breakdown. The esophagus moves partially digested food from the mouth to the stomach. *Tissue integrity, nutrition* status, and *gas exchange* can all be compromised by oral and esophageal problems. These disorders can also induce significant *pain*. The nurse plays an important role in maintaining and restoring oral and esophageal health through nursing interventions, including provision of patient and family education to restore optimal *nutrition* and comfort.

Oral cavity disorders can severely affect physiologic well-being, speech, body image, and self-esteem. Those at highest risk include people who (Radaic & Kapila, 2021; World Health Organization, 2023):

- Use tobacco and/or alcohol
- Eat food that is high in sugar content
- Have inadequate exposure to fluoride
- Have preexisting oral health disorders
- Have limited access to community oral health care
- Have systemic diseases (e.g., atherosclerosis, diabetes, Alzheimer's disease)

ORAL CAVITY CONDITIONS

✴ TISSUE INTEGRITY CONCEPT EXEMPLAR: STOMATITIS

Pathophysiology Review

Stomatitis is a broad term that refers to inflammation within the oral cavity. Painful, inflamed ulcerations (called *aphthous ulcers* or *canker sores*) (Fig. 46.1) that erode *tissue integrity* of the mouth are one of the most common forms of stomatitis. The sores cause *pain* and place the patient at risk for bleeding and infection. Treatment ranges from topical applicants to opioid analgesics and/or antifungal medication, depending on the source and degree of inflammation. Stomatitis is classified according to the cause of the inflammation.

Etiology and Genetic Risk

Primary stomatitis, the most common type, includes aphthous stomatitis (noninfectious stomatitis), herpes simplex

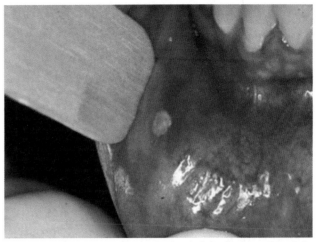

FIG. 46.1 Aphthous ulcer. (From Auerbach, P.S., Cushing, T.A., & Stuart H.N. [2017]. *Auerbach's wilderness medicine* [7th ed.]. Philadelphia: Elsevier.)

stomatitis, and traumatic ulcers. *Secondary stomatitis* generally results from infection by opportunistic viruses, fungi, or bacteria in patients who are immunocompromised or as a result of chemotherapy, radiation, or steroid drug therapy.

A common type of secondary stomatitis is caused by *Candida albicans,* which is sometimes present in small amounts in the mouth, especially in older adults. Long-term antibiotic therapy can destroy normal flora, which allows *Candida* to overgrow. The result can be candidiasis *(moniliasis),* a painful fungal infection.

👤 PATIENT-CENTERED CARE: OLDER ADULT HEALTH

Risk for Candidiasis

Older adults are at high risk for candidiasis because the immune system naturally declines during aging. The risk increases for those with diabetes or malnourishment or those under great stress. Taking multiple medications can contribute to oral dryness and decreased salivation. Teach proper mouth care to preserve *tissue integrity*, as prevention is much easier than treatment of this painful kind of stomatitis.

Stomatitis can result from infection, allergy, vitamin or mineral deficiency (complex B vitamins, folate, zinc, iron), systemic disease, and irritants such as tobacco and alcohol. Certain foods such as coffee, potatoes, cheese, nuts, citrus fruits, and gluten may trigger allergic responses that cause aphthous ulcers. Evidence suggests that activation of the cell-mediated immune system in some patients may be related to a genetic predisposition (Plewa & Chatterjee, 2021).

Incidence and Prevalence

The most common type of stomatitis, recurrent aphthous stomatitis (RAS), affects about 20% of the general population and is more commonly found in females (Bankvall et al., 2020).

Health Promotion/Disease Prevention

Proper oral hygiene can decrease the frequency and severity of stomatitis. Box 46.1 contains important teaching points to

BOX 46.1   Patient and Family Education

Maintaining a Healthy Oral Cavity

- Eat a well-balanced diet and stay hydrated by drinking water.
- Manage stress by using healthy coping mechanisms; stress can increase inflammation.
- Perform a weekly self-examination of your mouth; report changes or unusual findings to the primary health care provider or dentist.
- Report occlusion of teeth, mouth *pain*, or swelling to the primary health care provider.
- If you wear dentures, make sure that they are in good repair and fit properly.
- Thoroughly brush and floss your teeth (or brush dentures) consistently twice daily.
- Avoid mouthwashes that contain alcohol, which can damage *tissue integrity*.
- Avoid drugs that increase inflammation of the mouth or reduce saliva flow.
- See your dentist regularly; have dental problems addressed as soon as they are noted.

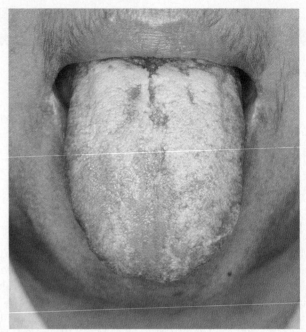

FIG. 46.2 Oral candidiasis. (From Millsop, J.W., & Fazel, N. [2016]. Oral candidiasis. *Clinics in Dermatology, 34*[4], 487–464. https://doi.org/10.1016/j.clindermatol.2016.02.022.)

provide to all adults, which will help them to improve and maintain oral health.

Interprofessional Collaborative Care

Care for the patient with stomatitis usually takes place in the community setting. The interprofessional team that collaborates to care for this patient includes the primary health care provider and nurse; a dentist and dental hygienist to provide care for the teeth, gums, and oral cavity; and an ear, nose, and throat specialist if needed.

Recognize Cues: Assessment

History. Ask about a history of recent infections, *nutrition* changes, oral hygiene habits, oral trauma, and stress. Also collect a drug history, including over-the-counter (OTC) drugs, herbal supplements, and nutrition. Document the course of current symptoms and determine whether stomatitis has occurred in the past. Ask whether the lesions interfere with swallowing, eating, or communicating. Severe stomatitis and edema have the potential to obstruct the airway. In cases of oral candidiasis, white plaquelike lesions appear on the tongue, palate, pharynx (throat), and buccal mucosa (inside the cheeks) (Fig. 46.2). When these patches are wiped away, the underlying surface is red, sore, and painful, and *tissue integrity* is compromised.

Physical Assessment/Signs and Symptoms. Assess for lesions, coating, and cracking. Document characteristics of the lesions, including location, size, shape, odor, color, and drainage. If lesions are seen along the pharynx and the patient reports dysphagia (difficulty with swallowing) or throat *pain*, the lesions might extend down the esophagus. To establish a definitive diagnosis, the primary health care provider may order additional swallowing studies.

Psychosocial Assessment. Severe stomatitis can be very painful, which can cause distress. Assess the patient's ability to cope with pain. Also determine whether the presence of stomatitis has an effect on the patient's body image or self-image.

Analyze Cues and Prioritize Hypotheses: Analysis

The priority collaborative problems for the patient with stomatitis include:

1. Impaired *tissue integrity* due to oral and/or esophageal lesions
2. *Pain* due to oral and/or esophageal lesions

▮ NURSING SAFETY PRIORITY

Action Alert

Airway obstruction, aspiration pneumonia, and malnutrition can result from dysphagia. Assess for signs and symptoms such as coughing or choking when swallowing, a sensation of food "sticking" in the pharynx, or difficulty swallowing. If dysphagia is suspected, use the PASS acronym for quick assessment: Is it **P**robable that the patient will have swallowing difficulty? **A**ccount for previous swallowing problems. **S**creen for signs and symptoms. Obtain a **S**peech-language pathologist (SLP) referral. Report signs and symptoms to the primary health care provider, and institute aspiration prevention interventions.

Generate Solutions and Take Actions: Planning and Implementation

Preserving Tissue Integrity

Planning: Expected Outcomes. The patient with stomatitis is expected to regain a healthy oral cavity with intact *tissue integrity*.

Interventions. Interventions for stomatitis are targeted toward health promotion and reduced risk for infection through careful oral hygiene and food selection. Delegate oral care to assistive personnel (AP), as this task falls within an

BOX 46.2 Best Practice for Patient Safety and Quality Care

Care of the Patient With Problems of the Oral Cavity

- Remove dentures if the patient has severe stomatitis or oral *pain*.
- Encourage the patient who is able to do so to perform oral hygiene twice daily, after meals, and as often as needed. Ensure that mouth care is provided if the client is unable.
- Increase oral care frequency to every 2 hours or more if stomatitis is not controlled.
- Teach patient to use a soft toothbrush or gauze, to use toothpaste free of sodium lauryl sulfate (SLS), and to avoid commercial mouthwashes and lemon glycerin swabs, which can irritate mucosa.
- Encourage frequent rinsing of the mouth with warm saline, sodium bicarbonate (baking soda) solution, or a combination of these solutions.
- Help the patient select soft, bland, and nonacidic foods.
- Apply topical analgesics or anesthetics as prescribed by the primary health care provider, and document effectiveness.

AP's skill set, and inspect the patient's oral cavity when the AP is done. Follow the procedures described in Box 46.2 for best oral care.

Drug therapy used for stomatitis includes solutions to address pain and infection. Commonly used drugs to address infection include (Brice, 2022):

- Clotrimazole troches
- Nystatin suspension (swish and spit)
- Chlorhexidine (swish and spit)

Minimizing Pain

Planning: Expected Outcomes. The patient with stomatitis is expected to experience minimized discomfort or absence of *pain*.

Interventions. Dietary changes may help decrease discomfort. Cool or cold liquids can be very soothing, whereas hard, spicy, salty, and acidic foods or fluids can further irritate the ulcers. Include foods high in protein to promote healing. Vitamin C may be recommended as a supplement; however, eating citrus fruits rich in vitamin C may be painful.

Over-the-counter (OTC) oral anesthetics can be recommended. Prescription drugs used as "swish and spit" agents for pain management include (Brice, 2022):

- 2% viscous lidocaine
- Diphenhydramine liquid
- Dyclonine lozenges
- Aluminum hydroxide, magnesium hydroxide, and simethicone suspension
- Attapulgite suspension

NURSING SAFETY PRIORITY

Drug Alert

Teach patients to use viscous lidocaine with extreme caution. Lidocaine causes a topical anesthetic effect, so patients may not easily feel burns from hot liquids. As sensation in the mouth and throat decreases, the risk for aspiration rises.

NCLEX Examination Challenge 46.1

Health Promotion and Maintenance

The nurse has provided teaching about maintaining a healthy oral cavity to people at a community health fair. Which of the following individuals would the nurse identify as being at high risk to develop an oral cavity disorder? **Select all that apply.**

A. Older adult with diabetes
B. Adult with a past medical history of skin cancer
C. Individual who is homeless and has no health insurance
D. Someone who has smoked a pack of cigarettes daily for 1 year
E. Person who uses the food pyramid to consume several small meals daily

Care Coordination and Transition Management

Remind the patient to take all medications as prescribed, especially antibiotics, even if the patient begins to feel better. If the patient has been prescribed medication for *pain*, teach about possible side effects, and discourage driving and activities that require concentration. Teach which drugs should be used to swish and swallow, which are to be used only as a rinse, and which are taken orally.

Teach about dietary choices that will not irritate the oral cavity and how to gently brush to promote good oral hygiene while preserving *tissue integrity* and minimizing *pain*.

Although most cases of stomatitis are self-limiting, some patients may experience persistent pain (e.g., for stomatitis related to ongoing treatment with chemotherapy and/or radiation). These patients may benefit from a support group related to their underlying illness or a group designated for those who are coping with persistent pain.

Evaluate Outcomes: Evaluation

Evaluate the care of the patient with stomatitis based on the identified priority patient problems. The expected outcomes include that the patient will:

1. Have healthy oral mucosa without inflammation or infection
2. Experience minimized discomfort or absence of *pain*

ORAL TUMORS: PREMALIGNANT LESIONS

Tumors of the mouth, whether benign, precancerous, or cancerous, can affect swallowing, chewing, and speaking. *Pain* can also limit daily activities and self-care. Oral tumors affect body image, especially if treatment involves removal of the tongue or part of the mandible (jaw) or requires a tracheostomy.

Erythroplakia

Erythroplakia, which is considered precancerous, appears as red, velvety mucosal lesions on the floor of the mouth, tongue, palate, and mandibular mucosa. It can be difficult to distinguish from inflammatory or immune reactions.

Leukoplakia

Leukoplakia causes thickened, white, firmly attached patches on the oral mucosa that cannot easily be scraped off. These

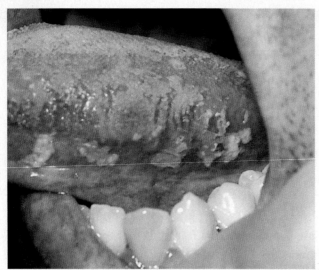

FIG. 46.3 Hairy leukoplakia. (From Sapp, J.P., Eversole, L.R., & Wysocki, G.P. [2004]. *Contemporary oral and maxillofacial pathology* [2nd ed.]. St. Louis: Elsevier.)

common oral lesions appear slightly raised and sharply rounded. Most of these lesions are benign; however, lesions on the lips or tongue can progress to cancer. Tobacco use increases the chance of development of leukoplakia.

> ◎ **CORE MEASURES**
>
> Always ask patients about current or historical tobacco use. The Joint Commission's Tobacco Treatment Measures (TOB) (2023b) requires offering practical counseling and treatment to people who use tobacco.

Long-term oral mucous membrane irritation (poorly fitting dentures, cheek chewing, broken teeth) can precede development of leukoplakia.

Oral hairy leukoplakia (Fig. 46.3) develops in people with immune compromise. It is often found in those with human immunodeficiency virus (HIV) (as an early symptom) or Epstein-Barr virus (EBV).

ORAL CANCER

Teach adults to visit a dentist at least twice a year for professional dental hygiene and an oral cancer screening, which includes inspecting and palpating the mouth for lesions (Fig. 46.4). Prevention strategies including stopping use of tobacco and alcohol, avoiding sun exposure to lips, and avoiding exposure to human papillomavirus (HPV), a sexually transmitted infection (see Chapter 65).

> 🧍 **PATIENT-CENTERED CARE: HEALTH EQUITY**
>
> **HPV-Related Oropharyngeal Cancer**
>
> White men have a much higher incidence of HPV-related oropharyngeal cancer than other men (Villalona et al., 2022). Advocate for men to be vaccinated for HPV and to have regular oral cancer screenings.

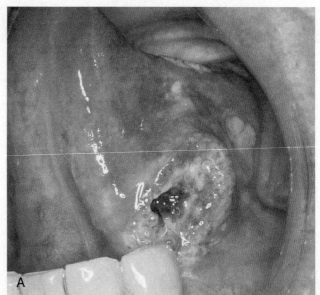

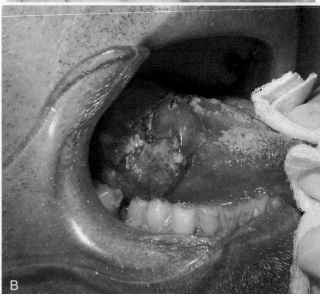

FIG. 46.4 Oral cancer. (A) Advanced squamous carcinoma. The classical ulcer with a rolled border and central necrosis is a late presentation. Note the surrounding areas of keratosis and erythema, which were present for many years before the carcinoma developed. (B) Clinical appearance of a squamous cell carcinoma of the posterolateral tongue shows an exophytic, ulcerated mass. (A from Odell, E. W. [2017]. *Cawson's Essentials of oral pathology and oral medicine* [9th ed.]. St. Louis: Elsevier. B from Ibsen, O.A., & Phelan, J.A. [2018]. *Oral pathology for the dental hygienist: With general pathology introductions* [7th ed.]. St. Louis: Elsevier.)

Industrial workers who have prolonged exposure to polycyclic aromatic hydrocarbons (PAH) are at high risk for development of oral and other cancers (Chang et al., 2021). The risk is compounded if the patient has human papillomavirus (HPV). People with *periodontal disease* (gum disease) (Fig. 46.5) in which mandibular (jaw) bone loss has occurred are also at risk.

Teach adults to follow the guidelines in Box 46.1 to maintain oral health.

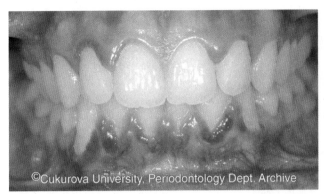

FIG. 46.5 Periodontal (gum) disease. (From Newman, M.G., Takei, H., Klokkevold, P.R., & Carranza, F.A. [2019]. *Newman and Carranza's Clinical periodontology* [13th ed.]. Philadelphia: Elsevier.)

Pathophysiology Review

Most oral cancers are squamous cell carcinomas that begin on the lips, tongue, buccal mucosa, and oropharynx in people over the age of 40. Oral lesions that are red, raised, and eroded are suspicious for cancer. A lesion that does not heal within 2 weeks or a lump or thickening in the cheek warrants further assessment (Oral Cancer Foundation [OCF], 2020).

Basal cell carcinoma of the mouth occurs primarily on the lips and is related most closely to sunlight exposure. The lesion is asymptomatic and resembles a raised scab. With time, it evolves into a characteristic ulcer with a raised, pearly border. Basal cell carcinomas in their early state rarely metastasize but can aggressively involve the skin of the face.

Kaposi sarcoma is a vascular tumor, appearing as a raised, purple, reddish, or brownish nodule or plaque, which is usually painless. It can be found on the hard palate, gums, tongue, or tonsils. It is most often associated with acquired immunodeficiency syndrome (AIDS [HIV-III]) (see Chapter 17).

PATIENT-CENTERED CARE: GENETICS/GENOMICS

Oral Cancer Risk

Ask about history of any cancer in patients who are at risk for, or may have, oral cancer. Genetic variations in patients with oral cancer have been found, especially the mutation of the *TP53* gene (Rogers, 2023). The tumor protein p53 (TP53) is essential for cell division regulation and prevention of tumor formation (National Library of Medicine, 2023).

NCLEX Examination Challenge 46.2

Health Promotion and Maintenance

The community nurse is assessing people at a health fair. Which person would the nurse encourage to seek a dental appointment for an oral cancer screening?

A. 28-year-old with Epstein-Barr virus
B. 36-year-old who recently traveled outside the country
C. 55-year-old with a slightly low body mass index (BMI)
D. 76-year-old with prolonged exposure to polycyclic aromatic hydrocarbons

BOX 46.3 Key Features

Oral Cancer

- Bleeding from the mouth
- Poor appetite, compromised **nutrition** status
- Difficulty chewing or swallowing
- Unplanned weight loss
- Thick or absent saliva
- Painless oral lesion that is red, raised, or eroded
- Thickening or lump in cheek

Interprofessional Collaborative Care

Care of the patient with oral cancer takes place in a variety of settings from the hospital to the community, depending on the degree of treatment needed. The interprofessional team that treats and cares for a patient with oral cancer may include the primary health care provider, dentist, surgeon, oncologist, nurse, speech therapist, registered dietitian nutritionist, social worker, and spiritual leader of the patient's choosing (if desired by the patient).

Recognize Cues: Assessment

Assess the patient's oral hygiene regimen and use of dentures or oral appliances. Ask about oral bleeding; alcohol or tobacco use; difficulty eating, chewing, or swallowing; and whether the patient has experienced unplanned recent weight loss (Box 46.3). Assess for educational, cultural, and/or spiritual needs that might affect health teaching or treatment, as well as the patient's self-image. Evaluate for the presence of a support system.

Thoroughly inspect the oral cavity for any lesions, **pain,** or restriction of movement; using gloves, a tongue blade, and penlight, examine all areas of the mouth. The primary health care provider will palpate for cervical nodes (Fig. 46.6).

A needle biopsy or an incisional biopsy of the abnormal tissue will be performed by the provider to assess for malignant or premalignant changes. In very small lesions, an excisional biopsy can permit complete tumor removal (OCF, 2020). CT or MRI may be performed to determine whether there is metastasis (or if staging is needed), and MRI is useful in detecting perineural involvement and evaluating thickness in cancers of the tongue.

Take Actions: Interventions

Oral cavity lesions can be treated by surgical excision; radiation and surgery; cryosurgery; or radiation, surgery, and chemotherapy. Multimodal therapy is most effective for major oral cancers (OCF, 2020). Mohs surgery is often used to remove basal cell carcinomas of the lip (Karen & Moy, 2021).

Airway maintenance to facilitate **gas exchange** is the priority of care for patients with oral cancer. Other nursing interventions focus on restoring and maintaining oral health to the best degree possible.

Nonsurgical Management. Implement interventions targeted to promote **gas exchange,** remove secretions, and prevent aspiration. Assess for dyspnea resulting from obstruction or excessive secretions. Assess the quality, rate, and depth of respirations. Auscultate the lungs for adventitious sounds, such

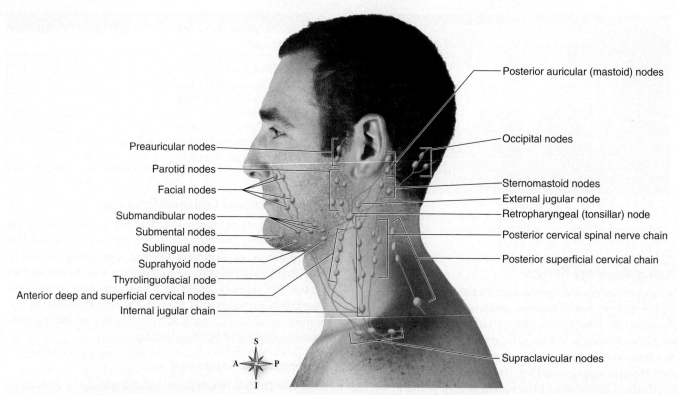

FIG. 46.6 The lymph nodes of the cervical region. (From Williamson, P., et. al. [2022]. *Anatomy & physiology* [11th ed.]. St. Louis: Elsevier.)

as wheezes caused by aspiration. Listen for stridor caused by partial airway obstruction. Promote deep breathing to help produce an effective cough and mobilize secretions.

Place the patient in semi-Fowler's or high-Fowler's position. If the patient is able to swallow and the gag reflex is intact, it is beneficial to encourage fluids to liquefy secretions for easier removal. Chest physiotherapy, often performed by the respiratory therapist, can be helpful. If needed, use oral suction equipment with a dental tip or a tonsil tip (Yankauer) to remove secretions. Teach the patient and family to use suction catheters as appropriate.

Steroids, which reduce inflammation, may be prescribed for edema associated with oral cavity lesions. Antibiotics may be prescribed for infection. A cool mist supplied by a face tent may help with oxygen transport and edema control.

⚠ NURSING SAFETY PRIORITY

Action Alert

Aspiration precautions must be instituted for patients with oral cancer. Assess the patient's level of consciousness (LOC), gag reflex (especially before giving fluids), and ability to swallow. Place the patient in a semi-Fowler's or high-Fowler's position, and keep suction equipment nearby. Remind assistive personnel to feed patients at risk for aspiration in small amounts. All family and visitors should be instructed to speak with the nurse before offering any type of food or drink to the patient. Thickened liquids may be needed; collaborate with the speech-language pathologist, who may recommend a swallow study.

Perform oral hygiene every 2 hours. Use a soft-bristle toothbrush or an ultrasoft "chemobrush," especially for patients with a low platelet count. Do not use oral swabs or disposable foam brushes, which do not adequately control bacteremia-promoting plaque and may further dry the oral mucosa. Water-based lubricant can be applied to moisten the lips and oral mucosa as needed.

The patient should avoid using commercial mouthwashes that contain alcohol and lemon-glycerin swabs, owing to their acidity. These substances can cause a burning sensation and contribute to dry oral mucous membranes. Encourage frequent rinsing of the mouth with sodium bicarbonate solution or warm saline (see Box 46.2). Follow agency or primary health care provider protocol.

Radiation therapy, chemotherapy, and/or targeted therapy may be used, depending on the tumor type, location, stage, and other recommended treatments. See Chapter 20 for information on these modalities.

Surgical Management. Depending on the type and stage of cancer, a different surgery may be recommended. Common surgeries that are used in the treatment of oral cancer include (Cancer Treatment Centers of America, 2021):

- Dental extracts and implants—teeth may need to be removed if radiation is used to treat oral cancer; prosthetic teeth can be inserted into a reconstructed mandible if necessary
- Glossectomy—removal of the tongue
- Gastrostomy tube—insertion of a feeding tube into the stomach if the oral cavity or oropharynx cannot be used to receive nutrition
- Laryngectomy—removal of the larynx and tumor

- Mandible resection (full or partial)—removal of part or all of the mandible
- Maxillectomy—removal of part or all of the hard palate
- Microsurgery—reconstruction of the mouth, throat, or mandible with body tissue from the patient (e.g., from the intestine, arm, abdomen)
- Neck dissection (partial, modified radical, or radical)—removal of lymph nodes in the neck, with or without muscle, nerve tissue, and veins
- Pedicle or free flap reconstruction—repair of the mouth, throat, or neck after a tumor is removed (often with the use of a skin graft)
- Tracheostomy—a hole created in the trachea for breathing purposes; may be permanent or temporary
- Tumor resection—removal of an entire oral tumor, with some surrounding normal tissue (known as the *margin*)

Preoperative Care. Preoperative care for patients undergoing significant head and neck cancer is discussed in Chapter 26. For patients undergoing same-day procedures on an ambulatory basis, such as the scalpel, laser, or cryoprobe removal of erythroplakia or leukoplakia, document the patient's level of understanding of the disease process, the rationale for the procedure, and the planned intervention. Evidence shows that preoperative oral health reduces postoperative inflammation and complications, so provide teaching and encourage the start of proper oral care before any procedure takes place.

Operative Procedures. The procedure chosen for isolated tumors is dependent on size, stage, and location. Removal may be done by scalpel, laser, or cryoprobe. Operative procedures for patients undergoing significant head and neck cancer are described in Chapter 23.

Postoperative Care. For small, local excisions, postoperative teaching includes planning for a liquid diet for a day, and then advancing the diet as tolerated. Activity can resume as tolerated, and *pain* is managed on a case-by-case basis. Remind the patient to keep any follow-up appointments and to continue meticulous oral care. Postoperative care for patients undergoing significant head and neck cancer is located in Chapter 23.

Care Coordination and Transition Management

Continuing care for the patient with an oral tumor depends on the severity of the tumor and the degree of treatment. Teach the patient who underwent a minor procedure for localized oral cancer about *nutrition* therapies to best restore oral and systemic health, drug therapy (if prescribed), and symptoms of infection to report. See Box 46.4 for more information. Also see Chapter 23 for the care of patients who undergo significant head and neck cancer surgery.

SIALADENITIS

Pathophysiology Review

Acute sialadenitis, inflammation of a salivary gland, can be associated with:

- Bacteria or viruses (commonly associated with cytomegalovirus)

BOX 46.4 Patient and Family Education

At-Home Care of the Patient With Oral Cancer

- Inspect the mouth daily for changes, such as redness/hyperpigmentation, lesions, or signs of infection.
- Continue meticulous oral hygiene at home.
- Use an ultrasoft toothbrush or chemobrush; clean brush after every use.
- Keep all follow-up appointments.
- Use a thickening agent for liquids if dysphagia is present.
- Eat soft foods if stomatitis occurs.
- Use saliva substitute as prescribed, if needed.

- Immunologic compromise (e.g., HIV infection, Sjögren syndrome)
- Decrease in saliva production (especially in patients undergoing radiation for head and neck cancer or thyroid cancer)
- Systemic drugs (phenothiazines, tetracyclines)

Acute sialadenitis most commonly affects the parotid or submandibular gland in adults. Although there is not a defining timeline to mark the transition, sialadenitis can become chronic if swelling persists over weeks to months (Hoffman, 2021).

Untreated infections of the salivary glands can evolve into an abscess, which can rupture and spread infection into the tissues of the neck and the mediastinum. The best prevention for acute sialadenitis is adherence to routine oral hygiene, which prevents infection from ascending to the salivary glands.

Interprofessional Collaborative Care

Assess for any predisposing factors for sialadenitis, such as ionizing radiation to the head or neck area. Collect a thorough drug history and ask about systemic illnesses, especially ones in which immunity is compromised.

Assess the oral cavity for dryness, *pain,* and swelling of the face in the area of the affected gland. Purulent drainage can sometimes be massaged from the affected area. Assess facial function, as the branches of cranial nerve VII (the facial nerve) are near the salivary glands. The patient may also report fever and general malaise.

Conservative care is directed at treating the underlying cause and increasing the flow of saliva. Teach the patient to stay hydrated, apply moist heat, and massage the gland by sweeping the fingers along the course of the gland with gentle pressure. *Pain* and inflammation can be managed with NSAIDs, and antibiotics will be prescribed if infection is suspected. *Sialagogues* (substances that stimulate the flow of saliva) may be recommended if saliva production has decreased.

The salivary glands are sensitive to ionizing radiation, such as from radiation therapy or radioactive iodine treatment of thyroid cancers. Radiation of the salivary glands can cause *pain* and edema, which generally subside after several days. Exposure of the glands to radiation produces a type of sialadenitis known as xerostomia (very dry mouth caused by a severe reduction in the flow of saliva) within 24 hours.

Xerostomia may be temporary or permanent, depending on the radiation dose and percentage of total salivary gland tissue irradiated. Frequent sips of water and frequent mouth care,

BOX 46.5   Factors Contributing to Decreased Lower Esophageal Sphincter Pressure

- Caffeinated beverages
- Coffee, tea, and cola
- Chocolate
- Nitrates
- Citrus fruits
- Tomatoes and tomato products
- Alcohol
- Peppermint, spearmint
- Smoking and use of other tobacco products
- Calcium channel blockers
- Anticholinergic drugs
- High levels of estrogen and progesterone
- Nasogastric tube placement

especially before meals, are the most effective interventions to address xerostomia. After the course of radiation therapy has been completed, saliva substitutes may provide moisture for short periods of time. Over-the-counter solutions are available.

ESOPHAGEAL CONDITIONS

✳ NUTRITION CONCEPT EXEMPLAR: GASTROESOPHAGEAL REFLUX DISEASE (GERD)

Pathophysiology Review

Gastroesophageal reflux disease (GERD), the most common upper gastrointestinal disorder in the United States, occurs most often in middle-age and older adults. Gastroesophageal reflux (GER) occurs as a result of backward flow of stomach contents into the esophagus, known as regurgitation. GERD is the chronic and more serious condition that arises from persistent GER.

Patients who are overweight or have obesity are at highest risk for GERD because excess weight increases intraabdominal pressure, which contributes to reflux. *Helicobacter pylori* may contribute to reflux (Rogers, 2023) by causing gastritis and thus poor gastric emptying. This increases frequency of GER events and acid exposure to the esophagus.

Etiology and Genetic Risk

There is not a single causative agent for GERD. Reflux produces symptoms by exposing the esophageal mucosa to the irritating effects of gastric or duodenal contents, resulting in inflammation. A patient with acute symptoms of inflammation is often described as having mild or severe reflux esophagitis (Rogers, 2023). When the lower esophageal sphincter (LES) is compromised (relaxed), gastric contents reflux into the esophagus. Eating large meals or certain foods, taking certain drugs, smoking, and using alcohol influence the tone function of the LES (Box 46.5). Reflux is generally sour or bitter. Although rare, a reflex salivary hypersecretion known

as *water brash* can occur in response to reflux. Water brash is different from regurgitation. The patient reports a sensation of fluid in the throat, but unlike with regurgitation, there is no bitter or sour taste.

Patients who have a nasogastric (NG) tube have decreased esophageal sphincter function. The tube keeps the cardiac sphincter open and allows acidic contents from the stomach to enter the esophagus. Other factors that increase intraabdominal and intragastric pressure (e.g., pregnancy, wearing tight belts or abdominal binders, bending over, ascites) overcome the gastroesophageal pressure gradient maintained by the LES and allow reflux to occur. Many patients with obstructive sleep apnea report frequent episodes of GERD. Nighttime reflux causes prolonged exposure of the esophagus to acid because the patient is usually in supine position, and secretions do not drain back down with gravity.

Studies have confirmed that there is a strong genetic connection that is associated with the development of GERD (Ong et al., 2022). As with many disorders, lifestyle choices contribute very significantly to this condition, as well.

During the process of healing, the body may substitute Barrett's epithelium (columnar epithelium) for the normal squamous cell epithelium of the lower esophagus; this becomes known as Barrett's esophagus. Although this new tissue is more resistant to acid and supports esophageal healing, it is premalignant and is associated with an increased risk for cancer in patients with prolonged GERD. The fibrosis and scarring that accompany the healing process can produce esophageal stricture (narrowing of the esophageal opening) (Fig. 46.7), which leads to progressive difficulty in swallowing. Uncontrolled esophageal reflux also increases the risk for other complications, such as asthma, laryngitis, dental decay, and cardiac disease, as well as serious concerns for hemorrhage and aspiration pneumonia.

Incidence and Prevalence

Between 18% and 28% of adults in North America have reflux disease (Locke, 2023). The population affected by GERD continues to get younger. Formerly considered a disorder that affected infants or middle-age and older adults, the proportion of people with GERD who are younger adults continues to rise. Do not assume that because a patient is younger, the patient is unlikely to have GERD.

 PATIENT-CENTERED CARE: HEALTH EQUITY

Advocacy for English Language Learners

Evidence shows health disparities in the recognition and treatment of GERD in Hispanic and Latino Americans (Kamal et al., 2023). Disparities increase when patients are not proficient in English and health care providers do not speak Spanish (Kamal et al., 2023). Advocate for the consistent use of professional medical translators for all patients who are English language learners.

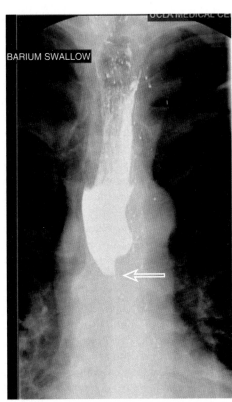

FIG. 46.7 Esophageal stricture. (From Chhetri, D. K., & Dewan, K. [2019]. *Dysphagia evaluation and management in otolaryngology.* St. Louis: Elsevier.)

Health Promotion/Disease Prevention

Adults with gastroesophageal reflux disease (GERD) may initially be asymptomatic. Teach patients to engage in healthy eating habits that include consuming small, frequent meals and limiting intake of fried, fatty, and spicy foods, and caffeine. Sitting upright for at least 1 hour after eating can promote proper digestion and reduce the risk for reflux.

Interprofessional Collaborative Care

Care for the patient with GERD usually takes place in the community setting. Seldom is surgery needed to correct the problem. The interprofessional team that collaborates to care for this patient typically includes the primary health care provider, nurse, and registered dietitian nutritionist (RDN).

Recognize Cues: Assessment

History. Ask the patient about a history of heartburn or atypical chest pain associated with the reflux of GI contents. Ask whether the patient has been newly diagnosed with asthma, has experienced morning hoarseness, or has coughing or wheezing, especially at night. These symptoms may indicate severe reflux reaching the pharynx or mouth or pulmonary aspiration.

Ask about dysphagia and *odynophagia* (painful swallowing), which can accompany chronic GERD.

Physical Assessment/Signs and Symptoms. Dyspepsia, also known as *indigestion,* and regurgitation are the main

NCLEX Examination Challenge 46.3

Physiological Integrity

The nurse has completed discharge teaching for a client with Barrett's esophagus. Which of the following client statements requires further nursing teaching? **Select all that apply.**

A. "I will be very careful when I eat or drink."
B. "I know that I am at a higher risk for cancer."
C. "I may experience stricture of the esophagus."
D. "I will now have a high sensitivity to acidic foods."
E. "I need to make sure to brush at least twice daily."

symptoms of GERD, although symptoms may vary in severity (Box 46.6). With severe GERD, this sensation generally occurs after each meal and lasts for 20 minutes to 2 hours. Discomfort may worsen when the patient lies down. Drinking fluids, taking antacids, or maintaining an upright posture usually provides prompt relief.

Other symptoms may include abdominal discomfort, feeling uncomfortably full, nausea, flatulence, eructation (belching), and bloating. Because indigestion might not be viewed as a serious concern, patients often delay seeking treatment. The symptoms typically worsen when the patient bends over, strains, or lies down. If the indigestion is severe, the *pain* may be felt in the chest and may radiate to the neck, jaw, or back, mimicking cardiac pain.

In addition to performing a gastrointestinal assessment, auscultate the patient's lung fields, assessing for crackles, which can be an indication of associated aspiration.

Psychosocial Assessment. Patients may come to the emergency department (ED), fearing that they are having a myocardial infarction. Stay with the patient as much as possible until a diagnosis is made, as worrying can create intense anxiety. Assess the client's ability to cope with stress and fear, and provide referrals as necessary.

PATIENT-CENTERED CARE: OLDER ADULT HEALTH

GERD Complications

Older adults are at risk for developing severe complications associated with GERD. They experience expected age-related physiologic changes, may have increased comorbidities due to multiple health conditions, and are prone to the effects of polypharmacy. Instead of the typical symptoms related to GERD, this population experiences dysphagia, vomiting, anorexia, anemia, cough, and respiratory concerns (Adanir et al., 2021). Collaborate with the primary health care provider when reporting these symptoms, as the patient may benefit from a workup for GERD.

Diagnostic Assessment. A definitive diagnostic test for GERD does not exist; however, the primary health care provider may use a clinical history or diagnostic tests that visualize the esophagus or measure the presence of gastric acid to establish a diagnosis when GERD is suspected (NIDDK, 2020). Usually, patients with classic GERD symptoms are diagnosed on the basis of clinical symptoms and history alone (Kahrilas, 2022). Those with atypical symptoms may benefit from an upper endoscopy (also called esophagogastroduodenoscopy [EGD]). This procedure involves insertion of an endoscope (a flexible plastic tube equipped with a light and lens) down the throat, which shows the esophagus and any associated abnormalities. A biopsy can be performed at the same time (see Chapter 45) (NIDDK, 2020). This test requires the use of moderate sedation during the procedure, and patients must have someone drive them home after recovery.

Ambulatory esophageal pH monitoring is the most accurate method of diagnosing GERD. In this procedure, a transnasally placed catheter or wireless, capsulelike device is affixed to the distal esophageal mucosa (Kahrilas, 2022). The patient is asked to keep a diary of activities and symptoms over 24 to 48 hours (depending on diagnostic method), and the pH is continuously monitored and recorded.

Although not as common, *esophageal manometry,* or motility testing, may be performed. Water-filled catheters are inserted in the patient's nose or mouth and slowly withdrawn while measurements of LES pressure and peristalsis are recorded. When used alone, manometry cannot establish a diagnosis of GERD; it is used to evaluate peristaltic function before considering surgery for GERD (Kahrilas, 2022).

Analyze Cues and Prioritize Hypotheses: Analysis

The priority collaborative problems for the patient with gastroesophageal reflux disease (GERD) include:

1. Potential for compromised *nutrition* status due to dietary selection
2. Acute *pain* due to reflux of gastric contents

Generate Solutions and Take Actions: Planning and Implementation

Balancing Nutrition

Planning: Expected Outcomes. The patient with imbalanced *nutrition* is expected to have improvement in nutrition status while the esophagitis heals.

Interventions. Interventions are designed to optimize *nutrition* status, decrease symptoms experienced with GERD, and prevent complications. Nursing care priorities include teaching the patient about proper dietary selections that provide optimum nutrients and that do not contribute to reflux.

Nonsurgical Management. For most patients, GERD can be controlled with **nutrition** therapy, lifestyle changes, and drug therapy. The most important role of the nurse is patient and caregiver education. Teach the patient that GERD is a chronic disorder that requires ongoing management. The disease should be treated more aggressively in older adults.

Ask about the patient's basic meal patterns and food preferences. Coordinate with the registered dietitian nutritionist (RDN), patient, and caregiver to adopt changes in eating that may decrease reflux symptoms.

Teach the patient to limit or eliminate foods that decrease LES pressure. Foods that irritate inflamed tissue and cause heartburn, such as peppermint, chocolate, fatty foods (especially fried), caffeine, and carbonated beverages, should be avoided. The patient should also restrict spicy and acidic foods (e.g., orange juice, tomatoes) until esophageal healing occurs. Recommend applications ("apps") that can help the patient follow a healthier diet, such as MyFitnessPal (www.myfitnesspal.com) or MyPlate (www.livestrong.com).

Explain that large meals increase volume and pressure within the stomach and delay gastric emptying. Recommend eating four to six small meals each day rather than three large ones. Advise the patient to eat slowly and chew thoroughly to facilitate digestion and prevent eructation (belching). Teach patients to avoid eating at least 3 hours before going to bed, because reflux episodes are most damaging at night. The risk for aspiration is increased if regurgitation occurs when the patient is lying down. Remind the patient to sleep propped up to promote **gas exchange**. This can be done by placing blocks under the head of the bed or by using a large, wedge-style pillow instead of a standard pillow.

Teach that alcohol and tobacco should be avoided, and make referrals to cessation groups and programs if needed. If weight management is needed, refer to the appropriate resources and community support groups.

Minimizing Pain

Planning: Expected Outcomes. The patient is expected to have relief of *pain* associated with GERD.

Interventions. Interventions are designed to minimize the patient's *pain*. Nursing care priorities focus on teaching the patient about lifestyle modifications that will improve comfort.

Nonsurgical Management. In addition to appropriate dietary selections that promote **nutrition** and allow esophageal tissues to heal, the patient should be encouraged to adhere to other methods of controlling symptoms to minimize **pain**.

Lifestyle changes. In addition to nutrition modifications, teach the patient about other lifestyle changes that decrease symptoms of GERD. Discourage heavy lifting, straining, and working in a position in which the patient bends at the abdomen. Encourage comfortable, nonrestrictive clothing.

Emphasize that these general adaptations are an essential and effective part of disease management and can produce prompt results in uncomplicated cases.

Patients with obesity often have obstructive sleep apnea in addition to GERD. Those who receive continuous positive airway pressure (CPAP) treatment report improved sleeping and decreased episodes of reflux at night. See Chapter 23 for a discussion of CPAP.

Drug therapy. Although not always possible, the elimination of drugs causing reflux should be explored with the primary health care provider. Some drugs lower LES pressure and cause reflux; these include oral contraceptives, anticholinergic agents, sedatives, NSAIDs (e.g., ibuprofen), nitrates, and calcium channel blockers.

Drug therapy for GERD management includes three major types: antacids, histamine blockers, and proton pump inhibitors (PPIs). These drugs, which are also used for peptic ulcer disease, have one or more of these functions:

- Inhibit gastric acid secretion
- Accelerate gastric emptying
- Protect the gastric mucosa

The stomach responds to these actions, and the *pain* that a patient experiences should decrease. See Table 47.1 in Chapter 47 for drug therapy used for GERD management and peptic ulcer disease.

Some PPIs, such as esomeprazole and pantoprazole, may be administered in IV form for short-term use to treat or prevent stress ulcers that can result from surgery. PPIs promote rapid tissue healing, but recurrence is common when the drug is stopped. Long-term use may mask reflux symptoms, and stopping the drug determines whether reflux has been resolved. Research has linked long-term PPI use to increased risk for development of kidney, liver, and cardiovascular disease, dementia, GI tumors, difficulty absorbing nutrients, and susceptibility to respiratory and GI infections (Yibirin et al., 2021). Evidence is still being gathered regarding several of these adverse effects, but it is important to acknowledge the need for monitoring during extended PPI use.

PATIENT-CENTERED CARE: OLDER ADULT HEALTH

PPIs and the Risk for Hip Fracture

Research has found that long-term use of proton pump inhibitors (PPIs) may increase the risk for hip fracture, especially in older adults. PPIs can interfere with calcium absorption and protein digestion and therefore reduce available calcium to bone tissue. Decreased calcium makes bones more brittle and likely to fracture, especially as adults get older (Lins Vieira, 2021).

Endoscopic therapies. The Stretta procedure, a nonsurgical method, can replace surgery for GERD when other measures are ineffective. In the Stretta procedure, the health care provider applies radiofrequency (RF) energy through the endoscope, using needles placed near the gastroesophageal junction. The RF energy decreases vagus nerve activity, thus reducing discomfort for the patient. Patients with obesity or those who have severe symptoms may not be candidates for this procedure. Postoperative instructions for patients who have undergone the Stretta procedure can be found in Box 46.7.

BOX 46.7 **Patient and Family Education**

Postoperative Instructions for Patients Having the Stretta Procedure

- Remain on clear liquids for 24 hours after the procedure.
- After the first day, consume a soft diet, such as custard, pureed vegetables, mashed potatoes, and applesauce.
- Avoid NSAIDs and aspirin for 10 days.
- Continue drug therapy as prescribed, usually proton pump inhibitors.
- Use liquid medications whenever possible.
- Do not allow nasogastric tubes to be inserted for at least 1 month because the esophagus could be perforated.
- Contact the primary health care provider immediately if these problems occur:
  - Abdominal *pain*
  - Bleeding
  - Chest *pain*
  - Dysphagia
  - Nausea or vomiting
  - Shortness of breath

Surgical Management. Surgical management is an option for clients with medically refractory GERD or those having a large hiatal hernia. Other clients may wish to have the surgery because of the required dependence on long-term medications that may be accompanied by side effects or a difficulty with adhering to the regimen (Antunes et al., 2022). A very small percentage of patients with GERD require antireflux surgery. It is usually indicated for patients who have not responded to medical treatment, have high-volume reflux, and intolerance or nonadherence to drug therapy; in some cases, it is also beneficial for patients with upper respiratory symptoms associated with GERD (Schwaitzberg, 2021). Various surgical procedures may be used through conventional open or laparoscopic techniques.

Laparoscopic Nissen fundoplication (LNF) is minimally invasive surgery (MIS) and is the standard surgical approach for treatment of severe GERD (Antunes et al., 2022). Information about this procedure can be found in the next section (Hiatal Hernias) in the Surgical Management discussion. Patients who have surgery are encouraged to continue following the basic antireflux regimen of antacids and *nutrition* therapy because the rate of recurrence is high.

The LINX Reflux Management System is a device that augments the LES with a ring composed of rare earth magnets (Schwaitzberg, 2021). The magnets attract to increase the closure pressure of the LES, yet still allow food passage with swallowing. The LINX can be effective for patients with typical GERD symptoms who have an abnormal pH study, only partially respond to daily PPI therapy, and do not have a hiatal hernia or severe esophagitis (Schwaitzberg, 2021). *Teach patients who have had LINX to talk with all health care providers before having an MRI.* Older LINX devices should *never* be in the presence of MRI, as serious injury could occur; newer devices, called *MR Conditional*, can undergo scanning under *certain* conditions (Schwaitzberg, 2021).

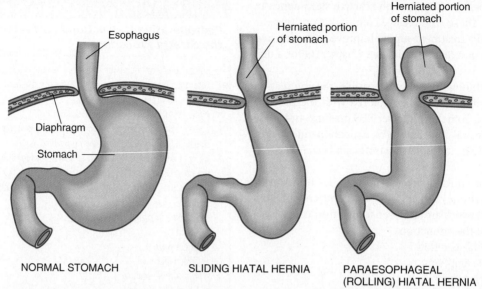

FIG. 46.8 Comparison of the normal stomach and sliding and paraesophageal (rolling) hiatal hernias.

For patients having surgery for GERD, follow preoperative and postoperative interventions presented in Chapter 9.

⚠ NURSING SAFETY PRIORITY
Action Alert

When caring for a patient who has had LINX device insertion, emphasize the importance of telling each health care provider about this procedure. If an MRI is recommended, only certain patients with more recent LINX devices *may* be eligible to undergo scanning. Patients with older LINX devices (which contain magnets) should *never* undergo MRI scanning. The health care provider can determine whether MRI is acceptable for the patient, given the date of LINX device insertion.

Care Coordination and Transition Management

Patients with GERD who do not require surgical intervention are managed in the community setting. Nursing interventions focus on helping the patient and family with current treatment and reducing risk for continuing symptoms and complications.

Remind the patient to make appropriate dietary selections that enhance **nutrition** and decrease symptoms associated with GERD. Teach how to properly adhere to drug therapy to minimize GERD-related **pain.**

For patients with nonsurgical GERD, teach about signs and symptoms of more serious complications, such as esophageal stricture and Barrett's esophagus.

Patients may find it helpful to work with a registered dietitian nutritionist (RDN) or a support group for meal-planning purposes. Give the patient information about local support groups for people with GERD and direct toward online communities that provide credible information and discussion for ongoing management of this condition.

Evaluate Outcomes: Evaluation

Evaluate the care of the patient with GERD based on the identified priority patient problem. The expected outcomes include

that the patient will:
- Adhere to appropriate dietary selections, medication therapy, and lifestyle modifications, which decrease signs and symptoms of GERD
- Experience minimized discomfort or absence of *pain*

HIATAL HERNIAS

Hiatal hernias, also called *diaphragmatic hernias,* involve the protrusion of the stomach through the esophageal hiatus of the diaphragm into the chest. The esophageal hiatus is the opening in the diaphragm through which the esophagus passes from the thorax to the abdomen.

Pathophysiology Review

Hiatal hernias are classified as type I (*sliding* hernias, which are most common) or types II through IV (paraesophageal, or *rolling,* hernias). In a type I (sliding) hernia, the esophago-gastric junction and a portion of the fundus of the stomach slide upward through the esophageal hiatus into the chest, usually as a result of weakening of the diaphragm (Fig. 46.8). The hernia generally moves freely and slides into and out of the chest during changes in position or intraabdominal pressure. Although volvulus (twisting of a GI structure) and obstruction do occur rarely, the major concern for a sliding hernia is the development of esophageal reflux and associated complications (see the section Nutrition Concept Exemplar: Gastroesophageal Reflux Disease [GERD] earlier in this chapter).

Types II through IV (paraesophageal) hernias are characterized as follows (Kahrilas, 2023):
- Type II—The gastroesophageal junction remains in its normal intraabdominal location, but the fundus (and possibly portions of the stomach's greater curvature) rolls through the esophageal hiatus and into the chest beside the esophagus (see Fig. 46.8).
- Type III—The gastroesophageal junction and the fundus both herniate through the hiatus, with the fundus lying above the gastroesophageal junction.

BOX 46.8 Key Features

Hiatal Hernias

Sliding Hiatal Hernias	Paraesophageal Hernias
• Heartburn	• Feeling of fullness (after eating)
• Regurgitation	• Breathlessness (after eating)
• Chest pain	• Feeling of suffocation (after eating)
• Dysphagia	• Chest pain that mimics angina
• Belching	• Worsening of symptoms in a recumbent position

- Type IV—The colon, spleen, pancreas, or small intestine is found in the hernia sac (instead of the stomach).

The risks for volvulus (twisting of a GI structure), obstruction (blockage), and strangulation (stricture) are high. The development of iron deficiency anemia is common because slow bleeding from venous obstruction causes the gastric mucosa to become engorged and ooze. Significant bleeding or hemorrhage is rare.

Interprofessional Collaborative Care

Care for the patient with a hiatal hernia takes place in the community setting unless surgery is needed to correct the problem. The interprofessional health care team includes the primary health care provider, nurse, surgeon, registered dietitian nutritionist, and spiritual leader of the patient's choice.

Recognize Cues: Assessment

Most patients with hiatal hernias are asymptomatic, but some experience symptoms similar to those with GERD (Rogers, 2023), as listed in Box 46.8. Symptoms usually worsen after a meal or when the patient is supine. Obtain a history and perform a physical assessment as you would for a patient with GERD (covered earlier in this chapter).

The *barium swallow study with fluoroscopy* is the most specific diagnostic test for identifying hiatal hernia. Rolling hernias are usually clearly visible, and sliding hernias can often be observed when the patient moves through a series of positions that increase intraabdominal pressure. To visualize sliding hernias, an esophagogastroduodenoscopy (EGD) may be performed to view both the esophagus and gastric lining (see Chapter 48). High-resolution manometry (HRM) with esophageal pressure topography (EPT) is used to identify larger sliding hiatal hernias (Kahrilas, 2023).

Take Actions: Interventions

Type I (sliding) hiatal hernias are usually treated medically. Treatment of types II through IV (paraesophageal) hiatal hernias are treated based on type, severity of symptoms, and risk of serious complications. When possible, medical management is favored over surgical intervention. For patients who have or are at risk for volvulus, bleeding, obstruction, strangulation, perforation, or respiratory compromise surgery is performed (Kahrilas, 2023).

Nonsurgical Management. Interventions for patients with a type I (sliding) hiatal hernia are similar to those

for GERD. These include drug therapy, *nutrition* therapy, and lifestyle changes. The primary health care provider typically recommends antacids or a proton-pump inhibitor to control reflux and its symptoms. *Nutrition* therapy is also important and follows the guidelines discussed earlier for GERD.

! NURSING SAFETY PRIORITY

Action Alert

When caring for a patient with hiatal hernia, education is one of the most important parts of nursing care. Follow health teaching as described for patients with GERD.

Surgical Management. Surgery may be required when the risk for complications is high or when damage from chronic reflux becomes severe.

Preoperative Care. If the surgery is not urgent, the surgeon may instruct a patient who is overweight to lose weight before surgery. Any patient who is to undergo surgery for hiatal hernia is advised to quit smoking. As part of preoperative teaching, reinforce the surgeon's instructions and prepare the patient for what to expect after surgery. See Chapter 9 for preoperative intervention.

Operative Procedures. Surgical repair can be done transabdominally or transthoracically. The transabdominal approach can be done as an open procedure or laparoscopically (Rosen & Blatnik, 2022). Surgery involves fundoplication, in which the stomach fundus is wrapped around the distal esophagus. The wrap is then closed with sutures to anchor the lower esophagus below the diaphragm (Fig. 46.9).

Laparoscopic Nissen fundoplication (LNF) is a minimally invasive surgical procedure commonly used for hiatal hernia repair. Complications after LNF occur less frequently compared with those seen in patients having the more traditional open surgical approach. A small percentage of patients are not candidates for LNF and therefore require a conventional open fundoplication.

Prepare the patient undergoing a transthoracic approach for a chest tube and a nasogastric tube, which will be present after surgery. These will be inserted during surgery and remain in place for several days.

Postoperative Care. Patients having the *LNF procedure* or paraesophageal repair via laparoscope are at risk for bleeding and infection, although these problems are not common. The nursing care priority is to observe for these complications and provide health teaching. See specific education in Box 46.9.

Postoperative care after *open repair* closely follows that required after any esophageal surgery. Carefully assess for complications of open surgery, as shown in Box 46.10. Report any unusual assessment findings to the surgeon.

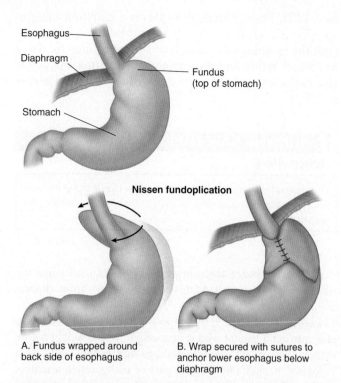

Esophagus
Diaphragm
Fundus (top of stomach)
Stomach

Nissen fundoplication

A. Fundus wrapped around back side of esophagus

B. Wrap secured with sutures to anchor lower esophagus below diaphragm

FIG. 46.9 Open surgical approach for Nissen fundoplication for gastroesophageal reflux disease or hiatal hernia repair.

BOX 46.9   Patient and Family Education

Postoperative Instructions for Patients Having Laparoscopic Nissen Fundoplication (LNF) or Paraesophageal Repair via Laparoscope

- Consume a soft diet for about a week; avoid carbonated beverages, tough foods, and raw vegetables that are difficult to swallow.
- Remain on antireflux medications as prescribed for at least a month or per your health care provider's recommendation.
- Do not drive for a week after surgery; do not drive if taking opioid pain medication.
- Walk every day, but do not do any heavy lifting.
- Remove small dressings 2 days after surgery, and shower; do not remove wound closure strips until 10 days after surgery.
- Wash incisions with soap and water, rinse well, and pat dry; report any redness or drainage from the incisions to your surgeon.
- Report fever above 101°F (38.3°C), nausea, vomiting, or uncontrollable bloating or *pain.* For patients older than 65 years, report temperature elevations above 100°F (37.8°C).
- Keep your follow-up appointment with your surgeon, usually 3 to 4 weeks after surgery.

❗ NURSING SAFETY PRIORITY

Action Alert

The primary focus of care after conventional surgery for a hiatal hernia repair is the prevention of respiratory complications. Elevate the head of the patient's bed at least 30 degrees to lower the diaphragm and promote lung expansion. Help the patient out of bed and begin ambulation as soon as possible. Be sure to support the incision during coughing to reduce *pain* and prevent excessive strain on the suture line, especially in patients with obesity.

BOX 46.10   Best Practice for Patient Safety and Quality Care

Assessment of Postoperative Complications Related to Fundoplication Procedures

Complication	Assessment Findings
Temporary dysphagia	Difficulty swallowing when oral feeding begins
Gas bloat syndrome	Difficulty belching to relieve distention
Atelectasis, pneumonia	Dyspnea, chest pain, or fever
Obstructed nasogastric tube	Nausea, vomiting, or abdominal distention and/or a nondraining nasogastric tube

---

For the patient who has undergone an open procedure, provide postoperative interventions presented in Chapter 9 regarding incentive spirometry, deep breathing, and prevention of venous thromboembolism. Patients with large hiatal hernias are at the highest risk for developing respiratory complications. The patient will have a large-bore (diameter) nasogastric (NG) tube to prevent the fundoplication wrap from becoming too tight around the esophagus. Initially the NG drainage should be dark brown with old blood. The drainage should become normal yellowish green within the first 8 hours after surgery. Check the NG tube every 4 to 8 hours for proper placement in the stomach. It should be properly anchored so that it does not become displaced, because reinsertion could perforate the fundoplication. Follow the surgeon's recommendations and agency policy for care of the patient with an NG tube.

Monitor patency of the NG tube to keep the stomach decompressed. This prevents retching or vomiting, which can strain or rupture the stomach sutures. The NG tube is irritating, so provide frequent oral hygiene to minimize *pain.* Assess hydration status regularly, and accurately assess and document intake and output. Adequate fluid replacement helps thin respiratory secretions.

Beginning with clear fluids, the patient gradually progresses to a near-normal diet during the first 4 to 6 weeks. Some foods, especially caffeinated or carbonated beverages and alcohol, are either restricted or eliminated. The food storage area of the stomach is reduced by the surgery, and meals need to be smaller and more frequent. *Carefully supervise the first oral feedings because temporary dysphagia is common.* Continuous dysphagia usually indicates that the fundoplication is too tight, and dilation may be required.

Other patients have *aerophagia* (air swallowing) from attempting to reverse or clear acid reflux. Teach them to relax consciously before and after meals, to eat and drink slowly, and to chew all food thoroughly. Air in the stomach that cannot be removed by belching can be extremely uncomfortable.

Some patients develop *gas bloat syndrome,* in which patients cannot voluntarily eructate (belch). The syndrome is usually temporary but may persist. Teach the patient to avoid drinking carbonated beverages and eating gas-producing foods (especially high-fat foods), chewing gum, and drinking with a straw. Frequent position changes and ambulation are often effective interventions for eliminating air from the GI tract. If gas *pain* is still present, it may be recommended that patients take simethicone, which relieves gas pressure.

Care Coordination and Transition Management

Patients undergoing open surgical repair require activity restrictions for 3 to 6 weeks postoperatively. For those who have undergone laparoscopic surgery, activity is typically restricted for a shorter time, and patients can return to their usual lifestyle more quickly, usually in about a week.

For long-term management, educate the patient on:
- Appropriate *nutrition* modifications
- Use of stool softeners or bulk laxatives to prevent constipation and straining
- Daily incisional inspection
- Conditions that require notification of the health care provider, including swelling, redness/hyperpigmentation, tenderness, discharge, or fever
- Avoidance of people with a respiratory infection; development of a respiratory infection with coughing can cause the incision or the fundoplication to dehisce.

ESOPHAGEAL TUMORS

Pathophysiology Review

Although esophageal tumors can be benign, most are malignant (cancerous), and the majority develop from the epithelium. Squamous cell carcinomas of the esophagus are located in the upper two-thirds of the esophagus. Adenocarcinoma, the most common type of esophageal cancer, usually occurs at the distal end of the esophagus and the upper portion of the stomach (Memorial Sloan Kettering Cancer Center, 2023). Esophageal tumors grow rapidly because there is no serosal layer to limit their extension. Because the esophageal mucosa is richly supplied with lymph tissue, there is typically early spread of tumors to lymph nodes. Esophageal tumors can protrude into the esophageal lumen and can cause thickening or invade deeply into surrounding tissue. In rare cases, the lesion may be confined to the epithelial layer (in situ). In most cases, the tumor is large and well established at diagnosis. More than half of esophageal cancers metastasize throughout the body.

Primary risk factors associated with the development of esophageal cancer include:
- Alcohol intake
- Diets chronically deficient in fresh fruits and vegetables
- Diets high in nitrates and nitrosamines (found in pickled and fermented foods)
- Malnutrition
- Obesity (especially with increased abdominal pressure)
- Smoking
- Untreated GERD

Interprofessional Collaborative Care

Care of the patient with esophageal tumors usually takes place in the hospital, followed by the community setting. The interprofessional team that collaborates to care for this patient generally includes the primary health care provider, nurse, surgeon, registered dietitian nutritionist (RDN), respiratory therapist, social worker, and spiritual leader of the patient's choice.

Recognize Cues: Assessment

Assess for risk factors related to symptoms or development of esophageal cancer. Men, regardless of race or ethnicity, have a higher incidence and higher mortality rates associated with esophageal cancer (American Cancer Society [ACS], 2020).

Cancer of the esophagus is a silent tumor in its early stages, with few observable signs. By the time the tumor causes symptoms, it usually has spread extensively. One of the most common symptoms of esophageal cancer is dysphagia. This symptom may not be present until the esophageal opening has narrowed. Weight loss often accompanies progressive dysphagia and can exceed 20 lb over several months. See Box 46.11 for more common clinical symptoms of esophageal tumors.

The diagnosis of esophageal cancer may cause significant anxiety. The disease is accompanied by distressing symptoms and is often terminal. The fear of choking can create unusual stress, especially at mealtimes. The loss of pleasure in eating and from its social aspects may affect relationships. Assess the patient's response to the diagnosis and prognosis. Ask about usual coping strengths and resources. Determine the availability of support systems and the potential impact of the disease and its treatment. Refer to psychological counseling, pastoral care, and/or the social worker or case manager as needed. Chapter 8 describes end-of-life care for patients in the terminal stage of the disease.

Diagnostic Assessment. An esophagogastroduodenoscopy (EGD) with biopsy is performed to inspect the esophagus and obtain tissue specimens for cell studies and disease staging. A complete cancer staging workup is performed, often by endoscopic ultrasound, to determine the extent of the disease and plan appropriate therapy.

Positron emission tomography (PET) may identify metastatic disease with more accuracy than a CT scan. PET can also help evaluate response to chemotherapy to treat the cancer.

BOX 46.11   Key Features

Esophageal Tumors

- Persistent and progressive dysphagia (most common feature)
- Feeling of food sticking in the throat
- Odynophagia (painful swallowing)
- Halitosis
- Chronic hiccups
- Chronic cough with increasing secretions
- Hoarseness
- Severe, persistent chest or abdominal pain or discomfort
- Anorexia
- Regurgitation
- Nausea and vomiting
- Weight loss (often more than 20 lb)
- Changes in bowel habits (diarrhea, constipation, bleeding)

NURSING SAFETY PRIORITY

Critical Rescue

When the patient with an esophageal tumor is eating or drinking, recognize that you must monitor for signs and symptoms of aspiration, which can cause airway obstruction, pneumonia, or both, especially in older adults. In coordination with the SLP, respond by teaching caregivers how to feed the patient, how to monitor for aspiration, and how to respond quickly if choking occurs.

Take Actions: Interventions

Treatment of patients with esophageal cancer depends on staging at diagnosis. Multimodal therapy is often necessary to treat esophageal cancer, as it is often advanced at diagnosis. Along with treatment of the cancer itself, patients with cancer of the esophagus experience many physical problems, and symptom management becomes essential.

Nonsurgical Management. Nonsurgical treatment options for cancer of the esophagus that can assist in disease and ***nutrition*** management may include:

- Nutrition and swallowing therapy
- Chemotherapy, radiation, and chemoradiation
- Photodynamic therapy and porfimer sodium
- Other therapies

Nutrition and Swallowing Therapy. Conduct a screening assessment to provide information about the patient's ***nutrition*** status. The registered dietitian nutritionist (RDN) determines the caloric needs of the patient to meet daily requirements. Perform weights daily before breakfast on the same scale each day. To keep the esophagus patent, position the patient upright for several hours after meals, and avoid allowing the patient to lie completely flat. Remind assistive personnel (AP) and other health care team members to keep the head of the bed elevated to a 30-degree angle or more to prevent reflux.

Semisoft foods and thickened liquids are preferred because they are easier to swallow. Document the amount of food and fluid intake every day to monitor progress in meeting desired ***nutrition*** outcomes. Liquid supplements are used between feedings to increase caloric intake. Ongoing efforts are made to preserve the ability to swallow, but enteral feedings (tube feedings) may be needed temporarily when dysphagia is severe. In patients with complete esophageal obstruction or life-threatening fistulas, the surgeon may create a gastrostomy or jejunostomy for feeding. Chapter 52 describes care for patients receiving enteral feeding.

Collaborate with the speech-language pathologist (SLP) to help the patient with oral exercises to improve swallowing (*swallowing therapy)* and with the occupational therapist (OT) for feeding techniques.

Chemotherapy and Radiation. *Chemotherapy* may be given preoperatively or in concurrence with other treatments. *Radiation therapy* can also be used alone but is used most frequently in combination with other treatments. *Chemoradiation* is a treatment for esophageal cancer that involves the use of chemotherapy at the same time as radiation therapy.

Photodynamic Therapy and Porfimer Sodium. *Photodynamic therapy (PDT)* is used as palliative treatment for patients with advanced esophageal cancer; it can relieve pain or make swallowing somewhat easier. PDT is sometimes used with *porfimer sodium* (Photofrin), a light-sensitive drug that collects in cancer cells, for palliation.

Other Therapies. *Esophageal dilation* (Fig. 46.10) may be performed as necessary throughout the course of the disease to achieve temporary but immediate relief of dysphagia. It is usually performed in an ambulatory care setting. Dilators are used to tear soft tissue, thereby widening the esophageal lumen (opening). In most cases, malignant tumors can be dilated safely, but perforation remains a significant risk.

Large metal stents may be used to keep the esophagus open for longer periods. These are placed via a procedure called *esophageal stenting*. A stent covered with graft material can be used to seal a perforation. Bacteremia can occur as a result of this procedure. To reduce the risk for sepsis and endocarditis, antibiotics are given. The treatment is repeated as often as needed to preserve the patient's ability to swallow. Complications associated with esophageal stenting include pain, stent migration, and recurrent dysphagia (Kumar et al., 2022).

Endoscopic therapies such as stenting can be offered as palliative care for patients who are not surgical candidates. Stenting can be performed with metal, plastic, or biodegradable mechanisms that are intended to relieve obstruction.

Targeted therapies such as trastuzumab, which targets the HER2 protein, may be given IV every 3 weeks (in addition to chemotherapy); at this time the optimal length of treatment is not known (American Cancer Society, 2021). This treatment can be used with chemotherapy or alone if chemotherapy has been ineffective.

Surgical Management. The purposes of different types of surgical resection vary from cure to palliation. *Esophagectomy* is the removal of all or part of the esophagus and is sometimes selected as the first line of therapy for esophageal cancer (Swanson, 2023). For patients with early-stage cancer, a laparoscopic-assisted minimally invasive esophagectomy (MIE) may be performed. However, most patients require

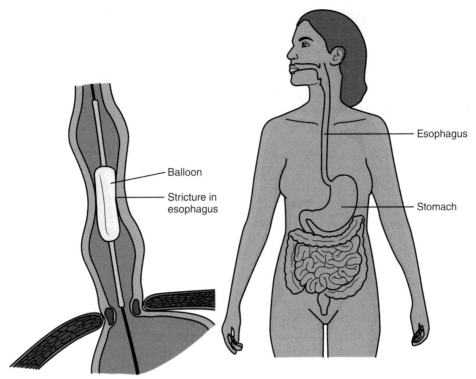

FIG. 46.10 Esophageal dilation.

conventional open surgery because of tumor size and metastasis by the time they are diagnosed with the disease.

Preoperative Care. Preoperative preparation for patients undergoing esophagectomy can be quite extensive. Advise the patient to stop smoking 2 to 4 weeks before surgery to enhance pulmonary function. Intensive preoperative respiratory rehabilitation and nutrition support may be ordered to strengthen the pulmonary system, which has been shown to decrease postoperative pulmonary complications (Swanson, 2023). Patient preparation may include lengthy *nutrition* support to decrease the risk for postoperative complications. Ideally this supplementation is given orally, but some patients require tube feeding or parenteral nutrition. Teach the patient and caregiver to monitor the patient's weight and intake and output. A preoperative evaluation may be required to treat dental disease. Instruct the patient to practice meticulous oral care four times daily to decrease the risk for postoperative infection.

Preoperative nursing care focuses on teaching and psychological support regarding the surgical procedure and preoperative and postoperative instructions. See Chapter 9 for specific preoperative teaching. On the day of surgery, the surgeon usually prescribes prophylactic antibiotics and supplemental oxygen.

Operative Procedures. There are numerous types of esophagectomies that can be performed based on the tumor location, length, extension, and adherence to surrounding structures (Swanson, 2023). The necessary extent of lymphadenectomy and the surgeon's preferences also influence surgical approach. Surgery may be minimally invasive or open.

Carefully review the specific type of procedure performed in order to optimize postprocedure nursing care.

Postoperative Care. Intensive postoperative care is necessary for the patient who has had an esophagectomy, because of the risk for multiple serious complications. Follow postoperative care as outlined in Chapter 9.

Remind all staff to keep the patient in a semi-Fowler's or high-Fowler's position to support ventilation and prevent reflux. *Ensure the patency of the chest tube drainage system, and monitor for changes in the volume or color of the drainage.*

> **⚠ NURSING SAFETY PRIORITY**
>
> **Action Alert**
>
> Respiratory care is the highest postoperative priority for patients having an esophagectomy. For those who had traditional surgery, intubation with mechanical ventilation is necessary for at least the first 16 to 24 hours. Pulmonary complications can arise, such as atelectasis and pneumonia. The risk for postoperative pulmonary complications is increased in the patient who has received preoperative radiation. Once the patient is extubated, support deep breathing, turning, and coughing every 1 to 2 hours. Assess the patient for decreased breath sounds and shortness of breath every 1 to 2 hours. Provide incisional support and adequate analgesia to enhance effective coughing.

Cardiovascular complications, particularly hypotension, can occur as a result of pressure placed on the posterior heart. Carefully monitor cardiovascular and pulmonary statuses in the postoperative period. See the Nursing Safety Priority boxes in this section.

! NURSING SAFETY PRIORITY

Action Alert

Monitor for symptoms of fluid volume overload, particularly in older patients and those who have undergone lymph node dissection. Assess for edema, crackles in the lungs, and increased jugular venous pressure. In the immediate postoperative phase, the patient is often admitted to the intensive care unit. Critical care nurses assess hemodynamic parameters such as cardiac output, cardiac index, and systemic vascular resistance every 2 hours to monitor for myocardial ischemia. Observe for atrial fibrillation, which can result from irritation of the vagus nerve during surgery, and manage according to agency protocol.

Wound management is a major postoperative concern with conventional surgery because the patient typically has multiple incisions and drains. *Provide direct support to the incision during turning and coughing to prevent dehiscence.* Wound infection can occur 4 to 5 days after surgery. Leakage from the site of anastomosis is a dreaded complication that can appear 2 to 10 days after surgery. If an anastomotic leak occurs, all oral intake is discontinued and does not resume until the site of the leak has healed. *Mediastinitis* (inflammation of the mediastinum) resulting from an anastomotic leak can lead to fatal sepsis.

✚ NURSING SAFETY PRIORITY

Critical Rescue

After esophageal surgery, recognize fever, fluid accumulation, signs of inflammation, and symptoms of early shock (e.g., tachycardia, tachypnea). Respond immediately by reporting any of these findings to the surgeon *and* the Rapid Response Team!

A nasogastric (NG) tube is placed intraoperatively to decompress the stomach to prevent tension on the suture line. Monitor the NG tube for patency, and carefully secure the tube to prevent dislodgment, which can disrupt the sutures at the anastomosis. *Do not irrigate or reposition the NG tube in patients who have undergone esophageal surgery unless ordered by the surgeon.* See Box 46.12 for best practices associated with managing the NG tube.

Nutrition management of the patient who has undergone esophageal surgery is an early postoperative concern. After conventional surgery, on the second postoperative day, initial feedings usually begin through the jejunostomy tube (J tube). Do not aspirate for residual because this increases the risk for mucosal tearing. Feedings are slowly increased over the next several days through the fifth postoperative day. A barium swallow is performed on the seventh postoperative day; if no anastomotic leaks are seen, the NG tube is discontinued (Swanson, 2023). A minimal liquid diet should be continued for the following 2 weeks. Further oral intake should be prescribed by the surgeon at the time of follow-up.

Care Coordination and Transition Management

Patients with esophageal cancer have many challenges to face once they are discharged home. Treatment regimens cause

BOX 46.12   Best Practice for Patient Safety and Quality Care

Managing the Patient With a Nasogastric Tube After Esophageal Surgery

- Check for tube placement every 4 to 8 hours.
- Ensure that the tube is patent and draining; drainage should turn from bloody to yellowish green by the end of the first postoperative day.
- Secure the tube well to prevent dislodgment.
- Do not irrigate or reposition the tube without a health care provider's order.
- Provide meticulous oral and nasal hygiene every 2 to 4 hours.
- Keep the head of the bed elevated to at least 30 degrees.
- When the patient is permitted to have a small amount of water, place the patient in an upright position and observe for dysphagia (difficulty swallowing).
- Observe for leakage from the anastomosis site (indicated by fever, fluid accumulation, and symptoms of early shock [tachycardia, tachypnea, altered mental status]).

long-lasting side effects, such as fatigue and weakness. These complex treatments also require the patient and caregiver to be knowledgeable about symptom management and to know when to report concerns.

Once the patient is discharged to home, ongoing respiratory care remains a priority. Give the patient and caregiver instructions for ambulation and incentive spirometer use. Encourage the patient to be as active as possible and to avoid excessive bed rest because this can lead to complications of immobility.

Nutrition support is important. Encourage the patient to continue increasing oral feedings as ordered by the surgeon. Teach to eat small, frequent meals containing high-calorie, high-protein foods that are soft and easily swallowed. Teach the value of using supplemental shakes. Emphasize the importance of sitting upright to eat and remaining upright after meals. Patients who have undergone esophageal resection can lose up to 10% of their body weight. Teach patients to monitor their weight at home and to report a weight loss of 5 lb or more in 1 month. If sufficient oral intake is not possible, tube feedings or parenteral nutrition at home at home may be needed.

📋 NATIONAL PATIENT SAFETY GOALS

Handwashing Guidelines

In accordance with The Joint Commission Home Care 2023 National Patient Safety Goals (2023a), teach the patient and family to protect themselves from infection in the home environment by following the World Health Organization (WHO) or the Centers for Disease Control and Prevention (CDC) handwashing guidelines. Remind them to contact the health care provider immediately if signs of respiratory infection develop. Patients should stay away from people with infections and avoid large crowds.

Teach the patient that dysphagia or odynophagia may recur because of stricture, reflux, or cancer recurrence. These symptoms should be reported to the health care provider promptly.

Despite radical surgery, the patient with cancer of the esophagus often still has a terminal illness and a relatively short life expectancy. This can cause significant anxiety

EVIDENCE-BASED PRACTICE

Effects of a Rehabilitation Program on Patients With Esophageal Cancer

Chen, H., et al. (2022). Effects of rehabilitation program on quality of life, sleep, rest-activity rhythms, anxiety, and depression of patients with esophageal cancer: A pilot randomized controlled trial. *Cancer Nursing, 45*(2), E582-E593.

This randomized controlled trial was performed with the understanding that many patients with esophageal cancer experience anxiety and depression, which contributes to a very poor quality of life. Often these psychological symptoms are impacted by reflux, which disturbs sleep and other activities of daily living (ADLs). The intention of this research was to determine whether a preplanned rehabilitation program, focused on improving quality of life through health-related activities, would have a favorable impact on patients with esophageal cancer.

Level of Evidence: 1
The research design was a randomized controlled trial, which represents a Level 1 type of evidence. Patients in this study were randomly assigned to an experimental group or a control group. The experimental group underwent 12 weeks of rehabilitation in the form of brisk walking and diet education, whereas the control group received routine care. Factors measured at baseline and postintervention included reflux severity, health-related quality of life, subjective and objective sleep quality, rest-activity rhythms, anxiety, and depression.

Commentary: Implications for Practice and Research
The data from this study confirmed that the patients receiving the intervention exhibited a significant improvement in reflux and a reported improvement in emotional regulation, socialization, difficulty eating, perceived anxiety, and sleep time. This type of intervention is manageable and cost-effective as a nonpharmacologic intervention for patients with esophageal cancer.

and depression in some patients (see the Evidence-Based Practice box). Emphasis is placed on maximizing quality of life. Realistic planning is important. Help family members in exploring sources of support and in arranging for hospice care when it becomes necessary. Chapter 8 describes end-of-life care.

ESOPHAGEAL TRAUMA

Trauma to the esophagus can result from blunt injuries, chemical burns, surgery or endoscopy (although rare), or the stress of continuous severe vomiting. Trauma may affect the esophagus directly, or it may create problems in the lungs or mediastinum. When excessive force is exerted on the esophageal mucosa, it may perforate or rupture, allowing the caustic acid secretions to enter the mediastinal cavity. These tears are associated with a high mortality rate related to shock, respiratory impairment, or sepsis.

Common causes of esophageal perforation include:
- Straining
- Seizures
- Trauma
- Foreign objects
- Instruments or tubes
- Complications of esophageal surgery
- Ulcers
- Chemical injury

Chemical injury is usually a result of the accidental or intentional ingestion of caustic substances. The damage to the mouth and esophagus is rapid and severe. Acid burns tend to affect the superficial mucosal lining, whereas alkaline substances cause deeper penetrating injuries. Strong alkalis can cause full perforation of the esophagus within 1 minute. Additional complications may include aspiration pneumonia and hemorrhage. Esophageal strictures may develop as scar tissue forms.

Patients with esophageal trauma are initially evaluated and treated in the emergency department. Assessment focuses on the nature of the injury and the circumstances surrounding it. *Assess for airway patency, breathing, chest pain, dysphagia, vomiting, and bleeding as the priorities for patient care.* If the risk for extending the damage is not excessive, an endoscopic study may be requested to evaluate tears or perforation. A CT scan of the chest can be done to assess for the presence of mediastinal air.

After the injury, keep the patient NPO to prevent further leakage of esophageal secretions. Esophageal and gastric suction can be used for drainage and to rest the esophagus. Esophageal rest is maintained for more than a week after injury to allow for initial healing of the mucosa. Total parenteral nutrition (TPN) is ordered to provide calories and protein for wound healing while the patient is not eating.

To prevent sepsis, the health care provider prescribes broad-spectrum antibiotics. High-dose corticosteroids may be administered to suppress inflammation and prevent strictures (esophageal narrowing). Opioid and nonopioid analgesics may be prescribed for *pain* management. When caustic burns involve the mouth, topical agents such as viscous lidocaine may be used.

If nonsurgical management is ineffective in healing injured esophageal tissue, the patient may need surgery to remove the damaged tissue. Those with severe injuries may require resection of part of the esophagus with a gastric pull-through and repositioning or replacement by a bowel segment. A gastrostomy tube (G-tube) placement may be needed to meet *nutrition* needs while healing.

GET READY FOR THE NEXT-GENERATION NCLEX® EXAMINATION!

Essential Nursing Care Points

Health Promotion/Disease Prevention	Chronic Disease Care
• Teach oral hygiene techniques, and remind adults to visit their dentist at least twice a year for preventative care. • Teach patients with nonhealing oral wounds to contact their primary health care provider or dentist. • Teach adults to avoid tobacco, alcohol, and sun exposure to decrease risk for oral cancer. • Discuss ways to change modifiable risk factors to decrease the chance of developing oral cancer.	• Stress the importance of controlling reflux through **nutrition** and drug therapy. • Teach the patient with GERD to elevate the head of the bed or sleep propped up. • Teach the patient and caregiver to recognize symptoms of dysphagia and appropriate ways to seek care if this condition occurs.
Regenerative or Restorative Care	**Hospice/Palliative/Supportive Care**
• Check the gag reflex and implement airway management interventions for patients having oral or esophageal surgery. • Assess for complications, and provide postoperative care for patients having surgical procedures for oral and esophageal problems. • Collaborate with the interprofessional team to design a plan of care for the patient with impaired swallowing and/or impaired **nutrition.**	• Collaborate with the registered dietitian nutritionist (RDN) to plan **nutrition** modifications for patients with GERD and undernutrition. • Refer patients to hospice, palliative care, and support groups as appropriate. • Provide support, education, and community referrals to patients with oral cancer and their significant others • Recognize that a diagnosis of oral cancer can be emotionally debilitating; refer patients who need ongoing psychosocial support to social services or mental health professionals who can provide long-term assistance.

Mastery Questions

1. A client who had the laparoscopic Nissen fundoplication (LNF) procedure is being discharged to home. Which of the following client statements requires further teaching by the nurse? **Select all that apply.**
   A. "I should eat a soft diet for at least 1 month."
   B. "My surgeon will remove my wound dressings after a week."
   C. "I should avoid any heavy lifting at this time."
   D. "A small amount of nausea and vomiting is normal after LNF."
   E. "I will need to take antireflux medications for the rest of my life."

2. A client is recovering from trauma to the esophagus. Which of the following actions would the nurse include in the plan of care? **Select all that apply.**
   A. Administer TPN per orders.
   B. Monitor secretions from gastric suction.
   C. Maintain NPO status and give ice chips.
   D. Maintain esophageal rest for at least 1 month.
   E. Determine the ongoing need for analgesia.

NGN Challenge 46.1

The nurse is reviewing the Nursing Flow Sheet for a 62-year-old client who is hospitalized for persistent vomiting associated with chemotherapy for breast cancer. The client reports throat pain and difficulty swallowing.

NURSING FLOW SHEET

Laboratory Test With Normal Values	October 12 0700	October 12 1910	October 13 0714
Sodium (136–145 mEq/L)	134 mEq/L	144 mEq/L	160 mEq/L
Potassium (3.5–5 mEq/L)	4.5 mEq/L	5.2 mEq/L	6 mEq/L
Chloride (98–106 mEq/L)	102 mEq/L	105 mEq/L	112 mEq/L
BUN (10–20 mg/dL)	18 mg/dL	19 mg/dL	22 mg/dL
Creatinine (0.3–0.6 mg/dL)	0.4 mg/dL	0.5 mg/dL	0.6 mg/dL

Which of the following actions would the nurse take to protect the client's oral cavity after reviewing these laboratory findings from the past 36 hours? **Select all that apply.**

○ Provide a very soft toothbrush.
○ Make the client NPO immediately.
○ Elevate the head of the bed at least 30 degrees.
○ Request an order for IV fluids to be administered.
○ Provide mouthwash to rinse out the oral cavity.
○ Ensure that dentures are clean and fit appropriately.
○ Regularly assess the mouth for lesions and redness.
○ Collaborate with the health care provider for a swallowing evaluation.

NGN Challenge 46.2

The nurse has documented an assessment for a 55-year-old client who is seeing the primary health care provider today for physical examination.

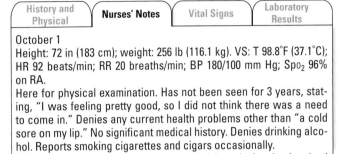

History and Physical	Nurses' Notes	Vital Signs	Laboratory Results

October 1
Height: 72 in (183 cm); weight: 256 lb (116.1 kg). VS: T 98.8°F (37.1°C); HR 92 beats/min; RR 20 breaths/min; BP 180/100 mm Hg; Spo₂ 96% on RA.
Here for physical examination. Has not been seen for 3 years, stating, "I was feeling pretty good, so I did not think there was a need to come in." Denies any current health problems other than "a cold sore on my lip." No significant medical history. Denies drinking alcohol. Reports smoking cigarettes and cigars occasionally.
In front of teeth 25 and 26 on lower lip is a 0.5-cm lesion that is raised 2 mm and red with signs of erosion. Reports that it arose about 4 weeks ago and hasn't gone away.

Complete the diagram by selecting from the choices below to specify what potential condition the client is likely experiencing, **2** nursing actions that are appropriate to take, and **2** parameters the nurse should monitor to assess the client's progress.

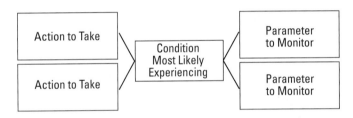

Actions to Take	Potential Conditions	Parameters to Monitor
Notify health care provider right away.	Aphthous ulcer	Teeth erosion
Teach client to clean the lesion with alcohol.	Oral hairy leukoplakia	New oral lesions or eruptions
Request a prescription for antibiotic ointment.	Basal cell carcinoma	Adherence to antiviral therapy
Explain the importance of tooth brushing to avoid spreading lesions.	Stomatitis	Signs of infection following removal
Encourage client to avoid excessive sunlight.		Metastasis to brain, bone, or lung

REFERENCES

Adanir, H., et al. (2021). Endoscopic findings of gastro-esophageal reflux disease in elderly and younger age groups. *Frontiers in Medicine, 8,* 606205. 1-6.

American Cancer Society (ACS). (2020). *Esophageal cancer risk factors.* https://www.cancer.org/cancer/esophagus-cancer/causes-risks-prevention/risk-factors.html.

American Cancer Society (ACS). (2021). *Targeted therapy for esophageal cancer*. https://www.cancer.org/cancer/esophagus-cancer/treating/targeted-therapy.html.

Antunes, C., Aleem, A., & Curtis, S. (2022 Jan-). Gastroesophageal Reflux Disease. [Updated 2022 Jul 4]. In *StatPearls [Internet]*. Treasure Island (FL): StatPearls Publishing. Available from: https://www.ncbi.nlm.nih.gov/books/NBK441938/.

Bankvall, M., et al. (2020). A family-based genome-wide association study of recurrent aphthous stomatitis. *Oral Diseases, 26*, 1696–1705.

Brice, S. (2022). Recurrent aphthous stomatitis. *UpToDate*. Retrieved May 20, 2023, from https://www.uptodate.com/contents/recurrent-aphthous-stomatitis.

Cancer Treatment Centers of America. (2021). *Surgery for oral cancer*. https://www.cancercenter.com/cancer-types/oral-cancer/treatments/surgery.

Chang, Y., Rager, J., & Tilton, S. (2021). Linking coregulated gene modules with polycyclic aromatic hydrocarbon-related cancer risk in the #d bronchial epithelium. *Chemical Research in Toxicology, 34*(6), 1445–1455.

Chen, H., et al. (2022). Effects of rehabilitation program on quality of life, sleep, rest-activity rhythms, anxiety, and depression of patients with esophageal cancer: A pilot randomized controlled trial. *Cancer Nursing, 45*(2), E582–E593.

Hoffman, H. (2021). Salivary gland swelling: Evaluation and diagnostic approach. *UpToDate*. Retrieved May 20, 2023, from https://www.uptodate.com/contents/salivary-gland-swelling-evaluation-and-diagnostic-approach.

Kahrilas, P. (2022). Clinical manifestations and diagnosis of gastroesophageal reflux in adults. *UpToDate* Retrieved May 20, 2023, from https://www.uptodate.com/contents/clinical-manifestations-and-diagnosis-of-gastroesophageal-reflux-in-adults.

Kahrilas, P. (2023). Hiatus hernia. *UpToDate*. Retrieved May 20, 2023, from https://www.uptodate.com/contents/hiatus-hernia.

Kamal, A., et al. (2023). Healthcare disparities in gastroesophageal reflux disease for Hispanic and Latino Americans: A solution-oriented approach for improvement. *American Journal of Gastroenterology, 118*(2), 193–196.

Karen, J., & Moy, R. (2021). Basal cell carcinoma treatment: Effective options for early and advanced BCC. *Skin Cancer Foundation*. https://www.skincancer.org/skin-cancer-information/basal-cell-carcinoma/bcc-treatment-options/.

Kumar, S., et al. (2022). How much progress have we made?: A 20-year experience regarding esophageal stents for the palliation of malignant dysphagia. *Diseases of the Esophagus, 35*(6), 1–7.

Lins Vieira, N. F., Da Silva Nascimento, J., Do Nascimento, C. Q., Barros Neto, J. A., & Oliveira Dos Santos, A. C. (2021). Association between bone mineral density and nutritional status, body composition and bone metabolism in older adults. *Journal of Nutrition, Health & Aging, 25*(1), 71–76.

Locke, R. (2023). *The prevalence and impact of gastroesophageal reflux disease*. https://aboutgerd.org/what-is/prevalence/.

Memorial Sloan Kettering Cancer Center. (2023). *Types of esophageal cancer*. https://www.mskcc.org/cancer-care/types/esophageal/types-esophageal.

National Institute of Diabetes and Digestive and Kidney Disease (NIDDK). (2020). *Diagnosis of GER and GERD*. https://www.niddk.nih.gov/health-information/digestive-diseases/acid-reflux-ger-gerd-adults/diagnosis.

National Library of Medicine. (2023). *TP53 tumor protein p53*. https://www.ncbi.nlm.nih.gov/gtr/genes/7157/.

Ong, J., An, J., Han, X., et al. (2022). Multitrait genetic association analysis identifies 50 new risk loci for gastro-oesophageal reflux, seven new loci for Barrett's oesophagus and provides insights into clinical heterogeneity in reflux diagnosis. *Gut, 71*, 1053–1061.

Oral Cancer Foundation (OCF). (2020). *April is oral cancer awareness month*. https://oralcancerfoundation.org/april-is-oral-cancer-awareness-month/.

Plewa, M. C., & Chatterjee, K. (2021). Aphthous stomatitis. [Updated 2022 Aug 7]. In: *StatPearls* [Internet]. Treasure Island, Florida: StatPearls Publishing; 2023 Jan-. Available from: https://www.ncbi.nlm.nih.gov/books/NBK431059/.

Radaic, A., & Kapila, Y. (2021). The oralome and its dysbiosis: New insights into oral microbiome-host interactions. *Computational and Structural Biotechnology Journal, 19*, 1335–1360.

Rogers, J. L. (2023). *McCance and Huether's Pathophysiology: The biologic basis for disease in adults and children* (9th ed.). St. Louis: Elsevier.

Rosen, M., & Blatnik, J. (2022). Surgical management of paraesophageal hernia. *UpToDate*. Retrieved May 20, 2023, from https://www.uptodate.com/contents/surgical-management-of-paraesophageal-hernia.

Schwaitzberg, S. (2021). Surgical management of gastroesophageal reflux in adults. *UpToDate*. Retrieved May 22, 2023, from https://www.uptodate.com/contents/surgical-management-of-gastroesophageal-reflux-in-adults.

Swanson, S. (2023). Surgical management of resectable esophageal and esophagogastric junction cancers. *UpToDate*. Retrieved May 20, 2023, from https://www.uptodate.com/contents/surgical-management-of-resectable-esophageal-and-esophagogastric-junction-cancers.

The Joint Commission. (2023a). *2023 Home Care National Patient Safety Goals*. https://www.jointcommission.org/-/media/tjc/documents/standards/national-patient-safety-goals/2023/ome-npsg-simplified-2023-july.pdf.

The Joint Commission. (2023b). *Tobacco use treatment: FDA-approved cessation medication. Specification manual for Joint Commission National Quality Measures (v2023B)*. https://manual.jointcommission.org/releases/TJC2023B/DataElem0322.html.

Villalona, S., et al. (2022). More than cervical cancer: Understanding racial/ethnic disparities in oropharyngeal cancer outcomes among males by HPV status. *Annals of Family Medicine, 20*(Supplement 1), 2625.

World Health Organization. (2023). *Oral health*. https://www.who.int/news-room/fact-sheets/detail/oral-health.

Yibirin, M., De Oliveira, D., Valera, R., Plitt, A. E., & Lutgen, S. (2021). Adverse effects associated with proton pump inhibitor use. *Cureus, 13*(1):e12759. https://doi.org/10.7759/cureus.12759.

47

Concepts of Care for Patients With Stomach Conditions

Keelin Cromar

http://evolve.elsevier.com/Iggy/

LEARNING OUTCOMES

1. Plan collaborative care with the interprofessional team to manage *infection* in patients with peptic ulcer disease (PUD).
2. Teach adults how to decrease the risk for gastric cancer.
3. Teach the patient and caregiver(s) about common drugs and other management strategies used for stomach conditions.
4. Plan patient- and family-centered nursing interventions to decrease the psychosocial impact caused by living with gastric cancer.
5. Apply knowledge of anatomy, physiology, and pathophysiology to provide evidence-based care for patients with stomach conditions.

6. Analyze assessment and diagnostic findings to generate solutions and prioritize nursing care for patients who have PUD.
7. Organize care coordination and transition management for patients having gastric surgery.
8. Use clinical judgment to plan evidence-based nursing care to promote *nutrition* and decrease *pain* and *inflammation* in patients with gastritis.
9. Incorporate factors that affect health equity into the plan of care for patients with gastric cancer.

KEY TERMS

dumping syndrome A postgastrectomy condition that refers to a group of vasomotor symptoms that occur after eating.

dyspepsia An epigastric burning sensation, often referred to as "heartburn."

gastrectomy Surgical removal of all (total gastrectomy) or part (subtotal gastrectomy) of the stomach.

gastritis The inflammation of gastric mucosa (stomach lining).

hematemesis Vomiting bright red or coffee-ground blood.

melena Dark, "tarry" (sticky) stool, indicating occult blood caused by digestion of blood within the small intestine.

peptic ulcer disease A condition that results when GI mucosal defenses become impaired and no longer protect the epithelium from the effects of acid and pepsin.

peritonitis An abdominal infection in which the abdomen is tender, rigid, and boardlike.

stress ulcer Acute gastric mucosal lesion occurring after an acute medical crisis or trauma, such as sepsis, a head injury, or surgery.

✳ PRIORITY AND INTERRELATED CONCEPTS

The priority concept for this chapter is:

- *Infection*
  The *Infection* concept exemplar for this chapter is Peptic Ulcer Disease (PUD).

The interrelated concepts for this chapter are:

- *Inflammation*
- *Nutrition*
- *Pain*

The stomach is part of the upper GI system that is responsible for a large part of the digestive process. Diseases that affect the stomach include gastritis, peptic ulcer disease (PUD), and cancer. These conditions can be very serious and sometimes life-threatening. Each of these health problems can result in impaired or altered *nutrition*. *Inflammation* and *infection* can cause *pain* and discomfort. Chapter 3 briefly reviews each of these health concepts.

GASTRITIS

Gastritis is the *inflammation* of gastric mucosa (stomach lining) (see complete discussion of inflammation in Chapter 16). Gastritis can be classified according to cause, cellular changes, or distribution of the lesions and can be erosive (causing ulcers) or nonerosive. Although the mucosal changes that result from *acute* gastritis typically heal after several months, this is not true for *chronic* gastritis.

Pathophysiology Review

Prostaglandins provide a protective mucosal barrier that prevents the stomach from digesting itself. If there is a disruption in the protective barrier, mucosal injury can occur. The resulting injury is worsened by histamine release and vagal nerve stimulation. Hydrochloric acid can then diffuse back into the mucosa and injure small vessels. This back-diffusion can cause edema, bleeding, and erosion of the lining of the stomach (Rogers, 2023).

Inflammation of the gastric mucosa or submucosa after exposure to local irritants or other causes can result in *acute gastritis.* The early pathologic manifestation of gastritis is a thickened, reddened mucous membrane with prominent rugae, or folds. Various degrees of mucosal necrosis and inflammation occur in acute disease. The diagnosis cannot be based solely on clinical symptoms. If the stomach muscle is not involved, complete recovery usually occurs in a few days with no residual evidence of gastric *inflammation.* If the muscle is affected, bleeding or hemorrhage may occur during an episode of acute gastritis.

The long-term use of nonsteroidal antiinflammatory drugs (NSAIDs) creates a high risk for acute gastritis. NSAIDs inhibit prostaglandin production in the mucosal barrier. Other risk factors include use of alcohol, coffee, and caffeine. Stress and cigarette smoking are considered risk factors for the development of acute gastritis (Rogers, 2023). Local irritation from radiation therapy and the accidental or intentional ingestion of corrosive substances, including acids or alkalis (e.g., lye and drain cleaners), may also cause acute gastritis. Steroids, aldosterone antagonists, and selective serotonin reuptake inhibitors can contribute to gastroduodenal *inflammation* and ulceration.

Chronic gastritis appears as a patchy, diffuse (spread out) *inflammation* of the mucosal lining of the stomach. As the disease progresses, the walls and lining of the stomach thin and atrophy. With progressive gastric atrophy from chronic mucosal injury, the function of the parietal (acid-secreting) cells decreases, and the source of intrinsic factor is lost. Intrinsic factor is critical for absorption of vitamin B_{12}. When body stores of vitamin B_{12} become depleted, pernicious anemia may result. The amount and concentration of acid in stomach secretions gradually decrease until the secretions consist of only mucus and water.

The most common form of chronic gastritis is caused by *Helicobacter pylori infection.* A direct correlation exists between the number of organisms and the degree of cellular abnormality present. The host response to the *H. pylori* infection is activation of lymphocytes and neutrophils. This results in a release of proinflammatory cytokines that damage the gastric mucosa (Dewayani et al., 2021).

Chronic gastritis causes persistent *inflammation* that extends deep into the mucosa, causing gastric gland destruction and cellular changes (Rogers, 2023). Chronic local irritation and toxic effects caused by alcohol ingestion, radiation therapy, and smoking have been linked to chronic gastritis. Surgical procedures that involve the pyloric sphincter, such as pyloroplasty, can lead to gastritis by causing reflux of alkaline secretions into the stomach. Other systemic disorders such as Crohn's disease, graft-versus-host disease, and uremia can also precipitate the development of chronic gastritis. Chronic *H. pylori* infection and autoimmune gastritis increase the risk of developing gastric cancer (Rogers, 2023).

BOX 47.1   Patient and Family Education

Gastritis Prevention

- Eat a well-balanced diet and exercise regularly, if possible.
- Avoid drinking excessive amounts of alcoholic beverages.
- Avoid long-term use of aspirin, other NSAIDs (e.g., ibuprofen), or corticosteroids.
- Avoid excessive intake of coffee (even decaffeinated).
- Be sure that foods and water are safe and free from contamination.
- Manage stress levels using complementary and integrative therapies, such as relaxation and meditation techniques.
- Stop smoking and/or using other forms of tobacco.
- Protect yourself against exposure to toxic substances in the workplace, such as lead and nickel.
- Seek medical treatment if you are experiencing symptoms of gastroesophageal reflux disease (GERD) (see Chapter 46).

Health Promotion/Disease Prevention

Gastritis is a very common health problem in the United States. A balanced diet, regular exercise, and stress-reduction techniques can help prevent it (Box 47.1). In addition, smoking and alcohol use should be avoided. Stress-reduction techniques can include aerobic exercise, meditation, and/or yoga, depending on individual preferences. Keep in mind that while these health promotion strategies may help reduce the incidence of gastritis, some individuals will not be able to practice them due to lack of resources, especially those who have financial difficulties or have family responsibilities that leave them little time to care for themselves. Respect each individual's situation and values to practice patient-centered care.

Interprofessional Collaborative Care

Care of the patient with gastritis usually takes place in the community setting. However, if symptoms are severe, the patient may be hospitalized.

Recognize Cues: Assessment

Symptoms of *acute gastritis* range from mild to severe. Patients typically report a rapid onset of epigastric **pain** and dyspepsia (an epigastric burning sensation, often referred to as "heartburn"). In some cases, gastric bleeding may occur and manifest as hematemesis (vomiting bright red or coffee-ground blood), or melena (dark, "tarry" [sticky] stool, indicating occult blood caused by digestion of blood within the small intestine).

Gastritis or food poisoning caused by endotoxins, such as staphylococcal endotoxin, has an abrupt onset. Severe nausea and vomiting occur within a few hours of ingestion of the contaminated food. *In some cases, gastric hemorrhage is the presenting symptom, which is a life-threatening emergency.*

Chronic gastritis causes few symptoms unless ulceration occurs. Patients may report nausea, vomiting, or upper abdominal discomfort. Periodic epigastric **pain** may occur after a meal. Some patients have anorexia.

Esophagogastroduodenoscopy (EGD) via an endoscope with biopsy is the gold standard for diagnosing gastritis. (See Chapter 45 for a discussion of nursing care associated with this procedure.) The primary health care provider performs a biopsy to establish a definitive diagnosis of the type of gastritis. If lesions are patchy and diffuse, biopsy of several suspicious areas may be necessary to avoid misdiagnosis. A *cytologic examination* of the biopsy specimen is performed to confirm or rule out gastric cancer. Tissue samples can also be taken to detect *H. pylori infection* using *rapid urease testing,* cultures, or molecular detection (PCR DNA) (Pagana et al., 2022). The results of these tests are more reliable if the patient has discontinued taking antacids and proton pump inhibitors (PPIs) for at least a week.

Take Actions: Interventions

Patients with gastritis are not often seen in the acute care setting unless they have an exacerbation ("flare-up") of acute or chronic gastritis that results in fluid and electrolyte imbalance, bleeding, or increased **pain.** Collaborative care is directed toward supportive care for relieving the symptoms and removing or reducing the cause of discomfort.

Acute gastritis is treated symptomatically and supportively because the healing process is spontaneous, usually occurring within a few days. When the cause is removed, **pain** and discomfort usually subside. If bleeding occurs, a blood transfusion and fluid replacement may be given. Surgery, such as partial gastrectomy, pyloroplasty, and/or vagotomy, may be needed for patients with major bleeding or ulceration. (See a discussion of gastric surgery procedures in this chapter later under Gastric Cancer.)

Eliminating the causative factor(s) is the primary treatment approach for *acute* gastritis. **Nutrition** and drug therapy may also be used. Teach the patient to limit intake of any foods that cause distress, such as those that contain caffeine or high acid content (e.g., tomato products, citrus juices). Bell peppers and onions are also commonly irritating foods. Most patients seem to progress better with a bland, nonspicy diet and smaller, more frequent meals. Alcohol and tobacco should also be avoided.

The primary health care provider often prescribes drugs that block and buffer gastric acid secretions to relieve **pain.** *H2-receptor antagonists,* such as famotidine, are typically used to block gastric secretions. Sucralfate, a *mucosal barrier fortifier,* may also be prescribed. Antisecretory agents *(proton pump inhibitors [PPIs]),* such as omeprazole or pantoprazole, may be prescribed to suppress gastric acid. *Antacids* used as buffering agents include aluminum hydroxide combined with magnesium hydroxide and aluminum hydroxide combined with simethicone and magnesium hydroxide (Table 47.1). Calcium carbonate (chewable or liquid) is also a potent antacid, but can trigger gastrin release, causing rebound acid secretion.

TABLE 47.1 Common Examples of Drug Therapy

Gastritis and Peptic Ulcer Disease

Class and Common Examples	Selected Nursing Implications
Antacids	
Increase pH of gastric contents by deactivating pepsin	
Magnesium hydroxide with aluminum hydroxide	Give 2 hr after meals and at bedtime. *Hydrogen ion load is high after ingestion of foods.* Use liquid rather than tablets. *Suspensions are more effective than chewable tablets.* Do not give other drugs within 1–2 hr of antacids. *Antacids interfere with absorption of other drugs.* Assess patients for a history of chronic kidney disease. *Hypermagnesemia may result, especially in patients with poorly functioning kidneys, thus causing toxicity.* Assess the patient for a history of heart failure. *Inadequate renal perfusion from heart failure decreases the ability of the kidneys to excrete magnesium, thus causing toxicity.* Observe the patient for the side effect of diarrhea. *Magnesium may cause diarrhea.*
Aluminum hydroxide	Give 1 hr after meals and at bedtime. *Hydrogen ion load is high after ingestion of food.* Use liquid rather than tablets if palatable. *Suspensions are more effective than chewable tablets.* Do not give other drugs within 1–2 hr of antacids. *Antacids interfere with absorption of other drugs.* Observe patients for the side effect of constipation. If constipation occurs, consider alternating with magnesium antacid. *Aluminum causes constipation, and magnesium has a laxative effect.* Use for patients with chronic kidney disease. *Aluminum binds with phosphates in the GI tract. This antacid does not contain magnesium.*
H2 Antagonists (Blockers)	
Decrease gastric acid secretions by blocking histamine receptors in parietal cells	
Famotidine Nizatidine **NOTE:** IV famotidine may also be given to prevent surgical stress ulcers.	Give single dose at bedtime for treatment of heartburn and PUD. *Bedtime administration suppresses nocturnal acid production.*
Mucosal Barrier Fortifiers	
Protect stomach mucosa	
Sucralfate	Give 1 hr before and 2 hr after meals and at bedtime. *Food may interfere with drug's adherence to mucosa.* Do not give within 30 min of giving antacids or other drugs. *Antacids may interfere with effect.*
Bismuth subsalicylate	Remind patient to refrain from taking aspirin while on this drug. *Aspirin is a salicylic acid and can lead to overdose.*

Continued

TABLE 47.1   Common Examples of Drug Therapy—cont'd

Gastritis and Peptic Ulcer Disease

Class and Common Examples	Selected Nursing Implications
Proton Pump Inhibitors	
Suppress HK–ATPase enzyme system of gastric acid secretion to suppress acid	
Omeprazole	Have patients take capsule whole; do not crush. *Delayed-release capsules allow absorption after granules leave the stomach.* Give 30 min before the main meal of the day. *The drug needs a chance to work before the patient eats, as the proton pump is activated by the presence of food.*
Lansoprazole	Give 30 min before the main meal of the day. *The drug needs a chance to work before the patient eats, as the proton pump is activated by the presence of food.*
Rabeprazole	Give after the morning meal. *This drug promotes healing and symptom relief of duodenal ulcers.* Do not crush capsule. *This drug is a sustained-release capsule.*
Pantoprazole	Do not crush. This drug is enteric coated. IV form must be given on a pump with a filter and in a separate line. *Given IV, this drug precipitates easily.* Do not give IV pantoprazole with other IV drugs. *The IV form is not compatible with most other drugs.* Monitor for adverse drug interactions if patient is on other medications. *This drug will alter how other drugs are metabolized, either increasing or decreasing their effectiveness.*
Esomeprazole	Assess for hepatic impairment. *Patients with severe hepatic problems need a low dose.* Do not give esomeprazole IV with other IV drugs. *The IV form is not compatible with most other drugs.* Monitor for adverse drug interactions if patient is on other medications. *This drug will alter how other drugs are metabolized, either increasing or decreasing the effectiveness.*
Prostaglandin Analogs	
Stimulate mucosal protection and decrease gastric acid secretions	
Misoprostol	Not commonly given but used for patients receiving NSAIDs to *protect the stomach mucosa.* Avoid magnesium-containing antacids. *Misoprostol and magnesium-containing antacids can cause diarrhea.* Do not administer to pregnant women. *This drug can cause abortion, premature birth, or birth defects.*
Antimicrobials	
Treat *H. pylori* infection	
Clarithromycin	Give with caution to patients with renal impairment; monitor renal function laboratory values. *This drug can increase the patient's BUN level and should be monitored.*
Amoxicillin	Teach patients to take the drug with food or immediately after a meal. *This drug can cause GI disturbances, including nausea, vomiting, and diarrhea.*
Tetracycline	Teach patients to take the drug at least 1 hr before meals or 2 hr after meals. *Dairy products and other foods may interfere with drug absorption.* Teach patients to avoid direct sunlight and wear sunscreen when outdoors. *This drug can cause the skin to burn as a result of photosensitivity.*
Metronidazole	Teach patients to take the drug with food. *This drug can cause GI disturbances, especially nausea.* Teach patients to avoid alcohol during drug therapy and for at least 3 days after therapy is completed. *The patient can experience a drug-alcohol reaction, including severe nausea, vomiting, and headache.*

BUN, Blood urea nitrogen; *PUD*, peptic ulcer disease.

Treatment of *chronic* gastritis varies with the cause. The approach to management includes the elimination of causative agents, treatment of any underlying disease (e.g., chronic kidney disease, Crohn's disease), avoidance of toxic substances (e.g., alcohol, tobacco), and health teaching.

Patients with *chronic* gastritis may have decreased absorption of vitamin B_{12} and sometimes require vitamin B_{12} injections for prevention or treatment of pernicious anemia. If *H. pylori* is present, the primary health care provider treats the **infection.** Current practice for infection treatment is described in the Drug Therapy discussion in the Peptic Ulcer Disease section.

✴ INFECTION CONCEPT EXEMPLAR: PEPTIC ULCER DISEASE (PUD)

Peptic ulcer disease (PUD) results when GI mucosal defenses become impaired and no longer protect the epithelium from the effects of acid and pepsin.

Pathophysiology Review

Many peptic ulcers are caused by *H. pylori* **infection.** The most common route of *H. pylori* infection transmission is either oral-to-oral (stomach contents are transmitted from mouth to mouth) or fecal-to-oral (from stool to mouth) contact.

As a response to the bacteria, cytokines, neutrophils, and other substances are activated and cause epithelial cell necrosis. Urease produced by *H. pylori* breaks down urea into ammonia, which neutralizes the acidity of the stomach. Additionally, the helical shape of *H. pylori* allows the bacterium to burrow into the mucous layer of the stomach and become undetectable by the body's immune cells. Although this bacterium does not cause illness in most people, it is a major risk factor for peptic ulcers and gastric cancer (Rogers, 2023).

Types of Ulcers

Three types of peptic ulcers may occur: duodenal ulcers, gastric ulcers, and stress ulcers (less common). *Duodenal ulcers* occur more often than other types. Most duodenal ulcers present in the upper portion of the duodenum. These ulcers are deep, sharply demarcated lesions that penetrate through the mucosa and submucosa into the muscularis propria (muscle layer). The floor of the ulcer consists of a necrotic area residing on granulation tissue and surrounded by areas of fibrosis (Rogers, 2023) (Fig. 47.1).

The main feature of a duodenal ulcer is high gastric acid secretion, although a wide range of secretory levels is found. Patients with duodenal ulcers have low pH levels (excess acid) in the duodenum for long periods. Protein-rich meals, calcium, and vagus nerve excitation stimulate acid secretion. Combined with hypersecretion, a rapid emptying of food from the stomach reduces the buffering effect of food and delivers a large acid bolus to the duodenum. Inhibitory secretory mechanisms and pancreatic secretion may be insufficient to control the acid load.

Gastric ulcers usually develop in the antrum of the stomach near acid-secreting mucosa (see Fig. 47.1). When a break in the mucosal barrier occurs (such as that caused by *H. pylori* **infection**), hydrochloric acid injures the epithelium. Gastric ulcers

may then result from back-diffusion of acid or dysfunction of the pyloric sphincter. When the pyloric sphincter does not function normally, bile refluxes (backs up) into the stomach. This reflux of bile acids may break the integrity of the mucosal barrier, which leads to mucosal **inflammation.** Toxic agents and bile then destroy the membrane of the gastric mucosa.

Gastric emptying is often delayed in patients with gastric ulceration. This causes regurgitation of duodenal contents, which worsens the gastric mucosal injury. Decreased blood flow to the gastric mucosa may also alter the defense barrier and thereby allow ulceration to occur.

Stress ulcers are acute gastric mucosal lesions occurring after an acute medical crisis or trauma, such as sepsis or a head injury. In the patient who is NPO for major surgery, gastritis may lead to stress ulcers. Patients who are critically ill, especially those with extensive burns (Curling ulcer), sepsis (ischemic ulcer), or increased intracranial pressure (Cushing ulcer), are also susceptible to these ulcers. Stress ulcers are associated with lengthened hospital stay and increased mortality rates.

Bleeding caused by gastric erosion is the main manifestation of acute stress ulcers. Multifocal lesions associated with stress ulcers occur in the stomach and proximal duodenum. These lesions begin as areas of ischemia and evolve into erosions and ulcerations that may progress to massive hemorrhage.

Complications of Ulcers

The most common complications of PUD are hemorrhage, perforation, pyloric obstruction, and intractable disease. *Hemorrhage is the most serious complication.* It tends to occur more often in patients with *gastric* and stress ulcers, and in older adults. Many patients have a second episode of bleeding if underlying **infection** with *H. pylori* remains untreated or if therapy does not include an H₂ antagonist or PPI. With massive bleeding the patient vomits bright red or coffee-ground blood (hematemesis). Gastric acid digestion of blood typically results in the coffee-ground appearance. Hematemesis usually indicates bleeding at or above the duodenojejunal junction (upper GI bleeding). Other signs and symptoms are listed in Box 47.2.

Minimal bleeding from ulcers manifests with occult blood in a dark, "tarry" stool (melena). Melena may occur in patients with gastric ulcers but is more common in those with duodenal ulcers.

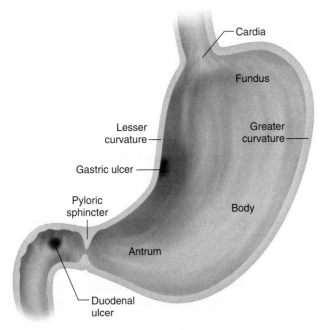

FIG. 47.1 Most common sites for peptic ulcers.

> ### BOX 47.2 Key Features
> #### *Upper GI Bleeding*
>
> - Bright red or coffee-ground vomitus (hematemesis)
> - Melena (tarry or dark, sticky stools)
> - Decreased hemoglobin and hematocrit
> - Decreased blood pressure
> - Increased heart rate
> - Weak peripheral pulses
> - Acute confusion (in older adults)
> - Vertigo
> - Dizziness or light-headedness
> - Syncope (loss of consciousness)

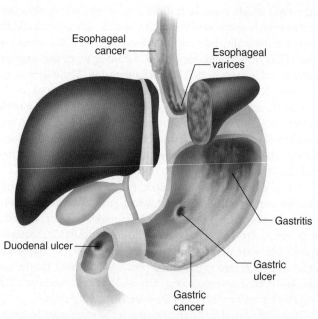

FIG. 47.2 Common causes of upper GI bleeding.

Gastric and duodenal ulcers can perforate and bleed (Fig. 47.2). Although not common, *perforation* occurs when the ulcer becomes so deep that the entire thickness of the stomach or duodenum is worn away. The stomach or duodenal contents can then leak into the peritoneal cavity. Sudden, sharp *pain* begins in the midepigastric region and spreads over the entire abdomen. The amount of pain correlates with the amount and type of GI contents spilled. The classic pain causes the patient to be apprehensive. The abdomen is tender, rigid, and boardlike as a result of this **infection** (**peritonitis**). The patient often assumes a "fetal" position to decrease the tension on the abdominal muscles. Patients can become severely ill within hours. Bacterial septicemia and hypovolemic shock can follow. Peristalsis diminishes and paralytic ileus can develop. *Peptic ulcer perforation is a surgical emergency and can be life-threatening!*

NCLEX Examination Challenge 47.1
Safe and Effective Care Environment

The nurse is caring for a client diagnosed with peptic ulcer disease (PUD). What would be the **priority** action for the nurse?
A. Irrigate the nasogastric tube (NGT) as needed.
B. Monitor vital signs frequently.
C. Provide supplemental oxygen.
D. Monitor bowel sounds.

Pyloric (gastric outlet) obstruction (blockage) occurs in a small percentage of patients and manifests with vomiting caused by stasis and gastric dilation. Obstruction occurs at the pylorus (the gastric outlet) and is caused by scarring, edema, inflammation, or a combination of these factors. Symptoms of obstruction include abdominal bloating, nausea, and vomiting. When vomiting persists, the patient may develop *metabolic alkalosis* from loss of large quantities of acid gastric juice (hydrogen and chloride ions) in the vomitus. *Hypokalemia* may also result from the vomiting or metabolic alkalosis.

Many patients with ulcers have a single episode with no recurrence. However, *intractability* may develop from complications of ulcers, excessive stressors in the patient's life, or an inability to adhere to long-term therapy. They no longer respond to conservative management, or recurrences of symptoms interfere with ADLs. In general, the patient continues to have recurrent **pain** despite treatment. Those who fail to respond to traditional treatments or who have a relapse after discontinuation of therapy are referred to a gastroenterology specialist.

Etiology and Genetic Risk

Peptic ulcer disease is caused most often by bacterial **infection** with *H. pylori* and long-term use of NSAIDs such as ibuprofen. NSAIDs break down the mucosal barrier and disrupt the mucosal protection mediated systemically by cyclooxygenase (COX) inhibition. Other risk factors for PUD are the same as for gastritis (see discussion earlier in this chapter). Patients with duodenal ulcers often have a positive family history of the disease.

Incidence and Prevalence

PUD affects about 4.5 million people in the United States annually (Anand & Katz, 2021). Primary health care provider visits, hospitalizations, and the mortality rate for PUD have decreased in the past few decades, in part because of the use of proton pump inhibitors and early detection and treatment of *H. pylori*.

Interprofessional Collaborative Care

Care of the patient with PUD generally takes place in the community setting, unless the patient develops a more serious condition such as upper GI bleeding, which requires acute management.

Recognize Cues: Assessment

History. A history of current or past medical conditions focuses on GI problems, particularly any history of diagnosis or treatment for *H. pylori* **infection.** Review all prescription and over-the-counter (OTC) drugs the patient is taking. Specifically inquire whether the patient is taking corticosteroids, chemotherapy, or NSAIDs. Also ask whether the patient has ever undergone radiation treatments. Assess whether the patient has had any GI surgeries, especially a partial gastrectomy or bariatric surgery, which can cause chronic gastritis.

Collect data related to the causes and risk factors for peptic ulcer disease (PUD). Question the patient about factors that can influence the development of PUD, including alcohol intake and tobacco use. Note whether certain foods such as tomatoes or caffeinated beverages precipitate or worsen symptoms. Information regarding actual or perceived daily stressors should also be obtained.

History and patterns of GI upset and pain are important to note, along with their relationship to eating and sleep patterns. Interventions and actions taken to relieve pain can also be significant. Inquire about any changes in the character of the pain because this may signal the development of complications.

For example, if *pain* that was once intermittent and relieved by food and antacids becomes constant and radiates to the back or upper quadrant, the patient may have ulcer perforation. However, many adults with active duodenal or gastric ulcers report having no ulcer symptoms.

Physical Assessment/Signs and Symptoms. Physical assessment findings may reveal epigastric tenderness and *pain*, usually located at the midline between the umbilicus and the xiphoid process. *If perforation into the peritoneal cavity is present, the patient typically has a rigid, boardlike abdomen accompanied by rebound tenderness and intense pain (peritonitis).* Initially, auscultation of the abdomen may reveal hyperactive bowel sounds, but these may diminish with progression of the *infection.* Perform a comprehensive pain assessment.

Dyspepsia is the most reported symptom associated with PUD. It is typically described as sharp, burning, or gnawing pain. Some patients may perceive discomfort as a sensation of abdominal pressure or of fullness or hunger. Specific differences between gastric and duodenal ulcers are listed in Table 47.2 (Rogers, 2023).

Document orthostatic blood pressures and monitor for signs and symptoms of dehydration to assess for fluid volume deficit that may occur from a bleeding ulcer. Dizziness when in an upright position is a specific symptom a patient with fluid volume deficit may experience. *Older adults may experience dizziness when they get out of bed and are at risk for falls.*

Psychosocial Assessment. Assess the impact of ulcer disease on the patient's lifestyle, occupation, family, and social and leisure activities. Evaluate the impact that lifestyle changes will have on the patient and family. This assessment may reveal information about the patient's ability to adhere to the prescribed treatment regimen and obtain the needed social support to make changes in lifestyle.

Laboratory Assessment. Three simple, noninvasive tests are available to detect *H. pylori* in the patient's blood, breath, or stool. Although the breath and stool tests are considered more accurate, *serologic testing* for *H. pylori* antibodies is the most common method to confirm *H. pylori* infection. The *urea breath test* involves swallowing a capsule, liquid, or pudding that contains radioactive carbon urea (^{13}C urea). After a few minutes the patient exhales; if the radioactive carbon is found, the bacterium is present. The *stool antigen test* is performed on a stool sample provided by the patient, which is tested for *H. pylori* antigens. Patients who have bleeding from a peptic ulcer may have *decreased hemoglobin and hematocrit* values. The *stool* may also be positive for occult (microscopic) blood if bleeding is present (Pagana et al., 2022).

Other Diagnostic Assessment. The most accurate diagnostic test for establishing the diagnosis of PUD is an esophagogastroduodenoscopy (EGD). Direct visualization of the ulcer crater by EGD allows the primary health care provider to take specimens for *H. pylori* testing and biopsy and cytologic studies for ruling out gastric cancer. The *rapid urease test* is used to quickly confirm the diagnosis, because urease is produced by the bacteria in the gastric mucosa. EGD may be repeated at 4- to 6-week intervals while the primary health care provider evaluates the progress of healing in response to therapy (Pagana et al., 2022). Chapter 45 describes this procedure in more detail.

GI bleeding may be confirmed using a *nuclear medicine scan.* No special preparation is required for this scan. The patient is injected with a contrast medium (usually technetium [^{99m}Tc]), and the GI system is scanned for the presence of bleeding after a waiting period. A second scan may be done 1 to 2 days after treatment for the bleeding to determine if the interventions were effective.

Analyze Cues and Prioritize Hypotheses: Analysis

The priority collaborative problems for patients with peptic ulcer disease (PUD) include:

- Acute or persistent **pain** due to gastric and/or duodenal ulceration
- Potential for upper GI bleeding due to gastric and/or duodenal ulceration or perforation

TABLE 47.2 Differential Features of Gastric and Duodenal Ulcers

Feature	Gastric Ulcer	Duodenal Ulcer
Age	50–70 yr	20–50 yr
Gender	Affects males and females equally	Affects males more often
Blood group	No differentiation	Most often type O
Stomach acid production	Normal secretion or hyposecretion	Hypersecretion
Occurrence	Mucosa exposed to acid-pepsin secretion	Mucosa exposed to acid-pepsin secretion; positive family history
Upper abdominal pain	Occurs 30–60 min after a meal; at night, rarely worsened by ingestion of food	Occurs 1½–3 hr after a meal; at night often awakens patient between 1 and 2 a.m. Relieved by ingestion of food
Response to treatment	Healing with appropriate therapy	Remissions and exacerbations
Hemorrhage	Hematemesis more common than melena	Melena more common than hematemesis
Cancer risk	Increased, but in less than 5%	Not increased
Recurrence	Tends to heal and recurs often in the same location	60% recur within 1 yr; 90% recur within 2 yr
Surrounding mucosa	Atrophic gastritis	No gastritis

Generate Solutions and Take Actions: Planning and Implementation

Managing Acute or Persistent Pain

Planning: Expected Outcomes. The patient with PUD is expected to report **pain** control as evidenced by no more than a 3 on a 0-to-10 pain intensity scale.

Interventions. PUD causes significant discomfort that impacts many aspects of daily living. Interventions to manage **pain** focus on drug therapy and dietary changes.

Drug Therapy. The primary purposes of drug therapy in the treatment of PUD are to (1) provide **pain** relief, (2) eliminate *H. pylori* **infection,** (3) heal ulcerations, and (4) prevent recurrence. Several regimens may be used. Although numerous drugs have been evaluated for the treatment of *H. pylori* infection, no single agent has successfully eradicated organism. A common drug regimen for *H. pylori* infection is PPI-based triple therapy, which includes a proton pump inhibitor (PPI), such as lansoprazole, plus two antibiotics such as metronidazole and tetracycline or clarithromycin and amoxicillin for 10 to 14 days. Some primary health care providers may prefer to use quadruple therapy, which contains a combination of a proton pump inhibitor (PPI), any two commonly used antibiotics as described previously, and the addition of bismuth. Bismuth therapy is often used in patients who are allergic to penicillin-based medications (Burchum & Rosenthal, 2022).

Bismuth subsalicylate inhibits *H. pylori* from binding to the mucosal lining and stimulates mucosal protection and prostaglandin production. Teach patients that they cannot take aspirin while on this drug because aspirin is a salicylic acid and could cause an overdose of salicylates. Patients should also be taught that bismuth may cause the stools and/or tongue to be discolored black. This discoloration is temporary and harmless.

👤 PATIENT-CENTERED CARE: OLDER ADULT HEALTH

Need for H. pylori *Screening*

> Many older adults have *H. pylori infection* that is undiagnosed because of vague symptoms associated with physiologic changes of aging and comorbidities that mask dyspepsia. Because the average age of gastric cancer diagnosis is 68 years, it is important to teach older adults about the symptoms of PUD and to consider *H. pylori* screening (American Cancer Society, 2023b). Early detection and aggressive treatment can prevent PUD and gastric cancer.

Hyposecretory drugs reduce gastric acid secretions and are therefore used for both peptic ulcer disease (PUD) and gastritis management. The primary prescribed drugs include proton pump inhibitors and H_2-receptor antagonists (see Table 47.1).

A *proton pump inhibitor (PPI) is the drug class of choice for treating patients with acid-related disorders.* Omeprazole, lansoprazole, dexlansoprazole, and esomeprazole are each available as delayed-release preparations designed to release their contents after they pass through the stomach. Omeprazole, lansoprazole, and dexlansoprazole may be dissolved in a sodium bicarbonate solution and given through any feeding tube. Bicarbonate protects the dissolved medication granules in gastric acid. This allows the drugs to be absorbed correctly. These capsules can

also be opened. The enteric-coated capsules can be put into apple juice or orange juice and given through a large-bore feeding tube. Esomeprazole, omeprazole, and pantoprazole are also available in oral suspension for feeding tube administration. Rabeprazole and pantoprazole are enteric-coated tablets that quickly dissolve after the tablet has moved through the stomach and should not be crushed before they are taken. Several of the PPIs, such as esomeprazole and pantoprazole, are also available in an IV form, which is useful for patients who are NPO (Burchum & Rosenthal, 2022).

Long-term use of PPIs has become more prevalent over the past two decades. This practice does not come without risks. Patients on PPIs should be assessed periodically to determine the necessity of PPI use. Recent studies have suggested there may be an increased risk of osteoporotic fractures related to long-term PPI use. PPIs should not be discontinued abruptly, to prevent rebound activation of the proton pump; a step-down approach over several days is recommended (Burchum & Rosenthal, 2022).

Nutrition Therapy. The role of diet in the management of ulcer disease is controversial. There is no evidence that dietary restriction reduces gastric acid secretion or promotes tissue healing, although a bland diet may assist in relieving symptoms. Food itself acts as an antacid by neutralizing gastric acid for 30 to 60 minutes. An increased rate of gastric acid secretion, called *rebound,* may follow.

Teach the patient to exclude any foods that cause discomfort. A bland, nonirritating diet is recommended during the acute symptomatic phase. Bedtime snacks are avoided because they may stimulate gastric acid secretion. Eating six smaller meals daily may help, but this regimen is no longer a regular part of therapy. No evidence supports the theory that eating six meals daily promotes healing of the ulcer. This practice may stimulate gastric acid secretion. Patients should avoid alcohol and tobacco because of their stimulatory effects on gastric acid secretion (Rogers, 2023).

Complementary and Integrative Health. Teach patients about complementary and integrative therapies that can reduce stress, including hypnosis and imagery. For example, the use of yoga and meditation techniques has demonstrated anxiety-reducing benefits. Many have suggested that GI disorders result from the dysfunction of both the GI tract itself and the brain. This means that emotional stress is thought to worsen GI disorders such as peptic ulcer disease (Page & Li, 2021). Yoga and meditation may alter the activities of the central and autonomic nervous systems. Herbs and other supplements may be used by some patients as discussed earlier in this chapter under Gastritis.

Managing Upper GI Bleeding

Planning: Expected Outcomes. The patient with upper GI bleeding (often called *upper GI hemorrhage, or UGH*) is expected to have bleeding promptly and effectively controlled and vital signs within normal limits.

Interventions. Blood loss from PUD results in high morbidity and mortality. Fluid volume loss secondary to vomiting can lead to dehydration and electrolyte imbalances. Interventions aimed at managing complications associated with PUD include prevention and/or management of bleeding, perforation, and gastric outlet obstruction. In some cases, surgical treatment of complications is necessary.

Nonsurgical Management. Because prevention or early detection of complications is needed to obtain a positive clinical outcome, monitor the patient carefully and immediately report changes to the primary health care provider.

Emergency: Upper GI Bleeding. The patient who is actively bleeding has a life-threatening emergency and needs supportive therapy to prevent hypovolemic shock and possible death (Pezzotti, 2020).

✚ NURSING SAFETY PRIORITY

Critical Rescue

> *Recognize that priority for care of the patient with upper GI bleeding is to maintain **a**irway, **b**reathing, and **c**irculation (ABCs). Respond to these needs by providing oxygen and other ventilatory support as needed, starting two large-bore IV lines for replacing fluids and blood, as well as monitoring vital signs, hematocrit, and oxygen saturation (Pezzotti, 2020).*

The purpose of managing hypovolemia is to expand intravascular fluid in a patient who is volume depleted. Carefully monitor the patient's fluid status, including intake and output. *Fluid replacement in older adults should be closely monitored to prevent fluid overload.* Serum electrolytes are also assessed because depletions from vomiting or nasogastric suctioning must be replaced. Volume replacement with isotonic solutions (e.g., 0.9% normal saline [NS] solution, lactated Ringer's solution) should be started immediately. The primary health care provider may prescribe blood products such as packed red blood cells (PRBCs) to expand volume and correct a low hemoglobin and hematocrit. For patients with active bleeding, fresh frozen plasma may be given if the prothrombin time is 1.5 times higher than the midrange control value (Pezzotti, 2020).

Continue to monitor the patient's hematocrit, hemoglobin, and coagulation studies for changes from the baseline measurements. With mild bleeding (less than 500 mL), slight feelings of weakness and mild perspiration may be present. When blood loss exceeds 1 L/24 hour, manifestations of hypovolemic shock may occur, including hypotension, chills, palpitations, diaphoresis, and a weak, thready pulse (see Chapter 31 for management of shock).

A combination of several different treatments, including nasogastric tube (NGT) placement, endoscopic therapy, interventional radiologic procedures, and acid suppression, can be used to control acute bleeding and prevent rebleeding. If the patient is actively bleeding at home, the patient will require hospital-based care. After the bleeding has stopped, proton pump inhibitors are the primary drugs utilized to aid ulcer healing (Pezzotti, 2020).

Nasogastric tube (NGT) placement. Upper GI bleeding or obstruction often requires the primary health care provider or nurse to insert a large-bore NGT to:

- Determine the presence or absence of blood in the stomach
- Assess the rate of bleeding
- Prevent gastric dilation
- Decompress to rest the GI system

Treatment of pyloric obstruction is directed toward restoring fluid and electrolyte balance and decompressing the dilated stomach. Obstruction related to edema and spasm generally responds to medical therapy. First, the stomach must be decompressed with nasogastric suction. Next, interventions are directed at correcting metabolic alkalosis and dehydration. The NGT is typically clamped after about 72 hours. Check the patient for retention of gastric contents. If the amount retained is not more than 50 mL in 30 minutes (or another prescribed parameter), the primary health care provider may allow oral fluids. In some cases, surgical intervention may be required to treat PUD.

Endoscopic therapy. Endoscopic therapy via an esophagogastroduodenoscopy (EGD) can assist in achieving homeostasis during an acute hemorrhage by isolating the bleeding artery to embolize (clot) it. During the EGD the health care provider will insert instruments through the endoscope to stop bleeding in three different ways: (1) inject chemicals into the bleeding site; (2) treat the bleeding area with heat, electric current, or laser; or (3) close the affected blood vessels with a band or clip (Pagana et al., 2022). During the EGD, a specialized endoscopy nurse and technician assist with the procedure.

Pre-EGD nursing care involves inserting one or two large-bore IV catheters if not already in place. A large catheter allows the patient to receive IV moderate sedation (e.g., midazolam [Versed] and an opioid) and possibly a blood transfusion. Keep the patient NPO for 4 to 6 hours before the procedure. This prevents the risk for aspiration and allows the endoscopist to view and treat the ulcer. A patient must sign a consent form for the EGD *after* the primary health care provider advises and educates the patient about the procedure.

❗ NURSING SAFETY PRIORITY

Action Alert

> After esophagogastroduodenoscopy (EGD), monitor vital signs, heart rhythm, and oxygen saturation frequently per agency protocol until the patient returns to baseline. In addition, frequently assess the patient's ability to swallow saliva. The patient's gag reflex may initially be absent after EGD because of anesthetizing (numbing) of the throat with a spray before the procedure. *After the procedure, do not allow the patient to have food or liquids until the gag reflex has returned!*

Endoscopic therapy is helpful for most patients with active bleeding. However, ulcers that continue to bleed or continue to rebleed despite endoscopic therapy may require an interventional radiologic procedure or surgical repair.

Interventional radiologic procedures. For patients with persistent, massive upper GI bleeding or those who are not surgical candidates, catheter-directed embolization may be performed. This endovascular procedure is usually done if endoscopic procedures are not successful or available. A femoral approach is most often used, but brachial access may be used. An arteriogram is performed to identify the arterial anatomy and find the exact location of the bleeding. The radiologist injects medication or other material into the blood vessels to stop the bleeding (Morgan et al., 2021). Nursing care of the patient following an arteriogram is similar to care following a percutaneous vascular intervention, which is described in Chapter 30.

Drug therapy. Aggressive acid suppression is used to prevent rebleeding. When acute bleeding is stopped and clot formation has taken place within the ulcer crater, the clot remains in contact with gastric contents. Acid-suppressive agents are used to stabilize the clot by raising the pH level of gastric contents. Typically, proton pump inhibitors are the drug of choice. These drugs prevent the transport of acid across the parietal cell membrane (Burchum & Rosenthal, 2022).

NCLEX Examination Challenge 47.2
Physiological Integrity

The nurse is caring for a client who just had an endoscopic procedure to treat GI bleeding resulting from a gastric peptic ulcer. Which action would be the **priority** for the nurse to take at this time?

A. Assess the client's gag reflex before offering any ice chips or fluids, if allowed.
B. Place the client in a flat supine position to maintain adequate blood pressure.
C. Monitor the client for a rigid, boardlike abdomen, which could indicate peritonitis.
D. Type and crossmatch at least 2 units of packed red blood cells in case of bleeding.

Surgical Management. Evidence-based guidelines for the treatment of PUD that include *H. pylori* treatment and the development of nonsurgical means of controlling bleeding have led to a decline in the need for surgical intervention. For some patients who have PUD, surgical intervention may be used to:

- Treat patients who do not respond to medical therapy or other nonsurgical procedures
- Treat a surgical emergency that develops as a complication of PUD, such as perforation

Two general surgical approaches are available for PUD: minimally invasive surgery and conventional open surgery. *Minimally invasive surgery (MIS)* via laparoscopy may be used to remove a chronic gastric ulcer or treat hemorrhage from perforation. Several small incisions allow access to the stomach and duodenum. The patient may have partial stomach removal (subtotal gastrectomy), pyloroplasty (to open the pylorus), and/or a vagotomy (vagus nerve cutting) to control acid secretion. Acid-reduction surgery may not be necessary because of the increased use of PPIs and endoscopic procedures in the treatment of PUD. The advantages of MIS over traditional open surgical procedures include a shorter hospital stay, fewer complications, less pain, and a quicker recovery (Pansa et al., 2020). Care of patients having gastric surgery is discussed later in this chapter under Gastric Cancer.

Care Coordination and Transition Management

Patients may be discharged from the hospital if there is no evidence of ongoing bleeding, orthostatic changes, or cardiopulmonary distress or compromise. Those discharged after treatment for peptic ulcer disease (PUD) and/or complications secondary to the disease face several challenges to manage the disease successfully. Long-term adherence to drug therapy may require the patient to take several drugs each day. Permanent lifestyle alterations in *nutrition* habits must also be made.

Home Care Management. Most patients are discharged to home to continue their recovery. Those who have had major surgery or complications, such as hemorrhage, may require one or two visits from a home care nurse to assess clinical progress, especially if the patient is an older adult (Box 47.3).

Self-Management Education. The primary focus of home care preparation is patient and family teaching regarding risk factors

BOX 47.3   Home Health Care
The Patient With Peptic Ulcer Disease

Assess gastrointestinal and cardiovascular status, including:
- Vital signs, including orthostatic vital signs
- Skin color
- Presence of abdominal pain (location, severity, character, duration, precipitating factors, and relief measures)
- Character, color, and consistency of stools
- Changes in bowel elimination pattern
- Hemoglobin and hematocrit
- Bowel sounds; palpate for areas of tenderness

Assess nutritional status, including:
- Dietary patterns and habits
- Intake of caffeine and alcohol
- Relationship of food ingestion to symptoms

Assess the patient's understanding of illness and ability to adhere to the therapeutic regimen:
- Symptoms to report to the primary health care provider
- Expected effects and side effects of medications
- Drugs to avoid, such as NSAIDs
- Need for smoking cessation, if applicable

for the recurrence of PUD. Teach patients and families how to recognize new complications and what to do if they occur.

Help the patient plan ways to make needed lifestyle changes. For postsurgical patients, especially those who have undergone partial stomach removal, smaller meals may be required. Other postoperative *nutrition* changes are described in the Self-Management Education discussion in the Gastric Cancer section.

! NURSING SAFETY PRIORITY
Action Alert

Teach the patient who has peptic ulcer disease to seek immediate medical attention if experiencing any of these symptoms:
- Sharp, sudden, persistent, and severe epigastric or abdominal pain
- Bloody or black stools
- Bloody vomit or vomit that looks like coffee grounds

Health Care Resources. If needed, refer the patient and family to the National Institute of Diabetes and Digestive and Kidney Diseases Health Information Center (https://www.niddk.nih.gov/health-information/digestive-diseases /) in the United States or to the Canadian Digestive Health Foundation (https://cdhf.ca/). These groups provide information and support to patients who have digestive disorders.

Evaluate Outcomes: Evaluation

Evaluate the care of the patient with peptic ulcer disease (PUD) based on the identified priority patient problems. The expected outcomes are that the patient:

- Does not have active PUD or *H. pylori* **infection**
- Verbalizes relief or control of **pain**
- Adheres to the drug regimen and lifestyle changes to prevent recurrence and heal the ulcer
- Does not experience upper GI bleeding; if bleeding occurs, it will be promptly and effectively managed

GASTRIC CANCER

Most cancers of the stomach are adenocarcinomas. This type of cancer develops in the mucosal cells that form the innermost lining of any portion or all of the stomach. In general, gastric cancer is more common in males than in females, and there is a sharp increase in adults over 65 years of age (American Cancer Society, 2023b). Often there are no symptoms in the early stages and the disease is advanced when diagnosed.

Pathophysiology Review

Gastric cancer usually begins in the glands of the stomach mucosa. Atrophic gastritis and intestinal metaplasia (abnormal tissue development) are precancerous conditions. Inadequate acid secretion in patients with atrophic gastritis creates an alkaline environment that allows bacteria (especially *H. pylori*) to multiply. This *infection* causes mucosa-associated lymphoid tissue (MALT) lymphoma, which starts in the stomach (Rogers, 2023).

Gastric cancers occur in either the upper portion of the stomach (cardia) or lower portion of the stomach (noncardia). In either location, they typically spread by direct extension through the gastric wall and into regional lymphatics, which carry tumor deposits to lymph nodes. Direct invasion of and adherence to adjacent organs (e.g., the liver, pancreas, and transverse colon) may also result. Hematogenous spread via the portal vein to the liver and via the systemic circulation to the lungs and bones is the most common mode of metastasis. Peritoneal seeding of cancer cells from the tumor areas to the omentum, peritoneum, ovary, and pelvic cul-de-sac can also occur.

In adults with *advanced* gastric cancer, there is invasion of the muscularis (stomach muscle) or beyond. These lesions are not cured by surgical resection. The overall 5-year survival rate of adults with stomach cancer in the United States is around 30% because most patients have no symptoms until the disease advances. If detected early, the 5-year survival rate is closer to 70% (American Cancer Society, 2023c).

Infection with *H. pylori* is the largest risk factor for gastric cancer because it carries the cytotoxin-associated gene A (*CagA*) gene. Patients with pernicious anemia, gastric polyps, chronic atrophic gastritis, and achlorhydria (absence of secretion of hydrochloric acid) are two to three times more likely to develop gastric cancer.

PATIENT-CENTERED CARE: HEALTH EQUITY

Gastric Cancer

All non-White groups, especially Blacks and Hispanics, have a higher incidence and mortality rate associated with noncardia gastric adenocarcinoma when compared with White groups; Korean and Japanese Americans have the highest incidence and mortality (Shah et al., 2020). A number of factors or social determinants of health may help explain these differences, including a higher percentage of non-White groups who smoke and have *H. pylori* that is not treated due to possible lack of health care access, poverty, and lack of guidelines for gastric cancer screening. Additionally, White groups are more likely than non-White groups to have chemotherapy prior to surgery for cancerous lesions, possibly due to lack of health care access or health care insurance (Shah et al., 2020).

The disease also seems to be positively correlated with eating excessive pickled foods, nitrates from processed foods, and salt added to food. The ingestion of these foods over a long period can lead to atrophic gastritis, a precancerous condition. A low intake of fruits and vegetables is also a risk factor for cancer (Rogers, 2023). Some patients may have food insecurity, owing to lack of finances, or may be unaware of the correlation between cancer and a lack of fruits and vegetables in the diet. Be sure to teach patients about the need for a healthy diet, and provide information regarding community food resources for those who are experiencing food insecurity.

Gastric surgery is also linked to an increased risk for gastric cancer because of the possible development of atrophic gastritis, which results in changes to the mucosa (Castagneto-Gissey et al., 2020). Patients with Barrett's esophagus from prolonged or severe gastroesophageal reflux disease (GERD) have an increased risk for cancer in the cardia (at the point where the stomach connects to the esophagus). Chapter 46 discusses GERD and esophageal cancer in detail.

Interprofessional Collaborative Care

Care of the patient with gastric cancer takes place in all settings, ranging from the home and community environment to the inpatient setting, including hospice, depending on the stage of disease and the outcomes of treatment.

Recognize Cues: Assessment

Although patients with *early* gastric cancer may be asymptomatic, dyspepsia and abdominal discomfort are the *most* common symptoms. However, these symptoms are often ignored, or a change in diet or use of antacids relieves them. As the tumor grows, these symptoms become more severe and do not respond to *nutrition* changes or drug therapy (Box 47.4).

In patients with advanced disease, anemia is evidenced by *low hematocrit* and hemoglobin values. Patients may have macrocytic or microcytic anemia associated with decreased iron or vitamin B_{12} absorption. *The stool may be positive for occult blood. Hypoalbuminemia* and *abnormal results of liver tests* (e.g., bilirubin and alkaline phosphatase) occur with advanced disease and hepatic metastasis. The level of carcinoembryonic antigen (CEA) is elevated in advanced cancer of the stomach (Pagana et al., 2022).

The primary health care provider uses esophagogastroduodenoscopy (EGD) with biopsy for definitive diagnosis of gastric cancer. (See Chapter 45 for a discussion of nursing care associated

BOX 47.4 Key Features

Early Versus Advanced Gastric Cancer

Early Gastric Cancer	Advanced Gastric Cancer
• Chronic dyspepsia	• Nausea and vomiting
• Abdominal discomfort initially relieved with antacids	• Iron deficiency anemia
	• Palpable epigastric mass
• Feeling of fullness	• Enlarged lymph nodes
• Epigastric, back, or retrosternal pain	• Weakness and fatigue
	• Progressive weight loss

with this diagnostic test.) The lesion can be viewed directly, and biopsies of all visible lesions can be performed to determine the presence of cancer cells. During the endoscopy, an endoscopic (endoluminal) ultrasound (EUS) of the gastric mucosa can also be performed. This technology allows the primary health care provider to evaluate the depth of the tumor and the presence of lymph node involvement, which permits more accurate staging of the disease. CT, positron emission tomography (PET), and MRI scans of the chest, abdomen, and pelvis are used in determining the extent of the disease and in planning therapy.

Take Actions: Interventions

Management of gastric cancer includes drug therapy, radiation, and/or surgery. Drug therapy and radiation may be used instead of surgery or as an adjunct before and/or after surgery.

Nonsurgical Management. Definitive treatment of gastric cancer depends on the stage of the disease. Radiation and chemotherapy commonly prolong survival of patients with advanced gastric disease.

Combination *chemotherapy* with multiple cycles of drugs such as oxaliplatin, fluorouracil, cisplatin, and epirubicin before and after surgery may be given (American Cancer Society, 2023a). Bone marrow suppression, nausea, and vomiting are common adverse drug effects. Chapter 18 discusses the general nursing care of patients receiving chemotherapy.

Although gastric cancers are somewhat sensitive to the effects of radiation, the use of this treatment is limited because the disease is often widely spread to other abdominal organs at diagnosis. Organs such as the liver, kidneys, and spinal cord can endure only a limited amount of radiation. Intraoperative radiotherapy (IORT) is available in large tertiary care health care systems.

Surgical Management. Surgical resection by removing the tumor is the preferred method for treating gastric cancer. The primary surgical procedures for the treatment of gastric cancer are total and subtotal (partial) gastrectomy. In early stages, laparoscopic surgery (minimally invasive surgery [MIS]) plus adjuvant chemotherapy or radiation may be curative. Patients having MIS have less pain, shorter hospital stays, rare postoperative complications, and recover more quickly. Over the past decade the use of MIS for gastric resections in the United States has increased from 18% to 37% (Khorfan et al., 2020). A classic study in a U.S. cancer center examined outcomes of MIS and an Enhanced Recovery After Surgery (ERAS) protocol. In addition to expected outcomes associated with laparoscopic surgery, patients in the study advanced their diets more quickly, experienced less weight loss, and increased their physical activity more quickly within the first week after the procedure when compared with patients having open traditional surgery (Desiderio et al., 2018).

Most patients with advanced disease are candidates for palliative surgical treatment. Metastasis in the supraclavicular lymph nodes, inguinal lymph nodes, liver, umbilicus, or perirectal wall indicates that the opportunity for cure by resection has been lost. Palliative resection may significantly improve the quality of life for a patient with obstruction, hemorrhage, or pain.

Preoperative Care. Before conventional open-approach surgery, a nasogastric tube (NGT) is often inserted and connected to suction to remove secretions and empty the stomach. This allows surgery to take place without contamination of the peritoneal cavity by gastric secretions. The NGT remains in place for a few days *after surgery* to prevent the accumulation of secretions, which may lead to vomiting or GI distention and pressure on the incision. Patients having laparoscopic surgery (minimally invasive surgery [MIS]) do not require an NGT.

Because weight loss is problematic for patients with gastric cancer, **nutrition** therapy is a vital aspect of preoperative and postoperative management. Before surgery, compression by the tumor can prevent adequate nutritional intake. To correct malnutrition before surgery, if present, the primary health care provider may prescribe enteral supplements to the diet and/or total parenteral nutrition (TPN). Vitamin, mineral, iron, and protein supplements are essential to correct nutritional deficits.

Other preoperative nursing measures for the patient undergoing open gastric surgery are the same as those for any patient undergoing abdominal surgery and general anesthesia (see Chapter 9).

Operative Procedures. The surgeon usually removes part or the entire stomach to take out the tumor. When the tumor is located in the midportion or distal (lower) portion of the stomach, a subtotal (partial) gastrectomy is typically performed. The omentum and relevant lymph nodes are also removed. The surgery may be performed as an MIS procedure or as an open conventional surgical technique, with or without robotic assistance.

For the patient with a removable growth in the proximal (upper) third of the stomach, a total gastrectomy is typically performed (Fig. 47.3). In this procedure the surgeon removes the entire stomach along with the lymph nodes and omentum. The surgeon sutures the esophagus to the duodenum or jejunum to reestablish continuity of the GI tract. More radical surgery involving removal of the spleen and distal pancreas is controversial, although the Whipple procedure may be used to prolong life. The complications of this drastic surgery are common and very serious (see Chapter 51). For patients with advanced disease, total gastrectomy is performed when gastric bleeding or obstruction is present.

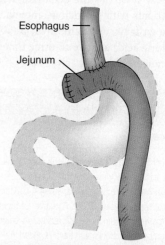

Esophagus

Jejunum

FIG. 47.3 Total gastrectomy with anastomosis of the esophagus to the jejunum (esophagojejunostomy) is the principal surgical intervention for extensive gastric cancer. (From Dorner, S., Stump, S. E., & Grodner, M. [2023]. *Nutritional foundations and clinical applications: A nursing approach* [8th ed.]. St. Louis: Elsevier.)

Patients with tumors at the gastric outlet who are not candidates for subtotal or total gastrectomy may undergo gastroenterostomy for palliation. The surgeon creates a passage between the body of the stomach and the small bowel, often the duodenum.

Postoperative Care. Provide evidence-based postoperative care for patients who have had general anesthesia to prevent atelectasis, paralytic ileus, wound *infection,* and peritonitis (see Chapter 9). Document and report any signs and symptoms of these complications immediately to the surgeon.

Auscultate the lungs for adventitious sounds (crackles or reduced breath sounds), and monitor for the return of bowel sounds. Take vital signs as appropriate to detect signs of infection or bleeding. Aggressive pulmonary exercises and early ambulation can help prevent respiratory complications and deep vein thrombosis. Inspect the operative site every 8 to 12 hours for the presence of redness/hyperpigmentation, swelling, or drainage, which indicate wound infection. Keep the head of the bed elevated to prevent aspiration from reflux.

Decreased patency caused by a clogged NGT can result in *acute gastric dilation* after surgery. This problem is characterized by epigastric pain and a feeling of fullness, hiccups, tachycardia, and hypotension. Notify the surgeon to obtain an order for irrigation or replacement of the NGT to relieve these symptoms.

Dumping syndrome is a term that refers to a group of vasomotor symptoms that occur after eating in patients who have had a gastrectomy. This syndrome is believed to occur as a result of the rapid emptying of food contents into the small intestine, which shifts fluid into the gut, causing abdominal distention. Observe for *early* manifestations of this syndrome, which typically occur within 20 minutes of eating. Symptoms include vertigo, tachycardia, syncope, sweating, pallor/ash gray skin, palpitations, and the desire to lie down. Report these manifestations to the surgeon, and encourage the patient to lie down. Monitor the patient for late symptoms.

Late dumping syndrome, which occurs 1 to 3 hours after eating, is caused by a release of an excessive amount of insulin. The insulin release follows a rapid rise in the blood glucose level that results from the rapid entry of high-carbohydrate food into the jejunum. Observe for manifestations, including dizziness, light-headedness, palpitations, diaphoresis, and confusion.

Dumping syndrome is managed by *nutrition* changes that include decreasing the amount of food taken at one time and eliminating liquids ingested with meals. In collaboration with the registered dietitian, teach the patient to eat a high-protein, high-fat, low- to moderate-carbohydrate diet. Acarbose may be used to decrease carbohydrate absorption. A somatostatin analog, octreotide two or four times daily 30 minutes before meals, may be prescribed in severe cases. This drug decreases gastric and intestinal hormone secretion and slows stomach and intestinal transit time (National Institute of Diabetes and Digestive and Kidney Diseases, 2019).

Delayed gastric emptying is often present after gastric surgery and usually resolves within 1 week. Edema at the anastomosis (surgical connection areas) or adhesions (scar tissue) obstructing the distal loop may cause mechanical blockage. Metabolic causes (e.g., hypokalemia, hypoproteinemia, or hyponatremia) should be considered. Edema at the anastomosis usually resolves

with nasogastric suction, maintenance of fluid and electrolyte balance, and proper *nutrition.*

Several problems related to *nutrition* develop related to partial removal of the stomach, including deficiencies of vitamin B_{12}, folic acid, and iron; impaired calcium metabolism; and reduced absorption of calcium and vitamin D. These problems are caused by a reduction of intrinsic factor. The decrease results from the resection and from inadequate absorption because of rapid entry of food into the bowel. In the absence of intrinsic factor, signs and symptoms of pernicious anemia may occur. Assess for the development of atrophic glossitis secondary to vitamin B_{12} deficiency. In atrophic glossitis, the tongue takes on a shiny, smooth, and "beefy" appearance. The patient may also have signs of anemia secondary to folic acid and iron deficiency. Monitor the complete blood count (CBC) for signs of megaloblastic anemia (low red blood cell [RBC] level) and leukopenia (low white blood cell [WBC] level). These manifestations are corrected by the administration of vitamin B_{12}. The primary health care provider may also prescribe folic acid or iron preparations. Anemias are discussed in Chapter 34.

Care Coordination and Transition Management

Patients who have undergone total gastrectomy and those who are debilitated with advanced gastric cancer are discharged to home with maximal assistance and support or to a transitional care unit or skilled nursing facility. Patients who have undergone subtotal gastrectomy and are not debilitated may be discharged to home with partial assistance for ADLs. Recurrence of cancer is common, and patients need regular follow-up examinations and imaging assessments. Collaborate with the case manager to ensure continuity of care and thorough follow-up with diagnostic testing.

Home Care Management. Gastric cancer is a life-threatening illness. Consequently, the patient and family members require physical and emotional care. Assess their ability to cope with the disease and the possible need for end-of-life care. The adverse effects of gastric cancer treatment can be debilitating, and patients need to learn symptom-management strategies. Hospice programs can help both the patient and the family cope with these physical and emotional needs.

Patients may fear returning home because of their inability for self-management. Enlisting family and health care resources for the patient may ease some of this anxiety. Provide the family with adequate information about community support systems to make the transition to home care easier. If the prognosis is poor, the patient and family will require continued professional support from case managers, social workers, and/or nurses to cope with death and dying. (See Chapter 8 for a discussion of end-of-life care.)

Self-Management Education. Educate the patient and family about any continuing needs, drug therapy, and nutrition therapy. If patients are discharged to home with surgical dressings, teach the patient and family how to change them. Review the manifestations of incisional infection (e.g., fever, redness/hyperpigmentation, and drainage) that they should report to the surgeon.

Patients who will be receiving radiation therapy or chemotherapy require instructions related to the side effects of these treatments. Nausea and vomiting are common side effects of chemotherapy, and instruction in the use of prescribed antiemetics may be needed. (See Chapter 18 for health teaching for patients receiving chemotherapy or radiation therapy.)

In collaboration with the registered dietitian nutritionist, teach the patient and family about the type and quantity of foods that will provide optimal nutritional value. Interventions to minimize dumping syndrome and decrease gastric stimulants are also emphasized. Remind the patient to:

- Eat small, frequent meals
- Avoid drinking liquids with meals
- Avoid foods that cause discomfort
- Eliminate caffeine and alcohol consumption
- Begin a smoking-cessation program, if needed
- Receive B_{12} injections, as prescribed
- Lie flat for a short time after eating

Health Care Resources. A home care referral provides continued assessment, assistance, and encouragement to the patient and family. A home care nurse can support care activities and provide valuable psychological support. Additional referrals to a registered dietitian, professional counselor, or clergy/spiritual leader may be necessary. Referral to a hospice agency can be of great assistance for the patient with advanced disease. Hospice care may be delivered in the home or in an institutional setting. Appropriate support groups (e.g., American Cancer Society Treatment and Support [https://www.cancer.org/treatment.html]) can be a major resource. Chapter 8 discusses end-of-life and palliative care in detail.

NCLEX Examination Challenge 47.3

Physiological Integrity

Which client statement regarding diet and nutrition after a total gastrectomy requires **further teaching** by the nurse?

A. "I should stay sitting up for an hour after I eat."
B. "I will avoid liquids with my meals."
C. "I need to eat small, frequent meals."
D. "I need to stay away from concentrated sweets."

GET READY FOR THE NEXT-GENERATION NCLEX® EXAMINATION!

Essential Nursing Care Points

Health Promotion/Disease Prevention

- Nurses need to teach individuals about how to prevent gastritis and promote gastric health by avoiding irritants such as smoking, excessive alcohol, high stress, and pickled and smoked foods.
- Nurses need to keep in mind that while these health promotion strategies may help reduce the incidence of gastritis, some individuals may not be able to practice them due to lack of resources, especially those who have financial difficulties or have family responsibilities that leave them little time to care for themselves.
- Nurses need to identify individuals who are at high risk for peptic ulcer disease (PUD) and gastric cancer and teach them about the need for *H. pylori* screening.
- Nurses should teach individuals to avoid long-term use of NSAIDs, which could cause a peptic ulcer.

Chronic Disease Care

- Esophagogastroduodenoscopy (EGD) with biopsy is the gold standard procedure for diagnosing gastric problems.
- The three most common types of peptic ulcers are duodenal, gastric, and stress ulcers.
- The most common classes of drugs used to manage gastritis and PUD are proton pump inhibitors (PPIs) and H_2 antagonists.
- Chemotherapy and radiation are commonly used to prolong survival of patients with advanced gastric cancer.
- Surgical resection by removing the tumor is the preferred method for treating gastric cancer.
- The primary surgical procedures for treating gastric cancer are total and partial gastrectomy.
- **Dumping syndrome** is a complication of gastrectomy that causes a group of vasomotor symptoms, causing vertigo, tachycardia, sweating, pallor/ash gray skin, and palpitations. Patients can minimize this problem by avoiding liquids with meals; eating small, frequent meals; and lying down after eating for a short period of time.

Regenerative or Restorative Care

- The most common complication of PUD is upper GI bleeding, or hemorrhage.
- Key features of upper GI bleeding are hematemesis and/or melena and symptoms associated with hypovolemia, including hypotension, tachycardia, dizziness, and decreased hemoglobin and hematocrit.
- Emergency management of upper GI bleeds includes oxygen therapy, airway support as needed, nasogastric tube (NGT) insertion, two large-bore IV lines, and lab test monitoring. Blood transfusions may also be needed.
- Treatments to diagnose and treat the source of GI bleeding include endoscopic therapies or interventional radiologic procedures.
- A common drug regimen to treat *H. pylori* infection is PPI-based triple therapy, which includes a PPI plus two antibiotics for 10–14 days.

Hospice/Palliative/Supportive Care

- Patients who have advanced gastric cancer and their families should be referred to a local palliative care program or hospice for symptom management at the end of life (see Chapter 8).

Mastery Questions

1. The nurse is reviewing the laboratory test results for a client recently diagnosed with peptic ulcer disease (PUD). Which result would the nurse report **immediately** to the primary health care provider?
   A. Blood urea nitrogen: 16 mg/dL (5.71 mmol/L)
   B. Serum creatinine: 0.9 mg/dL (79.6 mcmol/L)
   C. Hematocrit: 33% (0.33 volume fraction)
   D. Serum glucose: 102 mg/dL (5.66 mmol/L)

2. Which of the following statements to promote gastric health would the nurse include to educate an adult client? **Select all that apply.**
   A. "Stop smoking or using tobacco in any form."
   B. "Do not drink excessive amounts of alcohol."
   C. "Consume a healthy, well-balanced diet."
   D. "Exercise on a regular basis, if possible."
   E. "Avoid excessive amounts of pickled or smoked food."
   F. "Avoid taking large amounts of NSAIDs."

NGN Challenge 47.1
47.1.1

The nurse is caring for a 54-year-old client who was seen in the VA medical clinic.

History and Physical	Nurses' Notes	Vital Signs	Laboratory Results

1330: Presents to the clinic with report of worsening epigastric pain and anorexia that has continued for the past 2 weeks. Tries to avoid foods that make pain worse, such as onions and garlic; excessive alcohol also increases pain. States has not been eating very well for months since the client's partner "threw" the client out of the house after being discharged from military service with PTSD and depression. Has been living in the car most nights, but stays at the homeless shelter when the weather gets too cold. Is unemployed but the client's family members sometimes give the client money to buy food or gas. Alert and oriented × 4. No adventitious breath sounds; no shortness of breath. S_1 S_2 present; BS present × 4. VS: T 97.8°F (36.6°C), HR 84 beats/min, RR 18 breaths/min, BP 126/78 mm Hg. SpO_2 95% on RA. Current wt. 152 lb (68.9 kg), ht. 69 in (175.3 cm). States that weight has been about the same for 5 years. Confirmed *H. pylori +*.

Which of the following client findings require **immediate** follow up? **Select all that apply.**
- ○ Worsening epigastric pain
- ○ Anorexia
- ○ Avoids foods that make pain worse
- ○ Has PTSD and depression
- ○ Lives in a car
- ○ SpO_2 95% on RA
- ○ *H. pylori +*

47.1.2

The nurse is caring for a 54-year-old client who came to the VA clinic.

History and Physical	Nurses' Notes	Vital Signs	Laboratory Results

1330: Presents to the clinic with report of worsening episodic epigastric pain and anorexia that has occurred for the past 2 weeks. Tries to avoid foods that make pain worse, such as onions and garlic; excessive alcohol also increases pain. States has not been eating very well for months since the client's partner "threw" the client out of the house after being discharged from military service with PTSD and depression. Has been living in the car most nights, but stays at the homeless shelter when the weather gets too cold. Is unemployed but the client's family members sometimes give the client money to buy food or gas. Alert and oriented × 4. No adventitious breath sounds; no shortness of breath. S_1 S_2 present; BS present × 4. VS: T 97.8°F (36.6°C), HR 84 beats/min, RR 18 breaths/min, BP 126/78 mm Hg. SpO_2 95% on RA. Current wt. 152 lb (68.9 kg), ht. 69 in (175.3 cm). States that his weight has been about the same for 5 years. Confirmed *H. pylori +*.

1425: Started on PPI-based triple therapy for 10 days. Health teaching provided on how to take medications and need for adherence to drug regimen. Discharged with F/U appointment for clinic visit in 2 weeks.

Complete the following sentence by selecting from the list of word choices below.

The nurse analyzes the client findings and determines that they are consistent with [**Word Choice**] or [**Word Choice**].

Word Choices
Cholecystitis
Gastritis
Pancreatitis
Peptic ulcer disease

47.1.3

The nurse is caring for a 54-year-old client admitted to the ED.

History and Physical	Nurses' Notes	Vital Signs	Laboratory Results

1715: Client brought to ED by ambulance after falling in local homeless shelter. Was diagnosed with probable peptic ulcer disease last week at VA clinic. Admits lack of adherence with prescribed PPI-based triple therapy drug regimen. Currently drowsy but arousable; oriented × 2 and reporting pain of 8/10 in "stomach area." States has had several vomiting episodes during the day. One episode of 120 mL hematemesis while in ED. VS: T 100.2°F (37.9°C), HR 90 beats/min, RR 16 breaths/min, BP 98/56 lying position, Spo$_2$ 95% on RA.

Complete the following sentence by selecting from the lists of options below.

The nurse determines that the *priority* for care is to manage the

client's **1 [Select]** as evidenced by **2 [Select]** and **2 [Select]**.

Options for 1	Options for 2
Pain	Anemia
Hypovolemia	Disorientation
Vomiting	Hypotension
Fluid overload	Tachycardia

47.1.4

The nurse is caring for a 54-year-old client admitted to the ED.

History and Physical	Nurses' Notes	Vital Signs	Laboratory Results

1715: Client brought to ED by ambulance after falling in local homeless shelter. Was diagnosed with probable peptic ulcer disease last week at VA clinic. Admits lack of adherence with prescribed PPI-based triple therapy drug regimen. Currently drowsy but arousable; oriented × 2 and reporting pain of 8/10 in "stomach area." States has had several vomiting episodes during the day. One episode of 120 mL hematemesis while in ED. VS: T 100.2°F (37.9°C), HR 90 beats/min, RR 16 breaths/min, BP 98/56 mm Hg lying position, Spo$_2$ 92% on RA.

History and Physical	Laboratory Results	Vital Signs	Nurses' Notes

Laboratory Tests	Results	Reference Range
Blood urea nitrogen (BUN)	24 mg/dL (8.6 mmol/L)	10–20 mg/dL (2.9–8.2 mmol/L)
Creatinine (Cr)	1.2 mg/dL (106 μmol/L)	0.6–1.2 mg/dL (53–106 μmol/L)
Sodium (Na)	131 mEq/L (131 mmol/L)	136–145 mEq/L (136–145 mmol/L)
Potassium (K)	3.4 mEq/L (3.4 mmol/L)	3.5–5.0 mEq/L (3.5–5.0 mmol/L)
Glucose	74 mg/dL (3.9 mmol/L)	74–106 mg/dL (3.9–6.1 mmol/L)
Red blood cells (RBCs)	4.2 × 10^6 μL (4.2 × 10^9 /L)	4.7–6.1 × 10^6 μL (4.7–6.1 × 10^9 /L)
Hemoglobin (Hgb)	11.2 g/dL (6.95 mmol/L)	14–18 g/dL (8.7–11.2 mmol/L)
Hematocrit (Hct)	36% (0.36 volume fraction)	42%–52% (0.42–0.52 volume fraction)
White blood cells (WBCs)	13,500/mm^3 (13.5 × 10^9 /L)	5000–10,000/mm^3 (5.0–10.0 × 10^9 /L)

Select whether the following potential nursing actions are indicated or not indicated for the client at this time.

Potential Nursing Action	Indicated	Not Indicated
Give client clear liquids as tolerated		
Type and crossmatch 2 units packed RBCs		
Insert nasogastric tube and connect to suction		
Start IV infusion with NS and 20 mEq potassium via large-bore catheter		
Begin supplemental oxygen 3 L/min via NC		

47.1.5

The nurse is caring for a 54-year-old client admitted to the ED.

History and Physical	Nurses' Notes	Vital Signs	Laboratory Results

1715: Client brought to ED by ambulance after falling in local homeless shelter. Was diagnosed with probable peptic ulcer disease last week at VA clinic. Admits lack of adherence with prescribed PPI-based triple therapy drug regimen. Currently drowsy but arousable; oriented × 2 and reporting pain of 8/10 in "stomach area." States has had several vomiting episodes during the day. One episode of 120 mL hematemesis while in ED. VS: T 100.2°F (37.9°C), HR 90 beats/min, RR 16 breaths/min, BP 98/56 lying position, Spo$_2$ 92% on RA.

Select the **5** assessment parameters that would be essential for the nurse to monitor as part of the client's care.

○ Urinary output
○ Oxygen saturation
○ Oral intake
○ Blood pressure
○ Hematemesis
○ Pain intensity
○ Finger-stick blood glucose

47.1.6

A 54-year-old client is admitted to the medical unit following an endoscopic procedure. The nurse performs an admission assessment and compares current client findings with earlier findings when the client was admitted to the ED.

History and Physical	**Nurses' Notes**	Vital Signs	Laboratory Results

1715: Client brought to ED by ambulance after falling in local homeless shelter. Was diagnosed with probable peptic ulcer disease last week at VA clinic. Admits lack of adherence with prescribed PPI-based triple therapy drug regimen. Currently drowsy but arousable; oriented × 2 and reporting pain of 8/10 in "stomach area." States has had several vomiting episodes during the day. One episode of 120 mL hematemesis while in ED. VS: T 100.2°F (37.9°C), HR 90 beats/min, RR 16 breaths/min, BP 98/56 lying position, SpO_2 92% on RA.

History and Physical	**Laboratory Results**	Vital Signs	Nurses' Notes

Laboratory Tests	Results	Reference Range
Blood urea nitrogen (BUN)	24 mg/dL (8.6 mmol/L)	10–20 mg/dL mmol/L
Creatinine (Cr)	1.2 mg/dL (106 μmol/L)	0.6–1.2 mg/dL (53–106 μmol/L)
Sodium (Na)	131 mEq/L (131 mmol/L)	136–145 mEq/L (136–145 mmol/L)
Potassium (K)	3.4 mEq/L (3.4 mmol/L)	3.5–5.0 mEq/L (3.5–5.0 mmol/L)
Glucose	74 mg/dL (3.9 mmol/L)	74–106 mg/dL (3.9–6.1 mmol/L)
Red blood cells (RBCs)	4.2×10^6 μL (4.2×10^9 /L)	4.7–6.1×10^6 μL (4.7–6.1×10^9/L)
Hemoglobin (Hgb)	11.2 g/dL (6.95 mmol/L)	14–18 g/dL (8.7–11.2 mmol/L)
Hematocrit (Hct)	36% (0.36 volume fraction)	42%–52% (0.42–0.52 volume fraction)
White blood cells (WBCs)	$13,500$/mm³ (13.5×10^9/L)	5000–$10,000$/mm³ (5.0–10.0×10^9/L)

For each current client finding, indicate if the client's condition has improved or not improved.

Current Client Findings	Improved	Not Improved
BP 118/70 mm Hg		
SpO_2 97% on RA		
Pain 4/10		
Na 137 mEq/L (137 mmol/L)		
K 4.0 mEq/L (40 mmol/L)		
BUN 20 mg/dL (8.2 mmol/L)		

REFERENCES

American Cancer Society. (2023a). *Chemotherapy for stomach cancer.* https://www.cancer.org/cancer/stomach-cancer/treating/chemotherapy.html.

American Cancer Society. (2023b). *Key statistics about stomach cancer.* https://www.cancer.org/cancer/stomach-cancer/about/key-statistics.html.

American Cancer Society. (2023c). *Stomach cancer survival rates.* https://www.cancer.org/cancer/stomach-cancer/detection-diagnosis-staging/survival-rates.html.

Anand, B. S., & Katz, P. O. (2021). *Peptic ulcer disease.* Medscape. https://emedicine.medscape.com/article/181753-overview.

Burchum, J. R., & Rosenthal, L. D. (2022). *Lehne's pharmacology for nursing care* (11th ed.). St. Louis: Elsevier.

Castagneto-Gissey, L., Casella-Mariolo, J., Casella, G., & Mingrone, G. (2020). Obesity surgery and cancer: What are the unanswered questions? *Frontiers in Endocrinology, 11*(213). https://doi.org/10.3389/fendo.2020.00213.

*Desiderio, J., Stewart, C. L., Sun, V., Melstrom, L., Warner, S., Lee, B., et al. (2018). Enhanced recovery after surgery for gastric cancer improves clinical outcomes at a U.S. cancer center. *Journal of Gastric Cancer, 18*(3), 230–241.

Dewayani, A., Fauzia, K. A., Alfaray, R. I., Waskito, L. A., Doohan, D., Rezkitha, Y. A. A., et al. (2021). The roles of IL-17, IL-21, and IL-23 in the Helicobacter pylori infection and gastrointestinal inflammation: A review. *Toxins 2021, 13,* 315. https://doi.org/10.3390/toxins13050315.

Khorfan, R., Schlick, C., Yang, A. D., Odell, D. D., Bentrem, D. J., & Merkow, R. P. (2020). Utilization of minimally invasive surgery and its association with chemotherapy for locally advanced gastric cancer. *Journal of Gastrointestinal Surgery, 24*(2), 243–252. https://doi.org/10.1007/s11605-019-04410-x.

Morgan, T. G., Carlsson, T., Loveday, E., Collin, N., Collin, G., Mezes, P., et al. (2021). Needle or knife? The role of interventional radiology in managing uncontrolled gastrointestinal bleeding. *International Journal Gastrointestinal Intervention, 10*(17-22). https://doi.org/10.18528/ijgii200018.

National Institute of Diabetes and Digestive and Kidney Diseases. (2019). *Treatment of dumping syndrome.* https://www.niddk.nih.gov/health-information/digestive-diseases/dumping-syndrome/treatment.

Pagana, K., Pagana, T., & Pagana, T. (2022). *Mosby's manual of diagnostic and laboratory tests* (7th ed.). St. Louis: Elsevier.

Page, A. J., & Li, H. (2021). Molecular signaling in the gut-brain axis in stress. In G. Fink (Ed.), *Genetics, epigenetics, and genomics* (pp. 135–143). https://doi.org/10.1016/B978-0-12-813156-5.00012-1.

Pansa, A., Kurihara, H., & Memon, M. A. (2020). Updates in laparoscopic surgery for perforated peptic ulcer disease: State of the art and future perspectives. *Annals of Laparoscopic and Endoscopic Surgery, 5.* https://doi.org/10.21037/ales.2019.11.03.

Pezzotti, W. (2020). Understanding acute upper gastrointestinal bleeding in adults. *Nursing, 50*(5), 24–29. https://doi.org/10.1097/01.NURSE.0000659292.53003.39.

Rogers, J. L. (2023). *McCance and Huether's Pathophysiology: The biologic basis for disease in adults and children* (9th ed.). St. Louis: Elsevier.

Shah, S. C., McKinley, M., Gupta, S., Peek, R. M., Jr., Martinez, M. C., & Gomez, S. L. (2020). Population-based analysis of differences in gastric cancer incidence among races and ethnicities in individuals age 50 years and older. *Gastroenterology, 159,* 1705–1714.

48

Concepts of Care for Patients With Noninflammatory Intestinal Conditions

Keelin Cromar

http://evolve.elsevier.com/Iggy/

LEARNING OUTCOMES

1. Plan collaborative care with the interprofessional team to manage *elimination* in patients with intestinal obstruction.
2. Teach adults how to decrease the risk for colorectal cancer.
3. Teach the patient and caregiver(s) about common drugs and other management strategies used for colorectal cancer.
4. Plan patient- and family-centered nursing interventions to decrease the psychosocial impact caused by living with colorectal cancer.
5. Apply knowledge of anatomy, physiology, and pathophysiology to provide evidence-based care for patients with noninflammatory intestinal conditions.
6. Analyze assessment and diagnostic findings to generate solutions and prioritize nursing care for patients who have noninflammatory intestinal conditions.
7. Organize care coordination and transition management for patients with noninflammatory intestinal conditions.
8. Use clinical judgment to plan evidence-based nursing care to promote *elimination* and *fluid and electrolyte balance* and to decrease *pain* in patients with intestinal obstruction.
9. Incorporate factors that affect health equity into the plan of care for patients with colorectal cancer.

KEY TERMS

abdominal compartment syndrome A serious complication of abdominal trauma that causes end-organ dysfunction caused by intraabdominal hypertension (IAH).

abdominoperineal (AP) resection Surgical removal of the sigmoid colon, rectum, and anus through combined abdominal and perineal incisions.

borborygmi High-pitched bowel sounds that are proximal (above) an obstruction.

colectomy Surgical removal of the entire colon.

colon resection Surgical removal of part of the colon and regional lymph nodes.

colostomy The surgical creation of an opening of the colon (stoma) onto the surface of the abdomen to allow passage of stool.

exploratory laparotomy A surgical opening of the abdominal cavity.

fecal occult blood test (FOBT) A laboratory test to determine the presence of occult (microscopic) blood in the stool.

flatulence Excessive gas (flatus) in the intestines.

hemorrhoidectomy Surgical removal of hemorrhoids.

hemorrhoids Unnaturally swollen or distended veins in the anorectal region.

hernia A weakness in the abdominal muscle wall through which a segment of the bowel or other abdominal structure protrudes.

hernioplasty A surgical hernia repair procedure performed to reinforce the weakened outside abdominal muscle wall with a mesh patch.

herniorrhaphy Surgical repair of a hernia.

intussusception Telescoping of a segment of the intestine within itself.

irreducible (incarcerated) hernia A hernia that cannot be reduced or placed back into the abdominal cavity. Any hernia that is not reducible requires immediate surgical evaluation.

irritable bowel syndrome A functional GI disorder that causes chronic or recurrent diarrhea, constipation, and/or abdominal pain and bloating.

laparotomy A surgical procedure in which an abdominal incision allows direct visualization and repair of abdominal organs

mechanical obstruction A condition in which the bowel is physically blocked by problems outside the intestine (e.g., adhesions), in the bowel wall (e.g., Crohn's disease), or in the intestinal lumen (e.g., tumors).

minimally invasive inguinal hernia repair (MIIHR) Surgical hernia repair through a laparoscope.

nonmechanical obstruction A condition in which peristalsis is decreased or absent because of neuromuscular disturbance, resulting in a slowing of the movement or a backup of intestinal contents; also known as *paralytic ileus*.

obstipation No passage of stool.

polyps In the intestinal tract, small growths covered with mucosa and attached to the surface of the intestine; although most are benign, they are significant because some have the potential to become malignant.

reducible hernia A hernia that can be reduced or placed back into the abdominal cavity.

strangulated obstruction Bowel obstruction or hernia that has compromised blood flow (can be life-threatening).

volvulus Twisting of the intestine.

Without proper diagnosis and management, some intestinal problems can lead to inadequate absorption of vital nutrients and affect *elimination.* If these disorders become severe or progress, *pain* and problems with *fluid and electrolyte balance* may occur. Chapter 3 briefly reviews each of these health concepts. Intestinal health problems may be classified as inflammatory or noninflammatory; this chapter focuses on disorders that are noninflammatory in origin.

✷ ELIMINATION CONCEPT EXEMPLAR: INTESTINAL OBSTRUCTION

Pathophysiology Review

Intestinal obstruction can be partial or complete and classified as mechanical or nonmechanical. With either condition, *elimination* is compromised by this common and serious disorder.

Mechanical obstruction occurs when the bowel is physically blocked by problems outside the intestine (e.g., adhesions), in the bowel wall (e.g., Crohn's disease), or in the intestinal lumen (e.g., tumors). Nonmechanical obstruction (also known as *paralytic ileus* or *functional obstruction*) does not involve a physical obstruction in or outside the intestine. Instead, peristalsis is decreased or absent because of neuromuscular disturbance, resulting in a slowing of the movement or a backup of intestinal contents (Rogers, 2023).

Intestinal contents are composed of ingested fluid, food, and saliva; gastric, pancreatic, and biliary secretions; digestive enzymes; and swallowed air. In both mechanical and nonmechanical obstructions, the intestinal contents accumulate at and above the area of obstruction. Abdominal distention results due to inability of the intestine to absorb the contents and move the waste through the intestinal tract. To compensate for the delay, peristalsis increases to move the intestinal contents forward. This increase stimulates additional secretions, which then leads to further distention. The bowel then becomes edematous, and increased capillary permeability results. Plasma leaking into the peritoneal cavity and fluid trapped in the intestinal lumen decrease the absorption of fluid and electrolytes into the vascular space. Reduced circulatory blood volume (hypovolemia) and electrolyte imbalances may occur. Hypovolemia ranges from mild to extreme (hypovolemic shock) (Rogers, 2023).

Depending on the part of the intestine that is blocked, specific problems related to *fluid and electrolyte balance* and acid-base balance result. Obstruction high in the small intestine causes a loss of gastric hydrochloric acid, which can lead

to *metabolic alkalosis.* An obstruction below the duodenum but above the large bowel results in a loss of both acids and bases, so acid-base balance is usually compromised. Obstruction at the end of the small intestine and lower in the intestinal tract causes loss of alkaline fluids, which can lead to *metabolic acidosis* (Rogers, 2023).

If hypovolemia is severe, acute kidney injury or even death can occur. Bacterial peritonitis with or without perforation may also result. With *closed-loop obstruction* (blockage in two different areas) or a strangulated obstruction (obstruction with compromised blood flow that can be life-threatening), the risk for peritonitis (infection) is greatly increased. Bacteria in the intestinal contents remain stagnant in the obstructed intestine. This is not a problem unless the blood flow to the intestine is compromised. Bacteria without blood supply can form and release endotoxins into the peritoneal or systemic circulation and cause septic shock. The same process occurs when gangrene results from intestinal ischemia caused by mesenteric arterial occlusion.

With a strangulated obstruction, major blood loss into the intestine and the peritoneum may occur. Sepsis and bleeding can result in an increase in intraabdominal pressure (IAP) or acute compartment syndrome.

Etiology and Genetic Risk

Intestinal obstruction is caused by a variety of conditions and is associated with significant morbidity. Obstruction can occur anywhere in the intestinal tract, although the ileum in the small intestine (the narrowest part of the intestinal tract) is the most common site.

Mechanical obstruction can result from:
- Adhesions (scar tissue from surgeries or pathology)
- Benign or malignant tumor
- Complications of appendicitis
- Hernias
- Fecal impactions (especially in older adults)
- Strictures due to Crohn's disease (a chronic inflammatory bowel disease) or previous radiation therapy
- Intussusception (telescoping of a segment of the intestine within itself) (Fig. 48.1)
- Volvulus (twisting of the intestine) (see Fig. 48.1)
- Fibrosis due to disorders such as endometriosis

Postoperative ileus (POI) (paralytic ileus), or *nonmechanical* obstruction, is commonly caused by handling of the intestines during abdominal surgery. Patients with POI lose intestinal function for a few hours to several days. Electrolyte disturbances, especially hypokalemia, predispose the patient to this problem. POI can also be a consequence of peritonitis due to leakage of colonic contents, which causes severe irritation and triggers an inflammatory response and infection (see Peritonitis in Chapter 49). Vascular insufficiency to the bowel, also referred to as *intestinal ischemia,* is another potential cause of an ileus. It results when arterial or venous thrombosis or an embolus decreases blood flow to or in the mesenteric blood vessels surrounding the intestines. Severe insufficiency of blood supply can result in infarction of surrounding organs (e.g., bowel infarction), gangrene, and eventually sepsis and septic shock.

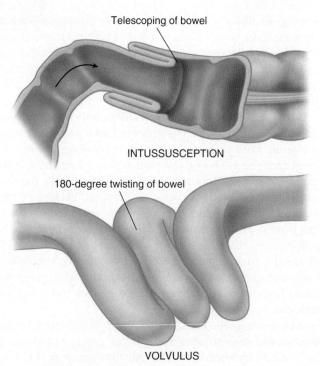

Telescoping of bowel

INTUSSUSCEPTION

180-degree twisting of bowel

VOLVULUS

FIG. 48.1 Two major types of mechanical obstruction.

Incidence and Prevalence

Because there are many causes of intestinal obstruction, the incidence and prevalence are not well known. However, obstruction occurs more commonly in patients who have had bowel surgery and in those with intestinal tumors. Older adults are the most likely group to have a bowel obstruction, often as a result of fecal impaction or malignant tumor.

Health Promotion/Disease Prevention

Individuals may be able to prevent intestinal obstruction, depending on the cause of the blockage. For example, physiologic changes associated with aging decrease peristalsis and cause constipation in older adults. If constipation is not treated or resolved, the older adult may develop a fecal impaction that causes an intestinal obstruction. Therefore, teach older adults ways to prevent constipation, including adequate fluid intake, regular exercise, a high-fiber diet, and, if needed, a stool softener. The box later in this chapter titled Patient-Centered Care: Older Adult Health lists interventions to prevent fecal impaction.

Other health promotion strategies to prevent intestinal obstruction include interventions that can aid in the prevention or early detection of colorectal cancer, including regular colon health screenings, a high-fiber diet, and a healthy lifestyle, if possible.

Interprofessional Collaborative Care

Care for the patient with an intestinal obstruction takes place in the hospital setting. The interprofessional team that primarily collaborates to care for this patient generally includes the primary health care provider, nurse, and registered dietitian nutritionist.

Recognize Cues: Assessment

History. Collect information about a history of GI disorders, surgeries, and treatments. Question the patient about recent nausea and vomiting and the color of emesis, noting whether vomitus is described as greenish-yellow, bilious, or hematemesis. Perform a thorough pain assessment, with particular attention to the onset, aggravating and alleviating factors, and patterns or rhythms of the *pain.* Severe pain that then stops and changes to tenderness on palpation may indicate perforation; this finding should be reported promptly to the primary health care provider. Ask about *elimination* patterns, including the passage of flatus and the time, character, and consistency of the last bowel movement. Singultus (hiccups) is common with all types of intestinal obstruction. When an obstruction is suspected, keep the patient NPO and contact the primary health care provider promptly for further direction.

Assess for a family history of colorectal cancer (CRC), and ask about blood in the stool or a change in bowel pattern. Body temperature with uncomplicated obstruction is rarely higher than 100°F (37.8°C). A temperature higher than this, with or without guarding and tenderness, and a sustained elevation in pulse may indicate a strangulated obstruction, peritonitis, or intestinal ischemia. Fever, tachycardia, hypotension, increasing abdominal pain, abdominal rigidity, or a change in the color of the skin overlying the abdomen should be reported to the primary health care provider immediately.

Physical Assessment/Signs and Symptoms. The patient with *mechanical* obstruction of the *small intestine* often has midabdominal *pain* or cramping. Pain can be sporadic, and the patient may feel comfortable between episodes. If strangulation is present, the pain will become more localized and persistent. Vomiting often accompanies obstruction and is more profuse with obstructions in the proximal small intestine. Vomitus may contain bile and mucus or be orange-brown and foul smelling because of bacterial overgrowth with low ileal obstruction. Prolonged vomiting can result in a disruption in *fluid and electrolyte balance.* Obstipation (no passage of stool) and failure to pass flatus are associated with complete obstruction; diarrhea may be present with partial obstruction.

Unlike small-bowel obstruction, *mechanical colonic obstruction* causes a mild, intermittent, colicky abdominal *pain.* Lower abdominal distention and obstipation may be present, or the patient may have ribbonlike stools if obstruction is partial. Alterations in bowel patterns and blood in the stools may accompany the obstruction if diverticulitis or colorectal cancer is the cause.

On examination of the abdomen, observe for abdominal distention, which is common in all forms of intestinal obstruction. Peristaltic waves may also be visible. Auscultate for proximal (above the obstruction) high-pitched bowel sounds (borborygmi), which are associated with cramping early in the obstructive process as the intestine tries to push the mechanical obstruction forward. During later stages of mechanical obstruction, bowel sounds are absent, especially distal to the obstruction. Abdominal tenderness and rigidity are usually minimal. The presence of a tense, fluid-filled bowel loop mimicking a palpable abdominal mass may signal a closed-loop, strangulating small-bowel obstruction.

In most types of *nonmechanical* obstruction, the pain is described as a constant, diffuse discomfort. Colicky cramping

BOX 48.1 Key Features
Small-Bowel and Large-Bowel Obstructions

Small-Bowel Obstructions	Large-Bowel Obstructions
• Abdominal discomfort or pain possibly accompanied by visible peristaltic waves in upper and middle abdomen	• Intermittent lower abdominal cramping
• Upper or epigastric abdominal distention	• Lower abdominal distention
• Nausea and early, profuse vomiting (may contain fecal material)	• Minimal or no vomiting
• Obstipation	• Obstipation or ribbonlike stools
• Severe fluid and electrolyte imbalances	• No major fluid and electrolyte imbalances
• Metabolic alkalosis (not always present)	• Metabolic acidosis (not always present)

BOX 48.2 Best Practice for Patient Safety and Quality Care
Nursing Care of Patients Who Have an Intestinal Obstruction

- Monitor vital signs, especially blood pressure and pulse, for indications of fluid balance.
- Assess the patient's abdomen at least twice a day for bowel sounds, distention, and passage of flatus.
- Monitor **fluid and electrolyte balance** status, including laboratory values.
- Manage the patient who has a nasogastric tube (NGT):
  - Monitor drainage.
  - Ensure tube patency.
  - Check tube placement.
  - Irrigate tube as prescribed.
  - Maintain the patient on NPO status.
  - Provide frequent mouth and nares care.
  - Maintain the patient in a semi-Fowler's position.
- Give analgesics for **pain** as prescribed.
- Maintain IV therapy for fluid and electrolyte replacement.
- Give alvimopan as prescribed for patients with a postoperative ileus.
- Maintain parenteral nutrition if prescribed.

is not characteristic of this type of obstruction. *Pain* associated with obstruction caused by vascular insufficiency or infarction is usually severe and constant. On inspection, abdominal distention is typically present. Note decreased bowel sounds when auscultating the abdomen in early obstruction and absent bowel sounds in later stages. Vomiting of gastric contents and bile is frequent, but the vomitus rarely has a foul odor and is rarely profuse. Obstipation may or may not be present. A comparison of small- and large-bowel obstructions is outlined in Box 48.1.

Laboratory Assessment. There is no definitive laboratory test to confirm a diagnosis of mechanical or nonmechanical obstruction. *White blood cell (WBC) counts* are normal unless there is a strangulated obstruction, infarction, and/or gangrene. *Hemoglobin, hematocrit,* and *blood urea nitrogen (BUN)* values are often elevated, indicating dehydration. Serum sodium, chloride, and potassium are typically decreased. Elevations in serum amylase levels may occur with strangulating obstructions, which can damage the pancreas (Pagana et al., 2022).

Other Diagnostic Assessment. The primary health care provider obtains imaging information from an *abdominal CT scan* or *MRI* as soon as an obstruction is suspected. Distention with fluid and gas in the small intestine with the absence of gas in the colon indicates an obstruction in the small intestine.

Choice of diagnostic tests depends on the suspected location of the obstruction. Initially, the primary health care provider may request an *abdominal ultrasound* to evaluate the potential cause of the obstruction. An endoscopy (sigmoidoscopy or colonoscopy) may also be performed to determine the cause of the obstruction, except when perforation or complete obstruction is suspected.

Analyze Cues and Prioritize Hypotheses: Analysis

The priority collaborative problem for patients with intestinal obstruction is potential for life-threatening complications due to reduced flow or blocked flow of intestinal contents.

Generate Solutions and Take Actions: Planning and Implementation

Interventions are intended to identify the cause and relieve the obstruction. Relieving the obstruction decreases the potential for medical complications and reduces *pain.* Intestinal obstructions can be relieved by nonsurgical or surgical management.

Reducing the Risk of Life-Threatening Complications

Planning: Expected Outcomes. The expected outcome is that the patient's obstruction will resolve to restore normal bowel *elimination,* prevent potentially life-threatening complications, and relieve *pain.*

Interventions. Collaborative and nursing interventions depend on the location, cause, type, and severity of the bowel obstruction.

Nonsurgical Management. If the obstruction is partial and there is no evidence of strangulation or ischemia, nonsurgical management may be the treatment of choice, as summarized in Box 48.2. Once the obstruction has been addressed effectively, *elimination* patterns are expected to resume.

Paralytic ileus responds very well to nonsurgical methods of relieving obstruction. Nonsurgical approaches are also preferred in the treatment of patients with terminal disease associated with bowel obstruction. In addition to being NPO, patients typically have a nasogastric tube (NGT) inserted to decompress the bowel by draining fluid and air. The tube is attached to suction.

Nasogastric tubes. Most patients with an obstruction have an NGT unless the obstruction is mild. A Salem sump tube is inserted through the nose and placed into the stomach. It is attached to low *continuous* suction. This tube has a vent ("pigtail") that prevents the stomach mucosa from being pulled away during suctioning.

⚠ NURSING SAFETY PRIORITY

Action Alert

At least every 4 hours, assess the patient with an NGT for proper placement of the tube, tube patency, and output (quality and quantity). Monitor the nasal skin around the tube for irritation. Use an approved device that secures the tube to the nose to prevent accidental removal. Assess for peristalsis by auscultating for bowel sounds with the suction disconnected (suction masks peristaltic sounds).

Monitor NGTs for proper functioning. Occasionally, NGTs move out of optimal drainage position or become plugged. In this case, a decrease in gastric output will be noted or stasis of the tube's contents. Assess the patient for nausea, vomiting, increased abdominal distention, and placement of the tube. If the NGT is repositioned or replaced, confirmation of proper placement may be obtained by x-ray before use. After appropriate placement is established, aspirate the contents, and irrigate the tube with 30 mL of normal saline every 4 hours or as requested by the primary health care provider.

NCLEX Examination Challenge 48.1

Safe and Effective Care Environment

The nurse is caring for a client recently admitted for a complete small-bowel obstruction. What would be the nurse's **priority** action for the client?
A. Prepare the client for abdominal surgery.
B. Provide frequent mouth and nares care.
C. Assess bowel sounds every 2 hours.
D. Monitor for fluid and electrolyte imbalances.

Other nonsurgical interventions. Most types of nonmechanical obstruction respond to nasogastric decompression with medical treatment of the primary disorder. Incomplete mechanical obstruction can sometimes be treated successfully without surgery. Obstruction caused by lower fecal impaction usually resolves after disimpaction and enema administration. Intussusception may respond to hydrostatic pressure changes during a barium enema.

For patients with a postoperative ileus (POI), alvimopan may be given for short-term use. This drug is an oral, peripherally acting mu opioid receptor antagonist that increases GI motility (Chamie et al., 2021).

IV fluid replacement and maintenance are indicated for all patients with intestinal obstruction because *fluid and electrolyte balance* is altered (particularly potassium and sodium) as a result of vomiting, NPO status, and nasogastric suction. The primary health care provider often prescribes aggressive fluid replacement with 2 to 4 L of an isotonic solution (normal saline or lactated Ringer's solution) with potassium added. These decisions are based on serum electrolytes and blood urea nitrogen (BUN) levels. Care should be used for patients who are susceptible to fluid overload (e.g., older adults with a history of heart or chronic kidney disease). Monitor lung sounds, weight, and intake and output daily. *Weight is the most reliable indicator of fluid balance.* Blood replacement may be indicated in strangulated obstruction because of blood loss into the bowel or peritoneal cavity.

Monitor vital signs and other measures of fluid status (e.g., urine output, skin turgor, mucous membranes) every 2 to 4 hours, depending on the severity of the patient's condition. In collaboration with the registered dietitian, the primary health care provider may prescribe parenteral nutrition (PN), especially if the patient has had chronic nutritional problems and has been NPO for an extended period. Chapter 52 discusses the nursing care of patients receiving PN.

The patient with intestinal obstruction is usually thirsty, although some older adults have a decreased thirst response. Remind assistive personnel to provide frequent mouth care to help maintain moist mucous membranes. A few ice chips may be allowed if the patient is not having surgery. Follow agency protocol or the primary health care provider's orders regarding ice chips.

Abdominal distention can cause severe *pain.* The colicky, crampy pain that comes and goes with mechanical obstruction, as well as the nausea, vomiting, dry mucous membranes, and thirst, contribute to the patient's discomfort. Continually assess the character and location of the pain and immediately report any *pain* that significantly increases or changes from colicky and intermittent to constant discomfort. These changes can indicate perforation of the intestine or peritonitis.

Analgesics may be temporarily withheld in the diagnostic workup period so that signs and symptoms of perforation or peritonitis are not masked. Explain to the patient and family the rationale for not giving analgesics. In addition, if analgesics such as morphine are given, they may slow intestinal motility and can cause vomiting. Be alert to this side effect because nausea and vomiting are also signs of NGT obstruction or worsening bowel obstruction. Consider the importance of nonpharmacologic pain control measures when withdrawing this type of medication (see Chapter 6 for detailed description of pain management).

Help the patient achieve a position of comfort, with frequent position changes to promote increased peristalsis. A semi-Fowler's position helps alleviate the pressure of abdominal distention on the chest and promotes thoracic excursion to facilitate breathing.

Pain is generally less with nonmechanical obstruction than with mechanical obstruction. With both types of obstruction, food or oral fluids aggravate the GI tract and increase pain (Rogers, 2023).

If strangulation is suspected, the primary health care provider prescribes IV broad-spectrum antibiotics. In cases of partial obstruction or paralytic ileus, drugs that enhance gastric motility (prokinetic agents) such as metoclopramide may be used.

Surgical Management. Patients with complete mechanical obstruction and in some cases of incomplete mechanical obstruction, surgical intervention is necessary to relieve the obstruction. Strangulated obstruction is complete, and surgical intervention is always required. If surgery is needed, an exploratory laparotomy (a surgical opening of the abdominal cavity) to investigate the cause of the obstruction is performed. More specific surgical procedures depend on the cause of the obstruction.

Provide general preoperative teaching for both the patient and family as discussed in Chapter 9. When the patient has a complete bowel obstruction, the patient may feel too ill to understand the information. In this case, reinforce the information with the family or other caregiver. Depending on the cause and severity of the obstruction and the expertise of the surgeon, patients have either minimally invasive surgery (MIS) via laparoscopy or a conventional open approach.

During a *conventional open surgical approach,* the surgeon makes a large incision, enters the abdominal cavity, and explores for obstruction and the cause, if possible (exploratory laparotomy). If adhesions are found, they are lysed (cut and released). Obstruction caused by a tumor or diverticulitis requires a colon resection with primary anastomosis or a temporary or permanent colostomy. When intestinal infarction is the cause of obstruction, an embolectomy, thrombectomy, or resection of the gangrenous small or large bowel may be necessary. Severe cases may require a colectomy (surgical removal of the entire colon).

Most patients have laparoscopic surgery (MIS) for mechanical intestinal obstructions and do *not* have an NGT. For the *MIS* approach, the specially trained surgeon makes several small incisions in the abdomen and places a video camera to view the abdominal contents to determine the extent of the obstruction. This procedure takes longer than the open approach, but blood loss is less, and healing is faster. Robotic assistance may be used, depending on the experience of the surgeon and available equipment.

General postoperative care for the patient undergoing an *exploratory laparotomy* is described in Chapter 9. For patients who have undergone an open surgical approach, an NGT is put into place until peristalsis resumes. A clear liquid diet may be prescribed to encourage return of peristalsis. As liquids are initiated, the NGT can be disconnected from suction and capped for 1 to 2 hours after consumption to determine whether the patient is able to tolerate them. If the patient vomits after liquids, the suction is resumed. When the patient has return of peristalsis, the NGT suction may be discontinued, and the tube is clamped for a scheduled amount of time. If the patient does *not* experience nausea while the NGT is clamped, the tube is removed.

The length of hospitalization for a patient having MIS to remove tumors, adhesions, and other obstructions may be as short as 1 to 2 days compared with 3 days or longer for patients undergoing a conventional open surgical approach. Recovery is shortened due to less *pain* and fewer postoperative complications among those who have laparoscopic surgery (MIS).

Care Coordination and Transition Management

All patients with intestinal obstruction are hospitalized for monitoring and treatment. The length of stay varies according to the type of obstruction, treatment, and presence of complications. Patients who have complicated obstruction, such as strangulation or incarceration, are at greater risk for peritonitis, sepsis, and shock.

Those with nonmechanical (functional) intestinal obstruction are less likely to require a lengthy hospitalization because of the obstruction alone. Nonmechanical obstruction generally responds to nasogastric suction and possible drug therapy within a few days. However, if an ileus occurs as a complication of an abdominal surgery, the hospital stay could be lengthy.

Home Care Management. Preparation for home care depends on the cause of the obstruction and the treatment required. Patients who have resolution of obstruction without surgical intervention are assessed for their knowledge of strategies to avoid obstruction recurrence. For example, if fecal impaction in an older adult is the cause of the obstruction, assessment of the patient's ability to carry out a bowel regimen independently may be necessary (see the Patient-Centered Care: Older Adult Health box).

PATIENT-CENTERED CARE: OLDER ADULT HEALTH

Preventing Fecal Impaction

- Teach the patient to eat high-fiber foods, including plenty of raw fruits and vegetables and whole-grain products. Keep in mind that these foods are expensive, making it difficult for some patients (especially those on a fixed or limited income) to eat healthy.
- Encourage the patient to drink adequate amounts of fluids, especially water.
- Teach the patient to avoid routine usage of laxatives; teach the patient that laxative overuse decreases abdominal muscle tone and contributes to an atonic colon.
- Encourage the patient to exercise regularly, if possible. Daily walks are an excellent exercise to promote intestinal motility.
- Use natural foods to stimulate peristalsis, such as warm beverages and prune juice.
- Take bulk-forming products to provide fiber and stool softeners to ease bowel *elimination.*

For patients who have had surgery, evaluate their ability to function at home with the added tasks of incision care and possibly colostomy care (see later discussion of colostomy care in the Colorectal Cancer section). If needed, identify a family caregiver who can help with patient care.

Self-Management Education. Instruct the patient to report any abdominal *pain* or distention, nausea, or vomiting, with or without constipation, because these symptoms might indicate recurrent obstruction. However, the patient should be reassured that recurrent paralytic ileus is not common.

Teach the patient who has had surgery about incision care, drug therapy, and activity limitations. Drug therapy may consist of oral opioid and nonopioid analgesics as needed for incisional discomfort. If opioid therapy is used, an over-the-counter laxative with a softener (e.g., docusate with senna) may be added to prevent constipation and possible recurrent obstruction.

Health Care Resources. The need for follow-up appointments depends on the cause of the obstruction and the treatment required. In collaboration with the case manager, arrange for a home health nurse if the patient or family needs help with incision or colostomy care.

Evaluate Outcomes: Evaluation

Evaluate the care of the patient with intestinal obstruction based on the identified priority patient problems. The expected outcomes are that the patient will:

- Have relief from the obstruction and no evidence of life-threatening complications.
- Report a return to usual bowel *elimination.*

COLORECTAL CANCER

Colorectal refers to the colon and rectum, which together make up the large intestine, also known as the *large bowel.* Colorectal cancer (CRC) is cancer of the colon or rectum. In the United States, it is the fourth most common malignancy and second most common cause of cancer-related death among adults (National Cancer Institute, 2021). Patients often consider a diagnosis of cancer as a "death sentence," but colon cancer is highly curable for many patients, especially if detected early.

Pathophysiology Review

Tumors occur in different areas of the colon, with more than half occurring within the rectosigmoid region as shown in Fig. 48.2. Most CRCs are adenocarcinomas, which are tumors that arise from the glandular epithelial tissue of the colon. Abnormal cellular regulation develops as a multistep process affecting immunity, resulting in several molecular changes. These changes include loss of key tumor suppressor genes and activation of certain oncogenes that alter colonic mucosa cell division. The increased proliferation of the colonic mucosa forms polyps that can become malignant tumors. Most CRCs are believed to arise from adenomatous **polyps** that present as small growths

covered with mucosa and attached to the surface of the intestine (Rogers, 2023).

CRC can metastasize by direct extension or by spreading through the blood or lymph. The tumor may spread locally into the four layers of the bowel wall and into neighboring organs. It may enlarge into the lumen of the bowel or spread through the lymphatics or the circulatory system. CRC enters the circulatory system directly from the primary tumor through blood vessels in the bowel or via the lymphatic system. The liver is the most common site of metastasis from circulatory spread. Metastasis to the lungs, brain, bones, and adrenal glands may also occur. Colon tumors can also spread by peritoneal seeding during surgical resection of the tumor. Seeding may occur when a tumor is excised, and cancer cells break off from the tumor into the peritoneal cavity. Chapter 18 discusses cancer pathophysiology in more detail.

The major risk factors for the development of colorectal cancer (CRC) include age older than 50 years, genetic predisposition, and/or personal or family history of cancer. However, recently an increasing number of adults under 50 years of age are being diagnosed with CRC without a clear cause. Some diseases also predispose the patient to cancer, such as familial adenomatous polyposis (FAP), Crohn's disease, and ulcerative colitis (American Cancer Society [ACS], 2023a).

PATIENT-CENTERED CARE: GENETICS/GENOMICS

Colorectal Cancer

People with a first-degree relative (parent, sibling, or child) diagnosed with colorectal cancer (CRC) have a three- to fourfold increase in the risk for developing the disease. Many genes are associated with CRC. An autosomal dominant inherited genetic disorder known as *familial adenomatous polyposis (FAP)* accounts for 1% of CRCs. FAP is the result of one or more mutations in the adenomatous polyposis coli *(APC)* gene. These patients develop thousands of adenomatous polyps over the course of 10 to 15 years. Adenomatous polyps have nearly a 100% chance of becoming malignant (Rogers, 2023). By 20 years of age, most patients require surgical intervention, usually a colectomy with ileostomy or ileoanal pull-through, to prevent cancer.

Lynch syndrome, also known as *hereditary nonpolyposis colorectal cancer (HNPCC),* is another autosomal dominant disorder and accounts for 3% to 5% of all CRCs. Lynch syndrome is also caused by gene mutations, including mutations in *MLH1, MSH2, MSH6, PMS1,* and *PMS2.* People with these mutations have an 80% chance of developing CRC at an average of 45 years of age. They also tend to have a higher incidence of endometrial, ovarian, stomach, small bowel, brain, and ureteral cancers (ACS, 2023b). Genetic testing is available for both familial CRC syndromes.

The role of infectious agents in the development of colorectal and anal cancer continues to be investigated. Some lower GI cancers are related to *Helicobacter pylori, Streptococcus bovis,* and human papillomavirus (HPV) infections.

There is also strong evidence that long-term smoking, obesity, physical inactivity, and heavy alcohol consumption are risk factors for CRC (ACS, 2023a). A high-fat diet, particularly animal fat from red meats, increases bile acid secretion and anaerobic bacteria, which are thought to be carcinogenic for the bowel.

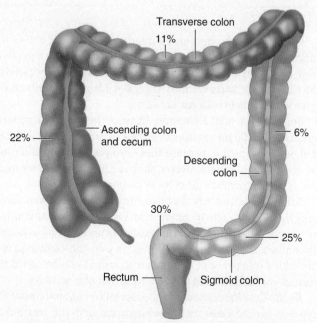

Transverse colon
11%

Ascending colon and cecum
22%

6%

Descending colon

30%

25%

Rectum

Sigmoid colon

FIG. 48.2 Incidence of cancer in relation to colorectal anatomy.

♥ BOX 48.3 MEETING *HEALTHY PEOPLE 2030* OBJECTIVES

Colorectal Cancer

To improve the health of adults, specific objectives related to colorectal cancer include:
- Reduce the colorectal cancer death rate.
- Increase the proportion of adults who get screened for colorectal cancer.

Diets with large amounts of refined carbohydrates that lack fiber decrease bowel transit time, which predisposes individuals to polyp formation.

Health Promotion/Disease Prevention

People at high risk can take action to decrease their chance of getting CRC. For example, teach patients whose family members have had hereditary CRC to get genetically tested for FAP and Lynch syndrome. If genetic mutations are present, the person at risk can collaborate with the health care team to decide which prevention or treatment plan to implement.

The *Healthy People 2030* initiative recognizes the need for national attention to the reduction of new cases of cancer and cancer-related illness, disability, and death (Box 48.3).

Teach adults about the need for diagnostic screening. Be aware that screening rates are lowest among uninsured and uneducated (less than high school education) adults (see the Patient-Centered Care: Health Equity box).

When adults turn 40 years of age, they should discuss with their primary health care providers the need for colon cancer screening. The interval depends on level of risk. Adults of average risk who are 45 years of age and older and without a family history should undergo regular CRC screening as recommended by the American Cancer Society (ACS, 2023a). The ACS screening options include stool-based testing, including fecal occult blood testing (FOBT) and multitargeted stool DNA (mt-sDNA) testing. FOBT should be completed yearly and mt-sDNA every 3 years. The ACS also recommends visual/structural exams, including a colonoscopy every 10 years or a flexible sigmoidoscopy or CT colonography every 5 years. Adults who have a personal or family history of the disease should begin frequent screening earlier (see the Legal/Ethical Considerations box).

⚖ LEGAL/ETHICAL CONSIDERATIONS

Screening for Colorectal Cancer

Regular screening for CRC is not recommended for individuals who are older than 85 years due to the risks associated with cancer treatment (ACS, 2023a). As a result, for those over 85 who are diagnosed with CRC, surgery is withheld. Screening for those between 75 and 85 years of age is optional, depending on predicted life expectancy. However, the incidence of CRC is increasing in people 80 years of age and older. These factors have raised ethical questions about when CRC screening should start and stop (Turshudzhyan et al., 2021).

Nurses need to play a role in ethical decisions that affect the quality of life. When all individuals have access to necessary CRC screening and cancer treatment, the ethical principle of justice is maintained.

Teach adults, regardless of risk, to modify their diets as needed to decrease fat, refined carbohydrates, and low-fiber foods. Obesity is a major risk factor for most types of cancer. Encourage baked or broiled foods, especially those high in fiber and low in animal fat. Remind adults to eat increased amounts of vegetables, including broccoli, cabbage, cauliflower, and sprouts. Assess the patient for food security, and refer the patient to community resources if needed.

Educate about the hazards of smoking, excessive alcohol, and physical inactivity. Refer patients as needed for smoking- or alcohol-cessation programs, and recommend ways to increase regular physical exercise, if possible. If cessation programs are offered online, assess whether the patient has access to high-speed Internet services and a digital device.

👤 PATIENT-CENTERED CARE: HEALTH EQUITY

Colorectal Cancer Disparities

Although deaths from colorectal cancer (CRC) have decreased over the past 30 years, the 5-year survival rates are lowest for Black individuals, especially those under 50 years of age, when compared to all other racial groups. Mortality is 30% to 40% higher among residents of poor regions, including those in Appalachia and in parts of the South and Midwest (ACS, 2023a). Social determinants of health that contribute to this health inequity include lack of access to CRC screening, lack of health insurance, low formal education (less than high school), and lack of innovative cancer care (ACS, 2023a). When working with individuals from poor geographic regions, be sure to teach them about the need for early CRC screening, and provide information about resources for screening and care.

Interprofessional Collaborative Care

Care for the patient with CRC usually takes place in a variety of health care settings. The interprofessional team that collaborates to care for this patient generally includes the surgeon, oncologist, and nurse and may include the registered dietitian, psychologist, social worker, and spiritual leader of the patient's choice.

Assessment: Recognize Cues

Physical Assessment/Signs and Symptoms. Ask the patient about vomiting and changes in bowel *elimination* habits, such as constipation or change in shape of stool with or without blood. The patient may also report fatigue (related to anemias), abdominal fullness, vague abdominal pain, or unintentional weight loss. These symptoms suggest advanced disease.

Additional signs and symptoms of CRC depend on the location of the tumor. *However, the most common signs are rectal bleeding, anemia, and a change in stool consistency or shape.* Stools may contain microscopic amounts of blood that are occult (hidden), or the patient may have mahogany (dark)-colored or bright red stools (Fig. 48.3). Gross blood is not usually detected with tumors of the ascending colon, but it is common (but not massive) with tumors of the descending colon and the rectum.

Tumors in the transverse and descending colon result in symptoms of obstruction as growth of the tumor blocks the passage of stool. The patient may report "gas pains," cramping,

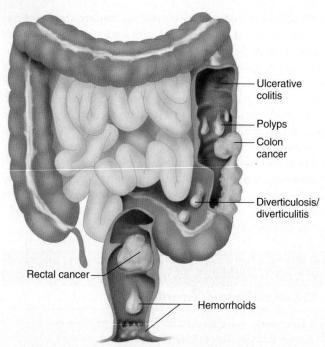

FIG. 48.3 Common causes of lower gastrointestinal bleeding.

Ulcerative colitis

Polyps

Colon cancer

Diverticulosis/ diverticulitis

Rectal cancer

Hemorrhoids

or incomplete evacuation. Tumors in the rectosigmoid colon are associated with hematochezia (the passage of red blood via the rectum), straining to pass stools, and narrowing of stools. Patients may report dull pain. Right-sided tumors can grow quite large without disrupting bowel patterns or appearance because the stool consistency is more liquid in this part of the colon. These tumors ulcerate and bleed intermittently; consequently, stools can contain mahogany (dark)-colored blood. A mass may be palpated in the lower right quadrant, and the patient often has anemia secondary to blood loss (Rogers, 2023).

Laboratory Assessment. A positive test result for occult (microscopic) blood in the stool (fecal occult blood test [FOBT] or fecal immunochemical test [FIT]) indicates bleeding in the GI tract. These tests can yield false-positive results if certain vitamins or drugs are taken before the test. Depending on the type of test being used, the patient may need to avoid aspirin, vitamin C, iron, and red meat for 48 hours before giving a stool specimen. Also assess whether the patient is taking antiinflammatory drugs (e.g., ibuprofen, corticosteroids, or salicylates). These drugs should be discontinued for a designated period before the test. For the FOBT, two or three separate stool samples should be tested on 3 consecutive days. Negative results do not completely rule out the possibility of CRC; for this reason, additional testing may be suggested (Pagana et al., 2022).

Carcinoembryonic antigen (CEA), an oncofetal antigen, is elevated in many people with CRC. The normal value is less than 5 ng/mL (Pagana et al., 2022). This protein is not specifically associated with CRC, and it may be elevated in the presence of other benign or malignant diseases and in smokers. CEA is often used to monitor the effectiveness of treatment and to identify disease recurrence.

Other Diagnostic Assessment. CT-guided virtual colonoscopy is a less invasive option for colorectal imaging. This test utilizes a CT scan and special computer software to examine the rectum and colon. It is thought to be more thorough than traditional invasive colonoscopy. However, treatments, biopsies, and surgeries cannot be performed when a virtual colonoscopy is used.

A *sigmoidoscopy* provides visualization of the lower colon using a fiberoptic scope. Polyps can be visualized, and tissue samples can be taken for biopsy. Polyps are usually removed during the procedure. A *colonoscopy* provides views of the entire large bowel from the rectum to the ileocecal valve. As with sigmoidoscopy, polyps can be seen and removed, and tissue samples can be taken for biopsy. *Colonoscopy is the definitive test for the diagnosis of colorectal cancer.* These procedures and associated nursing care are discussed in Chapter 45.

Take Actions: Interventions

The primary approach to treating CRC is to remove the entire tumor or as much of the tumor as possible to prevent or slow metastatic spread of the disease. A patient-centered collaborative care approach is essential to meet the desired outcomes.

Although surgical resection is the primary method used to control the disease, several adjuvant (additional) therapies are used. Adjuvant therapies are administered before or after surgery with a goal to cure and prevent recurrence, if possible.

Nonsurgical Management. The type of therapy used is based on the pathologic staging of the disease. The staging system used most often in colorectal cancer is the TNM (tumor, nodes, metastasis) classification; more information on the use of this system can be found in Chapter 18.

The administration of preoperative *radiation therapy* has not improved overall survival rates for colon cancer, but it has been effective in providing local or regional control of the disease. Postoperative radiation has not demonstrated any consistent improvement in survival or recurrence. However, as a palliative measure, radiation therapy may be used to control pain, hemorrhage, bowel obstruction, or metastasis to the lung in advanced disease. For rectal cancer, unlike colon cancer, radiation therapy is often a part of the treatment plan. Reinforce information about the radiation therapy procedure to the patient and family and monitor for possible side effects (e.g., diarrhea, fatigue). Chapter 18 describes the nursing care of patients undergoing radiation therapy.

Adjuvant *chemotherapy* after primary surgery is recommended for patients with stage II or stage III colorectal cancer to interrupt the DNA production of cells and destroy them. The drugs of choice are IV 5-fluorouracil with leucovorin (5-FU/LV), capecitabine, irinotecan hydrochloride, and oxaliplatin (Burchum & Rosenthal, 2022). These drugs can be used individually but are generally used in combination for the greatest treatment benefit. As with other chemotherapeutic drugs, these agents cannot discriminate between cancer and healthy cells. Therefore, common side effects are diarrhea, mucositis, leukopenia, mouth ulcers, and peripheral neuropathy. Some patients report that complementary and integrative therapies, including cannabis, are useful to minimize these side effects (Clark, 2021).

Bevacizumab is an angiogenesis inhibitor, also known as a *vascular endothelial growth factor (VEGF) inhibitor,* approved for metastatic CRC. This drug reduces blood flow to the growing tumor cells, thereby depriving them of necessary nutrients needed to grow (Burchum & Rosenthal, 2022). A VEGF inhibitor is usually given in combination with other chemotherapeutic agents.

Cetuximab and panitumumab are monoclonal antibodies known as *epidermal growth factor receptor (EGFR) inhibitors (EGFRIs)* and may also be given in combination with other drugs for metastatic disease (Burchum & Rosenthal, 2022). These drugs work by blocking factors that promote cancer cell growth.

Intrahepatic arterial chemotherapy, often with 5-fluorouracil (5-FU), may be administered to patients with liver metastasis. Patients with CRC also receive drugs for relief of symptoms, such as opioid analgesics and antiemetics. Chapter 18 describes the care of patients receiving chemotherapy in detail.

Surgical Management. Surgical removal of the tumor with margins free of disease is the best method of ensuring removal of CRC. Many factors help to determine the surgical approach for colorectal cancer; these include the size of the tumor, its location, the extent of metastasis, integrity of the bowel, and condition of the patient. During surgery a number of lymph nodes are removed and examined for the presence of cancer. The number of lymph nodes that contain cancer is a strong predictor of prognosis. The most common surgeries performed are colon resection (removal of part of the colon and regional lymph nodes) with reanastomosis, partial colectomy with a *colostomy (temporary or permanent)* or total colectomy with an *ileostomy/ileoanal pull-through,* and *abdominoperineal resection.* A colostomy is the surgical creation of an opening (stoma) of the colon onto the surface of the abdomen to allow passage of stool. An abdominoperineal (AP) resection is performed when rectal tumors are present. In this procedure, the surgeon removes the sigmoid colon, rectum, and anus through combined abdominal and perineal incisions.

For patients having a colon resection, minimally invasive surgery (MIS) via laparoscopy is a common surgical approach. MIS results in shorter hospital stays, less pain, fewer complications, and quicker recovery compared with the conventional open surgical approach (American Society of Colon & Rectal Surgeons [ASCRS], 2023b).

Preoperative Care. Reinforce the surgeon's explanation of the planned procedure. It is important that the patient understand the anatomic and physiologic changes that may occur with surgery. This includes the location and number of incision sites and drains.

Before evaluating the tumor and colon during surgery, the surgeon may be unable to determine whether a colostomy (or, less commonly, an ileostomy) will be necessary. The patient is told that a colostomy is a possibility. If a colostomy is planned, the surgeon consults a certified wound, ostomy, and continence nurse (CWOCN, sometimes referred to as the WOC nurse) to recommend optimal placement of the ostomy. The CWOCN teaches the patient about the rationale and general principles of ostomy care. In many settings, the CWOCN marks the patient's abdomen to indicate a potential ostomy site that will decrease the risk for complications, such as interference from

undergarments or a prosthesis with the ostomy appliance. Box 48.4 describes the preoperative role of the CWOCN.

The patient who requires low rectal surgery (e.g., abdominoperineal resection) is faced with the risk for postoperative sexual dysfunction and urinary incontinence after surgery due to nerve damage during surgery. The surgeon discusses the risk for these problems with the patient before surgery and allows the patient to verbalize concerns and questions related to this risk before giving informed consent. To reinforce teaching about abdominal surgery performed for the patient under general anesthesia and review the routines for turning and deep breathing, see Chapter 9. Teach the patient about the method of *pain* management to be used after surgery, such as IV patient-controlled analgesia (PCA), epidural analgesia, or other method.

If the bowel is not obstructed or perforated, elective surgery is planned. The patient may be instructed to complete a "bowel prep" to minimize bacterial growth and prevent complications. Mechanical cleaning is accomplished with laxatives and enemas or with "whole-gut lavage." The use of bowel preps is controversial, and some surgeons do not recommend it. For example, older adults may become dehydrated from this process.

To reduce the risk for infection, the surgeon may prescribe one dose of oral or IV antibiotics to be given before the surgical incision is made. Teach patients that a nasogastric tube (NGT) may be placed for decompression of the stomach after conventional open surgery. A peripheral IV or central venous catheter is also placed for fluid and electrolyte replacement while the patient is NPO after surgery. Patients who undergo minimally invasive surgery do not need an NGT.

The patient with colorectal cancer faces a serious illness with long-term consequences of the disease and treatment. A case manager or social worker can be very helpful in identifying patient and family needs and ensuring continuity of care and support.

BOX 48.4 Best Practice for Safety and Quality Care

Preoperative Assessment by the CWOCN Before Ostomy Surgery

Key Points of Psychosocial Assessment

Perform the following patient assessments:

- Knowledge level of disease and ostomy care
- Educational level
- Physical limitations (particularly sensory)
- Available support and resources
- Employment
- Involvement in hobbies and activities
- Financial concerns regarding purchase of ostomy supplies

Key Points of Physical Assessment

Before marking the placement for the ostomy, consider:

- Contour of the abdomen in lying, sitting, and standing positions
- Presence of skinfolds, creases, bony prominences, and scars
- Location of belt line
- Location that is easily visible to the patient
- Possible location in the rectus muscle

CWOCN, Certified wound, ostomy, and continence nurse.

Operative Procedures. For the conventional open surgical approach, the surgeon makes a large incision in the abdomen and explores the abdominal cavity to determine whether the tumor can be removed. For a colon resection, the portion of the colon with the tumor is excised, and the two open ends of the bowel are irrigated before anastomosis (reattachment) of the colon. If an anastomosis is not feasible because of the location of the tumor or inflammation of the bowel, a colostomy is created.

A temporary or permanent colostomy may be created in the ascending, transverse, descending, or sigmoid colon (Fig. 48.4). One of several techniques is used to construct a colostomy. A loop stoma (surgical opening) is made by bringing a loop of colon to the skin surface, severing, and everting the anterior wall, and suturing it to the abdominal wall. Loop colostomies are usually performed in the transverse colon and are usually temporary. An external rod may be used to support the loop until the intestinal tissue adheres to the abdominal wall. Care must be taken to avoid displacing the rod, especially during appliance changes.

An end stoma is often constructed, usually in the descending or sigmoid colon, when a colostomy is intended to be permanent. It may also be done when the surgeon oversews the distal stump of the colon and places it in the abdominal cavity, preserving it for future reattachment. An end stoma is constructed by severing the end of the proximal portion of the bowel and bringing it out through the abdominal wall.

The least common colostomy is the *double-barrel stoma*, which is created by dividing the bowel and bringing both the proximal and distal portions to the abdominal surface to create two stomas. The proximal stoma (closest to the patient's head) is the functioning stoma and eliminates stool. The distal stoma (farthest from the head) is considered nonfunctioning, although it may secrete some mucus. The distal stoma is sometimes referred to as a *mucous fistula*.

Laparoscopic (MIS) colon resection or total colectomy allows complete tumor removal with an adequate surgical margin and removal of associated lymph nodes. Several small incisions are made, and a miniature video camera is placed within the abdomen to help see the area that is involved. This technique takes longer than the conventional procedure and requires specialized training. However, blood loss and postoperative pain are reduced.

Postoperative Care. Patients who have an *open colon resection* without a colostomy receive care like those having any abdominal surgery (see Chapter 9). They typically have a nasogastric tube (NGT) after open surgery and receive IV PCA for the first 24 to 36 hours. After NGT removal, the diet is slowly progressed from liquids to solid foods as tolerated. The care of patients with an NGT is found in the Interventions discussion in the Intestinal Obstruction section earlier in this chapter.

By contrast, patients who have *laparoscopic surgery* (MIS) can eat solid foods very soon after the procedure. Because they

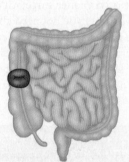

The **ascending colostomy** is done for right-sided tumors.

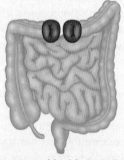

The **transverse (double-barrel) colostomy** is often used in such emergencies as intestinal obstruction or perforation because it can be created quickly. There are two stomas. The proximal one, closest to the small intestine, drains feces. The distal stoma drains mucus.

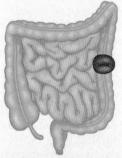

The **descending colostomy** is done for left-sided tumors.

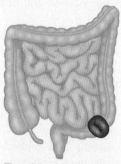

The **sigmoid colostomy** is done for rectal tumors.

FIG. 48.4 Different locations of colostomies in the colon.

usually have less *pain* and are at risk for fewer postoperative complications, they can ambulate and heal earlier than those who undergo the conventional approach. The hospital stay is usually shorter for the patient with MIS—typically 1 to 2 days, depending on the patient's age and general condition.

Colostomy Management. After a colostomy has been performed, the patient may return from surgery with a clear ostomy pouch system in place. A clear pouch allows the health care team to observe the stoma. If no pouch system is in place, a petrolatum gauze dressing is usually placed over the stoma to keep it moist. This is covered with a dry, sterile dressing. In collaboration with the CWOCN, place a pouch system as soon as possible. The colostomy pouch system, also called an *appliance,* allows more convenient and suitable collection of stool than a dressing does. Pouches are available in both one- and two-piece systems and are held in place by adhesive barriers or wafers.

Assess the color and integrity of the stoma frequently. A healthy stoma should be reddish pink (or dark red to pink) and moist and protrude about 1 to 3 cm from the abdominal wall but most commonly about 2 cm (Fig. 48.5). During the initial postoperative period, the stoma may be slightly edematous. A small amount of bleeding at the stoma is common. These minor problems tend to resolve within 6 to 8 weeks (Stelton, 2019).

> ### ⚠ NURSING SAFETY PRIORITY
> #### *Action Alert*
>
> Report any of these early postoperative stoma problems to the surgeon immediately:
> - Stoma ischemia and necrosis (dark red, purplish, or black color; dry)
> - Continuous heavy bleeding
> - Mucocutaneous separation (breakdown of the suture line securing the stoma to the abdominal wall)

Assess the condition of the peristomal skin (skin around the stoma), and frequently check the pouch system for proper fit and signs of leakage. The skin should be intact, smooth, and without redness/hyperpigmentation or excoriation. Monitor for common peristomal skin complications, including irritant dermatitis (from fecal content), skin stripping (from the adhesive barrier or wafer), and candidiasis (fungal infection under the barrier or wafer) (Stelton, 2019).

Teach patients that the colostomy typically starts to function 2 to 3 days after surgery. When it begins to function, the pouch may need to be emptied frequently because of excess gas collection. It should be emptied when it is one-third to one-half full of stool. Stool is typically more liquid immediately after surgery but becomes more solid, depending on where in the colon the stoma was placed. For example, stool from an ascending colon colostomy continues to be liquid, stool from a transverse colon colostomy becomes pasty, and stool from a descending colon colostomy becomes more solid (similar to stool expelled from the rectum).

Wound Management. For an AP resection, the perineal wound is generally surgically closed, and two bulb suction drains (Jackson-Pratt drains) are typically placed in the wound or through laparoscopic incisions near the wound. The drains help prevent drainage from collecting within the wound and are usually left in place for several days, depending on the character and amount of drainage. These drains are described in more detail in Chapter 9.

Monitoring drainage from the perineal wound and cavity is important because of the possibility of infection and abscess formation. Serosanguineous drainage from the perineal wound may be observed for 1 to 2 months after surgery. Complete healing of the perineal wound may take 6 to 8 months. This wound can be a greater source of *pain* than the abdominal incision and ostomy, and more care may be required. The patient may experience phantom rectal sensations because sympathetic innervation for rectal control has not been interrupted. Rectal pain and itching may occasionally occur after healing. Interventions may include use of antipruritic drugs, such as benzocaine, or warm compresses. Continually assess for signs of infection, abscess, or other complications, and implement methods for promoting wound drainage and comfort (Box 48.5).

> ### NCLEX Examination Challenge 48.2
> #### *Safe and Effective Care Environment*
>
> The nurse is planning care for a client who returned from PACU after an abdominoperineal (AP) resection of a rectal malignant tumor. What would the nurse anticipate as the client's **priority** problem?
> A. Nausea and vomiting
> B. Infection
> C. Pain
> D. Incontinence

Care Coordination and Transition Management

The patient and family are faced with a possible alteration in body functions. Medical and surgical interventions for the treatment of colorectal cancer may result in cure, disease control, or palliation. Nursing care is designed to help the patient and family plan effective strategies for expressing feelings of grief and to develop coping skills.

Collaborate with the case manager to help patients and their families cope with the immediate postoperative phase of recovery. After hospitalization for surgery, the patient is usually managed at

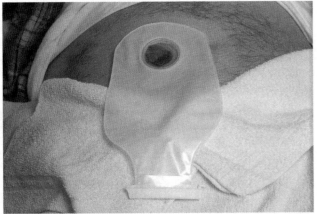

FIG. 48.5 Mature colostomy stoma. (From Stromberg, H. K. [2023]. *Medical-surgical nursing: Concepts and practice* [5th ed.]. St. Louis: Elsevier.)

BOX 48.5 Best Practice for Patient Safety and Quality Care

Perineal Wound Care

Wound Care
- Place an absorbent dressing (e.g., abdominal pad) over the wound.
- Instruct patients that they may:
  - Use a feminine napkin as a dressing
  - Wear jockey-type shorts rather than boxers

Comfort Measures
- If prescribed, soak the wound area in a sitz bath for 10 to 20 minutes three or four times per day, or use warm compresses.
- Administer an analgesic as prescribed and assess effectiveness.
- Instruct the patient about permissible activities. The patient should:
  - Assume a side-lying position in bed
  - Avoid sitting for long periods
  - Use foam pads or a soft pillow on which to sit whenever in a sitting position
  - Avoid the use of air rings or rubber donut devices

Prevention of Complications
- Maintain **fluid and electrolyte balance** by monitoring patient intake and output, including output from the perineal wound.
- Observe incision integrity and monitor wound drains; watch for erythema/hyperpigmentation, edema, bleeding, drainage, unusual odor, and excessive or constant **pain.**

home. Radiation therapy or chemotherapy is typically administered on an ambulatory care basis. For the patient with advanced cancer, hospice care may be an option (see Chapter 8).

Home Care Management. Assess all patients for their ability for self-management within limitations. For those requiring assistance with care, home health visits by nurses or assistive nursing personnel can be provided.

For the patient who has undergone a colostomy, review the home situation to help the patient arrange for care. Ostomy products should be kept in an area (preferably the bathroom) where the temperature is neither hot nor cold (skin barriers may become stiff or melt in extreme temperatures) to ensure proper functioning.

Self-Management Education. Before discharge, teach the patient to avoid lifting heavy objects or straining on defecation to prevent tension on the anastomosis site. If an open surgical approach is used, the patient should avoid driving and vigorous physical activity for 4 to 6 weeks while the incision heals. Patients who have undergone laparoscopy can usually return to all usual activities in 1 to 2 weeks.

Ongoing Colostomy Care. Rehabilitation after surgery requires that patients and family members or other caregivers learn how to perform colostomy care. Provide adequate opportunity before discharge for patients to learn the psychomotor skills involved in this care. Plan sufficient practice time for learning how to handle, assemble, and apply all ostomy equipment. Teach patients and families or other caregivers about:
- Appearance of a normal stoma
- Signs and symptoms of complications
- Measurement of the stoma
- Choice, use, care, and application of the appropriate appliance for the stoma
- Measures to protect the skin adjacent to the stoma
- Nutrition changes to control gas and odor
- What to expect in terms of stool consistency
- Resumption of normal activities, including work, travel, and sexual intercourse

The appropriate pouch system must be selected and fitted to the stoma. Patients with flat, firm abdomens may use either flexible (bordered with paper tape) or nonflexible (full skin barrier wafer) pouch systems. A firm abdomen with lateral creases or folds requires a flexible system. Patients with deep creases, flabby abdomens, a retracted stoma, or a stoma that is flush or concave to the abdominal surface can benefit from a convex appliance with a stoma belt. This type of system presses into the skin around the stoma, causing the stoma to protrude. Protrusion helps tighten the skin and prevents leaks around the stoma opening onto the peristomal skin.

Measurement of the stoma is necessary to determine the correct size of the stoma opening on the appliance. The opening should be large enough not only to cover the peristomal skin but also to avoid stoma trauma. The stoma shrinks within 6 to 8 weeks after surgery. Therefore, it needs to be measured at least once weekly during this time to gauge appliance fit and comfort. Measurements are also necessary if the patient gains or loses weight. Teach the patient and family caregiver to trace the pattern of the stoma area on the wafer portion of the appliance and to cut an opening about ⅛- to 1/16-inch larger than the stoma pattern to ensure that stoma tissue will not be constricted.

Skin preparation may include clipping peristomal hair or shaving the area (moving from the stoma outward) to achieve a smooth surface, prevent unnecessary discomfort when the wafer is removed, and minimize the risk for infected hair follicles. Advise the patient to clean around the stoma with mild soap and water before putting on an appliance. The patient should avoid using moisturizing soaps to clean the area because the lubricants can interfere with adhesion of the appliance.

❗ NURSING SAFETY PRIORITY

Action Alert

Stool softeners may be prescribed to keep stools soft in consistency for ease of passage. Teach patients to note the frequency, amount, and character of the stools. In addition to this information, teach those with colon resections to watch for and report signs and symptoms of intestinal obstruction and perforation (e.g., cramping, abdominal pain, nausea, vomiting). Advise the patient to avoid gas-producing foods and carbonated beverages. The patient may require 4 to 6 weeks to establish the effects of certain foods on bowel patterns.

❗ NURSING SAFETY PRIORITY

Action Alert

Teach the patient and family to use a skin sealant (preferably without alcohol) and allow it to dry before application of the appliance (colostomy pouch) to facilitate less painful removal of the tape or adhesive. If peristomal skin becomes raw (skin stripping), stoma powder or paste or a combination may also be applied. The paste or other filler cream is also used to fill in crevices and creases to create a flat surface for the flange of the colostomy bag. If the patient develops a fungal rash (candidiasis), an antifungal cream or powder should be used.

Control of gas and odor from the colostomy is often an important issue for patients with new ostomies. Although a leaking or inadequately closed pouch is the usual cause of odor, flatus can also contribute to it. Remind the patient with an ostomy that although, in general, no foods are forbidden, certain foods (such as vegetables) can cause flatus or contribute to odor when the pouch is open. Charcoal filters, pouch deodorizers, or placement of a breath mint in the pouch helps eliminate odors. The patient should be cautioned to not put aspirin tablets in the pouch because they may cause ulceration of the stoma. Vents that allow release of gas from the ostomy bag through a deodorizing filter are available and may decrease the patient's level of self-consciousness about odor.

The patient with a sigmoid colostomy may benefit from colostomy irrigation to regulate *elimination.* However, most patients with a sigmoid colostomy can become regulated through diet. Irrigation is similar to an enema but is administered through the stoma rather than the rectum.

Some patients require one or more home health visits by a nurse who assesses the patient for physical and psychosocial needs (Box 48.6).

Psychosocial Concerns. The diagnosis of cancer can be an emotional process for the patient and family or significant others, but treatment may be welcomed because it may provide hope for control of the disease. Explore reactions to the illness and perceptions of planned interventions.

The patient's reaction to ostomy surgery may include:

- Fear of not being accepted by others
- Feelings of grief related to disturbance in body image
- Concerns about sexuality (see the Evidence-Based Practice box)

🏠 BOX 48.6 Home Health Care

The Patient With a Colostomy

Assess gastrointestinal status, including:
- Dietary and fluid intake and habits
- Presence or absence of nausea and vomiting
- Weight gain or loss
- Bowel *elimination* pattern and characteristics and amount of effluent stool
- Bowel sounds

Assess condition of stoma at least weekly, including:
- Location, size, protrusion, color, and integrity (check for stoma retraction, prolapse, or stenosis)
- Presence of peristomal hernia
- Pain or swelling
- Signs of ischemia, such as dull coloring or dark or purplish bruising

Assess peristomal skin for:
- Presence or absence of excoriated skin, leakage underneath drainage system
- Presence of folliculitis (inflammation of hair follicles) or dermatitis (inflammation of skin)
- Fit of appliance and effectiveness of skin barrier and appliance

Assess the patient's and family's coping skills, including:
- Self-care abilities
- Acknowledgment of changes in body image and function
- Sense of loss

📄 EVIDENCE-BASED PRACTICE

Does Colorectal Cancer Surgery Affect Sexuality

Jakobson, J. (2021). State of recovery six months after rectal cancer surgery. *Gastroenterology, 44*(2), 98–105.

The researchers surveyed patients who had undergone several types of surgery (anterior resection and abdominoperineal [AP] resection) for colorectal cancer to determine what symptoms they might be experiencing 6 months after their procedures. Self-reported data were analyzed from 117 patients associated with one tertiary care center. All patients reported issues with sexual activity, but those who had anterior resections had more problems with mild GI symptoms when compared with those who had AP resection.

Level of Evidence: 4
This study was descriptive, or nonexperimental.

Commentary: Implications for Practice and Research
Few studies have been conducted to explore the quality of life for patients who have colorectal cancer surgery. This study indicates the need for nurses to prepare patients preoperatively for what they can expect after surgery, including sexuality problems. More research is needed to determine specific sexuality issues and how they may be managed.

Encourage the patient and family to verbalize their feelings. Education about how to physically manage the ostomy will empower both the family and patient to begin restoration of self-esteem and improvement of body image. Inclusion of family and significant others in the rehabilitation process may help preserve relationships and raise self-esteem. Anticipatory instruction includes information on leakage accidents, odor control measures, and adjustments to resuming sexual relationships.

Health Care Resources. Several resources are available to maintain continuity of care in the home environment and provide for patient needs that the nurse is not able to meet. Make referrals to community-based case managers or social workers who can provide further emotional counseling, aid in managing financial concerns, or arrange for services in the home or long-term care facility as needed.

Provide information about the United Ostomy Associations of America (UOAA) (www.ostomy.org), an advocacy group for people with ostomies. The UOAA website has literature, online resources, and information about local support groups. The organization conducts a visitor program that sends specially trained visitors (who have an ostomy ["ostomate"]) to talk with patients. After obtaining consent, make a referral to the visitor program so that the volunteer ostomate can see the patient both before and after surgery. A primary health care provider's consent for visitation may be necessary.

The local division or unit of the American Cancer Society (ACS) (www.cancer.org) can help provide necessary medical equipment and supplies, home care services, travel accommodations, and other resources for the patient who is having cancer treatment or surgery. Inform the patient and family of the programs available through the local division or unit. Other excellent Internet resources include Cancer Care (www.cancercare.org), the Colorectal Cancer Alliance (www.ccalliance.org), and the National Cancer Institute (www.cancer.gov).

The Canadian Cancer Society (www.cancer.ca) is an excellent resource for patients who live in Canada.

Because of short hospital stays, patients with new ostomies receive much health teaching from nurses who work for home health care agencies. This resource also helps provide physical care needs, medication management, and emotional support. If the patient has advanced colorectal cancer, a referral for hospice services in the home, nursing home, or other long-term care setting may be appropriate. The home health care nurse informs the patient and family about which ostomy supplies are needed and where they can be purchased. Price and location are considered before recommendations are made.

NCLEX Examination Challenge 48.3

Physiological Integrity

The nurse is teaching a postoperative client about ascending colostomy care. Which of the following statements would the nurse include in the health teaching? **Select all that apply.**

A. "Your stoma should remain reddish pink or dark red."
B. "Empty your appliance when it is completely full."
C. "You don't need to wear your appliance at all times."
D. "The stoma will shrink a little about 6 weeks after surgery."
E. "Be sure to use a skin sealant before applying your appliance."

IRRITABLE BOWEL SYNDROME

Irritable bowel syndrome (IBS) is a functional GI disorder that causes chronic or recurrent diarrhea, constipation, and/or abdominal *pain* and bloating. It is sometimes referred to as *spastic colon, mucous colon,* or *nervous colon.*

Pathophysiology Review

IBS is the most common digestive disorder seen in clinical practice and occurs in 10% to 15% of the population worldwide (Rogers, 2023). IBS causes GI motility changes, and increased or decreased bowel transit times result in changes in the normal *elimination* pattern to one of these classifications: diarrhea (IBS-D), constipation (IBS-C), or a mix of diarrhea and constipation (IBS-M). Symptoms of the disease typically begin to appear in young adulthood and continue throughout the patient's life.

The etiology of IBS remains unclear. Research suggests that a combination of environmental, immunologic, genetic, hormonal, and stress factors play a role in the development and course of the disorder. Examples of environmental factors include foods and fluids such as caffeinated or carbonated beverages and dairy products. Infectious agents have also been identified. Several studies have found that patients with IBS often have small-bowel bacterial overgrowth, which causes bloating and abdominal distention. Multiple normal flora and pathogenic agents have been identified, including *Pseudomonas aeruginosa.* Researchers believe that these agents are less causative and serve as measurable biomarkers for the disease (Rogers, 2023).

Immunologic and genetic factors have also been associated with IBS, especially cytokine genes, including proinflammatory interleukins (ILs), such as IL-6 and IL-1β, and tumor necrosis factor–alpha (TNF-α). These findings may provide the basis for targeted drug therapy for the disease (Mitselou et al., 2020).

In the United States, women are two times more likely to have IBS than are men. This difference may be the result of hormonal differences. However, in other areas of the world, this distribution pattern may not occur.

Considerable evidence relates stress and mental or behavioral illness, especially anxiety and depression, to IBS. Many patients diagnosed with IBS meet the criteria for at least one primary mental health disorder. However, the *pain* and other chronic symptoms of the disease may lead to secondary mental health disorders. For example, when diarrhea is predominant, patients fear that there will be no bathroom facilities available and can become very anxious. As a result, they may not want to leave their homes or travel on trips where bathrooms are not always available. The long-term nature of dealing with a chronic disease for which there is no cure can lead to secondary depression in some patients (Anxiety & Depression Association of America, 2021).

Interprofessional Collaborative Care

Care for the patient with IBS usually takes place in the outpatient setting, although patients with severe cases of IBS may need be hospitalized due to impaired *fluid and electrolyte balance*.

Recognize Cues: Assessment

Ask the patient about a history of fatigue, malaise, abdominal *pain,* changes in the bowel pattern (constipation, diarrhea, or an alternating pattern of both) or consistency of stools, and the passage of mucus. Patients with IBS do not usually lose weight. Ask whether the patient has had any GI infections. Collect information on all drugs that the patient is taking because some can cause symptoms similar to those experienced with IBS. Ask about the patient's nutritional history, including the use of caffeinated drinks or beverages sweetened with sorbitol or fructose, which can cause bloating or diarrhea.

The course of the illness is specific to each patient. Most patients can identify factors that cause exacerbations, such as diet, stress, or anxiety. Food intolerance may be associated with IBS. Dairy products (e.g., for those with lactose intolerance or milk protein), raw fruits, and grains can contribute to bloating, flatulence (excessive gas [flatus] in the intestines), and abdominal distention. Patients may keep a food diary to record possible triggers for IBS symptoms.

A flare-up of worsening cramps, abdominal *pain,* and diarrhea and/or constipation may bring the patient to the primary health care provider. One of the *most common concerns of patients with IBS is pain in the left lower quadrant of the abdomen, although it is not always present.* Assess the location, intensity, and quality of the *pain.* Some patients have internal visceral (organ) hypersensitivity that can cause or contribute to it. Nausea may be associated with mealtime and defecation. The constipated stools are small and hard and are generally followed by several softer stools. The diarrheal stools are soft and watery, and mucus is often present. Patients with IBS often report belching, gas, anorexia, and bloating.

The patient generally appears well, with a stable weight, and nutritional and fluid status is within normal ranges. Inspect and auscultate the abdomen. Bowel sounds vary but are generally within normal range. With constipation, bowel sounds may be hypoactive; with severe diarrhea, they may be hyperactive.

Routine laboratory values (including a complete blood count [CBC], serum albumin, erythrocyte sedimentation rate [ESR], and stools for occult blood) remain normal in IBS. Some health care providers request a *hydrogen breath test* or small-bowel bacterial overgrowth breath test. When small-intestinal bacterial overgrowth or malabsorption of nutrients is present, an excess of hydrogen is produced. Some of this hydrogen is absorbed into the bloodstream and travels to the lungs, where it is exhaled. Patients with IBS often exhale an increased amount of hydrogen.

Inform patients they will need to be NPO (may have water) for at least 12 hours before the hydrogen breath test. At the beginning of the test, the patient blows into a hydrogen analyzer for a baseline reading. Next, a dose of lactulose is ingested, and additional breath samples are taken every 20 minutes for 1 to 2 hours (Pagana et al., 2022).

Take Actions: Interventions

The patient with IBS is usually managed on an ambulatory care basis and learns self-management strategies. Interventions include health teaching, drug therapy, and stress reduction. Some patients also use complementary and integrative therapies. A holistic approach to patient care is essential for positive outcomes.

Dietary fiber and bulk help produce bulky, soft stools and establish regular bowel *elimination* habits. The patient should ingest about 30 to 40 Gm of fiber each day. Eating regular meals, drinking 8 to 10 glasses of water each day, and chewing food slowly help promote normal bowel function.

Drug therapy depends on the main symptom of IBS. The primary health care provider may prescribe bulk-forming or antidiarrheal agents and/or newer drugs to control symptoms.

For the treatment of *constipation-predominant IBS (IBS-C)*, bulk-forming laxatives, such as psyllium hydrophilic mucilloid, are generally taken at mealtimes with a glass of water. The hydrophilic properties of these drugs help prevent dry, hard, or liquid stools. Lubiprostone is an oral laxative approved for women with IBS-C; this drug increases fluid in the intestines to promote bowel *elimination.* Teach the patient to take the drug with food and water. Linaclotide is one of the newest drugs for IBS-C; it works by stimulating guanylate cyclase receptors in the intestines to increase fluid and promote bowel transit time. The drug also helps relieve *pain* and cramping that are associated with IBS. Teach patients to take this drug once a day about 30 minutes before breakfast (Burchum & Rosenthal, 2022).

Diarrhea-predominant IBS (IBS-D) may be treated with antidiarrheal agents, such as loperamide and psyllium (a bulk-forming agent). Alosetron, a selective serotonin (5-HT3) receptor antagonist, may be used with caution in *women* with IBS-D as a last resort when they have not responded to conventional therapy (Burchum & Rosenthal, 2022). Patients taking this drug must agree to report symptoms of colitis or constipation early because it is associated with potentially life-threatening bowel complications, including ischemic colitis (lack of blood flow to the colon).

NURSING SAFETY PRIORITY
Drug Alert

Before the patient begins alosetron, take a thorough drug history (including alternative treatments), both prescribed and over the counter, because alosetron interacts with many drugs in a variety of classes. Remind patients that they should not take psychoactive drugs or antihistamines while taking alosetron. Teach patients to report severe constipation, fever, increasing abdominal *pain,* increasing fatigue, darkened urine, bloody diarrhea, or rectal bleeding as soon as it occurs and to stop the drug immediately (Burchum & Rosenthal, 2022).

Patients with IBS who have bloating and abdominal distention *without constipation* have success with rifaximin, an antibiotic that works locally with little systemic absorption. The U.S. Food and Drug Administration (FDA) originally approved this drug for "traveler's diarrhea," and it now has been approved for use in IBS-D (Burchum & Rosenthal, 2022).

For IBS in which *pain* is the predominant symptom, tricyclic antidepressants such as amitriptyline have also been used successfully. Evidence remains unclear whether their effectiveness is the result of the antidepressant or anticholinergic effects of the drugs. If patients have postprandial (after eating) *pain,* they should take these drugs 30 to 45 minutes before mealtime.

Complementary and Integrative Health. In cases in which patients have increased intestinal bacterial overgrowth, recommend daily probiotic supplements. *Probiotics* have been shown to be effective for reducing bacteria and successfully alleviating GI symptoms of IBS. There is also evidence that peppermint oil capsules may be effective in reducing symptoms for patients with IBS (Burchum & Rosenthal, 2022).

Stress management is also an important part of holistic care. Relaxation techniques, meditation, and/or yoga may help the patient decrease GI symptoms. If the patient has a stressful work or family situation, personal counseling may be helpful. Based on patient preference, make appropriate referrals, or assist in making appointments if needed. The opportunity to discuss problems and attempt creative problem solving is often helpful. Teach the patient that regular exercise is important for managing stress and promoting regular bowel *elimination.*

NCLEX Examination Challenge 48.4
Health Promotion and Maintenance

A nurse is teaching a client about best practices to promote colon health and elimination. Which recommendation would the nurse include?

A. "Eat low-fiber foods to increase stool consistency."
B. "Drink at least 8 to 10 glasses of water each day."
C. "Eat soft foods to avoid excessive chewing."
D. "Take laxatives each night to promote elimination."

ABDOMINAL TRAUMA

Pathophysiology Review

The abdomen contains structures and organs that are vital to physiologic homeostasis. Trauma is an injury caused by external forces; abdominal injuries are the third leading cause of death

(Urden et al., 2022). Abdominal trauma typically occurs in one of two ways—blunt or penetrating. Blunt trauma happens when the abdomen has a direct impact with an object (punch or kick) or an abrupt deceleration (motor vehicle crash or fall) (O'Rourke et al., 2022). Penetrating trauma occurs when an object penetrates the abdominal wall (most often knife [stab] and gunshot wounds) and causes damage to the structures of the abdomen (Lotfollahzadeh & Burns, 2022).

Abdominal trauma can damage the structures in the abdomen, including the stomach, liver, spleen, bladder, and small and large intestines. The severity of abdominal trauma varies depending on the force, nature, and *mechanism of injury (MOI)*. Blunt and penetrating trauma may cause hematomas, lacerations, or ruptures of abdominal organs and structures. If untreated, these injuries put the patient at risk for severe complications, including intraabdominal hemorrhage, infection (peritonitis or abscess), paralytic ileus, abdominal compartment syndrome, hypovolemic shock, and bowel obstruction (Van, 2022).

Two of the most common life-threatening complications are hemorrhage, which leads to hypovolemic shock, and hollow viscus perforation, which leads to septic shock. *Hemorrhage* frequently occurs when the liver or spleen is damaged. Based on diagnostic testing, these injuries are graded from I to V (the worst) based on the extent of the injury, including the percentage of organ that is injured (Urden et al., 2022). *Hollow viscus injuries* cause perforation of the stomach, small intestine, and/or colon. Gastrointestinal contents leak into the peritoneal cavity, causing peritonitis and sepsis.

Abdominal compartment syndrome is a serious complication of abdominal trauma that causes end-organ dysfunction caused by intraabdominal hypertension (IAH). It arises when damage to the abdomen causes capillaries in the intestine and mesentery to become leaky, producing edema in the tissues of the abdomen. The edema causes increased intraabdominal pressure, pain, organ compression, and ischemia. Surgical intervention is often necessary to decompress organs and prevent permanent organ damage and failure (Van, 2022)

Interprofessional Collaborative Care

Care for the patient with abdominal trauma takes place in the emergency department (ED) and hospital setting. The interprofessional care team for this patient generally includes the ED team, surgical team, and specially trained trauma nurses. Trauma nursing principles are described in Chapter 10 of this book.

Recognize Cues: Assessment

Before specifically assessing the patient's abdominal injury, complete the primary survey and any resuscitation interventions (see Chapter 10 for a detailed description of these assessments). After the interprofessional team addresses immediate life-threatening issues, ask the patient to relay the history of the mechanism of injury (MOI), if possible. Understanding the MOI can provide insight into the instrument, force, and scope of possible damage.

> ### BOX 48.7 Key Features
> #### *Possible Assessment Findings in Patients With Blunt Abdominal Trauma*
>
> - Purplish or darkened areas in flank area or umbilicus (Cullen sign), which may indicate blood in the abdominal wall
> - Ecchymosis or darkened areas in flank area (Turner sign), which may indicate retroperitoneal bleeding or pancreatic injury
> - Hematoma in flank area, which may indicate kidney injury
> - Referred pain to left shoulder (Kehr sign), which may indicate ruptured spleen or diaphragm irritation or damage
> - Abdominal distention, which may indicate bleeding, ascites, or peritonitis from leakage of GI contents

Perform an abdominal assessment, keeping in mind that a specially trained practitioner (surgeon or emergency care provider) should perform any significant palpation and percussion. The abdominal assessment of a patient with abdominal trauma is completed at frequent intervals to detect changes or developing issues. Inspect the abdomen for abrasions, discoloration, or distention with the patient lying flat (Box 48.7). Bowel sounds may be decreased or absent due to bleeding, organ injury, peritonitis, or paralytic ileus.

Monitor the patient for gastrointestinal symptoms, including nausea and vomiting with or without blood. These symptoms may indicate organ damage or obstruction. Vital signs should be completed frequently to detect subtle or sudden changes that may indicate hemorrhage, shock, or sepsis. Have the patient describe experienced pain and determine quality, region, radiation, severity, and whether the pain is worsening. Worsening pain can be an indication of continued bleeding, perforation, or abdominal compartment syndrome, which will require immediate medical attention (Van, 2022).

During the primary survey in the ED, the patient with abdominal trauma usually has a bedside Focused Assessment with Sonography for Trauma (FAST) scan. A FAST scan can be completed rapidly to establish if there is any free fluid, such as blood or GI contents, in the abdomen. After the patient receives resuscitative care, an abdominal computed tomography (CT) scan is typically performed to better visualize fluid, blood, or structural damage.

Take Actions: Interventions

Management of abdominal trauma varies based on the severity and magnitude of injuries. Modalities of treatment may begin at any time during the primary or secondary survey completed by the ED team members (see Chapter 10 for a more detailed description of these surveys). Patients with active hemorrhage may have an immediate surgical intervention, while those with less life-threatening injuries may be closely monitored and receive symptom management.

Nonsurgical Management. Patients who do not require immediate surgical intervention are carefully monitored in the intensive care unit (ICU). The ICU team assesses the patient at frequent intervals. These assessments include focused assessment, pain, vital signs, and laboratory assessments, including hemoglobin and hematocrit to detect active bleeding (Urden et al., 2022). Blood transfusions are given to patients who experience active abdominal bleeding. Wound management is needed for patients who have penetrating trauma. If the patient's injuries cause impaired ventilation, the patient receives supplemental oxygen therapy or mechanical ventilation depending on the clinical presentation. Patients who have hollow viscus injuries receive antibiotic therapy to prevent sepsis from peritonitis. Deterioration of assessment and laboratory findings may indicate a need for surgical intervention (see Surgical Management later in this chapter). If patients remain stable for 24 to 48 hours in the ICU, they may be transferred to a less specialized nursing unit.

Surgical Management. The most common surgical procedure for abdominal trauma is a laparotomy, which is completed by making an incision into the abdominal cavity. This procedure allows visualization of abdominal organs of the abdomen and repair of any injuries that require surgical intervention. Some patients with abdominal trauma are taken directly to surgery for an exploratory laparotomy after the ED team's primary survey due to significant hemorrhage or decompensation. An exploratory laparotomy may also be performed if the patient shows signs of decompensation while under observation in the ICU.

Postoperative care of patients with a laparotomy requires close monitoring in the ICU for bleeding or infection. Patients who have hollow viscus injuries receive antibiotic therapy. Other postoperative care considerations are described in Chapter 9. Recovery times vary based on the extent of surgical intervention and the severity of the initial injury.

HERNIATION

A hernia is a weakness in the abdominal muscle wall through which a segment of the bowel or other abdominal structure protrudes. Hernias can also penetrate through any other defect in the abdominal wall, through the diaphragm, or through other structures in the abdominal cavity.

Pathophysiology Review

Two elements of hernia formation include congenital or acquired muscle weakness and increased intraabdominal pressure. The most significant factors contributing to increased intraabdominal pressure are obesity, pregnancy, and lifting heavy objects.

The most common types of abdominal hernias are indirect, direct, femoral, umbilical, and incisional.

- An *indirect inguinal hernia* is a sac formed from the peritoneum that contains a portion of the intestine or omentum. The hernia pushes downward at an angle into the inguinal canal. In males, indirect inguinal hernias can become large and often descend into the scrotum.
- *Direct inguinal hernias,* in contrast, pass through a weak point in the abdominal wall.
- *Femoral hernias* protrude through the femoral ring. A plug of fat in the femoral canal enlarges and eventually pulls the peritoneum and often the urinary bladder into the sac.
- *Umbilical hernias* are congenital or acquired. Congenital umbilical hernias appear in infancy. Acquired umbilical hernias directly result from increased intraabdominal pressure. They are most common in people who are obese.
- *Incisional,* or *ventral, hernias* occur at the site of a previous surgical incision. These hernias result from inadequate healing of the incision, which is usually caused by postoperative wound infections, inadequate nutrition, and obesity.

Hernias may also be classified as reducible, irreducible (incarcerated), or strangulated. A reducible hernia is one in which the contents of the hernial sac can be placed back into the abdominal cavity by application of gentle pressure. An irreducible (incarcerated) hernia cannot be reduced or placed back into the abdominal cavity. *Any hernia that is not reducible requires immediate surgical evaluation.*

A hernia is strangulated when the blood supply to the herniated segment of the bowel is cut off by pressure from the hernial ring (the band of muscle around the hernia). If a hernia is strangulated, ischemia and obstruction occur in the bowel loop. *This can lead to necrosis of the bowel, sepsis, and possibly bowel perforation. Signs of strangulation are abdominal distention, nausea, vomiting, pain, fever, and tachycardia.*

Indirect inguinal hernias, the most common type, occur mostly in men because they follow the tract that develops when the testes descend into the scrotum before birth. Direct hernias occur more often in older adults. Femoral and adult umbilical hernias are most common in pregnant women or those with obesity. Incisional hernias can occur in people who have undergone abdominal surgery (Rogers, 2023).

Interprofessional Collaborative Care

Care for the patient with a hernia usually takes place in the ambulatory outpatient setting. Patients with inguinal hernias often need surgery in a same-day surgical facility.

Recognize Cues: Assessment

The patient with a hernia typically comes to the primary health care provider's office, clinic, or the emergency department with a report of a "lump" or protrusion felt at the involved site. The development of the hernia may be associated with straining or lifting.

Perform an abdominal assessment, inspecting the abdomen when the patient is lying and again when standing. If the hernia is reducible, it may disappear when the patient is lying flat. The primary health care provider instructs the patient to strain or perform the Valsalva maneuver and observes for bulging. Auscultate for active bowel sounds. *Absent bowel sounds may indicate obstruction and strangulation, which are considered medical emergencies.*

To palpate an inguinal hernia, the primary health care provider gently examines the ring and its contents by inserting a finger in the ring and noting any changes when the patient coughs. *The hernia is never forcibly reduced; this maneuver could cause strangulated intestine to rupture.*

If a male patient suspects a hernia in his groin, the primary health care provider has him stand for the examination. Using the right hand for the patient's right side and the left hand for the patient's left side, the examiner pushes in the loose scrotal skin with the index finger, following the spermatic cord upward to the external inguinal cord. At this point, the patient is asked to cough, and any palpable herniation is noted.

Take Actions: Interventions

The type of treatment selected depends on patient factors such as age and the type and severity of the hernia.

Nonsurgical Management. Patients who are not surgical candidates (those with multiple health problems) may utilize a truss for an inguinal hernia. A truss is a pad made with firm material that is held in place over the hernia with a belt to help keep the abdominal contents from protruding into the hernial sac. If a truss is used, it is applied only after the primary health care provider has reduced the hernia if it is not incarcerated. The patient usually applies the truss on awakening. Teach the patient to assess the skin under the truss daily and to protect it with a light layer of powder.

Surgical Management. Most hernias are inguinal, and surgical repair is the treatment of choice. Surgery is usually performed on an ambulatory care basis for patients who have no preexisting health conditions that would complicate the operative course. In same-day surgery centers, anesthesia may be regional or general, and the procedure is typically laparoscopic. When bowel strangulation and tissue death occur, more extensive surgery, such as a bowel resection or temporary colostomy, may be necessary. Patients undergoing this extensive surgery are hospitalized for a longer period.

Surgical repair of a hernia is called **herniorrhaphy**. A **minimally invasive inguinal hernia repair (MIIHR)** through a laparoscope is the preferred surgical approach. A conventional open herniorrhaphy may be performed when laparoscopy is unsuitable. Patients having minimally invasive surgery (MIS) recover more quickly, have less pain, and develop fewer postoperative complications compared with those having a conventional open surgery.

In addition to patient education about the procedure, the most important preoperative preparation is to teach the patient to remain NPO for the number of hours before surgery that the surgeon specifies. If same-day surgery is planned, remind patients to arrange for someone to take them home and for that adult to be available for the rest of the day at home. For patients having a conventional open approach, provide general preoperative care as described in Chapter 9.

During an MIIHR, the surgeon makes several small incisions, identifies the defect, and places the intestinal contents back into the abdomen. An abdominal incision is used for a conventional open herniorrhaphy. When a **hernioplasty** is also performed, the surgeon reinforces the weakened outside abdominal muscle wall with a mesh patch.

The patient who undergoes MIIHR is discharged from the surgical center in 3 to 5 hours, depending on recovery from anesthesia. Teach the patient to avoid strenuous activity for several days before returning to work and a normal routine. A stool softener may be needed to prevent constipation. Caution patients who are taking oral opioids for pain management to not drive or operate heavy machinery. Teach them to observe incisions for redness/hyperpigmentation, swelling, heat, drainage, and increased pain and to promptly report their occurrence to the surgeon. Remind patients that soreness and discomfort (rather than severe, acute pain) are common after MIIHR. Be sure to make a follow-up telephone call on the day after surgery to check on the patient's status.

General postoperative care of patients who undergo a hernia repair is the same as that described in Chapter 9 *except that these patients should avoid coughing.* To promote lung expansion, encourage deep breathing and ambulation. With repair of an indirect inguinal hernia, the primary health care provider may suggest a scrotal support and ice bags applied to the scrotum to prevent swelling, which often contributes to pain. Elevation of the scrotum with a soft pillow helps prevent and control swelling.

Male patients who have undergone an inguinal hernia repair may have trouble voiding during the early postoperative period.

Encourage them to stand for a more natural position, allowing gravity to facilitate voiding and bladder emptying. Urine output of less than 30 mL/hr should be reported to the surgeon. Techniques to stimulate voiding such as allowing water to run may also be used. Fluid intake of at least 1500 to 2500 mL daily prevents dehydration, maintains urinary function, and minimizes constipation. A "straight" or intermittent ("in and out") catheterization is required if the patient cannot void. Box 48.8 summarizes best nursing practices for postoperative care after an MIIHR.

Most patients experience uneventful recoveries after a hernia repair. Surgeons generally allow them to return to their usual activities after surgery, with avoidance of straining and lifting for several weeks while subcutaneous tissues heal and strengthen.

On discharge, provide oral instructions and a written list of symptoms to be reported, including fever, chills, wound drainage, redness/hyperpigmentation or separation of the incision, or an increase in incisional pain. Teach the patient to keep the wound dry and clean with cleanser and water. Showering is usually permitted within a few days.

HEMORRHOIDS

Hemorrhoids are unnaturally swollen or distended veins in the anorectal region. The veins involved in the development of hemorrhoids are part of the normal structure of the anal region.

Pathophysiology Review

When functioning normally, anorectal veins function as a valve overlying the anal sphincter that assists in continence. Increased intraabdominal pressure causes elevated systemic and portal venous pressure, which is transmitted to the anorectal veins. Arterioles in

---

BOX 48.8 Best Practice for Patient Safety and Quality Care

Nursing Care of the Postoperative Patient Having a Minimally Invasive Inguinal Hernia Repair (MIIHR)

- Monitor vital signs, especially blood pressure and pulse, for indications of internal bleeding.
- Assess and manage incisional pain with oral analgesics; report and document severe *pain* that does not respond to drug therapy immediately.
- Encourage deep breathing and use of incentive spirometry after surgery; *teach the patient to avoid excessive coughing!*
- Encourage ambulation with assistance as soon as possible after surgery (within the first few hours).
- Apply ice packs as prescribed to the surgical area.
- Help the patient to void by standing the first time after surgery.
- Teach patients at discharge to:
  - Rest for several days after surgery.
  - Observe the incision sites for redness/hyperpigmentation or drainage and report these findings to the surgeon.
  - Shower 24 to 36 hours after removing any bandage, but do not remove wound closure strips; be aware that the strips will fall off in about a week.
  - Monitor temperature for the first few days and report the occurrence of a fever.
  - Do not lift more than 10 lb (4.5 kg) until allowed by the surgeon.
  - Avoid constipation by eating high-fiber foods and drinking extra fluids.
  - Return to work when allowed by the surgeon, usually in 1 to 2 weeks, depending on the patient's work responsibilities.

the anorectal region shunt blood directly to the distended anorectal veins, which increases the pressure. With repeated elevations in pressure from increased intraabdominal pressure and engorgement from arteriolar shunting of blood, the distended veins eventually separate from the smooth muscle surrounding them. This results in prolapse of the hemorrhoidal vessels.

Hemorrhoids can be internal or external (Fig. 48.6). *Internal hemorrhoids,* which cannot be seen on inspection of the perineal area, are above the anal sphincter. *External hemorrhoids* lie below the anal sphincter and can be seen on inspection of the anal region. *Prolapsed hemorrhoids* can become thrombosed or inflamed, or they can bleed (ASCRS, 2023a).

Hemorrhoids are common and insignificant unless they cause prolonged *pain* or bleeding. Because of the increase in abdominal pressure, the condition worsens during pregnancy or with constipation with straining, obesity, heart failure, prolonged sitting or standing, and strenuous exercise and weightlifting. Decreased fluid intake can also cause hemorrhoids because of the development of hard stool and subsequent constipation. Straining while evacuating stool causes hemorrhoids to enlarge.

Health Promotion/Disease Prevention

Prevention of constipation is the most essential measure to prevent hemorrhoids. Constipation can be prevented by eating more whole grains and raw vegetables and fruits to increase fiber in the diet. Encourage patients to drink plenty of water unless otherwise contraindicated (e.g., kidney disease, heart disease). Remind the patient to avoid straining at stool. Encourage regular exercise with a gradual buildup in intensity. Maintaining a healthy weight also helps prevent hemorrhoids.

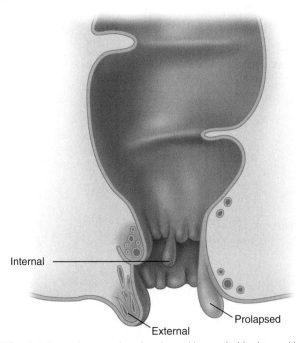

FIG. 48.6 Internal, external, and prolapsed hemorrhoids. *Internal hemorrhoids* lie above the anal sphincter and cannot be seen on inspection of the anal area. *External hemorrhoids* lie below the anal sphincter and can be seen on inspection of the anal region. Hemorrhoids that enlarge, fall down, and protrude through the anus are called *prolapsed hemorrhoids.*

Interprofessional Collaborative Care

Care of the patient with hemorrhoids usually takes place in the ambulatory care setting and is provided by the primary health care provider and nurse. If surgery is required, the patient will be admitted to an ambulatory (same-day) surgical center.

The most common symptoms of hemorrhoids are bleeding, swelling, and prolapse (bulging). Blood is characteristically bright red and is present on toilet tissue or streaked in the stool. *Pain* is a common symptom and is often associated with thrombosis, especially if thrombosis occurs suddenly. Other symptoms include itching and a mucous discharge. Diagnosis is usually made by inspection and digital examination.

Interventions are typically conservative and are aimed at reducing symptoms with minimal discomfort, cost, and time lost from usual activities. Cold packs applied to the anorectal region for a few minutes at a time beginning with the onset of pain and tepid sitz baths three or four times per day are often enough to relieve discomfort, even if the hemorrhoids are thrombosed.

Topical anesthetics, such as lidocaine, are useful for severe pain. Dibucaine ointment and similar products are available over the counter and may be applied for mild to moderate *pain* and itching. However, this ointment should only be used on a temporary basis because it can mask worsening symptoms and delay diagnosis of a severe disorder. When itching or inflammation is present, the primary health care provider may prescribe a steroid preparation, such as hydrocortisone. Cleansing the anal area with moistened cleansing tissues rather than standard toilet tissue helps avoid irritation. The anal area should be cleansed gently by dabbing rather than wiping.

Diets high in fiber and fluids are recommended to promote regular bowel movements without straining. Stool softeners, such as docusate sodium, can be used temporarily. Irritating laxatives should be avoided. Remind patients to avoid sitting for long periods. The primary health care provider may prescribe mild oral analgesics for pain if the hemorrhoids are thrombosed.

Conservative treatment should alleviate symptoms in 3 to 5 days. If symptoms continue or recur frequently, the patient may require surgical intervention.

The surgeon can perform several procedures in an ambulatory care setting to remove symptomatic hemorrhoids (hemorrhoidectomy). The type of surgery (e.g., ultrasound or laser removal) depends on the degree of prolapse, whether there is thrombosis, and the overall condition of the patient. Complications of these procedures include *pain,* thrombosis of other hemorrhoids, infection, bleeding, and abscess formation. A circular stapling device may be used if the hemorrhoid is prolapsed. This device is used to excise a band of mucosa above the prolapse and restore the hemorrhoidal tissue back into the anal canal.

Teach patients with hemorrhoids about the need to eat high-fiber, high-fluid diets to promote regular bowel patterns before and after surgery. Advise them to avoid stimulant laxatives, which can be habit forming.

For patients who undergo any type of surgical intervention, monitor for bleeding and *pain* after surgery and teach them to report these problems to their health care provider. Using moist heat (e.g., sitz baths or warm compresses) three or four times per day can help promote comfort.

! NURSING SAFETY PRIORITY

Action Alert

Tell the patient who has had surgical intervention for hemorrhoids that the first postoperative bowel movement may be very painful. Be sure that someone is with or near the patient when this happens. Some patients become light-headed and diaphoretic and may have syncope (temporary loss of consciousness) related to a vasovagal response.

The primary health care provider usually prescribes stool softeners such as docusate sodium to begin before surgery and continue after surgery. Analgesics and antiinflammatory drugs are prescribed. A mild laxative should be taken if the patient has not had a bowel movement by the third postoperative day.

▌GET READY FOR THE NEXT-GENERATION NCLEX® EXAMINATION!

Essential Nursing Care Points

Health Promotion/Disease Prevention

- Nurses should teach older adults ways to promote bowel *elimination*, including adequate fluid intake, regular exercise, a high-fiber diet, and, if needed, a stool softener.
- Constipation can result in an intestinal obstruction and/or development of hemorrhoids.
- Adults of average risk who are 45 years of age and older and without a family history should undergo regular colorectal cancer (CRC) screening as recommended by the American Cancer Society (ACS).

Chronic Disease Care

- The most common indications of colorectal cancer (CRC) are bleeding, anemia, and a change in stool consistency or shape.
- Adjuvant chemotherapy after stage II or III CRC surgery is used to prevent cancer cell growth or destroy any remaining cancer cells.
- Partial or total colectomy is the surgery of choice for patients who have CRC; a colostomy is often created for *elimination* of stool, which should start functioning 2 to 3 days after surgery.
- The healthy colostomy stoma should appear dark red or reddish pink; report changes in color or stoma retraction.
- Patients who have abdominoperineal (AP) resection surgery for their CRC can expect drainage for 1 to 2 months after surgery and painful wound healing to take as long as 6 to 8 months.
- Nurses should identify psychosocial concerns of patients who have CRC and help them plan how to manage them.
- Interventions for patients who have irritable bowel syndrome (IBS) include drug therapy (depending on the prominent IBS symptom), dietary fiber, adequate hydration, stress management, and chewing slowly.

Regenerative or Restorative Care

- Bowel obstructions can occur in the small or large bowel, and can either be mechanical or nonmechanical (paralytic ileus).
- Most patients who develop a small- or large-bowel obstruction have a nasogastric tube inserted and connected to low continuous suction for gastric decompression.
- Patients who have intestinal obstruction are at risk for impaired *fluid and electrolyte balance* and possible acid-base imbalance.
- Abdominal injuries are the result of blunt or penetrating trauma; hemorrhage and hollow viscus injuries (damage to the stomach or intestines) are two common complications for which nurses need to monitor.
- Any hernia that is not reducible requires immediate surgical evaluation.
- Signs of an inguinal hernia strangulation are abdominal distention, vomiting, pain, fever, and tachycardia; it is a potentially life-threatening condition that can result in bowel perforation and sepsis.
- The most common surgery for hernia repair is a minimally invasive inguinal hernia repair (MIIHR), which is typically performed in an ambulatory surgical center.
- General nursing care for a patient undergoing an MIIHR is similar to that for any surgical procedure except that patients should avoid coughing.
- Hemorrhoids are common and insignificant unless they cause prolonged *pain* or bleeding.
- Conservative treatment of hemorrhoids includes teaching patients to adhere to a high-fiber diet, stool softeners, and topical anesthetics.
- The nurse needs to tell the patient who has a hemorrhoidectomy that the first postoperative bowel movement will be very painful.

Hospice/Palliative/Supportive Care

- Nurses should refer patients who have advanced colorectal cancer with metastasis for palliative or hospice care.

Mastery Questions

1. The nurse is caring for an older adult who is admitted with a diagnosis of complete large bowel obstruction. What would the nurse anticipate as the likely cause of the obstruction?
   A. Fecal impaction
   B. Bowel volvulus
   C. Bowel intussusception
   D. Bowel polyp

2. The nurse is caring for a client who has a nasogastric tube (NGT) connected to low continuous suction for a paralytic ileus. Which of the following nursing interventions would be implemented when caring for this client? **Select all that apply.**
   A. Provide frequent mouth and nares care.
   B. Irrigate the NGT as needed to keep patent.
   C. Listen for the presence of bowel sounds every 4 to 8 hours.
   D. Measure NGT output and document.
   E. Limit the client's intake to full liquids.
   F. Monitor for skin integrity where the tube is inserted.

3. The nurse is planning care for a client recently diagnosed with a nonreducible inguinal hernia. Which primary health care provider order would the nurse anticipate?
   A. Insert a nasogastric tube connected to suction.
   B. Prepare the client for probable surgery.
   C. Administer supplemental oxygen therapy.
   D. Monitor vital signs every 1 to 2 hours.

NGN Challenge 48.1

The nurse is caring for a 43-year-old client admitted to the emergency department (ED).

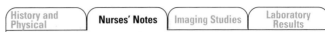

History and Physical	Nurses' Notes	Imaging Studies	Laboratory Results

0615: Brought to ED by college roommates, who state that the client has been "sick" since yesterday afternoon. Client states that cramping abdominal pain is currently 8/10. Has been nauseated and vomiting since yesterday. Abdomen distended; absent bowel sounds × 4. Vomited 115 mL foul-smelling greenish-brown emesis shortly after arriving to ED. Last BM 4 days ago. VS: T 100°F (37.8°C); HR 86 beats/min; RR 18 breaths/min; BP 110/58 mm Hg; Spo$_2$ 98%.

Complete the diagram below by selecting from the choices to specify what potential condition the client is likely experiencing, **2** nursing actions that are appropriate to take, and **2** parameters the nurse should monitor to assess the client's progress.

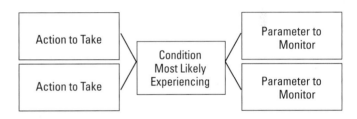

Actions to Take	Potential Conditions	Parameters to Monitor
Insert nasogastric tube connected to low continuous suction	Irritable bowel syndrome	Body temperature
Administer two enemas STAT	Bowel obstruction	Oxygen saturation levels
Prepare client for colectomy as soon as possible	Strangulated inguinal hernia	Serum electrolyte levels
Lay the client flat in a supine body position	Colorectal cancer	Intake and output
Start peripheral IV infusion of lactated Ringer's solution		Respiratory rate and rhythm

NGN Challenge 48.2

The nurse is caring for a 21-year-old client in the emergency department (ED).

History and Physical	Nurses' Notes	Imaging Studies	Laboratory Results

1430: Brought to ED via ambulance following motor vehicle crash. Alert and oriented × 4. Reports severe midabdomen pain of 9/10 with guarding. Lung fields clear; S_1 and S_2 present. Skin intact. Bruises noted around umbilicus with abdominal distention and active bowel sounds × 4. Able to move all extremities. Capillary refill less than 3 seconds. VS: T 98.6°F (37°C); HR 114 beats/min; RR 26 breaths/min; BP 94/50 mm Hg; Spo_2 90% on RA.

Complete the diagram below by selecting from the choices to specify what potential condition the client is likely experiencing, **2** nursing actions that are appropriate to take, and **2** parameters the nurse should monitor to assess the client's progress.

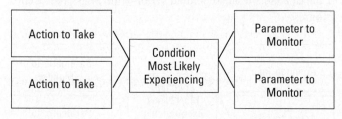

Actions to Take	Potential Conditions	Parameters to Monitor
Insert a nasogastric tube connected to low continuous suction	Abdominal compartment syndrome	Stool count
Initiate supplemental oxygen therapy	Abdominal sepsis	Vital signs
Place the client in a flat supine position	Intraabdominal hemorrhage	White blood cell count
Assist with performing a FAST scan	Intestinal obstruction	Abdominal pain level
Prepare for immediate surgery		Hemoglobin and hematocrit

REFERENCES

American Cancer Society (ACS). (2023a). *Colon cancer risk factors.* https://www.cancer.org/cancer/colon-rectal-cancer/causes-risks-prevention/risk-factors.html.

American Cancer Society (ACS). (2023b). *Family cancer syndromes.* https://www.cancer.org/cancer/cancer-causes/genetics/family-cancer-syndromes.html.

American Society of Colon & Rectal Surgeons (ASCRS). (2023a). *Hemorrhoids.* https://fascrs.org/patients/diseases-and-conditions/a-z/hemorrhoids.

American Society of Colon & Rectal Surgeons (ASCRS). (2023b). *Minimally invasive surgery.* https://fascrs.org/patients/diseases-and-conditions/a-z/minimally-invasive-surgery.

Anxiety & Depression Association of America. (2021). *Irritable bowel syndrome.* https://adaa.org/understanding-anxiety/related-illnesses/irritable-bowel-syndrome-ibs.

Burchum, J. L. R., & Rosenthal, L. D. (2022). *Lehne's pharmacology for nursing care* (11th ed.). St. Louis: Elsevier.

Chamie, K., Golla, V., Lenis, A. T., Lec, P. M., Rahman, S., & Viscusi, E. R. (2021). Peripherally acting μ-opioid receptor antagonists in the management of postoperative ileus: A clinical review. *Journal of Gastrointestinal Surgery, 25,* 293–302. https://doi.org/10.1007/s11605-020-04671-x.

Clark, C. S. (2021). *Cannabis: A handbook for nurses.* Philadelphia, PA: Wolters Kluwer.

Jakobson, J. (2021). State of recovery six months after rectal cancer surgery. *Gastroenterology, 44*(2), 98–105.

Lotfollahzadeh, S., & Burns, B. (2022). Penetrating abdominal trauma. *StatPearls.* Treasure Island, FL: StatPearls Publishing. https://www.ncbi.nlm.nih.gov/books/NBK459123/.

Mitselou, A., Grammeniatis, V., Varouktsi, A., Papadatos, S. S., Katsanos, K., & Galani, V. (2020). Proinflammatory cytokines in irritable bowel syndrome: A comparison with inflammatory bowel disease. *Intestinal Research, 18*(1), 115–120. https://doi.org/10.5217/ir.2019.00125.

National Cancer Institute. (2021). *Common cancer types.* https://www.cancer.gov/types/common-cancers.

O'Rourke, M. C., Landis, R., & Burns, B. (2022). Blunt abdominal trauma. *StatPearls.* Treasure Island, FL: StatPearls Publishing. https://www.ncbi.nlm.nih.gov/books/NBK431087.

Pagana, K., Pagana, T., & Pagana, T. (2022). *Mosby's manual of diagnostic and laboratory tests* (7th ed.). St. Louis: Elsevier.

Rogers, J. L. (2023). *McCance and Huether's Pathophysiology: The biologic basis for disease in adults and children* (9th ed.). St. Louis: Elsevier.

Stelton, S. (2019). Stoma and peristomal skin care: A clinical review. *American Journal of Nursing, 119*(6), 38–45.

Turshudzhyan, A., Trovato, A., & Tadros, M. (2021). Ethical dilemma of colorectal screening: What age should a screening colonoscopy start and stop? *World Journal of Gastrointestinal Endoscopy, 13*(9), 447–450.

Urden, L. D., Stacy, K. M., & Lough, M. E. (2022). *Critical care nursing: Diagnosis and management* (99th ed.). St. Louis: Elsevier.

Van, P. Y. (2022). *Overview of abdominal trauma.* Merck Manual: Professional Version. https://www.merckmanuals.com/professional/injuries-poisoning/abdominal-trauma/overview-of-abdominal-trauma.

49

Concepts of Care for Patients With Inflammatory Intestinal Conditions

Keelin Cromar

http://evolve.elsevier.com/Iggy/

LEARNING OUTCOMES

1. Plan collaborative care with the interprofessional team to manage *inflammation* in patients with chronic inflammatory bowel disease (IBD).
2. Teach adults how to decrease the risk for gastroenteritis.
3. Teach the patient and caregiver(s) about common drugs and other management strategies used for chronic IBD.
4. Plan patient- and family-centered nursing interventions to decrease the psychosocial impact caused by living with chronic IBD.
5. Apply knowledge of anatomy, physiology, and pathophysiology to provide evidence-based care for patients with acute and chronic inflammatory bowel conditions.
6. Analyze assessment and diagnostic findings to generate solutions and prioritize nursing care for patients who have acute intestinal *infection.*
7. Organize care coordination and transition management for patients having surgery for IBD.
8. Use clinical judgment to plan evidence-based nursing care to promote *elimination* and *nutrition* and decrease *pain* in patients with chronic IBD.
9. Incorporate factors that affect health equity into the plan of care for patients with chronic IBD.

KEY TERMS

abscess A localized infection in which there is a collection of pus.

appendectomy The removal of the inflamed appendix by using one of several surgical approaches.

appendicitis An acute inflammation of the vermiform appendix that occurs most often among young adults.

celiac disease A chronic inflammation of the small intestinal mucosa that can cause bowel wall atrophy, malabsorption, and diarrhea.

Crohn's disease (CD) A chronic inflammatory disease of the small intestine (most often), the colon, or both; the terminal ileum is most often affected.

diverticulitis The inflammation or infection of diverticula.

diverticulosis The presence of many abnormal pouchlike herniations (diverticula) in the wall of the intestine.

effluent Drainage.

fissure A tear, crack, or split in skin and underlying tissue.

fistula Abnormal opening (tract) between two organs or structures.

gastroenteritis A very common health problem worldwide that causes diarrhea and/or vomiting related to inflammation of the mucous membranes of the stomach and intestinal tract.

ileostomy A procedure in which a loop of the ileum is placed through an opening in the abdominal wall (stoma) for drainage of fecal material into a pouching system worn on the abdomen.

intestinal malabsorption (malabsorption syndrome) The inability of essential nutrients to be absorbed through a diseased intestinal wall, causing anemia and malnutrition (most common in Crohn's disease).

laparoscopy A minimally invasive surgery (MIS) with one or more small incisions near the umbilicus through which a small endoscope and tools are placed.

laparotomy An open surgical approach requiring a large abdominal incision.

ostomate A person who has an ostomy.

peritonitis A life-threatening, acute inflammation and infection of the visceral/parietal peritoneum and endothelial lining of the abdominal cavity.

progressive multifocal leukoencephalopathy (PML) A deadly infection that affects the brain.

steatorrhea Fatty diarrheal stools.

tenesmus An unpleasant and urgent sensation to defecate.

toxic megacolon Massive dilation of the colon and subsequent colonic ileus that can lead to gangrene and peritonitis.

ulcerative colitis (UC) A disease that creates widespread chronic inflammation of the rectum and rectosigmoid colon but can extend to the entire colon when the disease is extensive.

PRIORITY AND INTERRELATED CONCEPTS

The priority concepts for this chapter are:
- *Infection*
- *Inflammation*

The *Infection* concept exemplar for this chapter is Peritonitis.
The *Inflammation* concept exemplar for this chapter is Ulcerative Colitis.

The interrelated concepts for this chapter are:
- *Nutrition*
- *Elimination*
- *Pain*

The *intestinal tract* is made up of the small intestine and large intestine (colon). Digestion of food and absorption of nutrients occur primarily in the small intestine to meet the body's needs for energy. Water is reabsorbed in the large intestine to help maintain a fluid balance and promote the passage of waste products. When the intestinal tract and nearby structures become acutely inflamed, *pain* and *infection* can occur. Chronic bowel *inflammation* can affect *nutrition* and *elimination.* Chapter 3 briefly reviews each of these health concepts.

Appendicitis, gastroenteritis, and peritonitis are the most common *acute* inflammatory bowel disorders. These disorders can be potentially life-threatening and can have major systemic complications if not treated promptly. Ulcerative colitis (UC), Crohn's disease (CD), and diverticular disease are the three most common *chronic* inflammatory bowel diseases (IBDs) that affect adults.

INFECTION CONCEPT EXEMPLAR: PERITONITIS

The peritoneal cavity normally contains about 50 mL of sterile fluid (transudate), which prevents friction in the abdominal cavity during peristalsis. Peritonitis is a life-threatening, acute *inflammation* and *infection* of the visceral/parietal peritoneum and endothelial lining of the abdominal cavity.

Pathophysiology Review

When the peritoneal cavity is contaminated by bacteria, the body begins an inflammatory reaction, walling off a localized area to fight the infection. Vascular dilation and increased capillary permeability occur, allowing transport of leukocytes and subsequent phagocytosis of the offending organisms. If the process of walling off fails, the *inflammation* spreads and contamination becomes massive, resulting in diffuse (widespread) *infection* (Rogers, 2023).

Peritonitis is most often caused by contamination of the peritoneal cavity by bacteria or chemicals. Bacteria gain entry to the peritoneum by perforation (from appendicitis, diverticulitis, peptic ulcer disease) or from an external penetrating wound, a gangrenous gallbladder or bowel segment, bowel obstruction, or ascending infection through the genital tract. Less common causes include invasive tumors, leakage or contamination during surgery, or *infection* by skin pathogens in patients undergoing continuous ambulatory peritoneal dialysis (CAPD) (Sole et al., 2021).

When diagnosis and treatment of peritonitis are delayed, blood vessel dilation continues. The body responds to the continuing infectious process by shunting extra blood to the area of inflammation (hyperemia). Fluid is shifted from the extracellular fluid compartment into the peritoneal cavity, connective tissues, and GI tract *("third spacing").* This shift of fluid can result in a significant decrease in circulatory volume and *hypovolemic shock.* Severely decreased circulatory volume can result in insufficient perfusion of the kidneys, leading to acute kidney injury with impaired fluid and electrolyte balance (Sole et al., 2021).

Peristalsis slows or *stops* in response to severe peritoneal *inflammation* and *infection,* and the lumen of the bowel becomes distended with gas and fluid. Fluid that normally flows to the small bowel and the colon for reabsorption accumulates in the intestine in volumes of 7 to 8 L daily. The toxins or bacteria responsible for the peritonitis can also enter the bloodstream from the peritoneal area and lead to bacteremia, or septicemia (bacterial invasion of the blood), a life-threatening condition that can lead to systemic sepsis and septic shock (see Chapter 31).

Respiratory problems can occur due to increased abdominal pressure against the diaphragm from intestinal distention and fluid shifts to the peritoneal cavity. *Pain* can interfere with respirations at a time when the patient has an increased oxygen demand because of the infectious process.

Etiology and Genetic Risk

Common bacteria responsible for peritonitis include *Escherichia coli, Streptococcus, Staphylococcus,* pneumococci, and gonococci. Chemical peritonitis results from leakage of bile, pancreatic enzymes, and gastric acid. There are no genetic risks associated with this health problem.

Incidence and Prevalence

Peritonitis is a significant postoperative complication that has a mortality rate of up to 50% (Menz et al., 2021). This complication occurs most commonly in young adults with appendicitis and in older adults, whose immunity can be decreased.

Interprofessional Collaborative Care

Patients with peritonitis are hospitalized because of the severe nature of the illness. If complications are extensive, the patients are often admitted to a critical care unit.

Recognize Cues: Assessment

History. Ask the patient about abdominal *pain* and determine the character of the pain (e.g., cramping, sharp, aching), location of the pain, and if the pain is localized or generalized. Ask about a history of a low-grade fever or recent spikes in temperature.

Physical Assessment/Signs and Symptoms. Physical findings of peritonitis depend on several factors: the stage of the disease, the ability of the body to localize the process by walling off the *infection,* and whether the *inflammation* has progressed to generalized peritonitis (Box 49.1).

BOX 49.1 Key Features

Peritonitis

- Rigid, boardlike abdomen (classic)
- Abdominal *pain* (localized, poorly localized, or referred to the shoulder or chest)
- Distended abdomen
- Nausea, anorexia, vomiting
- Diminishing bowel sounds
- Inability to pass flatus or feces
- Rebound tenderness in the abdomen
- High fever
- Tachycardia
- Dehydration from high fever (poor skin turgor)
- Decreased urine output
- Hiccups
- Possible compromise in respiratory status

Patients most often appear acutely ill, lying still, possibly with the knees flexed. Movement is guarded, and they may report and show signs of *pain* (e.g., facial grimacing) with coughing or movement of any type. During inspection, observe for progressive abdominal distention, often seen when the *inflammation* and *infection* markedly reduce intestinal motility. Auscultate for bowel sounds, which usually disappear with progression of the inflammation.

The cardinal signs of peritonitis are abdominal pain, tenderness, and distention. Patients with *localized* peritonitis may have a tender abdomen with rebound tenderness on palpation in a well-defined area. With *generalized* peritonitis, tenderness is widespread.

Psychosocial Assessment. Patients with peritonitis may be very fearful and anxious about the implications of a diagnosis of peritonitis and may be distressed regarding the physical *pain* that they feel. Provide a calm presence and reassure patients that you will be there to help them during this time. Allow the patient to express feelings of fear and anxiety and provide nonjudgmental listening and presence.

Laboratory Assessment. White blood cell (WBC) counts are often elevated to $20,000/mm^3$ ($20 \times 10^9/L$) with a high neutrophil count (leukocytosis). The normal WBC count is 5000–10,000/mm^3 ($5–10 \times 10^9/L$) (Pagana et al., 2022). *Blood culture* studies may be done to determine whether septicemia has occurred and to identify the causative organism to determine appropriate antibiotic therapy. The primary health care provider may request laboratory tests to assess fluid and electrolyte balance and renal status, including blood urea nitrogen (BUN), creatinine, hemoglobin, and hematocrit. Oxygen saturation and arterial blood gases may be obtained to assess respiratory function and acid-base balance.

Imaging Assessment. Abdominal x-rays can assess for free air or fluid in the abdominal cavity, indicating perforation. The x-rays may also show dilation, edema, and *inflammation* of the small and large intestines. An *abdominal ultrasound* or *CT scan* may also be performed.

Analyze Cues and Prioritize Hypotheses: Analysis

The priority collaborative problems for patients with peritonitis include:

1. Acute *pain* due to abdominal *inflammation* and *infection*
2. Potential for fluid volume shift due to fluid moving into interstitial or peritoneal space

Generate Solutions and Take Actions: Planning and Implementation

The collaborative plan of care for the patient diagnosed with peritonitis focuses on treating the cause of the *infection* and managing the infectious process. Nonsurgical and/or surgical modalities may be required.

Managing Pain

Planning: Expected Outcomes. The patient is expected to report a *pain* level of 2 to 3 or what is acceptable to the patient on a 0-to-10 pain intensity scale as the *inflammation* and *infection* resolve.

Interventions. Interventions for peritonitis are usually nonsurgical, but surgery may be required to remove abscesses or other infectious material. Assess vital signs frequently, noting any change that may indicate septic shock, such as unresolved or progressive hypotension, decreased pulse pressure, tachycardia, fever, skin changes, and/or tachypnea. Monitor mental status changes for any sign of confusion or altered level of consciousness. Practice proper handwashing and maintain strict asepsis when caring for wounds, drains, and dressings to decrease chance of superimposed *infection.* If the patient has or requires a urinary catheter, maintain strict sterile technique and provide appropriate catheter care. Observe and document wound drainage; report any changes immediately to the primary health care provider. Administer broad-spectrum antibiotics as prescribed to treat known or potential pathogens. Provide oxygen if needed according to the patient's respiratory status and oxygen saturation via pulse oximetry.

Abdominal surgery may be needed to identify and repair the cause of the peritonitis. If the patient is critically ill and surgery could be life-threatening, it may be delayed. Surgery focuses on controlling the contamination, removing foreign material from the peritoneal cavity, and draining collected fluid.

An exploratory laparotomy (an open surgical approach requiring a large abdominal incision) or laparoscopy is used to remove or repair an inflamed or perforated organ (e.g., appendectomy for an inflamed appendix; a colon resection, with or without a colostomy, for a perforated diverticulum). Before the incision(s) is closed, the surgeon irrigates the peritoneum with antibiotic solutions. Several catheters may be inserted to drain the cavity and provide a route for irrigation after surgery.

If an *open* conventional surgical procedure is needed, the *infection* may slow healing of an incision, or the incision may be partially open to heal by second or third intention. These wounds require special care involving manual irrigation or packing as prescribed by the surgeon. If the surgeon requests peritoneal irrigation through a drain, *maintain sterile technique during manual irrigation* to prevent further risk for infection. Chapter 9 describes general preoperative and postoperative care.

! NURSING SAFETY PRIORITY

Action Alert

Monitor the patient's level of consciousness, vital signs, respiratory status (respiratory rate, respiratory effort, and breath sounds), and intake and output at least hourly immediately after abdominal surgery. Maintain the patient in a semi-Fowler's position to promote drainage of peritoneal contents into the lower region of the abdominal cavity. This position also helps increase lung expansion.

Restoring Fluid Volume Balance

Planning: Expected Outcomes. The patient will experience fluid volume balance.

Interventions. The primary health care provider prescribes hypertonic IV fluids and broad-spectrum antibiotics immediately after establishing the diagnosis of peritonitis. Remind assistive personnel to take a daily weight using the same scale each morning, and record intake and output carefully. A nasogastric tube (NGT) is inserted to decompress the stomach and the intestine if an open laparotomy is anticipated.

Multisystem complications can occur with peritonitis. Loss of fluids and electrolytes from the extracellular space to the peritoneal cavity, NGT suctioning, and NPO status require that the patient receive IV fluid replacement. Fluid rates may be changed frequently on the basis of laboratory values, assessment findings, and patient condition.

Assess whether the patient retains fluid used for irrigation by comparing and recording the amount of fluid returned with the amount of fluid instilled. Fluid retention could cause abdominal distention or pain.

Care Coordination and Transition Management

The length of hospitalization for a patient with peritonitis depends on the extent and severity of the infectious process. Patients who have a localized abscess (a localized *infection* in which there is a collection of pus) drained and who respond to antibiotics and IV fluids without multisystem complications are discharged in several days. Others may require mechanical ventilation or hemodialysis with longer hospital stays. Some patients may be transferred to a transitional care unit to complete their antibiotic therapy and recovery. Convalescence is often longer than after other surgeries because of multisystem involvement.

Before the patient is discharged home, assess the ability for self-management. Provide the patient and family with written and oral instructions to report the following problems to the primary health care provider immediately:

- Unusual or foul-smelling drainage
- Swelling, redness/hyperpigmentation, or warmth or bleeding from the incision site
- A temperature higher than 101°F (38.3°C)
- Abdominal *pain*
- Signs of wound dehiscence or ileus

Patients with large incisions that are left open heal by secondary or tertiary intention and require dressings, solution, and catheter-tipped syringes to irrigate the wound. A home care nurse may be needed to assess, irrigate, or pack the wound and change the dressing as needed until the patient and family feel comfortable with the procedure. If the patient needs assistance with ADLs, a home care aide or temporary placement in a skilled care facility may be indicated.

Review information about antibiotics and analgesics. For patients taking short-term oral opioid analgesics such as oxycodone with acetaminophen, a stool softener such as docusate sodium may be prescribed with a laxative. Older adults are especially at risk for constipation from codeine-based drugs. Remind patients to avoid taking additional acetaminophen to prevent liver toxicity.

Teach patients to refrain from any lifting of more than 5–10 lb (2.3–4.5 kg) for *at least* 6 weeks after an open surgical procedure. Other activity limitations are based on individual need and the primary health care provider's recommendation. Patients who have laparoscopic surgery can resume activities within a week or two and may not have any major restrictions.

NCLEX Examination Challenge 49.1

Safe and Effective Care Environment

The nurse is caring for a client who had surgery for an abdominal abscess that ruptured yesterday. What would be the nurse's **priority** assessment for the client at this time?

A. Continuous oxygen saturation
B. Fluid and electrolyte status
C. Nutritional status
D. Liver function

Evaluate Outcomes: Evaluation

Evaluate the care of the patient with peritonitis based on the identified priority patient problems. The expected outcomes are that the patient:

- Verbalizes relief or control of pain as *infection* resolves
- Experiences fluid and electrolyte balance

APPENDICITIS

The appendix usually extends off the proximal cecum of the colon just below the ileocecal valve. Appendicitis is an acute *inflammation* of the vermiform appendix that peaks in individuals between the ages of 15 and 19 but can occur in those who are younger or older.

Pathophysiology Review

Inflammation occurs when the lumen (opening) of the appendix is obstructed (blocked), leading to *infection* as bacteria invade the wall of the appendix. The initial obstruction is usually a result of fecaliths (very hard pieces of feces) (Rogers, 2023). When the lumen is blocked, the mucosa secretes fluid, increasing the internal pressure and restricting blood flow, which results in *pain.* This pain is typically felt in the right lower quadrant (RLQ). If the process occurs slowly, an abscess may develop, but a rapid process may result in peritonitis. *All complications of peritonitis are serious. Gangrene and sepsis can occur within 24 to 36 hours, are life-threatening, and are some of the most common indications for emergency surgery. Perforation may develop within 24 hours, but the risk rises rapidly after 48 hours.* Perforation of the appendix results in peritonitis with a temperature of greater than 101°F (38.3°C) and a rise in pulse rate.

Interprofessional Collaborative Care

Recognize Cues: Assessment

History taking and tracking the sequence of symptoms are important because nausea or vomiting before abdominal pain can indicate gastroenteritis. Abdominal pain followed by nausea and vomiting can indicate appendicitis. Classically, patients with appendicitis have cramping *pain* in the epigastric or periumbilical area. Anorexia is also a frequent symptom.

Perform a complete *pain* assessment. Initially pain can present anywhere in the abdomen or flank area. As the *inflammation* and *infection* progress, the pain becomes more severe and shifts to the RLQ between the anterior iliac crest and the umbilicus. This area is referred to as the *McBurney point* (Fig. 49.1). *Abdominal pain that increases with cough or movement and is relieved by bending the right hip or the knees suggests perforation and peritonitis.* The primary health care provider assesses for muscle rigidity and guarding on palpation of the abdomen. The patient may report pain after release of pressure. This sensation is referred to as *rebound* tenderness.

Laboratory findings do not establish the diagnosis, but often there is a moderate elevation of the *white blood cell (WBC) count* (leukocytosis) to 10,000 to 18,000/mm³ (10–18 × 10⁹/L) with a "shift to the left" (an increased number of immature WBCs). A WBC elevation to greater than 20,000/mm³ (20 × 10⁹/L) may indicate a perforated appendix. *Ultrasound* studies may show the presence of an enlarged appendix. If symptoms are recurrent or prolonged, a *CT scan* can be used to diagnose and may reveal the presence of a fecaloma (a small "stone" of feces) (Pagana et al., 2022).

Take Actions: Interventions

All patients with suspected or confirmed appendicitis are hospitalized, and most have surgery to remove the inflamed appendix. Keep the patient with suspected or known appendicitis NPO to prepare for the probability of surgery and to avoid

making the *inflammation* worse. Be sure that the patient's *pain* is adequately managed before surgical intervention.

> **! NURSING SAFETY PRIORITY**
> **Action Alert**
>
> For the patient with suspected appendicitis, administer IV fluids as prescribed to maintain fluid and electrolyte balance and replace fluid volume. Advise the patient to maintain a semi-Fowler's position as tolerated so that abdominal drainage can be contained in the lower abdomen. Once the diagnosis of appendicitis is confirmed and surgery is scheduled, administer opioid analgesics and antibiotics as prescribed. *The patient with suspected or confirmed appendicitis should not receive laxatives or enemas, which can cause perforation of the appendix. Do not apply heat to the abdomen because this may increase circulation to the appendix and result in increased* ***inflammation*** *and perforation!*

Surgery is required as soon as possible for most patients. An appendectomy is the removal of the inflamed appendix by one of several surgical approaches. Uncomplicated appendectomy procedures are done via laparoscopy. Laparoscopy is a minimally invasive surgery (MIS) with one or more small incisions near the umbilicus, through which a small endoscope and tools are inserted. Patients having this type of surgery for appendix removal have minimal postoperative complications (see Chapter 9). Patients having any type of laparoscopic procedure are typically discharged the same day of surgery with mild to moderate pain after discharge. Most patients can return to usual activities in 1 to 2 weeks.

If the diagnosis is not definitive but the patient is at high risk for complications from suspected appendicitis, the surgeon may perform an exploratory laparotomy. A laparotomy is an open surgical approach with a large abdominal incision.

Preoperative teaching is often limited because the patient is in *pain* or may be admitted quickly for emergency surgery. The patient is prepared for general anesthesia. After surgery, care of the patient who has undergone an appendectomy is the same as that required for anyone who has received general anesthesia (see Chapter 9).

If complications such as peritonitis or abscesses are found during *open* traditional surgery, wound drains are inserted and a nasogastric tube may be placed to decompress the stomach and prevent abdominal distention. Administer IV antibiotics and opioid analgesics as prescribed. Help the patient out of bed on the evening of surgery to help prevent respiratory complications, such as atelectasis. Patients may be hospitalized for as long as 3 to 5 days and return to usual activity in 4 to 6 weeks.

GASTROENTERITIS

Gastroenteritis is a very common health problem worldwide that causes diarrhea and/or vomiting related to *inflammation* of the mucous membranes of the stomach and intestinal tract. The small bowel is most commonly affected, and the condition can be caused by either viral (more common) or bacterial

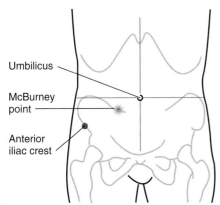

FIG. 49.1 The McBurney point is located midway between the anterior iliac crest and the umbilicus in the right lower quadrant. This is the classic area for localized tenderness during the later stages of appendicitis.

TABLE 49.1 Common Types of Gastroenteritis and Their Characteristics

Type of Gastroenteritis	Characteristics
Viral Gastroenteritis	
Epidemic viral	Caused by many parvovirus-type organisms
	Transmitted by the fecal-oral route in food and water
	Incubation period 10–51 hr
	Communicable during acute illness
Norovirus (Norwalk viruses)	Transmitted by the fecal-oral route and possibly the respiratory route (vomitus)
	Incubation in 48 hr
	Affects adults of all ages
	Older adults can become hypovolemic and experience electrolyte imbalances
Bacterial Gastroenteritis	
Campylobacter enteritis	Transmitted by the fecal-oral route or contact with infected animals or infants
	Incubation period 1–10 days
	Communicable for 2–7 wk
Escherichia coli diarrhea	Transmitted by fecal contamination of food, water, or fomites
Shigellosis	Transmitted by direct and indirect fecal-oral routes
	Incubation period 1–7 days
	Communicable during the acute illness to 4 wk after the illness
	Humans possibly carriers for months

infection. Table 49.1 lists common types of gastroenteritis and their primary characteristics.

Pathophysiology Review

Norovirus (also known as a *Norwalk-like virus*) is the leading foodborne disease that causes gastroenteritis. This virus occurs most often between November and April because it is resistant to low temperatures and has a long viral shedding before and after the illness. Due to COVID-19 restrictions including during the pandemic, the incidence of viral gastroenteritis in 2020 and 2021 decreased. Norovirus is transmitted (spread) through the fecal-oral route from person to person and from contaminated food and water. Infected individuals can also contaminate surfaces and objects in the environment. Vomiting may cause the virus to become airborne. The incubation time is 1 to 2 days.

In most cases of gastroenteritis, the illness is self-limiting and lasts about 3 days. However, in those who are immunosuppressed or in older adults, dehydration and hypovolemia can occur as complications requiring medical attention and possibly hospitalization.

Health Promotion/Disease Prevention

Outbreaks of norovirus have occurred in prisons, on cruise ships, and in nursing homes, college dormitories, and other places where large groups of people are in close proximity. Teach individuals that handwashing and sanitizing surfaces and other environmental items help prevent the spread of the illness. Hand sanitizers are often placed in public areas so that hands can be cleaned when washing with soap and water is inconvenient. Proper food and beverage preparation and storage is also important to prevent contamination.

Interprofessional Collaborative Care

Patients with gastroenteritis are generally cared for in the community setting and self-manage at home. Those who develop the more severe types of this condition or become extremely dehydrated during its course may be hospitalized.

Recognize Cues: Assessment

The patient history can provide information related to the potential cause of the illness. Ask about recent travel, especially to tropical regions of Asia, Africa, Mexico, or Central or South America, because these areas historically have been a source of gastroenteritis.

Inquire if the patient has eaten at any restaurant in the past 24 to 36 hours. Some people acquire gastroenteritis from eating in "fast food" restaurants or from food items purchased at a farmer's market or grocery store. Bacterial infections have caused large outbreaks that resulted from contaminated spinach and lettuce in the United States. Raw or undercooked food such as oysters, sushi, and rare or raw meat can also cause GI infections.

During the COVID-19 pandemic, many restaurants had difficulty obtaining their usual ingredients and food to maintain their usual menus. In addition, many restaurants were challenged to hire qualified employees. As a result, lack of adequate employee training and/or a tendency to keep food longer than usual may have caused an increased in bacterial gastroenteritis from contaminated food.

The patient who has gastroenteritis usually looks ill. Nausea and vomiting typically occur first, followed by abdominal cramping and diarrhea. For patients who are older or for those who have inadequate immune systems, weakness and cardiac dysrhythmias may occur from loss of potassium (hypokalemia) from diarrhea. Monitor for and document manifestations of hypokalemia and hypovolemia (dehydration).

! NURSING SAFETY PRIORITY

Action Alert

For patients with gastroenteritis, note any abdominal distention and listen for hyperactive bowel sounds. Depending on the amounts of fluids and electrolytes lost through diarrhea and vomiting, patients may have varying degrees of dehydration manifested by:

- Weight loss (unintentional)
- Poor skin turgor
- Fever (not common in older adults)
- Dry mucous membranes
- Orthostatic blood pressure changes (which can cause a fall, especially in older adults)
- Hypotension
- Oliguria (decreased or absent urinary output)

In some cases, dehydration may be severe and can occur very rapidly in older adults. Monitor mental status changes, such as acute confusion, that result from hypoxia due to dehydration in the older adult. These changes may be the only initial signs and symptoms of dehydration in older adults.

Take Actions: Interventions

For any type of gastroenteritis, encourage oral fluid replacement. The amount and route of fluid administration are determined by the patient's hydration status and overall health condition. Teach patients to drink extra fluids to replace fluid lost through vomiting and diarrhea. Oral rehydration therapy (ORT) may be needed for some patients to replace fluids and electrolytes. Examples of ORT solutions include sports drinks and Pedialyte. Depending on patients' age and severity of dehydration, they may be treated in the hospital with IV fluids to restore hydration.

Drugs that suppress intestinal motility may not be given for bacterial or viral gastroenteritis. *Use of these drugs can prevent the infecting organisms from being eliminated from the body.* If the primary health care provider determines that antiperistaltic/antidiarrheal agents are necessary, loperamide may be recommended.

⬤ NURSING SAFETY PRIORITY

Drug Alert

Diphenoxylate hydrochloride with atropine sulfate reduces GI motility but is used sparingly because of its habit-forming ability. *The drug should not be used in older adults because it also causes drowsiness and could contribute to falls.*

Treatment with antibiotics may be needed if the gastroenteritis is caused by bacterial *infection* with fever and severe diarrhea. Depending on the type and severity of the illness, examples of drugs that may be prescribed include ciprofloxacin or azithromycin. For gastroenteritis caused by shigellosis, antiinfective agents such as ciprofloxacin and azithromycin are prescribed (Burchum & Rosenthal, 2022).

Frequent stools that are rich in electrolytes and enzymes and frequent wiping and washing of the anal region can irritate the skin. Teach the patient to avoid toilet paper and to gently clean the area with warm water or an absorbent material, followed by thorough but gentle drying. Cream, oil, or gel can be applied to a damp, warm washcloth to remove stool that sticks to open skin. Special prepared skin wipes can also be used. Protective barrier cream can be applied to the skin between stools. Sitz baths for 10 minutes two or three times daily can also relieve discomfort.

If leakage of stool is a problem, the patient can use an absorbent cotton pad or liner and keep it in place with snug underwear. For patients who are incontinent, the use of incontinence pads at night instead of briefs allows air to circulate to the skin and prevents irritation. Remind assistive personnel to keep the perineal and buttock areas clean and dry and that frequent changes will be necessary.

During the acute phase of the illness, teach the patient and family about the importance of fluid replacement. Patient and family education regarding risk for transmission of gastroenteritis is also important (Box 49.2).

BOX 49.2 Patient and Family Education

Preventing Transmission of Gastroenteritis

Advise individuals to:
- Wash hands well for at least 30 seconds with soap, especially after a bowel movement, and maintain good personal hygiene.
- Restrict the use of glasses, dishes, eating utensils, and tubes of toothpaste for their own use. In severe cases, disposable utensils may be used.
- Maintain clean bathroom facilities to avoid exposure to stool.
- Inform the primary health care provider if symptoms persist beyond 3 days.
- Not prepare or handle food that will be consumed by others. If the patient is employed as a food handler, the public health department should be consulted for recommendations about the return to work.

✴ INFLAMMATION CONCEPT EXEMPLAR: ULCERATIVE COLITIS

Ulcerative colitis and Crohn's disease occur in about equal incidence. These chronic diseases have always been considered disorders that affect Whites. However, the incidence of chronic IBD in non-White populations is markedly increasing (Barnes et al., 2021).

Pathophysiology Review

Ulcerative colitis (UC) is a disease that creates widespread chronic *inflammation* of the rectum and rectosigmoid colon but can extend to the entire colon when the disease is extensive. Distribution of the disease can remain constant for years. UC is a disease that is associated with periodic remissions and exacerbations (flare-ups) and is often confused with Crohn's disease. Comparisons and differences are listed in Table 49.2.

Many factors can cause exacerbations, including intestinal *infection.* Most patients who are affected have mild to moderate disease, but a small percentage of patients experience severe symptoms. Older adults with UC are at high risk for impaired fluid and electrolyte balance due to diarrhea, including dehydration and hypokalemia (Rogers, 2023).

The intestinal mucosa becomes hyperemic (has increased blood flow), edematous, and reddened. In more severe inflammation, the lining can bleed and small erosions, or ulcers, occur. Abscesses can form in these ulcerative areas and result in tissue necrosis (cell death). Continued edema and mucosal thickening can lead to a narrowed colon and possibly a partial bowel obstruction. Table 49.3 lists the categories of the severity of UC.

The patient's stool typically contains blood and mucus. Patients report tenesmus (an unpleasant and urgent sensation to defecate) and lower abdominal colicky pain relieved with defecation. Malaise, anorexia, anemia, dehydration, fever, and weight loss are common. Extraintestinal manifestations such as migratory polyarthritis, ankylosing spondylitis, and erythema nodosum are present in a large number of patients. The common and extraintestinal complications of UC are listed in Table 49.4.

Etiology and Genetic Risk

The exact cause of UC is unknown, but a combination of genetic, immunologic, and lifestyle factors is thought to contribute to

TABLE 49.2 Differential Features of Ulcerative Colitis and Crohn's Disease

Feature	Ulcerative Colitis	Crohn's Disease
Location	Begins in the rectum and proceeds in a continuous manner toward the cecum	Most often in the terminal ileum, with patchy involvement through all layers of the bowel
Etiology	Unknown	Unknown
Peak incidence at age	15–35 yr and 55–70 yr	15–40 yr
Number of stools	10–20 liquid, bloody stools per day	5–6 soft, loose stools per day, nonbloody
Complications	Hemorrhage Nutritional deficiencies	Fistulas (common) Nutritional deficiencies
Patient need for surgery	25%–35%	65%–75%

TABLE 49.3 American College of Gastroenterologists Classification of Ulcerative Colitis Severity

Severity	Stool Frequency	Signs/Symptoms
Mild	<4 stools/day with/without blood	Asymptomatic Laboratory values usually normal
Moderate	>4 stools/day with/without blood	Minimal symptoms Mild abdominal pain Mild intermittent nausea Possible increased C-reactive protein[a] or ESR[b]
Severe	>6 bloody stools/day	Fever Tachycardia Anemia Abdominal pain Elevated C-reactive protein[a] and/or ESR[b]
Fulminant	>10 bloody stools/day	Increasing symptoms Anemia may necessitate transfusion Colonic distention on x-ray

[a]C-reactive protein is a sensitive acute-phase serum marker that is evident in the first 6 hours of an inflammatory process.
[b]ESR, Erythrocyte sedimentation rate; may be helpful but is less sensitive than C-reactive protein.
Adapted from Rubin, D. T., Ananthakrishnan, A. N., Siegel, C. A. et al. (2019). Clinical guideline: Ulcerative colitis in adults. *American Journal of Gastroenterology, 114*(3), 384–413. https://doi.org/10.14309/ajg.0000000000000152

TABLE 49.4 Complications of Ulcerative Colitis and Crohn's Disease

Complication	Description
Hemorrhage/perforation	Lower GI bleeding results from erosion of the bowel wall.
Abscess formation	Localized pockets of **infection** develop in the ulcerated bowel lining.
Toxic megacolon	Massive dilation of the colon and subsequent colonic ileus can lead to gangrene and peritonitis.
Intestinal malabsorption	Essential nutrients cannot be absorbed through the diseased intestinal wall, causing anemia and malnutrition (most common in Crohn's disease).
Nonmechanical bowel obstruction	Obstruction results from toxic megacolon or cancer.
Fistulas	In Crohn's disease in which the **inflammation** is transmural, fistulas can occur anywhere but usually track between the bowel and bladder, resulting in pyuria and fecaluria.
Colorectal cancer	Patients with ulcerative colitis with a history longer than 10 years have a high risk for colorectal cancer. This complication accounts for about one-third of all deaths related to ulcerative colitis.
Extraintestinal complications	Complications include arthritis, hepatic and biliary disease (especially cholelithiasis), oral and skin lesions, and ocular disorders, such as iritis. The cause is unknown.
Osteoporosis	Osteoporosis can occur, especially in patients with Crohn's disease.

disease development. A genetic basis of the disease has been supported because it is often found in families and twins. Immunologic causes, including autoimmune dysfunction, are likely the etiology of extraintestinal manifestations of the disease. Epithelial antibodies in the immunoglobulin G (IgG) class have been identified in the blood of some patients with UC (Rogers, 2023).

With long-term disease, cellular changes can occur that increase the risk for colon cancer. Damage from proinflammatory cytokines, such as interleukins (ILs) and tumor necrosis factor (TNF)-alpha, have cytotoxic effects on the colonic mucosa (Rogers, 2023).

Cigarette smoking can also increase the risk of developing UC. Individuals who consume diets high in animal fats and sugar but low in fruits and vegetables are also at risk for developing chronic IBD (Barnes et al., 2021).

Incidence and Prevalence

In the United States, about 3 million individuals are affected by chronic inflammatory bowel disease (IBD), with about half experiencing UC. Although diagnosis can occur at any age, most people are diagnosed between 20 and 35 years of age (Centers for Disease Control and Prevention [CDC], 2022).

Interprofessional Collaborative Care

Patients with UC may be managed at home, cared for in the community setting, or hospitalized, depending on their immediate condition related to this chronic bowel disease.

Recognize Cues: Assessment

History. Collect data on family history of IBD, previous and current therapy for the illness, and dates and types of surgery. Obtain a *nutrition* history, including intolerance of milk and milk products and fried, spicy, or hot foods. Ask about usual bowel *elimination* pattern (color, number, consistency, and character of stools); abdominal pain; tenesmus; anorexia; and fatigue. Note any relationship between diarrhea, timing of meals, emotional distress, and activity. Inquire about recent (past 2–3 months) exposure to antibiotics to rule out a *Clostridium difficile* infection. Has the patient traveled to or emigrated from tropical areas? Ask about recent use of NSAIDs because these can cause a flare-up of the disease. Inquire about any extraintestinal symptoms, such as arthritis, mouth sores, vision problems, and skin disorders.

Physical Assessment/Signs and Symptoms. Symptoms vary with an acuteness of onset. Vital signs are usually within normal limits in mild disease. In severe cases the patient may have a low-grade fever (99° to 100°F [37.2° to 37.8°C]). The physical assessment findings are usually nonspecific, and in milder cases the physical examination findings may be normal. Viral and bacterial infections can cause symptoms similar to those of UC.

Note any abdominal distention along the colon. Fever associated with tachycardia may indicate dehydration, peritonitis, and bowel perforation. Assess for signs and symptoms associated with extraintestinal complications, such as inflamed joints and lesions inside the mouth.

Psychosocial Assessment. Many patients are very concerned about the frequency of stools and the presence of blood. *The inability to control the disease symptoms, particularly diarrhea, can be disruptive and anxiety producing.* Severe illness may limit the patient's activities outside the home with fear of fecal incontinence, resulting in feeling "tied to the toilet." Anxiety and depression may result. Eating may be associated with pain and cramping and an increased frequency of stools. This can make mealtimes an unpleasant experience. Frequent visits to primary health care providers and close monitoring of the colon mucosa for abnormal cell changes can be anxiety provoking.

Assess the patient's understanding of the illness and the impact on lifestyle. Encourage and support the patient while exploring:

- The relationship of life events to disease exacerbations
- Stress factors that produce symptoms
- Family and social support systems
- Concerns regarding the possible genetic basis and associated cancer risks of the disease
- Internet access for reliable education information and possible telehealth

Laboratory Assessment. Hematocrit and hemoglobin levels may be low related to chronic blood loss, which indicates anemia and a chronic disease state. *An increased WBC count, C-reactive protein, or erythrocyte sedimentation rate (ESR) is consistent with inflammatory disease.* Blood levels of sodium, potassium, and chloride may be *low* related to frequent diarrheal stools and malabsorption through the diseased bowel. Hypoalbuminemia (decreased serum albumin) is found in patients with extensive disease from losing protein in the stool (Pagana et al., 2022).

Other Diagnostic Assessment. Magnetic resonance enterography (MRE) is the main examination used to study the bowel in patients who have chronic IBD. An MRE allows the primary health care provider to visualize the bowel lumen and wall, mesentery, and surrounding abdominal organs. Teach patients that they will need to fast for 4 to 6 hours before the test. As part of the test the patient drinks a large amount of contrast medium; this can cause abdominal discomfort and diarrhea. Be sure that the patient uses the restroom before positioning on the MRI table. The patient then lies prone while the first of two doses of glucagon are given subcutaneously. This substance helps to slow the bowel's activity and motility (Pagana et al., 2022).

An upper endoscopy and/or *colonoscopy* may be done to aid in diagnosis, but the bowel preparation ("prep") can be especially uncomfortable for patients with chronic inflammatory bowel disease (IBD). Frequent colonoscopies are recommended when patients have longer than a 10-year history of UC involving the entire colon because they are at high risk for colorectal cancer. In some cases, a *CT scan* may be done to confirm the disease or its complications. *Barium enemas* with air contrast can show differences between UC and Crohn's disease and identify complications, mucosal patterns, and the distribution and depth of disease involvement. During early disease, the barium enema may show incomplete filling as a result of *inflammation* and fine ulcerations along the bowel contour, which appear deeper in more advanced disease.

Analyze Cues and Prioritize Hypotheses: Analysis

The priority collaborative problems for patients with UC include:

1. Diarrhea due to *inflammation* of the bowel mucosa
2. Acute or persistent *pain* due to *inflammation* and ulceration of the bowel mucosa and skin irritation
3. Potential for lower GI bleeding and resulting anemia due to UC

Generate Solutions and Take Actions: Planning and Implementation

Managing Diarrhea

Planning: Expected Outcomes. The major concern for a patient with ulcerative colitis is the occurrence of frequent, bloody diarrhea and fecal incontinence from tenesmus. Therefore the expected outcome of treatment is for the patient to have decreased diarrhea, formed stools, and control of bowel movements, which allow for mucosal healing.

Interventions. Many measures are used to relieve symptoms and reduce intestinal motility, decrease *inflammation,* and promote intestinal healing. Nonsurgical and/or surgical management may be needed.

Nonsurgical Management. Nonsurgical management includes drug and *nutrition* therapy. Teach patients the need to consume a diet low in animal fats and sugars while increasing fruit and vegetable intake. Be aware that some patients may have food insecurity and do not have the financial resources to make these food purchases. For these patients, refer them to community resources, including food banks, that can provide nutritious foods at no cost.

Ask the patient about tobacco use, which is a risk factor for IBD. If appropriate, refer the patient to a smoking cessation program online or in person. Be aware that some programs have a cost associated with them and the patient may not be in a financial position to pay for this resource. Determine if there is a grant or financial assistance for the program.

The use of physical and emotional rest is also an important consideration. Teach the patient to record color, volume, frequency, and consistency of stools, either on paper or via an electronic app, to determine severity of the problem.

Monitor the skin in the perianal area for irritation and ulceration resulting from loose, frequent stools. Stool cultures may be sent for analysis if diarrhea continues. Have patients record their weight one or two times per week. If the patient is hospitalized, remind assistive personnel to weigh the patient on admission and daily in the morning before breakfast using the same scale and to document all weights.

Drug therapy. Common drug therapy for UC includes 5-aminosalicylates, glucocorticoids, immunosuppressants, immunomodulators, and antibiotics. Teach patients about side effects and adverse drug events (ADEs) and when to call their primary health care provider.

The *5-aminosalicylates* are drugs commonly used to treat mild to moderate UC and/or maintain remission. These drugs are thought to have an antiinflammatory effect on the lining of the intestine by inhibiting prostaglandins and are usually effective in 2 to 4 weeks.

Sulfasalazine is a 5-aminosalicylate metabolized by the intestinal bacteria into 5-ASA, which delivers the beneficial effects of the drug, and sulfapyridine, which is responsible for unwanted side effects. Teach patients to take a folic acid supplement because sulfasalazine decreases its absorption (Burchum & Rosenthal, 2022).

NURSING SAFETY PRIORITY

Drug Alert

Teach patients taking sulfasalazine to report nausea, vomiting, anorexia, rash, and headache to the health care provider. With higher doses, hemolytic anemia, hepatitis, male infertility, or agranulocytosis can occur. This drug is in the same family as sulfonamide antibiotics. *Therefore assess the patient for an allergy to sulfonamide or other drugs that contain sulfa before the patient takes the drug.* The use of a thiazide diuretic may be a contraindication for sulfasalazine (Burchum & Rosenthal, 2022).

Mesalamine is better tolerated than sulfasalazine because none of the preparations contain sulfapyridine. This may be given as a delayed-release drug in the terminal ileum and beyond within the colon, or as an extended-release drug that works throughout the colon and rectum. Mesalamine can also be given as an enema or a suppository. These preparations have minimal systemic absorption and therefore have fewer side effects (Crohn's and Colitis Foundation, 2022).

Glucocorticoids are corticosteroid therapies that may be prescribed during exacerbations of the disease. Prednisone is typically prescribed, and the dose may be increased as acute flare-ups occur. Once clinical improvement occurs, the corticosteroids are tapered because adverse effects commonly occur with long-term steroid therapy (e.g., hyperglycemia, osteoporosis, peptic ulcer disease, increased potential for infection, adrenal insufficiency). For patients with rectal *inflammation,* topical steroids in the form of small retention enemas or suppositories may be prescribed. Medications such as budesonide, steroids that are thought to work mostly in the bowel, produce fewer systemic side effects (Burchum & Rosenthal, 2022).

Immunomodulators are drugs that alter an individual's immune response. Alone, they are often not effective in the treatment of UC. However, in combination with steroids, they may offer a synergistic effect to a quicker response, thereby decreasing the steroid dose needed. Biological response modifiers (BRMs) used for UC (and Crohn's disease, discussed later in this chapter) include infliximab and adalimumab. Although not approved as a first-line therapy for UC, infliximab may be used for refractory disease or for severe complications, such as toxic megacolon and extraintestinal manifestations. Infliximab is an immunoglobulin G (IgG) monoclonal antibody that reduces the activity of tumor necrosis factor (TNF) to decrease *inflammation.* Adalimumab is another monoclonal antibody approved for refractory (not responsive to other therapies) cases. BRMs are used more commonly in management of Crohn's disease. These drugs cause immunosuppression and should be used with caution. Teach the patient to report any signs of a beginning *infection,* including a cold, and to avoid large crowds and others who are sick.

Several newer monoclonal antibodies have recently been approved by the U.S. Food and Drug Administration (FDA) for use in patients with chronic IBD. One of these drugs, vedolizumab, is an intestinal-specific leukocyte traffic inhibitor in that it prevents white blood cells from migrating to inflamed bowel tissue (Crohn's and Colitis Foundation, 2022).

NCLEX Examination Challenge 49.2

Physiological Integrity

The nurse is planning health teaching for a client starting adalimumab for ulcerative colitis. Which statement would the nurse include in the health teaching?
A. "You should not take this drug if you are allergic to sulfa drugs."
B. "Take a folic acid supplement while you are on this drug."
C. "This drug is a corticosteroid, so it will be slowly increased."
D. "You should avoid large crowds and anyone who has an infection."

Nutrition therapy and rest. Patients who are hospitalized with severe symptoms are kept NPO to ensure bowel rest. The primary health care provider may prescribe total parenteral *nutrition* (TPN) for severely ill and malnourished patients during severe exacerbations. Chapter 52 describes this therapy in detail. Patients with less severe symptoms may drink elemental formulas, which have components that are absorbed in the small bowel and reduce bowel stimulation.

Diet is not a major factor in the inflammatory process, but some patients with ulcerative colitis (UC) find that caffeine and alcohol increase diarrhea and cramping. For some patients, raw vegetables and other high-fiber foods can cause GI symptoms. Lactose-containing foods may be poorly tolerated and should be reduced or eliminated. Teach patients that carbonated beverages, pepper, nuts and corn, dried fruits, and smoking are common GI stimulants that could cause discomfort. Each patient differs in food and fluid tolerances.

During an exacerbation of the disease, patient activity is generally restricted because rest can reduce intestinal activity, provide comfort, and promote healing. Ensure that the patient has easy access to a bedpan, bedside commode, or bathroom in case of urgency or tenesmus.

Complementary and integrative health. In addition to dietary changes, complementary and integrative therapies may be used to supplement traditional management of UC. Examples include herbs (e.g., flaxseed), selenium, and vitamin C. Biofeedback, hypnosis, yoga, acupuncture, and ayurveda (a combination of diet, yoga, herbs, and breathing exercises) may be helpful. These therapies need further study to validate their effectiveness.

Surgical Management. Some patients with UC require surgery to help manage their disease when medical therapies alone are not effective. In some cases, surgery is performed for complications of UC such as toxic megacolon, hemorrhage, bowel perforation, dysplastic biopsy results, and colon cancer.

PATIENT-CENTERED CARE: CULTURE AND SPIRITUALITY

Health Equity Issues Related to Surgical Outcomes for Chronic Inflammatory Bowel Disease (IBD)

Surgical management for ulcerative colitis (UC) is more common and typically more successful than surgery to treat Crohn's disease. African Americans have worse surgical outcomes than do Whites, including a higher risk of sepsis and death (Barnes et al., 2021). Factors that may contribute to this inequity include social determinants of health such as delay in disease diagnosis, lack of health insurance coverage, and difficulty accessing an IBD specialist (gastroenterologist) (Barnes et al., 2021).

The development of Enhanced Recovery After Surgery (ERAS) protocols has helped to reduce the risk of sepsis and death for all patients by using evidence-based practices, focusing on nutrition, preventing postoperative paralytic ileus, and using nonopioid analgesia and goal-directed fluid therapy (Barnes et al., 2021; McCartney et al., 2023). Box 49.3 lists key components of the ERAS protocol for IBD surgery.

Preoperative care. General preoperative teaching related to abdominal surgery is described in Chapter 9. If a temporary or permanent ileostomy is planned, provide an in-depth explanation to the patient and family. An ileostomy is a procedure in which a loop of the ileum is placed through an opening in the abdominal wall (stoma) for drainage of fecal material into a pouching system worn on the abdomen. This external pouching system consists of a solid skin barrier (wafer) to protect the skin and a fecal collection device (pouch), similar to the system used for patients with colostomies (discussed in Chapter 48).

If an ileostomy is planned, the surgeon consults with a certified wound, ostomy, and continence nurse (CWOCN) before

---

BOX 49.3 Best Practice for Patient Safety and Quality Care

Key Components of the ERAS Protocol for IBD Surgery

Preoperative Care
- Patient education
- Frailty survey
- Reducing fasting time
- Carbohydrate loading
- Glucose control

Intraoperative Care
- Minimally invasive surgery
- Multimodal anesthesia
- Fluid administration

Postoperative Care
- Early ambulation
- Minimal IV
- Aggressive management of nausea and vomiting
- Nutritional consultation for early feeding
- Multimodal pain management
- Glucose control
- Early removal of indwelling urinary catheter

ERAS, Enhanced Recovery After Surgery; *IBD,* inflammatory bowel disease.
Data from Barnes, E. L., Loftus, E. V., Jr., & Kappelman, M. D. (2021). Effects of race and ethnicity on diagnoses and management of inflammatory bowel diseases. *Gastroenterology, 160,* 677–689.

---

surgery for recommendations on the best location for the stoma. A visit before surgery from an ostomate (a patient with an ostomy) may be helpful.

Operative procedures. Any one of several surgical approaches may be used for the patient with UC. Minimally invasive procedures, such as laparoscopic, laparoscopic-assisted, hand-assisted, and robotic-assisted surgery, are common for patients with UC in large tertiary care centers. Laparoscopic surgery usually involves several small incisions but often takes longer to perform than the open surgical approach. The natural orifice transluminal endoscopic surgery (NOTES) procedure can be performed via the anus or vagina in certain patients. The availability of this type of procedure depends greatly on the training of the surgeon. Patients may have moderate sedation or general anesthesia for minimally invasive surgical procedures. These patients are *not* typically admitted to critical care units for continuing postoperative care.

Patients who are obese, have had previous abdominal surgeries, or have dense scar tissue (adhesions) may not be candidates for laparoscopic procedures. A conventional open surgical approach involves general anesthesia and an abdominal incision. Patients with open procedures are initially admitted to critical care units for short-term stabilization.

RESTORATIVE PROCTOCOLECTOMY WITH ILEO POUCH–ANAL ANASTOMOSIS (RPC-IPAA). This procedure has become the gold standard for patients with UC. In some cases the surgery is performed via laparoscopy (laparoscopic RPC-IPAA). Typically it is a two-stage procedure that includes the removal of the colon and most of the rectum (Fig. 49.2); the anus and anal sphincter

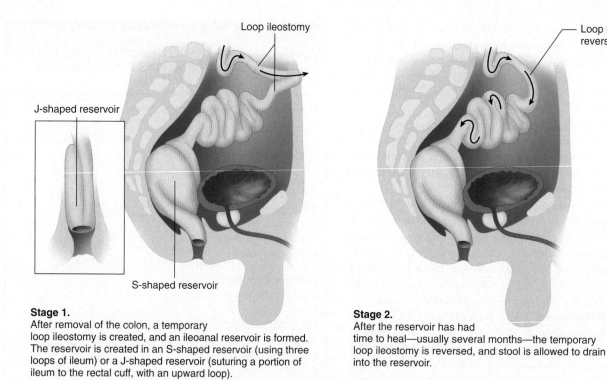

Stage 1.
After removal of the colon, a temporary
loop ileostomy is created, and an ileoanal reservoir is formed.
The reservoir is created in an S-shaped reservoir (using three
loops of ileum) or a J-shaped reservoir (suturing a portion of
ileum to the rectal cuff, with an upward loop).

Stage 2.
After the reservoir has had
time to heal—usually several months—the temporary
loop ileostomy is reversed, and stool is allowed to drain
into the reservoir.

FIG. 49.2 Creation of an ileoanal reservoir.

remain intact. The surgeon then surgically creates an internal pouch (reservoir) using the last 18 inches (45.7 cm) of the small intestine. The ileoanal pouch, sometimes called a J-pouch, S-pouch, or pelvic pouch, is then connected to the anus. A temporary ileostomy through the abdominal skin is created to allow healing of the internal pouch and all anastomosis sites. It also allows for an increase in the capacity of the internal pouch. In the second surgical stage, the temporary loop ileostomy is closed. The time interval between the first and second stages varies, but many patients have the second surgical stage to close the ileostomy within 1 to 2 months of the first surgery.

Usually, bowel continence is excellent after this procedure, but some patients report leakage of stool during sleep. They may take antidiarrheal drugs to help control this problem. Reassure patients that they might have frequent stools and urgency after this procedure.

TOTAL PROCTOCOLECTOMY WITH A PERMANENT ILEOSTOMY.
Total proctocolectomy with a permanent ileostomy is done for patients who are not candidates for or do not want the ileoanal pouch. The procedure involves the removal of the colon, rectum, and anus with surgical closure of the anus (Fig. 49.3A). The surgeon brings the end of the ileum out through the abdominal wall and forms a stoma, or permanent ostomy.

✚ NURSING SAFETY PRIORITY

Critical Rescue

The ileostomy stoma (Fig. 49.3B) is usually placed in the right lower quadrant of the abdomen below the belt line. It should not be prolapsed or retract into the abdominal wall. *Assess the stoma frequently after stoma placement. Recognize that it should be pinkish to cherry red to ensure an adequate blood supply. If the stoma looks pale, ash gray, bluish, or dark, report these findings to the surgeon immediately* (Stelton, 2019)!

Initially after surgery, the output from an ileostomy is a loose, dark green liquid that may contain some blood. Over time, a process called *ileostomy adaptation* occurs. The small intestine begins to perform some of the functions that had previously been done by the colon, including the absorption of increased amounts of sodium and water. Stool volume decreases, becomes thicker (pastelike), and turns yellow-green or yellow-brown. The **effluent** (fluid material) usually has little odor or a sweet odor. Any foul or unpleasant odor may be a symptom of a problem such as blockage or infection (McCartney et al., 2023).

The ileostomy drains frequently. Consequently the patient must always wear a pouch system. The stool from the small intestine contains many enzymes and bile salts, which can quickly irritate and excoriate the skin. Skin care around the stoma is a priority! A pouch system with a skin barrier (gelatin or pectin) provides sufficient protection for most patients. Other products are also available.

Postoperative Care. Provide general postoperative care after surgery, as described in Chapter 9. As part of the ERAS protocol, most patients have minimally invasive surgery (MIS) and therefore do *not* have a nasogastric tube (NGT). Patients who require open-approach surgery for UC have a large abdominal incision. Initially, they are NPO and an NGT is used for gastric decompression. The tube is removed in 1 to 2 days as the drainage decreases, and fluids and food are slowly introduced

In collaboration with the CWOCN, help the patient adjust and learn the required care. The ileostomy usually begins to drain stool within 24 hours after surgery at more than 1 L/day. Be sure that fluids are replaced by adding 500 mL or more each day to prevent dehydration. After about a week of high-volume output, the stool drainage slows and becomes thicker. During this period, patients may require antidiarrheal drugs.

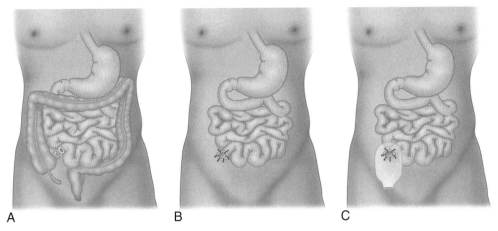

FIG. 49.3 (A) Total proctocolectomy with a permanent ileostomy. This involves removal of the colon, the rectum, and the anus with closure of the anus. (B) Ileostomy surgical stoma placement. (C) Ileostomy with ostomy appliance attached.

The hospital stay is usually from 1 to 4 days, depending on whether the patient has laparoscopic (MIS) or conventional open surgery. Patients having MIS have less pain from surgery, fewer complications, and faster restoration of bowel function when compared with other surgical patients.

For those who have the RPC-IPAA procedure, remind the patient that the internal pouch can become inflamed (pouchitis). This problem is usually treated effectively with metronidazole for 7 to 10 days. Teach patients that after the second stage of surgery they might have burning during bowel *elimination* because gastric acid cannot be absorbed well by the ileum. Also, instruct them to omit foods that can cause odors or gas, such as cabbage, asparagus, brussels sprouts, and beans. Teach patients to eliminate foods that cannot be digested well, such as nuts and corn. Food intolerances differ for each patient.

Surgery for UC may result in altered body image. However, it may decrease patients' symptoms and they may feel more comfortable than before the procedure. Patients must adjust to having an ostomy before they can resume their presurgery activities.

Managing Pain

Planning: Expected Outcomes. The desired outcome for patients is that they will verbalize decreased *pain* at a level of 2 to 3 or less on a 0-to-10 scale as a result of collaborative, evidence-based *pain* management interventions.

Interventions. *Pain* control requires multimodal pharmacologic and nonpharmacologic measures. Physical discomfort can contribute to emotional distress. A variety of symptom-reducing interventions and supportive measures are used. Surgery may reduce *pain* for some patients.

Increases in pain may indicate the development of complications such as peritonitis (see earlier discussion in this chapter). Assist patients in reducing or eliminating factors that can cause or increase the *pain* experience. For example, they may benefit from *nutrition* changes to decrease abdominal discomfort such as cramping and bloating.

Antidiarrheal drugs may be needed to control diarrhea, thus reducing the discomfort. However, they must be used with caution and for a short time because toxic megacolon can develop.

Perineal skin can be irritated by contact with loose stools and frequent cleaning. Explain special measures for skin care.

Use of medicated wipes is soothing if the rectal area is tender or sensitive from the use of toilet tissue. Several ostomy manufacturers produce a system for skin care that may help prevent and heal perineal skin irritation. These systems usually include a skin-cleaning solution, a moisturizing and healing cream, and a petroleum jelly–like barrier that prevents contact of moisture and stool with the skin.

Preventing or Monitoring for Lower GI Bleeding

Planning: Expected Outcomes. If possible, patients are expected to remain free of complications that can cause bleeding, such as perforation or anemia. For patients experiencing lower GI bleeding, they are expected to have a cessation of bleeding with prompt collaborative care.

Interventions. The nursing priority is to monitor the patient closely for signs and symptoms of GI bleeding resulting from the disease or its complications. If the patient has lower GI bleeding of more than 0.5 mL/min, a *GI bleeding scan* may be useful to localize the site of the bleeding (Pagana et al., 2022). However, this test cannot indicate the cause of the bleeding and may take several hours to administer. Patients in the critical care unit are not candidates for the test because they must leave the unit for it. *Keep in mind that GI bleeding is considered a medical emergency; therefore the patient should be monitored closely to detect this complication.*

✚ NURSING SAFETY PRIORITY

Critical Rescue

Recognize that it is important to monitor stools for blood loss in the patient with ulcerative colitis. The blood may be bright red (frank bleeding) or black and tarry (melena). Monitor hematocrit, hemoglobin, and electrolyte values and assess vital signs. Prolonged slow bleeding can lead to anemia. Observe for fever, tachycardia, and signs of fluid volume depletion. Changes in mental status may occur, especially among older adults, and may be the first indication of dehydration or anemia.

If symptoms of GI bleeding begin, respond by notifying the Rapid Response Team or primary health care provider immediately. Blood products are often prescribed for patients with severe anemia. Prepare for the blood transfusion by inserting two large-bore IV catheters if not already in place. Chapter 34 outlines nursing actions during blood transfusion.

Care Coordination and Transition Management

Home Care Management. The patient with ulcerative colitis provides self-management at home but may require hospitalization during severe exacerbations or after surgical intervention. In addition, those who have extraintestinal problems often need ongoing collaborative care for joint and/or skin problems.

Home care management focuses on controlling signs and symptoms and monitoring for complications. For patients returning home or transferring to nursing home or transitional care after surgery, ongoing respiratory care, incision care (if applicable), ostomy care, and pain management should be continued.

If the patient needs assistance with self-management at home, collaborate with the case manager or social worker to arrange the services of a home care aide or nurse. A home care nurse can provide assessment and guidance in integrating ostomy care into the patient's lifestyle. The nurse may also teach about wound care, including monitoring wound healing, if needed.

Self-Management Education. Teach the patient about the nature of ulcerative colitis, including its acute episodes, remissions, and symptom management. Stress that even though the cause is unknown, relapses can be prevented with proper health care. Teach patients taking immunosuppressive drugs, such as corticosteroids and biological response modifiers (biologics), to report signs of possible *infection* to the primary health care provider. Remind them to avoid crowds and anyone who has an infection. Review the purpose of drug therapy, when drugs should be taken, side effects, and adverse drug events.

Instruct the patient about measures to reduce or control abdominal *pain,* cramping, and diarrhea. Teach the patient and family about symptoms associated with disease exacerbation that should be reported to the primary health care provider, such as fever higher than 101°F (38.3°C), tachycardia, palpitations, and an increase in diarrhea, severe abdominal *pain,* or nausea/vomiting. Provide written information and contact numbers for the primary health care provider.

There is no special diet for a patient with an ileostomy. However, teach the patient to avoid any foods that cause gas. Examples include high-fiber foods such as nuts, raw cabbage, corn, celery, and popcorn. Patients need to learn which foods they tolerate best and adjust the diet accordingly. Some patients may require Vitamin B_{12} supplementation if the terminal ileum is removed (McCartney et al., 2023).

If the patient has undergone a temporary or permanent surgical diversion, collaborate with the CWOCN to explain and demonstrate required care so that the patient can self-manage or the family/caregiver can assist. Teach the importance of including adequate amounts of salt and water in the diet because the diversion can increase the loss of these substances. Urge the patient to be cautious in situations that lead to heavy sweating or fluid loss, such as strenuous physical activity, high environmental heat, and episodes of diarrhea and vomiting.

Finding the best ostomy pouching system is a major concern for many patients with an ileostomy. An effective system is one that:
- Protects the skin
- Contains the effluent (drainage) and reduces odor, if any
- Remains securely attached to the skin for a dependable period of time

Most patients desire an adhesive barrier that will last for 3 to 7 days. The barrier must create a solid seal to prevent the enzymes in the drainage from irritating the skin. Solid barriers are classified as "regular wear" or "extended wear." An adult with a high output may want an extended-wear barrier. A special cream can be used to help fill any uneven skin surfaces and provide a consistent seal. Pouches can also be individualized by the patient. Large pouches can hold more but are heavy when full. Patients must also consider the costs of the various systems and if or how much their insurance will help pay for them. Teach patients how to care for their ileostomy as described in Box 49.4.

A patient with an ileostomy may have many concerns about management at home and about sexual and social adjustments. Considering possible sexual issues helps the patient identify and discuss these concerns with the sex partner. For example,

---

BOX 49.4 Patient and Family Education
Ileostomy Care

Skin Protection
- Use a skin barrier to protect skin from contact with ostomy excretions.
- Use skin care products, such as skin sealants and ostomy skin creams. If skin continues to be exposed to ostomy contents, select a product to fill in problem areas and provide an even skin surface.
- Watch skin around the ostomy for any irritation or redness/hyperpigmentation.

Pouch Care
- Empty the pouch when it is one-third to one-half full.
- Change the pouch during inactive times, such as before meals, before retiring at night, on waking in the morning, and 2 to 4 hours after eating.
- Change the entire pouch system every 3 to 7 days.

Nutrition
- Chew food thoroughly.
- Be cautious about high-fiber and high-cellulose foods. These foods may need to be eliminated from the diet if they cause severe problems (diarrhea, constipation, or blockage). Examples include coconut, popcorn, tough-fiber meats, rice, cabbage, and vegetables with skins (tomatoes, corn, and peas).

Drug Therapy
- Avoid taking enteric-coated and capsule medications.
- Inform any primary health care provider who is prescribing medications about the ostomy. Before having prescriptions filled, inform the pharmacist about the ostomy.
- Do not take any laxative or enemas. Loose stools are normal. Contact your primary health care provider if no stool has passed in 6 to 12 hours.

Symptoms to Watch
- Report any drastic increase or decrease in drainage to the primary health care provider.
- If stomal swelling, abdominal cramping, or distention occurs or if ileostomy contents stop draining:
  - Remove the pouch with faceplate.
  - Lie down, assuming a knee-chest position.
  - Begin abdominal massage.
  - Apply moist towels to the abdomen.
  - Drink hot tea.
- If none of these maneuvers is effective in resuming ileostomy flow or if abdominal pain is severe, call the primary health care provider right away.

a change in positioning during intercourse may alleviate apprehension. Social situations may cause anxiety related to decreased self-esteem and a disturbance in body image. Encourage the patient to discuss possible concerns in addressing and resolving these potentially stressful events. Clinical depression is common among patients with ulcerative colitis. Refer patients to appropriate mental health resources if support is needed.

Some hospitals provide community support groups for their patients with chronic inflammatory bowel disease (IBD). These groups help patients and their families cope with the psychological impact of IBD and educate them about **nutrition** and complementary and integrative therapies.

Health Care Resources. For patients with a permanent ileostomy, locate a community ostomy support group by contacting the United Ostomy Associations of America (www.ostomy.org). The Ostomy Canada Society serves the needs of Canadian patients (www.ostomycanada.ca). A local support group or the Crohn's and Colitis Foundation (www.crohnscolitisfoundation.org) may be helpful in obtaining supplies and providing education for ostomates. Inform the patient and family members of available ostomy ambulatory care clinics and ostomy specialists. If the patient agrees, a visit from an ostomate can be continued after discharge.

Evaluate Outcomes: Evaluation

Evaluate the care of the patient with ulcerative colitis based on the identified priority patient problems. Expected outcomes may include that the patient will:

- Experience no diarrhea or a decrease in diarrheal episodes
- Verbalize decreased pain
- Have absence of lower GI bleeding
- Self-manage the ileostomy or ileoanal pouch (temporary or permanent)

CROHN'S DISEASE

Crohn's disease (CD) is a chronic inflammatory disease of the small intestine (most often), the colon, or both. It can affect the GI tract from the mouth to the anus but most commonly affects the terminal ileum. Non-White populations have more extensive intestinal inflammation when compared with Whites (Barnes et al., 2021). CD is a slowly progressive and unpredictable disease with involvement of multiple regions of the intestine with normal sections in between (called *skip lesions* on x-rays). Like ulcerative colitis (UC), this disease is recurrent, with remissions and exacerbations. However, patients with this IBD are more likely to have severe complications, which often lead to multiple hospital stays.

Pathophysiology Review

CD presents as **inflammation** that causes a thickened bowel wall. Strictures and deep ulcerations (cobblestone appearance) also occur, which put the patient at risk for developing a bowel fistula (abnormal opening [tract] between two organs or structures). The result is severe diarrhea and malabsorption of vital nutrients. Anemia is common, usually from iron deficiency or malabsorption issues (Rogers, 2023). Some Asian Americans carry a gene with an IBD-associated variation (*TNFSF15*) that causes more complex disease, including fistulas, strictures, and penetrating disease, when compared with other populations (Barnes et al., 2021).

The complications associated with CD are similar to those of UC (see Table 49.4). Hemorrhage is more common in UC, but it can occur in CD as well. Severe malabsorption by the small intestine is more common in patients with CD versus UC and may not involve the small bowel to any significant extent. Patients with CD can become very malnourished and debilitated due to intestinal malabsorption of dietary nutrients.

Rarely, cancer of the small bowel and colon develops but can occur after the disease has been present for 15 to 20 years. Fistula formation is a common complication of CD but is rare in UC. Fistulas can occur between segments of the intestine or manifest as cutaneous fistulas (opening to the skin) or perirectal abscesses. They can also extend from the bowel to other organs and body cavities, such as the bladder or vagina (Fig. 49.4). Some patients develop intestinal obstruction, which at first is secondary to **inflammation** and edema. Over time, fibrosis and scar tissue develop and obstruction results from a narrowing of the bowel. Most patients with CD require surgery at some point. Chapter 48 discusses surgical procedures for intestinal obstruction.

Almost a million individuals in the United States have Crohn's disease, and Canada has one of the highest incidences of Crohn's disease and colitis worldwide (Crohn's and Colitis

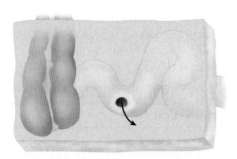
External enterocutaneous
(between skin and intestine)

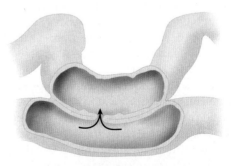
Enteroenteric
(between intestine and intestine)

FIG. 49.4 Types of fistulas that are complications of Crohn's disease.

Canada, 2020). Most patients experience symptoms and are diagnosed as adolescents or young adults between 15 and 35 years of age.

 ## PATIENT-CENTERED CARE: GENETICS/ GENOMICS

Genetics and Crohn's Disease (CD)

The exact cause of CD is unknown. A combination of genetic, immune, and life-style factors likely contributes to development of CD. About 20% of patients have a positive family history for the disease. The discovery of a mutation in the *NOD2* gene is associated with some patients who have CD. This gene is found in monocytes that normally recognize and destroy bacteria (Horowitz et al., 2021).

Proinflammatory cytokines, such as tumor necrosis factor (TNF)-alpha and interleukins (ILs), are immunologic factors that contribute to the etiology of CD. Many of the drugs used for the disease inhibit or block one or more of these factors.

Other risk factors include tobacco use (especially smoking) and living in urban areas (pollution). CD is most common in individuals of Ashkenazi Jewish background, but the incidence is increasing in non-White populations. Current research has found genetic markers in many populations that contribute to high rates of CD (Barnes et al., 2021). A diet high in animal fats and sugars and low in fruits and vegetables also places individuals at risk for IBD. Inadequate **nutrition** can also exacerbate the patient's symptoms.

Interprofessional Collaborative Care

Similar to patients with ulcerative colitis, patients with Crohn's disease may be self-managed at home, cared for in the community setting, or hospitalized depending on their immediate condition related to this chronic bowel disease.

Recognize Cues: Assessment

Crohn's disease can be exacerbated by bacterial infection. A detailed history is needed to identify manifestations specific to the disease. Ask about recent unintentional weight loss, the frequency and consistency of stools, the presence of blood in the stool, fever, and abdominal pain.

Perform a thorough abdominal assessment. Assess for manifestations of the disease and evaluate the patient's **nutrition** and hydration status.

When inspecting the abdomen, assess for distention, masses, or visible peristalsis. Inspection of the perianal area may reveal ulcerations, fissures (cracks, tears, or splits in skin), or fistulas. During auscultation, bowel sounds may be decreased or absent with severe **inflammation** or obstruction. An increase in high-pitched or rushing sounds may be present over areas of narrowed bowel loops. Muscle guarding, masses, rigidity, or tenderness may be noted on palpation by the primary health care provider.

The signs and symptoms associated with Crohn's disease vary greatly from person to person. Most patients report diarrhea, abdominal **pain,** and low-grade fever. Fever is common with fistulas, abscesses, and severe inflammation. If the disease occurs in only the ileum, diarrhea occurs five or six times per day, often

 ## EVIDENCE-BASED PRACTICE

What Is the Relationship of Fatigue and Clinical Symptoms of Crohn's Disease?

Kamp, K., Clark-Snustad, K., Barahimi, M., et al. (2022). Relationship between endoscopic and clinical disease activity with fatigue in inflammatory bowel disease. *Gastroenterology Nursing, 45*(1), 21–28.

Fatigue is a common symptom reported by patients who have inflammatory bowel disease (IBD) but has not been studied. The researchers conducted a retrospective medical record review of 160 patients with Crohn's disease to study the prevalence of fatigue based on clinical symptoms and endoscopic findings. Sixty-one percent of the study sample reported fatigue, which was significantly associated with clinical disease activity (symptoms) and anxiety. Fatigue was not significantly associated with endoscopic findings.

Level of Evidence: 4
The research was a descriptive study using a convenience sample.

Commentary: Implications for Practice and Research
This pilot study examined a symptom of Crohn's disease (fatigue) that had not been studied. Fatigue can affect a patient's quality of life and coping ability. Fatigue seemed to occur more in patients with high clinical disease activity (often diarrhea), which increased anxiety, as would be expected. Nurses need to recommend ways for patients to conserve their energy to self-manage and prepare them for this symptom. More research is needed on the relationship of psychosocial and physical aspects of IBD.

with a soft, loose stool. Steatorrhea (fatty diarrheal stools) is common. Stools may contain bright red blood. Fatigue is a very common symptom in patients experiencing systemic inflammation from active disease (see the Evidence-Based Practice box).

Abdominal pain from **inflammation** is usually constant and often located in the right lower quadrant. The patient also may have pain around the umbilicus before and after bowel movements. If the lower colon is diseased, pain is common in both lower abdominal quadrants.

Most patients with Crohn's disease have *weight loss*. Nutritional problems are the result of increased catabolism from chronic inflammation, anorexia, malabsorption, or self-imposed dietary restrictions. These problems result in impaired fluid and electrolyte balance and vital nutrient deficiencies (see Chapter 13 for more information on fluids and electrolytes).

The patient who has Crohn's disease (CD) needs a complete psychosocial assessment. The chronic nature of the disease process and the associated complications can greatly affect patients and their families. Lifestyle changes are necessary to cope with such a disruptive and painful chronic illness. Assess the patient's coping skills, and help identify support systems. Similar to problems associated with other chronic diseases, clinical depression and severe anxiety disorders are common among patients with CD.

! NURSING SAFETY PRIORITY

Action Alert

For the patient with Crohn's disease, be especially alert for signs and symptoms of peritonitis (discussed earlier in this chapter), small bowel obstruction, and nutritional and fluid imbalances. Early detection of a change in the patient's status helps reduce these life-threatening complications.

Anemia is common due to slow bleeding and poor nutrition. Serum levels of folic acid and vitamin B_{12} are generally low because of malabsorption, further contributing to anemia. Amino acid malabsorption and protein-losing enteropathy may result in *decreased albumin* levels. C-reactive protein and ESR may be elevated to indicate inflammation. White blood cells (WBCs) in the urine may show *infection* (pyuria), which is caused by ureteral obstruction or an enterovesical (bowel to bladder) fistula. If severe diarrhea or fistula is present, the patient may have fluid and electrolyte losses, particularly potassium and magnesium. Assess the patient for signs and symptoms that can occur related to electrolyte losses (see Chapter 13).

X-rays show the narrowing, ulcerations, strictures, and fistulas common with Crohn's disease. *Magnetic resonance enterography (MRE)* is performed to determine bowel activity and motility as discussed under the Other Diagnostic Assessment section in the Ulcerative Colitis concept exemplar.

Take Actions: Interventions

Collaborative care for patients with Crohn's disease is similar to that described in the discussion in the Ulcerative Colitis section. Specific interventions vary with the severity of disease and the complications that are present.

Nonsurgical Management

Drug Therapy. Drugs used to manage Crohn's disease (CD) are like those used in the treatment of ulcerative colitis (UC). For mild to moderate disease, 5-ASA drugs may be effective, although research shows that their use for CD has produced mixed results (see the Drug Therapy discussion in the Ulcerative Colitis section).

Most patients have moderate to severe disease and need stronger drug therapy to control their symptoms. Two agents that may be prescribed for CD are azathioprine and 6-mercaptopurine. These drugs suppress the immune system and can lead to serious infections.

A group of biological response modifiers (BRMs) are approved for use in CD when other drugs have been ineffective. These drugs inhibit tumor necrosis factor (TNF)-alpha, which decreases the inflammatory response. Examples of commonly used drugs for patients with CD include infliximab, adalimumab, natalizumab, and certolizumab pegol. These agents are not given to patients with a history of cancer, heart disease, or multiple sclerosis (Burchum & Rosenthal, 2022).

👤 PATIENT-CENTERED CARE: HEALTH EQUITY

Health Equity Issues Related to Drug Therapy for Crohn's Disease

As mentioned earlier in this chapter, clinical outcomes for non-White patients who have chronic inflammatory bowel disease (IBD) are worse than those for White patients. Some studies have demonstrated that Hispanic, African American, and Asian patients with Crohn's disease are less likely to receive biological response modifying drugs than White patients. This finding may contribute to less positive outcomes in non-White populations (Barnes et al., 2021).

💊 NURSING SAFETY PRIORITY

Drug Alert

Infliximab must be given in a health care setting, such as a medical office, via parenteral routes. Teach patients how to give themselves a subcutaneous injection for drugs that come in that form. Teach them to report injection site reactions, including redness/hyperpigmentation and swelling. Remind patients that headache, abdominal pain, and nausea and vomiting are common side effects. Teach them to avoid crowds and people with infection. Reinforce the need to report any *infection,* including a cold or sore throat, to the primary health care provider immediately (Burchum & Rosenthal, 2022).

Natalizumab is given intravenously under medical supervision every 4 weeks for moderate to severe Crohn's disease (CD) and when other drugs are not effective. Natalizumab can cause **progressive multifocal leukoencephalopathy (PML)**, a deadly infection that affects the brain. Before giving the drug, be sure that the patient is free of all infections. Teach patients the importance of reporting any cognitive, motor, or sensory changes immediately to the primary health care provider. Vedolizumab is used for treatment of moderate to severe CD. This drug is administered intravenously at weeks 0, 2, and 6, and then the first maintenance dose is given at 8 weeks. The maintenance doses continue every 8 weeks after that. Clinical trials confirm that vedolizumab does not increase the risk for PML, but because of its mechanism of action, the U.S. Food and Drug Administration (FDA) strongly encourages education regarding this possible complication (Bressler et al., 2021).

Although glucocorticoids can be effective for patients with CD, sepsis can result from abscesses or fistulas that may be present. These drugs mask the symptoms of *infection.* Therefore they must be used with caution and only on a short-term basis. Monitor the patient closely for signs of infection. Teach the patient not to stop the steroids abruptly because of the potential for adrenal insufficiency. Ciprofloxacin and metronidazole have been helpful in patients with fistulas, anorectal abscesses, and *infection* related to CD.

Nutrition Therapy. Long-standing nutritional deficits can have severe consequences for the patient with Crohn's disease. Poor *nutrition* can lead to inadequate fistula and wound healing, loss of lean muscle mass, decreased immune responses, and increased morbidity and mortality. During severe exacerbations of the disease, the patient may be hospitalized to provide bowel rest and nutritional support with total parenteral nutrition (TPN). Nutritional supplements such as Ensure or Sustacal can be given to provide nutrients and more calories. Teach the patient to avoid GI stimulants, such as caffeinated beverages and alcohol.

Fistula Management. Fistulas are common with acute exacerbations of Crohn's disease. They can be between the bowel and bladder (enterovesical), between two segments of bowel (enteroenteric), between the skin and bowel (enterocutaneous), or between the bowel and vagina (enterovaginal) (see Fig. 49.4). The patient with multiple fistulas often has complications such as systemic infections, skin problems (including abscesses and fissures), and malnutrition. Treatment of the patient with an abscess (a localized infection in which there is a collection of pus) requires an incision and drainage (I&D) local procedure. Management of the patient with a fistula is more complicated and includes *nutrition* and electrolyte therapy, skin care, and prevention of infection.

The patient requires at least 3000 calories daily to promote healing of the fistula. If the patient cannot take adequate oral fluids and nutrients, total enteral nutrition (TEN) or TPN may be prescribed. For patients who do not require TEN or TPN, consult with the registered dietitian nutritionist to:

- Carefully monitor the patient's tolerance of the prescribed diet
- Help the patient select high-calorie, high-protein, high-vitamin, low-fiber meals
- Offer enteral supplements
- Record food intake for accurate calorie counts

Prompt assistive personnel to provide enteral supplements, record accurate intake and output, and take daily weights while the patient is in the hospital.

INTERPROFESSIONAL COLLABORATION

Fistula Management

> Consult with the certified wound, ostomy, and continence nurse (CWOCN) to select the most appropriate wound management for each patient. According to the Interprofessional Education Collaborative (IPEC) Expert Panel's Competency of Roles and Responsibilities, interprofessional consultation with health care team members can help to identify additional problems that would benefit from their specialized knowledge and expertise (IPEC, 2016; Slusser et al., 2018).

Enzymes and bile in the stool contribute to the problem of skin irritation and excoriation. Skin irritation needs to be prevented. This may be accomplished by using skin barriers, pouching systems, and insertion of drains (Fig. 49.5). Skin barriers or dressings are used when the fistula drainage is less than 100 mL in 24 hours. A pouch is used for heavily draining fistulas to reduce the risk for skin breakdown and measure the effluent (output). However, they are very challenging because of location and drainage amount. Treatment with an antifungal

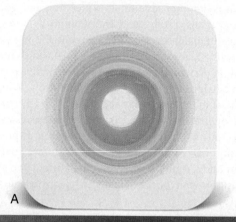

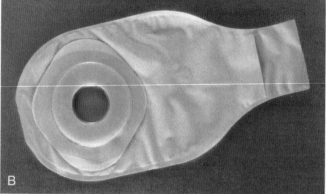

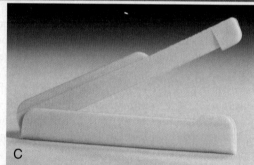

FIG. 49.5 Skin barriers, such as wafers (A), are cut to fit ⅛ inch around the fistula. A drainable pouch (B) is applied over the wafer and clamped (C) until the pouch is to be emptied. Effluent should drain into the bag and not contact the skin. (Courtesy ConvaTec, a Bristol-Myers Squibb Company, Princeton, NJ.)

powder applied to the skin around the fistula is often very helpful to prevent or treat *Candida* infection.

For some fistulas, pouching may not be possible because of their location. Drainage may need to be managed using regulated wall suction or a negative-pressure wound therapy device. Continuous low wall suction is attached to a suction catheter in the wound bed of the fistula, not into the fistula tract. These systems are not meant for long-term management.

Negative-pressure wound therapy (e.g., vacuum-assisted closure, or wound VAC therapy) promotes wound healing by secondary intention as it prepares the wound bed for closure, reduces edema, promotes granulation and perfusion, and removes exudate and infectious material. These systems should not be used in patients who are at risk for bleeding or only for the purpose of drainage containment.

Patients with fistulas are also at high risk for intraabdominal abscesses and sepsis. Antibiotic therapy is commonly prescribed. Observe for signs of sepsis (systemic infection), such as fever, abdominal pain, or a change in mental status. Monitor for increased WBC levels that could indicate a systemic infection.

Other Therapies. Other helpful interventions for the patient with CD are those that relax the patient and soothe the GI tract. Such therapies may include naturopathy, herbs (e.g., ginger), acupuncture, hypnotherapy, and ayurveda (a combination of diet, herbs, yoga, and breathing exercises). The evidence supporting the use of these substances for CD is lacking, but many patients find them helpful for overall physical and emotional health. Teach patients about the availability of these therapies, and support their use in the collaborative plan of care.

Surgical Management. Surgery for Crohn's disease may be performed in patients who have not improved with medical management or in those who have complications. Although commonly performed, surgery to manage Crohn's disease is generally not as successful as that for ulcerative colitis because of the extent of the disease. The patient with a fistula may undergo resection of the diseased area. Other indications for surgical treatment include perforation, massive hemorrhage, intestinal obstruction or strictures, abscesses, or cancer.

In some cases a resection (removal of part of the small bowel) can be performed via minimally invasive surgery (MIS) via laparoscopy. This surgical procedure involves one or more small incisions, less pain, and a quicker surgical recovery when compared with traditional open surgery. Both small bowel resection (usually the ileum) and ileocecal resection can be done using this procedure. For other patients, an open surgical approach is used to allow for better visual access to the bowel.

Stricturoplasty may be performed for bowel strictures related to Crohn's disease. This procedure increases the bowel diameter. Nursing care before and after each of these surgical procedures is similar to care for patients undergoing other types of abdominal surgery (see Chapter 9).

Care Coordination and Transition Management

The discharge care plan for the patient with Crohn's disease is similar to that for the patient with ulcerative colitis (see the Care Coordination and Transition Management discussion in the Ulcerative Colitis section). However, the number of hospitalizations and number of hospital readmissions is typically higher for patients with Crohn's disease when compared with those who have UC (see the Systems Thinking/Quality Improvement box).

Reinforce measures to control the disease and related symptoms and manage *nutrition.* Teach the patient and family to make arrangements for the patient to have easy access to the bathroom and privacy to perform fistula care, if needed.

The health teaching plan for Crohn's disease is similar to that for the patient with ulcerative colitis. Teach the patient about the usual progression of the disease, symptoms of complications, and when to notify the health care provider. Provide health teaching for drug therapy, including purpose, dose, and side effects. In addition to other drugs, vitamin supplements,

SYSTEMS THINKING/QUALITY IMPROVEMENT

Can Hospital Readmissions Be Reduced for Patients Who Have Crohn's Disease?

Choe, M., Van Graafeiland, B., & Parian, A. (2021). Improving follow-ups with gastroenterologists utilizing an appointment scheduling protocol in inflammatory bowel disease: A quality improvement project. *Gastroenterology Nursing, 44*(5), 91–100.

One in four patients who are hospitalized with inflammatory bowel disease (most often Crohn's disease) are readmitted in 90 days or less. The authors analyzed data to determine that patients discharged from the hospital experienced a lengthy wait time of over 40 days to have their outpatient follow-up gastroenterology appointment. A new appointment scheduling protocol was developed to ensure that patients who had recently been hospitalized or those recently diagnosed with Crohn's disease would have less wait time for the provider appointment. This protocol was piloted in 16 patients who met the criteria. For this group, appointment wait time was reduced from 40.4 days to 21.9 days.

Commentary: Implications for Practice and Research

The system in this quality improvement project was tertiary care for patients hospitalized with Crohn's disease in that reducing the wait time for follow-up provider appointments could possibly reduce hospital readmissions. A larger sample size would be needed to evaluate efficacy of the new appointment protocol and demonstrate a reduction in hospital admissions.

including monthly vitamin B_{12} injections, may be needed because of the inability of the ileum to absorb certain nutrients. In collaboration with the registered dietitian nutritionist, instruct the patient to follow a low-residue, high-calorie diet and to avoid foods that cause discomfort, such as milk, gluten (wheat products), and other GI stimulants such as caffeine.

Remind the patient to take rest periods, especially during exacerbations of the disease. If stress appears to increase symptoms of the disease, recommend stress-management techniques, counseling, and/or physical activity to improve quality of life. For long-term teaching, inform the patient about the increased risk for bowel cancer and the importance of frequent colorectal cancer screening (see Chapter 48).

If a patient has a fistula, explain and demonstrate wound care. Provide the opportunity for the patient to practice this care in the hospital. Ideally, patients should be independent in fistula care before leaving the hospital. However, because of location of the fistula (perirectal or vaginal) or a large abdomen, assistance may be needed. If this is the case, teach a family member or other caregiver how to manage the wound. Patients may be transferred to a transitional or skilled nursing unit for collaborative care.

In collaboration with the case manager, assist with obtaining the equipment and supplies for fistula care, such as skin barriers and wound drainage bags. A support group sponsored by the United Ostomy Associations of America (www.ostomy.org) or a local hospital in the community may also be available to help with meeting physical and psychosocial needs.

DIVERTICULAR DISEASE

Diverticula are pouchlike herniations of the mucosa through the muscular wall of any part of the gut, but most commonly the

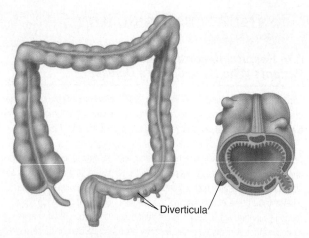

FIG. 49.6 Several abnormal outpouchings, or herniations, in the wall of the intestine, which are diverticula. These can occur anywhere in the small or large intestine but are found most often in the colon. Diverticulitis is the inflammation of a diverticulum that occurs when undigested food or bacteria become trapped in the diverticulum.

colon. Diverticulosis is the presence of many abnormal pouch-like herniations (diverticula) in the wall of the intestine. Acute diverticulitis is the inflammation or infection of diverticula.

Pathophysiology Review

Diverticula can occur in any part of the small or large intestine, but they usually occur in the sigmoid colon (Fig. 49.6). The muscle of the colon hypertrophies, thickens, and becomes rigid, and herniation of the mucosa and submucosa through the colon wall is seen. Diverticula seem to occur at points of weakness in the intestinal wall, often at areas where blood vessels interrupt the muscle layer. Muscle weakness develops as part of the aging process or because of a lack of fiber in the diet.

Diverticula *without* **inflammation** cause few problems. However, if undigested food or bacteria become trapped in a diverticulum, blood supply to that area is reduced. Bacteria invade the diverticulum, resulting in diverticulitis, which then can perforate and develop a local abscess. A perforated diverticulum can progress to an intraabdominal perforation with peritonitis. Lower GI bleeding may also occur (see earlier discussion in this chapter under Ulcerative Colitis).

High intraluminal pressure forces the formation of a pouch in the weakened area of the mucosa. Diets low in fiber that cause less bulky stool and constipation have been implicated in the formation of diverticula. Retained undigested food in diverticula is suggested to be one cause of diverticulitis. The retained food reduces blood flow to that area and makes bacterial invasion of the sac easier (Rogers, 2023).

The exact incidence of diverticulosis is unknown, but millions experience this problem, often without any symptoms or awareness of the disease. It is found in two-thirds of adults older than 80 years, with more men than women affected.

Interprofessional Collaborative Care

Patients with diverticular disease are self-managed at home, cared for in the community setting, or hospitalized if surgery is needed to correct a concern.

Recognize Cues: Assessment

The patient with *diverticulosis* usually has no signs or symptoms. Unless pain or bleeding develops, the condition may go undiagnosed. Diverticula are most often diagnosed during routine colonoscopy. Occasionally diverticulosis will cause symptoms. For the patient with uncomplicated diverticulosis, ask about intermittent **pain** in the left lower quadrant and a history of constipation. If diverticulitis is suspected, ask about a history of low-grade fever, nausea, and abdominal pain. Inquire about recent bowel **elimination** patterns because constipation may develop as a result of intestinal inflammation. Also, ask about any bleeding from the rectum.

The patient with *diverticulitis* may have abdominal **pain,** most often localized to the left lower quadrant. It is intermittent at first but becomes progressively steady. Occasionally, pain may be just above the pubic bone or may occur on one side. Abdominal pain is generalized if peritonitis develops. Nausea and vomiting are common. The patient's temperature is elevated, ranging from a low-grade fever to 101°F (38.3°C). Chills may be present. Often an increased heart rate (tachycardia) occurs with fever (Rogers, 2023).

Observe for abdominal distention. The patient may report tenderness over the involved area. Localized muscle spasm, guarded movement, and rebound tenderness may be present with peritoneal irritation. If generalized peritonitis is present, profound guarding occurs; rebound tenderness is more widespread; and sepsis, hypotension, or hypovolemic shock can occur. If the perforated diverticulum is close to the rectum, the health care provider may palpate a tender mass during the rectal examination. Blood pressure checks may show orthostatic changes. *If bleeding is massive, the patient may have hypovolemia and hypotension that result in shock.*

For the patient with uncomplicated diverticulosis, laboratory studies are not indicated. However, the patient with diverticulitis typically has an *elevated white blood cell (WBC) count. Decreased hematocrit and hemoglobin* values are common if chronic or severe bleeding occurs. Stool tests for occult blood, if requested, are sometimes positive. *Abdominal x-rays* may be done to evaluate for free air and fluid indicating perforation. A *CT scan* may be performed to diagnose an abscess or thickening of the bowel related to diverticulitis.

Abdominal ultrasonography, a noninvasive test, may also reveal bowel thickening or an abscess. The primary health care provider may recommend a colonoscopy 4 to 8 weeks *after the acute phase* of the illness to rule out a tumor in the large intestine, particularly if the patient has rectal bleeding.

Take Actions: Interventions

Patients are managed on an ambulatory care basis if the symptoms are mild. Monitor the patient for any prolonged or increased fever, abdominal **pain,** or blood in the stool. Patients with moderate to severe diverticulitis may be hospitalized, especially if they are older or have complications. Manifestations suggesting the need for admission are a temperature higher than 101°F (38.3°C), persistent and severe abdominal pain for more than 3 days, and/or lower GI bleeding.

A combination of drug and **nutrition** therapy with rest is used to decrease the **inflammation** associated with diverticular disease. Broad-spectrum antimicrobial drugs, such as metronidazole in conjunction with trimethoprim/sulfamethoxazole (TMP/SMZ) or ciprofloxacin, are often prescribed. A mild analgesic may be given for pain. The Patient-Centered Care: Older Adult Health—Diverticulitis box lists nursing interventions needed for care of older adults with diverticulitis.

The patient with more severe **pain** may be admitted to the hospital for IV fluids to correct dehydration and for IV drug therapy. For patients with moderate to severe diverticulitis, an analgesic may be prescribed to alleviate pain.

PATIENT-CENTERED CARE: OLDER ADULT HEALTH

Diverticulitis

- Provide antibiotics and analgesics as prescribed. Observe older patients carefully for side effects of these drugs, especially confusion (or increased confusion) and orthostatic hypotension.
- Do not give laxatives or enemas. Teach the patient and family about the importance of avoiding these measures.
- Encourage the patient to rest and to avoid activities that may increase intraabdominal pressure, such as straining and bending.
- While diverticulitis is active, provide a *low*-fiber diet. When the **inflammation** resolves, provide a *high*-fiber diet. Teach the patient and family about these diets and when they are appropriate.
- Because older patients do not always experience the typical **pain** or fever expected, observe carefully for other signs of active disease, such as a sudden change in mental status.
- Perform frequent abdominal assessments to determine distention and tenderness on palpation.
- Check stools for occult or frank bleeding.

Laxatives and enemas are avoided because they increase intestinal motility. Assess the patient on an ongoing basis for manifestations of impaired fluid and electrolyte balance.

Teach patients to rest during the acute phase of illness. Remind them to refrain from lifting, straining, coughing, or bending to avoid an increase in intraabdominal pressure, which can result in perforation of the diverticulum. **Nutrition** therapy should be restricted to low fiber or clear liquids based on symptoms. The patient with more severe symptoms is NPO. A nasogastric tube (NGT) is inserted if nausea, vomiting, or abdominal distention is severe. Infuse IV fluids as prescribed for hydration. In collaboration with a registered dietitian nutritionist, the patient increases dietary intake slowly as symptoms subside. When **inflammation** has resolved and bowel function returns to normal, a fiber-containing diet is introduced gradually.

Diverticulitis can result in rupture of the diverticulum with peritonitis, pelvic abscess, bowel obstruction, fistula, persistent fever or **pain**, or uncontrolled bleeding. The surgeon performs emergency surgery if peritonitis, bowel obstruction, or pelvic abscess is present. Colon resection, with or without a colostomy, is the most common surgical procedure for patients with diverticular disease. Chapter 48 discusses the nursing care for patients with this procedure.

Care Coordination and Transition Management

Discharge plans vary according to the treatment. The patient who has surgical intervention has the added responsibilities of incision care and possibly colostomy care with temporary activity limitations.

The patient should be instructed to avoid all fiber when symptoms of *diverticulitis* are present, because high-fiber foods can be irritating. As **inflammation** resolves, fiber can gradually be added until progression to a high-fiber diet is established. The patient who has undergone surgery is usually taking solid food by the time of discharge from the hospital.

Educate the patient regarding a high-fiber diet. Encourage the patient with *diverticulosis* to eat a diet high in cellulose and hemicellulose types of fiber. These substances can be found in wheat bran, whole-grain breads, and cereals. Teach the patient to eat at least 25 to 35 g of fiber per day. Fresh fruits and vegetables with high fiber content are added to provide bulk to stools.

If patients are not accustomed to eating high-fiber foods, teach them to add these foods to the diet gradually to avoid flatulence and abdominal cramping. A bulk-forming laxative, such as psyllium hydrophilic mucilloid, can be taken to increase fecal size and consistency. Teach the patient to drink plenty of fluids to help prevent bloating that may occur with a high-fiber diet. Alcohol should be avoided because it irritates the bowel. Foods containing seeds or indigestible material that may block a diverticulum, such as nuts, corn, popcorn, cucumbers, tomatoes, and figs, may need to be eliminated.

Provide oral and written instructions on incision care and the signs and symptoms to report to the health care provider for the patient who has had abdominal surgery. If a colostomy was created, reinforce and support ostomy care as needed. Encourage the patient to express concerns about body image. Allow time and address sexual concerns regarding the changed body image.

Instruct the patient with any type of diverticular disease about the manifestations of acute diverticulitis, including fever; abdominal pain; and bloody, mahogany, or tarry stools. Instruct patients to avoid the use of laxatives (other than bulk-forming types) and enemas. Reassure them that this disorder should not cause problems if a proper diet is followed.

In collaboration with the case manager, arrange for a home care nurse to assess wound healing and proper functioning of the ostomy and the appliance. If the patient is interested, arrange for a visit from an ostomy volunteer (ostomate) or an ostomy nurse. For information about other community resources, remind the patient to contact the United Ostomy Associations of America (www.ostomy.org).

NCLEX Examination Challenge 49.3

Physiological Integrity

The nurse is planning health teaching about nutrition for a client with a new ileostomy. Which of the following foods would the nurse recommend that the client **avoid**? **Select all that apply.**

A. Popcorn
B. Cabbage
C. Chicken
D. Egg
E. Peas
F. Banana

CELIAC DISEASE

Celiac disease is a multisystem chronic autoimmune bowel disease (Lebwohl & Rubio-Tapia, 2020). Patients who have other autoimmune diseases, such as rheumatoid arthritis and diabetes mellitus type 1, have an increased risk of developing celiac disease.

Pathophysiology Review

Celiac disease is a chronic *inflammation* of the small intestinal mucosa that can cause bowel wall atrophy, malabsorption, and diarrhea. Like many inflammatory disorders, it is thought to be caused by a combination of genetic, immunologic, and environmental or lifestyle factors. The primary complications of celiac disease are cancer, specifically non-Hodgkin lymphoma or GI cancers, and *nutrition* deficiencies.

Patients with celiac disease have varying signs and symptoms with cycles of remission and exacerbation (flare-up), usually related to how well they monitor their diet. Classic symptoms include anorexia, diarrhea and/or constipation, steatorrhea (fatty stools), abdominal pain, abdominal bloating and distention, and weight loss. Some patients have no symptoms. Still others have atypical symptoms that affect every body system, as listed in Box 49.5. Diagnosis is usually made by obtaining a screening blood test and endoscopy.

Interprofessional Collaborative Care

Dietary management is the only available treatment for achieving disease remission. In most cases, a gluten-free diet (GFD) results in healing of the intestinal mucosa after about 2 years. Gluten is the primary substance in wheat and wheat-based products. Teach patients to carefully check for hidden sources of gluten that are in foods, food additives, drugs, and cosmetics. Patients often take vitamin and mineral supplements to replace those lost from avoiding gluten foods. A registered dietitian nutritionist should be included in the patient's long-term planning and overall treatment.

PARASITIC INFECTION

Parasites can enter and invade the GI tract and cause *infection.* They commonly enter through the mouth (oral-fecal transmission) from contaminated food or water, oral-anal sexual practices, or contact with feces from a contaminated person.

Pathophysiology Review

Common parasites that cause infection in humans are *Giardia lamblia,* which causes giardiasis; *Entamoeba histolytica,* which causes amebiasis (amebic dysentery); and *Cryptosporidium.* The primary method for determining which parasitic infection is present is through stool analysis. The white blood cell (WBC) count can be very high when severe diarrhea (dysentery) is present. Table 49.5 differentiates these three common types of parasites.

A less common parasitic infection is increasing in the United States. Chagas disease is caused by the *Trypanosoma cruzi* parasite, which is most transmitted in impoverished areas of Latin America by the triatomine (kissing) bug. Patients first develop an acute *infection,* followed by an intermediate asymptomatic period and a chronic infection. Patients with chronic Chagas disease often develop cardiac dysrhythmias or heart failure and colon or esophagus dilation, causing impaired digestion and bowel *elimination.* An estimated 300,000 individuals in the United States have the

---

BOX 49.5 Key Features

Celiac Disease

Classic Symptoms
- Weight loss
- Anorexia
- Diarrhea and/or constipation
- Steatorrhea
- Abdominal pain and distention
- Vomiting

Atypical Symptoms
- Osteoporosis
- Joint pain and inflammation
- Lactose intolerance
- Iron deficiency anemia
- Depression
- Migraines
- Epilepsy
- Autoimmune disorders
- Stomatitis
- Early menopause
- Protein-calorie malnutrition

TABLE 49.5	Comparison of Common Parasitic Infections		
	Giardiasis (*Giardia lamblia*)	**Amebiasis (*Entamoeba histolytica*)**	**Cryptosporidium**
Description	Occurs in cysts and trophozoites Causes superficial invasion, destruction, and ***inflammation*** of small intestine mucosa	Occurs most commonly in crowded areas with poor sanitation Invades and ulcerates large intestinal mucosa	Occurs most commonly in immunosuppressed individuals Source is often contaminated swimming pools
Common assessment findings	Diarrhea Malabsorption syndrome Weight loss Nutrient deficiencies Acute phase is self-limiting Chronic phase can last for years	Can occur without symptoms May be mild or severe symptoms if they occur, including foul-smelling stools, abdominal cramping, and weight loss Can have extraintestinal symptoms	Primarily diarrhea Self-limiting health problem in individuals with normal immune system

disease (most in the southern areas of the United States), which can be transmitted through blood transfusions and organ transplantations. The Centers for Disease Control and Prevention (CDC) has targeted Chagas disease as one of five neglected parasitic infections that require public health action, as the number of cases is expected to increase (CDC, 2021).

Interprofessional Collaborative Care

Recognize Cues: Assessment

A thorough history can help determine potential sources of exposure to parasitic infection. A history of travel to parts of the world where such infections are prevalent increases suspicion for infection with parasites. GI symptoms related to travel might be delayed as long as 1 to 2 weeks after returning home. Immigrants (newcomers) may have the **infection** on entering a new country. A **nutrition** history is especially helpful if several people in a group become ill. Common water supplies or bodies of water may be infected with *Giardia* or *Cryptosporidium*. Trichinosis should be considered if the patient has eaten pork products.

Mild to moderate *E. histolytica* infestation causes the daily passage of several strongly foul-smelling stools, possibly with mucus but without blood, accompanied by abdominal cramping, flatulence (gas), fatigue, and weight loss.

The infected patient usually experiences remissions and recurrences. Severe amebic dysentery manifests with frequent, liquid, and foul-smelling stools with mucus *and* blood. Fever up to 104°F (40°C), tenesmus, generalized abdominal tenderness, and vomiting can also occur. The ulcerations of invading amebiasis that occur in the colon can cause pain, bleeding, and obstruction. Ulcerations can also occur in the rectum, resulting in formed stool with blood. Complications are rare but include appendicitis and bowel perforation.

Extraintestinal amebiasis can occur without symptoms of intestinal infection. The most common form is amebic liver abscess, which causes symptoms of fever, pain, and an enlarged liver. The abscess can rupture, and death can result if the infection and complications are not treated.

Take Actions: Interventions

Handwashing is the best way to prevent the spread of parasitic infections. Treatment for all types of *amebiasis* involves the use of amebicide drugs. Metronidazole followed by a luminal agent, such as paromomycin, is commonly prescribed for *amebiasis* (Burchum & Rosenthal, 2022). The patient with severe amebic dysentery requires IV fluid replacement and possibly an opiate-like drug, such as diphenoxylate hydrochloride and atropine sulfate, to control bowel motility. The patient with extraintestinal amebiasis or severe dehydration, especially the older adult, is hospitalized. The patient with asymptomatic, mild, or moderate disease is treated with drug therapy on an ambulatory care basis. Therapy effectiveness is based on the examination of at least three stools 2- to 3-day intervals, starting 2 to 4 weeks after drug therapy has been completed. *Teach patients the importance of keeping their follow-up appointments and taking all drugs as prescribed.*

Treatment for *giardiasis* is drug therapy. Metronidazole is the drug of choice. Tinidazole can be used as an alternative (Burchum & Rosenthal, 2022). Stools are examined 2 weeks after treatment to assess for drug effectiveness.

Infection with *Cryptosporidium* is usually self-limiting in adults who have normal immune function. Drug therapy for patients who are immunosuppressed may include paromomycin, an aminoglycoside antibiotic. Teach patients that this drug can cause dizziness.

> ## ! NURSING SAFETY PRIORITY
> ### *Action Alert*
>
> Explain modes of transmission of parasitic infections and means to avoid the spread of infection and recurrent contact with parasitic organisms. *Inform the patient that the infection can be transmitted to others until amebicides effectively kill the parasites. Teach the patient to:*
> - Avoid contact with stool
> - Keep toilet areas clean
> - Wash hands meticulously with an antimicrobial soap after bowel movements
> - Maintain good personal hygiene by bathing or showering daily
> - Avoid stool from dogs and beavers
>
> Advise the patient to avoid sexual practices that allow rectal contact until drug therapy is completed. *All household and sexual partners should have stool examinations for parasites.* If the water supply is suspected as the source, a sample is obtained and sent for analysis. Multiple infections are common in households, often as a result of contaminated shared water supplies. Well water and water from areas with inadequate or no filtration equipment can be sources of contamination.

GET READY FOR THE NEXT-GENERATION NCLEX® EXAMINATION!

Essential Nursing Care Points

Health Promotion/Disease Prevention	Chronic Disease Care
• Teach individuals that handwashing and sanitizing surfaces and other items help prevent the spread of gastroenteritis. • Proper food and beverage preparation is important to prevent gastroenteritis caused by contamination.	• Ulcerative colitis (UC) and Crohn's disease (CD) are the most common chronic inflammatory bowel diseases. • UC and CD are likely caused by a combination of genetic, immunologic, and lifestyle factors. • UC typically causes multiple diarrheal episodes each day. • Patients with UC are at risk for lower GI bleeding. • Patients with CD are at high risk for fistulas, which can cause major nutritional deficits and fluid and electrolyte imbalances. • Nurses need to consult with the registered dietitian nutritionist and wound specialist to effectively manage fistulas. • Diverticulosis is the presence of many abnormal pouchlike herniations (diverticula) in the wall of the intestine; acute diverticulitis is the inflammation or infection of diverticula. • Nurses should teach patients with diverticulosis to consume a high-fiber diet; patients with diverticulitis (inflammation) should consume a low-fiber diet. • CD is a chronic inflammatory disease that can be controlled with a gluten-free diet, which results in the healing of intestinal mucosa.
Regenerative or Restorative Care	**Hospice/Palliative/Supportive Care**
• Key features of peritonitis include a rigid, boardlike abdomen (classic), distended abdomen, abdominal pain, nausea and vomiting, fever, tachycardia, and diminishing bowel sounds. • Multisystem complications can occur from peritonitis, including loss of fluids and electrolytes. • Perforation of an inflamed appendix can cause peritonitis. • Surgical removal of the inflamed appendix is the treatment of choice for patients who have appendicitis.	• Patients who have inflammatory bowel problems usually are medically or surgically managed and do not die from their intestinal health problem unless there is a serious life-threatening complication such as sepsis.

Mastery Questions

1. The nurse is monitoring a postoperative client following abdominal surgery for peritonitis. For which of the following assessment findings would the nurse observe? **Select all that apply.**
   A. Bradycardia
   B. Severe abdominal pain
   C. Jaundice
   D. Boardlike abdomen
   E. Nausea and vomiting
   F. Fever

2. The nurse is evaluating health teaching for a client who recently had an ileostomy. Which statement by the client indicates a need for **further** teaching?
   A. "I will wear my pouch all of the time and change as needed."
   B. "I will watch my skin around the stoma for irritation or redness."
   C. "I will take a laxative every night to ensure that the ostomy works properly."
   D. "I will be careful and chew my food thoroughly so that it digests well."

3. The nurse is planning health teaching about how to follow an appropriate diet for a client recently diagnosed with celiac disease. What of the following foods would the nurse teach the client to **avoid**? **Select all that apply.**
   A. Wheat bread
   B. Broccoli
   C. Black beans
   D. Noodles
   E. Yogurt
   F. Cookies

NGN Challenge 49.1

49.1.1

The nurse is caring for a 24-year-old client in the emergency department (ED).

Highlight the findings that require **immediate** follow-up.

History and Physical	**Nurses' Notes**	Vital Signs	Diagnostic Results

1330: Client brought to ED by friend with report of severe abdominal pain and distention and nausea and vomiting since yesterday. Started with severe right abdominal lower quadrant pain that improved for about an hour before more diffuse pain occurred. Has not been able to eat or drink anything since last night. Alert and oriented × 4. No adventitious breath sounds. S_1 and S_2 present. Bowel sounds diminished in all quadrants. Currently reports 9/10 pain on a 0-to-10 pain scale. Pain lessens when changing positions. Has not voided since early this a.m. VS: T 102°F (38.9°C); HR 104 beats/min and regular; RR 22 breaths/min; BP 96/54 mm Hg; SpO_2 97% on RA.

49.1.2

The nurse is caring for a 24-year-old client in the ED.

History and Physical	**Nurses' Notes**	Vital Signs	Diagnostic Results

1330: Client brought to ED by friend with report of severe abdominal pain and distention and nausea and vomiting since yesterday. Started with severe right abdominal lower quadrant pain that improved for about an hour before more diffuse pain occurred. Has not been able to eat or drink anything since last night. Alert and oriented × 4. No adventitious breath sounds. S_1 and S_2 present. Bowel sounds diminished in all quadrants. Currently reports 9/10 pain on a 0-to-10 pain scale. Pain lessens when changing positions. Has not voided since early this a.m. VS: T 102°F (38.9°C); HR 104 beats/min and regular; RR 22 breaths/min; BP 96/54 mm Hg; SpO_2 97% on RA.

The nurse analyzes the client assessment findings. For each client finding listed below, determine if the finding is consistent with the health conditions of appendicitis, peritonitis, or diverticulitis. Each finding may support more than 1 condition.

Client Finding	Appendicitis	Peritonitis	Diverticulitis
Severe abdominal pain and distention			
Diminished bowel sounds			
Abdominal pain lessens with movement			
Nausea and vomiting			
Fever			
Rigid abdomen			
Anorexia			

49.1.3

The nurse reviews the results of a 24-year-old client's abdominal x-ray and compares them with the client's assessment findings as documented in the Nurses' Notes.

History and Physical	**Diagnostic Results**	Vital Signs	Nurses' Notes

1440: Moderate amount of free fluid in abdominal cavity. Small bowel dilated, indicating inflammation or ileus.

History and Physical	**Nurses' Notes**	Vital Signs	Diagnostic Results

1330: Client brought to ED by friend with report of severe abdominal pain and distention and nausea and vomiting since yesterday. Started with severe right abdominal lower quadrant pain that improved for about an hour before more diffuse pain occurred. Has not been able to eat or drink anything since last night. Alert and oriented × 4. No adventitious breath sounds. S_1 and S_2 present. Bowel sounds diminished in all quadrants. Currently reports 9/10 pain on a 0-to-10 pain scale. Pain lessens when changing positions. Has not voided since early this a.m. VS: T 102°F (38.9°C); HR 104 beats/min and regular; RR 22 breaths/min; BP 96/54 mm Hg; SpO_2 97% on RA.

Complete the following sentence by selecting from the lists of options below.

The *priority* for the client at this time is to **1 [Select]**, due to client findings of **2 [Select]**, **3 [Select]**, and **4 [Select]**.

Options for 1	Options for 2	Options for 3	Options for 4
Start antibiotic therapy	Tachycardia	Abdominal distention	Tachypnea
Replace fluids and electrolytes	Oxygen saturation	Possible ileus	Report of nausea and vomiting
Manage pain	Abdominal pain	Anorexia	Fever
Prepare the client for surgery	Free fluid in abdominal cavity	Hypotension	Less abdominal pain on movement

49.1.4

The nurse plans possible interventions for a 24-year-old client who was admitted to the ED with a probable diagnosis of peritonitis caused by a perforated appendix. Select the **4** nursing actions that would be appropriate for the client at this time.

○ Initiate IV access for fluid and electrolyte replacement.
○ Start supplemental oxygen therapy.
○ Maintain the client in a sitting position.
○ Administer antibiotic therapy.
○ Prepare for possible surgery.
○ Insert a nasogastric tube connected to suction.

49.1.5

The nurse is preparing to care for a 24-year-old client returning from the postanesthesia care unit (PACU) after an exploratory laparotomy to remove the perforated appendix, drain collected fluid, and irrigate the abdomen. The client has two abdominal drains and a large bulky surgical dressing. Which of the following nursing actions would the nurse take in the **immediate** postoperative period? **Select all that apply.**

○ Monitor the client's level of consciousness.

○ Assess respiratory status and oxygen saturation.

○ Maintain supplemental oxygen therapy until client is fully awake.

○ Discontinue IV fluids when returning to the surgical unit.

○ Monitor intake and output hourly.

○ Maintain the client in a semi-Fowler's position.

○ Encourage the use of incentive spirometry every 1 to 2 hours.

○ Maintain sequential compression stockings.

○ Administer oral antibiotic therapy as prescribed.

49.1.6

A 24-year-old client visits the surgeon for a follow-up visit after a hospital stay for peritonitis with surgical intervention. The nurse performs an initial assessment and compares the client's initial findings with findings today by reviewing the client's ED note.

History and Physical	Nurses' Notes	Vital Signs	Diagnostic Results

1330: Client brought to ED by friend with report of severe abdominal pain and distention and nausea and vomiting since yesterday. Started with severe right abdominal lower quadrant pain that improved for about an hour before more diffuse pain occurred. Has not been able to eat or drink anything since last night. Alert and oriented × 4. No adventitious breath sounds. S_1 and S_2 present. Bowel sounds diminished in all quadrants. Currently reports 9/10 pain on a 0-to-10 pain scale. Pain lessens when changing positions. Has not voided since early this a.m. VS: T 102°F (38.9°C); HR 104 beats/min and regular; RR 22 breaths/min; BP 96/54 mm Hg; Spo_2 97% on RA.

For each client finding listed below, determine if the finding is consistent with the client progressing or not progressing as a result of nursing and interprofessional collaborative actions.

Current Client Findings	Progressing	Not Progressing
Abdominal discomfort 2/10 on a 0-to-10 pain scale		
No nausea and vomiting since hospital discharge		
T 99°F (37.2°C)		
HR 84 beats/min and regular		
BP 112/68 mm Hg		

REFERENCES

Asterisk (*) indicates a classic or definitive work on this subject.

Barnes, E. L., Loftus, E. V., Jr., & Kappelman, M. D. (2021). Effects of race and ethnicity on diagnosis and management of inflammatory bowel diseases. *Gastroenterology, 160,* 677–689.

Bressler, B., Yarur, A., Silverberg, M. S., Bassel, M., Bellaguarda, E., Fourment, C., et al. (2021). Vedolizumab and anti-tumor necrosis factor α real-world outcomes in biologic-naïve inflammatory bowel disease patients: Results from the EVOLVE study. *Journal of Crohn's & Colitis, 15*(10), 1694–1706. https://doi.org/10.1093/ecco-jcc/jjab058.

Burchum, J. L. R., & Rosenthal, L. D. (2022). *Lehne's pharmacology for nursing care* (11th ed.). St. Louis: Elsevier.

Centers for Disease Control and Prevention (CDC). (2021). *Parasites-American trypanosomiasis.* http://www.cdc.gov/parasites/chagas

Centers for Disease Control and Prevention (CDC). (2022). *Inflammatory bowel disease (IBD): Data and statistics.* https://www.cdc.gov/ibd/data-statistics.htm.

Choe, M., Van Graafeiland, B., & Parian, A. (2021). Improving follow-ups with gastroenterologists utilizing an appointment scheduling protocol in inflammatory bowel disease: A quality improvement project. *Gastroenterology Nursing, 44*(5), 91–100.

Crohn's and Colitis Canada. (2020). *Canada leads the fight against IBD.* http://www.crohnsandcolitis.ca.

Crohn's and Colitis Foundation. (2022). *Irritable bowel disease (IBD) medication guide.* http://ibdmedicationguide.org.

Horowitz, J., Warne, N., Staples, J., Crowley, E., Gosalia, N., Murchie, R., et al. (2021). Mutation spectrum of NOD2 reveals recessive inheritance as a main driver of early onset Crohn's disease. *Scientific Reports, 11,* 5595. https://doi.org/10.1038/s41598-021-84938-8.

*Interprofessional Education Collaborative Expert Panel. (2016). *Core competencies for interprofessional collaborative practice: Report of an expert panel* (2nd ed.). Washington, DC: Interprofessional Education Collaborative.

Kamp, K., Clark-Snustad, K., Barahimi, M., & Lee, S. (2022). Relationship between endoscopic and clinical disease activity with fatigue in inflammatory bowel disease. *Gastroenterology Nursing, 45*(1), 21–28.

Lebwohl, B., & Rubio-Tapia, A. (2020). Epidemiology, presentation, and diagnosis of celiac disease. *Reviews and Perspectives Reviews in Basic and Clinical Gastroenterology and Hepatology, 160*(1), P63–75. https://doi.org/10.1053/j.gastro.2020.06.098.

McCartney, T., Markwell, A., Rauch-Pucher, M., & Cox-Reber, J. (2023). Caring for patients after ileostomy surgery. *American Journal of Nursing, 123*(2), 36–41.

Menz, J., Hundt, L., Schulze, T., Schmoeckel, K., Menges, P., & Domanska, G. (2021). Increased mortality and altered local immune response in secondary peritonitis after previous visceral operation in mice. *Scientific Reports, 11*(16175). https://doi.org/10.1038/s41598-021-95592-5.

Pagana, K., Pagana, T., & Pagana, T. (2022). *Mosby's manual of diagnostic and laboratory tests* (7th ed.). St. Louis: Elsevier.

Rogers, J. L. (2023). *McCance and Huether's Pathophysiology: The biologic basis for disease in adults and children* (9th ed.). St. Louis: Elsevier.

Slusser, M. M., Garcia, L. I., Reed, C.-R., & McGinnis, P. Q. (2018). *Foundations of interprofessional collaborative practice in health care.* St. Louis: Elsevier.

Sole, M. L., Klein, D. G., & Moseley, M. J. (2021). *Introduction to critical care nursing* (8th ed.). St. Louis: Elsevier.

Stelton, S. (2019). Stoma and peristomal skin care: A clinical review. *American Journal of Nursing, 119*(6), 38–45. https://doi.org/10.1097/01.NAJ.0000559781.86311.64.

50

Concepts of Care for Patients With Liver Conditions

Keelin Cromar

http://evolve.elsevier.com/Iggy/

LEARNING OUTCOMES

1. Plan collaborative care with the interprofessional team to manage *inflammation* and *infection* in patients with hepatitis.
2. Teach adults how to decrease the risk liver conditions.
3. Teach the patient and caregiver(s) about common drugs and other management strategies used for liver conditions.
4. Plan patient- and family-centered nursing interventions to decrease the psychosocial impact caused by living with chronic liver conditions.
5. Apply knowledge of anatomy, physiology, and pathophysiology to provide evidence-based care for patients with liver conditions.
6. Analyze assessment and diagnostic findings to generate solutions and prioritize nursing care for patients who have liver conditions.
7. Organize care coordination and transition management for patients having surgery for liver transplantation.
8. Use clinical judgment to plan evidence-based nursing care to promote *nutrition* and manage *cellular regulation* in patients with cirrhosis.
9. Incorporate factors that affect health equity into the plan of care for patients with liver cancer and cirrhosis.

KEY TERMS

alcohol withdrawal A condition that occurs after stopping heavy and prolonged alcohol intake; results in tremors, acute confusion, psychotic behaviors (such as delusions and hallucinations), and autonomic symptoms including tachycardia, elevated blood pressure, and diaphoresis.

ascites The collection of free fluid in the peritoneal cavity caused by increased hydrostatic pressure from portal hypertension.

asterixis A coarse tremor characterized by rapid, nonrhythmic extensions and flexions in the wrists and fingers (hand flapping).

cirrhosis A disease characterized by widespread fibrotic (scarred) bands of connective tissue that change the liver's anatomy and physiology.

ecchymoses Large purple, blue, or yellow bruises.

esophageal varices A complication of cirrhosis in which fragile, thin-walled esophageal veins become distended and tortuous from increased pressure (portal hypertension).

fetor hepaticus The distinctive breath odor of chronic liver disease and hepatic encephalopathy that is characterized by a fruity or musty odor.

hepatic encephalopathy (also called *portal-systemic encephalopathy [PSE]*) A complex cognitive syndrome that is caused by liver failure and cirrhosis.

hepatitis Widespread inflammation and infection of liver cells.

hepatomegaly Liver enlargement that commonly occurs in patients with early cirrhosis.

hepatopulmonary syndrome A complication of cirrhosis caused by excessive ascitic volume and manifested by dyspnea as a result of intraabdominal pressure, which limits thoracic expansion and diaphragmatic excursion.

hepatorenal syndrome A late complication of cirrhosis affecting the kidneys and manifested by oliguria, elevated blood urea nitrogen (BUN) and creatinine levels, and increased urine osmolarity.

icterus Yellow coloration of the eye sclerae.

jaundice Yellowish coloration of the skin caused by increased serum bilirubin.

nonalcoholic fatty liver disease (NAFLD) A liver disease associated with obesity, diabetes mellitus type 2, and metabolic syndrome that occurs when the liver stores excessive amounts of fat from the body unrelated to alcohol consumption.

nonalcoholic steatohepatitis (NASH) An advanced form of nonalcoholic fatty liver disease.

paracentesis An invasive procedure performed to remove abdominal fluid in patients who have massive ascites.

KEY TERMS—cont'd

petechiae Round, pinpoint, red-purple hemorrhagic lesions.

portal hypertension A major complication of cirrhosis resulting in persistent increase in pressure within the portal vein from 3 mm Hg to at least 10 mm Hg.

splenomegaly Spleen enlargement.

spontaneous bacterial peritonitis (SBP) An infection that results from bacteria collected in ascitic fluid.

transjugular intrahepatic portal-systemic shunt (TIPS) An interventional radiologic procedure performed in patients who have not responded to other modalities to manage hemorrhage or long-term ascites.

ultrasound transient elastography A noninvasive imaging test that measures liver stiffness, which helps the primary health care provider determine the amount of liver disease present.

 PRIORITY AND INTERRELATED CONCEPTS

The priority concepts for this chapter are:
- *Cellular Regulation*
- *Infection*

The **Cellular Regulation** concept exemplar for this chapter is Cirrhosis.
The **Infection** concept exemplar for this chapter is Hepatitis.

The interrelated concepts for this chapter are:
- *Inflammation*
- *Nutrition*

As the largest and one of the most vital internal organs, the liver performs more than 400 functions and affects all body systems. Common problems of the liver have an impact on *cellular regulation* and *nutrition.* Liver conditions range in severity from mild hepatic *inflammation* and *infection* to chronic end-stage cirrhosis. Chapter 3 briefly reviews these concepts.

CELLULAR REGULATION CONCEPT EXEMPLAR: CIRRHOSIS

Cirrhosis is extensive, irreversible scarring of the liver, usually caused by a chronic reaction to hepatic *inflammation* and necrosis. This scarring process directly impairs *cellular regulation.* Cirrhosis typically develops slowly and has a progressive, prolonged, destructive course resulting in end-stage liver disease.

Pathophysiology Review

Cirrhosis is characterized by widespread fibrotic (scarred) bands of connective tissue that change the liver's anatomy and physiology. *Inflammation* caused by toxins or disease results in extensive degeneration and destruction of hepatocytes (liver cells). As cirrhosis develops, the tissue becomes nodular. These nodules can block bile ducts and normal blood flow throughout the liver. Impairments in blood and lymph flow occur due to compression caused by excessive fibrous tissue. During early cirrhosis, the liver is usually enlarged and firm. As the pathologic process continues, the liver shrinks in size and becomes harder, resulting in decreased liver function over weeks to years. Some patients with cirrhosis have no symptoms until serious complications occur. Impaired liver function results in elevated serum liver enzymes.

Cirrhosis of the liver can be divided into several common types, depending on the cause of the disease (Rogers, 2023):
- Postnecrotic cirrhosis (caused by viral hepatitis [especially hepatitis C] and certain drugs or other toxins)
- Alcoholic (Laennec's) cirrhosis (caused by chronic alcoholism)
- Biliary cirrhosis (also called *cholestatic*; caused by chronic biliary obstruction or autoimmune disease)

Complications of Cirrhosis

Complications associated with hepatic cirrhosis depend on the amount of damage sustained by the liver. In *compensated* cirrhosis, the liver is scarred and *cellular regulation* is impaired, but the organ can still perform essential functions without causing major symptoms. In *decompensated* cirrhosis, liver function is impaired with obvious signs and symptoms of liver failure.

The loss of hepatic function contributes to development of metabolic abnormalities. Hepatic cell damage may lead to these common complications:
- Portal hypertension
- Ascites and esophageal varices
- Biliary obstruction
- Hepatic encephalopathy

Portal Hypertension. Portal hypertension is a persistent increase in pressure within the portal vein from 3 mm Hg to at least 10 mm Hg. This phenomenon is a major complication of cirrhosis. It results from increased resistance to or obstruction (blockage) of the flow of blood through the portal vein and its branches. The blood meets resistance to flow and seeks collateral (alternative) venous channels around the high-pressure area.

Blood flow backs into the spleen, causing splenomegaly (spleen enlargement). Veins in the esophagus, stomach, intestines, abdomen, and rectum become dilated. Portal hypertension can result in ascites (excessive abdominal [peritoneal] fluid), esophageal varices (distended veins), prominent abdominal veins (caput medusae), and hemorrhoids.

Ascites and Gastroesophageal Varices. Ascites is the collection of free fluid within the peritoneal cavity caused by increased hydrostatic pressure from portal hypertension. The collection of plasma proteins in the peritoneal fluid reduces the amount of circulating plasma proteins in the blood. When this decrease is combined with the inability of the liver to produce albumin because of impaired liver cell functioning, the serum colloid osmotic pressure is decreased in the circulatory system. The result is a fluid shift from the vascular system into the abdomen, a form of "third spacing." As a result, the patient may have hypovolemia and edema at the same time (Rogers, 2023).

Massive ascites may cause renal vasoconstriction, triggering the renin-angiotensin system. This results in sodium and water retention, which increases hydrostatic pressure and the vascular volume and leads to more ascites.

As a result of portal hypertension, the blood backs up from the liver and enters the esophageal and gastric veins. Esophageal varices occur when fragile, thin-walled esophageal veins become distended and tortuous from increased pressure. The potential for varices to bleed depends on size, which can be determined through direct endoscopic observation. Varices occur most often in the distal esophagus but can be present also in the stomach and rectum.

Decreased prothrombin production occurs with cirrhosis and puts the patient at risk for bleeding. Bleeding esophageal varices are a life-threatening medical emergency. Severe blood loss may occur, resulting in shock from hypovolemia. Bleeding may present as either hematemesis (vomiting blood) or melena (black, tarry stools). Loss of consciousness may occur before any observed bleeding. Variceal bleeding can occur spontaneously with no precipitating factors. However, any activity that increases abdominal pressure may increase the likelihood of variceal bleeding, including heavy lifting or vigorous physical exercise. In addition, chest trauma or dry, hard food in the esophagus can cause bleeding.

Patients with portal hypertension may have portal hypertensive gastropathy. This complication can occur with or without esophageal varices. Slow gastric mucosal bleeding occurs, which may result in chronic slow blood loss, occult-positive stools, and anemia.

Splenomegaly results from the backup of blood into the spleen. The enlarged spleen destroys platelets, causing thrombocytopenia (low serum platelet count) and increased risk for bleeding. Thrombocytopenia is often the first clinical sign of liver dysfunction.

Biliary Obstruction. Cirrhosis causes liver bile production to decrease. This prevents the absorption of fat-soluble vitamins (e.g., vitamin K). Without vitamin K, clotting factors II, VII, IX, and X are not produced in sufficient quantities, and the patient is susceptible to bleeding and easy bruising. These abnormalities are confirmed by coagulation studies. Some patients have a genetic predisposition to obstruction of the bile duct that leads to biliary cirrhosis—typically from gallbladder disease or an autoimmune disease called *primary biliary cirrhosis (PBC)*.

Jaundice (yellowish coloration of the skin) in cirrhosis is caused by one of two mechanisms: hepatocellular disease or intrahepatic obstruction (Fig. 50.1). Hepatocellular jaundice develops because the liver cells cannot effectively excrete bilirubin. This decreased excretion results in excessive circulating bilirubin levels. Intrahepatic obstructive jaundice results from edema, fibrosis, or scarring of the hepatic bile channels and bile ducts, which interferes with normal bile and bilirubin excretion. Patients with both types of jaundice often report pruritus (itching).

Hepatic Encephalopathy. Hepatic encephalopathy (also called *portal-systemic encephalopathy [PSE]*) is a complex cognitive syndrome caused by liver failure and cirrhosis. Early

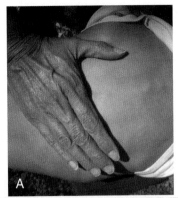

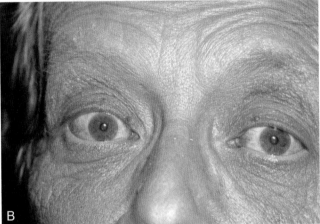

FIG. 50.1 (A and B) Jaundice as a result of liver dysfunction such as cirrhosis and hepatitis. (A from Leonard, P. C. [2020]. *Quick and easy medical terminology* [9th ed.]. St. Louis: Elsevier. B from Michelettie, R. G., James, W. D., Elston, D. M., & McMahon, P. J. [2023]. *Andrew's diseases of the skin clinical atlas* [2nd ed.]. St. Louis: Elsevier.)

symptoms of this complication include sleep disturbance, mood disturbance, mental status changes, and speech problems. Hepatic encephalopathy may be reversible with early intervention. Later neurologic symptoms include an altered level of consciousness, impaired thinking processes, and neuromuscular problems.

Hepatic encephalopathy may develop slowly in patients with chronic liver disease and go undetected until the later stages. Symptoms develop rapidly in acute liver dysfunction. Four stages of development have been identified (Box 50.1). The patient's symptoms may gradually progress to coma or fluctuate among the four stages.

Exact mechanisms of hepatic encephalopathy are not clearly understood, but likely are the result of shunting of portal venous blood into the central circulation, so the liver is bypassed. As a result, substances absorbed by the intestine are not broken down or detoxified and may lead to metabolic abnormalities, such as elevated serum ammonia and gamma-aminobutyric acid (GABA). Elevated serum ammonia results from the inability of the liver to detoxify protein by-products and is common in patients with hepatic encephalopathy. However, it is not a clear indicator of the presence of encephalopathy. Some patients may have major impairment without high elevations of serum ammonia, and elevations of ammonia can occur without evidence of encephalopathy.

BOX 50.1 Key Features

Stages of Hepatic Encephalopathy

Stage I: Subtle manifestations that may not be recognized immediately
- Personality changes
- Behavior changes (agitation, belligerence)
- Emotional lability (euphoria, depression)
- Impaired thinking
- Inability to concentrate
- Fatigue, drowsiness
- Slurred or slowed speech
- Sleep pattern disturbances

Stage II: Continuing mental changes
- Mental confusion
- Disorientation to person, place, time, or situation
- Asterixis (hand flapping)

Stage III: Progressive deterioration
- Marked mental confusion
- Stuporous, drowsy but arousable
- Abnormal electroencephalogram tracing
- Muscle twitching
- Hyperreflexia
- Asterixis (hand flapping)

Stage IV: Unresponsiveness, preceding death in patients who progress to this stage
- Unarousable, obtunded
- No response to painful stimulus
- No asterixis
- Positive Babinski sign
- Muscle rigidity
- Fetor hepaticus (characteristic liver breath—musty, sweet odor)
- Seizures

Factors that may contribute to or worsen hepatic encephalopathy in patients with cirrhosis include:
- High-protein diet
- Infection
- Hypovolemia (decreased fluid volume)
- Hypokalemia (decreased serum potassium)
- Constipation
- GI bleeding (causes a large protein load in the intestines)
- Drugs (e.g., hypnotics, opioids, sedatives, analgesics, diuretics, illicit drugs)

The prognosis depends on the severity of the underlying cause, precipitating factors, and degree of liver dysfunction (Rogers, 2023).

Other Complications. Development of hepatorenal syndrome indicates a poor prognosis for the patient with liver failure. This is often the cause of death in these patients. This syndrome is manifested by:

- A sudden decrease in urinary flow (<500 mL/24 hr) (oliguria)
- Elevated blood urea nitrogen (BUN) and creatinine levels with abnormally decreased urine sodium excretion
- Increased urine osmolarity

Hepatorenal syndrome often occurs after clinical deterioration from GI bleeding or the onset of hepatic encephalopathy. This may also complicate other liver diseases, including acute hepatitis and fulminant liver failure.

Patients with cirrhosis and ascites may develop acute spontaneous bacterial peritonitis (SBP). Those with very advanced liver disease are more susceptible to SBP. Bacteria responsible for SBP are typically from the bowel and reach the ascitic fluid after migrating through the bowel wall and the lymphatic system. Symptoms vary but may include malaise, fever, chills, ***pain*** (especially in the abdomen), and tenderness. However, symptoms can also be minimal with only mild indicators in the absence of fever. Worsening encephalopathy and increased jaundice may also be present without abdominal symptoms (Tholey, 2021).

Confirmation of SBP is typically made with paracentesis. During this procedure a sample of ascitic fluid is obtained by placing a needle into the peritoneal cavity. Following the procedure, the fluid is sent for diagnostic testing (cell count and culture). An ascitic fluid leukocyte count of more than 250 polymorphonuclear (PMN) leukocytes may indicate the need for treatment (Pagana et al., 2022).

Another major complication of cirrhosis is hepatopulmonary syndrome caused by excessive ascitic volume. The patient experiences dyspnea due to increased intraabdominal pressure, which limits thoracic expansion and diaphragmatic excursion.

Etiology and Genetic Risk

The most common causes of cirrhosis in the United States are chronic alcohol use, chronic viral hepatitis, and bile duct disease. Nonalcoholic fatty liver disease (NAFLD) and nonalcoholic steatohepatitis (NASH) can also lead to cirrhosis.

Hepatitis C is a bloodborne illness that usually causes chronic disease and compromises the body's immunity. This infection is the leading cause of cirrhosis and liver cancer in the United States (American Liver Foundation, 2023a). ***Inflammation*** caused by ***infection*** over time leads to progressive scarring of the liver. It usually takes decades for cirrhosis to develop, although alcohol use in combination with hepatitis C may speed the process.

PATIENT-CENTERED CARE: VETERAN HEALTH

Veterans and Hepatitis C

Veterans are at a high risk for hepatitis C viral infection, especially individuals who served during the Vietnam and post-Vietnam era due to exposures when assisting wounded comrades, sharing toothbrushes and razors, and using unsanitary tattoo equipment. In addition, the device used for military mandatory vaccinations in the late 1990s was a needleless "jet gun" that could have contributed to transmitting hepatitis C (Elliott et al., 2021). When caring for veterans, assess whether they have been tested for hepatitis C. If they have not been tested, provide information on how they can be tested or consult with the primary health care provider to arrange for testing in the health care setting.

Hepatitis B and hepatitis D are the most common causes of cirrhosis worldwide. Hepatitis B also causes *inflammation* and low-grade damage over decades that can ultimately lead to cirrhosis. Hepatitis D virus (HDV) can infect the liver but only in people who already have hepatitis B (see discussion in *Infection* Concept Exemplar: Hepatitis).

Cirrhosis may also occur due to nonalcoholic fatty liver disease (NAFLD). NAFLD is most closely tied to obesity, diabetes mellitus type 2, and metabolic syndrome and is covered later in this chapter.

Another common cause of cirrhosis is excessive and prolonged alcohol use. Alcohol has a direct toxic effect on the hepatocytes and causes liver *inflammation* (alcoholic hepatitis). The liver becomes enlarged, with cellular degeneration and infiltration by fat, leukocytes, and lymphocytes. Over time, the inflammatory process decreases and the destructive phase increases. Early scar formation is caused by fibroblast infiltration and collagen formation. Damage to the liver tissue progresses as malnutrition and repeated exposure to the alcohol continue. If alcohol is withheld, the fatty infiltration and *inflammation* are reversible. If alcohol use continues, widespread scar tissue formation and fibrosis infiltrate the liver due to cellular necrosis. The long-term use of illicit drugs, such as cocaine, has similar effects on the liver.

PATIENT-CENTERED CARE: GENDER HEALTH

Effect of Alcohol Related to Gender

The amount of alcohol necessary to cause cirrhosis varies widely from individual to individual, but notably there are gender differences. Two or three drinks per day over a minimum of 10 years may be all it takes for women to develop cirrhosis. For men, six drinks per day over the same time frame may cause the same level of liver damage. However, a smaller amount of alcohol over a long period of time can increase memory loss from alcohol toxicity of the cerebral cortex. Binge drinking can increase risk for hepatitis and fatty liver (Rogers, 2023).

Incidence and Prevalence

Chronic liver disease and cirrhosis combined account for a large number of deaths in the United States. About 2.7 million people in the United States have hepatitis C (American Liver Foundation, 2023c) and as many as 2.2 million American have hepatitis B (American Liver Foundation, 2023b). In Canada the estimated prevalence of hepatitis B is between 250,000 and 450,000 (Public Health Agency of Canada, 2021). It is more challenging to quantify the exact number of Canadians with liver disease, but it is thought that as many as 1 in 4 Canadians are affected by liver disease (Canadian Liver Foundation, 2021).

Health Promotion/Disease Prevention

Two of the most common causes of cirrhosis are chronic hepatitis C infection and chronic alcohol use. These problems are discussed later in this chapter. Objectives to improve the incidence and management of liver diseases are included as part of the *Healthy People 2030* initiative (Box 50.2).

♥ BOX 50.2   Meeting *Healthy People 2030* Objectives

Liver Diseases

Two objectives for individuals with liver diseases are included in the *Healthy People 2030* initiative:
- Reduce cirrhosis deaths.
- Increase the proportion of people who have cleared hepatitis C infection.
  Therefore it is essential that nurses teach individuals the importance of avoiding risk factors that contribute to or cause cirrhosis and hepatitis C (discussed later in this chapter).

Interprofessional Collaborative Care

Care for the patient with cirrhosis can take place in various settings by many members of the interprofessional health care team. These patients may, at different times, self-manage at home, be hospitalized for acute complications, need rehabilitative care, or be cared for in the community setting, including possible hospice care.

PATIENT-CENTERED CARE: HEALTH EQUITY

Health Equity Issues Related to Cirrhosis

When compared with White patients with cirrhosis, Black patients with cirrhosis have a higher rate of hospital admission, longer length of stay during each hospitalization, and a higher 90-day hospital readmission rate, even though the quality of care is the same for both groups. Factors contributing to these differences include a lower median outcome for Blacks, a lack of transportation or access to health care, and a higher incidence of coronary artery disease and diabetes mellitus, which contribute to the incidence of cirrhosis complications (Spiewak et al., 2020). Nurses need to be aware of these social determinants of health as part of the patient's plan of care. Provide information on community resources for transportation and health care access. Teach patients how to help ensure prevention or self-care management of comorbid chronic diseases.

Recognize Cues: Assessment

History. Obtain data from patients with suspected cirrhosis, including age, gender, and employment history, especially history of exposure to alcohol, drugs (prescribed and illicit), use of herbal preparations, and chemical toxins. Keep in mind that all exposures are important, regardless of how long ago they occurred. Determine whether there has ever been a needlestick injury. Sexual history and orientation may be important in determining an infectious cause for liver disease, because men having sex with men (MSM) are at high risk for hepatitis A, hepatitis B, and hepatitis C (Rogers, 2023).

Inquire about whether there is a family history of alcoholism and/or liver disease. Ask patients to describe their alcohol intake, including the amount consumed during a given period. Is there a history of illicit drug use, including oral, IV, and intranasal forms? Does the patient have tattoos? If so, ask about when and where they were obtained. Has the patient been in the military or in prison? Is the patient a health care worker, firefighter, or police officer? For patients previously or currently in an alcohol or drug recovery program, how long have they been sober? These questions can be difficult to answer and bring up sensitive topics. Be sure to establish why you are asking these questions and accept answers in a non-judgmental manner. Provide privacy during the interview. For many people, the behaviors causing the liver disease occurred years before the onset of their current illness, and they may be regretful or embarrassed.

Ask the patient about previous medical conditions, such as an episode of jaundice or acute viral hepatitis, biliary tract disorders (such as cholecystitis [gallbladder **inflammation**]), viral **infection,** surgery, blood transfusions, autoimmune disorders, obesity, altered lipid profile, heart failure, respiratory disorders, or liver injury.

Physical Assessment/Signs and Symptoms. Because cirrhosis has a slow onset, many of the *early* signs and symptoms are vague and nonspecific. Assess for:

- Fatigue
- Significant change in weight
- GI symptoms, such as anorexia and vomiting
- Pain in the abdominal area and liver tenderness (both of which may be ignored by the patient)

Liver function problems are often found during a routine physical examination or when laboratory tests are completed for an unrelated illness or problem. The patient with *compensated cirrhosis* may be completely unaware that there is a liver problem. The first sign may present before the onset of symptoms when routine laboratory tests, presurgical evaluations, or life and health insurance assessments show abnormalities. These tests could indicate abnormal liver function or thrombocytopenia (decreased serum platelet count), necessitating a more thorough diagnostic workup.

The development of late signs of *advanced cirrhosis* (also called *end-stage liver failure*) usually causes the patient to seek medical treatment. GI bleeding, jaundice, ascites, and spontaneous bruising indicate poor liver function and complications of cirrhosis.

Thoroughly assess all body systems of the patient with liver dysfunction or failure because it affects the entire body. The clinical picture and course vary from patient to patient, depending on the severity of the disease. Assess for the common late disease signs and symptoms outlined in Box 50.3.

Abdominal Assessment. *Massive ascites* can be detected as a distended abdomen with bulging flanks (Fig. 50.2). The umbilicus may protrude and dilated abdominal veins (caput medusae) may radiate from the umbilicus. Ascites can cause physical problems including orthopnea, and dyspnea from increased abdominal distention can interfere with lung expansion. The patient may have difficulty maintaining an erect body posture, and problems with balance may affect walking. Inspect and palpate for the presence of inguinal or umbilical hernias, which may develop because of increased intraabdominal pressure. *Minimal ascites* is often more difficult to detect, especially in the obese patient.

When performing an assessment of the abdomen, keep in mind that hepatomegaly (liver enlargement) occurs in many cases of early cirrhosis. Splenomegaly is common in

BOX 50.3   Key Features
Late-Stage Cirrhosis

- Jaundice and icterus (yellow coloration of the eye sclera)
- Dry skin
- Pruritus (itchy skin)
- Rashes
- Purpuric lesions, such as petechiae (round, pinpoint, red-purple hemorrhagic lesions) or ecchymoses (large purple, blue, or yellow bruises)
- Warm and bright red/hyperpigmented palms of the hands (palmar erythema)
- Vascular lesions with a red center and radiating branches, known as *spider angiomas* (also called *telangiectasias, spider nevi,* or *vascular spiders*), on the nose, cheeks, upper thorax, and shoulders
- Abdominal ascites
- Peripheral dependent edema of the extremities and sacrum
- Vitamin deficiency (especially fat-soluble vitamins A, D, E, and K)

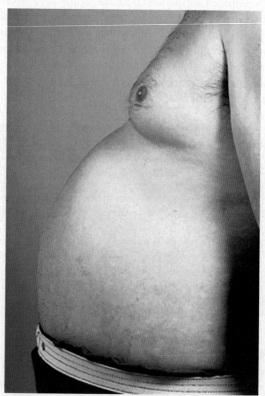

FIG. 50.2 Patient with abdominal ascites in late-stage cirrhosis. (From Leonard, P. C. [2020]. *Quick and easy medical terminology* [9th ed.]. St. Louis: Elsevier.)

nonalcoholic causes of cirrhosis. As the liver deteriorates, it usually becomes hard and smaller with nodules.

Measure the patient's abdominal girth to evaluate the progression of ascites (see Fig. 50.2). For measurement of abdominal girth, the patient lies flat while the examiner pulls a tape measure around the largest diameter (usually over the umbilicus) of the abdomen. The girth is measured at the end of exhalation. The abdominal skin and flanks should be marked to ensure the same tape measure placement on subsequent readings. *However, a rapid increase in body weight is the most reliable indicator of fluid retention.*

Other Physical Assessments. Observe any vomitus and stool for blood. This may be indicated by frank blood in the excrement or by a positive fecal occult blood test (FOBT). Gastritis, stomach ulceration, or oozing esophageal varices may be responsible for the blood in the stool. Note the presence of fetor hepaticus, which is the distinctive breath odor associated with chronic liver disease and hepatic encephalopathy and is characterized by a fruity or musty odor. Amenorrhea (no menstrual period) may occur in women. Men may exhibit testicular atrophy, gynecomastia (enlarged breasts), and impotence related to inactive hormones.

Continually assess the patient's neurologic function; it may also be helpful to include family members in conversations about the patient's baseline mental status if the patient is unable to effectively communicate. Subtle changes in mental status and personality often progress to coma—a late complication of hepatic encephalopathy. Monitor for asterixis—a coarse tremor characterized by rapid, nonrhythmic extensions and flexions in the wrists and fingers (hand flapping).

Psychosocial Assessment. Patients with hepatic cirrhosis may undergo subtle or obvious personality, cognitive, and behavior changes. They may experience sleep pattern disturbances or exhibit signs of emotional lability (fluctuations in emotions), euphoria (a very elevated mood), or depression. A psychosocial assessment identifies needs and helps guide care.

Repeated hospitalizations are common for patients with cirrhosis. It is a life-altering chronic disease that affects not only the patient but also the immediate and extended family members and significant others. There are significant emotional, physical, and financial changes. Substance use may continue even as health worsens. Use available community resources whenever possible. Collaborate with social workers, substance use counselors, and mental health/behavioral health care professionals as needed for patient assessment and management.

Part of the psychosocial assessment is to determine if the patient is alcohol dependent. If this is the case, the health care team should observe and prepare for alcohol withdrawal. Alcohol withdrawal occurs after stopping alcohol intake after heavy and prolonged use. Monitor for tremors, sometimes called the "jitters," which can begin as early as 6 to 8 hours after alcohol cessation. Cognitive and neurologic changes associated with delirium tremens (DTs) may include acute confusion, anxiety, and psychotic behaviors, such as delusions and hallucinations. Autonomic changes may include tachycardia, elevated blood pressure, and diaphoresis (Elliott, 2019). Care of the patient experiencing withdrawal can be a medical emergency. Consult professional resources for more information about caring for the alcohol-dependent patient.

Laboratory Assessment. Laboratory study abnormalities are common in patients with liver disease (Table 50.1). Serum levels of *aspartate aminotransferase* (AST), *alanine aminotransferase* (ALT), and *lactate dehydrogenase* (LDH) typically are elevated because these enzymes are released into the blood during hepatic **inflammation.** However, as the liver deteriorates, the hepatocytes may be unable to create an inflammatory response, and the AST and ALT levels may be normal. ALT levels are more specific to the liver, whereas AST can be found in muscle, kidney, brain, and heart. An AST/ALT ratio greater than 1.0 is usually found in alcoholic liver disease (Pagana et al., 2022).

TABLE 50.1 Significance of Abnormal Laboratory Findings in Liver Disease

Abnormal Finding	Significance
Serum Enzymes	
Elevated serum aspartate aminotransferase (AST)	Hepatic cell destruction, hepatitis
Elevated serum alanine aminotransferase (ALT)	Hepatic cell destruction, hepatitis (most specific indicator)
Elevated lactate dehydrogenase (LDH)	Hepatic cell destruction
Elevated serum alkaline phosphatase	Obstructive jaundice, hepatic metastasis
Elevated gamma-glutamyl transpeptidase (GGT)	Biliary obstruction, cirrhosis
Bilirubin	
Elevated serum total bilirubin	Hepatic cell disease
Elevated serum direct conjugated bilirubin	Hepatitis, liver metastasis
Elevated serum indirect unconjugated bilirubin	Cirrhosis
Elevated urine bilirubin	Hepatocellular obstruction, viral or toxic liver disease
Elevated urine urobilinogen	Hepatic dysfunction
Serum Proteins	
Increased serum total protein	Acute liver disease
Decreased serum total protein	Chronic liver disease
Decreased serum albumin	Severe liver disease
Elevated serum globulin	Immune response to liver disease
Other Tests	
Increased serum creatinine	Indication of kidney damage related to hepatorenal syndrome
Elevated serum ammonia	Advanced liver disease or hepatic encephalopathy
Prolonged prothrombin time (PT) or international normalized ratio (INR)	Hepatic cell damage and decreased synthesis of prothrombin

Increased *alkaline phosphatase* and gamma-glutamyl transpeptidase (GGT) levels are caused by biliary obstruction and therefore may increase in patients with cirrhosis. Alkaline phosphatase is a nonspecific bone, intestinal, and liver enzyme. Total serum *bilirubin* levels also rise. Indirect bilirubin levels increase in patients with cirrhosis because of the inability of the failing liver to excrete bilirubin. Because of this, bilirubin is present in the urine (urobilinogen) in increased amounts. Fecal urobilinogen concentration is decreased in patients with biliary tract obstruction. These patients have light- or clay-colored stools.

Total serum *albumin* levels are decreased in patients with severe or chronic liver disease as a result of decreased synthesis by the liver. Loss of osmotic "pull" proteins such as albumin promotes the movement of intravascular fluid into the interstitial tissues (e.g., ascites). *Prothrombin time/international normalized ratio (PT/INR)* is prolonged because the liver decreases the production of prothrombin. The platelet count is low, resulting in a characteristic thrombocytopenia of cirrhosis. Anemia may be reflected by decreased red blood cell (RBC), hemoglobin, and hematocrit values. The white blood cell (WBC) count may also be decreased. *Ammonia* levels are usually elevated in patients with advanced liver disease. Serum creatinine may be elevated in patients with deteriorating kidney function. Dilutional hyponatremia (low serum sodium) may occur in patients with ascites.

NCLEX Examination Challenge 50.1
Physiological Integrity

The nurse is assessing a client diagnosed with advanced liver cirrhosis. Which abnormal serum laboratory finding would the nurse anticipate for this client?

A. Elevated ammonia
B. Increased albumin
C. Decreased alkaline phosphatase
D. Decreased alanine aminotransferase

Imaging Assessment. Plain x-rays of the abdomen may show hepatomegaly, splenomegaly, or massive ascites. A CT scan may be requested. *MRI* is another test used to diagnose the patient with liver disease. This test can reveal mass lesions, giving additional specific information. MRI results are helpful in determining whether the condition is malignant or benign.

Other Diagnostic Assessments. Ultrasonography (US) of the liver is often the first assessment for an adult with suspected liver disease to detect ascites, hepatomegaly, and splenomegaly. It can also determine the presence of biliary stones or biliary duct obstruction. Liver US with Doppler is useful in detecting portal vein thrombosis and evaluating whether the direction of portal blood flow is normal.

Ultrasound transient elastography is a noninvasive test that measures liver stiffness, which helps the primary health care provider determine the amount of liver disease present. The normal amount of stiffness is 5.0 kilopascals (kPa). Higher degrees of stiffness indicate liver fibrosis. More than 13 kPa indicates that the patient has cirrhosis. The imaging study may not be as reliable in patients who have excessive ascites or obesity (Barr et al., 2020).

A liver biopsy may be necessary to determine the exact pathology and the extent of disease progression. This procedure can be problematic because patients with liver disease are at risk for bleeding. Even a percutaneous (through the skin) biopsy can pose a significant risk to the patient. To minimize this risk, an interventional radiologist can perform a liver biopsy by using a long sheath through a jugular vein, which then is threaded into the hepatic vein and liver. A tissue sample is obtained for microscopic evaluation. If a biopsy procedure is not possible, a radioisotope liver scan may be used to identify cirrhosis or other diffuse disease.

The primary health care provider may request arteriography if US is not conclusive in finding portal vein thrombosis. To evaluate the portal vein and its branches, a portal venogram may be performed instead by passing a catheter into the liver and portal vein.

The primary health care provider may perform an esophagogastroduodenoscopy (EGD) to directly visualize the upper GI tract to detect complications of liver failure. These complications may include bleeding or oozing esophageal varices, stomach irritation and ulceration, or duodenal ulceration and bleeding. EGD is performed by introducing a flexible fiberoptic endoscope into the mouth, esophagus, and stomach while the patient is under moderate sedation. The scope has a camera attached that permits direct visualization of the mucosal lining of the upper GI tract. In endoscopic retrograde cholangiopancreatography (ERCP), an endoscope is used to inject contrast material via the sphincter of Oddi to view the biliary tract and allow for stone removals, sphincterotomies, biopsies, and stent placements if required. These procedures are described in more detail in Chapter 45.

Analyze Cues and Prioritize Hypotheses: Analysis

The priority collaborative problems for patients with cirrhosis include:

1. Fluid overload due to third spacing of abdominal and peripheral fluid (ascites)
2. Potential for hemorrhage due to portal hypertension and subsequent GI varices
3. Acute confusion and other cognitive changes due to increased serum ammonia levels and/or alcohol withdrawal
4. Pruritus due to increased serum bilirubin and jaundice

Generate Solutions and Take Actions: Planning and Implementation

Managing Fluid Volume

Planning: Expected Outcomes. The patient with cirrhosis is expected to have less excess fluid volume as evidenced by decreased ascites and peripheral edema while maintaining an adequate circulatory volume.

Interventions. Fluid accumulations are minimal during the early stages of cirrhosis. During this stage nursing and interprofessional interventions are aimed at preventing the accumulation of additional fluid and decreasing any existing fluid collection. Nonsurgical treatment measures are used to treat ascites in most cases.

Supportive measures to control abdominal ascites include **nutrition** therapy, drug therapy, paracentesis, and respiratory support. The patient's fluid and electrolyte balance is carefully monitored during the treatment period.

Nutrition Therapy. The primary health care provider usually places the patient with early abdominal ascites on a low-sodium diet as an initial means of controlling fluid accumulation. The amount of daily sodium (Na$^+$) intake restriction varies, but a 1- to 2-g (2000 mg) Na$^+$ restriction may be tried first. Collaborate with a registered dietitian nutritionist to explain the purpose of the restriction and advise the patient and family to read the sodium content labels on all food and beverages. Table salt should be completely excluded. Low-sodium diets may be difficult to tolerate, so suggest alternative flavoring additives such as lemon, vinegar, parsley, oregano, and pepper. Remind patients that seasoned and salty food is an acquired taste; in time, they will become used to the decrease in dietary sodium.

Patients with *late-stage* cirrhosis are usually malnourished and have multiple dietary deficiencies. IV vitamin supplements such as thiamine, folate, and multivitamin preparations are typically given because the liver cannot store vitamins. For patients with biliary cirrhosis, bile may not be available for fat-soluble vitamin transport and absorption. A study by Chaney et al. (2020) found that malnutrition associated with end-stage cirrhosis caused patients to require multiple hospitalizations (see the Evidence-Based Practice box).

Drug Therapy. A *diuretic* is usually prescribed by the primary health care provider to reduce fluid accumulation and prevent cardiac and respiratory problems. Monitor the effect of diuretic therapy by weighing the patient daily, measuring daily intake and output, measuring abdominal girth, documenting

peripheral edema, and assessing electrolyte levels. Serious fluid and electrolyte imbalances, such as dehydration, hypokalemia (decreased potassium), and hyponatremia (decreased sodium), may occur with loop diuretic therapy. Depending on the diuretic selected, the provider may prescribe an oral or IV potassium supplement. Some clinicians prescribe furosemide and spironolactone as a combination diuretic therapy for the treatment of ascites. Because these drugs work differently, they are used for preservation of sodium and potassium balance.

All patients with ascites have the potential to develop spontaneous bacterial peritonitis (SBP) from bacteria in the collected ascitic fluid. Mild symptoms such as low-grade fever and loss of appetite occur may occur in some patients. In others, there may be abdominal pain, fever, and change in mental status. When performing an abdominal assessment, listen for bowel sounds and assess for abdominal wall rigidity. Treatment involves IV antibiotics including cephalosporins or fluroquinolones.

Paracentesis. Abdominal paracentesis may be needed if ascites affects a patient's respiratory effort. Paracentesis is an invasive procedure performed to remove abdominal fluid. The procedure is performed at the bedside, in an interventional radiology department, or in an ambulatory care setting. During this procedure the primary health care provider inserts a trocar catheter or drain into the abdomen to remove the ascitic fluid from the peritoneal cavity. This procedure is done using ultrasound for added safety. A short-term ascites drain catheter may be placed while the patient is awaiting surgical intervention, or tunneled ascites drains can allow a patient or family caregiver to drain ascitic fluid at home. Nursing implications associated with this procedure are described in Box 50.4.

If SBP is suspected, a sample of fluid is withdrawn and sent for cell count and culture. For the patient with symptoms of *infection,* the primary health care provider may prescribe antibiotics while awaiting the culture results.

Respiratory Support. Excessive ascitic fluid volume may cause patients to have respiratory problems. They may

---

📄 EVIDENCE-BASED PRACTICE

What Is the Effect of Malnutrition in Patients With Cirrhosis?

Chaney, A., Rawal, B., Harnois, D., et al. (2020). Nutritional assessment and malnutrition in patients with cirrhosis. Gastroenterology Nursing, 43(4), 284–291.

The purpose of this study was to determine the incidence and outcomes of malnutrition in patients with end-stage liver cirrhosis. A retrospective medical record review of 134 patients waiting for liver transplant was conducted using the Subjective Global Assessment score at the time of transplant evaluation, at follow-up nutritional visits, and at the time of transplant. Findings showed that malnutrition was present in 51.9% of patients at end-stage cirrhosis on their initial nutritional visit but increased to 61% by the time of transplant. Most patients had to wait over 180 days to obtain a transplant. During that wait time, increasing malnutrition led to more than 53% of patients being hospitalized.

Level of Evidence: 4
This was a descriptive study using a convenience sample.

Commentary: Implications for Practice and Research
This study demonstrated that malnutrition in patients who have end-stage cirrhosis leads to or contributes to hospitalizations, which increases health care costs and decreases quality of life. Nurses can help identify patients who have or are at risk for developing malnutrition and refer them to a registered dietitian nutritionist who can create an individualized plan of care to manage their nutritional status. More research is needed on the role of nurses in performing nutritional screening and the best evidence-based nutritional interventions that lead to more positive outcomes.

BOX 50.4 Best Practice for Patient Safety and Quality Care

The Patient Having a Paracentesis

- Explain the procedure and answer patient questions.
- Obtain vital signs, including weight, before the procedure.
- Ask the patient to void before the procedure to prevent injury to the bladder.
- Position the patient in bed with the head of the bed elevated.
- Monitor vital signs per protocol or primary health care provider request during the procedure.
- Measure the drainage and record precisely.
- Document the characteristics of the collected fluid.
- Label and send the fluid for laboratory analysis; document in the patient health record that specimens were sent.
- After the catheter has been removed, apply a dressing to the site; assess for leakage.
- Maintain bed rest per protocol.
- Take vital signs and weigh the patient after the paracentesis; document in the patient record the weight both before and after paracentesis. (The patient should experience a weight loss due to fluid removal.)

develop hepatopulmonary syndrome. Dyspnea develops due to increased intraabdominal pressure, which limits thoracic expansion and diaphragmatic excursion. Auscultate lungs every 4 to 8 hours for crackles or other adventitious breath sounds that could indicate pulmonary complications.

> ### ⚠ NURSING SAFETY PRIORITY
> #### *Action Alert*
>
> For patients with hepatopulmonary syndrome, monitor their oxygen saturation with pulse oximetry. If needed, notify the primary care provider and obtain an order for oxygen therapy to ease breathing. Elevate the head of the bed to at least 30 degrees or as high as the patient wants in order to improve breathing. This position with feet elevated to decrease dependent ankle edema often relieves dyspnea. Remind assistive personnel to weigh the patient daily every morning before breakfast using the same scale.

Fluid and electrolyte balance problems are common as a result of the disease or treatment. Laboratory tests, such as blood urea nitrogen (BUN), serum protein, hematocrit, and electrolytes, help determine fluid and electrolyte status. Elevated BUN, decreased serum proteins, and increased hematocrit may indicate hypovolemia.

When medical management fails to control ascites, the primary health care provider may choose to divert ascites into the venous system by creating a shunt. Patients with ascites are poor surgical risks. The transjugular intrahepatic portal-systemic shunt (TIPS) is a nonsurgical procedure that is used to control long-term ascites and reduce variceal bleeding. This procedure is described in the discussion of Interventions in the Preventing or Managing Hemorrhage section that follows.

Preventing or Managing Hemorrhage

Planning: Expected Outcomes. The patient is expected to be free of bleeding episodes. However, a hemorrhage is present, it is expected to be controlled by prompt, evidence-based interventions. Esophageal variceal bleeds are the most common cause of upper GI bleeding (also see Chapter 47 on management of upper GI bleeding).

Interventions. All patients with cirrhosis should be screened for esophageal varices by endoscopy to detect them early *before they bleed.* When patients have varices, they are placed on preventive therapy. If acute bleeding occurs, early interventions are used to manage it. *Because massive esophageal bleeding can cause rapid blood loss, emergency interventions are needed.*

The role of early drug therapy is to *prevent* bleeding and infection in patients who have varices. A nonselective *beta-blocking agent* such as propranolol is usually prescribed to prevent bleeding. Decreasing the heart rate and the hepatic venous pressure gradient may reduce the chance of bleeding. Monitor the patient's vital signs for bradycardia and hypotension.

Up to 20% of patients with cirrhosis who are admitted to the hospital as a result of upper GI bleeding have bacterial **infection,** and even more patients develop health care–associated infection. Infection is one of the most common indicators that patients will have an acute variceal bleed (AVB). Therefore patients with cirrhosis with GI bleeding should receive *antibiotics* when admitted to the hospital.

When bleeding occurs, the health care team intervenes quickly to control it by combining vasoactive drugs with endoscopic therapies. *Vasoactive* drugs, such as octreotide acetate and vasopressin, reduce blood flow through vasoconstriction to decrease portal pressure. Octreotide also suppresses secretion of gastrin, serotonin, and intestinal peptides, which decreases GI blood flow to help with pressure reduction within the varices. Vasopressin is rarely used because it is a very potent drug and has several adverse effects (Sole et al., 2021).

Endoscopic therapies include ligation of the bleeding veins or sclerotherapy. Both procedures are very effective in controlling bleeding and improving patient survival rates. Esophageal varices may be managed with *endoscopic variceal ligation (EVL) (banding).* This procedure involves the application of small "O" bands around the base of the varices to decrease their blood supply. The patient is unaware of the bands, and they cause no discomfort.

Endoscopic sclerotherapy (EST), also called *injection sclerotherapy,* is a method used to control bleeding. The varices are injected with a sclerosing agent via a catheter. Complications of this procedure include mucosal ulceration, which could result in further bleeding.

Rescue therapies may be warranted if bleeding recurs. These therapies include a second endoscopic procedure, balloon tamponade and esophageal stents, and shunting procedures. Short-term esophagogastric balloon tamponade with esophageal stents is a very effective way to control bleeding. However, the procedure can cause potentially life-threatening complications, such as aspiration, asphyxia, and esophageal perforation. Similar to a nasogastric tube (NGT), the tube is placed through the nose and into the stomach. An attached balloon is inflated to apply pressure to the bleeding variceal area. Before this tamponade, the patient is usually intubated and placed on a mechanical ventilator to protect the patient's airway. This therapy is used if the patient is not able to have a second endoscopy or TIPS procedure.

The transjugular intrahepatic portal-systemic shunt (TIPS) is a nonsurgical procedure performed by an interventional radiologist. This procedure is used for patients who have not responded to other modalities for hemorrhage or long-term ascites. When the procedure is preformed nonemergently, patients have an ultrasound exam to assess jugular vein anatomy and patency. IV sedation or general anesthesia is used for this procedure. During the procedure the radiologist places a large sheath through the jugular vein. A needle is guided through the sheath and pushed through the liver into the portal vein, a balloon enlarges this tract, and a stent is placed to keep it open. Most patients also have an ultrasound study of the liver after the TIPS procedure to verify blood flow through the shunt. Patients undergoing the TIPS procedure who have esophageal/gastric varices and hemorrhage problems may also require esophageal/gastric vein embolization as a part of the procedure. Patients with severe liver cirrhosis usually have little flow through the liver parenchyma. These patients develop large portal-esophageal (or portal-gastric) veins diverting blood away from the diseased liver. Even after a successful TIPS, the diverting veins may persist and must be embolized (intentionally blocked) so they will not rebleed.

Serious complications of the TIPS procedure are not common. Patients are usually discharged in 1 or 2 days and are followed up with ultrasound studies for the first year after the shunt is placed, to ensure continued patency. Patients must also be monitored for hepatic encephalopathy, which can be caused by a TIPS. After creation of the TIPS, blood now bypasses most of the liver's filtration processes, allowing toxins to circulate throughout the body. In some patients this can cause disturbances in consciousness and behavior. Lactulose or other medications are given to counteract this effect, and dietary modification may also be helpful. For severe cases a TIPS may have the flow reduced or closed completely to reverse the encephalopathy. This is done by deploying a smaller stent or occluding device inside the original TIPS. The decision can be a difficult one for the health care provider to make because reduction of flow through the shunt will likely cause the initial esophageal hemorrhaging to recur.

Patients receiving TIPS may have a significant elevation of their pulmonary artery pressure. This is a result of the sudden increase of blood flow to the right side of the heart. Diuretics help to treat this problem. For this reason, patients must be evaluated for right-sided heart failure before TIPS placement.

Depending on the procedure done to control esophageal bleeding, patients usually have a nasogastric tube (NGT) inserted to detect any new bleeding episodes. They often receive packed red blood cells, fresh frozen plasma, dextran, albumin, and platelets through large-bore IV catheters. Monitor vital signs every hour and check coagulation studies, including prothrombin time (PT), partial thromboplastin time (PTT), platelet count, and international normalized ratio (INR).

Preventing or Managing Confusion

Planning: Expected Outcomes. The patient is expected to be free of acute or chronic confusion. If it occurs, early intervention by the interprofessional health care team is the goal to maintain patient safety and prevent further health problems or death from encephalopathy.

Interventions. Collaborative interventions are planned around the management of slowing or stopping the accumulation of ammonia in the body to improve mental status and orientation. Assess the patient's neurologic status, and monitor during treatment.

Because ammonia is formed in the GI tract by the action of bacteria on protein, nonsurgical treatment measures to decrease ammonia production include dietary modifications and drug therapy to reduce bacterial breakdown. Patients with cirrhosis have increased nutritional requirements—high-carbohydrate, moderate-fat, and high-protein foods. However, the diet may be changed for those who have elevated serum ammonia levels with signs of encephalopathy. Patients should have a moderate amount of protein and fat foods and simple carbohydrates. Strict protein restrictions are not required because patients require protein for healing. In collaboration with the registered dietitian nutritionist, be sure to include family members or significant others in **nutrition** counseling. The patient is often weak and unable to remember complicated guidelines. Brief, simple directions regarding dietary modifications are recommended. Keep in mind any financial, cultural, or personal implications and the patient's food allergies when discussing food choices to provide optimal patient-centered care.

Drugs are used sparingly because they are difficult for a failing liver to metabolize. In particular, opioid analgesics, sedatives, and barbiturates should be limited, especially in the patient with a history of encephalopathy.

However, several types of drugs may eliminate or reduce ammonia levels in the body. These include lactulose or lactitol and nonabsorbable antibiotics. The primary health care provider may prescribe *lactulose* (or lactitol) to promote the excretion of ammonia in the stool. This drug is a viscous, sticky, sweet-tasting liquid that is given either orally or by NGT. This drug has a laxative effect. It works by increasing osmotic pressure to draw fluid into the colon and prevents absorption of ammonia in the colon. The drug may be prescribed to the patient who has manifested signs of encephalopathy, regardless of the stage (Burchum & Rosenthal, 2022). The desired effect of the drug is production of two or three soft stools per day and a decrease in patient confusion caused by increased ammonia.

Observe for response to lactulose and side effects including intestinal bloating and cramping. Serum ammonia levels are monitored but do not always correlate with symptoms. Hypokalemia and dehydration may result from excessive stools. Remind assistive personnel to support the patient's personal and skin care to prevent breakdown caused by excessive stools.

Several *nonabsorbable antibiotics* may be given if lactulose does not help the patient meet the desired outcome or if the patient is unable tolerate the drug. These drugs should not be given together. Older adults can become weak and dehydrated from multiple stools. Neomycin sulfate or rifaximin, both broad-spectrum antibiotics, may be given to act as intestinal antiseptics. These drugs destroy the normal flora in the bowel, diminishing protein breakdown and decreasing the rate of ammonia production. Maintenance doses of neomycin are given orally but may also be administered as a retention enema. Long-term use has the potential for kidney toxicity, and therefore this agent is not commonly used for an extended period. It is not used in patients with existing kidney disease (Sole et al., 2021).

Frequently assess for changes in level of consciousness and orientation. Check for asterixis and fetor hepaticus. These signs suggest worsening encephalopathy. Thiamine supplements and benzodiazepines may be needed if the patient is at risk for alcohol withdrawal.

NCLEX Examination Challenge 50.2

Physiological Integrity

The nurse is caring for a client who experiences upper GI bleeding due to esophageal varices caused by cirrhosis. Which of the following interventions would the nurse anticipate as appropriate to manage the client's bleeding? **Select all that apply.**

A. Administration of octreotide
B. Liver transplantation
C. Endoscopic sclerotherapy
D. Administration of lactulose
E. Administration of a beta-blocking agent

Managing Pruritus

Planning: Expected Outcomes. The patient is expected to experience decreased pruritus as a result of comfort measures and possibly drug therapy.

Interventions. Patients frequently report pruritus and dry skin due to jaundice from increased levels of serum bilirubin as cirrhosis progresses. Pruritus tends to increase in warmer conditions and in the early evening and at night. Comfort measures include avoiding being too warm, moisturizing the skin, and avoiding irritants to the skin. Some patients find that cool compresses and/or corticosteroid creams provide temporary relief. If these measures are not effective, drug therapy, including selective serotonin reuptake inhibitors such as sertraline, may be helpful.

Care Coordination and Transition Management

If patients with late-stage cirrhosis survive life-threatening complications, they are usually discharged to home or to a long-term care facility after treatment measures have managed acute medical problems. A home care referral may be needed if the patient is discharged to home. Chronically ill patients are often readmitted multiple times. Community-based care is aimed at optimizing comfort, promoting independence, supporting caregivers, and preventing rehospitalization.

INTERPROFESSIONAL COLLABORATION
Care of Patients With Cirrhosis

For patients with moderate to late-stage liver disease, collaborate with the case manager (CM) or other discharge planner to coordinate interprofessional continuing care. According to the Interprofessional Education Collaborative (IPEC) Expert Panel's Competency of Roles and Responsibilities, using the unique and complementary abilities of other team members optimizes health and patient care (IPEC Expert Panel, 2016). Collaborate with health care team members to help the patient to be as independent as possible, including physical and occupational therapists. Patients with end-stage disease may benefit from hospice care.

Assess physical adaptations needed to prepare the patient's home for recovery. The sleeping area needs to be close to a bathroom because diuretic and/or lactulose therapy increases the frequency of urination and stools. If the patient has difficulty reaching the toilet, additional equipment (e.g., bedside commode) is necessary. Special adult-size incontinence pads or briefs may be helpful if the patient has an altered mental status and incontinence. For the patient with shortness of breath from massive ascites, elevating the head of the bed and maintaining a semi-Fowler's to high-Fowler's position may help alleviate respiratory distress. Alternatively, a reclining chair with an elevated footrest may be used.

The patient who has a tunneled ascites drain is taught how to access the drain and remove excess fluid. Review the home care instructions that are provided with the drainage system with both the patient and family/caregiver. Remind them not to remove more than 2000 mL from the abdomen at one time to prevent hypovolemic shock.

The patient with encephalopathy often finds that small, frequent meals are best tolerated. If the nutritional intake or albumin/prealbumin is decreased after discharge, multivitamin and oral nutritional supplements are usually needed. Teach patients to avoid excessive vitamins and minerals that can be toxic to the liver, such as fat-soluble vitamins, excessive iron supplements, and niacin. Remind patients to check with their primary health care provider before taking any vitamin supplement.

Patients with bleeding from gastric ulcers may receive an H_2-receptor antagonist agent or proton pump inhibitor to reduce acid reflux (see Chapter 47). Those with episodes of spontaneous bacterial peritonitis (SBP) may be on a daily low-dose maintenance antibiotic.

Teach family members how to recognize signs of encephalopathy and to contact the primary health care provider if these signs develop. Reinforce that constipation, bleeding, and *infection* can increase the risk for encephalopathy.

One of the most important aspects of ongoing care for the patient with cirrhosis is health teaching about the need for the client to avoid alcohol, smoking, and illicit drugs. Advise the patient to avoid all over-the-counter drugs, especially acetaminophen, NSAIDs, and liver-toxic herbs, vitamins, and minerals. Reinforce the need to keep appointments for follow-up medical care. Remind the patient and family to notify the primary health care provider immediately if any GI bleeding (overt bleeding or melena) is noted so that reevaluation can begin quickly.

The patient is discharged to the home setting with an individualized teaching plan that includes *nutrition* therapy, drug therapy, and alcohol abstinence The encephalopathic patient may need to be monitored for adherence to drug therapy and alcohol abstinence, if appropriate. Individual and group therapy sessions may be arranged to help patients deal with alcohol abstinence if they are too ill to attend a formal treatment program. Because some patients may have alienated relatives over the years because of substance use, it may be necessary to help them identify a friend, neighbor, or sponsor in their recovery group for support. Refer the patient and family to self-help groups, such as Alcoholics Anonymous and Al-Anon. In Canada, SMART Recovery offers similar support, as well as additional services to manage addictions.

The patient with cirrhosis may also desire spiritual or other psychosocial support. Finances are frequently a problem for the chronically ill patient and family; social support and community services need to be identified. The American Liver Foundation (www.liverfoundation.org) and American Gastroenterological Association (www.gastro.org) are excellent sources for more information about liver disease.

Some patients may receive a liver transplant, which is discussed later in this chapter. For patients who are not candidates for liver transplantation, address end-of-life issues. Discuss options such as hospice care with patients and their families (see Chapter 8). Be aware and prepared that the patient and family may go through a grieving process.

Evaluate Outcomes: Evaluation

Evaluate the care of the patient with cirrhosis based on the identified priority patient problems. The expected outcomes include that the patient will:

- Have a decrease in or have no ascites

- Achieve fluid and electrolyte balance
- Not have hemorrhage or will be managed immediately if bleeding occurs
- Not develop encephalopathy or will be managed immediately if it occurs
- Successfully abstain from alcohol or drugs (if disease is caused by one or more of these substances) and have adequate **nutrition**

NONALCOHOLIC FATTY LIVER DISEASE

Pathophysiology Review

Nonalcoholic fatty liver disease (NAFLD) occurs when the liver stores excessive amounts of fat from the body unrelated to alcohol consumption. NAFLD is primarily related to obesity, increased levels of cholesterol and triglycerides, diabetes mellitus type 2, and metabolic syndrome. Therefore, preventing obesity and practicing a healthy lifestyle, if possible, can decrease the risk of NAFLD.

Individuals carrying the patatin-like phospholipase domain-containing 3 gene (PNPLA3) have an increased risk of developing NAFLD. People of Latino decent have this gene more often and are therefore at the highest risk for NAFLD (Salari et al., 2021). Over the past decade the prevalence of NAFLD has increase dramatically. Currently it is estimated that 100 million Americans have NAFLD (Vacca, 2020).

Nonalcoholic steatohepatitis (NASH) is a more severe form of NAFLD. NASH is defined by increased liver **inflammation,** hepatocyte injury, and liver fibrosis (Rogers, 2023). Nearly 20% of those diagnosed with NAFLD will develop NASH (American Liver Foundation, 2023d). As NAFLD and NASH progress they contribute to liver cancer, cirrhosis, or failure, causing premature death.

Interprofessional Collaborative Care

Recognize Cues: Assessment

When examining the patient's history, it is important to focus on risk factors for NAFLD. These include age, obesity, metabolic syndrome, and diabetes mellitus. Although risk factors may be present, many patients with NAFLD and NASH remain asymptomatic for years before they are diagnosed.

Physical Assessment. Initially these patients describe general symptoms including fatigue and malaise. Inquire about specific symptoms including right upper quadrant pain and pruritus (itching). Perform a comprehensive pain assessment if pain is present. Jaundice may also be present as the disease progresses.

Diagnostic Assessment. Laboratory findings for NAFLD and NASH include elevated ALT and AST, similar to those seen in other types of liver disease (see Table 50.1). Although important when establishing the presence of liver damage, increased liver enzymes cannot alone confirm the presence of NAFLD. The studies used to detect NAFLD are similar to those used for cirrhosis. Ultrasound transient elastography and liver biopsy are often used to gauge liver damage and level of liver fibrosis. These studies help to confirm the diagnosis of NAFLD and NASH (see Other Diagnostic Assessments in the Cirrhosis

section of this chapter for in-depth discussion regarding these diagnostic procedures).

Take Actions: Interventions

Currently there are no approved drugs to treat NAFLD. Patient management relies primarily on lifestyle modifications aimed at weight and fat loss including *nutrition,* exercise, and behavioral changes (Vacca, 2020). These adjustments can be challenging and have an impact on the physical and psychosocial aspects of the patient's life. With this in mind, it is important to use the interprofessional team approach including a registered dietitian nutritionist and qualified mental health practitioner.

INFECTION CONCEPT EXEMPLAR: HEPATITIS

Hepatitis is the widespread **inflammation** and **infection** of liver cells. *Viral* hepatitis, which can be acute or chronic, is the most common type. Less common types of hepatitis are caused by chemicals, drugs, and some herbs. This section discusses hepatitis caused by a virus. **Viral hepatitis** results from an infection caused by one of five categories of viruses:

- Hepatitis A virus (HAV)
- Hepatitis B virus (HBV)
- Hepatitis C virus (HCV)
- Hepatitis D virus (HDV)
- Hepatitis E virus (HEV)

Some cases of viral hepatitis are not caused by any of these viruses. These patients have non–A-E hepatitis. This section focuses on the most common viral types.

Pathophysiology Review

Liver injury with **inflammation** can develop after exposure to drugs and chemicals by inhalation, ingestion, or parenteral (IV) administration. *Toxic and drug-induced hepatitis* can result from exposure to hepatotoxins (e.g., industrial toxins, alcohol, and drugs). Hepatitis may also occur as a secondary **infection** during the course of infections with other viruses, such as Epstein-Barr, herpes simplex, varicella-zoster, and cytomegalovirus.

After the liver has been exposed to any causative agent (e.g., a virus), it becomes enlarged and congested with inflammatory cells, lymphocytes, and fluid, resulting in right upper quadrant pain and discomfort. As the disease progresses, the liver's normal lobular pattern becomes distorted as **cellular regulation** is compromised due to widespread **inflammation,** necrosis, and hepatocellular regeneration. This distortion increases pressure within the portal circulation, interfering with the blood flow into the hepatic lobules. Edema of the liver's bile channels results in obstructive jaundice.

Failure of the liver cells to regenerate, with progression of the necrotic process, results in a severe acute and often fatal form of hepatitis known as *fulminant hepatitis.* Hepatitis is considered chronic when liver **inflammation** lasts longer than 6 months. *Chronic hepatitis* usually occurs due to hepatitis B or hepatitis C. Superimposed infection with hepatitis D virus (HDV) in patients with chronic hepatitis B may also result in chronic hepatitis. Chronic hepatitis can lead to cirrhosis and liver cancer. Many patients have multiple infections, especially a combination of HBV with HCV, HDV, or human immunodeficiency virus (HIV) infections (Rogers, 2023).

Etiology and Genetic Risk

The five major types of acute viral hepatitis vary by etiology, mode of transmission, manner of onset, and incubation periods. Hepatitis cases must be reported to the local public health department, which then notifies the Centers for Disease Control and Prevention (CDC). Genetic factors do not play a major role in the cause of viral hepatitis.

Hepatitis A. The causative agent of hepatitis A, hepatitis A virus (HAV), is a ribonucleic acid (RNA) virus of the *Enterovirus* genus. *It is a hardy virus and survives on human hands.* The virus is resistant to detergents and acids but is destroyed by chlorine (bleach) and extremely high temperatures.

Hepatitis A usually has a mild course similar to a typical flulike infection and often goes unrecognized. It is spread most often by the fecal-oral route by fecal contamination either from person-to-person contact (e.g., oral-anal sexual activity) or by consuming contaminated food or water. Common sources of **infection** include shellfish caught in contaminated water and food contaminated by food handlers infected with HAV. The incubation period of hepatitis A is usually 15 to 50 days, with a peak of 25 to 30 days. The disease is usually not life-threatening, but it may be more severe in adults older than 40 years and those with preexisting liver disease such as hepatitis C (Rogers, 2023).

In a small percentage of hepatitis A cases, severe illness with extrahepatic signs and symptoms can occur. Advanced age and conditions such as chronic liver disease may cause widespread damage that requires a liver transplant. When the patient's immunity is decreased, death may occur. Incidence of hepatitis A is particularly high in countries where sanitation is poor; however, cases are diagnosed internationally across the globe. Some adults have hepatitis A and do not know it. The course is similar to that of a GI illness, and the disease and recovery are usually uneventful.

Hepatitis B. The hepatitis B virus (HBV) is not transmitted like HAV. It is a double-shelled particle containing DNA composed of a core antigen (HBcAg), a surface antigen (HBsAg), and another antigen found within the core (HBeAg) that circulates in the blood. HBV may be spread through these common modes of transmission (Rogers, 2023):

- Unprotected sexual intercourse with an infected partner
- Sharing needles, syringes, or other drug-injection equipment
- Sharing razors or toothbrushes with an infected individual
- Accidental needlesticks or injuries from sharp instruments, primarily in health care workers (low incidence)
- Blood transfusions (that have not been screened for the virus, before 1992)
- Hemodialysis
- Direct contact with the blood or open sores of an infected individual
- Birth (spread from an infected mother to baby during birth)

In addition, patients with compromised immunity from either disease or drug therapy are more likely to develop hepatitis B. The clinical course of hepatitis B may be varied. Symptoms usually occur within 25 to 180 days of exposure.

Blood tests confirm the disease, although many individuals with hepatitis B have no symptoms. Most adults who get hepatitis B recover and clear the virus from their body and develop immunity. However, a small percentage of people do not develop immunity and become carriers. Hepatitis carriers can infect others even though they are not sick and have no obvious signs of hepatitis B. Chronic carriers are at high risk for cirrhosis and liver cancer. Because of the high number of newcomers from endemic areas, the incidence of hepatitis B has increased in the United States.

Hepatitis C. The hepatitis C virus is an enveloped, single-stranded RNA virus that is genetically unstable and has at least six known major genotypes. Transmission is via blood to blood. The rate of sexual transmission is very low in a single-couple relationship but increases with multiple sex partners or in men who have unprotected sex with men. HCV is contracted by (Chaney, 2019):

- Illicit IV drug needle sharing (highest incidence)
- Blood, blood products, or organ transplants received before 1992
- Baby boomers (adults born between 1945 and 1965)
- Needlestick injury with HCV-contaminated blood (health care workers at high risk)
- Hemodialysis
- Health care workers
- People who are incarcerated (prisoners)
- Sharing of drug paraphernalia

The disease is *not* transmitted by casual contact or intimate household contact. However, those infected are advised to not share razors, toothbrushes, or pierced earrings because microscopic blood may be on these items.

The incubation period ranges from 2 weeks to 6 months. Acute infection and illness are not common. Most people are completely unaware that they have been infected. They may be asymptomatic and not diagnosed until many months or years after the initial exposure when an abnormality is detected during a routine laboratory evaluation or when liver complications occur. Unlike with hepatitis B, most people infected with hepatitis C do not clear the virus, and a chronic infection develops.

HCV does damage to the body's immunity over decades by causing a chronic **inflammation** in the liver that eventually causes the liver cells to scar. Scarring from chronic **infection** with either HBV or HCV frequently leads to cirrhosis, which is a risk factor for developing primary liver cancer (Rogers, 2023). Patients who develop liver cancer may have interventional radiologic procedures (such as transarterial chemoembolization [TACE]), cryotherapy, ablation, traditional chemotherapy, or selective internal radiation therapy (SIRT) (see Chapter 18 for more information on cancer management modalities and associated nursing care). Liver cancer can also occur as a metastatic disease process and is not associated with hepatitis or cirrhosis.

Hepatitis D. Hepatitis D (delta hepatitis) is caused by a defective RNA virus that needs the helper function of HBV. Therefore, it occurs only with HBV to cause viral replication. This usually develops into chronic disease. The incubation period is about 14 to 56 days. As with hepatitis B, the disease is transmitted primarily by parenteral routes, especially in patients who are IV drug users. Having sexual contact with someone with HDV is also a high-risk factor (Rogers, 2023).

Hepatitis E. The hepatitis E virus (HEV) causes a waterborne infection associated with epidemics in the Indian subcontinent, Asia, Africa, the Middle East, Mexico, and Central and South America. Many large outbreaks have occurred after heavy rains and flooding. Like hepatitis A, hepatitis E is caused by fecal contamination of food and water.

HEV is not commonly acquired in the United States. Most cases occur in those who have traveled to a country where HEV is endemic. Similar to hepatitis A, it is transmitted via the fecal-oral route with a similar clinical course. HEV has an incubation period of 15 to 64 days. There is no evidence at this time of a chronic form of the disease. The disease tends to be self-limiting and resolves on its own (CDC, 2020).

Incidence and Prevalence

The incidence of hepatitis A and hepatitis B is declining as a result of CDC recommendations for vaccination. However, hepatitis B and hepatitis C are a concern because of their association with cirrhosis and liver cancer. It is estimated that over 58 million people worldwide have chronic hepatitis C, with 1.5 million new cases occurring every year (World Health Organization [WHO], 2021).

Currently there is no vaccine for HCV. Patients may be treated with antiviral drug therapies. The desired outcome of treatment of HCV-infected patients is to reduce mortality and liver-related health adverse consequences, including end-stage liver disease and liver cancer. It is expected that the cases of HCV may rise over the next several decades due to increasing illicit drug use.

Health Promotion/Disease Prevention

Hepatitis vaccines for infants, children, and adolescents have helped to decrease the incidence of hepatitis A and hepatitis B. These vaccines are safe and not associated with major complications. Some adults are also advised to receive these immunizations.

Measures to prevent hepatitis A include:
- Proper handwashing, especially after handling shellfish
- Avoiding contaminated food or water (including tap water in countries with high incidence)
- Receiving immunoglobulin within 14 days if exposed to the virus
- Receiving the HAV vaccine before traveling to areas where the disease is common (e.g., Mexico, Caribbean)
- Receiving the vaccine if living or working in enclosed areas with others, such as college dormitories, correctional institutions, day-care centers, and long-term care facilities

Although there are also vaccines available to protect against hepatitis B virus (HBV) infection, objectives to improve the incidence and management of HBV and hepatitis C virus are included as part of the *Healthy People 2030* initiative (Box 50.5).

A combination HAV and HBV vaccine is also available for adults. Immunization against HBV is recommended for the following groups:

> **♥ BOX 50.5 Meeting *Healthy People 2030* Objectives**
>
> **Hepatitis A, B, and C**
>
> Several objectives to improve health related to liver infection include:
> - Reduce the rate of hepatitis A.
> - Reduce the rate of acute hepatitis B.
> - Reduce the rate of acute hepatitis C.
> - Increase the proportion of people who know they have chronic hepatitis B.
> - Reduce the rate of deaths with hepatitis B as a cause.
> - Increase the proportion of people who have cleared hepatitis C infection.
>
> Teach individuals how to prevent these liver infections, including obtaining vaccines as available.

> **BOX 50.6 Best Practice for Patient Safety and Quality Care**
>
> **Prevention of Viral Hepatitis in Health Care Workers**
>
> - Use Standard Precautions to prevent the transmission of disease between patients or between patients and health care staff (see Chapter 19).
> - Eliminate needles and other sharp instruments by substituting needleless systems (needlesticks are the major source of hepatitis B transmission in health care workers).
> - Receive the hepatitis B vaccine, which is given in a series of three injections. This vaccine also prevents hepatitis D by preventing hepatitis B.
> - For postexposure prevention of hepatitis A, seek medical attention immediately for immunoglobulin (Ig) administration.
> - Report all cases of hepatitis to the local health department.

- People who have sexual intercourse with more than one partner
- People with sexually transmitted infection (STI) or a history of sexually transmitted infection (STI)
- Men having unprotected sex with men (MSM)
- People with any chronic liver disease (such as hepatitis C or cirrhosis)
- Patients with HIV infection
- People who are exposed to blood or body fluids in the workplace, including health care workers, firefighters, and police
- People in correctional facilities (prisoners)
- Patients needing immunosuppressant drugs
- Family members, household members, and sexual contacts of people with HBV infection

Multiple hepatitis C virus (HCV) genotypes have made it difficult to develop an effective vaccine against hepatitis C. Teach baby boomer adults to have a one-time screening test for HCV due to the high risk of this infection in this population (Chaney, 2019).

Additional measures to prevent viral hepatitis for health care workers and others in contact with infected patients are listed in Box 50.6.

Interprofessional Collaborative Care

Care for the patient with hepatitis can take place in various settings. These patients may, at different times, self-manage at home, be hospitalized for immediate concerns, or be cared for in the community setting.

Recognize Cues: Assessment

History. Ask patients whether they have known exposure to a person with hepatitis. For the patient who presents with few or no symptoms of liver disease but has abnormal laboratory tests (e.g., elevated alanine aminotransferase [ALT] or aspartate aminotransferase [AST] level), the patient history may need to include additional questions regarding risk factors.

Physical Assessment/Signs and Symptoms. Assess whether the patient has any of the signs and symptoms associated with most types of vital hepatitis as listed in Box 50.7. Although HCV may be asymptomatic for most adults, some patients with a new HCV *infection* can experience some of the following signs and symptoms.

Lightly palpate the right upper abdominal quadrant to assess for liver tenderness. The patient may report right upper quadrant pain with jarring movements. Inspect the skin, sclerae, and mucous membranes for jaundice. The patient may present for medical treatment only after jaundice appears, believing that other vague symptoms are related to a flulike syndrome.

Jaundice in hepatitis results from intrahepatic obstruction and is caused by edema of the liver's bile channels. Dark urine and clay-colored stools are often reported by the patient. If possible, obtain a urine and stool specimen for visual inspection and laboratory analysis. The patient may also have skin abrasions from scratching because of pruritus (itching).

Patients with chronic HCV infection often have extrahepatic complications. Examples include:

- Depression
- Polyarthritis
- Myalgia
- Renal insufficiency
- Cognitive impairment
- Cardiovascular problems such as vasculitis and heart disease

Psychosocial Assessment. Viral hepatitis has various presentations; for most infected people the initial course is mild with few or no symptoms. The long-term complications of fibrosis and cirrhosis cause the more serious problem. This is especially true for patients who have chronic HBV and HCV infection.

Patients may experience emotional problems that center on their feeling sick and fatigued. General malaise, inactivity, and vague symptoms contribute to depression. Some patients often feel guilty and are remorseful about decisions made that caused the disease. These feelings are most likely to occur when the source of infection is from drug use.

Infectious diseases such as hepatitis continue to have a social stigma. The patient may feel embarrassed by the precautions that are imposed in the hospital and continue to be necessary at home. This embarrassment may cause the patient to limit social interactions. Patients may be afraid that they will spread the virus to family and friends.

Family members may be concerned about contracting the virus and may distance themselves from the patient. Allow them to verbalize these feelings and explore the reasons for these fears. Educate the patient and family members about modes of transmission and clarify information as needed.

Patients may be unable to return to work for several weeks during the acute phases of illness. The loss of wages and the cost of hospitalization for a patient without insurance coverage may produce great anxiety and financial burden. This situation may last for months or years if hepatitis becomes chronic.

Laboratory Assessment. Hepatitis A, hepatitis B, and hepatitis C are usually confirmed by acute elevations in levels of liver enzymes, indicating liver cellular damage, and by specific serologic markers.

Levels of ALT and AST may rise into the thousands in acute or fulminant cases of hepatitis. Alkaline phosphatase levels may be normal or elevated. Serum total bilirubin levels are elevated and are consistent with the clinical appearance of jaundice.

The presence of *hepatitis A* is established when hepatitis A virus (HAV) antibodies (HAV-Ab/IgM) are found in the blood. Ongoing *inflammation* of the liver by HAV is indicated by the presence of immunoglobulin M (IgM) antibodies, which persist in the blood for 3 to 6 weeks. Previous infection is identified by the presence of immunoglobulin G (IgG) antibodies. These antibodies persist in the serum and provide permanent immunity to HAV (Pagana et al., 2022).

The presence of the *hepatitis B virus* (HBV) is established when serologic testing confirms the presence of hepatitis B antigen-antibody systems in the blood and a detectable viral count (HBV polymerase chain reaction [PCR] DNA). Antigens located on the surface (shell) of the virus (HBsAg) and IgM antibodies to hepatitis B core antigen (HBcAg) are the most significant serologic markers. The presence of these markers establishes the diagnosis of hepatitis B. *The patient is infectious as long as hepatitis B surface antigen (HBsAg) is present in the blood.* Persistence of this serologic marker after 6 months or longer indicates a carrier state or chronic hepatitis. HBsAg levels normally decline and disappear after the acute hepatitis B episode. The presence of antibodies to HBsAg in the blood indicates recovery and immunity to hepatitis B. *People who have*

BOX 50.7 Key Features

Viral Hepatitis

- Abdominal pain
- Yellowish sclera (icterus)
- Arthralgia (joint pain) or myalgia (muscle pain)
- Diarrhea or constipation
- Light clay-colored stools
- Dark-yellow to brownish urine
- Jaundice
- Fever
- Fatigue
- Malaise
- Anorexia
- Nausea and vomiting
- Dry skin
- Pruritus (itching)

been vaccinated against HBV have a positive HBsAg because they also have immunity to the disease (Pagana et al., 2022).

To detect HCV infection, blood is tested for anti-HCV antibodies to HCV recombinant core antigen, *NS3 gene*, NS4 antigen, and NS5 antibody. The antibodies can be detected within 4 weeks of the infection (Pagana et al., 2022). To identify the actual circulating virus, the HCV RNA test is used. This confirms active virus and can measure the viral load. A diagnostic tool called the *OraQuick HCV Rapid Antibody Test* has the advantage of providing a quick diagnosis of the disease as a point-of-care test.

The presence of *hepatitis D* virus (HDV) can be confirmed by the identification of intrahepatic delta antigen or, more often, by a rise in the hepatitis D virus antibodies (HDV-Ab) titer. This increase can be seen within a few days of **infection** (Pagana et al., 2022).

Hepatitis E virus (HEV) testing is usually reserved for travelers with a history of hepatitis infection. HEV virus itself cannot be detected, so infection is identified by finding hepatitis E antibodies (HEV-Ab/IgM) in the patient's blood.

Other Diagnostic Assessment. *Liver biopsy* may be used to confirm the diagnosis of hepatitis and establish the stage and grade of liver damage or cancer. Characteristic changes help the pathologist distinguish among a virus, drug, toxin, fatty liver, iron, and other disease. This procedure is usually performed in an ambulatory care setting as a percutaneous procedure (through the skin) after a local anesthetic is given. If coagulation is abnormal, it may be done using either a CT-guided or transjugular route to reduce the risk for pneumothorax or hemothorax. *Ultrasound* also may be used.

Analyze Cues and Prioritize Hypotheses: Analysis

The priority collaborative problems for patients with hepatitis include:

1. Weight loss due to complications associated with **inflammation** of the liver
2. Fatigue due to **infection** and decreased metabolic energy production

Generate Solutions and Take Actions: Planning and Implementation

The patient with viral hepatitis can be mildly or acutely ill, depending on the severity of the **inflammation** and **infection.** Most patients are not hospitalized, although older adults and those with dehydration may be admitted for a short-term stay. The plan of care for all patients with viral hepatitis is based on measures to rest the liver, promote hepatic regeneration, strengthen immunity, and prevent complications, if possible.

Promoting Nutrition

Planning: Expected Outcomes. The patient will maintain appropriate weight and **nutrition** status.

Interventions. Patients with hepatitis, especially hepatitis A, may decline food because of general malaise, anorexia, abdominal discomfort, or nausea. The patient's diet should be high in carbohydrates and calories, with moderate amounts of fat and protein added after nausea and anorexia have subsided.

Small, frequent meals are often preferable to three standard meals daily. Ask the patient about appealing food preferences because favorite foods are tolerated better than randomly selected foods. High-calorie snacks may be needed. Supplemental vitamins are often prescribed.

Managing Fatigue

Planning: Expected Outcomes. The patient will progressively exhibit increasing energy as evidenced by participation in ADLs and self-reported decrease in level of fatigue.

Interventions. During the acute stage of viral hepatitis, interventions are aimed at resting the inflamed liver to promote hepatic cell regeneration. *Rest* is an essential intervention to reduce the liver's metabolic demands and increase its blood supply. Collaborative care is generally supportive. The patient is usually tired and expresses feelings of general malaise. Complete bedrest is usually not required, but rest periods alternating with periods of activity are indicated and are often enough to promote hepatic healing. Individualize the patient's plan of care and change it as needed to reflect the severity of symptoms, fatigue, and results of liver function tests and enzyme determinations. Activities such as self-care and ambulating are gradually added to the activity schedule as tolerated.

Drugs are used sparingly for patients with hepatitis to allow the liver to rest. An antiemetic to relieve nausea may be prescribed. However, because of the life-threatening nature of chronic hepatitis B and hepatitis C, several drugs are given, including antiviral and immunomodulating drugs.

Two groups of drugs are approved for management of hepatitis B—*interferon alfa preparations* and *nucleoside analogs.* Examples of interferon alfa drugs include interferon alfa-2b and peginterferon alfa-2a. These drugs are not used as often today because newer, more effective medications are available. Examples of nucleoside analogs include lamivudine and adefovir (Table 50.2).

For many years, the standard of care for hepatitis C was pegylated (PEG) interferon alfa plus ribavirin. In the past decade, new direct-acting antiviral (DAA) drugs such as second-generation protease inhibitors (PIs) that target specific steps in HCV replication are being used with much more success and fewer side or adverse effects. The current standard of practice for hepatitis C treatment is that a patient's drug regimen is determined by HCV viral genotype (American Association

---

⚠ NURSING SAFETY PRIORITY
Action Alert

Teach the patient with viral hepatitis and the family to use measures to prevent infection transmission. In addition, instruct the patient to avoid alcohol and check with the primary health care provider before taking any medication or vitamin, supplement, or herbal preparation.

Encourage the patient to increase activity gradually to prevent fatigue. Suggest that the patient eat small, frequent meals of high-carbohydrate foods and plan frequent rest periods.

Collaborate with the certified infection control practitioner and infectious disease specialist if needed in caring for these patients. These experts can suggest appropriate resources for the patient and family.

TABLE 50.2   Common Examples of Drug Therapy

Drug Therapy Used for Chronic Hepatitis B and Hepatitis C

Drug Category	Selected Nursing Implications
Chronic Hepatitis B: Nucleoside Analogs	
Tenofovir	Monitor kidney function. *Drug is excreted through kidneys; monitoring for renal impairment is important.* Teach risk for falls to prevent fractures. *Can cause bone demineralization.*
Adefovir	Monitor kidney function. *Drug is excreted through kidneys; monitoring for renal impairment is important.*
Lamivudine	Monitor kidney function. *Drug is excreted through kidneys; monitoring for renal impairment is important.* Remind patient to not discontinue drug without consulting with primary health care provider. *Discontinuation of drug can cause flareup of hepatitis B.*
Entecavir	Monitor kidney function. Teach the patient to avoid alcohol to prevent serious interaction. *Drug is excreted through kidneys; monitoring for renal impairment is important.*
Chronic Hepatitis C	
Second-generation protease inhibitors: • Glecaprevir • Grazoprevir • Simeprevir • Paritaprevir	Monitor CBC and chemistry panel. Instruct the patient on common reactions, such as rash, itching, nausea, and headache. *Kidney and liver function may become impaired, and electrolyte imbalances may occur when taking this drug.*
NS5A Inhibitor Drug Combinations	
Glecaprevir/pibrentasvir	Ask if the patient has had any other type of hepatitis or cirrhosis. *This combination drug can reactivate hepatitis B and cause liver failure.* Teach patient about monitoring liver enzymes, especially ALT. *The combination drug can cause liver toxicity, including an increase in liver enzymes.*
Elbasvir/grazoprevir	Ask patients if they have a history of or current hepatitis B. *The combination drug can reactivate hepatitis B and cause liver failure.* Teach patients about monitoring liver enzymes, especially ALT. *The combination drug can cause liver toxicity, including an increase in liver enzymes.*
Ledipasvir/sofosbuvir (for hepatitis C genotype 1 only)	Ask if the patient has had any other type of hepatitis or cirrhosis. *This combination drug can reactivate hepatitis B and cause liver failure.* Do not give this drug to patients receiving amiodarone. *If this drug combination is taken with amiodarone, the patient may experience severe symptomatic bradycardia and other cardiac problems, including chest pain.*
NS5A-NS5B Polymerase Inhibitor	
Sofosbuvir/velpatasvir (for almost all main types of hepatitis C)	Ask patients if they have a history of or current hepatitis B. *The combination drug can reactivate hepatitis B and cause liver failure.* Teach patients that their liver enzymes must be monitored, especially ALT elevation.

ALT, Alanine aminotransferase; *CBC,* complete blood count.

for the Study of Liver Diseases [AASLD], 2020). Examples of newer drugs, including second-generation PIs, are presented in Table 50.2. All these drugs can affect the immune system and make patients susceptible to **infection.** *Teach patients to avoid crowds and people who could be infectious.*

Care Coordination and Transition Management

Home care management varies according to the type of hepatitis and whether the disease is acute or chronic. A primary focus in any case is preventing the spread of the infection. For hepatitis transmitted by the fecal-oral route, careful handwashing and sanitary disposal of feces are important. Therefore patient and family education is very important.

Evaluate Outcomes: Evaluation

Evaluate the care of the patient with hepatitis based on the identified priority patient problems. The expected outcomes include that the patient will:

• Maintain adequate **nutrition** for body requirements

• Report increasing energy levels as the liver rests
• Achieve appropriate management of **infection** and **inflammation**

LIVER TRANSPLANTATION

The first liver transplant was performed in the United States the late 1960s. Over the past five decades this surgical procedure has become a common practice worldwide (Newman, 2020). Patients with end-stage liver disease or acute liver failure who have not responded to conventional medical or surgical intervention are potential candidates for liver transplantation.

Pathophysiology Review

Many diseases can cause liver failure. Cirrhosis (scarring of the liver) is the most common reason for liver transplants. Other common reasons include chronic hepatitis B and hepatitis C, bile duct diseases, autoimmune liver disease, alcoholic liver disease, and fatty liver disease.

A patient requiring transplantation has an extensive physiologic and psychological assessment and evaluation by primary health care providers and transplant coordinators. Alternative treatment should be extensively explored before designating a patient for a liver transplant. Patients who are *not* considered candidates for transplantation include those with:

- Severe cardiovascular instability with advanced cardiac disease
- Severe respiratory disease
- Metastatic tumors
- Inability to follow instructions regarding drug therapy and self-management

Liver transplantation has become the most effective treatment for an increasing number of patients with acute and chronic liver diseases. Inclusion and exclusion criteria vary among transplantation centers and are continually revised as treatment options change and surgical techniques improve.

Donor livers are obtained primarily from trauma victims who have not had liver damage. They are distributed through a nationwide program known as the United Network for Organ Sharing (UNOS). This system distributes deceased donor livers based on regional considerations and patient acuity. Candidates with the highest level of acuity receive highest priority.

The donor liver is transported to the surgery center in a solution that preserves the organ for up to 8 hours. During the deceased donor liver transplant (DDLT) surgery, the diseased liver is removed through an incision made in the upper abdomen. The new liver is carefully put in its place and attached to the patient's blood vessels and bile ducts. This procedure can take many hours to complete and requires a highly specialized team and large volumes of fluid and blood replacement.

Living donors have also been used and are usually a close family member or a spouse. Living donor liver transplant (LDLT) is done on a voluntary basis after careful psychological and physiologic preparation and testing. The donor's liver is resected (usually removal of one lobe) and implanted into the recipient after removal of the diseased liver. In both the donor and the recipient, the liver regenerates and grows to meet the demands of the body if there are no complications (see the Legal/Ethical Considerations box).

ⓘ LEGAL/ETHICAL CONSIDERATIONS

Legal/Ethical Issues Related to Liver Transplantation

A number of legal-ethical issues have surfaced as liver transplantation has become more common and the need for donors has increased. The primary issues include:

- Ensuring that living donors are provided complete information about the risks associated with transplantation surgery (informed consent)
- Increased use of hepatitis C virus–infected livers for transplantation since direct-acting antiviral (DAA) therapy has become more available
- More men than women receive liver transplants despite using the Model for End-Stage Liver Disease (MELD) score to determine the urgency of need for transplant
- Fewer liver transplants are performed for patients from Black and Hispanic populations when compared with the White population

These issues reflect the ethical principles of nonmaleficence and beneficence. Nurses need to advocate for patients who are potential living donors and assess their knowledge of the morbidity and mortality associated with LDLT to prevent patient harm. Nurses also need to advocate for all patients if they have an urgent need for liver transplantation regardless of their race, ethnicity, or gender. Nursing research is needed to explore these issues and how nurses can be the most effective advocates.

Interprofessional Collaborative Care

Care of the patient undergoing liver transplantation requires an interprofessional team approach. Receiving a transplant has a major psychosocial impact. Transplant complications cause patients to be very anxious. In collaboration with the members of the interprofessional health care team, assure them and their families that these problems can be managed and are often treated successfully.

In the immediate postoperative period, the patient is managed in the critical care unit and requires meticulous monitoring and care. Although liver transplantations are commonly performed, complications can occur. Some problems can be managed medically, whereas others require later hospitalizations or removal of the transplant. Monitor for signs and symptoms of complications of surgery and immediately report them to the surgeon (Table 50.3). The most common complications are acute graft rejection, vascular or biliary obstruction, and infection.

The success rate for transplantations has greatly improved since the introduction many years ago of cyclosporine (cyclosporin A), an immunosuppressant drug. Today, many other antirejection drugs are used. (See Chapter 16 for a discussion of rejection and preventive drug therapy for organ transplantation.)

❗ NURSING SAFETY PRIORITY

Action Alert

For the patient who has undergone liver transplantation, monitor for clinical signs and symptoms of rejection, which may include tachycardia, fever, pain in the right upper quadrant or flank, decreased bile pigment and volume, and increasing jaundice. Laboratory findings include elevated serum bilirubin, rising ALT and AST levels, elevated alkaline phosphatase levels, and increased prothrombin time/international normalized ratio (PT/INR) (Pagana et al., 2022).

TABLE 50.3   Assessment and Prevention of Common Postoperative Complications Associated With Liver Transplantation

Assessment	Prevention
Acute Graft Rejection	
Occurs from 7 to 14 days postoperatively. Manifested by tachycardia, fever, right upper quadrant (RUQ) or flank pain, diminished bile drainage or change in bile color, or increased jaundice	Prophylaxis with immunosuppressant agents, such as prednisone, tacrolimus, or cyclosporine (CSA)
Laboratory changes: (1) increased levels of serum bilirubin, transaminases, and alkaline phosphatase; (2) prolonged prothrombin time	Early diagnosis to treat with more potent antirejection drugs
Infection	
Can occur at any time during recovery	Antibiotic prophylaxis; vaccinations
Manifested by fever or excessive, foul-smelling drainage (urine, wound, or bile); other indicators depend on location and type of infection	Frequent cultures of tubes, lines, and drainage
	Early removal of invasive lines
	Good handwashing
	Early diagnosis and treatment with organism-specific antiinfective agents
Hepatic Complications (Bile Leakage, Abscess Formation, Hepatic Thrombosis)	
Manifested by decreased bile drainage, increased RUQ abdominal pain with distention and guarding, nausea or vomiting, increased jaundice, and clay-colored stools	If present, keep T-tube in dependent position and secure to patient; empty frequently, recording quality and quantity of drainage
Laboratory changes: increased levels of serum bilirubin and transaminases	Report signs and symptoms to surgeon immediately
	May need surgical intervention
Acute Kidney Injury	
Caused by hypotension, antibiotics, cyclosporine, acute liver failure, or hypothermia	Monitor all drug levels with nephrotoxic side effects
Indicators of hypothermia: shivering, hyperventilation, increased cardiac output, vasoconstriction, and alkalemia	Prevent hypotension
Early indicators of acute kidney injury: changes in urine output, increased blood urea nitrogen (BUN) and creatinine levels, and electrolyte imbalance	Observe for early signs of acute kidney injury and report them immediately to the surgeon

Transplant rejection is treated aggressively with immunosuppressive drugs. If therapy is not effective, liver function rapidly deteriorates. Multisystem organ failure, including respiratory and renal involvement, develops along with diffuse coagulopathies and portal-systemic encephalopathy (PSE). The only alternative for treatment is emergency retransplantation.

Infection is another potential threat to the transplanted graft and the patient's survival. Immunosuppressant therapy, which must be used to prevent and treat organ rejection, significantly increases the patient's risk for infection. Other risk factors include the presence of multiple tubes and intravascular lines, immobility, and prolonged anesthesia. Vaccinations and prophylactic antibiotics are helpful in protecting from infection.

In the early posttransplantation period, common infections include pneumonia, wound infections, and urinary tract infections. Opportunistic infections usually develop after the first postoperative month and include cytomegalovirus, mycobacterial infections, and parasitic infections. Latent infections such as tuberculosis and herpes simplex may be reactivated.

The primary health care provider prescribes broad-spectrum antibiotics for prophylaxis during and after surgery. Obtain culture specimens from all lines and tubes and collect specimens for culture at predetermined time intervals as dictated by the agency's policy. If an infection is detected, the primary health care provider prescribes organism-specific antiinfective agents. The patient should be taught to contact the primary health care provider at any time that signs of infection are present.

The biliary anastomosis is susceptible to breakdown, obstruction, and infection. If leakage occurs or if the site becomes necrotic or obstructed, an abscess can form or peritonitis, bacteremia, and cirrhosis may develop. Observe for potential complications, which are listed in Table 50.3.

! NURSING SAFETY PRIORITY
Action Alert

For the patient who has had a liver transplantation, monitor the temperature frequently per hospital protocol and report elevations, increased abdominal pain, distention, and rigidity, which are indicators of peritonitis. Nursing assessment also includes monitoring for a change in neurologic status that could indicate encephalopathy from a nonfunctioning liver. Report signs of clotting problems (e.g., bloody oozing from a catheter, petechiae, ecchymosis) to the surgeon immediately because they may indicate impaired function of the transplanted liver.

Teach patients to be aware of side effects of immunosuppressive drugs, such as hypertension, nephrotoxicity, drug-induced *infection,* and GI disturbances. Remind them that long-term management of care includes surveillance for malignancy, metabolic syndrome, and diabetes. Teaching the patient self-examination for skin, breast, and testicular malignancies and reminders for annual Papanicolaou (Pap) smears and other cancer screening tests are important. Posttransplant patients need to maintain lifestyle changes to increase their longevity after surgery.

GET READY FOR THE NEXT-GENERATION NCLEX® EXAMINATION!

Essential Nursing Care Points

Health Promotion/Disease Prevention

- The *Healthy People 2030* initiative recognizes the need for a reduction in deaths of patients who have liver cirrhosis.
- Two of the most common causes of cirrhosis are chronic hepatitis C infection and chronic alcohol use; therefore nurses need to teach people to avoid these risk factors.
- The *Healthy People 2030* initiative recognizes the need to decrease liver infections, particularly hepatitis A and B.
- Nurses should teach patients at risk to obtain vaccines to prevent hepatitis A and B.

Chronic Disease Care

- Cirrhosis is extensive, irreversible scarring of the liver, usually caused by a chronic reaction to hepatic *inflammation* and necrosis.
- Common complications of cirrhosis include portal hypertension, ascites, and esophageal varices.
- In the United States, hepatitis C is the most common cause of cirrhosis and liver cancer.
- Early symptoms of compensated cirrhosis include fatigue, anorexia, and possible abdominal pain.
- Symptoms of late-stage or end-stage cirrhosis include jaundice, ascites, vascular lesions, ecchymosis, and dry, itchy skin.
- There is no cure for cirrhosis; the nurse provides supportive care and manages complications associated with decompensated cirrhosis.
- Nonalcoholic fatty liver disease (NAFLD) occurs commonly in people who have obesity, increased lipid profile, diabetes mellitus type 2, and metabolic syndrome.
- Unlike with hepatitis B, people with hepatitis C virus (HCV) infection do not clear the infection, which becomes a chronic infection that can lead to cirrhosis and liver cancer.
- Second-generation protease inhibitors (PIs) are antiviral agents that are commonly used to manage chronic hepatitis C (see Table 50.2).
- Table 50.1 summarizes the significance of laboratory findings in patients with chronic liver disease.
- Patients who receive liver transplants may have a deceased donor liver or part of a liver from a living donor.
- Patients who receive a liver transplant are at risk for organ rejection and infection; these patients must take antirejection drugs for the rest of their lives.
- More men than women receive liver transplants despite use of the Model for End-Stage Liver Disease (MELD) score to determine the urgency of need for transplant.
- Fewer liver transplants are performed for patients from Black and Hispanic populations when compared with the White population.

Regenerative or Restorative Care

- Upper GI bleeding is an acute life-threatening complication of cirrhosis and is managed with drug therapy (octreotide), endoscopic therapies, and/or the transjugular intrahepatic portal-systemic shunt (TIPS) procedure.
- Hepatitis A is a common acute viral liver infection that is self-limiting and transmitted through the oral-fecal route; it most often results from consuming contaminated food.
- Common symptoms of acute hepatitis include jaundice, light clay-colored stools, dark urine, fatigue, fever, and GI symptoms.
- Most patients who contract hepatitis B clear the infection and do not have chronic disease.
- Commonly used drugs for hepatitis B include nucleotide analogs such as tenofovir and lamivudine (see Table 50.2).

Hospice/Palliative/Supportive Care

- Palliative and hospice care at home may be needed for patients who have end-stage liver failure and are not candidates for liver transplantation.

Mastery Questions

1. The nurse is caring for a client who is being prepared for a paracentesis. Which of the following actions is the **most** important for the nurse to take at this time?
   A. Place the client in a sitting position.
   B. Have the client void before the procedure.
   C. Weigh the client prior to the procedure.
   D. Provide supplemental oxygen.

2. The nurse is caring for a client who has stage II hepatic encephalopathy as a result of late-stage cirrhosis. Which of the following is the **priority** for the client's care at this time?
   A. Reorient the client to reality frequently.
   B. Monitor the client's serum bilirubin level.
   C. Keep the patient safe and free from injury.
   D. Administer antibiotic therapy.

3. The nurse is caring for a client who had a liver transplant yesterday. What is the **priority** nursing assessment for the client at this time?
   A. Monitor for symptoms of infection.
   B. Assess for neurologic status changes.
   C. Observe for signs of internal hemorrhage.
   D. Assess for indications of organ transplant rejection.

NGN Challenge 50.1

The nurse is caring for a 55-year-old client who had a liver transplant 7 days ago.

Laboratory Test	Today	Yesterday	2 Days Ago (Operative Day)	Reference Range
ALT	489 units/L (489 IU/L)	243 units/L (243 IU/L)	67 units/L (87 IU/L)	4–36 units/L (4–36 IU/L)
AST	315 units/L (5.23 mckat/L)	172 units/L (2.86 mckat/L)	54 units/L (0.9 mckat/L)	0–35 units/L (0–0.58 mckat/L)
Alkaline phosphatase	183 units/L (3.11 mckat/L)	157 units/L (2.67 mckat/L)	126 units/L (2.14 mckat/L)	30–120 units/L (0.5–2.0 mckat/L)
WBC count	9500/mm³/L (9.5 × 10⁹/L)	8000/mm³/L (8 × 10⁹/L)	7500/mm³/L (7.5 × 10⁹/L)	5000–10,000 /mm³ (5–10 × 10⁹/L)

*Tabs: History and Physical | **Laboratory Results** | Vital Signs | Nurses' Notes*

	Today	Yesterday	2 Days Ago (Operative Day)
Temperature	102.8°F (39.3°C)	101.6° F (38.7°C)	99.2°F (37.3°C)
Heart rate	101 beats/min	92 beats/min	86 beats/min
Respiratory rate	22 breaths/min	20 breaths/min	18 breaths/min
Blood pressure	145/78 mm Hg	134/72 mm Hg	128/70 mm Hg

*Tabs: History and Physical | **Vital Signs** | Laboratory Results | Nurses' Notes*

Complete the following sentence by selecting from the list of Word Choices below.

Based on the client findings, the nurse anticipates that the client is most likely experiencing [**Word Choice**], as evidenced by [**Word Choice**] and [**Word Choice**].

Word Choices
Increased liver enzymes
Bradycardia
Infection
Hypertension
Transplant rejection
Fever

NGN Challenge 50.2

The nurse is caring for a 62-year-old client admitted to the medical unit with a history of late-stage liver cirrhosis.

*Tabs: Health History | **Nurses' Notes** | Imaging Studies | Laboratory Results*

1430: Client reports shortness of breath unless sitting upright in bed. Also reports gaining 10 lb (4.5 kg) this week and feels very bloated due to constipation. Alert and oriented × 4. Lung sounds clear with no adventitious sounds. S₁ S₂ present; no murmurs. Bowel sounds distant × 4; abdomen very distended. VS: T 98°F (36.7°C); HR 82 beats/min and regular; RR 24 breaths/min; BP 158/90 mm Hg; Spo₂ 92% on RA.

Complete the diagram by identifying from the choices below to specify what potential condition the client is likely experiencing, **2** nursing actions that are appropriate to take, and **2** parameters the nurse should monitor to assess the client's progress.

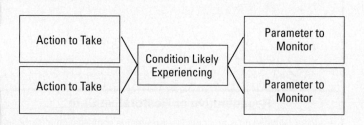

Actions to Take	Potential Conditions	Parameters to Monitor
Monitor bowel elimination	Irritable bowel syndrome	Body temperature
Anticipate paracentesis procedure	Intestinal obstruction	Oxygen saturation levels
Consult social worker about alcoholism	Abdominal ascites	Bowel sounds
Administer supplemental oxygen therapy	Colorectal cancer	Body weight
Weigh patient twice a day		Hemoglobin and hematocrit levels

REFERENCES

Asterisk (*) indicates a classic or definitive work on this subject.

American Association for the Study of Liver Diseases (AASLD). (2020). Hepatitis C guidance 2019 update: American Association for the Study of Liver Diseases–Infectious Diseases Society of America recommendations for testing, managing, and treating hepatitis C virus infection. *Hepatology, 71*(2), 686–721. https://doi.org/10.1002/hep.31060.

American Liver Foundation. (2023a). *Cirrhosis of the liver.* https://liverfoundation.org/for-patients/about-the-liver/diseases-of-the-liver/cirrhosis.

American Liver Foundation. (2023b). *Hepatitis B.* https://liverfoundation.org/for-patients/about-the-liver/diseases-of-the-liver/hepatitis-b/.

American Liver Foundation. (2023c). *Hepatitis C Information Center.* https://liverfoundation.org/for-patients/about-the-liver/diseases-of-the-liver/hepatitis-c/.

American Liver Foundation. (2023d). *Non-alcoholic fatty liver disease.* https://liverfoundation.org/for-patients/about-the-liver/diseases-of-the-liver/non-alcoholic-fatty-liver-disease.

Barr, R. G., Wilson, S. R., Rubens, D., Garcia-Tsao, G., & Ferraioli, G. (2020). Update to the society of radiologist in ultrasound liver elastography consensus statement. *Radiology, 296*(2), 263–274. https://doi.org/10.1148/radiol.2020192437.

Burchum, J. R., & Rosenthal, L. D. (2022). *Lehne's pharmacology for nursing care* (11th ed.). St. Louis: Elsevier.

Canadian Liver Foundation. (2021). *Your liver.* https://www.liver.ca/.

Centers for Disease Control and Prevention (CDC). (2020). *Hepatitis E.* https://www.cdc.gov/hepatitis/hev/index.htm.

Chaney, A. (2019). Caring for patients with chronic hepatitis C infection. *Nursing, 49*(3), 36–42. https://doi.org/10.1097/01.NURSE.0000553271.39804.a4.

Chaney, A., Rawal, B., Harnois, D., & Keaveny, A. (2020). Nutritional assessment and malnutrition in patients with cirrhosis. *Gastroenterology Nursing, 43*(4), 284–291.

Elliott, B., Chargualaf, K. A., & Patterson, B. (2021). *Veteran-centered care in education and practice.* New York, NY: Springer Publishing.

Elliott, D. Y. (2019). Caring for hospitalized patients with alcohol withdrawal syndrome. *Nursing Critical Care, 14*(5), 18–30. https://doi.org/10.1097/01.CCN.0000578828.37034.c2.

*Interprofessional Education Collaborative (IPEC) Expert Panel. (2016). *Core competencies for interprofessional collaborative practice: Report of an expert panel* (2nd ed.). Washington, D.C: Interprofessional Education Collaborative.

Newman, J. (2020). *Then and now: Living donor liver transplantation.* United Network for Organ Sharing (UNOS). https://unos.org/news/improvement/then-and-now-living-donor-liver-transplantation/.

Pagana, K., Pagana, T., & Pagana, T. (2022). *Mosby's manual of diagnostic and laboratory tests* (7th ed.). St. Louis: Elsevier.

Public Health Agency of Canada. (2021). *Report on Hepatitis B and C in Canada: 2018.* https://www.canada.ca/en/public-health/services/publications/diseases-conditions/report-hepatitis-b-c-canada-2018.html.

Rogers, J. L. (2023). *McCance and Huether's Pathophysiology: The biologic basis for disease in adults and children* (9th ed.). St. Louis: Elsevier.

Salari, N., Darvishi, N., Mansouri, K., Ghasemi, H., Hosseinian-Far, M., Darvishi, F., et al. (2021). Association between PNPLA3 rs738409 polymorphism and nonalcoholic fatty liver disease: a systematic review and meta-analysis. *BMC Endocrine Disorders, 21*(125). https://doi.org/10.1186/s12902-021-00789-4.

Sole, M. L., Klein, D. G., Moseley, M. J., Makic, M. B. F., & Morata, L. T. (2021). *Introduction to critical care nursing* (8th ed.). St. Louis: Elsevier.

Spiewak, T., Taefi, A., Patel, S., Li, C.-S., & Chak, E. (2020). Racial disparities of Black Americans hospitalized for decompensated liver cirrhosis. *BMC Gastroenterology, 20*, 245. https://doi.org/10.1186/s12876-020-01392-y.

Tholey, D. (2021). Spontaneous bacterial peritonitis. *Merck Manual: Professional Version.* https://www.merckmanuals.com/professional/hepatic-and-biliary-disorders/approach-to-the-patient-with-liver-disease/spontaneous-bacterial-peritonitis-sbp.

Vacca, V. M. (2020). Nonalcoholic fatty liver disease: What nurses need to know. *Nursing 2020, 50*(3), 32–39.

World Health Organization (WHO). (2021). *Hepatitis C.* https://www.who.int/news-room/fact-sheets/detail/hepatitis-c.

51

Concepts of Care for Patients With Conditions of the Biliary System and Pancreas

Lisa Vaira

http://evolve.elsevier.com/Iggy/

LEARNING OUTCOMES

1. Plan collaborative care with the interprofessional team to manage *inflammation* and *pain* in patients with pancreatitis.
2. Teach adults how to decrease the risk for acute pancreatitis.
3. Teach the patient and caregiver(s) about common drugs and other management strategies used for pancreatic cancer.
4. Plan patient- and family-centered nursing interventions to decrease the psychosocial impact caused by living with pancreatic disorders.
5. Apply knowledge of anatomy, physiology, and pathophysiology to provide evidence-based care for patients with cholecystitis.
6. Analyze assessment and diagnostic findings to generate solutions and prioritize nursing care for patients who have pancreatitis.
7. Organize care coordination and transition management for patients having surgery for cholecystitis.
8. Use clinical judgment to plan evidence-based nursing care to promote *nutrition* and manage *inflammation* in patients with pancreatitis.
9. Incorporate factors that affect health equity into the plan of care for patients with pancreatic cancer.

KEY TERMS

acute pancreatitis A serious, and at times life-threatening, inflammation of the pancreas.

biliary colic Severe right upper abdominal pain caused by obstruction of the cystic duct or movement of one or more gallstones.

cholecystectomy The surgical removal of the gallbladder.

cholecystitis An inflammation of the gallbladder that may be acute or chronic.

cholelithiasis Gallstones (also known as calculi).

chronic pancreatitis A progressive, destructive disease of the pancreas that has remissions and exacerbations (flare-ups).

dyspepsia An epigastric burning sensation, often referred to as "heartburn."

eructation Belching.

flatulence Gas (flatus) in the lower GI tract.

icterus Yellow coloration of the eye sclera.

jaundice Yellow coloration of the skin and mucous membranes.

pancreatic abscess Suppuration (pus formation) of pancreatic tissue caused by secondary bacterial invasion; often occurs in patients with acute or chronic pancreatitis.

pancreatic pseudocyst A condition in which infected pancreatic fluid becomes walled off by fibrous tissue.

partial pancreatectomy Surgical removal of part of the pancreas.

postcholecystectomy syndrome (PCS) A complication of cholecystectomy that causes increased abdominal or epigastric pain and vomiting and/or diarrhea weeks to months after surgery.

splenectomy Surgical removal of the spleen.

steatorrhea Fatty stools.

Whipple procedure (radical pancreaticoduodenectomy) Extensive surgical procedure used most often to treat cancer of the head of the pancreas; entails removal of the proximal head of the pancreas, the duodenum, a portion of the jejunum, the stomach (partial or total gastrectomy), and the gallbladder, with anastomosis of the pancreatic duct (pancreaticojejunostomy), the common bile duct (choledochojejunostomy), and the stomach (gastrojejunostomy) to the jejunum.

✳ **PRIORITY AND INTERRELATED CONCEPTS**

The priority concept for this chapter is:
- *Inflammation*
  The *Inflammation* concept exemplars for this chapter are Cholecystitis and Acute Pancreatitis.

The interrelated concepts for this chapter are:
- *Pain*
- *Nutrition*

The liver, gallbladder, and pancreas make up the biliary system. This chapter focuses on common problems of the gallbladder and pancreas. Liver disorders are described in Chapter 50. The biliary system secretes enzymes and other substances that promote food digestion in the stomach and small intestine. When these organs do not work properly, adults may experience impaired *digestion*, which can result in inadequate *nutrition.*

Disorders of the gallbladder and pancreas may extend to other organs because of the close anatomic location of these organs if the primary health problem is not treated early. *Inflammation* and obstruction (blockage) can occur in the biliary system from gallstones, edema, stricture, or tumors. These problems frequently cause the patient to have moderate to severe acute or persistent abdominal *pain.* These concepts are briefly reviewed in Chapter 3.

✳ INFLAMMATION CONCEPT EXEMPLAR: CHOLECYSTITIS

Pathophysiology Review

Cholecystitis is an *inflammation* of the gallbladder that affects many adults most commonly in affluent countries. It may be either acute or chronic, although most patients have the acute type. The inflammatory process often affects the client's *nutrition* status.

Acute Cholecystitis

Two types of acute cholecystitis can occur: calculous and acalculous cholecystitis. The most common type is *calculous* cholecystitis, in which chemical irritation and *inflammation* result from gallstones, or calculi (cholelithiasis), that obstruct the cystic duct (most often), gallbladder neck, or common bile duct (choledocholithiasis) (Fig. 51.1). About 95% of acute cholecystitis cases involve gallstones (Lindenmeyer, 2020). When the gallbladder is inflamed, trapped bile is reabsorbed and acts as a chemical irritant to the gallbladder wall. Reabsorbed bile, in combination with impaired circulation, edema, and distention of the gallbladder, causes ischemia and infection. The result is tissue sloughing with necrosis and gangrene within the gallbladder itself. The gallbladder wall may eventually perforate (rupture). If the perforation is small and localized, an abscess may form. Peritonitis (infection of the peritoneum) may result if the perforation is large (Rogers, 2023).

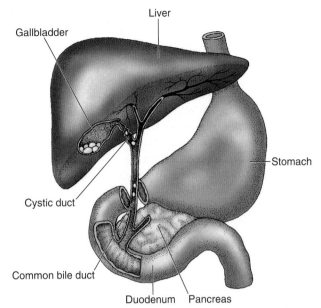

FIG. 51.1 Gallstones within the gallbladder and obstructing the common bile and cystic ducts.

The exact mechanism of gallstone formation is not clearly understood, but abnormal metabolism of cholesterol and bile salts plays an important role. The gallbladder provides an excellent environment for production of stones because it only occasionally mixes its normally abundant mucus with its highly viscous, concentrated bile. Impaired gallbladder motility can lead to stone formation by delaying bile emptying and causing biliary stasis.

Gallstones are composed of substances normally found in bile, such as cholesterol, bilirubin, bile salts, calcium, and various proteins. They are classified as cholesterol stones, pigmented stones, or mixed stones. Cholesterol calculi form because of metabolic imbalances of cholesterol and bile salts. They are the most common type found in adults in the United States (Rogers, 2023).

Bacteria can collect around the stones in the biliary system. Severe bacterial invasion can lead to life-threatening *suppurative* cholangitis when symptoms are not recognized quickly and pus accumulates in the ductal system.

Acalculous cholecystitis (*inflammation* occurring without gallstones) is typically associated with biliary stasis caused by any condition that affects the regular filling or emptying of the gallbladder. For example, a decrease in blood flow to the gallbladder or anatomic problems such as twisting or kinking of the gallbladder neck or cystic duct can result in pancreatic enzyme reflux into the gallbladder, causing *inflammation.* Sphincter of Oddi dysfunction (SOD) can also occur to cause reflux and inflammation. Most cases of this type of cholecystitis occur in patients with:

- Sepsis
- Severe trauma or burns
- Long-term total parenteral nutrition (TPN)
- Multiple organ dysfunction syndrome (MODS)
- Major abdominal surgery
- Hypovolemia

Chronic Cholecystitis

Chronic cholecystitis most often results when repeated episodes of cystic duct obstruction cause chronic *inflammation.* Calculi are often present. The gallbladder becomes fibrotic and atrophied, which results in decreased motility and deficient absorption. Chronic cholecystitis may also occur *without* calculi. In this case, the gallbladder atrophies and causes pain that is often misdiagnosed as gastritis. This problem is most likely to occur with consumption of a diet low in fat, such as a vegetarian diet. In some cases the atrophied gallbladder may adhere to nearby organs or the mesenteric wall if not surgically removed.

Pancreatitis and cholangitis (bile duct *inflammation*) can occur as chronic complications of cholecystitis. These problems result from the backup of bile throughout the biliary tract. Bile obstruction leads to jaundice (Rogers, 2023).

Jaundice (yellow coloration of the skin and mucous membranes) and icterus (yellow coloration of the eye sclera) can occur in patients with acute cholecystitis but are most commonly seen in those with the *chronic* form of the disease. Obstructed bile flow caused by edema of the ducts or gallstones contributes to *extrahepatic* obstructive jaundice. Jaundice in cholecystitis may also be caused by direct liver involvement. *Inflammation* of the liver's bile channels or bile ducts may cause *intrahepatic* obstructive jaundice, resulting in an increase in circulating levels of bilirubin, the major pigment of bile.

In an adult with obstructive jaundice, the normal flow of bile into the duodenum is blocked, and excessive bile salts accumulate in the skin. This accumulation of bile salts leads to pruritus (itching) or a burning sensation. The bile flow blockage also prevents bilirubin from reaching the large intestine, where it is converted to urobilinogen. Because urobilinogen accounts for the normal brown color of feces, clay-colored stools result. Water-soluble bilirubin is normally excreted by the kidneys in the urine. When an excess of circulating bilirubin occurs, the urine becomes dark (sometimes referred to as "tea-colored") because of the kidneys' effort to clear the bilirubin (Rogers, 2023).

Etiology and Genetic Risk

A familial or genetic tendency appears to contribute to the development of cholelithiasis, but this may be partially related to familial *nutrition* habits (excessive dietary cholesterol intake) and sedentary lifestyles. Gene-environment interactions may contribute to gallstone production. For example, some gene variations program some individuals to make and secrete more cholesterol into bile, leading to the increase in cholesterol-containing gallstones. Other risk factors for acute cholecystitis include:

- Type 2 diabetes mellitus
- Gastric bypass surgery
- Crohn's disease
- Rapid loss weight
- Sickle cell disease

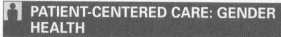

PATIENT-CENTERED CARE: GENDER HEALTH

Cholecystitis in Women

Obesity is a major risk factor for gallstone formation, especially in women. Pregnancy and drugs such as hormone replacements and birth control pills alter hormone levels and delay muscular contraction of the gallbladder, decreasing the rate of bile emptying. The incidence is higher in women who have had multiple pregnancies. Some clinicians continue to refer to the patient *most* at risk for acute cholecystitis and gallstones by the four *F*s: *F*emale, *F*orty, *F*at, and *F*ertile. However, cholecystitis often occurs in younger and older women and in those who are thin (Rogers, 2023).

Incidence and Prevalence

Cholecystitis and cholelithiasis most often occur in affluent countries throughout the world. Cholecystitis is more common in women than in men (Hassler et al., 2021).

Health Promotion/Disease Prevention

Teach individuals, especially women, to practice lifestyle habits that help prevent obesity, including avoiding excessive high-fat/high-cholesterol foods and exercising regularly. For patients who are obese, teach them about the need to lose weight slowly under the care of a qualified health care professional. Remember to assess for factors such as social determinants of health that could prevent individuals from following this advice. For example, some patients may experience food insecurity and cannot follow the recommended food choices. Other patients may lack transportation or adequate access to health care for a supervised weight loss plan. Provide information on health resources, including telehealth, to help patients access these needed services.

Interprofessional Collaborative Care

Care of the patient with cholecystitis primarily takes place by self-management at home, in the community, or within the same-day surgical center or hospital if surgery is required.

Recognize Cues: Assessment

History. Obtain the patient's height, weight, and vital signs, or ask that these activities be performed by assistive personnel (AP) with appropriate supervision. Ask about food preferences and determine whether excessive fat and cholesterol are part of the diet. Typically, diets high in fat, high in calories, low in fiber, and high in refined white carbohydrates place patients at high risk for developing gallstones. Consuming low-fat diets can contribute to chronic cholecystitis in young thin women.

Inquire if intake of certain foods causes pain. Question whether any GI symptoms occur when fatty food is eaten, such as flatulence (gas [flatus] in the lower GI tract), dyspepsia (an epigastric burning sensation, often referred to as "heartburn"), indigestion, eructation (belching), anorexia, nausea, vomiting, and abdominal *pain.*

Ask patients to describe their daily activity or exercise routines to determine whether they are sedentary, a risk factor for developing gallstones. Question whether there is a family history of gallbladder disease. Ask the patient about taking current or previous hormone replacement therapy (HRT). If the patient is biologically female, ask if she is taking or has recently been on oral contraceptives (birth control pills).

Physical Assessment/Signs and Symptoms. Patients with cholecystitis have abdominal ***pain,*** although symptoms vary in intensity and frequency. Ask the patient to describe the pain, including its intensity and duration, precipitating factors, and any measures that relieve it. Pain may be described as indigestion of varying intensity, ranging from a mild, persistent ache to a steady, constant pain in the right upper abdominal quadrant. It may radiate to the right shoulder or scapula. In some cases the abdominal ***pain*** of chronic cholecystitis may be vague and nonspecific. The usual pattern is episodic. Patients often refer to acute pain episodes as "gallbladder attacks."

PATIENT-CENTERED CARE: OLDER ADULT HEALTH

Older Adults and Cholecystitis

Older adults and patients with diabetes mellitus may have atypical symptoms of cholecystitis, including the absence of ***pain*** and fever. Localized tenderness may be the only presenting sign. The older patient may become acutely confused (delirium) as the first symptom of gallbladder disease.

Advanced physical assessment for rebound tenderness (Blumberg sign) and increased discomfort when the area is palpated (Murphy sign) is performed only by a primary health care provider (Jarvis & Eckhardt, 2024). To elicit rebound tenderness, the primary health care provider pushes the fingers deeply and steadily into the patient's abdomen and then quickly releases the pressure. Pain that results from the rebound of the palpated tissue may indicate peritoneal ***inflammation.*** To elicit inspiratory arrest, the primary health care provider performs palpation under the liver border while simultaneously instructing the patient to deep breathe. Pain on deep inhalation is a sign of cholecystitis. Deep palpation below the liver border in the right upper quadrant may reveal a sausage-shaped mass, representing the distended, inflamed gallbladder. Percussion over the posterior rib cage worsens localized abdominal ***pain.***

In *chronic* cholecystitis, patients may have slowly developing symptoms and may not seek medical treatment until late symptoms such as jaundice, clay-colored stools, and dark urine occur from biliary obstruction. Icterus may also be present. Steatorrhea (fatty stools) occurs because fat absorption is decreased as a result of the lack of bile. Bile is needed for the absorption of fats and fat-soluble vitamins in the intestine. As with any inflammatory process, the patient may have an elevated temperature of 99°F to 102°F (37.2°C to 38.9°C), tachycardia, and dehydration from fever and vomiting. The patient often will decline food intake because of the resulting ***pain*** or other symptoms that may occur. Box 51.1 highlights the most common signs and symptoms of cholecystitis.

BOX 51.1 Key Features

Cholecystitis

- Episodic or vague upper abdominal *pain* or discomfort that can radiate to the right shoulder
- Pain triggered by a high-fat or high-volume meal
- Anorexia
- Nausea and/or vomiting
- Dyspepsia
- Eructation
- Flatulence
- Feeling of abdominal fullness
- Rebound tenderness (Blumberg sign)
- Inspiratory arrest (Murphy sign)
- Fever
- Jaundice, clay-colored stools, dark urine

Laboratory Assessment. A differential diagnosis rules out other diseases that may cause similar symptoms, such as peptic ulcer disease, hepatitis, and pancreatitis. An increased *white blood cell (WBC)* count indicates ***inflammation.*** Serum levels of *alkaline phosphatase, aspartate aminotransferase (AST),* and *lactate dehydrogenase (LDH)* may be elevated, indicating abnormalities in liver function in patients with severe biliary obstruction. The direct (conjugated) and indirect (unconjugated) *serum bilirubin levels* are also elevated. If the pancreas is involved, serum amylase and lipase levels are elevated.

Other Diagnostic Assessments. Calcified gallstones are easily viewed on abdominal x-ray. Stones that are not calcified cannot be seen. *Ultrasonography (US) of the right upper quadrant is the best initial diagnostic test for cholecystitis* (Lindenmeyer, 2020). It is safe, accurate, and painless, although it may elicit an ultrasonic Murphy sign. Acute cholecystitis is seen as edema of the gallbladder wall and pericholecystic fluid.

A hepatobiliary scan (sometimes called a *hepatobiliary iminodiacetic acid [HIDA] scan*) can be performed to visualize the gallbladder and determine patency of the biliary system (Pagana et al., 2022). In this nuclear medicine test, a radioactive tracer or chemical is injected intravenously. About 20 minutes after the injection, a gamma camera tracks the flow of the tracer from the gallbladder to determine the ejection rate of bile into the biliary duct. A decreased bile flow indicates gallbladder disease with obstruction. Teach patients having this test to be NPO before the procedure. Remind the patient that the camera is large and close to the body for most of the procedure.

When the cause of cholecystitis or cholelithiasis is not known or the patient has symptoms of biliary obstruction (e.g., jaundice), *endoscopic retrograde cholangiopancreatography (ERCP)* may be performed. Some patients have the less invasive and safer *magnetic resonance cholangiopancreatography (MRCP),* which can be performed by an interventional radiologist. For this procedure the patient is given oral or IV contrast material (gadolinium) before having an MRI scan. Before the test, ask the patient about any history of urticaria (hives) or other allergy. MRI is also contraindicated in patients with a pacemaker or other incompatible devices. Gadolinium does not contain iodine, which decreases the risk for an allergic response. Chapter 45 discusses these tests in more detail.

Analyze Cues and Prioritize Hypotheses: Analysis

The priority collaborative problems for patients with cholecystitis include:

1. Acute or persistent *pain* due to gallbladder *inflammation* and/or gallstones
2. Weight loss due to decreased intake because of pain, nausea, and anorexia

Generate Solutions and Take Actions: Planning and Implementation

If cholecystitis and its associated pain cannot be managed medically, a laparoscopic cholecystectomy is the treatment of choice for patients with acute or long-term chronic cholecystitis. *Nutrition* status and *pain* control must be addressed before and after surgery.

Managing Acute Pain

Planning: Expected Outcomes. The patient with cholecystitis is expected to report a decrease in abdominal *pain* as evidenced by self-report of a level of 2 or 3 on a 0-to-10 pain intensity scale.

Interventions. The priorities for patient care include providing supportive care by relieving symptoms and decreasing *inflammation. Pain* assessment to measure the effectiveness of these interventions is an essential part of nursing care.

Nonsurgical Management. Most patients find that they need to avoid fatty foods to prevent further episodes of biliary colic. Withhold food and fluids if nausea and vomiting occur. IV therapy is used to prevent or manage dehydration. Many patients experience acute *pain* when gallstones partially or totally obstruct the cystic or common bile duct. Persistent pain may occur in patients with chronic cholecystitis without gallstones, and may be misdiagnosed as gastritis.

Acute biliary pain requires opioid analgesia, such as morphine or hydromorphone. All opioids may cause some degree of sphincter of Oddi spasm. Ketorolac, a potent NSAID, may be used for mild to moderate **pain.** Be sure to monitor the patient for increased pain, tachycardia, and hypotension because the drug can cause GI bleeding. The primary health care provider prescribes antiemetics to control nausea and vomiting. IV antibiotic therapy may also be given, depending on the cause of cholecystitis or as a one-time dose for surgery.

✚ NURSING SAFETY PRIORITY

Critical Rescue

The severe pain of **biliary colic** is produced by obstruction of the cystic duct of the gallbladder or movement of one or more gallstones. When a stone is moving through or is lodged within the duct, tissue spasm occurs in an effort to get the stone through the small duct. Biliary colic may be so severe that it occurs with tachycardia, pallor/ash gray skin, diaphoresis, and prostration (extreme exhaustion). Assess the patient for possible shock caused by biliary colic. *Notify the health care provider or Rapid Response Team if these symptoms occur.* Stay with the patient and keep the head of the bed flat if shock occurs.

An option for a small number of patients with cholelithiasis (gallstones) is the use of oral bile acid dissolution or gallstone-stabilizing agents. Drugs such as ursodiol and chenodiol may be given as long-term therapy to dissolve or stabilize gallstones (Burchum & Rosenthal, 2022). A gallbladder ultrasound is required every 6 months for the first year of therapy to determine the effectiveness of the drug. Teach patients taking this type of drug therapy to report diarrhea, vomiting, or severe abdominal pain, especially if it radiates to the shoulders, to their primary health care provider immediately. Remind them to take the medication with food and milk.

Another treatment option for patients who cannot have surgery is the insertion of a *percutaneous transhepatic biliary catheter* (drain) using CT or ultrasound guidance to open the blocked duct(s) so bile can flow (cholecystostomy). Catheters can be placed several ways, depending on the condition of the biliary ducts, in an internal, external, or internal/external drain. Biliary catheters usually divert bile from the liver into the duodenum to bypass a stricture. When all the bile enters the duodenum, it is called an *internal* drain. However, in some cases a patient has an *internal/external* drain in which part of the bile empties into a drainage bag. Patients who need this drain for an extended period may have the external drain capped. If jaundice or leakage around the catheter site occurs, teach the patient to reconnect the catheter to a drainage bag and have a follow-up cholangiogram injection done by an interventional radiologist. An *external*-only catheter is connected either temporarily or permanently to a drainage bag that should be *positioned lower than the catheter insertion site* to drain by gravity. A reduction in bile drainage indicates that the drain is no longer working.

Surgical Management. Cholecystectomy is the surgical removal of the gallbladder. One of two procedures is performed: the laparoscopic cholecystectomy or, in rare cases, the traditional open-approach cholecystectomy. A cholecystectomy is one of the most common surgeries in the United States (Zakko, 2020).

Laparoscopic cholecystectomy. Laparoscopic cholecystectomy, a minimally invasive surgery (MIS), is the gold standard and is performed far more often than the traditional open approach. The advantages of MIS when compared with the open approach include:

- Complications are not common.
- The death rate is very low.
- Bile duct injuries are rare.
- Patient recovery is quicker.
- Postoperative pain is less severe.

The laparoscopic procedure (often called a "lap chole") is commonly performed on an ambulatory care basis in a same-day surgery suite or agency. The surgeon explains the procedure, and the nurse answers questions and reinforces the instructions. Reinforce what to expect after surgery and review *pain* management, deep-breathing exercises, incisional care, and leg exercises to prevent deep vein thrombosis. There is no special preoperative preparation other than the routine preparation for surgery under general anesthesia described in Chapter 9.

During the surgery the surgeon makes a very small midline puncture at the umbilicus. Additional small incisions (less than an inch each) may be needed, although *single-incision* laparoscopic cholecystectomy (SILC) using a flexible endoscope is often done. The abdominal cavity is insufflated with 3 to 4 L of carbon dioxide. Gasless laparoscopic cholecystectomy using abdominal wall–lifting devices are used in some centers. This technique results in improved pulmonary and cardiac function. A trocar catheter is inserted, through which a laparoscope is introduced. The laparoscope is attached to a video camera, and the abdominal organs are viewed on a monitor. The gallbladder is dissected from the liver bed, and the cystic artery and duct are closed. The surgeon aspirates the bile and crushes any large stones, if present, and then extracts the gallbladder through the umbilical puncture site.

Removing the gallbladder with the laparoscopic technique reduces the risk for wound complications. Some patients have mild to severe discomfort from carbon dioxide retention in the abdomen, which may be felt throughout the thorax and shoulders.

> ## ! NURSING SAFETY PRIORITY
> ### Action Alert
>
> After a laparoscopic cholecystectomy, assess the patient's oxygen saturation level using pulse oximetry frequently until the effects of the anesthesia have passed. Remind the patient to perform deep-breathing and incentive spirometry exercises every hour.

Other postoperative care for the patient after a laparoscopic procedure is similar to that for any patient having minimally invasive endoscopic surgery (see Chapter 9). Offer the patient food and water when fully awake, and monitor for the nausea and/or vomiting that often results from anesthesia. If needed, administer an antiemetic drug such as ondansetron hydrochloride either IV push or as a disintegrating tablet. Several drug doses may be needed. Maintain an IV line to administer fluids until nausea and vomiting subside. Be sure to have the head of the bed elevated in the same-day surgery unit to prevent aspiration from vomiting. After nausea subsides, assist the patient to the bathroom to void. Early ambulation also promotes absorption of the carbon dioxide, which can decrease postoperative discomfort.

Administer an oral or IV push opioid and antiinflammatory drug as needed immediately after surgery. Continuous IV pain control is usually not required because there is only one or a few small incisions, which are covered with wound closure strips and small adhesive bandages or are surgically glued. The glue or closure strips lose their adhesiveness in about a week to 10 days and can be removed or fall off as the incision heals.

The patient is usually discharged from the hospital or surgery center the same day, although older and obese patients may stay overnight. Provide postoperative teaching regarding *pain* management, incision care, and follow-up appointments. Teach the patient to use ice and oral opioids for incisional pain, if needed, for a few days. For abdominal or thoracic discomfort from carbon dioxide retention, many patients report that heat application is helpful. The patient is typically allowed to bathe or shower the day after surgery.

After laparoscopic surgery the patient can return to usual activities much sooner than those having an open cholecystectomy. Instruct the patient to rest for the first 24 hours and then begin to resume usual activities. Most patients resume usual activities within a week.

The patient should be educated about possible intolerance to greasy foods. A large intake of fatty foods may result in abdominal *pain* and diarrhea, which could result in a *mild* postcholecystectomy syndrome (PCS) (see later discussion of PCS in the Traditional Cholecystectomy section). Teach patients to introduce foods high in fat one at a time to determine which foods are best tolerated.

A newer minimally invasive surgical procedure is *natural orifice transluminal endoscopic surgery (NOTES)* for removal or repair of organs. Surgery can be performed on many body organs through the mouth, vagina, and rectum. For removal of the gallbladder, the vagina is used most often in women because it can be easily decontaminated with an antiseptic and allows easy access into the peritoneal cavity. The surgeon makes a small internal incision through the cul-de-sac of Douglas between the rectum and uterine wall to access the gallbladder. The main advantages of this procedure are the lack of visible incisions, minimal pain, and decreased risk for postoperative complications (Roberts & Kate, 2020).

Traditional cholecystectomy. Use of the open surgical approach (abdominal laparotomy) has greatly declined during the past several decades. The few patients who have this type of surgical approach usually have severe biliary obstruction, and the ducts need to be explored to ensure patency. A surgeon may also choose to convert to an open cholecystectomy from laparoscopic due to poor visibility or suspected gallbladder cancer (Hassler et al., 2021).

The nurse provides the usual preoperative care and teaching in the operating suite on the day of surgery (see Chapter 9). The surgeon removes the gallbladder through a right upper quadrant incision and explores the biliary ducts for the presence of stones or other cause of obstruction. The surgeon may insert a drainage tube such as a Jackson-Pratt (JP) drain. This tube is placed in the gallbladder bed to prevent fluid accumulation. The drainage is usually serosanguineous (serous fluid mixed with blood) and is stained with bile in the first 24 hours after surgery. A one-dose IV antibiotic may be given to prevent infection before or during surgery.

Nursing care for a patient who has had a traditional open cholecystectomy is similar to the care for any patient who has had abdominal surgery under general anesthesia as described in Chapter 9. Postoperative incisional *pain* after a traditional cholecystectomy is controlled with opioids, IV acetaminophen, and/or IV antiinflammatory drug. Encourage the patient to use coughing and deep-breathing exercises when pain is controlled and the incision is splinted.

Antiemetics may be necessary for episodes of postoperative nausea and vomiting. Administer the antiemetic early, as prescribed, to prevent retching associated with vomiting and increased incisional *pain.*

Provide care for the incision and the surgical drain. The surgeon typically removes the surgical dressing within 24 hours after surgery.

Patients are NPO until fully awake after surgery. Document their level of consciousness, vital signs, and pain level. Assess the surgical incision for signs of infection, such as excessive redness/hyperpigmentation or purulent drainage. Report changes to the surgeon immediately. Begin ambulation as soon as possible to prevent deep vein thrombosis and promote peristalsis.

Advance the diet from clear liquids to solid foods as peristalsis returns. The patient usually resumes solid foods and is discharged to home 1 to 2 days after surgery, depending on any complications and the patient's general condition. In the early postoperative period, if bile flow is reduced, a low-fat diet may reduce discomfort and prevent nausea.

NCLEX Examination Challenge 51.1

Physiological Integrity

The nurse is reinforcing health teaching for a client preparing to have a laparoscopic cholecystectomy. Which of the following statements would the nurse include? **Select all that apply.**

A. "You should plan to be in the hospital for at least 2 days."
B. "You will likely have a surgical drain in place near the incision."
C. "We will give you a medication to help relieve nausea after surgery."
D. "The surgeon will use wound closure strips or skin glue on the incisions."
E. "We will monitor your oxygen level with the pulse oximeter on your finger."
F. "We may need to insert a nasogastric tube to help prevent nausea after surgery."

Promoting Nutrition

Planning: Expected Outcomes. The patient will not lose weight or will regain usual weight if indicated to meet metabolic needs.

Interventions. The patient with cholecystitis may decline food because of abdominal discomfort, nausea, and anorexia. The patient's diet should be high in fiber and low in fat. Teach patients to avoid gas-producing foods. Small, frequent meals are often preferable to three standard meals daily. Ask the patient about appealing food preferences because favorite foods are tolerated more readily than randomly selected foods. Teach the patient to weigh regularly to assess for stabilization of weight or report concerns associated with weight loss. If needed, monitor laboratory results such as blood urea nitrogen (BUN), prealbumin, albumin, and total protein and transferrin levels to assess ongoing *nutrition* and hydration status.

Care Coordination and Transition Management

Some patients with cholecystitis may have mild to moderate discomfort that can be managed by nutrition intervention; others may require surgery. Home care preparation is individual, based on each patient's circumstances.

Education needs to be started as soon as a patient has an initial experience with cholecystitis and has appropriate pain relief. Assess the patient's and family's knowledge of the disease and provide teaching as needed. The desired outcomes for discharge planning and education are to avoid further episodes of cholecystitis.

For most patients, a special diet is not required. Advise them to eat nutritious meals and avoid excessive intake of fatty foods, especially fried food, butter, and "fast food." If the patient is obese, recommend a weight-reduction program.

BOX 51.2   Key Features

Common Causes of Postcholecystectomy Syndrome

Biliary Causes	Nonbiliary Causes
Pseudocyst	Coronary artery disease
Common bile duct (CBD) leak	Intercostal neuritis
CBD or pancreatic duct stricture or obstruction	Unexplained pain syndrome
Sphincter of Oddi dysfunction	Psychiatric or neurologic disorder
Retained or new CBD gallstone	
Pancreatic or liver mass	
Primary sclerosing cholangitis	
Diverticular compression	

Remind the patient to report repeated abdominal or epigastric pain with vomiting and/or diarrhea that may occur several weeks to months after surgery. These symptoms indicate possible postcholecystectomy syndrome (PCS). There are multiple causes of PCS, some of which are related to the biliary system whereas others are not. Common causes of PCS are listed in Box 51.2.

Management depends on the exact cause but usually involves the use of endoscopic retrograde cholangiopancreatography (ERCP) to find the cause of the problem and repair it. This procedure and related nursing care are described in Chapter 45. Collaborative care includes *pain* management, antibiotics, *nutrition* and hydration therapy (possibly short-term parenteral nutrition), and control of nausea and vomiting.

Evaluate Outcomes: Evaluation

Evaluate the care of the patient with cholecystitis based on the identified priority patient problems. The expected outcomes include that the patient will:

- Report control of abdominal pain, as indicated by self-report and pain scale measurement
- Have adequate *nutrition* available to meet metabolic needs

✳ INFLAMMATION CONCEPT EXEMPLAR: ACUTE PANCREATITIS

The pancreas is unusual in that it functions as both an exocrine gland and an endocrine gland. The primary *endocrine* disorder is diabetes mellitus and is discussed in Chapter 56. The *exocrine* function of the pancreas is responsible for secreting enzymes that assist in the breakdown of starches, proteins, and fats. These enzymes are normally secreted in the inactive form and become activated once they enter the small intestine.

Pathophysiology Review

Acute pancreatitis is a serious and at times life-threatening *inflammation* of the pancreas. This inflammatory process is caused by a premature activation of excessive pancreatic enzymes that destroy ductal tissue and pancreatic cells, resulting in autodigestion and fibrosis of the pancreas. The pathologic changes occur in different degrees. The severity of pancreatitis depends on the extent of *inflammation* and tissue damage. Pancreatitis can range from mild involvement evidenced by edema and inflammation to *necrotizing hemorrhagic pancreatitis (NHP)*. NHP is diffuse bleeding pancreatic tissue with fibrosis and tissue death (Rogers, 2023).

Early activation (i.e., activation within the pancreas rather than the intestinal lumen) results in the inflammatory process of pancreatitis. Direct toxic injury to the pancreatic cells and the production and release of pancreatic enzymes (e.g., trypsin, lipase, elastase) result from the obstructive damage. After pancreatic duct obstruction, increased pressure may contribute to ductal rupture, allowing spillage of trypsin and other enzymes into the pancreatic parenchymal tissue. *Autodigestion* of the pancreas occurs as a result (Fig. 51.2). In *acute* pancreatitis, four major pathophysiologic processes occur: lipolysis, proteolysis, necrosis of blood vessels, and **inflammation.**

The hallmark of pancreatic necrosis is enzymatic fat necrosis of the endocrine and exocrine cells of the pancreas caused by the enzyme *lipase*. Fatty acids are released during this *lipolytic process* and combine with ionized calcium to form a soaplike product. The initial rapid lowering of serum calcium levels is not readily compensated for by the parathyroid gland. Because the body needs ionized calcium and cannot use bound calcium, hypocalcemia occurs (Rogers, 2023).

Proteolysis involves the splitting of proteins by hydrolysis of the peptide bonds, resulting in the formation of smaller polypeptides. Proteolytic activity may lead to thrombosis and gangrene of the pancreas. Pancreatic destruction may be localized and confined to one area or may involve the entire organ.

Elastase is activated by trypsin and causes elastic fibers of the blood vessels and ducts to dissolve. The *necrosis of blood vessels* results in bleeding, ranging from minor bleeding to massive hemorrhage of pancreatic tissue. Another pancreatic enzyme, kallikrein, causes the release of vasoactive peptides, bradykinin, and a plasma kinin known as kallidin. These substances contribute to vasodilation and increased vascular permeability, further compounding the hemorrhagic process. This massive destruction of blood vessels by necrosis may lead to generalized hemorrhage, with blood escaping into the retroperitoneal tissues. *Many deaths in patients with acute pancreatitis result from irreversible hypovolemic shock due to hemorrhage.*

The *inflammatory stage* occurs when leukocytes cluster around the hemorrhagic and necrotic areas of the pancreas. A secondary bacterial invasion may lead to suppuration (pus formation) of the pancreatic tissue called a pancreatic abscess. Pancreatic abscesses must be drained promptly to prevent sepsis. Mild infected lesions may be absorbed. When infected lesions are severe, calcification and fibrosis occur. If the infected fluid becomes walled off by fibrous tissue, a pancreatic pseudocyst develops. Pseudocysts often rupture spontaneously but may require surgical removal (Rogers, 2023).

Complications of Acute Pancreatitis

Acute pancreatitis may result in severe, life-threatening complications (Box 51.3). Jaundice occurs from swelling of the head of the pancreas, which slows bile flow through the common bile duct. The bile duct may also be compressed by calculi (stones)

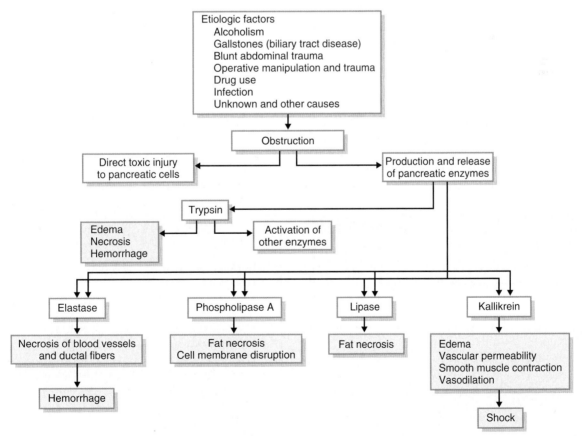

FIG. 51.2 The process of autodigestion in acute pancreatitis.

or a pancreatic pseudocyst. The resulting total bile flow obstruction causes severe jaundice. Intermittent hyperglycemia occurs from the release of glucagon, as well as the decreased release of insulin due to damage to the pancreatic islet cells. Total destruction of the pancreas may occur, leading to diabetes mellitus (Rogers, 2023).

Left lung pleural effusions frequently develop in the patient with acute pancreatitis. *Atelectasis and pneumonia may occur also, especially in older patients.*

Multisystem organ failure is caused by necrotizing hemorrhagic pancreatitis (NHP). NHP accounts for up to 10% of acute pancreatitis cases (Bartel, 2020). Acute pancreatitis also places the patient at risk for acute respiratory distress syndrome (ARDS). This severe form of pulmonary edema is caused by disruption of the alveolar-capillary membrane and is a serious complication of acute pancreatitis. (See Chapter 26 for a discussion of ARDS.) In acute pancreatitis, pulmonary failure accounts for more than half of all deaths that occur in the first week of the disease. Another severe complication of acute pancreatitis is acute kidney injury, which can occur due to a systemic inflammatory response (Bartel, 2020).

Coagulation defects are another major potential complication and may result in death. Complex physiologic changes in the pancreas cause the release of necrotic tissue and enzymes into the bloodstream, resulting in altered coagulation. Disseminated intravascular coagulation (DIC) involves hypercoagulation of the blood, with consumption of clotting factors and the development of microthrombi.

Shock in acute pancreatitis results from peripheral vasodilation from the released vasoactive substances and the retroperitoneal loss of protein-rich fluid from proteolytic digestion. Hypovolemia may result in decreased renal perfusion and acute renal failure. Paralytic (adynamic) ileus results from peritoneal irritation and seepage of pancreatic enzymes into the abdominal cavity.

Etiology and Genetic Risk

In many cases the cause of pancreatitis is not known, but many factors can injure the pancreas. Two of the most common causes are gallstones and alcohol use. Biliary disease due to gallstones accounts for up to 40% and alcohol use accounts for about 30% of cases of acute pancreatitis (Bartel, 2020). Additional factors that can cause or contribute to the development of acute pancreatitis are listed in Box 51.4.

Patients who have endoscopic retrograde cholangiopancreatography (ERCP) are at risk for experiencing direct damage to the pancreas and subsequently developing acute pancreatitis as a complication of the procedure. A retrospective medical record review of 824 patients who had ERCP to determine biliary duct obstruction found that almost 10% of the sample developed acute pancreatitis and 3% experienced bleeding (Hormati et al., 2020). Patients need to be fully informed about these common complications before consenting to the diagnostic procedure. Chapter 45 discusses this procedure and associated nursing care in detail.

Incidence and Prevalence

Although the exact number of cases is not known, the incidence of acute pancreatitis is increasing both in the United States and globally due to increased alcoholism and gallstones (Iannuzzi et al., 2022). Pancreatic "attacks" are especially common during holidays and vacations when alcohol consumption may be high, particularly among men. Women are affected most often after having cholelithiasis or childbirth (Rogers, 2023).

Death occurs in a small percentage of patients with acute pancreatitis, but with early diagnosis and treatment, mortality can be reduced. Mortality increases among hospitalized patients with pancreatitis and in *older adults.* The prognosis for recovery is usually good for pancreatitis associated with biliary tract disease and poor if pancreatitis accompanies alcoholism.

Health Promotion/Disease Prevention

Although there are a number of causes to acute pancreatitis, some of these causes can be avoided. For example, teach individuals about the need to avoid excessive alcohol, which is a common cause of acute pancreatitis. Obesity is a major risk factor for gallstones, another common cause of acute pancreatitis. Teach individuals, especially women, to practice lifestyle habits that help prevent obesity, including avoiding excessive high-fat/high-cholesterol foods and exercising regularly. For patients

---

BOX 51.3 Key Features

Potential Complications of Acute Pancreatitis

- Pancreatic infection (causes septic shock)
- Hemorrhage (necrotizing hemorrhagic pancreatitis [NHP])
- Acute kidney injury
- Paralytic ileus
- Hypovolemic shock
- Pleural effusion
- Acute respiratory distress syndrome (ARDS)
- Atelectasis
- Pneumonia
- Multiorgan system failure
- Disseminated intravascular coagulation (DIC)
- Diabetes mellitus

BOX 51.4 Key Features

Causes of Acute Pancreatitis

- Trauma: external (blunt trauma, stab wounds, gunshot wounds [GSWs])
- Endoscopic retrograde cholangiopancreatography (ERCP)
- Pancreatic obstruction: tumors, cysts, or abscesses; abnormal organ structure
- Metabolic problems: hyperlipidemia, hyperparathyroidism, or hypercalcemia
- Kidney involvement: chronic kidney disease or transplantation
- Familial, inherited pancreatitis
- Penetrating gastric or duodenal ulcers, resulting in peritonitis
- Viral infections such as coxsackievirus B and HIV infection
- Drug toxicities, including those associated with opiates, anticonvulsants, dipeptidyl peptidase–4 (DDP-4) inhibitors, glucagon-like peptide–1 (GLP-1) receptor agonists (gliptins), sulfonamides, thiazides, and steroids
- Cigarette smoking and tobacco use
- Cystic fibrosis
- Childbirth

who are obese, teach them about the need to lose weight slowly under the care of a qualified health care professional.

Remember to assess for factors such as social determinants of health that could prevent individuals from following this advice. For example, some patients may experience food insecurity and cannot follow the recommended food choices. Other patients may lack transportation or adequate access to health care for a supervised weight loss plan. Provide information on health resources, including telehealth, to help patients access these needed services.

Interprofessional Collaborative Care

Care for the patient with acute pancreatitis usually takes place in the hospital setting for *pain* control and possible surgical intervention.

Recognize Cues: Assessment

History. Most often the patient reports severe and constant abdominal *pain.* Conduct the interview *after pain is controlled.* Ask whether the abdominal pain occurs when drinking alcohol or eating a high-fat meal. Obtain information about alcohol use, including the amount of alcohol consumed during what period of time (i.e., years of consumption, how much usually consumed over a particular period). Question the patient about a family or personal history of alcoholism, pancreatitis, trauma, or biliary tract disease. Ask whether any abdominal surgical interventions such as cholecystectomy, or diagnostic procedures such as ERCP, have been performed recently.

Ask about other medical problems known to cause pancreatitis. Inquire about recent viral infections. Ask the patient or family member to list all prescription and over-the-counter (OTC) drugs taken recently, including nutritional and herbal supplements.

Physical Assessment/Signs and Symptoms. The diagnosis of acute pancreatitis is made based on the clinical presentation combined with the results of diagnostic studies, both laboratory and imaging assessments. Symptoms of acute pancreatitis vary widely and depend on the severity of the *inflammation.* Typically a patient is diagnosed after presenting with severe abdominal *pain* in the mid-epigastric area or left upper quadrant. Assess the intensity and quality of pain. The patient often states that the pain had a sudden onset and radiates to the back, left flank, or left shoulder. The pain is described as intense, *boring* (feeling that it is going through the body), and continuous, and is worsened by lying in the supine position. Often the patient finds relief by assuming the fetal position (with the knees drawn up to the chest and the spine flexed) or by sitting upright and bending forward. The patient may report weight loss resulting from nausea and vomiting. Obtain the patient's weight.

When performing an abdominal assessment, inspect for:
- Generalized jaundice
- Gray-blue discoloration of the abdomen and periumbilical area
- Gray-blue discoloration of the flanks, caused by pancreatic enzyme leakage to cutaneous tissue from the peritoneal cavity
Listen for bowel sounds; absent or decreased bowel sounds usually indicate paralytic (adynamic) ileus. On light palpation,

note abdominal tenderness, rigidity, and guarding as signs of peritonitis. Pancreatic ascites creates a dull sound on percussion.

Monitor and record vital signs frequently to assess for elevated temperature, tachycardia, and decreased blood pressure, or assign and closely supervise this activity. Auscultate the lung fields for adventitious sounds or diminished breath sounds and observe for dyspnea or orthopnea.

✚ NURSING SAFETY PRIORITY
Critical Rescue

For the patient with acute pancreatitis, monitor for significant changes in vital signs that may indicate the life-threatening complication of shock. Hypotension and tachycardia may result from pancreatic hemorrhage, excessive fluid volume shifting, or the toxic effects of abdominal sepsis from enzyme damage. Observe for changes in behavior and level of consciousness (LOC) that may be related to alcohol withdrawal, hypoxia, or impending sepsis with shock. Notify the provider or Rapid Response Team if vital sign changes, especially LOC, are significant.

Psychosocial Assessment. If excessive alcohol is a causative factor, tactfully explore the patient's alcohol intake history after the patient has adequate pain control. Provide patient privacy and establish a trusting relationship. Discuss the intake of alcohol and the reasons for excessive drinking. Use of the CAGE questionnaire or other alcohol use screening tool may be beneficial. Ask the patient when increased drinking episodes occur and whether binges occur during holidays, vacations, or weekends or revolve around particular activities, such as television viewing. Question the patient about any recent traumatic or stressful event that may have contributed to increased alcohol consumption, such as the death of a family member or a job loss.

Laboratory Assessment. Diagnostic laboratory abnormalities are typical in patients with acute pancreatitis (Table 51.1). A variety of pancreatic and nonpancreatic disorders can cause increased serum amylase levels. In patients with pancreatitis,

TABLE 51.1 Causes of Serum Laboratory Test Abnormalities in Acute Pancreatitis

Abnormal Laboratory Test Result	Cause
Elevated amylase	Pancreatic cell injury
Elevated lipase	Pancreatic cell injury
Elevated trypsin	Pancreatic cell injury
Elevated elastase	Pancreatic cell injury
Elevated glucose	Pancreatic cell injury resulting in impaired carbohydrate metabolism; decreased insulin release
Decreased calcium and magnesium	Fatty acids combined with calcium; seen in fat necrosis
Elevated bilirubin	Hepatobiliary obstructive process
Elevated alanine aminotransferase (ALT)	Hepatobiliary involvement/obstruction
Elevated aspartate aminotransferase (AST)	Hepatobiliary involvement
Elevated leukocyte count and presence of C-reactive protein	Inflammatory response

amylase levels usually increase within 12 to 24 hours and remain elevated for 2 to 3 days. Persistent elevations may be an indicator of duct obstruction or pancreatic duct leak (Pagana et al., 2022).

Lipase also helps determine the presence of acute pancreatitis. Although there be other reasons for increased serum lipase levels, pancreatitis is the most common cause (Pagana et al., 2022). Serum levels may rise later than amylase and remain elevated for up to 5 to 7 days. Because these levels stay elevated longer than amylase levels, the primary health care provider may find this test useful in diagnosing patients who are not examined until several days after the initial onset of symptoms. An increase in lipase and amylase in the urine is also expected (Pagana et al., 2022).

If pancreatitis is accompanied by biliary dysfunction (biliary pancreatitis), serum *bilirubin* is usually elevated. A sensitive indicator of biliary obstruction in acute pancreatitis is serum *alanine aminotransferase (ALT)*. A threefold or greater rise in concentration indicates that the diagnosis of acute biliary pancreatitis is valid. Elevated *white blood cell (WBC) count and differential, erythrocyte sedimentation rate (ESR)*, and serum *glucose* levels are also common in acute pancreatitis. The levels often correlate with disease severity.

Decreased serum *calcium* and *magnesium* levels are seen with fat necrosis. Calcium levels may fall and remain decreased for 7 to 10 days. Other tests include the basic metabolic panel (BMP), complete blood count (CBC), triglycerides, serum total protein, and albumin. The blood urea nitrogen (BUN), serum glucose, and triglycerides are usually elevated. Hemoconcentration is common because of third-space fluid loss. Leukocytosis (elevated WBC count) and thrombocytopenia (decreased platelets) are common. Albumin levels are decreased because cytokines (e.g., tumor necrosis factor [TNF]) released as part of the inflammatory response allow it to move from the bloodstream into the extravascular space. The presence of C-reactive protein suggests possible *inflammation* and necrosis (Pagana et al., 2022).

Imaging Assessment. Abdominal ultrasound may be used to diagnose causes of pancreatitis, such as gallstones, and can be performed at the bedside. However, it is not helpful in viewing the pancreas because of overlying bowel gas. Therefore *contrast-enhanced CT* provides a more reliable image and diagnosis of acute pancreatitis. This noninvasive technique may also be used to rule out pancreatic pseudocyst or ductal calculi.

An abdominal *x-ray* may also reveal gallstones. A chest x-ray may show elevation of the left side of the diaphragm or pleural effusion. Pancreatic stones are best diagnosed through ERCP.

Analyze Cues and Prioritize Hypotheses: Analysis

The priority collaborative problems for patients with acute pancreatitis include:

1. Severe acute *pain* due to pancreatic *inflammation* and enzyme leakage
2. Weight loss and inadequate *nutrition* due to inability to ingest food and absorb nutrients

---

Generate Solutions and Take Actions: Planning and Implementation

Managing Acute Pain

Planning: Expected Outcomes. The patient with acute pancreatitis is expected to experience a decrease in or absence of abdominal *pain,* as evidenced by self-report of a level of 2 or 3 on a 0-to-10 pain intensity scale.

Interventions. The priorities for care for the patient with acute pancreatitis are to provide supportive care by relieving symptoms, to decrease *inflammation,* and to anticipate or treat complications. *As for any patient, continually assess for and support the ABCs (airway, breathing, and circulation).* In collaboration with the respiratory therapist, if available, provide oxygen and other respiratory support as needed. The collaborative plan of care depends on the severity of the illness.

Severe continuous "boring" abdominal pain is the most common symptom of pancreatitis. The primary focus of nursing care is aimed at controlling *pain* by interventions that decrease GI tract activity, thus decreasing pancreatic stimulation. Pain assessment to measure the effectiveness of these interventions is an essential part of nursing care.

Nonsurgical Management. Mild pancreatitis requires hydration with IV fluids, *pain* control, and drug therapy. The interprofessional health care team initially attempts to relieve pain with nonsurgical interventions, which include fasting and rest, drug therapy, and comfort measures. If patients have a life-threatening complication or require frequent assessment, they are admitted to a critical care unit for invasive hemodynamic monitoring.

To rest the pancreas and reduce pancreatic enzyme secretion, withhold food and fluids (NPO) during the acute period. The primary health care provider prescribes IV isotonic fluid administration to maintain hydration. IV replacement of calcium and magnesium may also be needed. Measure and document intake and output. Some patients have an indwelling urinary catheter to obtain accurate measurements.

Nasogastric drainage and suction are reserved for more *severely ill* patients who have continuous vomiting or biliary obstruction. Gastric decompression using a nasogastric tube (NGT) prevents gastric juices from flowing into the duodenum.

Pain management for acute pancreatitis typically begins with the administration of opioids by patient-controlled analgesia (PCA). Drugs such as morphine or hydromorphone are typically given. Other options that have been used successfully to manage acute pain include IV or transdermal fentanyl and epidural analgesia (Burchum & Rosenthal, 2022).

In *mild* pancreatitis, the pain usually subsides in 2 to 3 days. However, with *severe* acute pancreatitis, the abdominal pain and tenderness may persist for up to 2 weeks. Drug dosages and intervals are individualized according to the severity of the disease and the symptoms.

Histamine receptor antagonists (e.g., famotidine) and proton pump inhibitors (e.g., pantoprazole) help decrease gastric acid secretion. Antibiotics may be prescribed, but they are indicated primarily for patients with acute necrotizing pancreatitis or pancreatic abscess.

Helping the patient assume a side-lying position (with the legs drawn up to the chest) may help decrease the abdominal *pain* of pancreatitis ("fetal position"). Sitting with the knees flexed toward the chest is also helpful.

If the patient is NPO or has an NGT, remind assistive personnel to implement frequent oral and nares hygiene measures to keep mucous membranes moist and free of inflammation or crusting. Because of the drying effect of drugs and the absence of oral fluids, the mouth and oral cavity may be extremely dry, resulting in considerable discomfort and possibly parotitis (inflammation of the parotid [salivary] glands).

Observe for signs and symptoms of hypocalcemia, such as muscle twitching, numbness, and irritability. Chapter 13 discusses assessment and care of patients with hypocalcemia in more detail.

Lowering the patient's anxiety level may also reduce *pain.* Explain all procedures and other aspects of patient care thoroughly. Provide reassurance, offer diversional activities such as music and reading material, and encourage visitors to direct attention away from the pain.

If pancreatitis was caused by gallstones, an ERCP with a sphincterotomy (opening of the sphincter of Oddi) may be performed on an urgent or emergent basis. If this procedure is not successful, surgery is required. ERCP is described in detail in Chapter 48.

Surgical Management. Surgical intervention for acute pancreatitis is usually not indicated. However, if an ERCP is not successful in removing gallstones, a laparoscopic cholecystectomy may be performed as described in the Surgical Management discussion in the section Inflammation Concept Exemplar: Cholecystitis.

Complications of pancreatitis, such as pancreatic pseudocyst and abscess, may also require surgical intervention. Laparoscopy (minimally invasive surgery [MIS]) may be done to drain an abscess or pseudocyst. For patients who are at high surgical risk, pseudocysts or abscesses can be treated with percutaneous drainage under CT guidance.

Promoting Nutrition

Planning: Expected Outcomes. The patient with acute pancreatitis is expected to have adequate *nutrition* to meet metabolic needs.

Interventions. The patient is maintained on NPO status in the early stages of pancreatitis. Antiemetics for nausea and vomiting are prescribed as needed. Patients who have severe pancreatitis and are unable to eat for 24 to 48 hours after illness onset may begin jejunal tube feeding unless paralytic ileus is present. *Early nutrition* intervention enhances immune system functioning and may prevent complications and worsening *inflammation* (Bartel, 2020). Enteral feeding is preferred over total parenteral nutrition (TPN) because it causes fewer episodes of glucose elevation and other complications associated with TPN. Be sure that the patient is weighed every day. Collaborate with the primary health care provider, registered dietitian nutritionist, and pharmacist to plan and implement the most appropriate nutrition intervention. Chapter 52 describes collaborative care of patients receiving enteral feeding and TPN.

When food is tolerated during the healing phase, the primary health care provider prescribes small, frequent, moderate- to high-carbohydrate, high-protein, low-fat meals. Food should be bland with little spice. GI stimulants such as caffeine-containing food (tea, coffee, cola, and chocolate), as well as alcohol, should be avoided. Monitor the patient beginning to resume oral food intake for nausea, vomiting, and diarrhea. *If any of these symptoms occur, notify the primary health care provider immediately.*

To boost caloric intake, commercial liquid nutritional preparations supplement the diet. The health care provider may also prescribe fat-soluble and other vitamin and mineral replacement supplements. Glutamine, omega-3 fatty acids, fiber, antioxidants, and/or nucleotides may be added to the patient's nutrition plan.

Care Coordination and Transition Management

Home care preparation is individualized for each patient's circumstances. Some patients may be severely weakened from their acute illness and need to confine activity to one floor, limiting stair climbing and other strenuous activities until they regain their strength. Collaborate with the case manager (CM) to plan the best place for the patient to recover and resources that may be needed. Patients may require several visits by a home care nurse if the hospitalization was complicated. In these cases, home care may be needed for wound care and rehabilitative services.

Education needs to be started early in the hospitalization period—as soon as the acute episodes of pain have subsided. Assess the patient's and family's knowledge of the disease.

The desired outcomes for discharge planning and education are to avoid further episodes of pancreatitis and prevent progression to a chronic disease. If the patient uses alcohol, instruct about the importance of abstaining from drinking to prevent further pain attacks and extension of *inflammation* and pancreatic insufficiency. Tell the patient that if alcohol is consumed, acute *pain* will return, and further autodigestion of the pancreas may lead to chronic pancreatitis.

Teach the patient to notify the primary health care provider after discharge to home if acute abdominal pain or biliary tract disease (as evidenced by jaundice, clay-colored stools, or darkened urine) occurs. These signs and symptoms are possible indicators of complications or disease progression.

The patient requires medical follow-up with the primary care provider to monitor the disease process. For those with alcoholism, provide information about groups such as Alcoholics Anonymous (AA). Family members may attend support groups such as Al-Anon and Alateen.

Evaluate Outcomes: Evaluation

Evaluate the care of the patient with acute pancreatitis based on the identified priority patient problems. The expected outcomes include that the patient will:

- Have control of abdominal *pain,* as indicated by self-report and pain scale measurement
- Have adequate *nutrition* available to meet metabolic needs

CHRONIC PANCREATITIS

Pathophysiology Review

Chronic pancreatitis is a progressive, destructive disease of the pancreas that has remissions and exacerbations (flare-ups). *Inflammation* and fibrosis of the tissue contribute to pancreatic insufficiency and diminished function of the organ.

Chronic pancreatitis can be classified into several categories. Chronic calcifying pancreatitis (CCP), the most common type, is primarily caused by alcoholism. In the early stages of the disease, pancreatic secretions precipitate as insoluble proteins that plug the pancreatic ducts and flow of pancreatic juices. As the protein plugs become more widespread, the cellular lining of the ducts changes and ulcerates. This inflammatory process causes fibrosis of the pancreatic tissue. Intraductal calcification and marked pancreatic tissue destruction (necrosis) develop in the late stages. The organ becomes hard and firm due to cell atrophy and pancreatic insufficiency (Rogers, 2023).

Chronic obstructive pancreatitis develops from *inflammation,* spasm, and obstruction of the sphincter of Oddi, often from cholelithiasis (gallstones). Inflammatory and sclerotic lesions occur in the head of the pancreas and around the ducts, causing an obstruction and backflow of pancreatic secretions. (See the Complications of Acute Pancreatitis section.)

Autoimmune pancreatitis is a chronic inflammatory process in which immunoglobulins invade the pancreas. Other organs may also be infiltrated, including the lungs and liver. Current research shows a correlation between the presence of autoimmune pancreatitis and cancers of other organs. This means that autoimmune pancreatitis may be a paraneoplastic syndrome (Okamoto et al., 2019).

Idiopathic and *hereditary chronic pancreatitis* may be associated with *SPINK1* and *CFTR* gene mutations and with mutations in the *BRCA2* gene. People with hereditary pancreatitis have been shown to have a 50- to 60-fold increased risk of pancreatic cancer (Rawla et al., 2019). The protein encoded by the *SPINK1* gene is a trypsin inhibitor. The *CFTR* gene is associated with cystic fibrosis. Research on these gene mutations can help in developing targeted drug therapy for treatment of these diseases.

Pancreatic insufficiency in any type of chronic pancreatitis causes loss of *exocrine* function. Most patients with chronic pancreatitis have decreased pancreatic secretions and bicarbonate. Pancreatic enzyme secretion must be greatly reduced to produce steatorrhea resulting from severe malabsorption of fats. These characteristic stools are pale, bulky, and frothy and have an offensive odor. The action of colonic bacteria on unabsorbed lipids and proteins is responsible for the extremely foul odor. On inspection of the stools, the fat content is visible.

Fat malabsorption also contributes to weight loss and muscle wasting (a decrease in muscle mass) and leads to general debilitation. Protein malabsorption results in a "starvation" edema of the feet, legs, and hands caused by decreased levels of circulating albumin.

The loss of pancreatic *endocrine* function is responsible for the development of diabetes mellitus in patients with chronic pancreatic insufficiency. (See Chapter 56 for a complete discussion of diabetes mellitus.)

The patient with chronic pancreatitis may have pulmonary complications, such as pleuritic pain, pleural effusions, and pulmonary infiltrates. Pancreatic ascites may decrease diaphragmatic excursion and lung expansion, resulting in impaired ventilation. In the ill patient with chronic pancreatitis, acute respiratory distress syndrome (ARDS) may develop (see Chapter 26).

Interprofessional Collaborative Care

Care for the patient with chronic pancreatitis takes place in the home or community setting but moves to the hospital setting for *pain* control and possible surgical intervention.

Recognize Cues: Assessment

Many symptoms of chronic pancreatitis differ from those of an acute *inflammation.* Abdominal pain is the major symptom for most types of pancreatitis. For those with chronic pancreatitis,

BOX 51.5 Key Features

Chronic Pancreatitis

- Intense abdominal **pain,** a major symptom, that is continuous and burning or gnawing
- Abdominal tenderness
- Ascites
- Possible left upper quadrant mass (if pancreatic pseudocyst or abscess is present)
- Respiratory compromise manifesting with adventitious or diminished breath sounds, dyspnea, or orthopnea
- Steatorrhea; clay-colored stools
- Weight loss
- Jaundice
- Dark urine
- Polyuria, polydipsia, polyphagia (diabetes mellitus)

pain is typically described as a continuous burning or gnawing dullness with periods of acute exacerbation (flare-ups). The pain is very intense and relentless. The frequency of acute exacerbations may increase as the pancreatic fibrosis develops. Box 51.5 lists the common symptoms of chronic pancreatitis.

Perform an abdominal assessment. Abdominal tenderness is less intense in patients with chronic pancreatitis than in those with acute pancreatitis. Massive pancreatic ascites may be present, producing dullness on abdominal percussion. Ascites may also be assessed by performing the fluid wave test (Jarvis & Eckhardt, 2024). Because respiratory complications can occur, auscultate the lung fields for adventitious sounds or decreased aeration and observe for dyspnea or orthopnea.

Ask the patient to collect a random stool specimen if able or ask about the appearance of stools. The specimen may show steatorrhea. Assess for unintentional weight loss; muscle wasting; jaundice; dark urine; and the symptoms of diabetes mellitus, such as polyuria (increased urinary output), polydipsia (excessive thirst), and polyphagia (increased appetite).

Diagnosis is based on the patient's symptoms and laboratory and imaging assessment. *Endoscopic retrograde cholangiopancreatography* (ERCP) is done to visualize the pancreatic and common bile ducts (Pagana et al., 2022). *Imaging studies* such as CT scanning, contrast-enhanced MRI, abdominal ultrasonography (US), and endoscopic ultrasonography (EUS) are also useful in making the diagnosis. In chronic pancreatitis, laboratory findings include normal or moderately elevated serum *amylase* and *lipase* levels (Pagana et al., 2022). Obstruction of the intrahepatic bile duct can cause elevated serum *bilirubin* and *alkaline phosphatase* levels. Intermittent elevations in serum *glucose* levels are common and can be detected by blood glucose monitoring, both fasting and nonfasting.

Take Actions: Interventions

The focus of caring for the patient with chronic pancreatitis is to manage acute or persistent **pain,** maintain adequate **nutrition,** and prevent disease recurrence.

Nonsurgical Management. The primary nonsurgical interventions include drug and **nutrition** therapy. The major

intervention for the pain of chronic pancreatitis is drug therapy. Medicate the patient as prescribed according to the assessment of the intensity of pain. Evaluate the effectiveness of the drug intervention. Initially opioid analgesia is used most frequently, but dependency may occur. Nonopioid analgesics may be tried to relieve pain. (See Chapter 6 for other interventions for acute and persistent pain.)

Pancreatic enzyme replacement therapy (PERT) is the standard of care to prevent malnutrition, malabsorption, and excessive weight loss. Pancreatic enzymes are usually prescribed in the form of capsules or tablets that contain varying amounts of amylase, lipase, and protease. Teach patients not to chew or crush pancreatic enzyme replacements that are available as delayed-release capsules or enteric tablets. Teach them to take the enzymes with all meals and snacks (Burchum & Rosenthal, 2022).

The dosage of pancreatic enzymes depends on the severity of the malabsorption. Record the number and consistency of stools per day to monitor the effectiveness of enzyme therapy. If pancreatic enzyme treatment is effective, the stools should become less frequent and less fatty.

! NURSING SAFETY PRIORITY

Action Alert

If the patient has diabetes, insulin or oral antidiabetic agents for glucose control are prescribed. Patients maintained on total parenteral nutrition (TPN) are particularly susceptible to elevated glucose levels and require regular insulin additives to the solution. Monitor blood glucose to control hyperglycemia. Check finger stick blood glucose (FSBG) or sugar (FSBS) levels every 2 to 4 hours. Chapter 52 describes in detail the care associated with TPN.

The primary health care provider may also prescribe drug therapy to decrease gastric acid. Gastric acid destroys the lipase needed to break down fats. Controlling the acidity of the stomach with H_2 blockers or proton pump inhibitors (Bartel, 2020), or neutralizing stomach acid with oral sodium bicarbonate, may enhance the effectiveness of PERT.

Protein and fat malabsorption results in significant weight loss and decreased muscle mass in the patient with chronic pancreatitis. Therefore the nutritional interventions for acute pancreatitis are also used for chronic pancreatitis. The patient often limits food intake to avoid increased pain. For this reason, nutrition maintenance is often difficult to achieve. Patients receive either total parenteral nutrition (TPN) or total enteral nutrition (TEN), including vitamin and mineral replacement.

Collaborate with the registered dietitian nutritionist to teach the patient about long-term dietary management. The patient needs an increased number of calories, up to 4000 to 6000 calories per day, to maintain weight. Food high in carbohydrates and protein also assists in the healing process. Food high in fat is avoided because it causes or increases diarrhea. Teach all patients to avoid alcohol. Alcohol-cessation programs may be recommended.

Surgical Management. Surgery is not a primary intervention for the treatment of chronic pancreatitis. However, it may be indicated for ongoing abdominal *pain*, incapacitating relapses of pain, or complications such as a pancreatic abscess or pancreatic pseudocyst (Bartel, 2020).

The underlying pathologic changes determine the procedure indicated. Using laparoscopy, the surgeon incises and drains an abscess or pseudocyst. Laparoscopic cholecystectomy or choledochotomy (incision of the common bile duct) may be indicated if biliary tract disease is an underlying cause of pancreatitis. If the pancreatic duct sphincter is fibrotic, the surgeon performs a sphincterotomy (incision of the sphincter) to enlarge it. Endoscopic sphincterotomy may be used for patients who are poor surgical candidates.

In some cases, laparoscopic distal pancreatectomy may be appropriate for resection of the distal pancreas or pancreas head. Endoscopic pancreatic necrosectomy and natural orifice transluminal endoscopic surgery (NOTES) may be used to remove necrosed pancreatic tissue. Both procedures are performed through the GI wall without a visible skin incision. The NOTES procedure is discussed in Surgical Management in the Inflammation Concept Exemplar: Cholecystitis section.

Auto islet transplantation may be used to treat chronic pancreatitis (Bartel, 2020). In this surgical procedure, the entire pancreas is removed, then the insulin-producing cells are isolated and infused into the liver. Pancreas transplantation is performed most often for patients with severe, uncontrolled diabetes. Chapter 56 discusses pancreas transplantation.

Care Coordination and Transition Management

Collaborate with the hospital-based case manager (CM) or discharge planner about home care or follow-up in another setting. A community-based CM may continue to follow the patient after hospital discharge. Teach patients and families that toilet facilities must be easily accessible because of chronic steatorrhea and frequent defecation. If they are not easily accessible, a bedside commode is obtained for the home.

Chronic illnesses are devastating for families. The high costs of medical insurance, medical treatment, and drug therapy cause serious financial problems. Often the patient with chronic pancreatitis is unable to work. Collaborate with the CM about ways to assist the patient with resources for financial help.

The patient may require several home visits by nurses, depending on the severity of the chronic health problems and home maintenance and support needs. The nurse assesses the patient for pain, enzyme therapy, and psychosocial adaptation to a chronic illness.

Because there is no known cure for chronic pancreatitis, patient and family education is aimed at preventing acute episodes of the disease, providing long-term care, and promoting health maintenance. Box 51.6 outlines self-management to help prevent exacerbations of the disease.

The frequency of defecation (whether continent or incontinent) poses challenging skin care problems. Instruct the patient to keep the skin dry and free of the abrasive fatty stools, which damage the skin. The skin should be cleaned thoroughly after each stool, and a moisture barrier applied to prevent breakdown and maintain skin integrity. Many products on the market actively repel stool from the skin. Remind the patient to report

---

BOX 51.6   Patient and Family Education

How to Prevent Exacerbations of Chronic Pancreatitis

- Avoid things that make your symptoms worse, such as drinking caffeinated beverages.
- Avoid alcohol ingestion; seek a self-help group for assistance.
- Avoid nicotine.
- Eat bland, low-fat, high-protein, and moderate-carbohydrate meals; avoid gastric stimulants such as spices.
- Eat small meals and snacks high in calories.
- Take the pancreatic enzymes that have been prescribed for you with meals.
- Rest frequently; restrict your activity to one floor until you regain your strength.

---

any skin breakdown so therapeutic interventions to promote skin integrity can be started.

If the patient develops diabetes mellitus due to chronic pancreatitis, management of elevated glucose levels after discharge from the hospital may require oral antidiabetic agents or insulin injections. If this is the case, collaborate with the certified diabetes educator (CDE) to provide in-depth teaching concerning diabetes, its signs and symptoms, medical management, drug therapy, nutrition therapy, blood glucose monitoring, and general care.

Refer the patient and family to a counselor or a self-help group, such as Alcoholics Anonymous (www.aa.org) and Al-Anon (www.al-anon.org), if appropriate.

PANCREATIC CANCER

Cancer of the pancreas is a leading cause of cancer deaths each year in the United States. Early diagnosis is difficult because the pancreas is hidden and surrounded by other organs. Most often the tumor is discovered in the late stages of development and may be a well-defined mass or diffusely spread throughout the pancreas. Treatment has limited results, and the overall 5-year survival rates are very low (American Cancer Society [ACS], 2023b).

Pathophysiology Review

The tumor may be a primary cancer, or it may result from metastasis from cancers of the lung, breast, thyroid, kidney, or skin. Primary tumors are generally adenocarcinomas and grow in well-differentiated glandular patterns. They grow rapidly and spread to surrounding organs (stomach, duodenum, gallbladder, and intestine) by direct extension and invasion of lymphatic and vascular systems. This highly metastatic lesion may eventually invade the lung, peritoneum, liver, spleen, and lymph nodes.

Signs and symptoms depend on the site of origin or metastasis. The head of the pancreas is the most common site. The tumors are usually small lesions with poorly defined margins. Jaundice results from tumor compression and obstruction of the common bile duct and from gallbladder dilation, causing the organ to enlarge.

Cancers of the body and tail of the pancreas are usually large and invade the entire tail and body. These tumors may be palpable abdominal masses, especially in the thin patient. Through metastatic spread via the splenic vein, metastasis to the liver may cause hepatomegaly (enlargement of the liver). Regardless of where it originates, it spreads rapidly through the lymphatic and venous systems to other organs.

Venous thromboembolism is a common complication of pancreatic cancer. Necrotic products of the pancreatic tumor are believed to have thromboplastic properties resulting in the blood's hypercoagulable state. In addition, the patient is at high risk because of decreased mobility and extensive surgical manipulation.

The exact cause of pancreatic cancer is unknown. The major risk factors associated with the disease include:

- Smoking and tobacco use
- Obesity
- Chronic pancreatitis
- Cirrhosis
- Older age (over 65 years)
- Genetic syndromes

PATIENT-CENTERED CARE: HEALTH EQUITY

Health Outcomes for Pancreatic Cancer

Pancreatic cancer occurs more often in men than in women and more often in Blacks than Whites (Rawla et al., 2019). Black patients are diagnosed later in their disease and often have less insurance coverage when compared with White patients (Noel & Fiscella, 2019). Patients are likely not to seek health care if they are not able to pay or do not have health insurance.

Interprofessional Collaborative Care

Care for the patient with pancreatic cancer usually takes place in the hospital setting, and eventually with hospice support.

Recognize Cues: Assessment

Pancreatic cancer often presents in a slow and vague manner. The presenting symptoms depend somewhat on the location of the tumor. The first sign may be jaundice, which suggests late, advanced disease (Box 51.7).

No specific blood tests are diagnostic of pancreatic cancer. Serum *amylase* and *lipase* levels and *alkaline phosphatase* and *bilirubin* levels are increased. The degree of elevation depends on the acuteness or chronicity of the pancreatic and biliary damage. Elevated *carcinoembryonic antigen* (CEA) levels occur in most patients with pancreatic cancer. This test may provide early information about the presence of tumor cells. The tumor marker CA 19-9 has been found to be a useful serologic test for monitoring a proven diagnosis and continuing surveillance for potential spread or recurrence (Pagana et al., 2022).

Endoscopic ultrasonography (EUS) is now considered the gold standard for tumor detection and diagnosis (Kurihara et al., 2020). *Endoscopic retrograde cholangiopancreatography* (ERCP) and CT also provide visual diagnostic data. An alternative to ERCP is a percutaneous transhepatic cholangiography

BOX 51.7 Key Features
Pancreatic Cancer

- Jaundice
- Icterus
- Clay-colored (light) stools
- Dark urine
- Abdominal *pain,* usually vague, dull, or nonspecific, that radiates into the back
- Weight loss
- Anorexia
- Nausea or vomiting
- Glucose intolerance
- Splenomegaly (enlarged spleen)
- Flatulence
- GI bleeding
- New-onset diabetes mellitus
- Ascites (abdominal fluid)
- Leg or calf pain (from thrombophlebitis)
- Weakness and fatigue

(PTC) with placement of a percutaneous transhepatic biliary drain (PTBD). This drain decompresses the blocked biliary system by draining bile internally, externally, or both. Aspiration of pancreatic ascitic fluid by means of abdominal paracentesis may reveal cancer cells and elevated amylase levels. Pancreatic fluid cytology may also be performed using an endoscopic nasopancreatic drainage (ENPD) catheter (Kurihara et al., 2020).

Take Actions: Interventions

Management of the patient with pancreatic cancer is geared toward preventing tumor spread and decreasing pain. These measures are not curative, only palliative. The cancers are often metastatic and recur despite treatment.

Nonsurgical Management. As in other types of cancer, chemotherapy or radiation is used to relieve pain by shrinking the tumor. It may be used before, after, or instead of surgery. *Chemotherapy* has had limited success in increasing survival time. In most cases, combining agents has been more successful than single-agent chemotherapy. The current standard for chemotherapy is 6 months of treatment with FOLFORINOX, a combination of folinic acid, 5-fluorouracil (5-FU), irinotecan, and oxaliplatin. If a patient is unable to tolerate the FOLFORINOX protocol, then 6 months of gemcitabine and capecitabine or gemcitabine and nab-paclitaxel (for patients with metastatic disease) is the second choice (Springfield et al., 2019). Gemcitabine alone may still provide benefit to those who are unable to tolerate combination chemotherapy. Observe for adverse drug effects, such as fatigue, rash, anorexia, and diarrhea.

Other targeted therapies being investigated include growth factor inhibitors, antiangiogenesis factors, and kinase inhibitors. Kinase inhibitors are a newer group of drugs that focus on cancer cells with little or no effect on healthy cells. Chapter 18 discusses nursing implications of chemotherapy in detail.

To control pain, the patient takes high doses of opioid analgesics (usually morphine) as prescribed before the pain escalates and peaks. Because of the poor prognosis, drug dependency is not a consideration. Chapter 6 describes in detail the care of the patient with chronic cancer pain.

Intensive external beam *radiation* therapy to the pancreas may be used to treat resectable or borderline resectable pancreatic cancer. It also may offer pain relief for people with advanced pancreatic cancer by shrinking tumor cells, alleviating obstruction, and improving food absorption (ACS, 2023a). For people with advanced cancer, it does not improve survival rates. The patient may experience discomfort during and after the radiation treatments. Chapter 18 describes radiation therapy in more detail, including associated nursing care.

For patients experiencing biliary obstruction who are at high surgical risk, biliary stents can ensure patency to relieve pain. These stents are devices made of plastic materials that keep the ducts of the biliary system open. A biliary stent may be placed endoscopically during an endoscopic retrograde cholangiopancreatography (ERCP) or can be placed through the skin during a percutaneous transhepatic cholangiography (PTC).

Surgical Management. Complete surgical resection of the pancreatic tumor offers the patient with pancreatic cancer the only effective treatment, but it is done only in patients with small tumors. Partial pancreatectomy is the preferred surgery for resectable or borderline resectable tumors, depending on length of time since diagnosis. Types of partial pancreatectomy include Whipple procedure (pancreaticoduodenectomy), pylorus-preserving pancreaticoduodenectomy (PPPD), and distal pancreatectomy. Whereas the Whipple procedure and PPPD are used for treatment of tumors in the pancreatic head and neck, a distal pancreatectomy is for resection of tumors in the body and tail (National Cancer Institute, 2023). Recent technologic advances have expanded the role of *minimally invasive surgery (MIS)* via laparoscopy in the staging, palliation, and removal of pancreatic cancers. The procedure selected depends on the purpose of the surgery and stage of the disease. For example, if the patient has a biliary obstruction, a laparoscopic procedure to relieve it is performed. This procedure diverts bile drainage into the jejunum.

For locally advanced tumors, the surgeon may perform *radical pancreatectomy.* Most pancreatic surgical procedures have traditionally been done using an open surgical approach. Because of new advances in laparoscopic technology using a hand-assisted or robotic-assisted device, this method is beginning to replace the conventional method. Some surgeons are not yet trained in how to perform this technique. Therefore the traditional open surgical approach remains a common method of performing these surgeries.

Preoperative Care. The patient with pancreatic cancer may be at poor surgical risk because of malnutrition and debilitation. Specific care depends on the type of surgical approach being used.

Often, in the late stages of pancreatic cancer or before the Whipple procedure, the primary health care provider inserts a small catheter into the jejunum (jejunostomy) so enteral feedings may be given. This feeding method is preferred to prevent reflux and facilitate absorption. Feedings are started in low concentrations and volumes and gradually increased as tolerated. Provide feedings using a pump to maintain a constant volume, and assess for diarrhea frequency to determine tolerance. Chapter 52 provides additional information about enteral feeding.

For optimal **nutrition,** TPN may be necessary in addition to tube feedings or as a single measure. When central venous access is required, a peripherally inserted central catheter (PICC) or other type of IV catheter may be necessary. Meticulous IV line care is an important nursing measure to prevent catheter sepsis. Sterile dressing changes and site observation are extremely important. Additional nursing care measures for the patient receiving TPN are given in Chapter 52. Monitor nutrition indicators such as serum prealbumin and albumin.

For the laparoscopic procedure, no bowel preparation is needed. However, either approach requires that the patient be NPO for at least 6 to 8 hours before surgery. Surgeon preference and agency policy determine the preferred protocol for preoperative preparation.

Operative Procedures. The Whipple procedure (radical pancreaticoduodenectomy) is an extensive surgical procedure used most often to treat cancer of the head of the pancreas. The procedure entails removal of the proximal head of the pancreas, the duodenum, a portion of the jejunum, the stomach (partial or total *gastrectomy*), and the gallbladder, with anastomosis of the pancreatic duct (*pancreaticojejunostomy*), the common bile duct (*choledochojejunostomy*), and the stomach (*gastrojejunostomy*) to the jejunum (Fig. 51.3). In addition, the surgeon may remove the spleen (splenectomy).

Postoperative Care. In addition to routine postoperative care measures, the patient who has undergone an *open* radical pancreaticoduodenectomy requires intensive nursing care and

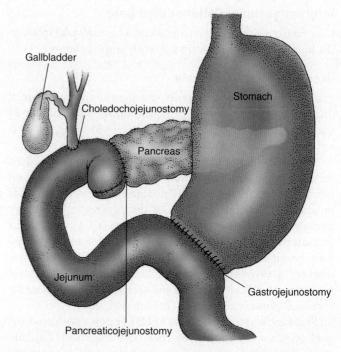

FIG. 51.3 The three anastomoses that constitute the Whipple procedure: choledochojejunostomy, pancreaticojejunostomy, and gastrojejunostomy.

TABLE 51.2 Potential Complications of the Whipple Procedure

Body System	Potential Complications
Cardiovascular system	Hemorrhage at anastomosis sites with hypovolemia Myocardial infarction Heart failure Thrombophlebitis
Pulmonary system	Atelectasis Pneumonia Pulmonary embolism Acute respiratory distress syndrome Pulmonary edema
Endocrine/renal complications	Unstable diabetes mellitus Chronic kidney disease
GI system	Adynamic (paralytic) ileus Gastric retention Gastric ulceration Bowel obstruction from peritonitis Acute pancreatitis Hepatic failure Thrombosis to mesentery
Integumentary system	Infection Dehiscence Fistulas: pancreatic, gastric, and biliary

is typically admitted to a surgical critical care unit. Observe for multiple potential complications of the open Whipple procedure as listed in Table 51.2.

PATIENT-CENTERED CARE: HEALTH EQUITY

Pancreatic Cancer Treatment and Outcomes

Be aware that Black patients have higher rates of surgical complications and mortality after pancreatic resection for cancer when compared with other populations. One factor that may help explain these differences is that Blacks tend to have their surgery more often in low-volume hospitals, meaning that the surgical team is less specialized or experienced than those in a high-volume hospital (Noel & Fiscella, 2019). Another factor is that some Black patients may not have adequate insurance coverage or the same access to health care when compared with other patients.

The primary benefits of *MIS* for the patient are a shorter postoperative recovery and less pain than with traditional open procedure. The patient having the laparoscopic Whipple surgery or radical pancreatectomy is also less at risk for severe complications. For patients having one of these procedures, observe for and implement preventive measures for these common surgical complications:

- Diabetes (Check blood glucose often.)
- Hemorrhage (Monitor pulse, blood pressure, skin color, and mental status [e.g., level of consciousness (LOC)].)
- Wound infection (Monitor temperature and assess wounds for redness/hyperpigmentation and induration [hardness].)

- Bowel obstruction (Check bowel sounds and stools.)
- Intraabdominal abscess (Monitor temperature and patient's report of severe pain.)

Immediately after surgery the patient is NPO and usually has a nasogastric tube (NGT) to decompress the stomach. Monitor GI drainage and tube patency. In open surgical approaches, biliary drainage tubes are placed during surgery to remove drainage and secretions from the area and prevent stress on the anastomosis sites. Assess the tubes and drainage devices for tension or kinking and maintain them in a dependent position.

Monitor the drainage for color, consistency, and amount. The drainage should be serosanguineous. The appearance of clear, colorless, bile-tinged drainage or frank blood with an increase in output may indicate disruption or leakage of an anastomosis site. Most of the disruptions of the site occur within 7 to 10 days after surgery. Hemorrhage can occur as an early or late complication.

Place the patient in the semi-Fowler's position to reduce tension on the suture line and anastomosis site and to optimize lung expansion. Stress can be decreased by maintaining NGT drainage at a low continuous or high intermittent suction level to keep the remaining stomach (if a partial gastrectomy is done) or the jejunum (if a total gastrectomy is done) free of excessive fluid buildup and pressure. The NGT also reduces stimulation of the remaining pancreatic tissue.

✚ NURSING SAFETY PRIORITY

Critical Rescue

The development of a fistula (an abnormal passageway) is the most common and most serious postoperative complication (Gupta & Yelamanchi, 2021). Biliary, pancreatic, or gastric fistulas result from partial or total breakdown of an anastomosis site. The secretions that drain from the fistula contain bile, pancreatic enzymes, or gastric secretions, depending on which site is ruptured. *These secretions, particularly pancreatic fluid, are corrosive and irritating to the skin; and internal leakage causes chemical peritonitis.* Peritonitis (inflammation and infection of the peritoneum causing boardlike abdominal rigidity) requires treatment with multiple antibiotics. *If you suspect any postoperative complications resulting from minimally invasive surgery (MIS) or open surgical approaches, call the surgeon or Rapid Response Team immediately and provide assessment findings that support your concerns.*

Because the *open* Whipple procedure is extensive and can take many hours to complete, maintaining fluid and electrolyte balance can be difficult. Patients often have significant intraoperative blood loss and postoperative bleeding. The intestine is exposed to air for long periods, and fluid evaporates. Significant losses of fluid and electrolytes occur from the NGT and other drainage tubes. In addition, these patients may be malnourished and have low serum levels of protein and albumin, which maintain colloid osmotic pressure within the circulating system. Reduction in the serum osmotic pressure makes the patient likely to develop third spacing of body fluids, with fluid moving from the vascular to the interstitial space, resulting in shock. These problems are less likely to occur when MIS is used. Therefore, when possible, the trained surgeon prefers to perform laparoscopic Whipple procedures to prevent the many complications that can occur.

! NURSING SAFETY PRIORITY

Action Alert

To detect early signs of hypovolemia and prevent shock, closely monitor vital signs for decreased blood pressure and increased heart rate, decreased vascular pressures with a pulmonary artery catheter (Swan-Ganz catheter) (in the ICU setting), and decreased urine output. Be alert for pitting edema of the extremities, dependent edema in the sacrum and back, and an intake that far exceeds output. Maintain sequential compression devices to prevent deep vein thrombosis.

Maintenance of IV isotonic fluid replacement with colloid replacements is important. Monitor hemoglobin and hematocrit values to assess for blood loss and the need for blood transfusions. Review electrolyte values for decreased serum levels of sodium, potassium, chloride, and calcium. IV fluid concentrations must be altered to correct these electrolyte imbalances. The physician prescribes replacement of electrolytes as needed.

Immediately after the Whipple procedure, the patient may have hyperglycemia or hypoglycemia resulting from stress and surgical manipulation of the pancreas. Most of the endocrine cells (responsible for insulin and glucagon secretion) are located in the body and tail of the pancreas. In some patients, up to half of the gland remains, and diabetes does not develop. However, a large number of patients have diabetes before surgery. For patients having a radical pancreatectomy, administer insulin as prescribed because the entire pancreas is removed. Monitor glucose levels frequently during the early postoperative period and administer insulin injections as prescribed.

NCLEX Examination Challenge 51.3

Physiological Integrity

The nurse is planning care for a client who had a laparoscopic Whipple surgery. For which of the following complications would the nurse assess?
Select all that apply.
A. Bleeding
B. Wound infection
C. Intestinal obstruction
D. Diabetes mellitus
E. Abdominal abscess

Care Coordination and Transition Management

The patient with pancreatic cancer is usually followed by a case manager (CM), both in the hospital and in the home or other community-based setting. Collaborate with the CM to ensure that the patient receives cost-effective treatment and that needs are met.

The stage of progression of pancreatic cancer and available home care resources determine whether the patient can be discharged to home or whether additional care is needed in a skilled nursing facility or with a hospice provider. Home care preparations depend on the patient's physical and activity limitations and should be tailored to personal needs. Coordinate care with the patient, family, or whoever will be providing care after discharge from the hospital (i.e., home care provider, hospice care provider, or extended-care provider).

The patient and family need compassionate emotional support to deal with issues related to this illness. The diagnosis of pancreatic cancer can frighten and overwhelm the patient and family. Help family members look realistically and objectively at the amount of physical care required. Tell family members that their own physical and emotional health is at risk during this stressful period and that supportive counseling may be needed. If the family does not have a religious affiliation or a spiritual leader (e.g., a minister or a rabbi) to provide support, suggest alternative counseling options. Refer patients and families to the certified hospital chaplain if desired. It is appropriate for the nurse to make the initial contact or appointment according to the patient's or family's wishes.

When the patient is discharged to home, many interventions are palliative and aimed at managing symptoms such as pain. In many cases the diagnosis of pancreatic cancer is made a few months before death occurs. The patient needs time to adjust to the diagnosis, which is usually made too late for cure or prolonged survival. Help the patient identify what needs to be done to prepare for death, including end-of-life care. For example, the patient may want to write a will or see family members and friends not seen recently. The patient needs to make known to family members or others any specific requests for the funeral or memorial service. These actions help prepare for death in a dignified manner. Chapter 8 discusses in detail anticipatory grieving and preparation for death, as well as symptom management during the end of life.

Regular home care nursing and assistive personnel visits may be scheduled to assist the patient and family by providing physical, psychological, and supportive care. Provide information about local palliative and hospice care (see Chapter 8) and cancer support groups.

GET READY FOR THE NEXT-GENERATION NCLEX® EXAMINATION!

Essential Nursing Care Points

Health Promotion/Disease Prevention

- To help prevent biliary and pancreatic disorders, nurses need to teach individuals, especially women, to practice lifestyle habits that help prevent obesity, including avoiding excessive high-fat/high-cholesterol foods and exercising regularly.
- Nurses should teach individuals about the need to avoid excessive alcohol, which is a common cause of acute pancreatitis.

Chronic Disease Care

- Chronic pancreatitis is a progressive, destructive disease of the pancreas that has remissions and exacerbations.
- To prevent exacerbations of chronic pancreatitis, patients should avoid alcohol, nicotine, high-fat gastric-stimulating foods, and large meals.
- Patients who have chronic pancreatitis need to take pancreatic enzyme replacements with every meal.
- The Whipple procedure is an extensive surgery used most often to treat cancer of the head of the pancreas; many life-threatening complications can result from this surgery, including heart failure, myocardial infarction, pulmonary embolism, pulmonary edema, and acute respiratory distress syndrome (ARDS).
- Nurses need to be aware that Black patients have higher rates of surgical complications and mortality after pancreatic resection for cancer when compared with other populations.
- The 5-year survival rate for patients who have pancreatic cancer is very low.

Regenerative or Restorative Care

- Key features of cholecystitis (*inflammation* of the gallbladder) include upper abdominal *pain*, nausea and/or vomiting, dyspepsia, eructation, flatulence, and possibly fever. If biliary obstruction occurs, jaundice, clay-colored stools, and dark urine may also be present.
- The most common treatment for cholecystitis is a laparoscopic cholecystectomy (gallbladder removal); this minimally invasive surgery (MIS) is usually performed in a same-day ambulatory surgical center with minimal surgical complications or restrictions.
- Biliary colic may occur when the cystic duct is obstructed or gallstones move, causing symptoms of shock. If this occurs, the nurse notifies the Rapid Response Team immediately and stays with the patient.
- Acute pancreatitis is a serious, and at times life-threatening, *inflammation* of the pancreas; the two most common causes of this disease are gallstones and alcoholism.
- The pain described by patients who have acute pancreatitis is severe and "boring;" nurses need to manage pain with opioids, rest, and possible nasogastric decompression if an ileus occurs.
- Potentially life-threatening complications of acute pancreatitis include necrotizing hemorrhagic pancreatitis, acute kidney injury, hypovolemic shock, ARDS, and multiorgan system failure.
- Pancreatic injury from inflammation or cancer causes an elevation in pancreatic enzymes (amylase, lipase, trypsin, and elastase). Serum glucose is also increased because cells that usually secrete insulin are damaged.

End-of-Life Care/Hospice/Palliative Care

- Every patient needs time and support to adjust to the diagnosis of pancreatic cancer, which is usually made too late for cure or prolonged survival. Help each patient identify what needs to be done to prepare for death, including end-of-life care.
- Nurses need to provide information about local palliative and hospice care (see Chapter 8) and cancer support groups for patients who have pancreatic cancer.

Mastery Questions

1. The nurse is caring for a client who is experiencing obstructive jaundice cause by gallstones. Which of the following client assessment findings would the nurse anticipate? **Select all that apply.**
   A. Icterus
   B. Peritonitis
   C. Clay-colored stools
   D. Urinary retention
   E. Dark urine

2. The nurse is caring for a client diagnosed with acute pancreatitis. Which of the following serum laboratory test findings would the nurse expect for this client? **Select all that apply.**
   A. Elevated amylase
   B. Decreased glucose
   C. Elevated lipase
   D. Increased leukocytes
   E. Decreased elastase
   F. Decreased trypsin

3. The nurse is caring for a client who had a laparoscopic Whipple surgery. Which of the following postoperative complications would be the **priority** for the nurse to manage?
   A. Hyperglycemia
   B. Wound infection
   C. Deep vein thrombosis
   D. Respiratory distress

NGN Challenge 51.1

The nurse reviews the Nurses' Notes for a 45-year-old client admitted to the medical unit from the emergency department (ED).

Health History	**Nurses' Notes**	Imaging Studies	Laboratory Results

1945: Client presented to ED with report of moderate to severe LUQ abdominal pain that radiates to back and is worse when lying flat for the last 2 days. Has had new episodes of nausea and vomiting for almost a week. Alert and oriented × 4. Lung sounds clear with no adventitious sounds. S_1 and S_2 present; no murmurs. Decreased bowel sounds × 4; abdomen distended with ascites. VS: T 99.8°F (37.7°C); HR 96 beats/min and regular; RR 20 breaths/min; BP 102/56 mm Hg; SpO_2 95% on RA. H/O type 2 diabetes mellitus; reports substance use for 30 years including street drugs (primarily cocaine) and alcohol.

Complete the diagram by selecting from the choices below to specify what potential condition the client is likely experiencing, **2** nursing actions that are appropriate to take, and **2** parameters the nurse should monitor to assess the client's progress.

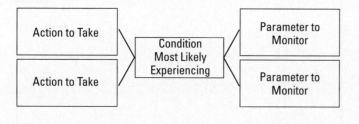

Actions to Take	Potential Conditions	Parameters to Monitor
Insert an indwelling urinary catheter	Acute cholecystitis	Abdominal pain
Keep NPO and start isotonic IV fluids	Acute pancreatitis	Oxygen saturation levels
Consult social worker about alcoholism	Chronic pancreatitis	Heart rate
Administer supplemental oxygen therapy	Pancreatic cancer	Serum amylase
Manage pain with analgesics		Blood pressure

NGN Challenge 51.2

The nurse reviews the Nurses' Notes for a 37-year-old client admitted to the ED.

Health History	**Nurses' Notes**	Imaging Studies	Laboratory Results

1620: Well-nourished client presented to ED with report of moderate RUQ abdominal pain, excessive burping and passing flatus, and anorexia for 3 days. Nausea and vomiting last night following dinner. Alert and oriented × 4. Lung sounds clear with no adventitious sounds. S_1 and S_2 present; no murmurs. Bowel sounds present × 4; abdomen soft without distention. VS: T 99°F (37.2°C); HR 85 beats/min and regular; RR 20 breaths/min; BP 118/64 mm Hg; SpO_2 95% on RA. H/O gastric bypass surgery 3 months ago; H/O diabetes mellitus type 2 for 17 years due to early obesity. Denies any history of or current substance use.

Complete the diagram by selecting from the choices below to specify what potential condition the client is likely experiencing, **2** nursing actions that are appropriate to take, and **2** parameters the nurse should monitor to assess the client's progress.

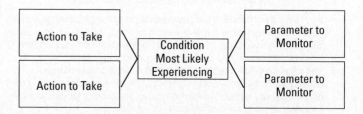

Actions to Take	Potential Conditions	Parameters to Monitor
Manage client's pain and nausea	Acute pancreatitis	Episodes of nausea and vomiting
Insert a nasogastric tube to continuous low suction	Chronic pancreatitis	Oxygen saturation levels
Prepare client for abdominal ultrasound	Cholecystitis	Blood pressure
Administer supplemental oxygen therapy	Pancreatic cancer	Body weight
Prepare for abdominal surgery		Abdominal pain

REFERENCES

American Cancer Society (ACS). (2023a). *Pancreatic cancer.* https://www.cancer.org/cancer/pancreatic-cancer.html.

American Cancer Society (ACS). (2023b). *Survival rates for pancreatic cancer.* https://www.cancer.org/cancer/pancreatic-cancer/detection-diagnosis-staging/survival-rates.

Bartel, M. (2020). *Pancreatitis. Merck Manual Professional Version.* https://www.merckmanuals.com/professional/gastrointestinal-disorders/pancreatitis.

Burchum, J. L. R., & Rosenthal, L. D. (2022). *Lehne's pharmacology for nursing care* (11th ed.). Elsevier.

Gupta, N., & Yelamanchi, R. (2021). Pancreatic adenocarcinoma: A review of recent paradigms and advances in epidemiology, clinical diagnosis and management. *World Journal of Gastroenterology,* 27(23), 3158–3181. https://doi.org/10.3748/wjg.v27.i23.3158.

Hassler, K. R., Collins, J. T., Philip, K., & Jones, M. W. (2021). Laparoscopic Cholecystectomy. In *StatPearls.* StatPearls Publishing.

Hormati, A., Alemi, F., Mohammadbeigi, A., Sarkeshikian, S. S., & Saeidi, M. (2020). Prevalence of endoscopic cholangiopancreatography complications and amylase sensitivity for predicting pancreatitis in ERCP patients. *Gastroenterology Nursing,* 43(5), 350–354.

Iannuzzi, J. P., King, J. A., Leong, J. H., Quan, J., Windsor, J. W., Tanyingoh, D., et al. (2022). Global incidence of acute pancreatitis in increasing over time: A systematic review and meta-analysis. *Gastroenterology,* 162(1), 122–134.

Jarvis, C., & Eckhardt, A. (2024). *Physical examination & health assessment* (9th ed.). Elsevier Saunders.

Kurihara, K., Hanada, K., & Shimizu, A. (2020). Endoscopic Ultrasonography Diagnosis of Early Pancreatic Cancer. *Diagnostics (Basel, Switzerland), 10*(12), 1086. https://doi.org/10.3390/diagnostics10121086.

Lindenmeyer, C. C. (2020). *Acute cholecystitis. Merck Manual Professional Version.* https://www.merckmanuals.com/professional/hepatic-and-biliary-disorders/gallbladder-and-bile-duct-disorders/acute-cholecystitis?query=Cholecystitis.

National Cancer Institute. (2023). National Institute of Health. Pancreatic cancer treatment (Adult)(PDQ)-Health Professional Version. https://www.cancer.gov/types/pancreatic/hp/pancreatic-treatment-pdq.

Noel, M., & Fiscella, K. (2019). Disparities in pancreatic cancer treatment and outcomes. *Health Equity, 3*(1), 532–540.

Okamoto, A., Watanabe, T., Kamata, K., Minaga, K., & Kudo, M. (2019). Recent Updates on the Relationship between Cancer and Autoimmune Pancreatitis. *Internal Medicine (Tokyo, Japan), 58*(11), 1533–1539. https://doi.org/10.2169/internalmedicine.2210-18.

Pagana, K. D., Pagana, T. J., & Pagana, T. N. (2022). *Mosby's Manual of diagnostic and laboratory tests* (7th ed.). Elsevier Health Sciences (US).

Rawla, P., Sunkara, T., & Gaduputi, V. (2019). Epidemiology of pancreatic cancer: global trends, etiology and risk factors. *World Journal of Oncology, 10*(1), 10–27. https://doi.org/10.14740/wjon1166.

Roberts, K. E., & Kate, V. (2020). *Transvaginal cholecystectomy.* http://emedicine.medscape.com/article/1900692.

Rogers, J. L. (2023). *McCance and Huether's Pathophysiology: The biologic basis for disease in adults and children* (9th ed.). St. Louis: Elsevier.

Springfeld, C., Jäger, D., Büchler, M. W., Strobel, O., Hackert, T., Palmer, D. H., & Neoptolemos, J. P. (2019). Chemotherapy for pancreatic cancer. *Presse medicale (Paris, France : 1983), 48*(3 Pt 2), e159–e174. https://doi.org/10.1016/j.lpm.2019.02.025.

Zakko, S. F. (2020). Patient education: Gallstones (beyond the basics). *UpToDate.* Retrieved September 15, 2022, from https://www.uptodate.com/contents/gallstones-beyond-the-basics#H8.

52

Concepts of Care for Patients With Malnutrition: Undernutrition and Obesity

Cherie R. Rebar

http://evolve.elsevier.com/Iggy/

LEARNING OUTCOMES

1. Plan collaborative care with the interprofessional team to promote **nutrition** in patients with malnutrition.
2. Teach adults how to decrease the risk for malnutrition.
3. Teach the patient and caregiver(s) about common drugs and other management strategies used for malnutrition.
4. Plan patient- and family-centered nursing interventions to decrease the psychosocial impact caused by living with malnutrition.
5. Apply knowledge of anatomy, physiology, and pathophysiology to provide evidence-based care for patients with malnutrition affecting **fluid and electrolyte balance** and **nutrition.**
6. Analyze assessment and diagnostic findings to generate solutions and prioritize nursing care for patients with malnutrition.
7. Organize care coordination and transition management for patients with malnutrition.
8. Use clinical judgment to plan evidence-based nursing care to promote **fluid and electrolyte balance** and **nutrition** and prevent complications in patients with malnutrition.
9. Incorporate factors that affect health equity into the plan of care for patients with malnutrition.

KEY TERMS

anorexia Loss of appetite for food.

anorexia nervosa Eating disorder of self-induced starvation resulting from a fear of fatness, even though the patient is underweight.

bariatrics Branch of medicine that manages patients with obesity and its related diseases.

binge eating disorder Eating disorder that involves eating in binges with a feeling of loss of control over the eating behavior.

body mass index (BMI) Measure of nutritional status that does not depend on frame size; indirectly estimates total fat stores within the body by the relationship of weight to height.

body surface area (BSA) Calculated estimate of a person's total body surface area reflecting physiologic and metabolic processes including heat exchange, blood volume, and size of vital organs. Used as an indicator for appropriate dosage calculation, especially for anticancer agents.

bolus feeding Method of tube feeding that involves intermittent feeding of a specified amount of enteral product at specified times during a 24-hour period, typically every 4 hours.

bulimia nervosa Eating disorder characterized by episodes of binge eating in which the patient ingests a large amount of food in a short time, followed by purging behavior, such as self-induced vomiting or excessive use of laxatives and diuretics.

cachexia Extreme body wasting and malnutrition that develop from an imbalance between food intake and energy use.

continuous feeding Method of tube feeding in which small amounts of enteral product are continuously infused (by gravity drip or by a pump or controller device) over a specified time.

cyclic feeding Method of tube feeding similar to continuous feeding (see definition of continuous feeding) except the infusion is stopped for a specified time in each 24-hour period ("down time"); the down time typically occurs in the morning to allow bathing, treatments, and other activities.

dietary reference intakes (DRIs) Nutritional guide developed by the Institute of Medicine of the National Academies that provides a scientific basis for food guidelines in the United States and Canada.

dumping syndrome Vasomotor symptoms that typically occur within 30 minutes after eating, including vertigo, tachycardia, syncope, sweating, pallor/ash gray skin, and palpitations.

enterostomal feeding tube Tube used for patients who need long-term enteral feeding.

food allergy Reaction to a food (or multiple foods), rooted in the immune system, that can cause a life-threatening complication such as anaphylaxis.

food intolerance Inability to tolerate a food (or multiple foods), rooted in the gastrointestinal system when a food cannot be properly broken down.

gastric bypass Type of gastric restriction surgery in which gastric resection is combined with malabsorption surgery. The patient's stomach, duodenum, and part of the jejunum are bypassed so that fewer calories can be absorbed. Also known as a *Roux-en-Y gastric bypass,* or *RNYGB.*

gastrostomy Stoma created from the abdominal wall into the stomach.

jejunostomy Surgical creation of an opening between the jejunum and surface of the abdominal wall.

knee height caliper Device that uses the distance between the patient's patella and heel to estimate height.

kwashiorkor Lack of protein quantity and quality in the presence of adequate calories. Body weight is more normal, and serum proteins are low.

lactose intolerance Type of food intolerance when a patient has an inadequate amount of lactase enzyme, which converts lactose into absorbable glucose.

malnutrition Deficiencies, excesses, or imbalances in a person's intake of energy and/or nutrients.

marasmus Calorie malnutrition in which body fat and protein are wasted and serum proteins are often preserved.

medical nutrition supplements Enteral products (e.g., Ensure, Boost) taken by patients who cannot or do not consume enough nutrients in their usual diet.

nasoduodenal tube (NDT) Tube inserted through a nostril and into the small intestine.

nasoenteric tube (NET) Feeding tube inserted nasally and then advanced into the gastrointestinal tract.

nasogastric (NG) tube Tube inserted through a nostril and into the stomach for liquid feeding or for withdrawing gastric contents.

nutrition screening Assessment of nutrition status that includes inspection, measured height and weight, weight history, usual eating habits, ability to chew and swallow, and any recent changes in appetite or food intake.

obesity Increase in body weight at least 20% above the upper limit of the normal range for ideal body weight, with an excess amount of body fat; in an adult, a body mass index greater than 30. Subdivided into Class I, II, or III.

overweight Increase in body weight for height compared with a reference standard (e.g., the Metropolitan Life height and weight tables) or 10% greater than ideal body weight. However, the weights listed in such tables may not reflect excess body fat, which in an adult is a body mass index of 25 to 29.9.

panniculectomy Surgical removal of the abdominal apron (panniculus).

percutaneous endoscopic gastrostomy (PEG) Stoma created from the abdominal wall into the stomach for insertion of a short feeding tube.

protein-energy undernutrition (PEU) Nutritional disorder that may present in three forms: marasmus, kwashiorkor, and marasmic-kwashiorkor. Also called *protein-calorie malnutrition.*

refeeding syndrome Life-threatening metabolic complication that can occur when nutrition is restarted for a patient who is in a starvation state.

skinfold measurements Estimation of body fat, usually calculated through measurement of the triceps and subscapular skinfolds with a special caliper.

starvation Complete lack of nutrients.

total parenteral nutrition (TPN) Provision of intensive nutritional support for an extended time; delivered to the patient through access to central veins, usually the subclavian or internal jugular veins.

undernutrition State of wasting, stunting, and being underweight.

⁂ PRIORITY AND INTERRELATED CONCEPTS

The priority concept for this chapter is:
- *Nutrition*

The interrelated concept for this chapter is:
- *Fluid and Electrolyte Balance*

  The *Nutrition* concept exemplars for this chapter are Undernutrition and Obesity.

To function well, the body needs adequate *nutrition* to grow; maintain temperature, approximate respirations, and cardiac output; and facilitate muscle strength, protein synthesis, and storage and metabolism. In healthy adults, most energy supplied by carbohydrates, protein, and fat undergoes digestion and is absorbed from the GI tract. The relationship between energy used and energy stored is referred to as *energy balance.* Weight is gained when food intake is more than energy used, and weight loss occurs when energy used is more than intake. The body attempts to meet its calorie requirements even if it is at the expense of protein needs; when calorie intake is insufficient, body proteins are used for energy.

Influenced by personal preference, demographic location, cultural norms, spiritual observations, financial feasibility, and availability of nutritional sources, *nutrition* status varies for each patient. Further influencing factors include age, height, weight, gender, speed of metabolism, influence of exercise or activity, medications taken, substances used (e.g., alcohol or illicit drugs), and types of fluids consumed. The estimated energy requirement (EER) ranges from 1600 to 3200 calories per day for healthy adults; age, sex, height, weight, and level of activity are considered when a personalized eating plan is created (U.S. Department of Agriculture, 2023; U.S. Department of Agriculture and U.S. Department of Health and Human Services, 2020). The caloric requirement may decrease if a patient needs to lose weight or increase if the patient needs to gain weight or promote healing.

> ### BOX 52.1   2020–2025 Dietary Guidelines for Americans
>
> - Follow a healthy eating pattern at every life stage.
> - Customize and enjoy nutrient-dense food and beverage choices to reflect personal preferences, cultural traditions, and budgetary considerations.
> - Focus on meeting food group needs with nutrient-dense foods and beverages, and stay within calorie limits.
> - Limit foods and beverages higher in added sugars, saturated fat, and sodium, and limit alcoholic beverages.

From U.S. Department of Agriculture and U.S. Department of Health and Human Services. (2020). *Dietary Guidelines for Americans 2020-2025* (9th ed.). https://www.dietaryguidelines.gov/sites/default/files/2020-12/Dietary_Guidelines_for_Americans_2020-2025.pdf.

GENERAL NUTRITION RECOMMENDATIONS FOR HEALTH PROMOTION/DISEASE PREVENTION

Current attention on *nutrition* is focused on health promotion and the prevention of disease by healthy eating and exercise. Dietary reference intakes (DRIs) based on age, gender, and life stage serve as a *nutrition* guide for more than 40 nutrients and provide a scientific basis for food guidelines in the United States and Canada (National Academies of Sciences, Engineering, & Medicine, n.d.). In the United States, the *Dietary Guidelines for Americans* are revised by the U.S. Department of Agriculture (USDA) and the U.S. Department of Health and Human Services (USDHHS) every 5 years. Examples of the *2020-2025 Guidelines* (9th edition) are listed in Box 52.1.

"Start Simple with MyPlate" is an initiative that reminds users about building healthy eating habits into a lifestyle (U.S. Department of Agriculture, 2022) (Fig. 52.1). This pictorial demonstrates how to build a healthy plate of food, consisting of the right proportions of fruits, vegetables, grains, proteins, and dairy products. Canada publishes Canada's Food Guide (Government of Canada, 2023), a similar visual reference.

Common Diets

Given the variance in people's preferences, place of residence, availability of foods, financial means, cultural or spiritual observations, and financial circumstances, there is not a specific "typical (or common) diet." Some people consume a highly nutrient-rich diet and remain adequately hydrated with water. Others eat excess foods heavy in fats or carbohydrates and choose to drink soda or juice on a regular basis, which can lead to obesity. Others do not have adequate access to nutrient-dense food and hydration and may experience undernutrition. Individuals with obesity or undernutrition both experience malnutrition in different ways, as the state of malnutrition occurs on a continuum.

In ideal circumstances, patients should consume a diet containing complex carbohydrates, lean proteins, and monounsaturated or polyunsaturated fats that also contains necessary vitamins and minerals. The specific foods you recommend to patients to meet their nutritional needs depends on the variances mentioned earlier.

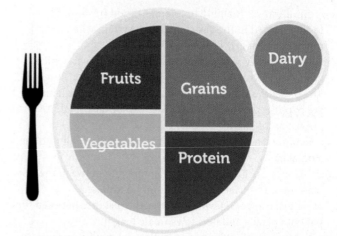

FIG. 52.1 The U.S. Department of Agriculture MyPlate. (From U.S. Department of Agriculture, 2023, www.ChooseMyPlate.gov; https://www.myplate.gov/eat-healthy/what-is-myplate; https://myplate-prod.azureedge.us/sites/default/files/2022-01/SSwMP%20Mini-Poster_English_Final2022.pdf.)

Some adults follow vegetarian diet patterns for health, environmental, religious, cultural, or spiritual reasons (Box 52.2).

People who eat a vegan diet can develop anemia as a result of a vitamin B_{12} deficiency. Teach people who are vegans to include a daily source of vitamin B_{12} in their diets, such as a fortified breakfast cereal, fortified soy beverage, or meat substitute. Refer those interested in vegetarianism to www.eatright.org, which contains many credible resources regarding vegetarian health (Academy of Nutrition and Dietetics, 2023).

> ### 🔲 PATIENT-CENTERED CARE: CULTURE AND SPIRITUALITY
> #### Food Preferences
>
> Many adults have specific food preferences based on their ethnicity or race. Health teaching about *nutrition* should incorporate any cultural preferences voiced by the patient. Never assume what a patient's preferences will be. Always ask the patient when providing care.

FOOD SENSITIVITIES

Some adults have food allergies or intolerances. A true food allergy differs from a food intolerance in the sense that an allergy to a food can cause life-threatening complications such as anaphylaxis. A food allergy is rooted in the immune system. The most common food allergies are nuts, peanuts, and shellfish (Rogers, 2023). A food intolerance involves the gastrointestinal system and occurs when the system cannot properly break down food (American Academy of Allergy, Asthma, and Immunology, 2023).

An example of a food allergy is shellfish, which can cause coughing; edema (face, lips, tongue, throat); shortness of breath; or anaphylaxis in certain patients. An example of a food intolerance is lactose intolerance, in which a patient has an inadequate amount of the lactase enzyme, which converts lactose into absorbable glucose. Ingesting a milk product causes bloating,

BOX 52.2 Vegetarian Types

Lacto-vegetarian—allows dairy[a]; avoids meat, poultry, seafood, eggs, and foods that contain those items
Ovo-vegetarian—allows eggs; avoids meat, poultry, seafood, and dairy[a]
Lacto-ovo vegetarian—allows eggs and dairy[a]; avoids meat, poultry, seafood
Pescatarian—allows fish; avoids meat, poultry, dairy,[a] eggs
Vegan—consumes a plant-based diet only; avoids meat, poultry, seafood, dairy,[a] eggs, and foods that contain those items. (**NOTE:** Some people who eat a vegan diet also avoid honey.)

[a] Dairy = milk, cheese, yogurt, butter, etc.

PATIENT-CENTERED CARE: OLDER ADULT HEALTH

Preventing Constipation

The USDA (2022) recommends that older adults consume plenty of water and fiber to prevent or manage constipation. In addition to water, beverage choices can include unsweetened fruit or vegetable juice, low-fat or fat-free milk, or fortified soy beverages.

diarrhea, abdominal discomfort, and flatulence. When taking a history, ask patients specifically what kind of reaction they have to certain foods; document and plan care accordingly.

NUTRITION ASSESSMENT

Nutrition status reflects the balance between nutrient requirements and intake. Evaluation of nutritional status is an important part of total patient assessment and includes:
- Review of the nutritional history
- Food and fluid intake record
- Notation of access to appropriate sources of nutrition
- Laboratory data
- Food-drug interactions
- Health history and physical assessment
- Anthropometric measurements
- Psychosocial assessment

Monitor the *nutrition* status of a patient during hospitalization as an important part of your initial assessment. Collaborate with the interprofessional health care team to identify patients at risk for nutritional problems.

Initial Nutrition Screening

The Joint Commission Patient Care Standards require that a nutrition screening occur within 24 hours of the patient's hospital admission, with a full nutritional assessment for patients identified as being at risk (The Joint Commission, 2022). The initial screening includes inspection, measured height and weight, weight history, usual eating habits, ability to chew and swallow, and any recent changes in appetite or food intake.

The Full MNA® Form (Mini Nutritional Assessment) (Fig. 52.2) is a helpful and brief screening tool that can assist in identifying older adults who are malnourished or at risk for undernutrition. An even shorter version—the MNA®, which refers

BOX 52.3 Best Practice for Patient Safety and Quality Care

Nutrition Screening Assessment

General
- Does the patient have conditions that cause nutrient loss (e.g., malabsorption syndromes, wounds, prolonged diarrhea)
- Does the patient have conditions that increase the need for nutrients (e.g., fever, burns, injury)
- Has the patient been NPO for 3 days or more?
- Is the patient receiving a modified diet or a diet restricted in one or more nutrients?
- Is the patient being enterally or parenterally fed?
- Does the patient describe food allergies, lactose intolerance, or limited food preferences?
- Has the patient experienced a recent unexplained weight loss?
- Is the patient on drug therapy, including prescription, over-the-counter, or herbal/natural products?

Gastrointestinal
- Does the patient have glossitis, stomatitis, or esophagitis?
- Does the patient have difficulty chewing or swallowing or have poor dentition?
- Does the patient have a partial or total GI obstruction?
- Does the patient report nausea, indigestion, vomiting, diarrhea, or constipation?
- Does the patient have an ostomy?

Cardiovascular
- Does the patient have ascites or edema?
- Is the patient able to perform ADLs?
- Does the patient have heart failure?

Genitourinary
- Is fluid intake about equal to fluid output?
- Is the patient hemodialyzed or peritoneally dialyzed?

Respiratory
- Is the patient receiving oxygen or on mechanical ventilatory support?
- Does the patient have chronic obstructive pulmonary disease (COPD) or asthma?

Integumentary
- Does the patient have abnormal skin, nail, or hair changes?
- Does the patient have rashes or dermatitis?
- Does the patient have dry or pale mucous membranes or decreased skin turgor?
- Does the patient have pressure injuries?

Musculoskeletal
- Does the patient have cachexia?

Modified Courtesy Ross Products Division, Abbott Laboratories, Columbus, OH.

to the Mini Nutritional Assessment–Short Form (formerly the MNA®-SF) (Nestle Nutrition Institute, n.d.)—is also available for use in the clinical setting. Another tool that is available is the Adult Malnutrition Screening and Nutrition Intervention (Fig. 52.3).

See Box 52.3 for examples of questions to consider as part of the initial assessment.

Mini Nutritional Assessment
MNA®

Nestlé
NutritionInstitute

Last name:	First name:

Sex:	Age:	Weight, kg:	Height, cm:	Date:

Complete the screen by filling in the boxes with the appropriate numbers.
Add the numbers for the screen. If score is 11 or less, continue with the assessment to gain a Malnutrition Indicator Score.

Screening

A Has food intake declined over the past 3 months due to loss of appetite, digestive problems, chewing or swallowing difficulties?
0 = severe decrease in food intake
1 = moderate decrease in food intake
2 = no decrease in food intake ☐

B Weight loss during the last 3 months
0 = weight loss greater than 3kg (6.6lbs)
1 = does not know
2 = weight loss between 1 and 3kg (2.2 and 6.6 lbs)
3 = no weight loss ☐

C Mobility
0 = bed or chair bound
1 = able to get out of bed / chair but does not go out
2 = goes out ☐

D Has suffered psychological stress or acute disease in the past 3 months?
0 = yes   2 = no ☐

E Neuropsychological problems
0 = severe dementia or depression
1 = mild dementia
2 = no psychological problems ☐

F Body Mass Index (BMI) = weight in kg / (height in m)^2
0 = BMI less than 19
1 = BMI 19 to less than 21
2 = BMI 21 to less than 23
3 = BMI 23 or greater ☐

Screening score (subtotal max. 14 points) ☐☐

12-14 points:	Normal nutritional status
8-11 points:	At risk of malnutrition
0-7 points:	Malnourished

For a more in-depth assessment, continue with questions G-R

Assessment

G Lives independently (not in nursing home or hospital)
1 = yes   0 = no ☐

H Takes more than 3 prescription drugs per day
0 = yes   1 = no ☐

I Pressure sores or skin ulcers
0 = yes   1 = no ☐

J How many full meals does the patient eat daily?
0 = 1 meal
1 = 2 meals
2 = 3 meals ☐

K Selected consumption markers for protein intake
• At least one serving of dairy products (milk, cheese, yoghurt) per day   yes ☐ no ☐
• Two or more servings of legumes or eggs per week   yes ☐ no ☐
• Meat, fish or poultry every day   yes ☐ no ☐
0.0 = if 0 or 1 yes
0.5 = if 2 yes
1.0 = if 3 yes ☐.☐

L Consumes two or more servings of fruit or vegetables per day?
0 = no   1 = yes ☐

M How much fluid (water, juice, coffee, tea, milk...) is consumed per day?
0.0 = less than 3 cups
0.5 = 3 to 5 cups
1.0 = more than 5 cups ☐.☐

N Mode of feeding
0 = unable to eat without assistance
1 = self-fed with some difficulty
2 = self-fed without any problem ☐

O Self view of nutritional status
0 = views self as being malnourished
1 = is uncertain of nutritional state
2 = views self as having no nutritional problem ☐

P In comparison with other people of the same age, how does the patient consider his / her health status?
0.0 = not as good
0.5 = does not know
1.0 = as good
2.0 = better ☐.☐

Q Mid-arm circumference (MAC) in cm
0.0 = MAC less than 21
0.5 = MAC 21 to 22
1.0 = MAC greater than 22 ☐.☐

R Calf circumference (CC) in cm
0 = CC less than 31
1 = CC 31 or greater ☐

Assessment (max. 16 points) ☐☐.☐
Screening score ☐☐.☐
Total Assessment (max. 30 points) ☐☐.☐

Malnutrition Indicator Score

24 to 30 points	☐	Normal nutritional status
17 to 23.5 points	☐	At risk of malnutrition
Less than 17 points	☐	Malnourished

References
1. Vellas B, Villars H, Abellan G, *et al.* Overview of the MNA® - Its History and Challenges. *J Nutr Health Aging.* 2006; **10:456**-465.
2. Rubenstein LZ, Harker JO, Salva A, Guigoz Y, Vellas B. Screening for Undernutrition in Geriatric Practice: Developing the Short-Form Mini Nutritional Assessment (MNA-SF). *J. Geront.* 2001; **56A**: M366-377
3. Guigoz Y. The Mini-Nutritional Assessment (MNA®) Review of the Literature - What does it tell us? *J Nutr Health Aging.* 2006; **10:**466-487.

For more information: www.mna-elderly.com

FIG. 52.2 Full MNA® Form (Mini Nutritional Assessment). (Société des Produits Nestlé S.A., Vevey, Switzerland, Trademark Owners.)

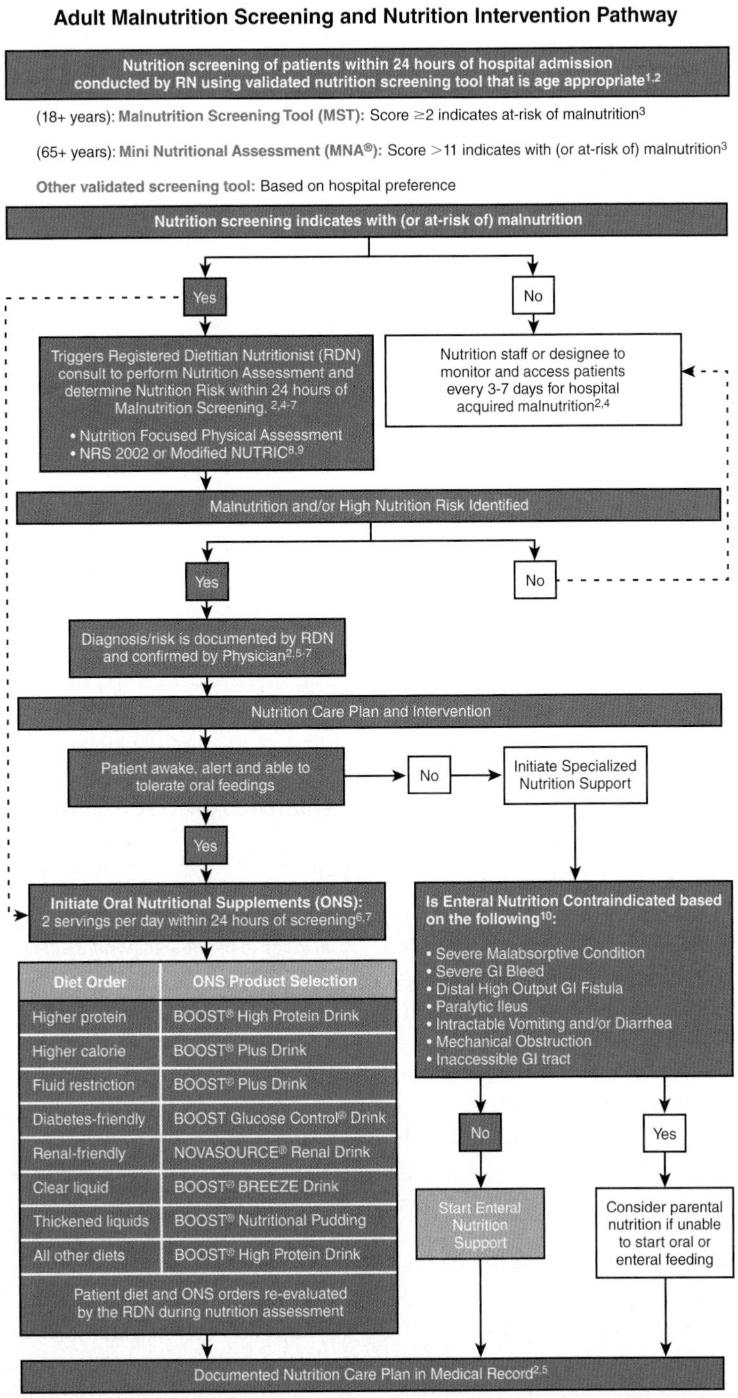

Adult Malnutrition Screening and Nutrition Intervention Pathway

FIG. 52.3 Adult Malnutrition Screening and Nutrition Intervention Pathway. (From Nestle Health Science. Copyright © 2019. https://www.nestlemedicalhub.com/sites/site.prod.nestlemedicalhub.com/files/2020-04/Adult%20Malnutrition%20Screening%20and%20Intervention%20PATHWAY_122019%20FINAL.pdf.)

Anthropometric Measurements

Anthropometric measurements are noninvasive methods of evaluating **nutrition** status. These measurements include obtaining height and weight and assessment of body mass index (BMI). You may delegate the task of obtaining height and weight to assistive personnel (AP) under your supervision, as this is within their scope. Be sure to instruct the AP to follow up with measurements as soon as this activity is completed, as this information affects the plan of care.

Obtaining accurate measurements is important because patients tend to overestimate height and underestimate weight. Measurements taken days or weeks later may indicate an early change in **nutrition** status. Follow agency policy or the primary health care provider's orders for frequency of measurement.

Measure and weigh patients with the same scale and with the same amount of clothing (without shoes) each time. A sliding-blade knee height caliper, which uses the distance between the patient's patella and heel to estimate height, can be used for those who cannot stand. It is especially useful for patients who have knee or hip contractures.

The type of scale used depends on the patient's ability to stand or sit; wheelchair scales or bed scales can be used for nonambulatory individuals. When using a bed scale, document the number of sheets, pillows, and blankets on the bed at the time of measurement. Lines, devices, and equipment should be lifted off the bed when the measurement is taking place. Normal weights for adult men and women are available from several reference standards, such as the Metropolitan Life tables. Online calculators are also available to calculate ideal body weight. *An unintentional weight loss of 5% in a month or 10% over a 6-month period significantly affects **nutrition** status and should be evaluated.*

> ### ! NURSING SAFETY PRIORITY
> **Action Alert**
>
> Obtain weight at the same time each day, if possible, preferably before breakfast. Conditions such as heart failure and renal disease cause weight gain; dehydration and conditions such as cancer cause weight loss. *Weight is the most reliable indicator of fluid gain or loss!*

Assessment of body fat is usually calculated by the registered dietitian nutritionist (RDN) if in a hospital setting or by a fitness trainer or physical therapist in the community setting. The body mass index (BMI) indirectly estimates total fat stores within the body by the relationship of weight to height (Table 52.1). *For this reason, obtaining an accurate height is as important as an accurate weight.* Online calculators can perform this computation, which divides a patient's weight in kilograms by the square of height in meters. The least risk for malnutrition is associated with scores between 18.5 and 24.9. BMIs above and below these values are associated with increased health risks (CDC, 2022a).

Limitations of BMI calculations include (Harvard T.H. Chan School of Public Health, 2023b; Simpson, 2021):

- Indirect and imperfect measurements, as it does not distinguish between body fat and lean body mass
- Inability to accurately predict body fat in older adults
- Inability to account for sex assigned at birth and racial differences (e.g., women usually have more body fat than men; people of Asian ethnicity usually have more body fat than people of other races [Harvard T.H. Chan School of Public Health, 2023a])

Body surface area (BSA) is an estimate of a patient's total body surface area. It reflects multiple physiologic and metabolic processes (Flint & Hall, 2022). BSA can be used as an indicator for appropriate dosage calculation for medication and IV administration, especially for anticancer agents, and to estimate the degree of severity in patients who have been significantly burned (Eaton & Lyman, 2022; Flint & Hall, 2022).

BSA is calculated in meters squared, combining a patient's weight and height and reflecting an estimate of their total surface (outside body layer) area (Eaton & Lyman, 2022). If a

TABLE 52.1   Body Mass Index (BMI) Ranges

BMI	Weight Status
Below 18.5	Underweight
18.5–24.9	Normal or healthy weight
25.0–29.9	Overweight
30.0 and above	Obese

From Centers for Disease Control and Prevention (CDC). (2022b). *Defining adult overweight & obesity.* https://www.cdc.gov/obesity/basics/adult-defining.html.

> ### 👤 PATIENT-CENTERED CARE: OLDER ADULT HEALTH
> **Eating Habits**
>
> Body weight and BMI usually increase throughout adulthood until about 60 years of age. As some adults get older, they often become less hungry and eat less, even if they are healthy. Others continue usual eating patterns and are at higher risk for obesity—especially older adult females (CDC, 2022a). Do not assume that an older adult automatically eats less; personalize the nutritional assessment to accurately assess eating patterns for every patient.

> ### NCLEX Examination Challenge 52.1
> **Health Promotion and Maintenance**
>
> An older adult is admitted to the hospital. The client's height is 5 feet, 8 inches (1.73 m), and weight is 272 lb (123.4 kg). The nurse calculates the client's current body mass index (BMI) as _____. **Fill in the blank. Round your answer to the nearest whole number.**

patient has a BSA of 3 m², it means that the patient's skin surface could be placed into a 3-meter × 3-meter box.

Calculate BSA by the Mosteller formula, which takes the square root of the height in centimeters, multiplied by the weight in kilograms, divided by 3600. The average BSA is 1.9 m² for males and 1.6 m² for females (Omni, 2022). Be aware that accurate calculation of weight is imperative, as height is unlikely to change significantly, but weight is variable.

Skinfold measurements estimate body fat. The *triceps and subscapular* skinfolds are most commonly measured with a special caliper. Both are compared with standard measurements and recorded as percentiles. The *midarm circumference (MAC) and calf circumference (CC)* are needed if the full MNA® or the MNA® tool is used. Place a flexible tape around the upper arm (or calf) at the midpoint; wrap gently to avoid compressing the tissue, and record the findings in centimeters in the electronic health record.

✴ NUTRITION CONCEPT EXEMPLAR: UNDERNUTRITION

Pathophysiology Review

Undernutrition is a multinutrient problem. If a patient does not, or cannot, consume calories and protein, intake of healthy nutrients is compromised. Inadequate nutrient intake can also result when an adult is admitted to the hospital or long-term

PATIENT-CENTERED CARE: CULTURE AND SPIRITUALITY

Meals in the Health Care Setting

In some cases, undernutrition results when meals provided in the health care setting differ from what the patient usually eats. Be sure to identify specific food preferences that the patient can eat and enjoy that are in keeping with personal cultural practices.

BOX 52.4 Common Complications of Undernutrition

Cardiovascular
- Reduced cardiac output

Endocrine
- Cold intolerance

Gastrointestinal
- Anorexia
- Diarrhea
- Impaired protein synthesis
- Malabsorption
- Vomiting
- Weight loss

Immunologic
- Susceptibility to infectious disease

Integumentary
- Dry, flaky skin
- Various types of dermatitis
- Poor wound healing

Musculoskeletal
- Cachexia
- Decreased activity tolerance
- Decreased muscle mass
- Impaired functional ability

Neurologic
- Weakness

Psychiatric
- Substance misuse

Respiratory
- Reduced vital capacity

care facility. For example, decreased staffing may not allow time for patients who need to be fed, especially older adults, who may eat slowly. Many diagnostic tests, surgery, trauma, and unexpected medical complications require a period of NPO in which nutrients are not being consumed or cause anorexia (loss of appetite). See Box 52.4 for common complications of undernutrition and Table 52.2 for common signs and symptoms of nutrient deficiencies. See Box 52.5 for concerns when assessing undernutrition in the older adult.

Etiology and Genetic Risk

The etiology of undernutrition is multifactorial and dependent on the specific type of undernutrition experienced. Protein-energy undernutrition (PEU), formerly protein-calorie malnutrition (PCM), has two common forms (Morley, 2022):

- Marasmus: A calorie malnutrition in which body fat and protein are wasted. Serum proteins are often preserved.
- Kwashiorkor: A lack of protein quantity and quality in the presence of adequate calories. Body weight is more normal, and serum proteins are low.

Starvation, a complete lack of nutrients, is an acute and severe form of PEU, which usually occurs when food is unavailable (e.g., during a time of famine or exposure to the

TABLE 52.2 Signs and Symptoms of Nutrient Deficiencies

Sign/Symptom	Potential Nutrient Deficiency
Hair	
Alopecia	Zinc
Easy to remove	Protein
Lackluster hair	Protein
"Corkscrew" hair	Vitamin C
Decreased pigmentation	Protein
Eyes	
Dryness of conjunctiva	Vitamin A
Corneal vascularization	Riboflavin
Keratomalacia	Vitamin A
Bitot spots (keratin buildup in the conjunctiva)	Vitamin A
GI Tract	
Nausea, vomiting	Pyridoxine
Diarrhea	Zinc, niacin
Stomatitis	Pyridoxine, riboflavin, iron
Cheilosis	Pyridoxine, iron
Glossitis	Pyridoxine, zinc, niacin, folic acid, vitamin B_{12}
Magenta tongue	Vitamin A, riboflavin
Swollen, bleeding gums	Vitamin C
Fissured tongue	Niacin
Hepatomegaly	Protein
Skin	
Dry and scaling	Vitamin A
Petechiae/ecchymoses	Vitamin C
Follicular hyperkeratosis	Vitamin A
Nasolabial seborrhea	Niacin
Bilateral dermatitis	Niacin
Musculoskeletal	
Subcutaneous fat loss	Calories
Muscle wastage	Calories, protein
Edema	Protein
Osteomalacia, bone pain, rickets	Vitamin D
Hematologic	
Anemia	Vitamin B_{12}, iron, folic acid, copper, vitamin E
Leukopenia, neutropenia	Copper
Low prothrombin time, prolonged clotting time	Vitamin K, manganese
Neurologic	
Disorientation	Niacin, thiamine
Confabulation	Thiamine
Neuropathy	Thiamine, pyridoxine, chromium
Paresthesia	Thiamine, pyridoxine, vitamin B_{12}
Cardiovascular	
Heart failure, cardiomegaly, tachycardia	Thiamine
Cardiomyopathy	Selenium
Cardiac dysrhythmias	Magnesium

Courtesy Ross Products Division, Abbott Laboratories, Columbus, OH.

BOX 52.5 Assessing the Older Adult for Undernutrition

Ask the older adult about signs or symptoms that could indicate undernutrition.

Physical Concerns

- Chronic conditions/illnesses
- Constipation
- Decreased appetite
- Dentition—poor dental health; poor-fitting dentures; lack of teeth or dentures
- Drugs—prescription and OTC drugs that may impair taste or appetite
- Dry mouth
- "Failure to thrive" (a combination of three of five symptoms, including weakness, slow walking speed, low physical activity, unintentional weight loss, exhaustion)
- Impaired eyesight
- Pain that is acute or persistent
- Weight loss

Psychosocial Concerns

- Inability to prepare meals due to functional decline, fatigue, knowledge deficit, memory
- Decrease in enjoyment of meals
- Depression
- Income (ability to afford food)
- Loneliness
- Proximity to sources of nutrient-dense foods (e.g., grocery store)
- Transportation access to get to sources of nutrient-dense foods

elements) (Morley, 2022). Unrecognized or untreated PEU can lead to dysfunction or disability and increased morbidity and mortality.

Acute PEU may develop in patients who were adequately nourished before hospitalization but experience starvation while in a catabolic state from infection, stress, or injury. *Chronic* PEU can occur in those who have a chronic health condition such as cancer, end-stage kidney or liver disease, or chronic neurologic disease.

Eating disorders such as anorexia nervosa, bulimia nervosa, and binge eating disorder are psychiatric diagnoses with causative agents of psychiatric origin. These conditions can lead to a state of undernutrition. Anorexia nervosa is a self-induced state of starvation resulting from a fear of fatness, even though the patient is underweight. This condition is often accompanied by a psychiatric diagnosis of *body dysmorphic disorder* (BDD). BDD is an obsessive-compulsive condition in which patients spend an abnormal amount of time attempting to reach what they consider to be body perfection. In the case of a patient with anorexia nervosa, perfection is found in being thin. The condition affects the patient's ability to carry out normal ADLs and significantly impacts quality of life (Phillips, 2022; Perkins, 2019). If this condition is suspected, collaborate with the primary health care provider to determine whether a psychiatric consultation is needed. Bulimia nervosa is characterized by episodes of binge eating in which the patient ingests a large amount of food in a short time. The binge eating is followed by some form of purging behavior, such as self-induced vomiting

or excessive use of laxatives and diuretics. If not treated, death can result from starvation, infection, or suicide. Binge eating disorder is a separate psychiatric diagnosis from bulimia nervosa. It resembles bulimia nervosa in terms of binge-eating episodes, and it involves a feeling of loss of control over the eating behavior (Office on Women's Health, 2022); however, it is not accompanied by purging. Again, collaborate with the primary health care provider if this condition is suspected. Further information about eating disorders can be found in mental health nursing textbooks.

Incidence and Prevalence

Globally, there are about 462 million people who are underweight (World Health Organization, 2021). Data are difficult to collect regarding patients who are malnourished, as they are seen in a variety of settings for multiple concerns, many of which are perceived to be unrelated to *nutrition*.

PATIENT-CENTERED CARE: OLDER ADULT HEALTH

Protein-Energy Undernutrition

Older adults are most at risk for poor *nutrition*, especially PEU. Risk factors include physiologic changes of aging, environmental factors, and health problems. See Box 52.5, Assessing the Older Adult for Undernutrition, which lists some of the major factors for which you will assess. If psychosocial concerns are present, collaborate with mental health or social work professionals who can assist. Chapter 4 discusses nutrition for older adults in more detail.

INTERPROFESSIONAL COLLABORATION

Care of Older Adults at Risk for Undernutrition

For older adults with undernutrition or at risk for undernutrition, assess for psychosocial concerns that can impact their desire or ability to consume nutrient-rich foods. If any of these concerns is rooted in mental health, such as depression or loneliness, collaborate with a mental health professional, such as a counselor or psychiatric–mental health nurse practitioner, who can work with the patient to enhance emotional well-being. If the concerns are economic or access-related, collaborate with the case manager or social worker, who can help identify ways to facilitate better access to sources of nutrition. According to the Interprofessional Education Collaborative (IPEC) Expert Panel's Competency of Roles and Responsibilities, using the unique and complementary abilities of other team members optimizes health and patient care (IPEC, 2016; Slusser et al., 2019).

Health Promotion/Disease Prevention

It is estimated that 50% to 71% of older adult patients are malnourished before hospital admission (Bellanti et al., 2022; Ritchie & Yukawa, 2023). It is also thought that one-third of nourished older adults who are admitted will develop some degree of malnutrition during hospitalization (Bellanti et al., 2022).

Status of *nutrition* may vary based on prehospitalization status, intake during a current illness or injury, and accurate assessment and intervention of health care professionals. Malnourishment can increase the length of the patient's stay and contribute to the rate of readmission. Nurses can have a significant impact on a patient's length of stay when adequately advocating for the patient's nutritional status. (See the Systems Thinking/Quality Improvement box.)

 INTERPROFESSIONAL COLLABORATION

The Patient With Undernutrition

For patients with undernutrition, consult with a registered dietitian nutritionist (RDN), who can assist with meeting nutritional needs while the patient is hospitalized, as well as help with planning for continued nutritional health after discharge. According to the Interprofessional Education Collaborative (IPEC) Expert Panel's Competency of Roles and Responsibilities, using the unique and complementary abilities of other team members optimizes health and patient care (IPEC, 2016; Slusser et al., 2019).

⊳⊳ **SYSTEMS THINKING/QUALITY IMPROVEMENT**

An Interprofessional Focus on Preventing Readmissions for Patients at High Risk for Malnutrition

Beckett, C., & Walsh, S. (2019). The malnutrition readmission prevention protocol. *American Journal of Nursing, 119*(12):60–64.

Reflecting on the fact that malnutrition affects one in three hospitalized patients, the authors of this study desired to put an evidence-based protocol in place to improve patient outcomes and avoid reduced reimbursement associated with 30-day malnutrition-related readmissions. Nurses, the clinical manager of nutritional services, physicians, care coordination staff, physical therapists, quality staff, and informatics experts were tasked together as an interprofessional team to address high hospital readmission rates due to patient malnourishment.

After a comprehensive review of evidence was accomplished, the team developed the evidence-based Malnutrition Readmission Prevention Protocol, which identifies three stages of risk for malnutrition. The protocol was used first in one facility and then implemented across a hospital system. Informatics specialists worked to create automatic alerts within the electronic health record to flag health care professionals to use the protocol. Using this tool, patients were identified for inpatient management of nutritional supplementation, and then referral to a registered dietitian nutritionist (RDN) was made. The RDN coordinated availability of 30-day supplementation to be used in the home environment following discharge. An important part of protocol use was involving the patient (and caregiver, as appropriate) in conversations regarding inpatient and outpatient nutritional management. Follow-up calls were made by care management nurses; home visits were conducted by paramedics; and primary care providers were notified to coordinate care after discharge.

Over a 5-year period, readmissions due to malnutrition decreased from 42% to 13.3%.

Commentary: Implications for Practice and Research

Coordinating an effort in which all professions involved in patient care had input into the protocol well before implementation facilitated a collaborative effort created with best practice and favorable patient outcomes in mind. Using the protocol together and meeting the patient's nutritional needs in the inpatient and outpatient settings greatly decreased the readmission rate related to malnutrition. Working together facilitates better outcomes when all stakeholders, including the patient and caregiver, are involved in care processes and planning.

Interprofessional Collaborative Care

Care for the patient with undernutrition takes place in a variety of settings, such as the home, the community, and in the hospital setting if more comprehensive management is needed.

Recognize Cues: Assessment

History. See Box 52.3 to complete the initial history. For older adults, also see Box 52.5, Assessing the Older Adult for Undernutrition. Keep in mind that an unintentional weight loss of 5% in 30 days, or 10% over a 6-month period, significantly affects *nutrition* status and should be further evaluated.

In collaboration with the registered dietitian nutritionist (RDN), also obtain information about the patient's:
- Usual daily food intake and timing of eating
- Food preferences (including cultural considerations)
- Eating behaviors/patterns
- Change in appetite
- Recent weight changes
- Economic status that may influence access to, or purchase of, food

A full *nutrition* history usually includes a 24-hour recall of food intake and the frequency with which foods are consumed. The adequacy of the diet can be evaluated by comparing the amount and types of foods consumed daily with the established standards. The registered dietitian nutritionist (RDN) then provides a more detailed analysis of nutritional intake.

Be aware that patients who live in food deserts (i.e., urban areas where fresh, healthy food is in low supply or unaffordable) may have difficulty obtaining food that is densely nutritious.

Physical Assessment/Signs and Symptoms. Assess for signs and symptoms of various nutrient deficiencies (see Table 52.2). Inspect hair, eyes, oral cavity, nails, and musculoskeletal and

 PATIENT-CENTERED CARE: HEALTH EQUITY

Access to Nutritional and Activity Resources

The Centers for Disease Control and Prevention's Division of Nutrition, Physical Activity, and Obesity (DNPAO) (2023) are working to promote good *nutrition*, regular physical activity, and a healthy weight for everyone. When collecting a nutritional history, ask whether patients feel they can regularly identify, obtain, and afford nutritious foods. Also ask whether they have access to physical areas where they can be active, such as local parks. Collect information that identifies the knowledge patients have about healthy eating and movement and that helps to determine which teaching will be most beneficial. As needed, refer patients who can benefit from nutritional support to local organizations that can assist with resources and education.

❗ **NURSING SAFETY PRIORITY**

Action Alert

Assess for difficulty or pain with chewing or swallowing. Unrecognized dysphagia is a common problem among older adults and can cause undernutrition, dehydration, and aspiration pneumonia. See Chapter 46 for more information.

neurologic systems. Examine the condition of the skin, including any reddened or open areas. Anthropometric measurements may also be obtained. Monitor all food and fluid intake. A three-day caloric intake may be collected and then calculated by the registered dietitian nutritionist (RDN). Delegate this activity to assistive personnel (AP) under your ongoing supervision, and direct AP to report the intake and output values back after obtaining them. Ask AP to report any signs of choking while the patient eats. Document the presence of mouth pain, difficulty chewing, nausea, vomiting, heartburn, or any other symptoms of discomfort with eating.

Psychosocial Assessment. The psychosocial history provides information about the patient's economic status, occupation, educational level, ethnicity/race, living and cooking arrangements, and emotional status. Determine whether financial resources are adequate for providing the necessary food. If resources are inadequate, the social worker or case manager may refer the patient and caregiver to available community services.

Laboratory Assessment. Interpret laboratory data carefully with regard to the total patient; focusing on an isolated value may yield an inaccurate conclusion. In general, laboratory values that may be decreased in the presence of undernourishment include (Pagana et al., 2022):
- Cholesterol
- Hemoglobin
- Hematocrit
- Serum albumin
- Thyroxine-binding prealbumin (PAB)
- Transferrin

Analyze Cues and Prioritize Hypothesis: Analysis

The priority collaborative problem for the patient with undernutrition is:
1. Weight loss due to inability to access, ingest, or digest food or absorb nutrients

Generate Solutions and Take Actions: Planning and Implementation

Improving Nutrition

Planning: Expected Outcomes. The patient with undernutrition is expected to have nutrients available to meet the patient's metabolic needs.

Interventions. The preferred route for food intake is orally through the GI tract because it enhances the immune system and is safer, easier, less expensive, and more enjoyable.

Meal Management. Following the primary health care provider's and RDN's recommendation, provide high-calorie, nutrient-rich foods (e.g., milkshakes, cheese, and supplement drinks such as Boost or Ensure). A feeding schedule of six small meals may be tolerated better than three large ones. A pureed or dental soft diet may be easier for those who have problems chewing or do not have teeth. Follow recommendations in Box 52.6 to provide a more enjoyable and productive eating experience for patients with undernutrition.

Nutritional Supplementation. If the patient cannot take in enough nutrients in food, fortified medical nutrition

---

BOX 52.6 Best Practice for Patient Safety and Quality Care

Promoting Nutrition Intake

Environment
- Remove bedpans, urinals, and emesis basins from the environment.
- Eliminate or decrease offensive odors as much as possible.
- Decrease environmental distractions as much as possible.
- Administer pain medication and/or antiemetics for nausea at least 1 hour before mealtime.

Comfort
- Allow the patient to toilet before mealtime.
- Provide mouth care before mealtime.
- Ensure that eyeglasses and hearing aids are in place, if appropriate, during meals.
- Remind assistive personnel (AP) to have the patient sit in a chair, if possible, at mealtime.

Function
- Ensure that meals are visually appealing, appetizing, and at appropriate temperatures.
- If needed, open cartons and packages and cut up food.
- Observe during meals for food intake, and document the percentage consumed.
- Encourage self-feeding (if able), or feed the patient slowly (delegate to AP, if desired).
- Eliminate or minimize interruptions during mealtime for nonurgent procedures or rounds.

---

supplements (MNS) (e.g., Ensure, Sustacal, Carnation Instant Breakfast [also available as a lactose-free supplement]) may be given, especially to older adults. For patients with liver and renal disease or diabetes, special products that meet these needs are available (e.g., Glucerna for patients with diabetes).

Nutrition supplements are supplied as liquid formulas, powders, soups, coffee, and puddings in a variety of flavors. Examples include Duocal for carbohydrates and fats, and Beneprotein for protein. Follow the primary health care provider's prescription for nutritional supplementation.

Drug Therapy. Multivitamins, zinc, and an iron preparation are often ordered to treat or prevent anemia in patients who are malnourished. Monitor the patient's hemoglobin and hematocrit levels for efficacy of treatment, and assess for side effects. For example, iron can cause constipation, and zinc can cause nausea and vomiting.

Total Enteral Nutrition. If a patient cannot achieve adequate *nutrition* via oral intake, total enteral nutrition (TEN) may be needed. Enteral tube feedings may be necessary to supplement oral intake or to provide total nutrition.

Patients likely to receive TEN can be divided into three groups:
- Those who can eat but cannot maintain adequate *nutrition* by oral intake of food alone
- Those with permanent neuromuscular impairment who cannot swallow
- Those who do not have permanent neuromuscular impairment but cannot eat because of their condition

Patients in the first group are often older adults or patients receiving cancer treatment. In some cases, artificial nutrition and hydration may not be desired. Check for advance directives stating whether the patient desires artificial nutrition and hydration if certain conditions exist. If advance directives are not in place, yet the patient has a designated durable power of attorney, that individual can make health-related decisions when the patient is unable to do so. Legal and ethical questions often arise when patients do not have advance directives, are unable to make their wishes known, and do not have a designated durable power of attorney. *The decision to feed or not to feed is complex, and there is no clear right or wrong answer.* See the Legal/Ethical Considerations box for more information.

LEGAL/ETHICAL CONSIDERATIONS

Ethics Committees and Feeding

Decisions about legal/ethical situations regarding feeding benefit from the involvement of interprofessional ethics committees in health care facilities. When clinicians are making decisions about the desirability of tube feedings for patients who cannot express their own wishes and who do not have an advance directive in place, the focus should be on achieving consensus by:

- Reviewing what is known about tube feedings, especially their risks and benefits
- Reviewing the medical facts about the patient
- Investigating any available evidence that would help understand the patient's wishes
- Obtaining the input of all stakeholders in the situation
- Delaying any action until consensus is achieved

Those in the second group of patients likely to receive TEN usually have permanent swallowing problems due to a condition such as brain attack, severe head trauma, or advanced multiple sclerosis. These patients require some type of feeding tube for delivery of the enteral product on a long-term basis.

Patients in the third group receive enteral *nutrition* for as long as their illness lasts. The feeding is discontinued when the patient's condition improves and oral intake can resume.

A therapeutic combination of carbohydrates, fat, vitamins, minerals, and trace elements is available in liquid form. A prescription from the health care provider is required for enteral nutrition, but the RDN usually makes the recommendation and computes the amount and type of product needed for each patient.

NCLEX Examination Challenge 52.2

Safe and Effective Care Environment

A client with terminal cancer who is comatose has a durable power of attorney but no advance directive. When total enteral nutrition (TEN) is prescribed, which nursing action would be appropriate?

A. Contact the durable power of attorney.
B. Begin administration of TEN immediately.
C. Consult the interprofessional ethics committee.
D. Ask the health care provider whether to start nutritional therapy.

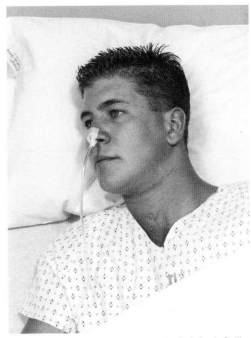

FIG. 52.4 Nasoduodenal tube. (From Lilley, L., Rainforth Collins, S., Harrington, S., & Snyder, J. [2011]. *Pharmacology and the nursing process* [6th ed.]. St. Louis: Mosby.)

Methods of administering total enteral nutrition. TEN is administered as a "tube feeding" through a nasoenteric or enterostomal tube. It can be used in the patient's home or any health care setting.

A **nasoenteric tube (NET)** is a feeding tube inserted nasally and then advanced into the GI tract, such as a Dobbhoff tube. Commonly used NETs include the **nasogastric (NG) tube,** the smaller (small-bore) **nasoduodenal tube (NDT)** (Fig. 52.4), and the nasojejunal tube (NJT), which is used less often. All of these types of tubes are used for less than 4 weeks to provide short-term feeding.

Enterostomal feeding tubes are used for patients who need *long-term* enteral feeding. The surgeon directly accesses the GI tract using various surgical, endoscopic, and laparoscopic techniques. Under sedation, a **gastrostomy**—a stoma created from the abdominal wall into the stomach—is created. Then a **percutaneous endoscopic gastrostomy (PEG)** or dual-access gastrostomy-jejunostomy (PEG/J) tube (Fig. 52.5) is placed. A **jejunostomy** is used for long-term feedings when it is desirable to bypass the stomach, such as with gastric disease, upper GI obstruction, and abnormal gastric or duodenal emptying. This can be accomplished via a direct percutaneous endoscopic jejunostomy (DPEJ) (see Fig. 52.5) (DeLegge, 2021).

Tube feedings are administered by bolus feeding, continuous feeding, or cyclic feeding. **Bolus feeding** is an intermittent feeding of a specified amount of enteral product at set intervals during a 24-hour period, typically every 4 hours. This method can be accomplished manually or by infusion through a mechanical pump or controller device. **Continuous feeding** is similar to IV therapy in that small amounts are continuously infused (by gravity drip or a pump or controller device) over a specified time. **Cyclic feeding** is the same as continuous feeding

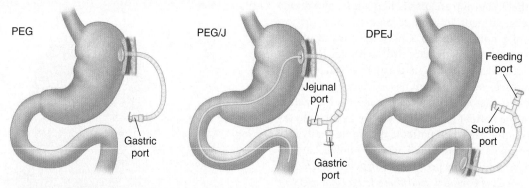

FIG. 52.5 Percutaneous endoscopic gastrostomy (PEG), dual-access gastrostomy-jejunostomy (PEG/J) tube, and direct percutaneous endoscopic jejunostomy (DPEJ). (Redrawn from Zhu, Y., Shi, L., Tang, H., & Tao, G. [2012]. Current considerations of direct percutaneous endoscopic jejunostomy. *Canadian Journal of Gastroenterology 26*[2], 92–96.)

except that the infusion is stopped for a specified time in each 24-hour period, usually 6 hours or longer ("down time"). Down time typically occurs in the morning to allow bathing, treatments, and other activities. Follow the health care provider's prescription for type, rate, and method of tube feeding, as well as the amount of additional water ("free water") needed. If the patient can swallow small amounts of food, the patient may also eat orally while the tube is in place.

The nurse is responsible for the care and maintenance of the feeding tube and the enteral feeding. See Box 52.7.

! NURSING SAFETY PRIORITY
Action Alert

If a gastrostomy or jejunostomy tube cannot be moved while you are performing your regular assessment, notify the health care provider immediately because the retention disk may be embedded in the tissue. Cover the site with a dry, sterile dressing and change the dressing at least once a day.

Complications of total enteral nutrition. The nursing priority for care of a patient receiving TEN is safety, which includes preventing, assessing, and managing complications associated with tube feeding. Some complications of therapy result from the type of tube used to administer the feeding, and others result from the enteral product itself. The most common problem is the development of an obstructed ("clogged") tube. Use the information in Box 52.8 to address this concern (Drummond Hayes & Drummond Hayes, 2018).

Patients receiving TEN are at risk for several other complications, including refeeding syndrome; tube misplacement and dislodgment; abdominal distention and nausea/vomiting; and problems with *fluid and electrolyte balance,* often associated with diarrhea. These problems can be prevented if the patient is monitored carefully and complications are detected early.

TUBE MISPLACEMENT AND DISLODGMENT. Misplacement or dislodgment of the tube can cause aspiration and possible death. Immediately remove any tube that you suspect is dislodged! An x-ray is the most accurate confirmation method and should always be done on initial tube insertion. If a larger bore NG tube

is used, after the initial placement is confirmed, check gastric residual before each intermittent feeding or drug administration, or at least every 6 hours during feeding (Hodin & Bordeianou, 2023). Do not rely on traditional methods for checking tube placement such as auscultation; pH testing of GI contents; testing of biochemical markers, such as bilirubin, trypsin, or pepsin; or assessment for carbon dioxide using capnometry. Once x-ray confirmation has been made, mark the tube exit point as a baseline for visual reevaluation of placement at each assessment.

! NURSING SAFETY PRIORITY
Action Alert

If enteral tubes are misplaced or become dislodged, the patient is likely to aspirate. *Aspiration pneumonia is a life-threatening complication associated with TEN, especially for older adults.* Observe for fever and signs of dehydration, such as dry mucous membranes and decreased urinary output. Auscultate lungs every 4 to 8 hours to check for diminishing breath sounds, especially in lower lobes. Patients may become short of breath and report chest discomfort. If a chest x-ray confirms this diagnosis, treatment with antibiotics is started.

ABDOMINAL DISTENTION AND NAUSEA/VOMITING. Abdominal distention, nausea, and vomiting during tube feeding are often caused by overfeeding. To *prevent* overfeeding, check gastric residual volumes every 6 hours, depending on agency policy and patient assessment. If residual feeding is obtained, check with the health care provider for the appropriate intervention (usually to slow or stop the feeding for a time) or consult the American Society of Parenteral and Enteral Nutrition (ASPEN) (2023) best practice recommendations (ASPEN, 2023). Follow agency policy regarding holding feeding if necessary. After a period of rest, the feeding can be restarted, usually at a lower flow rate.

FLUID AND ELECTROLYTE IMBALANCES. Patients receiving enteral nutrition therapy, especially older adults and those with cardiac or renal problems, are at an increased risk for fluid imbalances. Some electrolyte imbalances can be avoided. For example, a patient with renal problems and existing high potassium levels may be given a special formula lower in potassium.

Fluid imbalances associated with enteral nutrition are usually related to the body's response to increased serum osmolarity,

BOX 52.7 Best Practice for Patient Safety and Quality Care

Tube-Feeding Care and Maintenance

- If nasogastric or nasoduodenal feeding is ordered, use a soft, flexible, small-bore feeding tube (smaller than 12 Fr).
- Recognize that tubes with ports minimize contamination by eliminating the need to open the feeding system to administer drugs.
- **The initial placement of the tube should be confirmed by x-ray study** even if another method of confirmation is available, such as electromagnetic feeding tube–placement device (ETPD). Evidence shows that radiographic confirmation is essential (Hodin & Bordeianou, 2023).
- If correct tube placement is ever in question, a chest x-ray should again be performed.
- Secure the tube with tape or a commercial attachment device after applying a skin protectant; change the tape regularly.
- If a gastrostomy or jejunostomy tube is used, assess the insertion site for signs of infection or excoriation (e.g., excessive redness/hyperpigmentation, drainage). Rotate the tube 360 degrees each day, and check for in-and-out play of about ¼ inch (0.6 cm).
- Check and document residual volume every 6 hours or per agency policy by aspirating stomach contents into a syringe. If residual feeding is obtained, check with the health care provider for the appropriate intervention (usually to slow or stop the feeding for a time), or consult the American Society of Parenteral and Enteral Nutrition's best practice recommendations (ASPEN, 2023).
- Check the feeding pump to ensure proper mechanical operation.
- Ensure that the enteral product is infused at the ordered rate (mL/hr).
- Change the feeding bag and tubing every 24 to 48 hours; label the bag with the date and time of the change with your initials. Use an irrigation set for no more than 24 hours.
- For continuous or cyclic feeding, add only 4 hours of product to the bag at a time to prevent bacterial growth. *A closed system is preferred, and each set should be used no longer than 24 hours.*
- Wear clean gloves when changing or opening the feeding system or adding product; wipe the lid of the formula can with clean gauze; wear sterile gloves when caring for patients who are critically ill or immunocompromised.
- Label open cans with date and time opened; cover and keep refrigerated. Discard any unused open cans after 24 hours.
- Do not use any color of food dye in formula because it can cause serious complications.
- To prevent aspiration, keep the head of the bed elevated at least 30 degrees during the feeding and for at least 1 hour after the feeding for bolus feeding; continuously maintain the semi-Fowler's position for patients receiving cyclic or continuous feeding.
- Monitor laboratory values, especially blood urea nitrogen (BUN), serum electrolytes, hematocrit, prealbumin, and glucose.
- Monitor for complications of tube feeding, especially diarrhea.
- Monitor and document the patient's weight and intake and output per the health care provider's order or agency policy.

BOX 52.8 Best Practice for Patient Safety and Quality Care

Maintaining a Patent Feeding Tube

- Recognize that a tube occlusion is more easily prevented than corrected.
- Specific risks for tube occlusion include delivering multiple medications without flushing between administration, not flushing before and after overall medication administration, using longer tubes, and using tubes of smaller diameter.
- Consult with the pharmacist to be sure the prescribed medications are compatible with the enteral **nutrition** formula.
- Consult with the pharmacist to confirm that medications and formula can be cleared from the tube with appropriate flushing.
- Collaborate with the health care provider to use liquid medications instead of crushed tablets when possible, unless the liquid form of medication causes diarrhea.
- Do not mix drugs with the feeding product before giving. Crush tablets as finely as possible and dissolve in warm water. *(Check to see which tablets are safe to crush. For example, do not crush slow-acting [SA] or slow-release [SR] drugs.)*
- Flush the tube with 30 mL of water, using at least a 30-mL syringe to prevent tube rupture:
  - At least every 4 hours
  - Before and after medication administration
  - After any interruption of enteral nutrition
- If the tube becomes clogged, use 30 mL of water for flushing, applying gentle pressure with a 50-mL piston syringe.
- *Do not* instill a carbonated beverage or cranberry juice; these have an acidic pH that can worsen the occlusion by causing enteral nutrition formula proteins to precipitate in the tube.
- Use warm water as the best choice for unclogging.
- Attach a 30- or 60-mL piston syringe to the feeding tube; retract the plunger to facilitate dislodging the clog. Then fill the flush with warm water, reattach it to the tube, and attempt flushing. If continued resistance is experienced, move the plunger gently back and forth. Then clamp the tube to allow the warm water to penetrate the clog for about 20 minutes.
- If water does not unclog the tube, an experienced nurse can use an activated pancreatic enzyme solution ordered by the health care provider, following agency policy.
- As a final attempt, commercially available enzyme declogging kits or devices can be used by an experienced nurse, again following agency policy.
- If unclogging is unsuccessful, replacement of the tube is recommended.

Data from Boullata, J., Carrera, A., Harvey, L., et al. (2017). ASPEN safe practices for enteral nutrition therapy. *Journal of Parenteral and Enteral Nutrition, 41*(1), 15–103; Drummond Hayes, K., & Drummond Hayes, D. (2018). Best practices for unclogging feeding tubes in adults. *Nursing2018, 48*(6), 66; Guenter, P., & Lyman, B. (2021). Evidence-based strategies to prevent enteral nutrition complications: Follow these tips to keep your patients safe. *American Nurse Journal, 16*(6), 18–22; Jackson, K., & Tomlinson, S. (2021). *Essential procedures: Acute care.* Philadelphia, PA: Wolters Kluwer.

but fluid overload from too much tube feeding can also occur. If patients do *not* have normal renal and cardiac function, expansion of the plasma volume can lead to circulatory overload and pulmonary edema, especially in older adults. Assess for signs and symptoms, such as peripheral edema, sudden weight gain, crackles, dyspnea, increased blood pressure, and bounding pulse; report these to the health care provider.

Excessive diarrhea and/or dehydration may develop when hyperosmolar enteral preparations are delivered quickly and excessive water loss is experienced. A more iso-osmolar formula may be needed. If diarrhea continues, and especially if it has a very foul odor, evaluate for *Clostridium difficile* or other infectious organisms. Contamination can occur because of repeated and often faulty handling of the feeding solution and system.

In some cases, diarrhea may follow the administration of multiple liquid medications, such as elixirs and suspensions that have a very high osmolarity. Examples include acetaminophen, furosemide, and phenytoin. Discuss this with the health care provider to determine whether the patient's drug regimen can be changed to prevent diarrhea or if dilution is possible.

The two most common electrolyte imbalances associated with enteral nutrition therapy are hyperkalemia and hyponatremia. Both of these conditions may be related to hyperglycemia-induced hyperosmolarity of the plasma and the resultant osmotic diuresis. Risks for disturbances in *fluid and electrolyte balance* are discussed in detail in Chapter 13.

REFEEDING SYNDROME. Refeeding syndrome is a potentially life-threatening complication related to fluid and electrolyte shifts during aggressive nutritional rehabilitation of the patient in a state of starvation. Prevent this complication by carefully assessing and managing nutritional needs early before a patient is severely malnourished.

✚ NURSING SAFETY PRIORITY

Critical Rescue

> Recognize signs of refeeding syndrome, which include hypophosphatemia and hypokalemia noted in laboratory values, heart failure, peripheral edema, rhabdomyolysis, seizures, hemolysis, and respiratory insufficiency (Mehler, 2023). Respond by contacting the health care provider immediately. More information on *fluid and electrolyte balance* can be found in Chapter 13.

Parenteral Nutrition. When a patient cannot effectively use the GI tract for *nutrition,* either partial or total parenteral nutrition therapy may be needed. This form of nutrition is introduced into the veins and differs from standard IV therapy in that any or all nutrients (carbohydrates, proteins, fats, vitamins, minerals, electrolytes, and trace elements) can be given. Parenteral nutrition can be mixed by the pharmacist using compounded bags or delivered from a multichamber bag in which commercially premixed solutions are used (King, 2019). In a multichamber bag, dextrose, amino acids, electrolytes, and lipids are preloaded in separate chambers that are mixed together right before administration. The benefit of compounding is that mixtures can be highly personalized to each patient. However, a downfall is the rate of human error that can take place in the compounding, labeling, and administration processes (King, 2019). A benefit of the multichamber bag is that shelf life is 12 months or more (compared with a 7- to 9-day shelf life for individually compounded formulations). The downfall is lack of customization to the individual patient, as multichamber bags usually contain less protein and fewer electrolytes than personalized formulations (King, 2019). At the time of publication, the American Society for Parenteral and Enteral Nutrition (ASPEN) recommends using premixed formulations or multichamber bag solutions.

Peripheral parenteral nutrition (PPN). Peripheral parenteral nutrition (PPN) is administered through a cannula or catheter in a large distal vein of the arm on a short-term basis. It is usually used for patients who can eat but are not able to take in enough nutrients to meet their needs. PPN is fat-based and does not contain all of the carbohydrates a patient needs, so it is not used on a long-term basis (Baiu & Spain, 2019). The patient must have adequate peripheral vein access and be able to tolerate large volumes of fluid to have this type of nutritional therapy. PPN has an osmolarity lower than conventional parenteral nutrition and must be administered in a high volume and/or with a high fat formulation to deliver adequate nutrients (Seres, 2021). Monitor for irritation at the site of the cannula or catheter insertion, as infusion of large volumes of PPN can be irritating to tissue.

✚ NURSING SAFETY PRIORITY

Critical Rescue

> Recognize that you must monitor patients receiving fat emulsions for fever, increased triglycerides, clotting problems, and multisystem organ failure, which may indicate fat overload syndrome, especially in patients who are critically ill. Respond to any of these signs and symptoms by discontinuing the IV fat emulsion infusion and reporting the changes to the health care provider immediately.

Total parenteral nutrition. When the patient requires intensive *nutrition* support for an extended time, the health care provider orders centrally administered total parenteral nutrition (TPN). TPN (Fig. 52.6) is delivered through a temporary central line inserted in the neck or chest, a long-term tunneled catheter or implanted part inserted in the chest, or via a PICC line (Baiu & Spain, 2019). (See Chapter 15 for care.) This type of nutrition is hypertonic and contains a high glucose content.

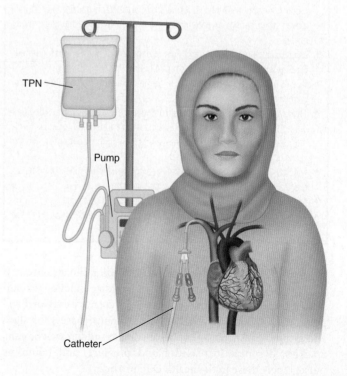

FIG. 52.6 Total parenteral nutrition.

TPN solutions are administered with an infusion pump. The osmolarity of the fluid and the concentrations of the specific components make controlled delivery essential. See Box 52.9 for appropriate nursing interventions.

Patients receiving parenteral nutrition fluids are at risk for a wide variety of serious and potentially life-threatening complications. Complications may result from the solutions or from the peripheral or central venous catheter (see Chapter 15).

The patient with cardiac or renal dysfunction can develop problems with *fluid and electrolyte balance,* including fluid overload, heart failure, and pulmonary edema. The health care provider usually requests frequent serum electrolyte levels to detect imbalances. Potassium and sodium imbalances are common, especially when insulin is also administered as part of the therapy. Calcium imbalances, particularly hypercalcemia, are associated with TPN. The risk for metabolic and electrolyte complications is reduced when the administration rate is carefully controlled and patients are closely observed. Monitor for any of these imbalances, and report any major changes or abnormalities to the health care provider immediately.

Care Coordination and Transition Management

The patient with undernutrition, once stabilized, can be cared for in an acute care hospital, transitional care unit, long-term care agency, or their home.

BOX 52.9 Best Practice for Patient Safety and Quality Care

Care and Maintenance of Total Parenteral Nutrition

- Follow the Infusion Nurses Society's Infusion Therapy Standards of Practice (Gorski et al., 2021).
- Check each bag of total parenteral nutrition (TPN) solution for accuracy by comparing it with the original prescription.
- Administer insulin as ordered.
- Monitor the IV pump for accuracy in delivering the ordered hourly rate.
- If the TPN solution is temporarily unavailable, collaborate with the health care provider so that 10% dextrose/water ($D_{10}W$) or 20% dextrose/water ($D_{20}W$) can be administered until the TPN solution can be obtained.
- If the TPN administration is not on time ("behind"), do not attempt to "catch up" by increasing the rate.
- Monitor and document the patient's weight daily or according to facility protocol.
- Monitor serum electrolytes and glucose daily or per facility protocol.
- Monitor for, report, and document complications, including problems with *fluid and electrolyte balance.*
- Monitor and carefully record the patient's intake and output.
- Assess the patient's IV site for signs of infection or infiltration (see Chapter 15).
- Change the IV tubing every 24 hours or per facility protocol.
- Change the dressing every 48 hours for a gauze dressing change and 7 days for a transparent dressing change (see Chapter 15).
- Before administering TPN, have a second nurse check the prescription and solution to increase patient safety.

Home Care Management. The patient with undernutrition needs a variety of resources at home to continue consistent *nutrition* support. If food can be consumed orally, the case manager or other discharge planner can determine whether financial resources are available for nutritional supplements. If the hospital provides ambulatory nutrition counseling services, the patient may be scheduled for follow-up after discharge for assessment of weight gain.

Self-Management Education. The registered dietitian nutritionist (RDN) teaches the patient with undernutrition (and family, as indicated) about a high-calorie, high-protein diet and *nutrition* supplements. It is important for you, as the nurse, to:
- Reinforce the importance of adhering to the ordered diet.
- Review any drugs the patient may be taking.
- Teach the importance of taking iron immediately before or during meals.
- Caution the patient that iron tends to cause constipation.
- Emphasize ways to prevent constipation, including adequate fiber intake, adequate fluids, and exercise.

Health Care Resources. The patient with undernutrition discharged to home on enteral or parenteral nutrition support needs the specialized services of a home nutritional therapy team. This team generally consists of the health care provider, nurse, registered dietitian nutritionist (RDN), pharmacist, and case manager or social worker. Several commercial companies supply these services to patients at home in addition to the feeding supplies and formulas and health teaching.

Evaluate Outcomes: Evaluation

Evaluate the care of the patient with undernutrition based on the identified priority patient problem. The primary expected outcome is that the patient consumes available nutrients to meet the metabolic demands for maintaining weight and total protein and has adequate hydration.

✳ NUTRITION CONCEPT EXEMPLAR: OBESITY

Pathophysiology Review

The pathophysiology of obesity is complex. Numerous chemicals in the body, including hormones known as *adipokines,* work together to affect appetite and fat metabolism. Dysregulation of these chemicals can result in conditions such as appetite increase, overstimulation of the autonomic nervous system, blood vessel inflammation, and ventricular hypertrophy. Complications of obesity can affect many organ systems (Box 52.10).

The terms *obesity* and *overweight* are often used interchangeably, but they refer to different health problems. In both problems, the patient often has not consumed enough *healthy* nutrients to achieve adequate *nutrition* and has an abnormal or excessive amount of fat accumulation (World Health Organization, 2023). Overweight is reflected by a body mass index (BMI) of 25 to 29. Obesity is reflected by a BMI of 30 or above (CDC, 2022b).

BOX 52.10 Common Complications of Obesity

Cardiovascular
- Coronary artery disease (CAD)
- Hyperlipidemia
- Hypertension
- Peripheral artery disease (PAD)

Endocrine
- Insulin resistance
- Metabolic syndrome
- Type II diabetes

Gastrointestinal
- Cholelithiasis

Genitourinary/ Reproductive
- Erectile dysfunction in men
- Menstrual irregularities in women
- Urinary incontinence

Integumentary
- Delayed wound healing
- Susceptibility to infections

Musculoskeletal
- Chronic back and/or joint pain
- Early onset of osteoarthritis

Neurologic
- Stroke

Psychiatric
- Depression

Respiratory
- Obesity hypoventilation syndrome
- Obstructive sleep apnea

Obesity is subdivided into three categories (CDC, 2022b):
- Class I—BMI of 30 to <35
- Class II—BMI of 35 to <40
- Class III—BMI of 40 or higher (sometimes called "extreme" or "severe" obesity)

The distribution of excess body fat rather than the degree of obesity has been used to predict increased health risks. The waist circumference (WC) is a stronger predictor of coronary artery disease (CAD) than is the BMI. A WC greater than 35 inches (89 cm) in women and greater than 40 inches (102 cm) in men indicates central obesity (National Heart, Lung, and Blood Institute; National Institutes of Health; U.S. Department of Health and Human Services, n.d.). Central obesity is a major risk factor for CAD, brain attack, type 2 diabetes, some cancers (e.g., colon, breast), sleep apnea, and early death.

The waist-to-hip ratio (WHR) is also a predictor of CAD. This measure differentiates peripheral lower body obesity from central obesity. A WHR of 0.95 or greater in men (0.8 or greater in women) indicates android obesity with excess fat at the waist and abdomen.

Etiology and Genetic Risk

The causes of obesity involve complex interrelationships of many environmental, genetic, and behavioral factors. One of the most common causes of being overweight or obese is eating *high-fat and high-cholesterol diets.* Obesity is associated with diet when it contains a significant amount of *saturated* fat, which increases low-density lipoproteins (LDL, or LDL-C for low-density lipoproteins cholesterol). *Trans fatty acids* (TFAs), saturated fats, and cholesterol are linked to a higher risk for heart disease (Oteng & Kersten, 2020). By contrast, monounsaturated and polyunsaturated fats are healthy fats.

Physical inactivity has been identified as another cause of overweight and obesity. The major barriers to increasing physical activity include lack of time, comfort level in a sedentary lifestyle, and decreased mobility due to health conditions.

Drug therapy also contributes to obesity when prescribed medications cause weight gain when they are taken on a long-term basis. Examples include:
- Corticosteroids
- Estrogens and certain progestins
- NSAIDs
- Antihypertensives
- Antidepressants and other psychoactive drugs
- Antiepileptic drugs
- Certain oral antidiabetic agents

👤 PATIENT-CENTERED CARE: GENETICS/ GENOMICS

Genetic Classifications of Obesity

Evidence shows that genetic classifications of obesity can be (Loos & Yeo, 2022; Lin & Li, 2021):
1. Monogenic (caused by a single gene);
2. Syndromic (severe obesity associated with other phenotypes, including neurodevelopmental abnormalities such as Prader-Willi syndrome);
3. Oligogenic (due to the absence of a certain phenotype); or
4. Polygenic (caused by a cumulative effect of numerous genes whose effect is increased in the environment where weight gain is prominent)

Polygenic obesity is most common. In any predisposition to obesity, environment (lifestyle) is also a strong influence. Encourage patients to focus on lifestyle modifications that are within their control, even if they believe genetics is the root cause of obesity.

Incidence and Prevalence

Worldwide, the prevalence of overweight and obesity has doubled since 1980 (Chooi et al., 2019). About one-third of the world's population is now classified as overweight or obese (Chooi et al., 2019). *This problem is a leading cause of preventable death.*

Health Promotion/Disease Prevention

Obesity is a major public health problem and is associated with many complications, including death. As a result of this continuing concern, one of the *Healthy People 2030* nutrition objectives is to reduce the proportion of adults with obesity (U.S. Department of Agriculture and U.S. Department of Health and Human Services, 2020). See Box 52.11 for more.

In collaboration with the registered dietitian nutritionist (RDN), teach the importance of weight management and physical activity to improve health. Even a 5% weight loss can drastically decrease the risk for coronary artery disease (CAD) and diabetes mellitus. Teach patients that physical activity can be as simple as walking 20 minutes a day.

Interprofessional Collaborative Care

Care for the patient with obesity takes place in a variety of settings—from the home to the community to a hospital setting

BOX 52.11 Meeting *Healthy People 2030* Select Objectives and Targets for Adults: Nutrition and Healthy Eating

Increase consumption of these items in people aged 2 years and over:
- Calcium
- Dark green vegetables, red and orange vegetables, and beans and peas
- Fruit
- Potassium
- Vegetables (overall vegetables)
- Vitamin D
- Whole grains

Decrease consumption of these items in people aged 2 years and over:
- Added sugars
- Saturated fats
- Sodium

General:
- Reduce household food insecurity and hunger

Data from Office of Disease Prevention and Health Promotion. (2023). *Healthy People 2023: Nutrition and healthy eating.* U.S. Department of Health and Human Services. https://health.gov/healthypeople/objectives-and-data/browse-objectives/nutrition-and-healthy-eating.

(if more comprehensive management or surgery is needed). Members of the interprofessional team who collaborate most closely to care for this patient include the primary health care provider, the surgeon (if surgery is required), the nurse, the social worker, and the registered dietitian nutritionist (RDN). For patients who experience psychological impact related to obesity, a psychologist or therapist will also have an important role in care.

NCLEX Examination Challenge 52.3

Health Promotion and Maintenance

A client states, "I keep trying to lose weight, but I can't because I am genetically obese." Which nursing responses would be appropriate? **Select all that apply.**

A. "Genes can contribute to obesity."
B. "Have you considered bariatric surgery?"
C. "Let's talk about your family history with weight."
D. "What are your feelings about increasing physical activity?"
E. "It would be good for us to discuss your usual nutritional intake."

Recognize Cues: Assessment

History. Patients with obesity may be embarrassed or reluctant to talk about their weight or fear judgment because of the stigma that can be attached to this condition. Approach patients with obesity by using the acronym RESPECT, created by The Ohio State University (Aycock et al., 2017). Create a **r**apport with them in an **e**nvironment that is **s**afe. Ensure their safety and **p**rivacy, **e**ncourage them to set realistic goals (in the planning phase), provide **c**ompassion, and use **t**act in conversation.

See Box 52.3 to complete the initial history. In collaboration with the registered dietitian nutritionist (RDN), also obtain the information as noted in the History section under the concept exemplar of Undernutrition.

Additionally, ask about:
- Appetite
- Attitude toward food
- Presence of any chronic diseases
- Drugs taken (prescribed and over-the-counter [OTC], including herbal preparations)
- Physical activity/functional ability
- Family history of obesity
- What forms of weight loss have been tried in the past and their results

Physical Assessment/Signs and Symptoms. Obtain an accurate height and weight measurement. Anthropometric measurements may also be obtained.

Examine the skin for reddened or open areas. Lift skinfold areas, such as pendulous breasts and abdominal aprons (*panniculus*), to observe for *Candida* (yeast) (a condition called *intertrigo*) or other infections or lesions. Infection of the panniculus is referred to as *panniculitis*.

Psychosocial Assessment. Obtain a psychosocial history to determine the patient's circumstances and emotional factors that might prevent successful weight loss or that might be worsened by intervention. Ask about the perception of current weight and weight reduction. Some patients do not view weight as a problem, which affects planning, treatment, and outcome. Ask patients questions about their health beliefs related to being overweight, such as:
- What does food mean to you?
- Do you want to lose weight?
- What prevents you from losing weight?
- What do you think will motivate you to lose weight?
- How do you think you might benefit from losing weight?
- Do you have a support system in place that will encourage you during weight loss?

Some patients become very depressed regarding their weight and/or failure of weight loss efforts. If the patient reports depressed symptoms that have occurred consistently for more than 2 weeks that impact performing ADLs, referral to a mental health professional can be helpful.

Analyze Cues and Prioritize Hypothesis: Analysis

The priority collaborative problem for the patient with obesity is:
1. Weight gain, which stresses all vital organs due to excessive intake of calories

Generate Solutions and Take Actions: Planning and Implementation

If the patient with obesity is to be hospitalized, an appropriate bariatric care room is important in the provision of high-quality, patient-centered care whether nonsurgical or surgical management is planned. Ensure that the patient has the right room so that care can be maximized to the very best benefit. See Table 52.3 for criteria for these types of rooms.

Improving Nutrition

Planning: Expected Outcomes. The patient with obesity is expected to return to a normal BMI while consuming dense nutrients that meet metabolic needs without overeating.

Nonsurgical Management. Weight loss may be accomplished by *nutrition* modification with or without the aid of drugs and in

TABLE 52.3	**Criteria for a Bariatric Room**
Criterion	**Specifications**
Location	Designation specifically for bariatric care
Capacity	Single patient
Area	Minimum clear floor area of 18 m²
Entry	At least 60 inches (1500 mm) wide
Clearance	Minimum distance of 5 feet (1.5 m) between sides and foot of bed and wall
Bedding	Bariatric bed with low air loss mattress
Handwashing station	Mounted on wall; able to withstand downward static force of a predetermined maximum patient weight
Toilet room	Toilet with weight capacity of 1000 lb (453 kg)
	Toilet mounted to floor with at least 24 inches (61 cm) from wall to center of toilet line, and 3 feet, 8 inches (112 cm) of clear space on the opposite side of the toilet for wheelchair and caregiver access
	Grab bars on the side of the toilet that can withstand 1000 lb (453 kg) of downward force
Bathing facilities	Shower stall—4 feet × 5 feet (1.2 m × 1.5 m) with turning radius of 71 inches (1800 mm) (separate area from washing station and toilet room)
	Grab bars in the shower stall that support 1000 lb (453 kg) of downward force
	Handheld spray nozzles mounted on a side wall
	Enclosure for privacy
	Portable shower chair
Patient lift system	Built-in mechanical lift system that accommodates up to 1000 lb (453 kg)
Airborne isolation room	At least one airborne isolation room per bariatric unit should be available
General	Gowns of appropriate size
	Equipment of appropriate size (e.g., bedpans, blood pressure cuffs, antiembolus stockings, sequential compression devices, gait and transfer belts, stretchers)
	Furnishings of accommodative size (e.g., recliners, chairs)

Data from Diabetes, Obesity and Nutrition Strategic Clinical Network, Alberta Health Services, Bariatric Care and Rehabilitation Research Group, Faculty of Rehabilitation Medicine – University of Alberta, & Obesity Canada. (2022). *Guidelines for the care of hospitalized patients with bariatric needs.* https://www.albertahealthservices.ca/assets/about/scn/ahs-scn-don-guidelines-for-hospitalized-patients-bariatric-needs.pdf; Dockrell, S., & Hurley, G. (2021). Moving and handling care of bariatric patients: A survey of clinical nurse managers. *Journal of Research in Nursing, 26*(3), 194-204; Lim, R. (2022). Hospital accreditation, accommodations, and staffing for care of the bariatric surgical patient. *UpToDate.* Retrieved May 23, 2023, from https://www.uptodate.com/contents/hospital-accreditation-accommodations-and-staffing-for-care-of-the-bariatric-surgical-patient.

combination with a regular exercise program. Patients who may be candidates for surgical treatment include those who have:

- Repeated failure of nonsurgical interventions
- A BMI equal to or greater than 40
- Weight more than 100% above ideal body weight

Diet programs. Diets for helping adults lose weight include fasting, very-low-calorie diets, nutritionally balanced diets, and unbalanced low-energy diets.

Short-term fasting programs and *very-low-calorie diets* (usually 200 to 800 calories/day) require an initial cardiac evaluation and supervision by the interprofessional health care team. Neither diet is ideal due to risks involved and the likelihood of regaining weight after completion of the diet. Ketosis is a risk of short-term fasting.

Nutritionally balanced diets generally provide about 1200 to 1800 calories/day with a conventional distribution of carbohydrate, protein, and fat. Vitamin and mineral supplements may be used. These diets adhere to conventional foods that are economical and easy to obtain.

Unbalanced low-energy diets, such as the low-carbohydrate diet, restrict one or more nutrients. Protein and vegetables are encouraged, but certain carbohydrates and high-fat foods are not. Although results are mixed per health research, these diets are extremely popular.

Nutrition therapy. Nutrition recommendations for each patient are developed through close interaction among the patient, caregiver, primary health care provider, nurse, and registered dietitian nutritionist (RDN). The diet must meet the patient's needs, habits, and lifestyle and should be realistic. At a minimum, the diet should:

- Be evidence based
- Be nutritionally balanced (see Diet Programs section)
- Have a low risk-benefit ratio
- Be practical and conducive to long-term success

Calorie estimates are easily calculated. Resting metabolic rate is determined using a gender-specific formula that incorporates the appropriate activity factor. This figure reflects the total calories needed daily for maintaining current weight. To encourage a weight loss of 1 lb (0.45 kg) a week, the registered dietitian nutritionist (RDN) subtracts 500 calories each day. To encourage a weight loss of 2 lb (0.9 kg) a week, 1000 calories each day are subtracted. The amount of weight lost varies with the patient's food intake, level of physical activity, and water losses. A reasonable expected outcome of 5% to 10% loss of body weight has been shown to improve glycemic control and reduce cholesterol and blood pressure. These benefits continue if the weight loss is sustained.

Exercise program. For most adults, adding physical activity to a healthy diet produces more weight loss than dieting alone. More of the weight lost is fat, which preserves lean body mass. An increase in exercise can reduce the waist circumference and the waist-to-hip ratio. Even a small loss of 5% to 10% of overall

TABLE 52.4 Common Examples of Drug Therapy

Overweight and Obesity Treatment

Drug	Selected Nursing Implications
Bupropion-naltrexone (combines the antidepressant bupropion with the opioid antagonist naltrexone)	Patients with uncontrolled hypertension, seizures, anorexia nervosa, or bulimia nervosa or patients who are withdrawing from drugs or alcohol should not take this drug; *this medication is contraindicated in these populations.* Patients taking bupropion should not take this drug; *cumulative doses can increase risks for side effects.* Monitor for suicidal ideation; *this can develop due to the antidepressant effect.*
Liraglutide (activates appetite regulation in the brain)	Given by injection; *ensure that patient knows how to properly administer this medication.* Monitor ALT and AST; *there is an increased risk for pancreatitis when taking this drug.* Patients taking insulin should not take this drug; *hypoglycemia can develop.* Teach to report taking this drug to all health care providers; *alpha$_1$-adrenergic antagonists can increase or decrease the side effects of other drugs such as beta-blockers, calcium channel blockers, or medications used to treat erectile dysfunction.*
Orlistat (inhibits lipase; thus, fats are only partially digested and absorbed)	Monitor liver enzymes; *rare cases of liver injury have been reported.* Teach to take a multivitamin daily; *the body may not normally absorb enough vitamins found in foods due to the effect of the drug.* Teach that loose stools, abdominal cramps, and nausea can occur unless fat intake is reduced to less than 30% of the daily intake; *the drug mechanism facilitates GI symptoms since fats are only partially digested and absorbed.*
Phentermine-topiramate (combines short-term weight loss drug phentermine with seizure medication topiramate)	Patients with glaucoma or hyperthyroidism should not take this medication; *this medication can increase eye pressure and thyroid activity.* Determine whether patient is pregnant or planning pregnancy; *this medication can cause birth defects.* (**NOTE:** Patient should also refrain from using this medication if breastfeeding).
Semaglutide (increases resting metabolism and feeling of fullness; reduces appetite)	Given by injection; *ensure that patient knows how to properly administer this medication.* Monitor ALT, AST, and thyroid panels; *this medication can increase the risk for developing pancreatitis and (in rare cases) thyroid tumor.*
Setmelanotide (targets impaired MC4R pathway, the underlying hunger)	Given by injection; *ensure that patient knows how to properly administer this medication.* Teach that sexual function may change while taking this medication; *priapism, spontaneous penile erection, and changes in sexual arousal that occur without sexual activity are side effects.* Teach to report any feelings of depression, mood changes, or suicidal thoughts; *this medication can cause these symptoms.* Recommend the patient have a full body skin examination before and during treatment; *this medication can cause skin changes.* Teach that increasing skin pigmentation and darkening of moles or nevi can occur; *these are side effects associated with this medication.*

From the National Institute of Diabetes and Digestive and Kidney Disorders. (2021). *Prescription medications to treat overweight and obesity.* https://www.niddk.nih.gov/health-information/weight-management/prescription-medications-treat-overweight-obesity.

weight is beneficial to blood pressure and to cholesterol and glucose levels (Centers for Disease Control and Prevention, 2022c).

A minimum-level workout should be developed so that consistency can be achieved and maintained. Encourage walking 20 minutes a day and increasing the time as endurance increases. The activity may be performed all at once or divided over the course of the day.

Drug therapy. Four medications are FDA-approved for overweight and obesity treatment. The primary health care provider will work with the patient to determine which, if any, of these drugs are appropriate. See Table 52.4 for information about select types of drug therapy used for treatment of overweight and obesity.

Cryolipolysis. Cryolipolysis is a nonsurgical procedure also known as "fat freezing." This procedure is used to reduce fat deposits in certain body areas (American Society for Dermatological Surgery, 2023). However, it is not meant for people with overweight and obesity; it is used primarily for removal of small amounts of excess fatty tissue that cannot be changed by diet or exercise (American Society for Dermatological Surgery,

2023). Redirect patients requesting cryolipolysis to the primary health care provider for further discussion.

Behavioral management. Behavioral management of obesity helps the patient change daily eating habits to lose weight. Self-monitoring techniques include keeping a journal of foods eaten (food diary), exercise or activity patterns, and emotional and situational factors. Stimulus control involves controlling the external cues that promote overeating. Reinforcement techniques are used to self-reward the behavior change. Cognitive restructuring involves modifying negative beliefs by learning positive coping self-statements. Counseling by health care professionals must continue before, during, and after treatment. The 12-step program offered by Overeaters Anonymous (www.oa.org) has helped many adults lose weight, especially those who eat compulsively.

Oral superabsorbent hydrogel. FDA-cleared to be a medical device instead of drug therapy, this type of treatment comes in the form of a small capsule taken orally with water before meals. The capsule disintegrates in the stomach and releases superabsorbent hydrogel particles that absorb water, which expand to take up 25% of total gastric volume (Anasari & Miras, 2022). The particles also absorb food, which contributes to fullness. They break down in the colon, release water that is reabsorbed into the body, and are then excreted in feces (Anasari & Miras, 2022).

The average patient in a recent study of this type of treatment decreased daily intake by 300 calories and lost (and maintained the loss of) about 5% of total weight over a 6-month period (Greenway et al., 2019). Side effects include fullness, bloating, abdominal cramping, and flatulence (Gelesis, Inc., 2023).

Complementary and integrative health. Many complementary and integrative therapies have been tested and used for obesity. These modalities aim to suppress appetite and therefore limit food intake to lose weight:

- Acupuncture
- Acupressure
- Ayurveda (a combination of holistic approaches)
- Hypnosis

Evidence about the effectiveness of each of these therapies varies. Encourage the patient to speak to the primary health care provider to determine whether any of these methods are recommended.

Surgical Management. Some patients seek to improve their appearance by reducing the amount of adipose tissue in selected areas of the body. A typical example of this type of surgery is *liposuction*, which can be done in a health care provider's office or ambulatory surgery center. Although the patient's appearance may improve, if weight gain continues, the fatty tissue will return. This procedure is not a solution for adults with obesity.

Bariatrics is a branch of medicine that manages patients with obesity and its related diseases. Certain adults may be considered for this type of weight loss surgery. These include patients who:

- Do not respond to traditional interventions
- Have a body mass index (BMI) of 40 or greater
- Have a BMI of 35 or greater, with other health risk factors

Surgical procedures include gastric bypass, sleeve gastrectomy, adjustable gastric band, biliopancreatic diversion with duodenal switch (BPD/DS), and single anastomosis duodeno-ileal bypass with sleeve gastrectomy (SADI-S) (American Society for Metabolic and Bariatric Surgery [ASMBS], 2023). Another procedure, gastrointestinal electrical stimulation (GES), involves the implantation of a vagal-blocking device (vBloc) into the abdomen (Anasari & Miras, 2022) that causes early satiety, and thus, reduced intake (Shikora et al., 2019).

Depending on the procedure, the surgeon may choose to use a conventional open approach or perform minimally invasive surgery (MIS). Many patients have MIS via either the laparoscopic adjustable gastric band (LAGB) procedure or laparoscopic sleeve gastrectomy (LSG). Both procedures are classified as restrictive surgeries. The decision of whether the patient is a candidate for the MIS is based on weight, body build, history of abdominal surgery, and coexisting medical complications. With any surgical approach, patients must agree to modify their lifestyle and follow stringent protocols to lose weight and keep the weight off. After successful bariatric surgery, many patients no longer have complications of obesity, such as diabetes mellitus, hypertension, depression, or sleep apnea.

Preoperative care. Preoperative care is similar to that for any patient undergoing abdominal surgery or laparoscopy (see Chapter 9). However, patients with obesity are at increased surgical risks of pulmonary and thromboembolitic complications, as well as death. Some surgeons require a specific amount of weight loss before bariatric surgery to minimize complications. Patients also have a thorough psychological assessment and testing to detect depression, substance abuse, or other mental health/behavioral health problems that could interfere with success after surgery. Cognitive ability, coping skills, development, motivation, expectations, and support systems are also assessed. Patients who are not alert and oriented or do not have sufficient strength and mobility are not considered for bariatric surgery. *The primary role of the nurse is to reinforce health teaching in preparation for surgery.* Most bariatric surgical centers provide educational sessions for groups of patients who plan to have the procedure.

Operative procedures. *Gastric restriction* surgeries, the easiest to perform, allow for normal digestion without the risk of nutrition deficiencies. In a banding procedure, the surgeon places an adjustable band to create a small proximal stomach pouch through a laparoscope (Fig. 52.7A–B). The band may or may not be inflatable.

In the vertical sleeve *gastroplasty* (see Fig. 52.7C), about three-fourths of the stomach is removed, with the sleevelike remaining stomach having a much-reduced capacity. In the *biliopancreatic diversion with duodenal switch* (see Fig. 52.7D), a less common bariatric surgery, almost 80% of the stomach is removed. The remaining pouch is connected to the bottom of the small intestine (bypassing the upper portion). Therefore, most calories and nutrients are routed into the colon, where they are not absorbed (Phillips & Zieve, 2022).

The most common bariatric surgery performed in the United States is the *Roux-en-Y gastric bypass (RNYGB),* which is often done as a robotic-assistive surgical procedure. Most commonly called a gastric bypass, this procedure results in quick weight loss, but it is more invasive with a higher risk for postoperative complications. In this procedure, gastric resection is combined with malabsorption surgery. The patient's stomach, duodenum, and part of the jejunum are bypassed so that fewer calories can be absorbed (see Fig. 52.7E).

Postoperative care. Postoperative care depends on the type of surgery performed. Patients having one of the MIS procedures have less pain, scarring, and blood loss. They typically have a faster recovery time and a faster return to daily activities. However, even patients having MIS are considered to have had major abdominal surgery along with all its risks, and their care is planned accordingly. These patients may require less than 24 hours in the hospital; some may need 1 to 2 days. Patients with open procedures may need several days to recover.

A major focus of postoperative care must be placed on patient and staff safety. Patients should be placed in a bariatric room (see Table 52.3). Always use additional personnel when moving the patient. Ensure that side rails are not touching the body because they can cause pressure injuries. Pressure between skinfolds and tubes and catheters can also cause skin breakdown. Monitor the skin in these areas, and keep the skin clean and dry.

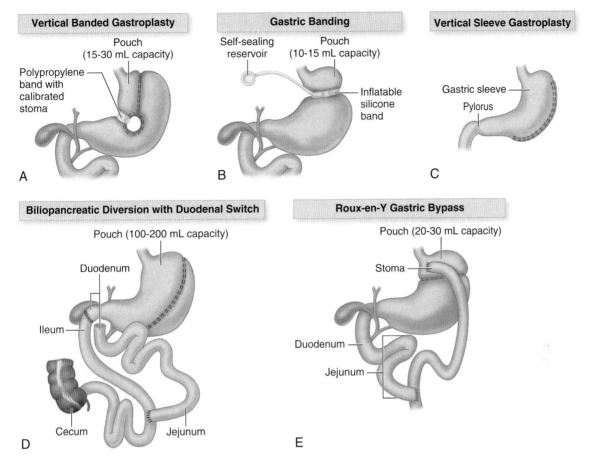

FIG. 52.7 Bariatric surgical procedures. (A) Vertical banded gastroplasty. (B) Gastric banding. (C) Vertical sleeve gastroplasty. (D) Biliopancreatic diversion with duodenal switch. (E) Roux-en-Y gastric bypass (RNYGB). (From Silvestri, L., & Silvestri, A. [2020]. *Saunders Comprehensive review for the NCLEX-RN examination* [8th ed.]. St. Louis: Elsevier.)

Care of the patient who has undergone any type of bariatric surgery is similar to that of any patient having abdominal or laparoscopic surgery (see Chapter 9). *The priority for postoperative care is airway management.* Patients with short and thick necks often have compromised airways and need aggressive respiratory support—possibly mechanical ventilation in the critical care unit.

In addition to the postoperative complications typically associated with abdominal and laparoscopic surgeries, patients who have undergone bariatric surgery are at risk for anastomotic leaks (a leak of digestive juices and partially digested food through an anastomosis). Implement measures to prevent complications as noted in Box 52.12.

All patients experience some degree of pain, but it is usually less severe when MIS is performed. Patients may use patient-controlled analgesia (PCA) with morphine for up to the first 24 hours. All patients receive oral opioid analgesic agents (liquid form when possible) as prescribed after the PCA is discontinued. Acute pain management is discussed in detail in Chapter 6.

Clear liquids are introduced slowly if the patient can tolerate water, and 1-ounce cups are used for each serving. A full liquid diet follows tolerance of the clear liquid diet; usually patients are discharged on full liquids. Pureed foods follow in about a week, with each meal consisting of about 5 tablespoons of food.

! NURSING SAFETY PRIORITY

Action Alert

Some patients who undergo bariatric surgery have a nasogastric (NG) tube put in place, especially after open surgical procedures. In gastroplasty procedures, the NG tube drains both the proximal pouch and the distal stomach. Closely monitor the tube for patency. *Never reposition the tube because its movement can disrupt the suture line!* The NG tube is removed on the second day if the patient is passing flatus.

After several weeks of pureed foods, soft foods are introduced. Around the eighth postoperative week, solid, nutrient-dense foods are incorporated. Remind the patient to eat and drink slowly, to consume only small meals, to stop eating before feeling full, to choose foods high in protein, and to avoid foods that are fatty or have high sugar content.

Care Coordination and Transition Management

Obesity can be a chronic, lifelong problem if weight loss is not accomplished. Diets, drug therapy, exercise, and behavioral

BOX 52.12 Best Practice for Patient Safety and Quality Care

Care of the Patient After Bariatric Surgery

Cardiovascular/Respiratory Care
- Place the patient in semi-Fowler's position to improve breathing and decrease risk for sleep apnea, pneumonia, or atelectasis.
- Monitor oxygen saturation; provide oxygen, bilevel, or continuous positive airway pressure (BiPAP or CPAP) ventilation per orders.
- Apply sequential compression stockings and administer prophylactic anti-coagulant therapy as prescribed to prevent venous thromboembolisms, including pulmonary embolism (PE).

Gastrointestinal Care
- Apply an abdominal binder to prevent wound dehiscence for open surgical procedures.
- Observe for signs and symptoms of **dumping syndrome** (caused by food entering the small intestine too quickly) after *gastric bypass,* such as tachy-cardia, nausea, diarrhea, and abdominal cramping. If this occurs, treatment ranges from dietary adjustments, to administration of antidiarrheal agents and/or acarbose depending on symptom severity, to surgical intervention.
- Provide six small feedings (clear and then full liquids as ordered) and plenty of fluids to prevent dehydration in collaboration with the registered dieti-tian nutritionist (RDN).
- Measure and record abdominal girth daily or as per orders.

Genitourinary Care
- Remove urinary catheter within 24 hours after surgery to prevent urinary tract infection.

Integumentary Care
- Observe skin areas and folds for redness/hyperpigmentation, excoriation, or breakdown, and treat these problems early.
- Use absorbent padding between folds to prevent pressure areas and skin breakdown.
- Ensure that tubes and catheters are not causing pressure on the skin.

Musculoskeletal Care
- Collaborate with the physical therapist for transfers or ambulation assistive devices, such as walkers.
- Encourage and assist with turning every 2 hours, using an appropriate weight-bearing overhead trapeze.

✚ NURSING SAFETY PRIORITY

Critical Rescue

Anastomotic leaks are the most common serious complication and cause of death after gastric bypass surgery. Recognize that you must monitor for symptoms of this life-threatening problem, which includes increasing back, shoulder, or abdominal pain; restlessness; and unexplained tachycardia and oliguria. If any of these findings is present, respond by contacting the surgeon immediately!

BOX 52.13 Patient and Family Education

Discharge Teaching Topics for the Patient After Bariatric Surgery

Nutrition: Diet progression, nutrient (including vitamin and mineral) supple-ments, hydration guidelines

Drug therapy: Analgesics and antiemetic drugs, if needed; drugs for other health problems

Wound care: Clean procedure for open or laparoscopic wounds; cover during shower or bath

Activity level: Restrictions, such as avoiding lifting; activity progression; return to driving and work

Signs and symptoms to report: Fever; excessive nausea or vomiting; epi-gastric, back, or shoulder pain; red, hot, or draining wound(s); pain, red-ness/hyperpigmentation, or swelling in legs; chest pain; difficulty breathing

Follow-up care: Health care provider office or clinic visits, support groups and other community resources, counseling for patient (and caregiver, if needed)

Continuing education: Nutrition and exercise classes; follow-up visits with registered dietitian nutritionist (RDN)

---

modification can produce short-term weight losses with reason-able safety. However, many patients who do lose weight often regain it. Treatment of obesity should focus on the long-term reduction of health risks and problems associated with obe-sity, improvements in quality of life, and the promotion of a health-oriented lifestyle.

Home Care Management. In collaboration with the registered dietitian nutritionist (RDN), counsel the patient on a healthful eating pattern. The physical therapist or exercise physiologist recommends an appropriate exercise program. A psychologist may recommend cognitive restructuring approaches that help alter dysfunctional eating patterns.

For patients who have surgery, additional discharge teach-ing is needed. Box 52.13 lists the important areas that should be reviewed. Patients are usually followed closely by the surgeon and registered dietitian nutritionist (RDN) for several years. Encourage patients to keep all appointments and to adhere to the treatment plan to ensure success. Plastic surgery, such as **panniculectomy** (removal of the abdominal apron, or pannic-ulus), may be performed if needed after weight is stabilized, usually in about 18 to 24 months.

For patients with Type 2 diabetes mellitus who have undergone bariatric surgery, shared medical appointments (SMAs) can be valuable (Reigel et al., 2021). This type of appointment involves a group of patients who have under-gone the same surgery. The group meets periodically for an extended amount of time with the health care provider and interprofessional team for follow-up care. Group members have individual time with the health care provider and then interact with each other and other health care professionals in an effort to improve self-management following surgery (Reigel et al., 2021).

Self-Care Management. Remind patients to coordinate with their surgeon or primary health care provider to create a manageable and appropriate physical activity plan. For patients having nonsurgical management, emphasize the need to decrease overall fat intake and to avoid reliance on appetite-reducing drugs. Keeping a food journal that documents mood and events that take place with eating can be helpful to identify eating patterns.

Teach patients who have had bariatric surgery that postsur-gical bowel changes are common. Vitamin and mineral sup-plements are prescribed after surgery, especially vitamin D,

B-complex vitamins, iron, and calcium, and adherence to this regimen is important for surgical success.

Health Care Resources. Provide the patient with a list of available community resources, such as Overeaters Anonymous (www.oa.org). For patients who have had or are contemplating surgery, the American Society for Metabolic and Bariatric Surgery (www.asmbs.org) may be helpful.

Evaluate Outcomes: Evaluation

Evaluate the care of the patient with obesity based on the identified priority patient problem. The primary expected outcome is that the patient consumes appropriate, nutrient-dense foods to meet metabolic demands without overeating. For surgical patients, an additional expected outcome is that the patient remains free of infection after bariatric surgery.

GET READY FOR THE NEXT-GENERATION NCLEX® EXAMINATION!

Essential Nursing Care Points

Health Promotion/Disease Prevention

- Perform *nutrition* screening for all patients to determine those at risk.
- Calculate BMI as a measure of *nutrition* status and/or BSA for dosage calculation purposes.

Chronic Disease Care

- Teach patients how to successfully manage food allergies or food intolerances.
- Ensure that the patient with food allergies has an epinephrine autoinjector in case of emergency.
- Teach patients receiving enteral or parenteral nutrition at home (and family, as appropriate) how to obtain *nutrition* while avoiding complications.
- Teach patients who are undernourished to eat high-protein, high-calorie foods and to take nutritional supplements.
- Teach patients prescribed injectable drugs for obesity how to self-administer this medication.

Regenerative or Restorative Care

- Ensure that feeding tube placement is verified by x-ray before use for feeding or medication administration.
- Maintain feeding tube patency for patients receiving total enteral nutrition.
- Place patients receiving tube feeding in a semi-Fowler's position at all times to prevent aspiration; check residual contents every 6 hours or as designated per agency policy.
- Collaborate with the interprofessional health care team, especially the registered dietitian nutritionist (RDN), when caring for patients with malnutrition.
- Use gloves when changing feeding system tubing or adding product; use sterile gloves when working with patients who are critically ill or immunocompromised.

Hospice/Palliative/Supportive Care

- Advocate for properly constructed and supplied bariatric rooms, and for supplies that are made to provide dignified care to patients with bariatric needs.
- Recognize that the choice to provide feeding at the end of life can be a complex legal and ethical matter if the patient doesn't have an advance directive or a durable power of attorney.
- Seek input from the interprofessional legal and ethics committee if questions arise regarding tube feeding for a patient who doesn't have an advance directive or a durable power of attorney.

Mastery Questions

1. The nurse is caring for a client who underwent bariatric surgery. Which information would the nurse include in discharge teaching? **Select all that apply.**
   A. Stay hydrated by drinking fruit juice.
   B. Solid food can be introduced into the diet in a week.
   C. Report back, shoulder, or abdominal pain to the surgeon.
   D. It is not unusual to have little urine output for the first few weeks.
   E. Each reintroduced meal should contain about 5 tablespoons of food.

2. The nurse has performed a Mini Nutritional Assessment on a client. When the Malnutrition Indicator Score is 15, which action would the nurse take?
   A. Discuss weight loss strategies with the client.
   B. Contact the health care provider for a nutrition consultation.
   C. Document the findings as demonstrating adequate nourishment.
   D. Ask the registered dietitian nutritionist (RDN) for a lower-calorie diet.

NGN Challenge 52.1

The nurse is caring for a client in the emergency department who reports having Roux-en-Y gastric bypass surgery 2 months ago. Today, soon after eating, the client began to experience nausea, diarrhea, abdominal cramping, and pain that they rated at a 7 on a 0-to-10 scale. Vital signs include T 99.4°F (37.4°C), blood pressure 158/98 mm Hg, heart rate 92 beats/min, and respirations 20 breaths/min.

Complete the diagram by selecting from the choices below to specify what potential condition the client is likely experiencing, **2** nursing actions that are appropriate to take, and **2** parameters the nurse should monitor to assess the client's progress.

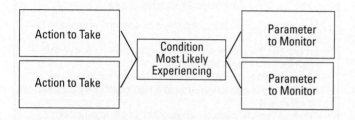

Actions to Take	Potential Conditions	Parameters to Monitor
Administer antihypertensive drug	Dumping syndrome	Temperature for fever
Notify the health care provider	Viral gastroenteritis	Resolution of diarrhea
Prepare for emergency surgery	Myocardial infarction	Dressing saturation following surgery
Provide dietary teaching	Surgical suture disruption	EKG results
Obtain STAT ECG.		Adherence to dietary recommendations

NGN Challenge 52.2

The nurse is monitoring laboratory results for a client with peripheral edema who is receiving total parenteral nutrition (TPN).

Parameters	Results Today (0630)	Results Yesterday (0545)	Results 2 Days Prior (Admission)
Serum sodium (Reference range 136 mEq/L–145 mEq/L [136 mmol/L–145 mmol/L])	145 mEq/L (145 mmol/L)	144 mEq/L (144 mmol/L)	145 mEq/L (145 mmol/L)
Serum potassium (Reference range 3.5–5 mEq/L [3.5–5 mmol/L])	2.9 mEq/L (2.9 mmol/L)	3.2 mEq/L (3.2 mmol/L)	3.3 mEq/L (3.3 mmol/L)
Serum phosphate (Reference range 3–4.5 mg/dL [0.97–1.45 mmol/L])	1.9 mg/dL (0.61 mmol/L)	2.4 mg/dL (0.77 mmol/L)	3.0 mg/dL (0.97 mmol/L)
Serum magnesium (Reference range 1.2–2.1 mEq/L [0.65–1.05 mmol/L])	1.4 mEq/L (0.7 mmol/L)	1.2 mEq/L (0.6 mmol/L)	1.1 mEq/L (0.55 mmol/L)

Complete the following sentence by selecting from the lists of options below.

Based on recent assessment findings and medical history, the client most likely has **1 [Select]** as evidenced by **2 [Select]** and **3 [Select]**.

Options for 1	Options for 2 and 3
Kwashiorkor	Hypokalemia
Bulimia nervosa	Hyperphosphatemia
Refeeding syndrome	Hyponatremia
Obesity	Peripheral edema

REFERENCES

Academy of Nutrition and Dietetics. (2023). *Vegetarianism: The basic facts.* https://www.eatright.org/health/wellness/vegetarian-and-plant-based/vegetarianism-the-basic-facts.

American Academy of Allergy, Asthma, and Immunology. (2023). *Food intolerance versus food allergy.* Retrieved from https://www.aaaai.org/conditions-and-treatments/library/allergy-library/food-intolerance.

American Society for Dermatological Surgery. (2023). *Cryolipolysis for excess fat.* https://www.asds.net/skin-experts/skin-treatments/cryolipolysis/cryolipolysis-for-excess-fat.

American Society for Metabolic and Bariatric Surgery (ASMBS). (2023). *Bariatric surgery procedures.* https://asmbs.org/patients/bariatric-surgery-procedures.

American Society for Parenteral and Enteral Nutrition. (2023). *Parenteral and enteral nutrition (ASPEN).* Malnutrition solution center. https://www.nutritioncare.org/Malnutrition/.

Anasari, S., & Miras, A. (2022). Clinical efficacy and mechanism of action of medical devices for obesity and type 2 diabetes. *Current Opinion in Endocrine and Metabolic Research, 23,* 1–11.

*Aycock, D., et al. (2017). Language sensitivity, the RESPECT model, and continuing education. *The Journal of Continuing Education in Nursing, 48*(11), 517–524.

Baiu, I., & Spain, D. (2019). Parenteral nutrition. *Journal of the American Medical Association, 321*(21), 2141.

Bellanti, F., et al. (2022). Malnutrition in hospitalized old patients: Screening and diagnosis, clinical outcomes, and management. *Nutrients, 14*(4), 910. https://doi.org/10.3390/nu14040910.

Centers for Disease Control and Prevention (CDC). (2022a). *About adult BMI.* www.cdc.gov/healthyweight/assessing/bmi/adult_bmi/

Centers for Disease Control and Prevention (CDC). (2022b). *Defining adult overweight and obesity.* Retrieved from https://www.cdc.gov/obesity/basics/adult-defining.html.

Centers for Disease Control and Prevention (CDC). (2022c). *Losing weight.* https://www.cdc.gov/healthyweight/losing_weight/index.html.

Centers for Disease Control and Prevention's Division of Nutrition. (2023). *Physical Activity, and Obesity (DNPAO)Health equity.* . https://www.cdc.gov/nccdphp/dnpao/health-equity/index.html.

Chooi, Y., Ding, C., & Magkos, F. (2019). The epidemiology of obesity. *Metabolism Clinical and Experimental, 92,* 6–10.

DeLegge, M. (2021). Gastrostomy tubes: Uses, patient selection, and efficacy in adults. *UpToDate.* Retrieved May 24, 2023, from https://www.uptodate.com/contents/gastrostomy-tubes-uses-patient-selection-and-efficacy-in-adults.

Drummond Hayes, K., & Drummond Hayes, D. (2018). Best practices for unclogging feeding tubes in adults. *Nursing 2018, 48*(6), 66.

Eaton, K., & Lyman, G. (2022). Dosing of anticancer agents in adults. *UpToDate.* Retrieved May 24, 2023, from https://www.uptodate.com/contents/dosing-of-anticancer-agents-in-adults.

Flint, B., & Hall, C. (2022). Body surface area. [Updated 2022 Mar 26]. In *StatPearls [Internet].* Treasure Island (FL): StatPearls Publishing. 2022 Jan-. Available from: https://www.ncbi.nlm.nih.gov/books/NBK559005/.

Gelesis, Inc. (2023). *Plenity FAQ.* https://www.myplenity.com/faq#

Gorski, L. A., Hadaway, L., Hagle, M. E., et al. (2021). Infusion therapy standards of practice. (8th ed.). *Journal of Infusion Nursing, 44*(1S), S1–S224.

Government of Canada. (2023). *Canada's food guide.* Retrieved from https://food-guide.canada.ca/en/.

Greenway, F., Aronne, L., Raben, A., et al. (2019). A randomized, double-blind, placebo-controlled study of Gelesis100: A novel nonsystemic oral hydrogel for weight loss. *Obesity, 27,* 205–216. https://doi.org/10.1002/oby.22347.

Harvard, T. H. Chan School of Public Health. (2023a). *Ethnic differences in BMI and disease risk.* https://www.hsph.harvard.edu/obesity-prevention-source/ethnic-differences-in-bmi-and-disease-risk/.

Harvard, T. H. Chan School of Public Health. (2023b). *Measuring obesity.* https://www.hsph.harvard.edu/obesity-prevention-source/obesity-definition/how-to-measure-body-fatness/.

Hodin, R., & Bordeianou, L. (2023). Inpatient placement of nasogastric and nasoenteric tubes in adults. *UpToDate.* Retrieved March 7, 2023, from https://www.uptodate.com/contents/inpatient-placement-and-management-of-nasogastric-and-nasoenteric-tubes-in-adults.

Interprofessional Education Collaborative (IPEC). (2016). *Core competencies for interprofessional collaborative practice: 2016 update.* Retrieved from https://nebula.wsimg.com/2f68a39520b-03336b41038c370497473?AccessKeyId=DC06780E69ED19E-2B3A5&disposition=0&alloworigin=1.

King, K. (2019). Trends in parenteral nutrition. *Today's Dietician, 21*(1), 36–39.

Lin, X., & Li, H. (2021). Obesity: Epidemiology, pathophysiology, and therapeutics. *Frontiers in Endocrinology, 12:*706978.

Loos, R., & Yeo, G. (2022). The genetics of obesity: from discovery to biology. *Genetics, 23,* 120–133. https://doi.org/10.1038/s41576-021-00414-z.

Mehler, P. (2023). Anorexia nervosa in adults and adolescents: The refeeding syndrome. *UpToDate.* Retrieved May 24, 202, from https://www.uptodate.com/contents/anorexia-nervosa-in-adults-and-adolescents-the-refeeding-syndrome.

Morley, J. (2022). *Protein-energy undernutrition: Merck manual professional version.* https://www.merckmanuals.com/professional/nutritional-disorders/undernutrition/protein-energy-undernutrition-peu.

National Academies of Sciences, Engineering, & Medicine. (n.d.). *Summary report of dietary reference intakes.* https://www.nationalacademies.org/our-work/summary-report-of-the-dietary-reference-intakes.

National Heart, Lung, and Blood Institute; National Institutes of Health; U.S. Department of Health and Human Services (n.d.). Assessing your weight and health risk https://www.nhlbi.nih.gov/health/educational/lose_wt/risk.htm.

Nestle Nutrition Institute (n.d.). Mini nutritional assessment - short form (MNA-SF). https://www.mna-elderly.com/forms/mini/mna_mini_english.pdf.

Office of Disease Prevention and Health Promotion. (2023). *Healthy People 2030: Nutrition and healthy eating.* U.S. Department of Health and Human Services. https://health.gov/healthypeople.

Office on Women's Health. (2022). *Binge eating disorder.* https://www.womenshealth.gov/mental-health/mental-health-conditions/eating-disorders/binge-eating-disorder.

Omni. (2022). *BSA calculator – Body surface area.* https://www.calctool.org/other/bsa.

Oteng, A., & Kersten, S. (2020). Mechanisms of actions of trans fatty acids. *Advances in Nutrition, 11*(3), 697–708.

Pagana, K. D., Pagana, T. J., & Pagana, T. N. (2022). *Mosby's manual of diagnostic and laboratory tests* (7th ed.). St. Louis: Elsevier.

Perkins, A. (2019). Body dysmorphic disorder: *The drive for perfection. Nursing 2019, 49*(3), 28–33.

Phillips, K. (2022). Body dysmorphic disorder. In *Ferri's Clinical Advisor* 268.e9-268.e10.

Phillips, M., & Zieve, D. (2022). *Biliopancreatic diversion (BPD).* https://medlineplus.gov/ency/imagepages/19499.htm.

Reigel, J., Glasenapp, K., & Haglund, K. (2021). Optimizing the perioperative process for the bariatric surgery candidate. *MedSurg Nursing, 30*(3), 192–196.

Ritchie, C., & Yukawa, M. (2023). Geriatric nutrition: Nutritional issues in older adults. *UpToDate.* Retrieved May 24, 2023, from https://www.uptodate.com/contents/geriatric-nutrition-nutritional-issues-in-older-adults.

Rogers, J. L. (2023). *McCance and Huether's Pathophysiology: The biologic basis for disease in adults and children* (9th ed.). St. Louis: Elsevier.

Seres, D. (2021). Nutrition support in critically ill patients: Parenteral nutrition. *UpToDate.* Retrieved May 24, 2023, from https://www.uptodate.com/contents/nutrition-support-in-critically-ill-patients-parenteral-nutrition.

Shikora, S., et al. (2019). *Neurologic metabolic surgery: A review Bulletin of the American College of surgeons.* https://bulletin.facs.org/2019/03/neurologic-metabolic-surgery-a-review/.

Simpson, I. (2021). *BMI and Body Composition in Division I Athletes [Master's thesis].* OhioLINK Electronic Theses and Dissertations Center. Ohio State University. http://rave.ohiolink.edu/etd-c/view?acc_num=osu16189252323773.

Slusser, M., et al. (2019). *Foundations of interprofessional collaborative practice* (1st ed.). St. Louis: Elsevier.

The Joint Commission. (2022). *Nutritional and functional screening.* https://www.jointcommission.org/standards/standard-faqs/critical-access-hospital/provision-of-care-treatment-and-services-pc/000001652/.

U.S. Department of Agriculture. (USDA). (2022). *Start simple with MyPlate.* https://myplate-prod.azureedge.us/sites/default/files/2022-01/SSwMP%20Mini-Poster_English_Final2022.pdf.

U.S. Department of Agriculture (USDA). (2023). *MyPlate.* https://www.myplate.gov/myplate-plan.

U.S. Department of Agriculture and U.S. Department of Health and Human Services. (2020). *Dietary Guidelines for Americans, 2020-2025* (9th ed.). DietaryGuidelines.gov.

World Health Organization. (2021). *Malnutrition.* https://www.who.int/news-room/fact-sheets/detail/malnutrition.

World Health Organization. (2023). *Obesity.* Retrieved from https://www.who.int/topics/obesity/en/.

Assessment of the Endocrine System

Cherie R. Rebar

http://evolve.elsevier.com/Iggy/

LEARNING OUTCOMES

1. Use knowledge of anatomy and physiology to perform a focused assessment of the endocrine system.
2. Teach evidence-based health promotion activities to help prevent endocrine health problems or trauma.
3. Identify factors that affect health equity for patients with health problems related to the endocrine system.
4. Explain how genetic implications and physiologic aging of the endocrine system affect cellular regulation.
5. Interpret assessment findings for patients with a suspected or actual endocrine problem.
6. Plan evidence-based care and support for patients undergoing diagnostic testing of the endocrine system.

KEY TERMS

aldosterone Mineralocorticoid that maintains extracellular fluid volume and electrolyte composition; promotes sodium and water reabsorption and potassium excretion in the kidney.

antidiuretic hormone (ADH) Vasopressin.

catecholamines Epinephrine and norepinephrine.

cortisol Glucocorticoid that affects the body's response to stress, nutrition metabolism, emotional stability, immune function, and sodium and water balance.

gonads The male and female reproductive endocrine glands.

hormones Natural chemicals that exert their effects on specific tissues known as target tissues.

insulin Hormone that increases glucose uptake by the cells, causing a decrease in blood glucose levels.

negative feedback mechanism Signals to an endocrine gland to secrete a hormone in response to a body change to cause a reaction that will result in actions to oppose the action of the initial condition change and restore homeostasis.

target tissues Tissues that have receptors corresponding to different hormones that when bound to the hormones respond by changing their activity.

thyroxine (T_4) Thyroid hormone that contributes to metabolism with triiodothyronine (T_3).

triiodothyronine (T_3) Thyroid hormone that contributes to metabolism with thyroxine (T_4).

✵ PRIORITY AND INTERRELATED CONCEPTS

The priority concepts for this chapter are:
- *Fluid and Electrolyte Balance*
- *Glucose Regulation*

The interrelated concepts for this chapter are:
- *Nutrition*
- *Reproduction*
- *Sexuality*

The ductless glands of the endocrine system secrete hormones—natural biochemicals—into the bloodstream that contribute to maintenance of homeostasis in the body. They serve to facilitate a delicate *fluid and electrolyte balance* and influence *glucose regulation* and multiple other processes within the body.

Endocrine glands are located in many areas (Fig. 53.1) and affect all other body systems. There is no direct anatomic connection between the glands and their target tissues, which have receptors corresponding to different hormones. Instead, endocrine glands secrete hormones into the bloodstream for transportation to the target tissues (Rogers, 2023). When bound to hormones, the target tissues respond by changing their activity.

The endocrine glands include:
- Adrenal glands
- Gonads (testes and ovaries)

ENDOCRINE SYSTEM

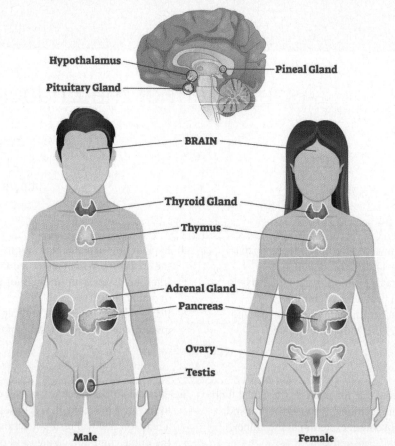

FIG. 53.1 Locations of various glands within the endocrine system. (Used with permission from istockphoto.com, 2020, VectorMine.)

- Hypothalamus (a neuroendocrine gland)
- Pancreas
- Parathyroid
- Pineal gland
- Pituitary gland
- Thymus (part of the lymphatic system as well; functions primarily in childhood)
- Thyroid

Body functions controlled by the endocrine system for homeostasis and regulation include temperature, metabolism, growth, *nutrition,* elimination, *fluid and electrolyte balance,* and *reproduction.* Many interactions must occur between the endocrine system and all other body systems to ensure that each system maintains homeostasis in response to environmental changes. For example, the endocrine system keeps the internal body temperature at or near 98.6°F (37°C), even when environmental temperatures vary. Other actions keep the serum sodium level between 136 and 145 mEq/L (mmol/L), whether a healthy adult eats 2 g or 12 g of sodium per day.

Table 53.1 lists hormones secreted by various endocrine glands. Although circulating hormones travel through the blood to all body areas, they exert their actions only on target tissues. Hormones recognize their target tissues and exert their actions by binding to receptors on or within the target tissue cells. In general, each receptor site type is specific for only one hormone. Hormone-receptor actions work in a "lock and key" manner in that a receptor site (lock) can only be activated by the correct hormone (key) (Fig. 53.2). Once the hormone has unlocked its receptor, the target tissue creates a specific response.

Endocrine system problems and disorders are influenced by:
- An excess of a specific hormone
- A deficiency of a specific hormone
- Poor hormone-receptor interactions, which decrease target tissue responsiveness

ANATOMY AND PHYSIOLOGY REVIEW

The normal blood level range of each hormone is well defined. Excesses or deficiencies of hormone secretion can lead to pathologic conditions affecting many body systems.

Hormones maintain homeostasis of cellular function through a series of one or more negative feedback control mechanisms. A negative feedback mechanism signals an endocrine gland to secrete a hormone in response to a body change to *oppose* the action of the initial condition change and restore homeostasis.

Hormone secretion depends on the body's need. When a body condition starts to deviate from the normal range and a specific response is needed to correct this change, secretion of

TABLE 53.1 Principal Hormones of the Endocrine Glands

Gland	Hormones
Hypothalamus	Corticotropin-releasing hormone (CRH)
	Gonadotropin-releasing hormone (GnRH)
	Growth hormone–inhibiting hormone (somatostatin GHIH)
	Growth hormone–releasing hormone (GHRH)
	Melanocyte-inhibiting hormone (MIH)
	Prolactin-inhibiting hormone (PIH)
	Thyrotropin-releasing hormone (TRH)
Anterior pituitary	Adrenocorticotropic hormone (ACTH, corticotropin)
	Follicle-stimulating hormone (FSH)
	Growth hormone (GH)
	Luteinizing hormone (LH)
	Melanocyte-stimulating hormone (MSH)
	Prolactin (PRL)
	Thyroid-stimulating hormone (TSH), also known as *thyrotropin*
Posterior pituitary	Oxytocin
	Vasopressin (antidiuretic hormone [ADH])
Thyroid	Calcitonin
	Thyroxine (T$_4$)
	Triiodothyronine (T$_3$)
Parathyroid	Parathyroid hormone (PTH)
Adrenal cortex	Glucocorticoids (cortisol)
	Mineralocorticoids (aldosterone)
Ovary	Estrogen
	Progesterone
Testes	Testosterone
Pancreas	Glucagon
	Insulin
	Somatostatin

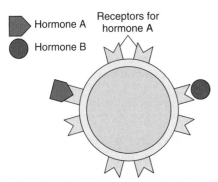

FIG. 53.2 "Lock and key" hormone-receptor binding. Hormone A fits and binds to its receptors, causing a change in cell action. Hormone B does not fit or bind to receptors; no change in cell action results.

the specific hormone capable of starting the correcting action or response is stimulated until the need (demand) is met and the body returns to homeostasis. As the correction occurs, hormone secretion decreases (and may halt).

An example of a simple negative feedback hormone response is the control of insulin secretion. When blood glucose levels start to rise above normal, the hormone insulin is secreted. Insulin increases glucose uptake by the cells, causing a *decrease* in blood glucose levels. The action of insulin (decreasing blood glucose levels) is the *opposite of* or *negative to* the condition that stimulated insulin secretion (elevated blood glucose levels).

Some hormones have more complex interactions for negative feedback. These interactions involve a series of reactions in which more than one endocrine gland, as well as the final target tissues, is stimulated. In this situation, the first hormone in the series may have another endocrine gland or glands as the target tissue. The final result of complex negative feedback for endocrine function is still opposite of the initiating condition.

An example of complex control is the interaction of the hypothalamus and the anterior pituitary with the adrenal cortex (Fig. 53.3). Low blood levels of cortisol from the adrenal cortex stimulate the secretion of corticotropin-releasing hormone (CRH) in the hypothalamus. CRH stimulates the anterior pituitary gland to secrete adrenocorticotropic hormone (ACTH). ACTH then triggers the release of cortisol from the adrenal cortex, the final endocrine gland in this series. The rising blood levels of cortisol inhibit CRH release from the hypothalamus. Without CRH, the anterior pituitary gland stops secretion of ACTH. In response, normal blood cortisol levels are maintained.

Adrenal Glands

The adrenal glands are vascular, tent-shaped organs on the top of each kidney (see Fig. 53.1). They have an outer cortex and an inner medulla. Adrenal hormones affect the entire body.

Adrenal Cortex

The adrenal cortex makes up about 90% of the adrenal gland and has cells divided into three layers. The main hormone types secreted by the cortex are the mineralocorticoids and the glucocorticoids. In addition, the cortex also secretes small amounts of sex hormones.

Mineralocorticoids are produced and secreted by the adrenal cortex to help control **fluid and electrolyte balance**. Aldosterone is the mineralocorticoid that maintains extracellular fluid volume and electrolyte composition. It promotes sodium and water reabsorption and potassium excretion in the kidney. Aldosterone secretion is regulated by the renin-angiotensin-aldosterone system (RAAS), serum potassium ion level, and adrenocorticotropic hormone (ACTH).

Renin is produced by specialized cells of the kidney arterioles. Its release is triggered by a decrease in extracellular fluid volume from blood loss, sodium loss, or postural changes. Hypoxemia also triggers renin release. Renin converts renin substrate (angiotensinogen), a plasma protein, to angiotensin I. Angiotensin I is then converted by an enzyme to form angiotensin II, the active form of angiotensin. In turn, angiotensin II stimulates the secretion of aldosterone. Chapter 13 (see Fig. 13.6) further explains the RAAS functions. Aldosterone causes the kidney to reabsorb sodium and water to bring the plasma volume and osmolarity back to normal.

Serum potassium level also controls aldosterone secretion. It is secreted whenever the serum potassium level increases above normal by as little as 0.1 mEq/L (mmol/L). Aldosterone then enhances kidney excretion of potassium to reduce the blood potassium level back to normal, correcting even the smallest **fluid and electrolyte balance**.

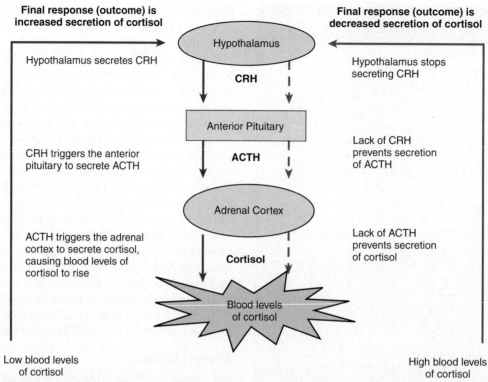

FIG. 53.3 Examples of positive and negative feedback control of hormone secretion. *ACTH,* Adrenocorticotropic hormone; *CRH,* corticotropin-releasing hormone.

Glucocorticoids are produced by the adrenal cortex and are essential for life. The main glucocorticoid produced by the adrenal cortex is cortisol. Cortisol affects:

- The body's response to stress
- Carbohydrate, protein, and fat metabolism
- Emotional stability
- Immune function
- Fluid and electrolyte balance (sodium)

Cortisol also influences other important body processes. For example, it must be present for action of the catecholamines (epinephrine, norepinephrine [NE]) and maintenance of the normal excitability of the heart muscle cells (Rogers, 2023). Glucocorticoid functions are listed in Box 53.1.

Glucocorticoid release is regulated directly by the anterior pituitary hormone *ACTH* and indirectly by the hypothalamic corticotropin-releasing hormone *(CRH).* The release of ACTH and CRH is affected by the serum level of free cortisol, the normal sleep-wake cycle, and stress.

As described earlier and shown in Fig. 53.3, when blood cortisol levels are low, the hypothalamus secretes CRH, which triggers the pituitary to release ACTH. Then ACTH triggers the adrenal cortex to secrete cortisol. Adequate or elevated blood levels of cortisol *inhibit* the release of CRH and ACTH. This inhibitory effect is another example of a negative feedback system.

Glucocorticoid release peaks in the morning and reaches its lowest level 12 hours after the peak. Emotional, chemical, or physical stress increases the release of glucocorticoids.

Sex hormones (androgens and estrogens) are secreted in low levels by the adrenal cortex. Adrenal secretion of these hormones is usually not significant because the gonads (ovaries and

testes) secrete much larger amounts of estrogens and androgens. However, in women, the adrenal gland is the major source of androgens.

Adrenal Medulla

The adrenal medulla is a sympathetic nerve ganglion that has secretory cells. Stimulation of the sympathetic nervous system causes the release of adrenal medullary hormones, the catecholamines (epinephrine and norepinephrine [NE]). These hormones travel to all areas of the body through the blood and exert their effects on target cells. The adrenal medullary hormones are not essential for life because they also are secreted by other body tissues, but they do play a role in the stress response.

The adrenal medulla secretes about 15% NE and 85% epinephrine. Hormone effects vary with the specific receptor in the cell membranes of the target tissue.

BOX 53.1   Functions of Glucocorticoid Hormones in Adults

Glucocorticoid hormones function to:

- Prevent hypoglycemia by increasing liver glucose production (gluconeogenesis) and inhibiting peripheral glucose use
- Maintain excitability and responsiveness of cardiac muscle
- Increase lipolysis, releasing glycerol and free fatty acids
- Increase protein catabolism
- Degrade collagen and connective tissue
- Increase the number of mature neutrophils released from bone marrow
- Exert antiinflammatory effects that decrease the migration of inflammatory cells to sites of injury
- Maintain behavior and cognitive functions

These receptors are of two types: alpha adrenergic and beta adrenergic, which are further classified as alpha$_1$ and alpha$_2$ receptors and beta$_1$, beta$_2$, and beta$_3$ receptors. NE acts mainly on alpha-adrenergic receptors, and epinephrine acts mainly on beta-adrenergic receptors.

Catecholamines exert their actions on many target organs (Table 53.2). Activation of the sympathetic nervous system, which then releases adrenal medullary catecholamines, is an important part of the stress response. Catecholamines are secreted in small amounts at all times to maintain homeostasis. Stress triggers increased secretion of these hormones, resulting in the "fight-or-flight" response, a state of heightened physical and emotional awareness.

Gonads

The gonads are the male and female reproductive endocrine glands. Male gonads are the testes, and female gonads are the ovaries. Function of the gonads is dormant until puberty when, under the influence of gonadotropic hormones secreted by the anterior pituitary, the glands and external genitalia mature. The testes are stimulated to produce testosterone, and the ovaries are stimulated to produce estrogen. These changes are responsible for the development of secondary sexual characteristics. The structure and function of the gonads are described in Chapter 61.

Hypothalamus and Pituitary Glands

Parts of the hypothalamus are composed of glandular tissues that have many control functions for the rest of the endocrine system. It is located beneath the thalamus in the brain, and nerve fibers connect the hypothalamus to the rest of the central nervous system. The hypothalamus shares a small, closed circulatory system with the anterior pituitary gland, the *hypothalamic-hypophysial portal system.* This system allows hormones produced in the hypothalamus to travel directly to the anterior pituitary gland, so only very small amounts are present in systemic circulation where they are not needed.

The function of the hypothalamus is to produce regulatory hormones (see Table 53.1). Some of these hormones are released into the blood and travel to the anterior pituitary, where they either stimulate or inhibit the release of anterior pituitary hormones.

The pituitary gland is located at the base of the brain in a protective pocket of the sphenoid bone (see Fig. 53.1). It is divided into the anterior lobe *(adenohypophysis)* and the posterior lobe *(neurohypophysis).* Nerve fibers in the hypophysial stalk directly connect the hypothalamus to the posterior pituitary (Fig. 53.4).

In response to the releasing hormones of the hypothalamus, the anterior pituitary secretes some tropic (trophic) hormones that have as their target tissues other endocrine glands. Other pituitary hormones, such as prolactin, produce their effect directly on final target tissues (Table 53.3).

The hormones of the posterior pituitary—vasopressin (antidiuretic hormone [ADH]) and oxytocin—are produced in the hypothalamus and delivered to the posterior pituitary, where they are stored. These hormones are released from the posterior pituitary into the blood when needed.

Other factors such as drugs, diet, lifestyle, and pathologic conditions can affect hormone release from the pituitary gland.

Pancreas

The pancreas has exocrine and endocrine functions. The exocrine function of the pancreas involves the secretion of digestive enzymes through ducts that empty into the duodenum. The cells in the islets of Langerhans perform the pancreatic endocrine functions. About 1 million to 2 million islet cells are found throughout the pancreas (Seiron et al., 2019).

The islets have three distinct cell types: alpha cells, which secrete glucagon; beta cells, which secrete insulin (Fig. 53.5); and delta cells, which secrete somatostatin. Glucagon and insulin affect carbohydrate, protein, and fat metabolism.

Glucagon is a hormone that increases blood glucose levels as a part of *glucose regulation.* It is triggered by decreased blood glucose levels and increased blood amino acid levels. This

TABLE 53.2 Catecholamine Receptors and Effects of Adrenal Medullary Hormone Stimulation on Selected Organs and Tissues		
Organ or Tissue	**Receptors**	**Effects**
Eyes	Alpha	Dilation of pupils
Heart	Beta$_1$	Increased heart rate Increased contractility
Blood vessels	Alpha	Vasoconstriction
	Beta$_2$	Vasodilation
Bronchioles	Beta$_2$	Relaxation; dilation
GI tract	Alpha	Increased sphincter tone
	Beta	Decreased motility
Fat cells	Beta	Increased lipolysis
Liver	Alpha	Increased gluconeogenesis and glycogenolysis
Pancreas	Alpha	Decreased glucagon and insulin release
	Beta	Increased glucagon and insulin release
Skin	Alpha	Increased sweating
Fat cells	Beta	Increased lipolysis
Liver	Alpha	Increased gluconeogenesis and glycogenolysis
Pancreas	Alpha	Decreased glucagon and insulin release
	Beta	Increased glucagon and insulin release

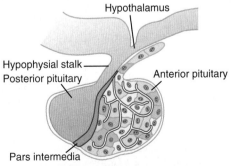

FIG. 53.4 Hypothalamus, hypophysial stalk, anterior pituitary gland, and posterior pituitary gland. (From Guyton, A., & Hall, J. [2006]. *Textbook of medical physiology* [11th ed.]. Philadelphia: Saunders.)

TABLE 53.3   Pituitary Hormones: Target Tissues and Subsequent Actions

Hormone	Target Tissue	Actions
Anterior Pituitary		
Adrenocorticotropic hormone, corticotropin (ACTH)	Adrenal cortex	Stimulates synthesis and release of corticosteroids and adrenocortical growth
Follicle-stimulating hormone (FSH) (known as *interstitial cell–* or *Sertoli cell–stimulating hormone* in males)	Ovary	Stimulates estrogen secretion and follicle maturation
	Testis	Stimulates spermatogenesis
Growth hormone (GH)	Bone and soft tissue	Promotes growth through lipolysis, protein anabolism, and insulin antagonism
Luteinizing hormone (LH)	Ovary	Stimulates ovulation and progesterone secretion
	Testes	Stimulates testosterone secretion
Melanocyte-stimulating hormone (MSH)	Melanocytes	Promotes pigmentation
Prolactin (PRL)	Mammary glands	Stimulates breast development and milk production (no known function in men)
Thyroid-stimulating hormone (TSH) or thyrotropin	Thyroid	Stimulates synthesis and release of thyroid hormone
Posterior Pituitary[a]		
Oxytocin	Uterus and mammary glands	Stimulates uterine contractions and breast milk secretion
Vasopressin (antidiuretic hormone [ADH])	Kidney	Promotes water reabsorption

[a]These hormones are synthesized in the hypothalamus and are stored in the posterior pituitary gland. They are transported from the hypothalamus down the hypothalamic stalk to the posterior pituitary while bound to proteins known as *neurophysins*.

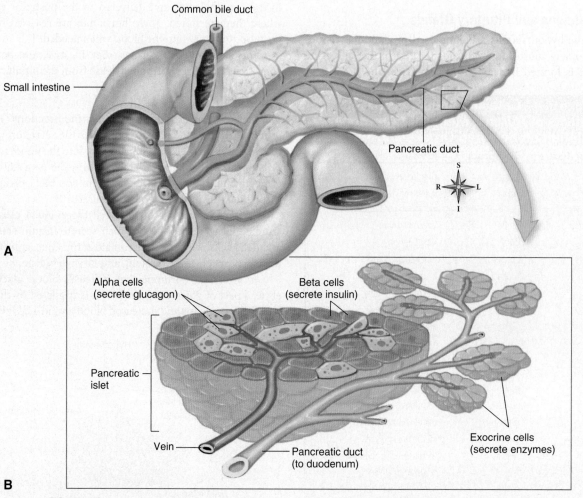

FIG. 53.5 Structure of the pancreas. (From Patton, K. T., & Thibodeau, G. A. [2020]. *Structure & function of the body* [16th ed.]. St. Louis: Elsevier.)

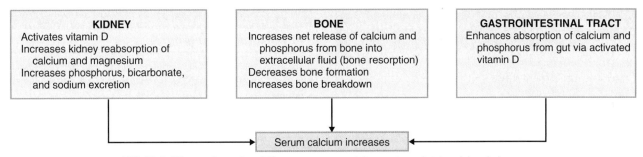

KIDNEY	BONE	GASTROINTESTINAL TRACT
Activates vitamin D Increases kidney reabsorption of calcium and magnesium Increases phosphorus, bicarbonate, and sodium excretion	Increases net release of calcium and phosphorus from bone into extracellular fluid (bone resorption) Decreases bone formation Increases bone breakdown	Enhances absorption of calcium and phosphorus from gut via activated vitamin D

Serum calcium increases

FIG. 53.6 Effects of parathyroid hormone on target tissues to maintain calcium balance.

hormone helps prevent hypoglycemia. Chapter 56 discusses glucagon function and *glucose regulation* in more detail.

Insulin promotes the movement and storage of carbohydrate, protein, and fat. It lowers blood glucose levels by enhancing glucose movement across cell membranes and into the cells of many tissues. Insulin secretion rises in response to an increase in blood glucose levels. More information on insulin is presented in Chapter 56.

Somatostatin, which is secreted in the pancreas, intestinal tract, and brain, inhibits the release of glucagon and insulin from the pancreas. It also inhibits the release of gastrin, secretin, and other GI peptides.

Parathyroid Glands

The parathyroid glands consist of four small glands located close to or within the back surface of the thyroid gland (see Fig. 53.1). These cells secrete parathyroid hormone (PTH).

PTH regulates calcium and phosphorus metabolism by acting on bones, the kidneys, and the GI tract (Fig. 53.6). Bone is the main storage site of calcium. PTH increases *bone resorption* (bone release of calcium into the blood from bone storage sites), thus increasing serum calcium. In the kidneys, PTH activates vitamin D, which then increases the absorption of calcium and phosphorus from the intestines. In the kidney tubules, PTH allows calcium to be reabsorbed and put back into the blood.

Serum calcium levels determine PTH secretion. Secretion decreases when serum calcium levels are high, and it increases when serum calcium levels are low. PTH and calcitonin work together to maintain normal calcium levels in the blood and extracellular fluid.

Pineal Gland

The cone-shaped pineal gland in the brain is approximately the size of a grain of rice. It is located at the base of the brain in the corpus callosum. It secretes melatonin when it is dark, thereby helping to regulate circadian rhythm and the sleep-wake cycle.

Thyroid Gland

The thyroid gland is in the anterior neck, directly below the cricoid cartilage (Fig. 53.7). It has two lobes joined by a thin strip of tissue *(isthmus)* in front of the trachea.

The thyroid gland is composed of follicular and parafollicular cells. Follicular cells produce the thyroid hormones thyroxine (T_4) and triiodothyronine (T_3). Parafollicular cells produce *thyrocalcitonin (TCT, or calcitonin),* which helps regulate serum calcium levels.

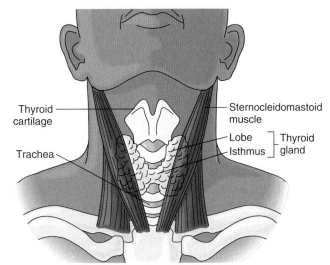

FIG. 53.7 Anatomic location of the thyroid gland.

Control of metabolism occurs through T_3 and T_4. Both hormones increase metabolism, which causes an increase in oxygen use and heat production in all tissues. Most circulating T_4 and T_3 are bound to plasma proteins. The free hormone moves into the cell, where it binds to its receptor in the cell nucleus. Once in the cell, T_4 is converted to T_3, the most active thyroid hormone. Conversion of T_4 to T_3 is impaired by stress, starvation, dyes, and some drugs. Cold temperatures increase the conversion. Box 53.2 lists the functions of thyroid hormones in adults.

Secretion of T_3 and T_4 is controlled by the hypothalamic-pituitary-thyroid gland axis negative feedback mechanism. The hypothalamus secretes thyrotropin-releasing hormone (TRH). TRH triggers the anterior pituitary gland to secrete thyroid-stimulating hormone (TSH), which then stimulates the thyroid gland to make and release thyroid hormones. If thyroid hormone levels are high, release of TRH and TSH is inhibited. If thyroid hormone levels are low, TRH and TSH release is increased. Cold and stress are two factors that cause the hypothalamus to secrete TRH, which then stimulates the anterior pituitary to secrete TSH.

Dietary intake of protein and iodine is needed to produce thyroid hormones. Iodine is absorbed from the intestinal tract as iodide. The thyroid gland draws iodide from the blood and concentrates it. After iodide is in the thyroid, it combines with the amino acid *tyrosine* to form T_4 and T_3. These hormones bind to thyroglobulin and are stored in thyroid follicular cells. When stimulated, T_3 and T_4 are released into the blood. They enter

BOX 53.2   Functions of Thyroid Hormones in Adults

Thyroxine (T_4) and triiodothyronine (T_3) function to:
- Regulate metabolic rate of all cells
- Regulate body heat production
- Serve as insulin antagonists
- Maintain growth hormone secretion and skeletal maturation
- Affect central nervous system development
- Influence muscle tone and vigor
- Maintain calcium mobilization
- Affect RBC production
- Maintain cardiac rate, force, and output
- Affect respiratory rate and oxygen utilization
- Maintain secretion of the GI tract
- Regulate protein, carbohydrate, and fat metabolism
- Stimulate lipid turnover, free fatty acid release, and cholesterol synthesis

Calcitonin functions to:
- Lower serum calcium
- Lower serum phosphate levels

Data from Rogers, J. L. (2023). *McCance and Huether's Pathophysiology: The biologic basis for disease in adults and children* (9th ed.). St. Louis: Elsevier.

NCLEX Examination Challenge 53.1
Physiological Integrity

The nurse is caring for an older adult female who has experienced two fractures in the past year. Which laboratory value would the nurse monitor as the **priority**?

A. Calcium
B. Cortisol
C. Thyroxine (T_4)
D. Triiodothyronine (T_3)

all cells, where they bind to DNA receptors and activate genes important in metabolism to regulate basal metabolic rate (BMR).

Calcium and phosphorus balance occurs partly through the actions of calcitonin (thyrocalcitonin [TCT]), which also is produced in the thyroid gland. Calcitonin lowers serum calcium and serum phosphorus levels by reducing bone resorption (release) of these minerals. Its actions are opposite of parathyroid hormone (PTH).

The serum calcium level determines calcitonin secretion. Low serum calcium levels suppress the release of calcitonin. Elevated serum calcium levels increase its secretion.

Endocrine Changes Associated With Aging

The effects of aging on the endocrine system vary but usually result in reduced glandular function and decreased hormone secretion. A notable exception is the prostate gland, which increases in size, producing hyperplasia and higher concentrations of adrenal steroids (Touhy & Jett, 2023). For women, reduced function of the ovaries is somewhat faster with more noticeable changes; it can also be dramatic if the individual undergoes a hysterectomy, which prompts an immediate surgical menopause.

It can be challenging to distinguish normal from abnormal endocrine activity in older adults because of chronic illness, changes in diet and activity, sleep disturbances, decreased metabolism, and the use of drug therapy that may affect hormone function. Consider these factors when assessing the older adult with endocrine dysfunction.

Encourage older adults to participate in regular screening examinations based upon their primary health care provider's recommendation. The box titled Patient-Centered Care: Older Adult Health: Age-Related Endocrine System Changes lists the common endocrine changes that occur in the older adult.

PATIENT-CENTERED CARE: OLDER ADULT HEALTH
Age-Related Endocrine System Changes

Change	Nursing Considerations
Decreased Antidiuretic Hormone (ADH) Production	
Urine is more dilute and may not concentrate when fluid intake is low.	The patient is at greater risk for dehydration; assess frequently for this condition.
	If not contraindicated by another health condition, teach assistive personnel (AP) to offer fluids at least every 2 hours while the patient is awake.
Decreased Ovarian Production of Estrogen	
Bone density decreases.	Teach about the importance of regular exercise and weight-bearing activity to maintain bone density.
Skin is thinner, drier, and at greater risk for injury.	
Perineal and vaginal tissues become drier, and the risk for cystitis increases.	Encourage the intake of healthy foods with adequate protein and 2 L of fluid daily (if not contraindicated by another health condition).
	Protect skin integrity, as noted in Chapter 21.
	Perform or assist the patient to perform perineal care at least twice daily.
	Teach sexually active older women to urinate immediately after sexual intercourse, and teach how vaginal lubricants can reduce discomfort and tissue damage during intimacy.

Age-Related Endocrine System Changes

Change	Nursing Considerations
Decreased Glucose Tolerance Weight becomes greater than ideal, along with: • Elevated fasting blood glucose level • Elevated random blood glucose level • Slow wound healing • Frequent yeast infections • Polydipsia • Polyuria	Assess for family history of obesity and T2DM. Teach about the importance of regular exercise and maintenance of a healthy weight. Teach the signs and symptoms of diabetes that should be reported to the primary health care provider. Suggest diabetes testing for any patient with: • Persistent vaginal candidiasis • Failure of a wound to heal in 2 weeks or less (especially of the leg or foot) • Increased and persistent hunger and thirst • Noticeable and persistent decrease in energy level
Decreased General Metabolism Patient has less tolerance for cold. Appetite is decreased. Heart rate and blood pressure (BP) are decreased.	Teach patients to dress in layers so that layers can be added or removed based upon temperature. Assess for additional signs and symptoms of an endocrine disorder, including for: • Lethargy • Constipation (as a change from usual bowel habits) • Decreased cognition • Slowed speech • Body temperature consistently below 97°F (36°C) • Heart rate consistently below 60 beats/min

Endocrine Changes Associated With COVID-19

The endocrine system, like all other body systems, is vulnerable to the effects of COVID-19. Numerous studies and reports demonstrate that hyperglycemia arose frequently in patients not previously diabetic (Clarke et al., 2022). This is likely due to the ability of the SARS-CoV-2 virus to infect and replicate in pancreatic cells.

Ketoacidosis was often diagnosed in older patients of non-White ethnic groups with a history of type 2 diabetes mellitus (T2DM) (Clarke et al., 2022). An international registry has been established to continue long-term research about the relationship between new-onset diabetes and COVID-19.

Disruptions in thyroid function, such as subacute thyroiditis that developed during infection with COVID-19, were noted by several studies. However, these studies also demonstrate that thyroid function appeared to return to normal within several months following infection with no lasting alteration in thyroid hormones (Clarke et al., 2021; Khoo et al., 2021).

Little data exists on the impact of COVID-19 on ovarian function. However, an international survey of 3762 participants from 56 countries demonstrated that 36.1% of respondents reported changes in menses after COVID-19 (Davis et al., 2021). Variations included a new onset of period irregularity, abnormally heavy periods, and postmenopausal bleeding (Davis et al., 2021).

RECOGNIZE CUES: ASSESSMENT

Patient History

Baseline endocrine assessment data must include age because certain disorders are more common in older than in younger patients, such as diabetes mellitus, loss of ovarian function, and decreased thyroid function. Sex assigned at birth is also important to know, as some disorders appear more frequently in one sex versus another. For example, thyroid problems are more common in women (Rogers, 2023).

Assess for a history of endocrine problems, symptoms that could indicate a disorder, and hospitalizations. Ask women at which age menarche began and whether menopause has occurred. Ask about past and current drugs, such as cortisone, levothyroxine, oral contraceptives, and antihypertensive agents. The use of exogenous hormone drugs, when not needed for hormone replacement, can cause serious dysfunction in many endocrine glands. Use the opportunity to teach patients about the dangers of misusing hormone-based drugs such as androgens and thyroid hormones (Burchum & Rosenthal, 2022).

Endocrine Assessment

Type 2 diabetes (T2DM) occurs when the pancreas, a gland within the endocrine system, cannot effectively use insulin. This condition is common among some racial and ethnic minority groups and people of lower socioeconomic status (Centers for Disease Control and Prevention [CDC], 2022).

The CDC's Division of Diabetes Translation (DDT) program exists to reduce and one day eliminate health disparities for people in the United States who have or are at risk for T2DM (CDC, 2022). Carefully assess all patients for endocrine dysfunction and advocate for early intervention. Provide health teaching to all patients with, or at risk for, T2DM so that diabetes-related disparities are reduced.

Nutrition History

Nutrition or GI tract changes can be associated with numerous different endocrine problems. For example, moderate to severe arginine vasopressin deficiency (AVP-D) or arginine vasopressin resistance (AVP-R) triggers excessive thirst, and adrenal hypofunction triggers salt craving. Persistent increases in hunger and thirst also are associated with diabetes mellitus. Rapid changes in weight without diet changes can be associated with a thyroid or hypothalamic disorder.

Iodine, a substance that is not produced by the body, is needed to produce thyroid hormone. People get iodine through dietary intake. Common sources of dietary iodine are located in Box 53.3. Ask whether the patient consumes these foods, and in what type of quantity.

Family History and Genetic Risk

Ask the patient about any family history of obesity, growth or developmental difficulties, diabetes mellitus, infertility, or thyroid disorders. These problems may have an autosomal dominant, autosomal recessive, or cluster pattern of inheritance.

Current Health Problems

Focus on the patient's reason for seeking health care. Ask questions such as those listed in Box 53.4.

Physical Assessment

Inspection

An endocrine problem can change physical features because of its effect on growth and development, sex hormone levels, *fluid and electrolyte balance*, and metabolism.

Observe the patient's general appearance, and assess height, weight, fat distribution, and muscle mass in relationship to age.

Assess scalp and body hair growth patterns. When examining the head, focus on abnormalities of facial structure, features, and expression, such as:
- Prominent forehead or jaw
- Round or puffy face
- Dull or flat expression
- Exophthalmos (protruding eyeballs and retracted upper lids)

Check the lower neck for a visible enlargement of the thyroid gland. Normally the thyroid tissue cannot be observed. The isthmus may be noticeable when the patient swallows. While standing in front of the patient, ask the patient to swallow. Under normal circumstances, the thyroid is usually not visible; however, it can be visualized moving upward when someone swallows (Jarvis & Eckhardt, 2024). Jugular vein distention may be seen on inspection of the neck and can indicate fluid overload.

Observe skin color, and look for areas of pigment loss (*hypopigmentation*) or excess (*hyperpigmentation*). Fungal skin infections, slow wound healing, bruising, and petechiae are often seen in patients with adrenal hyperfunction. Skin infections, foot ulcers, and slow wound healing often occur with diabetes mellitus. With some types of adrenal gland dysfunction, the skin over the joints, as well as any scar tissue, may show increased pigmentation due to increased levels of adrenocorticotropic hormone (ACTH) and melanocyte-stimulating hormone.

Vitiligo (patchy areas where pigment is lost) is seen with primary hypofunction of the adrenal glands and is caused by

---

BOX 53.3 Common Sources of Dietary Iodine

- Dairy products
  - Cheese
  - Milk
  - Yogurt
- Other sources
  - Eggs
  - Iodine-containing multivitamins
  - Iodized table salt
  - Saltwater fish (e.g., salmon, sardines, tuna)
  - Seaweed (e.g., kelp, nori)
  - Shellfish (e.g., scallops, shrimp)

Data from American Thyroid Association. (2023). Iodine deficiency. https://www.thyroid.org/iodine-deficiency/.

BOX 53.4 Collecting a Systems History Related to Endocrine Problems

General
- When did symptoms begin?
- Did symptoms occur gradually or start suddenly?
- Have you been treated for this problem in the past? (If so, was treatment effective?)
- How have the current problems affected your activities of daily living?
- Has your energy level changed since the symptoms began?
- Do you find that you are hot or cold much of the time?
- Do you notice that you are sleeping the same, more, or less since the symptoms began?
- Have you noticed a change in your hair distribution (e.g., less hair on the head, shaving more or less than usual)?
- Have you noticed a chance in your facial contour or body proportions, or have you experienced eye protrusion?
- Has the quality of your voice changed?

Nutrition and Elimination
- Would you rate your **nutrition** intake as healthy, unhealthy, or needs work? Please explain.
- Have you been eating differently (more, less, or different foods) since symptoms began?
- Have you noticed a significant change in your weight in the last 6 months?
- Have you noticed any difference in urinary or bowel elimination since symptoms began?
- How often do you urinate, and do you feel you urinate large amounts?
- Do you have to wake up from sleep to urinate? If so, how often?
- How often do you have a bowel movement, and can you describe them?

Reproduction
- (Women): Do you still have menstrual cycles, and if so, when was your last period?
- (Women): Have you noticed a change in flow, duration, or frequency of your menses since symptoms began?
- Has your libido changed since symptoms began?
- Do you have concerns about how your symptoms impact **sexuality** or **reproduction**?

autoimmune destruction of melanocytes in the skin. It is seen most often on the face, neck, arms, hands, legs, and fold areas (Jarvis & Eckhardt, 2024). Mucous membranes may have large areas of uneven pigmentation. Document the location, color, distribution, and size of skin color changes that have occurred since the last visit or since the patient noticed differences from a baseline appearance.

Inspect the fingernails for malformation, thickness, or brittleness, all of which may suggest thyroid gland problems. Examine the extremities and the base of the spine for edema, which occurs with impaired *fluid and electrolyte balance*.

Check the trunk for any abnormalities in chest size and symmetry. Truncal obesity and the presence of a "buffalo hump" between the shoulders on the back may indicate adrenocortical excess. Hormonal imbalances can also change secondary sexual characteristics. Inspect the breasts of men as well as women for size, symmetry, pigmentation, and discharge. Low testosterone levels in men induce breast enlargement (*gynecomastia*). *Striae* (reddish-purple "stretch marks") on the breasts or abdomen are often seen with adrenocortical excess.

Assess the patient's hair distribution for signs of endocrine gland dysfunction. Changes can include *hirsutism* (excessive body hair growth, especially on the face, the chest, and the center abdominal line of women), excessive scalp hair loss, or changes in hair texture (Jarvis & Eckhardt, 2024). Differentiate between this type of hair loss versus normal hair loss that occurs with aging.

Examination of the genitalia may reveal a dysfunction in hormone secretion. The distribution and quantity of pubic hair are often affected in hypogonadism. Ask whether a change in the size of the scrotum and penis (or of the labia and clitoris) has occurred.

Auscultation

Auscultate the chest to assess cardiac rate and rhythm to obtain a baseline assessment. Some endocrine problems induce dysrhythmias, while others cause dehydration and volume depletion. Document any difference in the patient's blood pressure and pulse in the lying, standing, or sitting positions (orthostatic vital signs).

When an enlarged thyroid gland is palpated, the area of enlargement is auscultated for bruits. Hypertrophy of the thyroid gland causes an increase in vascular flow, which may result in bruits.

Palpation

The thyroid gland and the testes can be examined by palpation. Sometimes these examinations are done by the primary health care provider, and other times they are done by the nurse. Chapters 61 and 64 discuss examination of the testes.

The thyroid gland is palpated for size, shape, symmetry, and the presence of nodules, tenderness, or other irregularities. The examiner stands behind the patient, and asks the patient to sit straight and bend the head slightly forward. With both thumbs on the back of the patient's neck, the examiner's fingers are curved around to the front of the neck on either side of the trachea. When the patient swallows, the thyroid is felt as it rises.

The right lobe is examined with the patient's head turned to the right and with the trachea gently displaced by the examiner's left fingers. The right lobe is palpated with the examiner's right hand. This procedure is reversed to examine the left lobe (Jarvis & Eckhardt, 2024).

> ⚠ **NURSING SAFETY PRIORITY**
> *Action Alert*
>
> Avoid applying pressure on or palpating the thyroid in a patient who has or is suspected to have hyperthyroidism. These actions can stimulate a sudden release of thyroid hormones and cause a thyroid storm.

Psychosocial Assessment

Many endocrine problems can change a patient's behaviors, personality, psychological responses, and self-image. Assess the patient's coping skills, support systems, and health-related beliefs. Ask whether the patient has noticed a change in how stress is handled, frequency of crying, or degree of patience and anger expression. Patients may not recognize these changes in themselves. If the patient is agreeable, ask a family member about changes in behaviors or personality.

A number of endocrine disorders affect the patient's perception of self. Body features can change greatly in disorders of the pituitary, adrenal, and thyroid glands. Infertility, impotence, and other changes that affect *sexuality* and *reproduction* may result from endocrine problems. Encourage the patient to express feelings and concerns about a change in appearance or in function.

Patients with endocrine problems may require lifelong drug therapy and follow-up care. Assess their readiness to learn and their ability to carry out specific self-management skills. Determine whether the patient has resources to cover prolonged health treatment, and make referrals as necessary.

> **NCLEX Examination Challenge 53.2**
> *Physiological Integrity*
>
> The nurse is caring for a 42-year-old client. Which finding would require the nurse to further assess for a possible endocrine problem?
> A. Thyroid gland visible upon inspection
> B. Recently was prescribed bifocal eyeglasses
> C. Reports noticing a receding hairline over the past year
> D. 10-lb weight loss in 6 months after decreasing sugar intake

Diagnostic Assessment
Laboratory Assessment

Laboratory tests are an essential part of the diagnostic process when assessing for endocrine problems. Fluids commonly used for these tests include blood, urine, and saliva. Salivary levels of steroid hormones (cortisol, testosterone, progesterone, and estradiol) accurately reflect blood levels of these hormones (Pagana et al., 2022). Protein hormones, such as those from the pituitary gland and thyroid gland, are not assessed using saliva.

Always check with the agency's laboratory for proper collection and handling of the specimen. Specialized testing for specific endocrine disorders is described in Chapters 54 to 56. Box 53.5 lists correct techniques for collection of specimens for general endocrine testing.

Assays. An assay measures the level of a specific hormone in blood or other body fluid. The most common assays for endocrine testing are antibody-based immunologic assays and chromatographic assays, which include mass spectrometry that measures the presence of a hormone(s) based on its molecular mass and chemical composition. These assays are very sensitive and can detect even minute quantities of a given hormone. Many different hormone concentrations can be analyzed at the same time by the mass spectrometry method.

Provocative/Suppression Tests. Measurement of specific hormone blood levels does not always distinguish between the normal and the abnormal. The wide normal range for some hormones makes it necessary to trigger responses by provocative ("stimulation") or suppression tests.

For the patient who might have an underactive endocrine gland, a stimulus may be used to determine whether the gland is capable of normal hormone production. This method is called *provocative testing.* Measured amounts of selected hormones are given to stimulate the target gland to maximum production. Hormone levels are then measured and compared with expected normal values. Failure of the hormone level to rise with provocation indicates hypofunction.

Suppression tests are used when hormone levels are high or in the upper range of normal. Drugs or other substances known to normally suppress hormone production are administered. Failure of suppression of hormone production during testing indicates hyperfunction.

Urine Tests. The levels of hormones and their metabolites in the urine can be measured to determine endocrine function. Because many of the endocrine hormones are secreted in a pulsatile fashion, measurement of a specific hormone in a 24-hour urine collection, rather than as a single blood or urine sample, better reflects the function of a specific gland, such as the adrenal gland. Teach the patient how to collect a 24-hour urine sample (see also Box 53.5).

Certain hormones require additives in the container at the beginning of the collection. Instruct the patient not to discard the preservative from the container and to use caution when handling it because some are caustic. Teach that this collection is timed for *exactly* 24 hours. Instruct the patient to talk with their health care provider before taking new prescribed or over-the-counter drugs during endocrine testing because some drugs can interfere with the assay.

Glucose Tests. Tests for functions of the islet cells of the pancreas measure the result of pancreatic islet cell function. Blood glucose values and the oral glucose tolerance test help diagnose diabetes mellitus. The glycosylated hemoglobin (A1C) value indicates the *average* blood glucose level over a period of 100 to 120 days prior to the test (Pagana et al., 2022). (See Chapter 56 for testing associated with diabetes mellitus.)

Genetic Tests. When some hormone levels are too low to be measured, genetic testing may be performed. Advances in DNA sequencing technology have resulted in opportunities for genetic testing in the clinical setting that did not previously exist (Newey, 2019). This type of testing is particularly useful when the patient has limited knowledge of family history.

Imaging Assessment

Anterior, posterior, and lateral skull x-rays may be used to view the sella turcica, the bony pocket in the skull where the pituitary gland rests. Erosion of the sella turcica indicates invasion of the wall from an abnormal growth.

MRI with contrast is the most sensitive method of imaging the pituitary gland, although CT scans can also be used to evaluate it. CT scans are usually used to evaluate the adrenal glands, ovaries, and pancreas. The thyroid, parathyroid glands, ovaries, and testes can be evaluated by ultrasound.

A thyroid scan, a type of nuclear medicine assessment, can be done to determine the nature of thyroid problems. The patient takes a pill containing radioactive iodine; it collects in the thyroid, which is then imaged 4 to 6 hours later (UCLA Health, 2023).

Other Diagnostic Assessment

Ultrasound-guided fine needle aspiration is a safe and quick ambulatory procedure used to indicate the composition of thyroid nodules. It is used to determine whether surgical intervention is needed.

BOX 53.5 | Patient and Family Education

Endocrine Testing

For Blood Tests

- Check your laboratory's method of handling hormone test samples for tube type, timing, drugs to be administered as part of the test, and any other specifications. For example, blood samples drawn for catecholamines must be placed on ice and taken to the laboratory immediately.
- Explain the procedure and any restrictions to the patient.
- If you are drawing blood samples from an IV line, clear the line thoroughly. Do not use a double- or triple-lumen line to obtain samples; contamination or dilution from another port is possible.
- Emphasize the importance of taking a drug prescribed for the test on time. Tell the patient to set an alarm if the drug is to be taken during the night.

For Urine Tests

- Check with the laboratory to determine any special handling of the urine specimen (e.g., Is a preservative needed? Does the container need to be kept cold?).
- If needed, make sure that the preservative has been added to the collection container at the beginning of the collection.
- Tell the patient about any preservative and the need to avoid splashing urine from the container because some preservatives make the urine caustic.
- If the specimen must be kept cool or cold, instruct the patient to place the container in an inexpensive cooler with ice. The specimen container should not be kept with food or drinks.
- Instruct the patient to begin the urine collection (whether for 2, 4, 8, 12, or 24 hours) by first emptying the bladder and NOT using this specimen as part of the collection. The timing for the urine collection begins *after* this specimen is discarded.
- Tell the patient to note the time of the discarded specimen and to plan to collect all urine from this time until the end of the urine collection period.
- To end the collection, instruct the patient to empty the bladder at the end of the timed period, even if the urge to urinate is not felt, and to add that urine to the collection.

GET READY FOR THE NEXT-GENERATION NCLEX® EXAMINATION!

Essential Assessment Points

- Understand that endocrine problems can have a slow and insidious onset or an abrupt onset.
- Ask whether there is a family history of endocrine disorders, as some problems have a genetic component.
- Ask the patient what prescribed and over-the-counter drugs are taken on a regular basis, because some drugs can alter endocrine function.
- Differentiate endocrine changes associated with aging from abnormal findings.
- Provide support to the patient who expresses concerns about appearance or functional changes associated with an endocrine problem.
- Use effective communication when teaching patients and caregivers what to expect during tests and procedures associated with endocrine assessment.
- Interpret laboratory results related to endocrine assessment, and report abnormal findings to the health care provider.
- Identify and report complications of endocrine testing to the health care provider.
- Teach all patients that abusing or misusing hormones or steroids can have an adverse effect on endocrine function.

Mastery Questions

1. The nurse is preparing to assess endocrine function in an older adult. Which of the following assessment findings would be anticipated? **Select all that apply.**
   A. Anorexia
   B. Heat intolerance
   C. Slow wound healing
   D. Diminished urination
   E. Elevated fasting glucose

2. A client is asked to collect a 24-hour urine specimen while at home. Which teaching would the nurse provide?
   A. Keep the collection container in the refrigerator.
   B. Collect only morning and evening urine specimens for this test.
   C. Gently swirl the urine in the container to mix with the preservative.
   D. Begin the 24-hour timing after emptying the bladder and discarding that urine.

REFERENCES

Burchum, J., & Rosenthal, L. (2022). *Lehne's pharmacology for nursing care* (11th ed.). St. Louis: Elsevier.

Centers for Disease Control and Prevention. (2022). *National Center for Chronic Disease Prevention and Health Promotion (NCCDPHP): Division of Diabetes Translation at a Glance.* https://www.cdc.gov-/chronicdisease/resources/publications/aag/diabetes.htm.

Clarke, S., et al. (2021). Normal adrenal and thyroid function in patients who survive COVID-19 infection. *Journal of Clinical Endocrinology and Metabolism, 106*(8), 2208–2220.

Clarke, S., et al. (2022). Impact of COVID-19 on the endocrine system: A mini-review. *Endocrinology, 163*(1), bqb203.

Davis, H., et al. (2021). Characterizing long COVID in an international cohort: 7 months of symptoms and their impact. *E Clinical Medicine, 38*:101019.

Jarvis, C., & Eckhardt, A. (2024). *Physical examination & health assessment* (9th ed.). St. Louis: Elsevier.

Khoo, B., et al. (2021). Thyroid function before, during, and after COVID-19. *Journal of Clinical Endocrinology and Metabolism, 106*(2), e803–e811.

Newey, P. (2019). Clinical genetic testing in endocrinology: Current concepts and contemporary challenges. *Clinical Endocrinology, 91,* 587–607.

Pagana, K. D., Pagana, T. J., & Pagana, T. N. (2022). *Mosby's manual of diagnostic and laboratory tests* (7th ed.). St. Louis: Elsevier.

Rogers, J. L. (2023). McCance and Huether's *Pathophysiology: The biologic basis for disease in adults and children* (9th ed.). St. Louis: Elsevier.

Seiron, P., et al. (2019). Characterisation of the endocrine pancreas in type 1 diabetes: Islet size is maintained but islet number is markedly reduced. *The Journal of Pathology Clinical Research, 5*(4), 248–255.

Touhy, T., & Jett, K. (2023). *Ebersole and Hess' toward healthy aging: Human needs and nursing response* (11th ed.). St. Louis: Elsevier.

UCLA Health. (2023). *Endocrine surgery: Thyroid scan.* https://www.uclahealth.org/medical-services/surgery/endocrine-surgery/patient-resources/patient-education/endocrine-surgery-encyclopedia/thyroid-scan.

54

Concepts of Care for Patients With Pituitary and Adrenal Gland Conditions

Cherie R. Rebar and Russell Worthen

http://evolve.elsevier.com/Iggy/

http://evolve.elsevier.com/Iggy/

LEARNING OUTCOMES

1. Plan collaborative care with the interprofessional team to promote *fluid and electrolyte balance* in patients with pituitary and adrenal gland problems.
2. Teach adults how to decrease the risk for pituitary and adrenal gland problems.
3. Teach the patient and caregiver(s) about common drugs and other management strategies used for pituitary and adrenal gland problems.
4. Plan patient- and family-centered nursing interventions to decrease the psychosocial impact caused by living with pituitary and adrenal gland problems.
5. Apply knowledge of anatomy, physiology, and pathophysiology to provide evidence-based care for patients with pituitary and adrenal gland problems affecting *fluid and electrolyte balance.*
6. Analyze assessment and diagnostic findings to generate solutions and prioritize nursing care for patients with pituitary and adrenal gland problems.
7. Organize care coordination and transition management for patients with pituitary and adrenal gland problems.
8. Use clinical judgment to plan evidence-based nursing care to promote *fluid and electrolyte balance* and prevent complications in patients with pituitary and adrenal gland problems.
9. Incorporate factors that affect health equity into the plan of care for patients with pituitary and adrenal gland problems.

KEY TERMS

acute adrenal insufficiency Life-threatening event in which the need for cortisol and aldosterone is greater than the body's supply. Also known as *adrenal crisis* or *Addisonian crisis.*

AVP deficiency (AVP-D) Central diabetes insipidus.

AVP resistance (AVP-R) Nephrogenic diabetes insipidus.

Cushing disease Type of Cushing syndrome in which a pituitary gland tumor secreting adrenocorticotropic hormone (ACTH) stimulates the overproduction of cortisol in the body.

Cushing syndrome Set of symptoms caused by an excess of cortisol; usually related to taking ongoing corticosteroid therapy.

diabetes insipidus (DI) Disorder in which water loss is caused by a deficiency in vasopressin (antidiuretic hormone [ADH]) or an inability of the kidneys to respond to vasopressin. *Now known as AVP-D or AVP-R.*

gynecomastia Male breast tissue development.

hyperaldosteronism Increased secretion of aldosterone with mineralocorticoid excess.

hypercortisolism Clinical state arising from excessive tissue exposure to cortisol and/or other glucocorticoids; over time, it results in Cushing syndrome.

hyperpituitarism Hormone oversecretion that occurs with anterior pituitary tumors or tissue hyperplasia.

hypophysectomy Surgical removal of the pituitary gland.

hypopituitarism Deficiency of one and sometimes more than one pituitary hormone.

syndrome of inappropriate antidiuretic hormone (SIADH) (also known as *Schwartz-Bartter syndrome*) Problem in which vasopressin (antidiuretic hormone [ADH]) is secreted even when plasma osmolarity is low or normal, resulting in water retention and fluid overload.

virilization Presence of male secondary sex characteristics.

✦ PRIORITY AND INTERRELATED CONCEPTS

The priority concept for this chapter is:
- *Fluid and Electrolyte Balance*
  The *Fluid and Electrolyte Balance* concept exemplar for this chapter is Cushing Syndrome (Hypercortisolism)

The interrelated concepts for this chapter are:
- *Cellular Regulation*
- *Immunity*

Fluid and electrolyte balance is greatly affected by the pituitary and adrenal glands, which function to secrete hormones that affect the **cellular regulation** of the entire body. When these hormones are secreted in excessive or insufficient amounts, physical and psychological changes result. Anterior pituitary hormones regulate growth, appetite, metabolism, temperature regulation, and sexual development. The posterior pituitary hormone *vasopressin* (antidiuretic hormone [ADH]) helps maintain **fluid and electrolyte balance.** Adrenal gland hormones are life sustaining.

A complete assessment is performed to detect specific clinical findings. The patient also often undergoes many diagnostic tests and relies on the nurse for explanations. Surgical intervention may be indicated to treat disorders of the pituitary or adrenal glands. Priority nursing care includes assessment, patient education, evaluating patient response to therapy, and providing support.

DISORDERS OF THE PITUITARY GLAND

HYPOPITUITARISM

Pathophysiology Review

Hypopituitarism is a deficiency of one or more of the pituitary hormones. It is most commonly caused by pituitary tumors. If only one pituitary hormone is deficient, the condition is known as *selective hypopituitarism*. When two or more of the anterior pituitary hormones are decreased, it is known as *panhypopituitarism* (PHP) and becomes much more serious (National Cancer Institute, n.d.).

The cause of hypopituitarism varies. A tumor on the hypothalamus can induce hypopituitarism. Benign or malignant pituitary tumors can compress and destroy pituitary tissue. Pituitary function can be impaired by malnutrition or rapid loss of body fat. Shock or severe hypotension reduces blood flow to the pituitary gland, leading to hypoxia, infarction, and reduced hormone secretion. Other causes of hypopituitarism include head trauma, brain tumors or infection, radiation or surgery of the head and brain, and HIV-III (AIDS). *Idiopathic hypopituitarism* has an unknown cause.

Deficiencies of *adrenocorticotropic hormone (ACTH)* or *thyroid-stimulating hormone (TSH)* are the *most* life-threatening because they cause a decrease in the secretion of vital hormones from the adrenal and thyroid glands. Adrenal gland hypofunction is discussed later in this chapter; hypothyroidism is discussed in Chapter 56. See Table 54.1 for hormones secreted by the anterior pituitary and posterior pituitary glands and their major actions.

TABLE 54.1 Hormones Secreted and Their Action

Source	Hormone Secreted	Action
Anterior pituitary	Adrenocorticotropic hormone (ACTH)	Stimulates synthesis and adrenal cortical hormones
	Follicle-stimulating hormone	*Females:* Stimulates ovarian follicle growth and ovulation
		Males: Stimulates sperm production
	Growth hormone (GH)	Stimulates bone and muscle growth, promotes protein synthesis and fat metabolism, decreases carbohydrate metabolism
	Luteinizing hormone (LH)	*Females:* Stimulates corpus luteum development, release of oocyte, and estrogen and progesterone production
		Males: Stimulates secretion of testosterone and development of the interstitial tissue of the testes
	Prolactin (PRL)	Prepares female breasts for lactation
	Thyroid-stimulating hormone (TSH)	Stimulates synthesis and secretion of thyroid hormone
Posterior pituitary	Vasopressin (antidiuretic hormone [ADH])	Increases water reabsorption by the kidneys
	Oxytocin	Simulates uterine contractions; stimulates milk ejection from the breasts after birth

Data from Carmichael, J. (2023). *Overview of the pituitary gland. Merck Manual Professional Version.* https://www.merckmanuals.com/home/hormonal-and-metabolic-disorders/pituitary-gland-disorders/overview-of-the-pituitary-gland; Sadiq, N., & Tadi, P. (2022). *Physiology, pituitary hormones.* Treasure Island, FL: StatPearls Publishing. https://www.ncbi.nlm.nih.gov/books/NBK557556/; and Rawindraraj, A. D., Basit, H., & Jialal, I. (2022). Physiology, anterior pituitary. [Updated 2022 May 8]. In: StatPearls [Internet]. Treasure Island, FL: StatPearls Publishing; 2023 Jan-. Available from https://www.ncbi.nlm.nih.gov/books/NBK499898/.

BOX 54.1 Key Features

Pituitary Hypofunction

Deficient Hormone	Signs and Symptoms
Anterior Pituitary Hormones	
Adrenocorticotropic hormone (ACTH)	Anorexia
	Decreased axillary and pubic hair (women)
	Decreased serum cortisol levels
	Headache
	Hypoglycemia
	Hyponatremia
	Malaise and lethargy
	Pale/ash gray complexion
	Postural hypotension
Gonadotropins • Luteinizing hormone (LH) • Follicle-stimulating hormone (FSH)	Women: • Amenorrhea • Anovulation • Beast atrophy • Decreased axillary and pubic hair • Decreased libido • Loss of bone density • Low estrogen levels Men: • Decreased body hair • Decreased facial hair • Decreased ejaculate volume • Decreased libido • Impotence • Loss of bone density • Reduced muscle mass
Growth hormone (GH)	Decreased bone density
	Decreased muscle strength
	Increased serum cholesterol levels
	Pathologic fractures
Thyroid-stimulating hormone (TSH, thyrotropin)	Alopecia
	Decreased libido
	Decreased thyroid hormone levels
	Hirsutism
	Intolerance to cold
	Lethargy
	Menstrual abnormalities
	Slowed cognition
	Weight gain
Posterior Pituitary Hormones	
Vasopressin (antidiuretic hormone [ADH])	AVP-D (diabetes insipidus) • Dehydration • Greatly increased urine output • Hypotension • Increased plasma osmolarity • Increased plasma electrolyte levels, especially sodium • Increased thirst • Low urine specific gravity (<1.005) • Urine output that does not decrease when fluid intake decreases

Interprofessional Collaborative Care

Patients with hypopituitarism require lifelong hormone replacement therapy (HRT). Such patients can be found in the community and in any care setting. It is important that HRT continue when they are admitted to an acute care setting for any reason.

Recognize Cues: Assessment

Deficiencies of specific pituitary hormones cause changes in target organ function and even physical appearance. See the specific changes outlined in Box 54.1.

Gonadotropin (luteinizing hormone [LH] and follicle-stimulating hormone [FSH]) deficiency changes secondary sex characteristics in men and women. Men may have facial and body hair loss. Ask about impotence and decreased libido. Women may report amenorrhea, *dyspareunia* (painful intercourse), infertility, and decreased libido. Women may also have dry skin, breast atrophy, and a decrease or absence of axillary and pubic hair.

Neurologic symptoms of hypopituitarism as a result of tumor growth often first occur as changes in vision. Assess for changes in the patient's vision, especially peripheral vision. Headaches, diplopia, and limited eye movement are common.

Laboratory findings vary widely. Some pituitary hormone levels may be measured directly. Laboratory assessment of some pituitary hormones involves measuring the *effects* of the hormones rather than the actual hormone levels. For example, blood levels of triiodothyronine (T_3) and thyroxine (T_4) from the thyroid, testosterone and estradiol from the gonads, and prolactin (PRL) levels are measured easily. If levels of any of these hormones are low, further pituitary evaluation is necessary.

Pituitary problems may cause changes in the *sella turcica* (the bony nest where the pituitary gland rests) (Rogers, 2023). Changes include enlargement, erosion, and calcifications as a result of pituitary tumors, as well as soft tissue lesions, seen most distinctly with CT and MRI. An angiogram can help rule out an aneurysm or any other vascular problems in the area before surgery.

Take Actions: Interventions

Management of hypopituitarism focuses on replacement of all deficient hormones to ensure appropriate **cellular regulation.** Men who have gonadotropin deficiency receive replacement therapy with androgens (testosterone), usually by the parenteral or transdermal route. Therapy begins with high-dose testosterone and is continued until virilization (presence of male secondary sex characteristics) is achieved. Positive responses include increases in penis size, libido, muscle mass, bone size, and bone strength, as well as increases in facial and body hair. After virilization is achieved the dose may be decreased, but therapy continues throughout life. Therapy to increase fertility requires gonadotropin-releasing hormone (GnRH) injections, not testosterone therapy (Kaiser & Ho, 2020).

Androgen therapy is avoided in men with prostate cancer to prevent enhancing tumor cell growth. Side effects of therapy include gynecomastia (male breast tissue development), acne, baldness, and prostate enlargement.

Women who have gonadotropin deficiency receive HRT with a combination of estrogen and progesterone. The risk for hypertension or thrombosis is increased with estrogen therapy, especially among smokers and those who use nicotine in any form. Emphasize measures to reduce risk and the need for regular health visits. For inducing pregnancy, specific hormones may be given to trigger ovulation.

Adults with growth hormone (GH) deficiency may be treated with subcutaneous injections of human growth hormone (hGH). Injections are given at night, after the last meal of the day, to mimic normal GH release (Kaiser & Ho, 2020).

HYPERPITUITARISM

Pathophysiology Review

Hyperpituitarism is hormone oversecretion. This occurs with anterior pituitary tumors or tissue *hyperplasia* (tissue overgrowth). Tumors occur most often in the anterior pituitary cells that produce growth hormone (GH), prolactin (PRL), and adrenocorticotropic hormone (ACTH). Overproduction of PRL also may occur in response to tumors that overproduce GH and ACTH. Excess ACTH may occur with increased secretion of melanocyte-stimulating hormone (MSH).

 ## PATIENT-CENTERED CARE: GENETICS/ GENOMICS

Multiple Endocrine Neoplasia Type 1

One cause of hyperpituitarism is multiple endocrine neoplasia, type 1 (MEN1), in which there is inactivation of the suppressor gene *MEN1* (Online Mendelian Inheritance in Man [OMIM], 2017). MEN1 has an autosomal dominant inheritance pattern and may result in a benign tumor of the pituitary, parathyroid glands, or pancreas. In the pituitary, excessive production of growth hormone occurs and leads to acromegaly. Ask a patient with acromegaly whether either parent also has this problem or has had a tumor of the pancreas or parathyroid glands.

Most often hyperpituitarism is caused by a benign pituitary adenoma (Gounden et al., 2022). Adenomas are classified by the hormone secreted. As an adenoma gets larger and compresses brain tissue, neurologic changes, as well as endocrine problems,

may occur. Symptoms may include vision changes, headache, and increased intracranial pressure (ICP). It can also be caused by a hypothalamic problem of excessive production of releasing hormones, which then overstimulate a normal pituitary gland.

Prolactin (PRL)-secreting tumors are the most common type of pituitary adenoma. Excessive PRL inhibits the secretion of gonadotropins and sex hormones in men and women, resulting in *galactorrhea* (breast milk production), amenorrhea, and infertility.

PATIENT-CENTERED CARE: HEALTH EQUITY

Pituitary Adenoma

Evidence shows a disparity in treatment of pituitary adenomas for patients of low income, particularly for patients who are Black and urban residents (Ghaffari-Rafi et al., 2022). There is also a significant dichotomy in the time to surgery following diagnosis (Gordon et al., 2022). Fully advocate for all patients to receive high-quality, timely, evidence-based care when pituitary adenoma is suspected or diagnosed.

Overproduction of GH in adults results in *acromegaly* (Fig. 54.1). The onset is gradual with slow progression, and changes may remain unnoticed for years before diagnosis. Early detection and treatment are essential to prevent irreversible enlargement of the face, hands, and feet. Other changes include increased skeletal thickness, hypertrophy of the skin, and enlargement of many organs such as the liver and heart. Some changes may be reversible after treatment, but skeletal changes are permanent.

Bone thinning and bone cell overgrowth occur slowly. Breakdown of joint cartilage and hypertrophy of ligaments, vocal cords, and eustachian tubes are common. Nerve entrapment and *hyperglycemia* (elevated blood glucose levels) are common.

Excess ACTH overstimulates the adrenal cortex. The result is excessive production of glucocorticoids, mineralocorticoids, and androgens, which leads to the development of Cushing disease or syndrome (see Fluid and Electrolyte Balance Concept Exemplar: Cushing Syndrome [Hypercortisolism]).

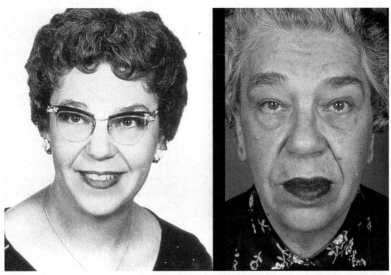

FIG. 54.1 Progression of acromegaly. (Courtesy Group for Research in Pathology Education [GRIPE], Oklahoma City, OK.)

Interprofessional Collaborative Care

Most care of a patient with hyperpituitarism occurs on an outpatient basis. When surgical intervention is required, hospitalization is necessary.

Recognize Cues: Assessment

Symptoms of hyperpituitarism vary with the hormone produced in excess. Obtain the patient's age, gender, and family history. Ask about any change in hat, glove, ring, or shoe size and the presence of fatigue. The patient with high GH levels may have backache and joint pain from bone changes. Ask specifically about headaches and changes in vision.

The patient with hypersecretion of PRL often reports sexual function difficulty. Ask women about menstrual changes, decreased libido, painful intercourse, and any difficulty in becoming pregnant. Men may report decreased libido and impotence.

Usually only one hormone is produced in excess because the cell types within the pituitary gland are so individually organized and distinct. The most common hormones produced in excess with hyperpituitarism are PRL, ACTH, and GH. Changes in appearance and target organ function occur with excesses of specific anterior pituitary hormones as described in Box 54.2.

Suppression testing can help diagnose hyperpituitarism. High blood glucose levels usually suppress the release of GH. A prescribed dose of oral glucose is given and then followed by serial GH level measurements. GH levels that do not fall below 5 ng/mL (mcg/L) indicate a positive (abnormal) result associated with hyperpituitarism.

Take Actions: Interventions

The expected outcomes of management for hyperpituitarism are to return hormone levels to normal or near normal, reduce or eliminate headache and visual disturbances, prevent complications, and reverse as many of the body changes as possible.

Nonsurgical Management. Encourage the patient to express concerns about altered physical appearance, such as galactorrhea, gynecomastia, and reduced sexual functioning. Reassure the patient that treatment may reverse some of these problems.

NCLEX Examination Challenge 54.1

Physiological Integrity

A 25-year-old female client presents for an annual physical, reporting health changes over the past year. Which of the following findings require the nurse to conduct further assessment? **Select all that apply.**
A. Visual changes
B. 15-lb weight gain
C. Persistent low energy
D. Irregular menstrual cycle
E. Recent sprained ankle due to sports injury

Drug therapy may be used alone or with surgery and/or radiation. Common drugs used are the dopamine agonists bromocriptine and cabergoline. These drugs stimulate dopamine receptors in the brain and inhibit the release of GH and PRL. Usually, small tumors decrease in size until the pituitary gland is of normal size, and larger tumors decrease in size to some extent.

 BOX 54.2   Key Features

Anterior Pituitary Hyperfunction

Prolactin (PRL)
- Hypogonadism (loss of secondary sexual characteristics)
- Decreased gonadotropin levels
- Galactorrhea
- Increased body fat
- Increased serum prolactin levels

Growth Hormone (GH), Acromegaly
- Thickened lips
- Coarse facial features
- Increasing head size
- Lower jaw protrusion
- Enlarged hands and feet
- Joint pain
- Barrel-shaped chest
- Hyperglycemia
- Sleep apnea
- Enlarged heart, lungs, and liver

Adrenocorticotropic Hormone (ACTH): Pituitary Cushing Syndrome
- Elevated plasma cortisol levels
- Weight gain
- Truncal obesity
- Moon face
- Extremity muscle wasting
- Loss of bone density
- Hypertension
- Hyperglycemia
- Striae and acne

Thyrotropin (Thyroid-Stimulating Hormone [TSH])
- Elevated plasma TSH and thyroid hormone levels
- Weight loss
- Tachycardia and dysrhythmias
- Heat intolerance
- Increased GI motility
- Fine tremors

Gonadotropins (Luteinizing Hormone [LH], Follicle-Stimulating Hormone [FSH])
Men
- Elevated LH and FSH levels
- Hypogonadism or hypergonadism

Women
- Normal LH and FSH levels

NURSING SAFETY PRIORITY

Drug Alert

Teach patients taking bromocriptine to seek medical care immediately if chest pain, dizziness, or watery nasal discharge occurs because of the possibility of serious side effects, including cardiac dysrhythmias, coronary artery spasms, and fibrotic changes.

A

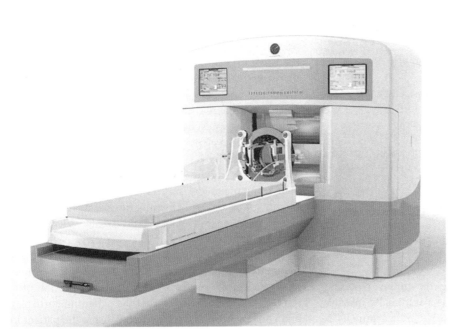

B

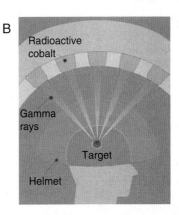

FIG. 54.2 Gamma Knife radiosurgery. (A) The Gamma Knife device consists of an 18,000-kg shield surrounding a hemispheric array of 201 cobalt-60 sources. (B) The sources are oriented such that all 201 beams converge at a single point (also known as the isocenter of the Gamma Knife). (From Newton, H. B. [2022]. *Handbook of neuro-oncology neuroimaging* [3rd ed.]. St. Louis: Elsevier.)

Side effects of bromocriptine include orthostatic (postural) hypotension, headaches, nausea, abdominal cramps, and constipation. Give bromocriptine with a meal or a snack to reduce GI side effects. Treatment starts with a low dose and is gradually increased until the desired level is reached. *If pregnancy occurs, the patient should speak with their health care provider immediately to determine whether the drug can be continued at this time.*

The most common and effective agents used for acromegaly are the somatostatin analogs and growth hormone (GH) receptor blocker. Most often used are the somatostatin analogs octreotide and lanreotide, and a GH receptor blocker, pegvisomant (Burchum & Rosenthal, 2022). Octreotide inhibits GH release through negative feedback. Pegvisomant blocks GH receptor activity and blocks production of insulin-like growth factor (IGF). Combination therapy with monthly injections of a somatostatin analog and weekly injections of pegvisomant has provided good control of the disease.

Radiation therapy does not have immediate effects in reducing pituitary hormone excesses, and months to years may pass before a therapeutic effect can be seen. When used, it is generally considered third-line therapy following medication and surgery (Melmed & Katznelson, 2023). The use of the Gamma Knife or stereotactic confocal radiotherapy method of delivering radiation to pituitary tumors has reduced the long-term side effects of this therapy (Fig. 54.2).

Surgical Management. Surgical removal of the pituitary gland (**hypophysectomy**) along with any tumor is the most common treatment for hyperpituitarism (Fig. 54.3). Successful surgery decreases hormone levels, relieves headaches, and may reverse changes in sexual functioning. This is most commonly

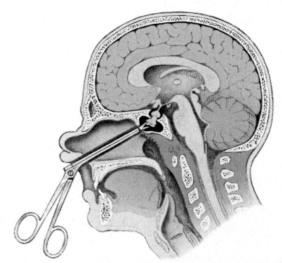

FIG. 54.3 Hypophysectomy. (From Urden, L. D., Stacy, K. M., & Lough, M. E. [2022]. *Critical care nursing: diagnosis and management* [9th ed.]. St. Louis: Elsevier.)

performed transnasally or transsphenoidally and uses a bone or fat patch to close the hole and prevent cerebrospinal fluid (CSF) leakage.

Preoperative Care. Explain that nasal packing may be present for 2 to 3 days after surgery, it will be necessary to breathe through the mouth, and a "mustache" dressing ("drip" pad) may be placed under the nose. It is very critical that the patient be instructed to *not* cough, sneeze, blow the nose, or bend forward after surgery. These activities can increase intracranial pressure (ICP) and delay healing.

Operative Procedures. Depending on tumor size and location, a transsphenoidal approach or a minimally invasive endoscopic transnasal approach with smaller instruments is used with the patient under general anesthesia instead of a more invasive procedure. Nasal packing is sometimes inserted after the transsphenoidal incision is closed, and a mustache dressing is sometimes applied. These are not needed for the minimally invasive transnasal procedure.

Postoperative Care. Monitor the patient's neurologic response every hour and document any changes in vision or mental status, altered level of consciousness, or decreased extremity strength. Observe for complications such as transient diabetes insipidus (DI; discussed later in this chapter), cerebrospinal fluid (CSF) leakage, infection, and increased ICP.

Teach the patient to report any postnasal drip or increased swallowing, which may indicate leakage of CSF. Keep the head of the bed elevated. Assess nasal drainage for quantity, quality, and the presence of glucose (present in CSF). A light yellow color at the edge of the clear drainage on the dressing is called the *halo sign* and indicates CSF. If the patient has persistent, severe headaches, CSF fluid may have leaked into the sinus area. Most CSF leaks resolve with bed rest, and surgical intervention is rarely needed.

Teach the patient to avoid coughing early after surgery because it increases pressure in the incision area and may lead to a CSF leak. Remind the patient to perform deep breathing hourly while awake to prevent pulmonary problems. Instruct the patient to rinse the mouth frequently and to apply a lubricating jelly to dry lips to manage the dryness from mouth breathing.

Assess for indications of infection, especially meningitis, such as headache, fever, and nuchal rigidity. The surgeon may prescribe antibiotics, analgesics, and antipyretics.

If the entire pituitary gland has been removed, replacement of thyroid hormones and glucocorticoids is lifelong. See Box 54.3 for specific nursing actions after hypophysectomy.

After surgery the patient needs daily self-management regimens and frequent checkups. Advise the patient to avoid activities that might interfere with healing or increase intracranial pressure (ICP). Teach the patient to avoid bending over from the waist to pick up objects or tie shoes because this position increases ICP. Teach the patient to bend the knees and then lower the body to pick up fallen objects. ICP also increases when the patient strains to have a bowel movement. Suggest techniques to prevent constipation, such as eating high-fiber foods, drinking plenty of fluids, and using stool softeners or laxatives as prescribed.

Teach the patient to avoid toothbrushing for about 2 weeks after transsphenoidal surgery. Frequent mouth care with oral mouth rinses and daily flossing provide adequate oral hygiene. A decreased sense of smell is expected after surgery and usually lasts 3 to 4 months.

Hormone replacement with vasopressin may be needed to maintain fluid balance (see discussion of Interventions in the Diabetes Insipidus section). If the anterior portion of the pituitary gland is removed, instruct the patient in cortisol, thyroid, and gonadal hormone replacement. Teach the patient to report the return of any symptoms of hyperpituitarism immediately to the primary health care provider.

ARGININE VASOPRESSIN DEFICIENCY AND ARGININE VASOPRESSIN RESISTANCE/ DIABETES INSIPIDUS

Pathophysiology Review

Diabetes insipidus (DI) is a disorder of the posterior pituitary gland in which water loss is caused by a deficiency in vasopressin (antidiuretic hormone [ADH]) or an inability of the kidneys to respond to vasopressin. In early 2023, new terminology for diabetes insipidus was adopted globally. Arginine vasopressin deficiency (AVP-D) refers to central diabetes insipidus, and arginine vasopressin resistance (AVP-R) refers to nephrogenic diabetes insipidus. The result is the excretion of large volumes of dilute urine because the distal kidney tubules and collecting ducts do not reabsorb water; this leads to *polyuria*, dehydration, and disturbed *fluid and electrolyte balance*.

Massive water loss increases plasma osmolarity and serum sodium levels, which stimulate the sensation of thirst. Thirst promotes increased fluid intake and aids in maintaining hydration. A compromised thirst mechanism can lead to dehydration, particularly in older adults. *Severe dehydration can lead to death.*

! NURSING SAFETY PRIORITY

Action Alert

Ensure that no patient suspected of having AVP-D or AVP-R is deprived of fluids for more than 4 hours because these patients cannot reduce urine output, and severe dehydration can result.

PATIENT-CENTERED CARE: GENETICS/GENOMICS

Nephrogenic Diabetes Insipidus

AVP-R can be caused by a mutation in the gene encoding arginine vasopressin (OMIM, 2022). AVP-R is a genetic disorder in which the vasopressin (antidiuretic hormone [ADH]) receptor has a defect that prevents kidney tubules from interacting with vasopressin. The result is poor water reabsorption by the kidney, although the actual amount of hormone produced is not deficient. This problem is most commonly inherited as an X-linked recessive disorder affecting males (OMIM, 2022). When assessing a patient with AVP-R, always ask whether anyone else in the family has ever had this disorder.

Interprofessional Collaborative Care

Recognize Cues: Assessment

Most patients with moderate to severe AVP-D or AVP-R report polyuria, nocturia, and polydipsia (Bichet, 2023b). Symptoms include an increase in urination and excessive thirst. Ask about a history of recent surgery, head trauma, or drug use (e.g., lithium), which can cause AVP-R. Although increased fluid intake prevents serious volume depletion, the patient who is deprived of fluids or who cannot increase oral fluid intake may develop shock from fluid loss. Symptoms of dehydration (e.g., poor skin turgor, dry or cracked mucous membranes) may be present. (See Chapter 13 for discussion of dehydration.)

Water loss changes blood and urine tests. Hypernatremia can quickly develop. The 24-hour fluid intake and output is measured without restricting food or fluid intake. AVP-D or AVP-R are considered if urine output is more than 3 L during this period and is greater than the volume ingested (Bichet, 2023b). The amount of urine excreted in 24 hours may vary from 4 to 30 L/day. Urine is dilute with a low specific gravity (less than 1.005) and low osmolality (<300 mOsm/L) (Hui et al., 2023).

Take Actions: Interventions

Management of AVP-D focuses on controlling symptoms using drug therapy with desmopressin (Bichet, 2023a; Burchum & Rosenthal, 2022). As a synthetic drug, it serves to replace natural vasopressin (ADH). It is available orally, as a sublingual "melt," subcutaneously, or intranasally in a metered spray. The frequency of dosing varies with patient responses. Ulceration of the mucous membranes, allergy, a sensation of chest tightness, and lung inhalation of the spray may occur with use of the intranasal preparations. If side effects occur or if the patient has an upper respiratory infection, oral or subcutaneous vasopressin is used.

Drug therapy induces water retention and can cause fluid overload (see Chapter 13). *Teach patients to weigh themselves daily to identify weight gain.* Stress the importance of using the same scale and weighing at the same time of day while wearing a similar amount and type of clothing. If weight gain of more than 2.2 lb (1 kg) along with other signs of water toxicity occurs (e.g., persistent headache, acute confusion, nausea, vomiting), instruct the patient to go immediately to the emergency department or call 911. Instruct the patient to wear a medical alert bracelet identifying the disorder and drug.

NURSING SAFETY PRIORITY

Drug Alert

Desmopressin can induce hyponatremia, which can lead to seizures, coma, respiratory failure, or death. Carefully monitor serum sodium for patients being treated with this drug.

Treatment of AVP-R is selected based on cause. Urine output can be lowered with a low-salt, low-to-normal protein diet and diuretics (Bichet, 2023c). In adults, restricting sodium intake to less than 2.3 g/day and reducing protein intake to <1.0 mg/kg daily diminishes urine output (Bichet, 2023c). A thiazide diuretic induces mild volume depletion; even a weight loss of 1 to 1.5 kg can reduce urine output significantly (Bichet, 2023c). Other treatments are dependent on the patient's individualized needs.

For the hospitalized patient, nursing management focuses on early detection of dehydration and maintaining adequate hydration. Actions include accurately measuring fluid intake and output, checking urine specific gravity, and recording the patient's weight daily.

Urge the patient to drink fluids in an amount equal to urine output. If fluids are given intravenously, ensure the patency of the access catheter and accurately monitor the amount infused hourly.

Some patients may require lifelong drug therapy. Check their ability to assess symptoms, and adjust dosages as prescribed for changes in conditions. Teach that polyuria and polydipsia indicate the need for another dose.

SYNDROME OF INAPPROPRIATE ANTIDIURETIC HORMONE

Pathophysiology Review

The syndrome of inappropriate antidiuretic hormone (SIADH) or *Schwartz-Bartter syndrome* is a problem in which antidiuretic hormone (ADH, vasopressin) is secreted even when plasma osmolarity is low or normal, resulting in water retention and fluid overload. A decrease in plasma osmolarity normally inhibits ADH production and secretion. SIADH occurs with many conditions (e.g., cancer therapy, pulmonary infection or impairment) and can be caused by select drugs (Sterns, 2021) as noted in Box 54.4.

In SIADH, ADH continues to be released when not needed, leading to water retention and disturbances of *fluid and electrolyte balance.* Water retention results in dilutional *hyponatremia* (a decreased serum sodium level) and fluid overload. The increase in blood volume increases the kidney filtration and inhibits the release of renin and aldosterone, which increase urine sodium loss and results in greater hyponatremia.

Interprofessional Collaborative Care

Recognize Cues: Assessment

Ask patients about their medical history, which may reveal conditions that can cause SIADH (see Box 54.4). Early symptoms of SIADH are related to the water retention causing dilution of serum sodium levels *(hyponatremia).* GI disturbances, such as

BOX 54.4   Conditions Causing the Syndrome of Inappropriate Antidiuretic Hormone

Malignancies
- Small cell lung cancer
- Pancreatic, duodenal, and GU carcinomas
- Thymoma
- Hodgkin lymphoma
- Non-Hodgkin lymphoma

CNS Disorders
- Trauma
- Infection
- Tumors (primary or metastatic)
- Strokes
- Porphyria
- Systemic lupus erythematosus

Pulmonary Disorders
- Viral and bacterial pneumonia
- Lung abscesses
- Active tuberculosis
- Pneumothorax
- Chronic lung diseases
- Mycoses
- Positive-pressure ventilation

Select Drug Examples
- Antidepressants (SSRIs, tricyclics, MAOIs, venlafaxine)
- Antiseizure medications (carbamazepine, sodium valproate, lamotrigine)
- Antipsychotics (phenothiazines, butyrophenones)
- Anticancer agents (cyclophosphamide, methotrexate, vincristine)
- Antidiabetic drugs (chlorpropamide, tolbutamide)
- Vasopressin analogs (desmopressin, oxytocin, vasopressin)
- Exogenous ADH
- Opiates

ADH, Antidiuretic hormone; *CNS,* central nervous system; *GU,* genitourinary.

loss of appetite, nausea, and vomiting, may occur first, as discussed in Chapter 13. Weigh the patient and document any recent weight gain. Use this information to monitor responses to therapy. In SIADH, free water (not salt) is retained and dependent edema is not usually present, even though water is retained.

Water retention, hyponatremia, and fluid shifts affect central nervous system function, especially when the serum sodium level is below 115 mEq/L (mmol/L). The patient may have lethargy, headaches, hostility, disorientation, and a change in level of consciousness. Lethargy and headaches can progress to decreased responsiveness, seizures, and coma. Assess deep tendon reflexes, which are usually decreased.

Vital sign changes include full and bounding pulse (caused by the increased fluid volume) and hypothermia (caused by central nervous system disturbance). Chapter 13 presents other findings that occur with hyponatremia.

Water retention causes urine volume to decrease and urine osmolarity to increase. At the same time, plasma volume increases, and plasma osmolarity decreases. Elevated urine sodium levels and specific gravity reflect increased urine concentration. Serum sodium levels decrease, sometimes to as low as 110 mEq/L (mmol/L), because of fluid retention and sodium loss.

Take Actions: Interventions

Interventions for SIADH focus on restricting fluid intake, promoting the excretion of water, replacing lost sodium, and

interfering with the action of ADH. Nursing interventions include monitoring response to therapy, preventing complications, teaching the patient and family about fluid restrictions and drug therapy, and preventing injury.

Fluid restriction is essential because fluid intake further dilutes plasma sodium levels. In some cases, fluid intake may be restricted to as little as 500 to 1000 mL/24 hr. Use saline instead of water to dilute tube feedings, irrigate GI tubes, and give drugs by GI tube.

Measure intake, output, and daily weights to assess the degree of fluid restriction needed. A weight gain of 2.2 lb (1 kg) or more per day or a gradual increase over several days is cause for concern. A 2.2-lb (1-kg) increase is equal to a 1000-mL fluid retention (1 kg = 1 L). Prevent mouth dryness with frequent oral rinsing (warn patients to not swallow the rinses).

Drug therapy with vasopressin receptor antagonists (vaptans) such as conivaptan or tolvaptan is used to treat SIADH when hyponatremia is present in hospitalized patients (Burchum & Rosenthal, 2022). These drugs promote water excretion without causing sodium loss. Tolvaptan is an oral drug, and conivaptan is given intravenously. Tolvaptan is used much less frequently (Sterns, 2022). It contains a black box warning that rapid increases in serum sodium levels (greater than 12 mEq/L [mmol/L] increase in 24 hours) have been associated with central nervous system demyelination that can lead to serious complications and death (Otsuka America Pharmaceutical, 2021). There is also a black box warning that indicates that liver failure and death are possible (Otsuka America Pharmaceutical, 2022).

💊 NURSING SAFETY PRIORITY
Drug Alert

> Administer tolvaptan or conivaptan only in the hospital setting so that serum sodium levels can be monitored closely for the development of hypernatremia and other complications.

Diuretics may be used on a limited basis to manage SIADH when sodium levels are near normal and heart failure is present. With diuretics, sodium loss can be potentiated, further contributing to the problems caused by SIADH. For milder SIADH, demeclocycline, an oral antibiotic, may help reach **fluid and electrolyte balance,** although the drug is not approved for this problem and is no longer available in most countries, making it a rarely used treatment.

Hypertonic saline (i.e., 3% sodium chloride [3% NaCl]) is used for SIADH when the serum sodium level is very low (Robinson & Verbalis, 2016). Give IV saline cautiously because it may add to existing fluid overload and promote heart failure. If the patient needs routine IV fluids, a saline solution is ordered to prevent further sodium dilution.

Monitor the patient's response to therapy to prevent the fluid overload from becoming worse, leading to pulmonary edema and heart failure. Any patient with SIADH, regardless of age, is at risk for these complications. The older adult or one who also has cardiac, kidney, pulmonary, or liver problems is at greater risk.

Monitor for increased fluid overload (bounding pulse, increasing neck vein distention, lung crackles, dyspnea, increasing peripheral edema, reduced urine output) at least every 2 hours. *Pulmonary edema can occur very quickly and can lead to death.* Notify the primary health care provider of any change that indicates the fluid overload is not responding to therapy or is worse.

Providing a safe environment is needed when the serum sodium level falls below 120 mEq/L (mmol/L). The risk for neurologic changes and seizures increases as a result of osmotic fluid shifts into brain tissue. Observe for and document changes in the patient's neurologic status. Assess for subtle changes, such as muscle twitching, increasing irritability, or restlessness, before these progress to seizures or coma. Check orientation to time, place, and person every 2 hours because disorientation or confusion may be present as an early indication. Reduce environmental noise and lighting to prevent overstimulation.

The frequency of neurologic checks depends on the patient's status. For the patient being treated for SIADH who is hyponatremic but alert, awake, and oriented, checks every 2 to 4 hours may be sufficient. For the patient who has had a change in level of consciousness, perform neurologic checks at least every hour or as per orders. Inspect the environment every shift, making sure that basic safety measures, such as side rails being securely in place, are observed.

DISORDERS OF THE ADRENAL GLAND

ADRENAL GLAND HYPOFUNCTION

Pathophysiology Review

Adrenal cortex production of steroid hormone may decrease as a result of inadequate secretion of adrenocorticotropic hormone (ACTH), dysfunction of the hypothalamic-pituitary control mechanism, or direct problems of adrenal gland tissue (Cole, 2018). Symptoms may develop gradually or occur quickly with stress.

Insufficiency of adrenocortical steroids causes problems through the loss of aldosterone and cortisol action. Decreased cortisol levels result in hypoglycemia. Gastric acid production and glomerular filtration decrease. Decreased glomerular filtration leads to excessive blood urea nitrogen (BUN) levels, which cause anorexia and weight loss.

Reduced aldosterone secretion causes disturbances of *fluid and electrolyte balance.* Potassium excretion is decreased, causing hyperkalemia. Sodium and water excretion are increased, causing hyponatremia and hypovolemia. Potassium retention also promotes reabsorption of hydrogen ions, which can lead to acidosis.

Low adrenal androgen levels decrease body, axillary, and pubic hair, especially in women, because the adrenals produce most of the androgens in females. The severity of symptoms is related to the degree of hormone deficiency.

Acute adrenal insufficiency (*adrenal crisis* or *Addisonian crisis*) is a medical emergency in which the need for cortisol and aldosterone is greater than the body's supply

(Nieman, 2022c; Rogers, 2023). Life-threatening symptoms can appear without warning. It often occurs in response to a stressful event (e.g., surgery, trauma, severe infection), especially when the adrenal hormone output is already reduced. Problems are the same as those of chronic insufficiency but are more severe. However, unless intervention is initiated promptly, sodium levels fall, and potassium levels rise rapidly (Nieman, 2022c). Severe hypotension results from the blood volume depletion that occurs with the loss of aldosterone.

Adrenal insufficiency is classified as primary (called Addison disease) or secondary. Causes of primary and secondary adrenal insufficiency are listed in Box 54.5. In primary adrenal insufficiency, glucocorticoids, mineralocorticoids, and androgens are reduced. In secondary adrenal insufficiency, mineralocorticoid function is preserved. A common cause of secondary adrenal insufficiency is the sudden cessation of long-term glucocorticoid therapy. This therapy suppresses production of glucocorticoids through negative feedback and causes atrophy of the adrenal cortex. Glucocorticoid drugs must be withdrawn gradually to allow for pituitary production of ACTH and activation of adrenal cells to produce cortisol. This can often be an underlying cause of shock in patients withdrawn from steroids too quickly.

Interprofessional Collaborative Care

Acute adrenal insufficiency is an emergency and is managed in an acute care setting. Without appropriate management, death ensues (Nieman, 2022c). Chronic adrenal insufficiency is usually managed in the outpatient environment.

Recognize Cues: Assessment

History. For patients who are not experiencing acute adrenal insufficiency, ask about symptoms and factors that cause adrenal hypofunction. Ask about any change in activity level because lethargy, fatigue, and muscle weakness are often present. Include questions about salt intake, as salt craving often occurs with hypofunction.

GI problems, such as anorexia, nausea, vomiting, diarrhea, and abdominal pain, often occur (Grossman, 2022). Ask about weight loss during the past months. Women may have menstrual changes related to weight loss, and men may report impotence.

BOX 54.5 Causes of Primary and Secondary Adrenal Insufficiency

Primary Causes	Secondary Causes
• Autoimmune disease[a]	• Pituitary tumors
• Tuberculosis	• Postpartum pituitary necrosis
• Metastatic cancer	• Hypophysectomy
• HIV-III (AIDS)	• High-dose pituitary or whole-brain radiation
• Hemorrhage	• Cessation of long-term corticosteroid drug therapy[a]
• Gram-negative sepsis	
• Adrenalectomy	
• Abdominal radiation therapy	
• Drugs (mitotane) and toxins	

[a]Most common cause.

BOX 54.6   Key Features

Adrenal Insufficiency

Cardiovascular Symptoms
- Anemia
- Hypercalcemia
- Hyperkalemia
- Hyponatremia
- Hypotension

GI Symptoms
- Abdominal pain
- Anorexia
- Constipation or diarrhea
- Nausea, vomiting
- Salt craving
- Weight loss

Integumentary Symptoms
- Hyperpigmentation
- Vitiligo

Neuromuscular Symptoms
- Fatigue
- Joint pain
- Muscle pain
- Muscle weakness

Ask whether the patient has had radiation to the abdomen or head. Abdominal radiation could directly damage the adrenal glands, whereas cranial radiation could interfere with hypothalamic or pituitary influences on adrenal function. Document medical problems (e.g., tuberculosis or previous intracranial surgery) and all past and current drugs, especially steroids, anticoagulants, opioids, and cancer drugs.

Inquire about whether the patient has had or been exposed to COVID-19. Evidence shows that the SARS-CoV-2 virus targets the adrenal glands and can induce insufficiency in some patients (Hamazaki et al., 2022; Kanczkowski et al., 2022).

Physical Assessment/Signs and Symptoms. Symptoms of adrenal insufficiency vary, and the severity is related to the degree of hormone deficiency as listed in Box 54.6. In patients with primary insufficiency (problem with adrenal gland function), plasma ACTH and melanocyte-stimulating hormone (MSH) levels are elevated in response to the adrenal-hypothalamic-pituitary feedback system. (Both ACTH and MSH are made from the same prehormone molecule. Anything that stimulates increased production of ACTH often also leads to increased production of MSH.) Elevated MSH levels result in areas of *increased* pigmentation. In primary autoimmune disease, patchy areas of *decreased* pigmentation *(vitiligo)* may occur because of destruction of skin melanocytes. Body hair may also be decreased. In secondary adrenal insufficiency (problem in the hypothalamus or pituitary gland leading to decreased ACTH and MSH levels), skin pigmentation is not changed.

Assess for hypoglycemia (e.g., sweating, headaches, tachycardia, and tremors) and fluid depletion (postural hypotension and dehydration). Hyperkalemia can cause dysrhythmias with an irregular heart rate and can result in cardiac arrest. Hyponatremia leading to hypotension and decreased cognition can occur.

Psychosocial Assessment. Depending on the degree of imbalance, patients may appear lethargic, depressed, confused, and even psychotic. Assess the patient's orientation to person, place, time, and situation. Families may report that the patient has wide mood swings and is forgetful.

Diagnostic Assessment. Laboratory findings are listed in Table 54.2 and include low serum sodium and low salivary cortisol levels, low fasting blood glucose, elevated potassium, and increased blood urea nitrogen (BUN) levels. In primary disease, the eosinophil count and ACTH level are elevated. Plasma cortisol levels do not rise during provocation tests (see Chapter 56).

Urinary 17-hydroxycorticosteroids are the glucocorticoid metabolites, and 17-ketosteroid levels reflect the adrenal androgen metabolites. Both levels are in the low or low-normal range in adrenal hypofunction.

An ACTH stimulation (provocative) test is the most definitive test for adrenal insufficiency. ACTH is given intravenously, and plasma cortisol levels are obtained at 30-minute and 1-hour intervals. In primary insufficiency, the cortisol response is absent or very decreased. In secondary insufficiency, it is increased. When acute adrenal insufficiency is suspected, treatment is started without stimulation testing.

Imaging Assessment. CT and MRI are most helpful in determining the cause of pituitary problems leading to adrenal insufficiency. CT and MRI can show adrenal gland atrophy but not its cause.

Take Actions: Interventions

Nursing interventions focus on promoting fluid balance, monitoring for fluid deficit, and preventing hypoglycemia. Because hyperkalemia can cause dysrhythmias with an irregular heart rate and result in cardiac arrest, assessing cardiac function is a nursing priority. Assess vital signs every 1 to 4 hours, depending on the patient's condition and the presence of dysrhythmias or postural hypotension. Weigh the patient daily and record intake and output. Monitor laboratory values to identify hemoconcentration (e.g., increased hematocrit or BUN). Chapter 13 discusses dehydration in detail.

Cortisol and aldosterone deficiencies are corrected by hormone replacement therapy described in Table 54.3. Hydrocortisone corrects glucocorticoid deficiency. Oral cortisol replacement regimens and dosages vary. The most common drug used for this purpose is prednisone. In general, divided doses are given, with two-thirds given on arising in the morning and one-third at 6:00 p.m. to mimic the normal release of this hormone.

⬭ NURSING SAFETY PRIORITY

Drug Alert

Prednisone and prednisolone are sound-alike drugs, and care is needed to avoid confusion. Although they are both corticosteroids, they are not interchangeable because prednisolone is more potent than prednisone.

An additional mineralocorticoid hormone, such as fludrocortisone, may be needed to maintain or restore *fluid and electrolyte balance* (especially sodium and potassium). Dosage

TABLE 54.2   LABORATORY PROFILE
Adrenal Gland Assessment

Test	Normal Range	Hypofunction	Hyperfunction
Sodium	136–145 mEq/L (mmol/L)	Low	High
Potassium	3.5–5.0 mEq/L (mmol/L)	High	Low
Glucose (fasting)	70–110 mg/dL (4-6 mmol/L)	Normal to low	Normal to high
Calcium	Total: 9–10.5 mg/dL (2.25–2.75 mmol/L) Ionized: 4.5–5.6 mg/dL (1.05–1.30 mmol/L)	High	Low
Bicarbonate	23–30 mEq/L (mmol/L)	High	Low
Blood urea nitrogen (BUN)	10–20 mg/dL (3.6–7.1 mmol/L)	High	Normal
Cortisol (serum)	6 a.m. to 8 a.m.: 5–23 mcg/dL (138–635 nmol/L) 4 p.m. to 6 p.m.: 3–13 mcg/dL (83–359 nmol/L)	Low	High
Cortisol (salivary)	7 a.m. to 9 a.m.: 100–750 ng/dL 3 p.m. to 5 p.m.: <401 ng/dL	Low	High

Data from Pagana, K. D., Pagana, T. J., & Pagana, T. N. (2022). *Mosby's manual of diagnostic and laboratory tests* (7th ed.). St. Louis: Elsevier.

TABLE 54.3   COMMON EXAMPLES OF DRUG THERAPY
Adrenal Hypofunction

Drug	Selected Nursing Implications
Cortisone	Instruct the patient to take the drug with meals or a snack *to avoid gastric irritation.*
Hydrocortisone	Instruct the patient to report signs or symptoms of excessive drug therapy (e.g., rapid weight gain, round face, fluid retention), *which indicate Cushing syndrome and a possible need for a dosage adjustment.*
Prednisone	Instruct the patient to report illness *because the usual daily dosage may not be adequate during periods of illness or severe stress.*
Fludrocortisone	Monitor the patient's blood pressure *to assess for the potential side effect of hypertension.* Instruct the patient to report weight gain or edema *because sodium intake may need to be restricted.*

adjustment may be needed, especially in hot weather when more sodium is lost because of excessive perspiration. *Salt restriction or diuretic therapy should not be started without considering whether it might lead to an adrenal crisis.*

Emergency nursing care actions for patients experiencing acute adrenal insufficiency are listed in Box 54.7.

NCLEX Examination Challenge 54.2
Physiological Integrity

The nurse is monitoring laboratory values for a client with adrenal insufficiency undergoing IV therapy with hydrocortisone. Which finding demonstrates that treatment has been effective? (Reference ranges: sodium = 136–145 mEq/L [mmol/L]; potassium = 3.5–5.0 mEq/L [mmol/L])
A. Serum sodium 150 mEq/L (mmol/L); serum potassium 7.16 mEq/L (mmol/L)
B. Serum sodium 138 mEq/L (mmol/L); serum potassium 4.2 mEq/L (mmol/L)
C. Serum sodium 122 mEq/L (mmol/L); serum potassium 2.8 mEq/L (mmol/L)
D. Serum sodium 118 mEq/L (mmol/L); serum potassium 6.7 mEq/L (mmol/L)

FLUID AND ELECTROLYTE BALANCE CONCEPT EXEMPLAR: CUSHING SYNDROME (HYPERCORTISOLISM)
Pathophysiology Review

Hypercortisolism is a clinical state arising from excessive tissue exposure to cortisol and/or other glucocorticoids

(Uwaifo & Hura, 2023). This condition is also called Cushing syndrome, a set of symptoms caused by the excess of cortisol in the body (Box 54.8). Patients with disorders that require ongoing therapy with drugs such as prednisone are at risk for development of this condition. In uncommon cases, a benign, hormone-secreting tumor of the adrenal glands causes too much cortisol to be produced, which can also cause Cushing syndrome (Findling et al., 2022).

Some patients have a benign pituitary gland tumor that secretes adrenocorticotropic hormone (ACTH), which stimulates the overproduction of cortisol in the body (American Association of Neurological Surgeons, 2023). This condition is called Cushing disease, which is a specific type of Cushing syndrome (Findling et al., 2022). Pituitary hyperplasia can also cause this disorder (Findling et al., 2022). Women are more likely than men to develop Cushing disease.

The body's metabolism and all body systems are affected in Cushing syndrome. An increase in total body fat results from slow turnover of plasma fatty acids. This fat is redistributed, producing truncal obesity, "buffalo hump," and "moon face" (Fig. 54.4) (Jarvis & Eckhardt, 2024). Increases in the breakdown of tissue protein result in decreased muscle mass and muscle strength, thin skin, and fragile capillaries. Effects on minerals lead to bone density loss.

High levels of corticosteroids reduce lymphocyte production and shrink organs containing lymphocytes, such as the spleen and the lymph nodes. White blood cell (WBC) cytokine

Emergency Management of the Patient With Acute Adrenal Insufficiency

Hormone Replacement
- Start rapid infusion of normal saline or dextrose 5% in normal saline.
- Initial higher doses of hydrocortisone sodium or dexamethasone are administered as an IV bolus.
- Administer additional hydrocortisone sodium by continuous IV infusion over the next 8 hours.
- Give an additional dose of hydrocortisone intramuscularly concomitantly with hydration every 12 hours.
- Initiate an IV H_2 histamine blocker (e.g., cimetidine) for ulcer prevention.

Hyperkalemia Management
- Administer insulin and dextrose intravenously to shift potassium into cells. Dosing is often based on renal function.
- Give potassium binding and excreting resin.
- Give loop or thiazide diuretics.
- Avoid potassium-sparing diuretics.
- Cardiac cell membrane stabilization with IV calcium.
- Initiate potassium restriction.
- Monitor intake and output.
- Monitor heart rate, rhythm, and ECG for signs and symptoms of hyperkalemia (slow heart rate; heart block; tall, peaked T waves; fibrillation; asystole).

Hypoglycemia Management
- Administer IV glucose as per orders.
- Prepare to administer glucagon as needed and as per orders.
- Maintain IV access.
- Monitor blood glucose level hourly.

Endogenous Secretion (Cushing Disease)
- Bilateral adrenal hyperplasia[a]
- Pituitary adenoma increasing the production of ACTH (pituitary Cushing disease)
- Malignancies: Carcinomas of the lung, GI tract, pancreas
- Adrenal adenomas or carcinomas

Exogenous Administration (Cushing Syndrome)
- Therapeutic use of ACTH or glucocorticoids—most commonly for treatment of:
  - Asthma
  - Autoimmune disorders
  - Organ transplantation
  - Cancer chemotherapy
  - Allergic responses
  - Chronic fibrosis

[a]Most common cause.
ACTH, Adrenocorticotropic hormone.

production is decreased. These changes reduce immunity and increase the risk for infection.

In most cases, increased androgen production also occurs and causes acne, *hirsutism* (increased body hair growth), and

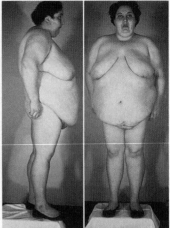
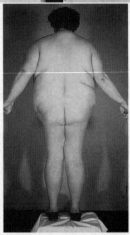

FIG. 54.4 Typical appearance of a patient with Cushing disease or syndrome. Note truncal obesity, moon face, buffalo hump, thinner arms and legs, and abdominal striae. (From Wenig, B. M., Heffess, C.S ., & Adair, C. F. [1997]. *Atlas of endocrine pathology.* Philadelphia: Saunders.)

occasionally clitoral hypertrophy. Increased androgens disrupt the normal ovarian hormone feedback mechanism, decreasing the ovaries' production of estrogens and progesterone. *Oligomenorrhea* (scant or infrequent menses) occurs as a result.

Etiology and Genetic Risk

As noted earlier, the most common exogenous cause of Cushing syndrome is taking a glucocorticoid medication such as prednisone (Findling et al., 2022) to control serious chronic inflammatory conditions (Nieman, 2018). Research shows a genetic link is involved in the development of adrenocortical tumors (Kamilaris et al., 2021).

Incidence and Prevalence

The incidence and prevalence of Cushing syndrome is difficult to determine, as many people take prescribed glucocorticoids, milder cases may go undiagnosed, and most cases are not reported (Nieman, 2023a).

Health Promotion/Disease Prevention

Encourage patients on glucocorticoid therapy to talk directly with their primary health care provider or specialist to determine if dosage adjustments need to be made. There is no known way to prevent the formation of tumors related to Cushing syndrome and Cushing disease.

Interprofessional Collaborative Care
Recognize Cues: Assessment

History. Ask about the patient's other health problems and drug therapies because glucocorticoid drug therapy is common. Regardless of cause, patients have many changes because of the widespread effect of excessive cortisol. They may report weight gain and an increased appetite. Ask about changes in activity or sleep patterns, fatigue, and muscle weakness. Ask about bone pain or a history of fractures, because osteoporosis results from hypercortisolism. Ask about a history of frequent infections and easy bruising. Women often stop menstruating. GI problems include ulcer formation from increased hydrochloric acid secretion and decreased production of protective gastric mucus.

Physical Assessment/Signs and Symptoms. The patient with hypercortisolism has specific, predictable physical changes, although all body systems are affected as described in Box 54.9 (see Fig. 54.4). These body changes are opposite to those seen in primary adrenal insufficiency (Addison disease). (Box 54.10). Changes in fat distribution may result in fat pads on the neck, back, and shoulders (buffalo hump); an enlarged trunk

---

BOX 54.10 Comparison of Symptoms Seen in Addison Disease and Cushing Syndrome

Addison Disease	Cushing Syndrome
• Personality changes	• Thinning hair
	• Acne
	• Moon face
	• Hirsutism
	• Emotional instability
• Hyperpigmentation of skin	• "Buffalo hump" and easy bruising
	• Striae on abdomen, thighs, upper arms
• Cardiac insufficiency	• Cardiac hypertrophy
• Hypotension	• Hypertension
	• Edema
• Anorexia	• Increased appetite
• Nausea and vomiting	• Weight gain
• Diarrhea	
• Muscle weakness	• Muscle wasting
• Adrenal atrophy	• Bone thinning, osteoporosis
	• Reduced immunity

---

with thin arms and legs; and a round face (moon face). Other changes include muscle wasting and weakness. Assess for and document changes and use these findings to prioritize patient problems.

Skin changes result from blood vessel fragility and include bruises, thin or translucent skin, and wounds that have not healed. Reddish-purple *striae* (stretch marks) occur on the abdomen, thighs, and upper arms because of the destructive effect of cortisol on collagen.

Acne and a fine coating of hair may occur over the face and body. In women, look for the presence of hirsutism, clitoral hypertrophy, and male pattern balding related to androgen excess.

Cardiac changes occur as a result of disturbed **fluid and electrolyte balance.** Both sodium and water are reabsorbed and retained, leading to hypervolemia and edema formation. Blood pressure is elevated, and pulses are full and bounding.

Musculoskeletal changes occur as a result of nitrogen depletion and mineral loss. Muscle mass decreases, especially in arms and legs (see Fig. 54.4). Muscle weakness increases the risk for falls. Bone is thinner, and osteoporosis is common, increasing the risk for fractures.

Glucose metabolism is affected by hypercortisolism. Fasting blood glucose levels are high because the liver releases glucose and the insulin receptors are less sensitive; therefore blood glucose does not move as easily into the tissues.

Immune changes caused by excess cortisol result in reduced **immunity.** Excess cortisol reduces the number of circulating lymphocytes, inhibits macrophage activity, reduces antibody synthesis, and inhibits production of cytokines and inflammatory chemicals (e.g., histamine). Infection risk is increased; and the patient may not have fever, purulent exudate, or redness/hyperpigmentation in the affected area when an infection is present.

Psychosocial Assessment. Hypercortisolism can result in emotional instability, and patients often say that they do not

---

 ### BOX 54.9 Key Features

Cushing Syndrome/Cushing Disease (Hypercortisolism)

General Appearance
- Moon face
- Buffalo hump
- Truncal obesity
- Weight gain

Cardiovascular Symptoms
- Hypertension
- Frequent dependent edema
- Bruising
- Petechiae

Immune System Symptoms
- Increased risk for infection
- Reduced immunity
- Decreased inflammatory responses
- Signs and symptoms of infection and inflammation possibly masked

Musculoskeletal Symptoms
- Muscle atrophy (most apparent in extremities)
- Osteoporosis with:
  - Fragility fractures
  - Decreased height and vertebral collapse
  - Aseptic necrosis of the femur head
  - Slow or poor healing of bone fractures

Skin Symptoms
- Thinning skin
- Increased facial and body hair
- Striae and increased pigmentation

feel like themselves. Ask about mood swings, irritability, new-onset confusion, or depression. Ask patients whether they have been crying or laughing inappropriately or have had difficulty concentrating. The excess hormones stimulate the central nervous system, heightening the awareness of and responses to sensory stimulation. The patient often reports sleep difficulties and fatigue. All of these changes along with the physical changes strongly suggest hypercortisolism (Nieman, 2018).

Laboratory Assessment. Laboratory tests include blood, salivary, and urine cortisol levels. These are high in patients with any type of hypercortisolism. Plasma ACTH levels vary, depending on the cause of the problem. In pituitary Cushing disease, ACTH levels are elevated. In adrenal Cushing disease or when Cushing syndrome results from chronic steroid use, ACTH levels are low.

Salivary cortisol levels may be used to detect hypercortisolism because these levels accurately reflect blood levels, especially late-night specimens. Higher levels indicate hypercortisolism.

A urine cortisol test is usually also collected as a 24-hour specimen (Pagana et al., 2022). In Cushing disease, or Cushing syndrome caused by a tumor, levels of urine cortisol are expected to be elevated (Pagana et al., 2022).

To screen for Cushing disease, an overnight dexamethasone suppression testing can be used (Nieman, 2022a) after a baseline 24-hour urine test has been completed (Pagana et al., 2022). A dose of dexamethasone is given at bedtime. A fasting blood draw is performed the next morning at 8 a.m. to assess the plasma cortisol level, followed by another 24-hour urine collection (Pagana et al., 2022). When cortisol levels are suppressed by dexamethasone, Cushing disease is *not* present.

Additional laboratory findings that accompany hypercortisolism include:

- Increased blood glucose level
- Decreased lymphocyte count
- Increased sodium level
- Decreased serum calcium level

Imaging Assessment. Imaging for hypercortisolism is done only after a diagnosis of hypercortisolism is made; this is done to avoid unnecessary testing and possible misdiagnosis (Uwaifo & Hura, 2023). CT or MRI may be ordered to assess adrenal glands; MRI is more common for assessing the pituitary gland (Bell, 2021).

Analyze Cues and Prioritize Hypotheses: Analysis

The priority problems for patients with Cushing disease or Cushing syndrome are:

1. Fluid overload due to hormone-induced water and sodium retention
2. Potential for injury due to skin thinning, poor wound healing, and bone density loss
3. Potential for infection due to hormone-induced reduced *immunity*

Generate Solutions and Take Actions: Planning and Implementation

Expected outcomes if hypercortisolism management are the reduction of plasma cortisol levels, removal of tumors, and restoration of normal or acceptable body appearance. When the disorder is caused by pituitary or adrenal problems, cure is possible. When caused by drug therapy for another health problem, the focus is to prevent complications from hypercortisolism.

Restoring Fluid Volume Balance

Planning: Expected Outcomes. The patient with hypercortisolism is expected to achieve and maintain a normal or near-normal *fluid and electrolyte balance.*

Interventions. Interventions for patients with fluid volume excess focus on ensuring patient safety, restoring *fluid and electrolyte balance,* and providing supportive care. Depending on the cause, surgical management may be used to reduce cortisol production.

Nonsurgical Management. Nonsurgical interventions focus on patient safety, drug therapy, nutrition therapy, and monitoring; these interventions are the basis of nonsurgical action for hypercortisolism and fluid overload.

Patient safety includes preventing fluid overload from becoming worse, leading to pulmonary edema and heart failure. Any patient with fluid overload, regardless of age, is at risk for these complications. The older adult or one who has coexisting cardiac problems, kidney problems, pulmonary problems, or liver problems is at greater risk.

Monitor for indicators of fluid overload (bounding pulse, increasing neck vein distention, lung crackles, increasing peripheral edema, reduced urine output) at least every 2 hours. *Pulmonary edema can occur quickly and lead to death.* Notify the primary health care provider of any change indicating that fluid overload either is not responding to therapy or is worse.

The patient with fluid volume excess and dependent edema is at risk for skin breakdown. Use a pressure-reducing or pressure-relieving overlay on the mattress. Assess skin pressure areas, especially the coccyx, elbows, hips, and heels, daily for redness/hyperpigmentation or open areas. For patients receiving oxygen by mask or nasal cannula, check the skin around the mask, nares, and ears and under the elastic band. Help the patient change positions every 2 hours or ensure that others assigned to perform the intervention are diligent in this action.

Drug therapy involves the use of drugs that interfere with adrenocorticotropic hormone (ACTH) production or adrenal hormone synthesis for temporary relief and are categorized as *steroidogenesis inhibitors.* Ketoconazole and levoketoconazole are commonly used oral medications used to inhibit one or more steps in cortisol synthesis (Nieman, 2022b). Ketoconazole can cause reversible liver damage, so liver function tests must be closely followed (Nieman, 2022b).

For patients with hypercortisolism resulting from increased ACTH production, cyproheptadine may be used because it interferes with ACTH production. For adults with increased ACTH production who have type 2 diabetes and who do not respond to other drug therapies, mifepristone may be used, a synthetic steroid that blocks glucocorticoid receptors. Osilodrostat can be used in patients with ongoing disease following transsphenoidal surgery or who are not candidates for pituitary surgery (Nieman, 2022b).

NURSING SAFETY PRIORITY
Drug Alert

Ketoconazole is teratogenic. Advise anyone who is pregnant or plans to become pregnant to report this to their primary health care provider before taking this drug (Nieman, 2022b).

A drug to manage hypercortisolism resulting from a pituitary adenoma is pasireotide. This subcutaneous drug binds to somatostatin receptors on the adenoma and inhibits tumor production of corticotropin. Lower levels of corticotropin lead to lower levels of cortisol production in the adrenal glands. The drug is ineffective for patients whose tumors do not have somatostatin receptors.

Monitor the patient for response to drug therapy, especially weight loss and increased urine output. Observe for symptoms of problems with *fluid and electrolyte balance,* especially changes in ECG patterns. Assess laboratory findings, especially sodium and potassium values, whenever samples are drawn.

Nutrition therapy for the patient with hypercortisolism may involve restrictions of both fluid and sodium intake to control fluid volume. Often sodium restriction involves only "no added salt" to ordinary table foods when fluid overload is mild. For more pronounced fluid overload, the patient may be restricted to anywhere from 2 to 4 g of sodium per day. When sodium restriction is ongoing, teach the patient and family how to check food labels for sodium content and how to keep a daily record of sodium ingested. Explain to the patient and family the reason for any fluid restriction and the importance of adhering to the prescribed restriction.

Monitor intake and output and weight to assess therapy effectiveness. Ensure that assistive personnel (AP) understand that these measurements need to be accurate, not just estimated, because treatment decisions are based on the findings. Schedule fluid offerings throughout the 24 hours. Teach AP to check urine for color and character and to report these findings. Check the urine specific gravity (a specific gravity below 1.005 may indicate fluid overload). If IV therapy is used, infuse only the amount ordered.

Fluid retention may not be visible. Rapid weight gain is the best indicator of fluid retention and overload. Each 1 lb (about 500 g) of weight gained (after the first ½ lb) equates to 500 mL of retained water. Weigh the patient at the same time daily (before breakfast), using the same scale. Have the patient wear the same type of clothing for each weigh-in.

Surgical Management. Surgical management of adrenocortical hypersecretion depends on the cause of the problem. When adrenal hyperfunction is due to increased pituitary secretion of ACTH, removal of a pituitary adenoma using minimally invasive techniques may be attempted. Sometimes a total *hypophysectomy* (surgical removal of the pituitary gland) is needed. (See earlier discussion of Hypophysectomy in the Hyperpituitarism section.) If hypercortisolism is caused by an adrenal tumor, an *adrenalectomy* (removal of the adrenal gland) may be needed.

Preoperative care. Preoperative care starts with correcting disturbances of *fluid and electrolyte balance* before surgery. Continue to monitor blood potassium, sodium, and chloride levels. Dysrhythmias from potassium imbalance may occur, and cardiac monitoring is needed. Hyperglycemia is controlled before surgery.

The patient with hypercortisolism is at risk for complications of infections and fractures. Prevent infection with handwashing and aseptic technique. Decrease the risk for falls by raising top side rails and encouraging the patient to ask for assistance when getting out of bed. A high-calorie, high-protein diet is ordered before surgery.

Glucocorticoid preparations are given before surgery. The patient continues to receive glucocorticoids during surgery to prevent adrenal crisis because the removal of the tumor results in a sudden drop in cortisol levels. Before surgery, discuss the need for long-term hormone replacement therapy (HRT).

Operative procedures. Operative procedures include a unilateral adrenalectomy when one gland is involved or a bilateral adrenalectomy when ACTH-producing tumors cannot be treated by other means or when both adrenal glands are diseased. The surgical procedure most often performed is laparoscopic adrenalectomy, a minimally invasive surgical approach (Nieman, 2023b). If necessary, open surgery through the abdomen or the lateral flank can be performed.

Postoperative care. Postoperative care after adrenalectomy includes monitoring in an ICU. Immediately after surgery, assess the patient every 15 minutes for shock (e.g., hypotension; a rapid, weak pulse; and a decreasing urine output) resulting from insufficient glucocorticoid replacement. Monitor vital signs, central venous pressure, pulmonary wedge pressure, intake and output, daily weights, and serum electrolyte levels.

After a bilateral adrenalectomy, patients require lifelong glucocorticoid and mineralocorticoid HRT, starting immediately after surgery. In unilateral adrenalectomy, HRT continues until the remaining adrenal gland increases hormone production. This therapy may be needed for up to 2 years after surgery.

Preventing Injury. The patient is at risk for injury from skin breakdown, bone fractures, and GI bleeding. Prevention of these injuries is a major nursing care focus.

Planning: Expected Outcomes. The patient with hypercortisolism is expected to avoid injury.

Interventions. Priority nursing interventions for prevention of injury focus on skin assessment and protection, coordinating care to ensure gentle handling, and patient teaching regarding drug therapy for prevention of GI ulcers.

Skin injury is a continuing risk even after surgery has corrected the cortisol excess because the changes induced in the skin and blood vessels remain for weeks to months. Assess the skin for reddened areas, excoriation, breakdown, and edema. If mobility is decreased, turn the patient every 2 hours and pad bony prominences.

Instruct patients to avoid activities that can result in skin trauma. Teach them to use a soft toothbrush and an electric shaver. Instruct patients to keep the skin clean and dry it thoroughly after washing. Excessive dryness can be prevented by using a moisturizing lotion.

Adhesive tape often causes skin breakdown. Use tape sparingly and remove it carefully. After venipuncture, the patient may have increased bleeding because of blood vessel fragility. Apply pressure over the site until bleeding has stopped.

Fragility fractures from bone density loss and osteoporosis are possible for months to years after cortisol levels have returned to normal. When helping patients move in bed, use a lift sheet instead of grasping them. Remind the patient to call for help when walking. Review the use of walkers or canes, if needed. Teach AP to use a gait belt when walking with a patient who has bone density loss.

Collaborate with a registered dietitian nutritionist (RDN) to teach the patient about nutrition therapy. A high-calorie diet that includes increased amounts of calcium and vitamin D is needed. Milk, cheese, yogurt, and green leafy and root vegetables add calcium to promote bone density. Advise the patient to avoid caffeine and alcohol, which increase the risk for GI ulcers and reduce bone density.

GI bleeding is common with hypercortisolism. Cortisol (1) inhibits production of the thick, gel-like mucus that protects the stomach lining, (2) decreases blood flow to the area, and (3) triggers the release of excess hydrochloric acid. Although surgery reduces cortisol levels, the normal mucus and increased blood flow may take weeks to return. Interventions focus on drug therapy to reduce irritation, protect the GI mucosa, and decrease secretion of hydrochloric acid.

Antacids buffer stomach acids and protect the GI mucosa. Teach the patient that these drugs should be taken on a regular schedule rather than on an as-needed basis.

Some agents block the H_2 receptors in the gastric mucosa. When histamine binds to these receptors, a series of actions release hydrochloric acid. Drugs that block the H_2-receptor site include cimetidine, famotidine, and nizatidine. Omeprazole and esomeprazole inhibit the gastric proton pump and prevent the formation of hydrochloric acid.

Instruct the patient to reduce alcohol or caffeine consumption, smoking, and fasting because these actions cause gastric irritation. NSAIDs and drugs that contain aspirin or other salicylates can cause gastritis and intensify GI bleeding. These should be avoided or limited.

Preventing Infection. Glucocorticoids reduce both the inflammation and the immune responses of **immunity**, increasing the risk for infection. For the patient who is taking glucocorticoid replacement therapy, the risk is ongoing. For the patient who is recovering from surgery to prevent hypercortisolism, the infection risk continues for weeks after surgery.

Planning: Expected Outcomes. The patient with hypercortisolism is expected to remain free from infection and avoid situations that increase the risk for infection.

Interventions. Protect the patient with reduced **immunity** from infection. All personnel must use extreme care during all nursing procedures. Thorough handwashing is important. Anyone with an upper respiratory tract infection who enters the patient's room must wear a mask. Observe strict aseptic technique when performing dressing changes or any invasive procedure.

Continually assess the patient for possible infection. Symptoms may not be obvious because excess cortisol suppresses infection indicators caused by inflammation. Fever and pus formation depend on the presence of white blood cells (WBCs). The patient who has reduced **immunity** may have a severe infection without pus and with only a low-grade fever.

Monitor the patient's daily complete blood count (CBC) with differential WBC count, especially neutrophils. Inspect the mouth during every shift for lesions and mucosa breakdown. Assess the lungs every 8 hours for crackles, wheezes, or reduced breath sounds. Assess all urine for odor and cloudiness. Ask about any urgency, burning, or pain on urination.

Take vital signs at least every 4 hours to assess for fever. A temperature elevation of even 1°F (0.5°C) above baseline is significant for a patient who has reduced **immunity** and indicates infection until otherwise proven.

Perform pulmonary hygiene every 2 to 4 hours. Listen to the lungs for crackles, wheezes, or reduced breath sounds. Urge the patient to deep breathe or use an incentive spirometer every hour while awake.

NCLEX Examination Challenge 54.3
Physiological Integrity

The nurse is caring for a client with Cushing syndrome who must remain on continued glucocorticoid therapy for another health problem. Which intervention would the nurse include when designing the plan of care?

A. Increase intake of sodium.
B. Encourage drinking extra fluids.
C. Secure IV access with nonadhesive bandaging.
D. Massage areas where skin is under pressure.

Care Coordination and Transition Management

Home Care Management. The patient with hypercortisolism usually has muscle weakness and fatigue for some weeks after surgery and remains at risk for falls and other injuries. These problems may necessitate one-floor living for a short time; and a home health aide may be needed to assist with hygiene, meal preparation, and maintenance.

Self-Management Education. Patients taking exogenous glucocorticoids who are discharged to home remain at continuing risk for impaired **fluid and electrolyte balance,** especially fluid volume excess. Teach them and their family to monitor and record the patient's weight daily to show the primary health care provider at any checkups. Also instruct the patient to call the primary health care provider for weight gain of more than 3 lb (1.36 kg) in a week or more than 1 to 2 lb (0.45 to 0.91 kg) in a 24-hour period.

After bilateral adrenalectomy, lifelong HRT is needed to prevent adrenal insufficiency. Without the adrenal glands the patient completely depends on the exogenous drug. If the drug is stopped, even for a day or two, no other glands will produce the glucocorticoids and the patient will develop acute adrenal insufficiency, a life-threatening condition.

Management of this problem is described in the Adrenal Gland Hypofunction section. Teach the patient and family about adherence to the drug regimen and its side effects as described in Box 54.11.

Protecting patients with reduced *immunity* from infection at home is important. Urge them to use proper hygiene and social distancing and to avoid crowds and others with infections. Encourage the patient and all people living in the same home to have yearly influenza vaccinations. Stress that the patient should immediately notify the primary health care provider if a fever or any other sign of infection develops.

Health Care Resources. Immediately after returning home, the patient may need a support person to stay and provide more attention than could be given by a visiting nurse or home care aide. Contact with the interprofessional health care team is needed for follow-up and identification of potential problems. The patient taking corticosteroid therapy may have symptoms of adrenal insufficiency if the dosage is inadequate. Suggest that the patient obtain and wear a medical alert bracelet listing the condition and the drug replacement therapy.

Evaluate Outcomes: Evaluation

Evaluate the care of the patient with Cushing syndrome (hypercortisolism) based on the identified priority patient problems. The expected outcomes of interventions are that the patient will:

- Maintain *fluid and electrolyte balance* as indicated by blood pressure at or near the normal range, stable body weight, and normal serum sodium and potassium levels
- Remain free from injury as indicated by having intact skin, minimal bruising, absence of bone fractures, and no occult blood in vomitus, stools, or GI secretions
- Remain free from infection as indicated by absence of fever, purulent drainage, cough, or pain or burning on urination

---

BOX 54.11   Patient and Family Education

Cortisol Replacement Therapy

- Take your medication in divided doses, as prescribed (e.g., the first dose in the morning and the second dose between 4 p.m. and 6 p.m.) for best effects.
- Take your medication with meals or snacks to prevent stomach irritation.
- Weigh yourself daily and keep a record to show your primary health care provider.
- Increase your dosage as directed by your primary health care provider for increased physical stress or severe emotional stress.
- Never skip a dose of medication. If you have persistent vomiting or severe diarrhea and cannot take your medication by mouth for 24 to 36 hours, call your primary health care provider. If you cannot reach your primary health care provider, go to the nearest emergency department. You may need an injection to take the place of your usual oral medication.
- Always wear your medical alert bracelet or necklace.
- Make regular visits for health care follow-up.
- Learn (and have a family member learn) how to give yourself an IM injection of hydrocortisone in case you cannot take your oral drug.

HYPERALDOSTERONISM

Pathophysiology Review

Hyperaldosteronism is an increased secretion of aldosterone with mineralocorticoid excess. Primary hyperaldosteronism (Conn syndrome) in adults results from excessive secretion of aldosterone from one or both adrenal glands, usually caused by an adrenal adenoma. In secondary hyperaldosteronism, excessive secretion of aldosterone is caused by the high levels of angiotensin II that are stimulated by high plasma renin levels. Some causes include kidney hypoxia, diabetic nephropathy, and excessive use of some diuretics.

Increased aldosterone levels cause disturbances of *fluid and electrolyte balance,* which then trigger the kidney tubules to retain sodium and excrete potassium and hydrogen ions. Hypernatremia, hypokalemia, and metabolic alkalosis result. Sodium retention increases blood volume, which raises blood pressure, increasing the risk for strokes, heart attacks, and kidney damage. (See Chapter 13 for discussion of specific electrolyte imbalances.)

Hypokalemia and elevated blood pressure are the most common problems that patients with hyperaldosteronism develop. They may have headache, fatigue, muscle weakness, dehydration, and loss of stamina. *Polydipsia* and *polyuria* occur less frequently. *Paresthesias* may occur if potassium depletion is severe.

Hyperaldosteronism is diagnosed on the basis of laboratory studies and imaging with CT or MRI. Serum potassium levels are decreased, and sodium levels are elevated. Plasma renin levels are low, and aldosterone levels are high. Hydrogen ion loss leads to metabolic alkalemia (elevated blood pH). Urine has a low specific gravity and high aldosterone levels.

Interprofessional Collaborative Care

Surgery is a common treatment for hyperaldosteronism, and one or both adrenal glands may be removed. The patient's potassium level must be corrected before surgery. Drugs used to increase potassium levels include spironolactone, a potassium-sparing diuretic and aldosterone antagonist. Potassium supplements may be used to increase potassium levels before surgery.

The patient who has undergone a unilateral adrenalectomy may need temporary glucocorticoid replacement; replacement is lifelong when both adrenal glands are removed. Glucocorticoids are given before surgery to prevent adrenal crisis.

When surgery cannot be performed, spironolactone therapy is continued to control hypokalemia and hypertension. Because spironolactone is a potassium-sparing diuretic, hyperkalemia can occur in patients who have impaired kidney function or excessive potassium intake. Advise the patient to avoid potassium supplements and foods rich in potassium, such as meat, fish, and many (but not all) vegetables and fruits. Hyponatremia can occur with spironolactone therapy, and the patient may need increased dietary sodium. Instruct patients to report symptoms of hyponatremia, such as muscle weakness, dizziness, lethargy, or drowsiness. Instruct them to report any additional side effects of spironolactone therapy, including gynecomastia, diarrhea, headache, rash, urticaria (hives), confusion, erectile dysfunction, hirsutism, and amenorrhea. Additional drug therapy to control hypertension is often needed.

GET READY FOR THE NEXT-GENERATION NCLEX® EXAMINATION!

Essential Nursing Care Points

Health Promotion/Disease Prevention	Chronic Disease Care
• Encourage the patient with adrenal insufficiency to wear a medical alert bracelet and to always carry simple carbohydrates. • Instruct patients who are taking a corticosteroid for more than a week to refrain from stopping the drug suddenly.	• Teach all patients to take antithyroid drugs or thyroid hormone replacement therapy (HRT) as prescribed. Emphasize which medications are prescribed as lifelong therapy. • Monitor ongoing laboratory results, as well as patient signs and symptoms, as indicators of long-term therapy effectiveness. • Instruct patients taking bromocriptine to seek medical care immediately if chest pain, dizziness, or watery nasal discharge develops. • Teach patients who have permanent endocrine hypofunction the proper techniques and timing of HRT. • Teach patients with AVP-D how to take or self-administer desmopressin orally, subcutaneously, or by nasal spray as prescribed. • Ensure that patients know symptoms of infection and when to seek medical care. • Remind patients with AVP-R or AVP-D about the symptoms of dehydration.
Regenerative or Restorative Care	**Hospice/Palliative/Supportive Care**
• During the immediate period after a hypophysectomy, remind the patient to avoid activities that increase intracranial pressure (ICP). • Accurately measure intake and output in patients with DI or syndrome of inappropriate antidiuretic hormone (SIADH). • Ensure that patients with or suspected of having DI have fluids at least every 4 hours.	• Although thyroid cancer is rarely fatal, provide referrals appropriately for patients who may be in need of palliative care or hospice.

Mastery Questions

1. The nurse is preparing to assess a client with AVP-D. Which assessment would the nurse perform **first**?
   A. Assess serum sodium level.
   B. Determine degree of fatigue.
   C. Evaluate IV site for possible phlebitis.
   D. Quantify how much of meals was consumed.

2. Which of the following instructions would the nurse provide to a client who just underwent pituitary removal surgery? **Select all that apply.**
   A. "Monitor the drip pad under your nose for drainage type."
   B. "A mild amount of confusion is normal several days later."
   C. "Blow your nose and cough hourly to keep the airway clear."
   D. "You will take glucocorticoid therapy for 1 week following surgery."

NGN Challenge 54.1

The nurse is caring for a client who underwent hypophysectomy earlier in the day. The client uses the call light. When the nurse enters the room, the client says, "I feel like I can't stop swallowing." The dressing under the client's nose appears to be damp, and the lips and mucous membranes are dry.

Complete the diagram by selecting from the choices below to specify what potential condition the client is likely experiencing, **2** nursing actions that are appropriate to take, and **2** parameters the nurse should monitor to determine the effectiveness of nursing actions.

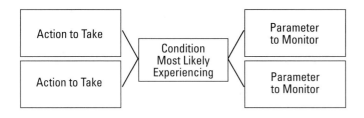

Actions to Take	Potential Conditions	Parameters to Monitor
Brush teeth to moisten mucous membranes	Sinusitis	Dressing under the nose
Remind to cough to loosen secretions	Evisceration	Temperature
Administer antiviral medication	Cerebrospinal fluid leakage	Signs of increased intracranial pressure
Assess for halo sign	Syndrome of inappropriate antidiuretic hormone	Low-fiber dietary intake
Ensure head of bed is elevated		Return of sense of smell

NGN Challenge 54.2

The nurse is monitoring select laboratory results for a 56-year-old client who has been hospitalized with pneumonia.

Parameters	Results Today (0702)	Results 12 Hours Ago (0736)	Results 24 Hours Ago (0714)
Serum sodium (Reference range 136–145 mEq/L [136–145 mmol/L])	129 mEq/L (129 mmol/L)	138 mEq/L (138 mmol/L)	140 mEq/L (140 mmol/L)
Serum potassium (Reference range 3.5–5 mEq/L [3.5–5 mmol/L])	6.5 mEq/L (6.5 mmol/L)	5.8 mEq/L (5.8 mmol/L)	4.6 mEq/L (4.6 mmol/L)
Glucose (Reference range 74–106 mg/dL [4.1–5.9 mmol/L])	67 mg/dL (3.7 mmol/L)	73 mg/dL (4.05 mmol/L)	81 mg/dL (4.5 mmol/L)

After the health care provider has examined the client and assigned a diagnosis, which of the following actions would the nurse take at this time? **Select all that apply.**

○ Assess orientation.
○ Apply cardiac monitor.
○ Discourage fluid intake.
○ Plan to take daily weights.
○ Record intake and output.
○ Prepare to administer cortisol replacement therapy.
○ Ensure informed consent for hypophysectomy is signed.

REFERENCES

American Association of Neurological Surgeons. (2023). *Cushing's syndrome/disease*. https://www.aans.org/en/Patients/Neurosurgical-Conditions-and-Treatments/Cushings-Disease.

Bell, D. (2021). Cushing syndrome. https://radiopaedia.org/articles/cushing-syndrome?lang=us.

Bichet, D. (2023a). Arginine vasopressin deficiency (Central diabetes insipidus): Treatment. *UpToDate*. Retrieved May 22, 2023, from https://www.uptodate.com/contents/arginine-vasopressin-deficiency-central-diabetes-insipidus-treatment.

Bichet, D. (2023b). Arginine vasopressin resistance (Nephrogenic diabetes insipidus): Clinical manifestations and causes. *UpToDate*. Retrieved May 22, 2023, from https://www.uptodate.com/contents/arginine-vasopressin-resistance-nephrogenic-diabetes-insipidus-clinical-manifestations-and-causes.

Bichet, D. (2023c). Arginine vasopressin resistance (Nephrogenic diabetes insipidus): Treatment. *UpToDate*. Retrieved May 22, 2023, from https://www.uptodate.com/contents/arginine-vasopressin-resistance-nephrogenic-diabetes-insipidus-treatment.

Burchum, J., & Rosenthal, L. (2022). *Lehne's pharmacology for nursing care* (11th ed.). St. Louis: Elsevier.

Cole, S. (2018). Evaluation and treatment of adrenal dysfunction in the primary care environment. *Nursing Clinics of North America*, 54, 385–394.

Findling, J., et al. (2022). *Cushing's syndrome and Cushing disease*. https://www.endocrine.org/patient-engagement/endocrine-library/cushings-syndrome-and-cushing-disease.

Ghaffari-Rafi, A., et al. (2022). Demographic and socioeconomic disparities of pituitary adenomas and carcinomas in the United States. *Journal of Clinical Neuroscience*, 98, 96–102.

Gordon, A., et al. (2022). Health care disparities in transsphenoidal surgery for pituitary tumors: An experience from neighboring urban public and private hospitals. *Journal of Neurological Surgery: Skull Base*. https://doi.org/10.1055/s-0042-1757613.

Gounden V, Anastasopoulou C, & Jialal I. Hypopituitarism. [Updated 2022 Jul 24]. In *StatPearls [Internet]*. Treasure Island (FL): StatPearls Publishing; 2023. Available from: https://www.ncbi.nlm.nih.gov/books/NBK470414/.

Grossman, A. (2022). *Addison disease. Merck Manual Professional Version*. https://www.merckmanuals.com/professional/endocrine-and-metabolic-disorders/adrenal-disorders/addison-disease.

Hamazaki, K., Nishigaki, T., Kuramoto, N., et al. (2022). Secondary adrenal insufficiency after COVID-19 diagnosed by insulin tolerance test and corticotropin-releasing hormone test. *Cureus*, 14(3):e23021. https://doi.org/10.7759/cureus.23021.

Hui, C., et al. (2023). Diabetes insipidus. [Updated 2023 Jan 2]. In: *StatPearls [Internet]*. Treasure Island, FL: StatPearls Publishing; 2023 Jan-. Available from: https://www.ncbi.nlm.nih.gov/books/NBK470458/.

Jarvis, C., & Eckhardt, A. (2024). *Physical examination & health assessment* (8th ed.). St. Louis: Elsevier.

Kaiser, U., & Ho, K. (2020). Pituitary physiology and diagnostic evaluation. In S. Melmed, R. J. Auchus, A. B. Goldfine, R. J. Koenig, & C. J. Rosen (Eds.), *Williams' textbook of endocrinology* (14th ed.). Philadelphia: Elsevier.

Kamilaris, C., Stratakis, C., & Hannah-Shmouni, F. (2021). Molecular genetic and genomic alterations in Cushing syndrome and primary aldosteronism. *Frontiers in Endocrinology: Cancer Endocrinology*, 12. https://www.frontiersin.org/articles/10.3389/fendo.2021.632543/full.

Kanczkowski, W., Beuschlein, F., & Bornstein, S. R. (2022). Is there a role for the adrenal glands in long COVID? *Endocrinology*, 18, 451–452. https://doi.org/10.1038/s41574-022-00700-8.

Melmed, S., & Katznelson, L. (2023). Treatment of acromegaly. *UpToDate*. Retrieved May 21, 2023, from https://www.uptodate.com/contents/treatment-of-acromegaly.

National Cancer Institute. (n.d.). *Panhypopituitarism*. https://www.cancer.gov/publications/dictionaries/cancer-terms/def/panhypopituitarism

Nieman, L. (2018). Diagnosis of Cushing's syndrome in the modern era. *Endocrinology and Metabolism Clinics*, 47(2), 259–273.

Nieman, L. (2022a). Establishing the diagnosis of Cushing's syndrome. *UpToDate*. Retrieved May 21, 2023, from https://www.uptodate.com/contents/establishing-the-diagnosis-of-cushings-syndrome.

Nieman, L. (2022b). Medical treatment of hypercortisolism (Cushing disease). *UpToDate*. Retrieved May 21, 2023, from https://www.uptodate.com/contents/medical-therapy-of-hypercortisolism-cushings-syndrome.

Nieman, L. (2022c). Treatment of adrenal insufficiency in adults. *UpToDate*. Retrieved May 21, 2023, from https://www.uptodate.com/contents/treatment-of-adrenal-insufficiency-in-adults.

Nieman, L. (2023a). Epidemiology and clinical manifestations: Cushing's syndrome. *UpToDate*. Retrieved May 22, 2023, from https://www.uptodate.com/contents/epidemiology-and-clinical-manifestations-of-cushings-syndrome.

Nieman, L. (2023b). Persistent or recurrent Cushing's disease: Surgical adrenalectomy. *UpToDate*. Retrieved May 21, 2023, from https://www.uptodate.com/contents/persistent-or-recurrent-cushings-disease-surgical-adrenalectomy.

Online Mendelian Inheritance in Man (OMIM). (2017). *Multiple endocrine neoplasia type 1*. www.omim.org/entry/131100.

Online Mendelian Inheritance in Man (OMIM). (2022). *Diabetes insipidus, nephrogenic, X-linked*. www.omim.org/entry/304800.

Otsuka America Pharmaceutical. (2021). *Samsca (tolvaptan)*. https://www.samsca.com/.

Otsuka America Pharmaceutical. (2022). *Jynarque (tolvaptan)*. https://www.jynarquehcp.com/.

Pagana, K. D., Pagana, T. J., & Pagana, T. N. (2022). *Mosby's manual of diagnostic and laboratory tests* (7th ed.). St. Louis: Elsevier.

Rogers, J. L. (2023). *McCance and Huether's Pathophysiology: The biologic basis for disease in adults and children* (9th ed.). St. Louis: Elsevier.

Sterns, R. (2021). Pathophysiology and etiology of the syndrome of inappropriate antidiuretic hormone secretion (SIADH). *UpToDate*. Retrieved May 21, 2023, from https://www.uptodate.com/contents/pathophysiology-and-etiology-of-the-syndrome-of-inappropriate-antidiuretic-hormone-secretion-siadh.

Sterns, R. (2022). Treatment of hyponatremia: Syndrome of inappropriate antidiuretic hormone secretion (SIADH) and reset osmostat. *UpToDate*. Retrieved May 21, 2023, from https://www.uptodate.com/contents/treatment-of-hyponatremia-syndrome-of-inappropriate-antidiuretic-hormone-secretion-siadh-and-reset-osmostat.

Uwaifo, G., & Hura, D. Hypercortisolism. [Updated 2023 Jan 8]. In *StatPearls [Internet]*. Treasure Island, FL: StatPearls Publishing; 2023. Available from: https://www.ncbi.nlm.nih.gov/books/NBK551526/

55

Concepts of Care for Patients With Thyroid and Parathyroid Gland Conditions

Melanie N. Luttrell

http://evolve.elsevier.com/Iggy/

LEARNING OUTCOMES

1. Plan collaborative care with the interprofessional team to promote *cellular regulation, nutrition,* and *gas exchange* in patients with thyroid and parathyroid problems.
2. Teach adults how to decrease the risk for thyroid and parathyroid problems.
3. Teach the patient and caregiver(s) about common drugs and other management strategies used for thyroid and parathyroid problems.
4. Plan patient- and family-centered nursing interventions to decrease the psychosocial impact caused by living with thyroid and parathyroid problems.
5. Apply knowledge of anatomy, physiology, and pathophysiology to provide evidence-based care for patients

with thyroid and parathyroid problems affecting *cellular regulation, nutrition,* and *gas exchange.*
6. Analyze assessment and diagnostic findings to generate solutions and prioritize nursing care for patients with thyroid and parathyroid problems.
7. Organize care coordination and transition management for patients with thyroid and parathyroid problems.
8. Use clinical judgment to plan evidence-based nursing care to promote *cellular regulation, nutrition,* and *gas exchange* and prevent complications in patients with thyroid and parathyroid problems.
9. Incorporate factors that affect health equity into the plan of care for patients with thyroid and parathyroid problems.

KEY TERMS

euthyroid A condition of having normal or near-normal thyroid function.

exophthalmos Abnormal protrusion of the eyes.

goiter Visibly enlarged thyroid gland.

Graves disease Autoimmune disorder in which the production of autoantibodies (thyroid-stimulating immunoglobulins [TSIs]) that attach to the thyrotropin (TRAb) receptor on the thyroid gland greatly increases thyroid hormone production.

Hashimoto thyroiditis (HT) Autoimmune disorder in which infection and inflammation of the thyroid gland causes the production of autoantibodies to thyroglobulin (Tg) or thyroid peroxidase (TPO), which results in extensive tissue destruction and reduced secretion of thyroid hormones.

hyperparathyroidism Disorder in which parathyroid secretion of parathyroid hormone is increased, resulting in hypercalcemia and hypophosphatemia.

hyperthyroidism Excessive thyroid hormone secretion from the thyroid gland.

hypoparathyroidism A rare disorder in which parathyroid function is decreased and serum calcium levels cannot be maintained.

hypothyroidism Reduced or absent hormone secretion from the thyroid gland that results in whole-body decreased metabolism from inadequate cellular regulation.

myxedema coma A serious complication of untreated or poorly treated hypothyroidism with dangerously reduced cardiopulmonary and neurologic functioning, although few affected adults become comatose.

pretibial myxedema Dry, waxy swelling of the front surfaces of the lower legs that resembles benign tumors or keloids; associated with hyperthyroidism.

tetany Hyperexcitability of nerves and muscles.

thyroid storm A life-threatening event that occurs in patients with uncontrolled hyperthyroidism, most often with Graves disease.

thyroiditis An inflammation of the thyroid gland.

Problems of the thyroid and parathyroid gland can affect numerous body systems, and range in severity from mild to life-threatening. The thyroid gland and parathyroid glands secrete hormones that affect whole-body metabolism, *cellular regulation, nutrition, gas exchange,* electrolyte balance, and excitable membrane activity.

CELLULAR REGULATION CONCEPT EXEMPLAR: HYPOTHYROIDISM

Hypothyroidism is reduced or absent hormone secretion from the thyroid gland that results in decreased metabolism from inadequate *cellular regulation.* In its early stages, the disorder can be missed because the onset is gradual and symptoms can mimic those of multiple other disease processes.

Pathophysiology Review

Symptoms of hypothyroidism are widespread and reflect overall decreased metabolism from low levels of thyroid hormones (THs). Thyroid cells may fail to produce sufficient levels of THs for several reasons. For example, sometimes the cells themselves are damaged and no longer function normally. At other times, the thyroid cells are functional, but the adult does not ingest enough of the substances needed to make thyroid hormones, especially iodine and tyrosine. Aging can also affect thyroid function, as shown in the Patient-Centered Care: Older Adult Health—Thyroid Function and Aging box.

When the production of thyroid hormones is too low or absent, the blood levels of THs are also very low, resulting in a decreased metabolic rate. This lower metabolism causes the hypothalamus and anterior pituitary gland to make stimulatory hormones, especially thyroid-stimulating hormone (TSH), in an attempt to trigger hormone release from the poorly responsive thyroid gland. The TSH binds to thyroid cells and causes the thyroid gland to enlarge, forming a **goiter** (visibly enlarged thyroid gland [Fig. 55.1]), although thyroid hormone production itself does not increase. The presence of a goiter is common in several thyroid issues and does not definitively indicate either hypothyroidism or hyperthyroidism.

Most tissues and organs are affected by the low metabolic rate and reduced *cellular regulation* caused by hypothyroidism. Cellular energy is decreased, and metabolites that are compounds of proteins and sugars called *glycosaminoglycans (GAGs)* build up inside cells. This GAG buildup increases mucus and water, forming cellular edema referred to as *myxedema.* This

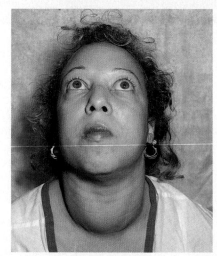

FIG. 55.1 Goiter.

condition changes the patient's appearance (Fig. 55.2) The tongue can thick and substantially enlarge (called *macroglossia*). Nonpitting edema can form in multiple places, especially in the pretibial areas or on top of the feet bilaterally. The hands, elbows, and face can also be affected rarely.

Myxedema coma is a rare but serious complication of untreated or poorly treated hypothyroidism with dangerously reduced cardiopulmonary and neurologic functioning.

👤 **PATIENT-CENTERED CARE: OLDER ADULT HEALTH**

Thyroid Function and Aging

Age-Related Change	Nursing Considerations
Thyroid hormone secretion decreases with age, resulting in reduced circulating hormone levels.	• Do not rely solely on laboratory values to assess whether and to what degree hypothyroidism may be present (or the effects of therapy). Although secretion is reduced, clearance is also reduced, allowing circulating hormones to be present longer. • Patient symptom changes may help to evaluate hormone replacement therapy (HRT) effectiveness; remember that symptoms may be less pervasive in older patients than in younger patients. • Be aware that some medications (such as amiodarone) can cause changes in thyroid hormone levels.
Muscle mass decreases and body fat increases from age-related decreased metabolism.	• Avoid using change in muscle strength as an indicator of reduced thyroid function.
Age-related changes in cardiovascular and neurologic function make the older adult more sensitive to HRT.	• When hypothyroidism is present and thyroid HRT is started, doses should be started low with increases made slowly to avoid inducing cardiovascular and neurologic toxicities. • Always assess older adults on thyroid HRT for chest pain, shortness of breath, and mental status changes including confusion and changes in sleep habits (American Thyroid Association, 2023).

Decreased metabolism causes the heart muscle to become flabby and the chamber sizes to increase. The result is decreased cardiac output with decreased perfusion and *gas exchange* in the brain and other vital organs, causing tissue and organ failure. *The mortality rate for myxedema coma is extremely high, and this condition is a life-threatening emergency.* Early recognition of symptoms is essential (Ross, 2023a). Myxedema coma can be caused by a variety of events, drugs, or conditions.

Etiology and Genetic Risk

Most cases of hypothyroidism in the United States occur because of an autoimmune problem called Hashimoto thyroiditis (HT). In HT, the body produces autoantibodies that attack thyroid tissue, resulting in inflammation, extensive tissue destruction, and reduced secretion of thyroid hormones (Davies, 2022). In North America, other common causes include thyroid surgery and radioactive iodine (RAI) treatment of hyperthyroidism. Worldwide, hypothyroidism is common in areas where the soil and water have little natural iodide, causing endemic goiter. Hypothyroidism is also caused by a variety of other conditions (Box 55.1).

There is a genetic basis for a condition called congenital hypothyroidism; this condition is present at birth when the thyroid gland does not function properly. There are also genetic connections between thyroid dysfunction and conditions such as Down syndrome and Turner syndrome, and between thyroid function and atrial fibrillation (Ellervik et al., 2019; Gavryutina et al., 2022). However, not all cases of hypothyroidism are genetic in nature.

Incidence and Prevalence

Hypothyroidism occurs in about 4% to 10% of adults, with women being affected five to eight times more often than men (Ross, 2022a).

Health Promotion/Disease Prevention

There is no known way to prevent hypothyroidism. It is recommended that patients stay alert for symptoms associated with this disorder, as it is more easily treated when it is early in development.

BOX 55.1 Causes of Hypothyroidism

Primary Causes

Decreased Thyroid Tissue
- Surgical or radiation-induced thyroid destruction
- Autoimmune thyroid destruction
- Congenital (poor thyroid development)
- Cancer (thyroidal or metastatic)

Decreased Synthesis of Thyroid Hormone
- Endemic iodine deficiency
- Drugs:
  - Amiodarone
  - Guaifenesin
  - Lithium

Secondary Causes

Inadequate Production of Thyroid-Stimulating Hormone
- Congenital pituitary defects
- Pituitary tumors, trauma, infections, or infarcts
- Hypothalamic tumors, trauma, infections, or infarcts

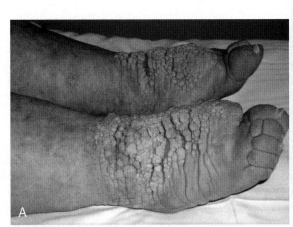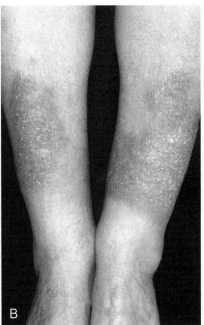

FIG. 55.2 Myxedema. (A) Elephantiasic pretibial myxedema. (B) Pretibial myxedema. (A from Preedy, V. R. [2020]. *Pathology: Oxidative stress and dietary antioxidants.* St. Louis: Elsevier. B from Michelettie, R. G., James, W. D., Elston, D. M., et al. [2023]. *Andrew's diseases of the skin clinical atlas* [2nd ed.]. St. Louis: Elsevier.)

BOX 55.2   Key Features

Hypothyroidism

Cardiovascular Symptoms
- Bradycardia
- Decreased activity tolerance
- Diastolic hypertension
- Pericardial effusion

Respiratory Symptoms
- Dyspnea
- Hypoventilation
- Pleural effusion

GI Symptoms
- Abdominal distention/ascites
- Constipation
- Weight gain

Metabolic Symptoms
- Decreased basal metabolic rate
- Decreased body temperature
- Cold intolerance

Reproductive Symptoms
Women
- Anovulation
- Decreased libido
- Menstrual changes (amenorrhea or prolonged periods)

Men
- Decreased libido
- Impotence

Psychosocial Symptoms
- Apathy
- Depression

Integumentary Symptoms
- Cool, pale/ash gray, dry, coarse, scaly skin
- Decreased hair growth, with loss of eyebrow hair
- Dry, coarse, brittle hair
- Poor wound healing
- Thick, brittle nails

Neuromuscular Symptoms
- Confusion
- Decreased tendon reflexes
- Hearing loss
- Impaired memory
- Inattentiveness
- Lethargy or somnolence
- Muscle aches and pain
- Paresthesia of the extremities
- Slowing of intellectual functions
- Slowness or slurring of speech

Other Symptoms
- Facial puffiness
- Goiter (enlarged thyroid gland)
- Hoarseness
- Nonpitting edema of the hands and feet
- Periorbital edema
- Thick tongue
- Weakness, fatigue

Interprofessional Collaborative Care

Depending on the severity of the symptoms at the time of diagnosis, initial therapy for hypothyroidism may start in an acute care environment or in the outpatient setting. When symptoms are severe or if myxedema coma is present, an intensive care environment may be required. Drug therapy is lifelong, and patients must learn to manage their disorder.

Recognize Cues: Assessment

History. A decrease in thyroid hormones produces many symptoms related to slowed metabolism from inadequate *cellular regulation.* Ask the patient to compare activity now with that of a year ago. The patient often reports an increase in time spent sleeping. Generalized weakness, muscle aches, and paresthesia may also be present. Constipation and cold intolerance are common. Ask whether more blankets at night or extra clothing, even in warm weather, has been needed. Some changes may be subtle, occurring slowly over time, and are often missed, especially in older adults.

Patients may report a decreased libido. Women may have had difficulty becoming pregnant or have changes in menses (heavy, prolonged bleeding or amenorrhea). Men may have problems with impotence and infertility.

Ask about current or previous use of drugs, such as lithium or amiodarone, both which can impair thyroid hormone production. In addition, ask whether the patient has ever been treated for hyperthyroidism and what specific treatment was used.

Inquire about whether the patient has a history of COVID-19. Studies have shown that the SARS-CoV-2 virus can affect the thyroid. COVID-19 can aggravate existing autoimmune thyroid disease (Duntas & Jonklaas, 2021). Research continues to evaluate the potential long-term effects of COVID-19 on the endocrine system.

Physical Assessment/Signs and Symptoms. Observe the patient's overall appearance, keeping in mind that symptoms range from mild to severe. Common changes seen with hypothyroidism include coarse skin, edema around the eyes and face, weight gain, dyspnea on exertion, and hoarseness. Patients' overall muscle movement is slow. They may not speak clearly because of tongue thickening and may take a longer time to respond to questions because of reduced cognitive functioning. Box 55.2 lists common signs and symptoms of the disorder.

Cardiac and respiratory functions are decreased, leading to reduced *gas exchange.* The heart rate may be below 60 beats/min, and the respiratory rate may be slow. Body temperature is often lower than 97°F (36.1°C).

Weight gain is very common, even when the adult is not overeating. Weigh the patient and assess whether the result is the same or different from the weight a year ago.

Depending on the cause of hypothyroidism, the patient may have a goiter. The presence of a goiter *suggests* a thyroid problem but does not indicate whether the problem is excessive hormone secretion or too little hormone secretion.

Psychosocial Assessment. Hypothyroidism can contribute to mood. If depression is severe, family members may bring the patient in for the initial evaluation. Patients may be too lethargic, apathetic, or drowsy to recognize changes in their condition. Families may report that the patient is withdrawn and has reduced cognition. Assess attention span and memory, both of which can be impaired by hypothyroidism. The resulting mental slowness can contribute to social isolation.

Laboratory Assessment. Laboratory findings for hypothyroidism show a reduction of serum triiodothyronine (T_3) and thyroxine (T_4) levels. TSH levels are high in primary hypothyroidism but can be decreased or near normal in patients with secondary hypothyroidism (Table 55.1). Older patients tend to have higher TSH levels (Ross, 2022c).

Analyze Cues and Prioritize Hypotheses: Analysis

The priority problems for patients who have hypothyroidism are:
1. Decreased *gas exchange* due to decreased energy, muscle weakness, and fatigue

2. Reduced perfusion due to decreased cardiac output
3. Potential for the complication of myxedema coma

Generate Solutions and Take Actions: Planning and Implementation

Respiratory and cardiac problems are serious, and their management is a priority. The most common cause of death among patients with myxedema coma is respiratory failure.

Improving Gas Exchange
Planning: Expected Outcomes. With appropriate management, the patient with hypothyroidism is expected to have improved *gas exchange.*

Interventions. Observe and record the rate and depth of respirations and adequacy of *gas exchange.* Measure oxygen saturation by pulse oximetry, and apply oxygen if the patient has hypoxemia. Auscultate the lungs for a decrease in breath sounds or presence of crackles. If hypothyroidism is severe, the patient may require ventilatory support. Severe respiratory distress occurs with myxedema coma.

Sedating a patient with hypothyroidism can make gas exchange worse and should be avoided if possible. When sedation is needed, the dosage may be reduced because hypothyroidism increases sensitivity to these drugs. For the patient receiving sedation, assess for adequate gas exchange.

Supporting Cardiac Output
Planning: Expected Outcomes. The patient is expected to have adequate cardiac output and perfusion.

Interventions. The patient may have increased blood pressure and dysrhythmias. Nursing priorities include monitoring blood pressure, heart rate, and rhythm for changes and preventing complications. If hypothyroidism is

---

⚡ TABLE 55.1 **Laboratory Profile**			

Thyroid Function

Test	Normal Range (Will Vary by Laboratory)	Hypothyroidism	Hyperthyroidism
Serum T_3	Age >50 years: 40–180 ng/dL (0.6–2.8 nmol/L) Age 20–50 years: 70–205 ng/dL (1.2–3.4 nmol/L)	Decreased	Increased
Serum T_4 (total)	Males: 4–12 mcg/dL (59–135 nmol/L) Females: 5–12 mcg/dL (71–142 nmol/L) Older adults >60 years old: 5–11 mcg/dL (64–142 nmol/L)	Decreased	Increased
"Direct" free T_4	0.8–2.8 ng/dL (10–36 pmol/L)	Decreased	Increased
TSH	0.3–5 µU/mL (0.3–5 mU/L)	High (primary hypothyroidism) Low (secondary or tertiary hypothyroidism)	High (secondary or tertiary hyperthyroidism) Low (Graves disease)

Data from Pagana, K. D., Pagana, T. J., & Pagana, T. N. (2022). *Mosby's manual of diagnostic and laboratory tests* (7th ed.). St. Louis: Elsevier.

chronic, the patient may have cardiovascular disease. *Instruct the patient to report episodes of chest pain or chest discomfort immediately.*

The patient with hypothyroidism requires lifelong thyroid hormone replacement. Synthetic hormone preparations are usually prescribed, such as levothyroxine. Therapy is started at a dose selected by the health care provider and gradually increased over a period of weeks if needed. *Patients with more severe symptoms of hypothyroidism, older adults, patients with coronary disease, and patients in which the degree of hypothyroidism is unknown are started on the lowest dose of thyroid hormone replacement* (Ross, 2023b). This precaution is especially important when the patient has known cardiac problems. Starting at too high a dose or increasing the dose too rapidly can cause abnormal heart rhythms, heart failure, and myocardial infarction. With myxedema coma, the drug may need to be given intravenously because of severely reduced motility and absorption of the GI tract.

NURSING SAFETY PRIORITY

Drug Alert

Teach patients who are beginning thyroid replacement therapy to take the drug *exactly* as prescribed and not to change the dose or schedule without consulting the primary health care provider. Levothyroxine should be taken with water on an empty stomach, 30 to 60 minutes before a meal in the morning. Teach the patient that there are several drugs that can reduce the absorption of this medication, such as iron, calcium supplements, and antacids. These drugs should be taken separately from levothyroxine by at least 4 hours.

Assess for chest pain and dyspnea during initiation of therapy. The final dosage is determined by blood levels of TSH and the patient's physical response. The dosage and time required for symptom relief vary with each patient. Monitor for and teach the patient and family about the symptoms of hyperthyroidism, which can occur with replacement therapy.

Preventing Myxedema Coma

Planning: Expected Outcomes. The patient will not experience myxedema coma.

Interventions. Any patient with hypothyroidism who has other health problems or who is newly diagnosed is at risk for myxedema coma. Although myxedema coma is now a rare effect of hypothyroidism, the nurse must be able to recognize signs of this medical emergency. Factors leading to myxedema coma include acute illness, surgery, chemotherapy, discontinuation of thyroid replacement therapy, and use of sedatives or opioids. Problems that often occur with this condition include:

- Greatly reduced level of consciousness and cognition
- Respiratory failure
- Hypotension
- Hyponatremia
- Hypothermia
- Hypoglycemia
- Bradycardia

BOX 55.3   Best Practice for Patient Safety and Quality Care

Emergency Care of the Patient With Myxedema Coma

- Maintain a patent airway.
- Replace fluids with IV normal or hypertonic saline as per orders.
- Replace T_3 and/or T_4 intravenously as prescribed.
- Give IV glucose as prescribed.
- Administer corticosteroids as prescribed.
- Check the patient's temperature hourly.
- Monitor blood pressure hourly.
- Cover the patient with warm blankets.
- Monitor for changes in mental status.
- Turn every 2 hours.
- Institute Aspiration Precautions.

! NURSING SAFETY ALERT

Action Alert

Myxedema coma can lead to shock, organ damage, and death. Assess the patient with hypothyroidism at least every 8 hours for changes that indicate increasing severity, especially changes in mental status, and report these promptly to the primary health care provider.

Treatment is instituted quickly according to the patient's symptoms and without waiting for laboratory confirmation. Management interventions are listed in Box 55.3.

Care Coordination and Transition Management

Hypothyroidism is usually chronic. Patients usually continue life in the community setting and are managed on an outpatient basis. Patients in acute care settings, subacute care settings, and rehabilitation centers may have long-standing hypothyroidism in addition to other health problems. Ensure that whoever is responsible for overseeing the patient's daily care is aware of the condition and understands its management.

Home Care Management. Patients with hypothyroidism do not usually require changes in the home unless cognition has decreased to the point that they are a danger to themselves or others. Activity intolerance and fatigue may necessitate one-floor living for a period of time.

The patient may need help with medication administration. Discuss this issue with the family and patient and develop a plan for drug therapy. One person should be clearly designated as responsible for drug preparation and delivery so that doses are neither missed nor duplicated. If home health care is needed, facilitate this connection.

Self-Management Education. The most important educational need for the patient with hypothyroidism is about hormone replacement therapy and its side effects. Emphasize the need for lifelong medication, and review the symptoms of both hyperthyroidism and hypothyroidism. If symptoms have not improved before discharge, discuss the need for extra heat or clothing because of cold intolerance.

Teach the patient to wear a medical alert bracelet. Teach the patient and family when to seek medical interventions for dosage adjustment and the need for periodic blood tests of hormone levels. Instruct the patient not to take any over-the-counter drugs without consulting the primary health care provider because thyroid hormone preparations interact with many other medications and supplements.

Advise the patient to maintain **nutrition** by consuming a well-balanced diet with adequate fiber and fluid intake to prevent constipation. Caution that use of fiber supplements may interfere with the absorption of thyroid hormone. Thyroid hormones should be taken on an empty stomach, at least 30 to 60 minutes before breakfast. Remind the patient about the importance of adequate rest.

Teach the patient to self-monitor for therapy effectiveness. The two easiest parameters to check are need for sleep and bowel elimination. When the patient requires more sleep and is constipated, thyroid hormone levels may need to be checked by the primary health care provider for potential dose adjustment. When the patient has difficulty getting to sleep and has more bowel movements than usual, the dose may need to be decreased.

Health Care Resources. Refer patients who desire support groups to credible resources. Various endocrine organizations offer access in person, as well as online.

Evaluate Outcomes: Evaluation

Evaluate the care of the patient with hypothyroidism based on the identified priority patient problems. The expected outcomes are that with proper management the patient should:

- Maintain normal cardiovascular function with a pulse above 60 beats/min and a blood pressure within normal limits for age and general health
- Maintain adequate respiratory function and **gas exchange** with SpO_2 above 93%
- Demonstrate improvement in cognition

NCLEX Examination Challenge 55.1

Physiological Integrity

A client taking levothyroxine for hypothyroidism reports fatigue and wearing a sweater regularly despite warm weather. Which of the following actions would the nurse take? **Select all that apply.**

A. Obtain vital signs.
B. Check body temperature.
C. Review medication record.
D. Measure intake and output.
E. Assess swallowing reflex.

HYPERTHYROIDISM

Pathophysiology Review

Hyperthyroidism is excessive thyroid hormone secretion from the thyroid gland. The same symptoms and terms are used even if the cause is ingestion of synthetic thyroid hormones when thyroid function is normal. Excessive thyroid hormones reduce **cellular regulation** by increasing metabolism in all body organs, which then produces many different symptoms. Hyperthyroidism can be temporary or permanent, depending on the cause.

 BOX 55.4   Key Features

Hyperthyroidism

Cardiovascular Symptoms
- Chest pain
- Dysrhythmias
- Increased systolic blood pressure
- Palpitations
- Rapid, shallow respirations
- Tachycardia

GI Symptoms
- Increased appetite
- Increased stools
- Weight loss

Metabolic Symptoms
- Fatigue
- Heat intolerance
- Increased basal metabolic rate

Reproductive Symptoms
Women
- Amenorrhea

Men
- Erectile dysfunction
- Gynecomastia

Psychosocial Symptoms
- Anxiety
- Hyperactivity
- Restlessness

Integumentary Symptoms
- Diaphoresis (excessive sweating)
- Fine, soft, silky body hair
- Smooth, warm, moist skin
- Thinning of scalp hair

Neuromuscular Symptoms
- Eyelid retraction, eyelid lag
- Hyperactive deep tendon reflexes
- Insomnia
- Muscle weakness
- Tremors

Other Symptoms
- Goiter
- Wide-eyed or startled appearance (exophthalmos)[a]

[a] Present in Graves disease only.

The excessive thyroid hormones stimulate most body systems, causing hypermetabolism and increased sympathetic nervous system activity. Symptoms are listed in Box 55.4.

Thyroid hormones stimulate the heart, increasing rate and stroke volume. These responses increase cardiac output, blood pressure, and blood flow.

Elevated thyroid hormone levels affect protein, fat, and glucose metabolism. Protein buildup and breakdown are increased, but breakdown exceeds buildup. Glucose tolerance is decreased, and the patient has *hyperglycemia* (elevated blood glucose levels). Fat metabolism is increased, and body fat decreases. Although the patient has an increased appetite, the increased metabolism causes weight loss and **nutrition** deficits.

Thyroid hormones are produced in response to the stimulation hormones secreted by the hypothalamus and anterior pituitary glands. Oversecretion of thyroid hormones changes the secretion of hormones from the hypothalamus and the anterior pituitary gland through negative feedback (see Chapter 53). Thyroid hormones also have some influence over sex hormone production. Women often experience menstrual problems and decreased fertility. Men can experience gynecomastia and reduced libido.

Etiology and Genetic Risk

Hyperthyroidism has many causes. The most common form of the disease is Graves disease, which is an autoimmune disorder (Cleveland Clinic, 2023). It often occurs after an episode of thyroid inflammation in which the production of autoantibodies (thyroid-stimulating immunoglobulins [TSIs]) that attach to the thyroid-stimulating hormone (TSH) receptors on the thyroid gland greatly increases thyroid hormone production (Davies, 2021). This increases the number of glandular cells, which enlarges the gland, forming a goiter, and overproduces thyroid hormones.

In Graves disease, all the general symptoms of hyperthyroidism are present. In addition, other changes specific to Graves disease may occur, including exophthalmos (abnormal protrusion of the eyes) and pretibial myxedema (dry, waxy swelling of the front surfaces of the lower legs that resembles benign tumors or keloids) (Fig. 55.3). (Davies, 2023). Graves disease can also be aggravated by COVID-19 (Duntas & Jonklaas, 2021).

Hyperthyroidism caused by multiple thyroid nodules is termed *toxic multinodular goiter (TMNG)*. The nodules may be enlarged thyroid tissues or benign tumors (adenomas). These patients usually have had a goiter for years. The symptoms are milder than those seen in Graves disease, and the patient does not have exophthalmos or pretibial myxedema.

Hyperthyroidism can also be caused by excessive use of thyroid replacement hormones. This type of problem is called *exogenous hyperthyroidism.*

PATIENT-CENTERED CARE: GENETICS/ GENOMICS

Susceptibility to Graves Disease

Susceptibility to Graves disease is associated with several gene mutations. In addition, Graves disease is associated with other autoimmune disorders, such as diabetes mellitus, vitiligo, and rheumatoid arthritis and often occurs in both members of identical twins (Davies, 2021). Ask the patient with Graves disease whether any other family members also have the problem.

Incidence and Prevalence

Hyperthyroidism is a common endocrine disorder. Graves disease can occur at any age but is diagnosed most often in women between 30 and 50 years of age (Cleveland Clinic, 2023). Toxic multinodular goiter primarily affects women until 50 years of age. At that time, it is equally prevalent in men and women (Khalid & Can, 2023).

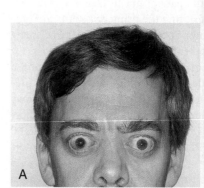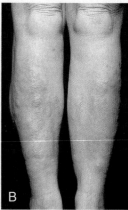

FIG. 55.3 (A) Exophthalmos. (B) Pretibial myxedema. (From Belchetz, P., & Hammond, P. [2003]. *Mosby's color atlas and text of diabetes and endocrinology.* Edinburgh: Mosby.)

Interprofessional Collaborative Care
Recognize Cues: Assessment

History. Confirm age and usual weight. Many changes and problems occur because the reduced **cellular regulation** of hyperthyroidism affects all body systems; however, changes can occur over such a long period that patients may be unaware of them. The increased metabolic rate affects **nutrition.** The patient may report recent unplanned weight loss, an increased appetite, and an increase in the number of bowel movements per day.

Heat intolerance is often the first symptom the patient notices. The patient may have increased sweating even when environmental temperatures are comfortable for others and may even wear lighter clothing in cold weather. The patient may also report palpitations or chest pain as a result of cardiovascular effects. Ask about changes in breathing patterns because dyspnea (with or without exertion) is common, as well.

Visual changes may also be an early problem that the patient or family notices, especially exophthalmos with Graves disease (see Fig. 55.3). Ask about changes in vision such as blurring or double vision and eye fatigue.

Ask about changes in energy level or in the ability to perform normal ADLs. Fatigue and insomnia are common. Families may report that the patient can be restless or anxious.

Ask women about changes in libido and whether they have had changes in menses because amenorrhea or a decreased menstrual flow is common. Ask men whether there has been a decrease in libido.

Ask about previous thyroid surgery or radiation therapy to the neck, because some adults remain hyperthyroid after surgery or are resistant to radiation therapy. Ask about past and current drug use, especially the use of thyroid hormone replacement or antithyroid medications.

Physical Assessment/Signs and Symptoms. Exophthalmos is common in patients with Graves disease. The wide-eyed or "startled" look is due to edema in the extraocular muscles and increased fatty tissue behind the eye, which pushes the eyeball forward and may cause problems with focusing. Pressure on the optic nerve may impair vision. If the eyelids fail to close completely and the eyes are unprotected, they may become dry and corneal ulcers may develop. Observe the eyes for excessive tearing and a bloodshot appearance. Ask about sensitivity to light (*photophobia*).

Two other eye problems are common in all types of hyperthyroidism: eyelid retraction (eyelid lag) and globe (eyeball) lag. In eyelid lag, the upper eyelid fails to descend when the patient gazes slowly downward. In globe lag, the upper eyelid pulls back faster than the eyeball when the patient gazes upward. During assessment ask the patient to look down and then up, and document the response.

Observe the size and symmetry of the thyroid gland. The generalist medical-surgical nurse does not palpate the thyroid gland even though it is superficially located. If the patient has a goiter, the thyroid gland may be up to four times its normal size (see Fig. 55.1). *Not all patients with a goiter have hyperthyroidism.* Bruits (turbulence from increased blood flow) may be heard within the gland with a stethoscope.

> ## ❗ NURSING SAFETY PRIORITY
> ### *Action Alert*
>
> Do not palpate a goiter or thyroid tissue in a patient with hyperthyroid symptoms. This action can stimulate the sudden release of excessive thyroid hormones and trigger a life-threatening episode of thyroid storm.

The cardiovascular problems associated with hyperthyroidism include increased systolic blood pressure, tachycardia, and dysrhythmias (such as atrial fibrillation). Usually the diastolic pressure is decreased, causing a widened pulse pressure.

Inspect the hair and skin. Fine, soft, silky hair and smooth, warm, moist skin are common. Many patients notice thinning of scalp hair. Muscle weakness and hyperactive deep tendon reflexes are common. Observe motor movements of the hands for tremors. The patient may appear restless and irritable.

Psychosocial Assessment. Wide mood swings, decreased attention span, and anxiety are common. Hyperactivity often leads to fatigue because of the inability to sleep well. Some patients describe their activity as having two modes (i.e., either "full speed ahead" or "completely stopped"). Ask whether they cry or laugh without cause or have difficulty concentrating. Family members often report a change in the patient's mental or emotional status.

Laboratory Assessment. Testing for hyperthyroidism involves measurement of blood levels for triiodothyronine (T_3), thyroxine (T_4), and thyroid-stimulating hormone (TSH). Antibodies to the TSH receptor (thyrotropin receptor [TRAb]) can also be measured to diagnose Graves disease. The most common changes in laboratory tests for hyperthyroidism are listed in Table 55.1.

Other Diagnostic Assessments. Evaluate the position, size, and functioning of the thyroid gland. Radioactive iodine (RAI [^{123}I]) is given by mouth, and the uptake of iodine by the thyroid gland (radioactive iodine uptake [RAIU]) is measured. The half-life of ^{123}I is short, and radiation precautions are not needed. Pregnancy should be ruled out before the scan is performed. RAIU is increased in hyperthyroidism and can be used to

identify active nodules in the patient with suspected nodular thyroid disease.

Ultrasonography of the thyroid is common and can determine its size and the general composition of any masses or nodules. This outpatient procedure takes about 30 minutes to perform and is painless. An *ECG* may show supraventricular tachycardia, atrial fibrillation, and premature ventricular contractions.

Take Actions: Interventions

Because Graves disease is the most common form of hyperthyroidism, the interventions discussed in the following sections include those specific for the problems that occur with this disease. Interventions include drug therapy, radioiodine ablation, and surgery. Medical management is used to decrease the effect of thyroid hormone on cardiac function and to reduce thyroid hormone secretion. Surgery is an option for those with severe disease or a large goiter, or for those patients who are unable to tolerate other forms of management. The priorities for nursing care focus on monitoring for complications, reducing stimulation, promoting comfort, and teaching the patient and family about therapeutic drugs and procedures.

Nonsurgical Management. Monitoring includes measuring the patient's apical pulse, blood pressure, and temperature at least every 4 hours. Instruct the patient to immediately report any palpitations, dyspnea, vertigo, or chest pain. Increases in temperature may indicate a rapid worsening of the patient's condition and the onset of thyroid storm, a rare, life-threatening event that occurs in patients with uncontrolled hyperthyroidism. It presents with symptoms of hyperthyroidism that are more intense than normal and is characterized by high fever and tachycardia. *Immediately report a temperature increase of even 1°F (1.8°C).* If this task of collecting temperature is delegated to assistive personnel (AP), instruct them to report the patient's temperature as soon as it has been obtained. If temperature is elevated, immediately assess the patient's cardiac status. If the patient has a cardiac monitor, check for dysrhythmias.

Reducing stimulation helps prevent increasing the symptoms of hyperthyroidism and the risk for cardiac complications. Encourage the patient to rest. Keep the environment quiet by closing the door to the room, limiting visitors, and postponing non-essential care or treatments.

Promoting comfort includes reducing the room temperature to decrease discomfort caused by heat intolerance. Instruct AP to ensure that the patient always has a fresh pitcher of ice water and to change the bed linen whenever it becomes damp from diaphoresis. Suggest that the patient take a cool shower or sponge bath several times each day. For patients with exophthalmos, prevent eye dryness by encouraging the use of artificial tears.

Drug therapy with antithyroid medication is the initial treatment for hyperthyroidism. Remission is possible for some patients when using these drugs, especially in those with mild disease and with a small goiter. Table 55.2 lists teaching priorities for the patient receiving drug therapy for hyperthyroidism. The preferred drugs are the thionamides, especially methimazole, because of its ease of use (Ross, 2022b). Propylthiouracil is used much less commonly because of its toxic effects on the liver. These drugs block thyroid hormone production by preventing

TABLE 55.2   Common Examples of Drug Therapy

Hyperthyroidism

Drug	Selected Nursing Implications
Methimazole (first-line therapy) *or* propylthiouracil	Teach patients to avoid crowds and people who are ill; *this drug reduces the immune response, increasing the risk for infection.*
	Teach patients to check for weight gain, slow heart rate, and cold intolerance; *these symptoms are associated with hypothyroidism and the potential need for a lower drug dose.*
	Teach women taking methimazole to notify their primary health care provider if they become pregnant; *this drug causes birth defects and should not be used during pregnancy.*
	Teach patients taking propylthiouracil to report darkening of the urine or a yellow appearance to the skin or whites of the eyes; *these symptoms can indicate possible liver toxicity or failure, a serious side effect of propylthiouracil.*
Iodine (saturated solution of potassium iodine [SSKI])	Administer orally, diluted in a glass of water or beverage; *this controls its transport into the thyroid.*
	Give 1 hour after thionamides or 1 week later than radioiodine; *this decreases the risk for an exacerbation of hyperthyroidism.*

iodide binding in the thyroid gland. The response to these drugs is delayed because the patient may have large amounts of stored thyroid hormones that continue to be released.

Iodine preparations may be used for short-term therapy for surgery. They decrease blood flow through the thyroid gland, reducing the production and release of thyroid hormone. Improvement usually occurs within 2 weeks, but it may be weeks before metabolism returns to normal. This treatment can result in hypothyroidism, and the patient is monitored closely for the need to adjust the drug regimen.

Beta-adrenergic blocking drugs such as atenolol or propranolol may be used as supportive therapy. These drugs relieve symptoms such as diaphoresis, anxiety, tachycardia, and palpitations but do not inhibit thyroid hormone production. See Chapters 29 and 30 for a discussion of the actions and nursing implications of these agents.

NURSING SAFETY PRIORITY

Drug Alert

Although similar in action, methimazole and propylthiouracil are *not* interchangeable. The dosages for propylthiouracil are much higher than those for methimazole.

NURSING SAFETY PRIORITY

Drug Alert

Methimazole can cause birth defects and may need to be changed to a different medication during the first trimester of pregnancy. Instruct women to notify their primary health care provider if pregnancy occurs.

The patient with hyperthyroidism may receive *radioactive iodine (RAI) therapy* in the form of oral ^{131}I. The dosage depends on the thyroid gland's size and sensitivity to radiation. The thyroid picks up the RAI, and some of the cells that produce thyroid hormone are destroyed by the local radiation. Because the gland stores thyroid hormones to some degree, the patient may

BOX 55.5   Patient and Family Education

Safety Precautions for the Patient Receiving an Unsealed Radioactive Isotope

- Sit to urinate (males and females) to avoid splashing urine on the seat, walls, and floor.
- Flush the toilet (with the lid closed) two to three times after each use.
- Men with urinary incontinence should use condom catheters and a drainage bag rather than absorbent gel-filled briefs or pads.
- Women with urinary incontinence should use facial tissue layers in their clothing to catch the urine rather than absorbent gel-filled briefs or pads. These tissues should then be flushed.
- Avoid close contact with pregnant women, infants, and young children for the prescribed amount of time (usually at least a week) after therapy (this is dose dependent). Remain at least 6 feet away from these people, including avoiding sleeping in the same bed.
- Patients may need to delay returning to work and travel for a few days depending on the dose of therapy given.
- Some radioactivity will be in your saliva during the first week after therapy. Precautions to avoid exposing others to this contamination include:
  - Not sharing toothbrushes or toothpaste tubes
  - Not preparing food or sharing beverages

not have symptom relief until 6 to 8 weeks after RAI therapy. As a result, if symptoms are severe, additional drug therapy for hyperthyroidism may still be needed during the first few weeks after RAI treatment. This drug is not used in pregnant women because ^{131}I crosses the placenta and can damage the fetal thyroid gland.

RAI therapy is performed on an outpatient basis. One dose may be sufficient, although some patients need a second dose. The radiation dose is low and is usually completely eliminated within a month; however, the source is unsealed, and some radioactivity is present in the patient's body fluids and stool for a few days after therapy. Radiation precautions are needed to prevent exposure to family members and other people. Teach patients the precautions listed in Box 55.5 to use during the first few days after receiving ^{131}I.

The degree of thyroid destruction varies. Some patients become hypothyroid as a result of treatment. The patient then

Thyroid gland with thyroid cancer. Removal of one lobe of the thyroid. Total removal of the thyroid gland.

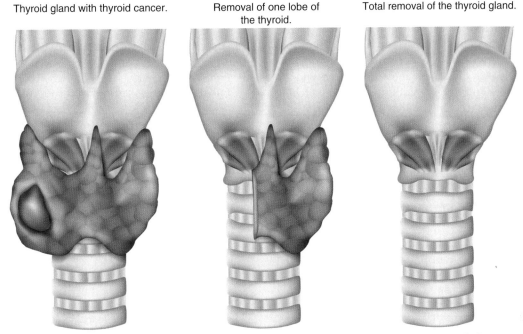

FIG. 55.4 **Thyroidectomy.** (Used with permission from istockphoto.com, 2019, medialstocks.)

needs lifelong thyroid hormone replacement. All patients who have undergone RAI therapy should be monitored regularly for changes in thyroid function.

Surgical Management. Surgery to remove all or part of the thyroid gland is used to manage Graves and other types of hyperthyroidism that do not respond to nonsurgical management strategies. It is also used when a large goiter causes tracheal or esophageal compression. Removal of all *(total thyroidectomy)* or part *(subtotal thyroidectomy)* (Fig. 55.4) of the thyroid tissue decreases the production of thyroid hormones. After a total thyroidectomy, patients must take lifelong thyroid hormone replacement.

Preoperative Care. The patient is treated with thionamide drug therapy first to have near-normal thyroid function (euthyroid) before thyroid surgery. Iodine preparations may be used to decrease thyroid size and vascularity, thereby reducing the risk for hemorrhage and the potential for thyroid storm during surgery. (Thyroid storm is discussed earlier in the Nonsurgical Management section, and later in the Thyroid Storm section of Hyperthyroidism.)

Explain the surgery and the care after surgery to the patient. Hypertension, dysrhythmias, and tachycardia must be controlled before surgery. Remind the patient to coordinate with the surgeon if modification needs to be made to help the patient be physiologically ready for surgery.

Teach the patient to perform deep-breathing exercises. Stress the importance of supporting the neck when coughing or moving by placing both hands behind the neck to reduce strain on the incision. Also teach that a drain and a dressing may be in place after surgery.

Operative Procedures. Many thyroidectomies are now performed as minimally invasive surgeries. With these surgeries,

as with the traditional open approach, the parathyroid glands and recurrent laryngeal nerves are avoided to reduce the risk for complications and injury.

Postoperative Care. *Monitoring the patient for complications is the most important nursing action after thyroid surgery.* Monitor vital signs every 15 minutes until the patient is stable and then every 30 minutes thereafter. Increase or decrease the monitoring of vital signs based on changes in the patient's condition.

Assess the patient's level of discomfort and administer prescribed drugs for pain control as needed. Use pillows to support the head and neck. Place the patient, while awake, in a semi-Fowler's position. Avoid positions that cause neck extension.

Help the patient deep-breathe every 30 minutes to 1 hour. Suction oral and tracheal secretions when necessary.

Thyroid surgery can cause hemorrhage, respiratory distress with reduced ***gas exchange,*** parathyroid gland injury (resulting in *hypocalcemia* [low serum calcium levels] and tetany [hyperexcitability of nerves and muscles]), damage to the laryngeal nerves, and thyroid storm. Remain alert to the potential for complications and identify symptoms early.

Hemorrhage is most likely to occur during the first 24 hours after surgery. Inspect the neck dressing and behind the patient's neck for blood. If a drain is present, a moderate amount of serosanguineous drainage is normal. Hemorrhage may be seen as bleeding at the incision site or as respiratory distress caused by tracheal compression.

*Respiratory distress and reduced **gas exchange*** can result from swelling, tetany, or damage to the laryngeal nerve, resulting in spasms. Laryngeal *stridor* (harsh, high-pitched respiratory sounds) is heard in acute respiratory obstruction. Keep emergency tracheostomy equipment in the patient's room. Check that oxygen and suctioning equipment are nearby and in working order.

Hypocalcemia and tetany may occur if the parathyroid glands are removed or damaged or if their blood supply is impaired during thyroid surgery, resulting in decreased parathyroid hormone (PTH) levels. Ask the patient about tingling around the mouth or of the toes and fingers. Assess for muscle twitching as a sign of calcium deficiency. Calcium gluconate for IV use should be available in an emergency situation. (For information on the later signs of hypocalcemia, see the Assessment discussion in the Hypoparathyroidism section. Hypocalcemia is also discussed in Chapter 13.)

✚ NURSING SAFETY PRIORITY

Critical Rescue

Monitor the patient to identify symptoms of obstruction and poor **gas exchange** (stridor, dyspnea, falling oxygen saturation, inability to swallow, drooling) after thyroid surgery. If any indications are present, respond by immediately initiating the Rapid Response Team.

Laryngeal nerve damage may occur during surgery. This problem results in hoarseness and a weak voice. Assess the patient's voice at 2-hour intervals and document any changes. Reassure the patient that hoarseness is usually temporary.

Thyroid storm is a life-threatening event that occurs in patients with uncontrolled hyperthyroidism, most often with Graves disease. Symptoms develop quickly, and the problem is fatal if left untreated. It is often triggered by stressors such as trauma, infection, diabetic ketoacidosis, and pregnancy. Other conditions that can lead to thyroid storm include vigorous palpation of the goiter, exposure to iodine, and radioactive iodine (RAI) therapy. Thyroid storm after surgery is now uncommon because of drug therapy before the procedure.

Symptoms of thyroid storm are caused by excessive thyroid hormone release, which dramatically increases metabolic rate. *Key symptoms include fever and tachycardia.* The patient may have abdominal pain, nausea, vomiting, and diarrhea. Often, anxiety and tremors are reported. As the crisis progresses, the patient may become restless, confused, or psychotic and may have seizures, leading to coma. *Even with treatment, thyroid storm may lead to death.*

✚ NURSING SAFETY PRIORITY

Critical Rescue

When caring for a patient with hyperthyroidism, even after a thyroidectomy, assess temperature often because an increase of even 1°F (1.8°C) may indicate an impending thyroid crisis. If a temperature increase occurs, respond by reporting it immediately to the primary health care provider.

Emergency measures vary with the intensity and type of changes observed. Interventions focus on maintaining airway patency, promoting adequate ventilation and **gas exchange,**

BOX 55.6 Best Practice for Patient Safety and Quality Care

Emergency Care of the Patient During Thyroid Storm

- Maintain a patent airway and adequate ventilation.
- Give oral antithyroid drugs as prescribed: methimazole or propylthiouracil.
- If antithyroid drugs cannot be used, a bile acid sequestrant such as cholestyramine may be ordered to help reduce thyroid levels.
- Administer iodide solution, nonsalicylate antipyretic drugs, and glucocorticoids as prescribed.
- Give oral propranolol as prescribed to control heart rate.
- Monitor continually for cardiac dysrhythmias.
- Monitor vital signs every 15 to 30 minutes.
- Provide comfort measures, including a cooling blanket.
- Correct dehydration with normal saline infusions per orders.
- Apply cooling blanket or ice packs to reduce fever.

reducing fever, and stabilizing the hemodynamic status. Box 55.6 outlines interventions for emergency management of thyroid storm.

Eye and vision problems associated with Graves disease are not usually fully corrected by treatment for hyperthyroidism. Management is symptomatic. Teach the patient with mild problems to elevate the head of the bed at night and use artificial tears. If photophobia is present, dark glasses may be helpful. For those who cannot close the eyelids completely, recommend gently taping the lids closed at bedtime to prevent irritation and injury.

If pressure behind the eye continues and forces the eye forward, blood supply to the eye can be compromised, leading to ischemia and blindness. In severe cases, short-term glucocorticoid therapy is prescribed to reduce swelling and halt the infiltrative process. Prednisone is given in high doses at first and then is tapered down according to the patient's response. Other management strategies include selenium and teprotumumab. Surgical intervention in the form of orbital decompression may be needed if loss of sight or damage to the eyeball is possible.

Health teaching includes reviewing with the patient and family the symptoms of hyperthyroidism and instructing the patient to report any increase or recurrence of these. Also teach about the symptoms of hypothyroidism (discussed previously) and the need for lifelong thyroid hormone replacement. Reinforce the need for regular follow-up because hypothyroidism can occur several years after radioactive iodine therapy completion. This is especially important for young adults, as most patients need 1 or 2 dosage adjustments postsurgery to achieve optimal maintenance (Ross, 2022d).

NCLEX Examination Challenge 55.2

Physiological Integrity

The nurse is caring for a client 4 hours after a total thyroidectomy. Which assessment finding would alert the nurse to a possible complication?

A. Temperature 98.0°F (36.7°C)
B. Absence of bowel movement
C. Report of tingling around the mouth and in the hands
D. Small amount of serosanguineous drainage on dressing

THYROIDITIS

Thyroiditis is a group of conditions that cause inflammation of the thyroid gland. Some of these conditions can cause pain, whereas others do not. Thyroiditis can also be acute or chronic.

Infectious thyroiditis is caused by bacterial invasion of the thyroid gland. It can be acute or chronic. Acute symptoms include sudden pain and tenderness on one side of the neck, malaise, and fever (Burman, 2021). It usually resolves with IV antibiotic therapy. Chronic infections usually are less painful and can occur with symptoms present bilaterally.

Subacute or granulomatous thyroiditis results from a viral infection of the thyroid gland after a cold or other upper respiratory infection. The patient experiences neck pain and the thyroid gland feels hard and enlarged on palpation (goiter). Thyroid function can remain normal, although the typical pattern is hyperthyroidism, then hypothyroidism, followed by return to euthyroid levels.

Radiation thyroiditis occurs 5 to 10 days after treatment with radioiodine. Symptoms are typically mild and transient, disappearing within a week.

Palpation/trauma-induced thyroiditis can also occur during physical examination, biopsy, neck surgery, or trauma.

Chronic autoimmune thyroiditis (Hashimoto thyroiditis [HT]) is a common type of hypothyroidism. The thyroid is invaded by antithyroid antibodies and lymphocytes, causing selective thyroid tissue destruction. When large amounts of the gland are destroyed, hypothyroidism results.

Symptoms of Hashimoto thyroiditis include dysphagia and painless enlargement of the gland. Diagnosis is based on circulating antithyroid antibodies. Serum thyroid hormone levels and TSH levels vary with disease stage and type. An antithyroid peroxidase antibody (anti-TPO, or TPO-Ab) test is elevated with Hashimoto thyroiditis.

THYROID CANCER

Pathophysiology Review

The four major types of thyroid cancer are papillary, follicular, medullary, and anaplastic (National Cancer Institute, 2023b). Papillary and follicular thyroid cancers are sometimes referred to as *differentiated thyroid cancer* (National Cancer Institute, 2023a). The initial sign of thyroid cancer is typically a single, painless lump or nodule in the thyroid gland. Additional signs and symptoms depend on the presence and location of *metastasis* (spread of cancer cells).

Papillary carcinoma, the most common type of thyroid cancer, occurs most often in women around 50 years of age (Limaiem et al., 2023). It is a slow-growing tumor that can be present for years before spreading to nearby lymph nodes. When the tumor is confined to the thyroid gland, the chance for cure is possible with a partial or total thyroidectomy.

Follicular carcinoma occurs most often in adults between the ages of 40 to 60 and in countries where iodine is not found readily in the diet (American Cancer Society, 2019). It invades blood vessels and spreads to bone and lung tissue. When it adheres to the trachea, neck muscles, great vessels, and skin, dyspnea and dysphagia result. When the tumor involves the recurrent laryngeal nerves, the patient may have a hoarse voice.

Medullary carcinoma can occur occasionally due to multiple endocrine neoplasia type 2 (MEN2), a familial endocrine disorder (Tuttle, 2022). It is often found in children and young adults. More common is the sporadic type of medullary carcinoma, which is not inherited and typically affects adults aged 40 to 60 (American Cancer Society, 2019).

Anaplastic carcinoma is a rapidly growing, aggressive tumor that invades nearby tissues. It is rare and difficult to treat (American Cancer Society, 2019). Symptoms include shortness of breath, hoarseness, and dysphagia.

PATIENT-CENTERED CARE: HEALTH EQUITY

Thyroid Cancer in African Americans

African Americans are at a higher risk for anaplastic thyroid cancer than other racial groups (African American Wellness Project, 2023). This type of cancer is very aggressive. Advocate for all patients to have access to health care (including telehealth) and transportation to appointments to improve early recognition and intervention (Haymart, 2022).

Interprofessional Collaborative Care

Surgery is the treatment of choice for most types of thyroid cancer. If the cancer is small and contained, removing just one lobe may be possible. A total thyroidectomy is usually performed with dissection of lymph nodes in the neck if regional lymph nodes are involved. (See the postoperative care discussion in the Surgical Management section for Hyperthyroidism). Radioactive iodine (RAI) may be given after surgery to help destroy remaining tissue. If this is not successful, targeted drugs called kinase inhibitors may be available for use.

External beam radiation and/or chemotherapy is used most often for anaplastic carcinoma because this cancer has usually metastasized at diagnosis, making it difficult to remove completely (Tuttle & Sherman, 2023). Radiation can be used to shrink the tumor prior to surgery or can be implemented after surgery to treat cancer that persists. RAI is not used to treat anaplastic carcinoma.

The patient is hypothyroid after treatment for thyroid cancer. Nursing interventions then focus on teaching about the management of hypothyroidism. (See the discussion of patient-centered collaborative care in the Cellular Regulation Concept Exemplar: Hypothyroidism section.) Very rarely is thyroid cancer fatal. For patients who may need palliative care or hospice, provide referrals appropriately.

HYPOPARATHYROIDISM

Pathophysiology Review

The parathyroid glands maintain calcium and phosphate balance. Serum calcium level is normally maintained within a narrow range. Parathyroid secretion of parathyroid hormone

TABLE 55.3   Laboratory Profile

Parathyroid Function

Test	Normal Range	Hypoparathyroidism	Hyperparathyroidism
Serum calcium	Total: 9.0–10.5 mg/dL (2.25–2.62 mmol/L) **NOTE:** Values may be slightly lower in older adults.	Decreased	Increased in primary hyperparathyroidism
Serum magnesium **Critical levels <0.5 or >3 mEq/L mg/dL**	1.3–2.1 mEq/L (0.65–1.05 mmol/L)	Decreased	Increased
Serum parathyroid hormone	10–65 pg/mL (10–65 ng/L)	Decreased	Increased
Serum phosphorus **Critical level <1 mg/dL**	3–4.5 mg/dL (0.97–1.45 mmol/L)	Increased	Decreased
Vitamin D	25–80 ng/mL (62.5–200 nmol/L)	Decreased	Variable

Data from Pagana, K. D., Pagana, T. J., & Pagana, T. N. (2022). *Mosby's manual of diagnostic and laboratory tests* (7th ed.). St. Louis: Elsevier.

(PTH) acts directly on the kidney, causing increased kidney reabsorption of calcium and increased phosphorus excretion.

Hypoparathyroidism is a rare disorder in which parathyroid function is decreased and serum calcium levels cannot be maintained, resulting in *hypocalcemia* (low serum calcium levels). Problems are directly related to a lack of parathyroid hormone (PTH) secretion or to decreased effectiveness of PTH on target tissue.

Hypoparathyroidism occurs most often postsurgically after removal of the thyroid or parathyroid glands, or after surgery for head or neck cancers.

This disorder can also occur as a result of an autoimmune or genetic process.

Interprofessional Collaborative Care

Recognize Cues: Assessment

Ask about any head or neck surgery or radiation therapy because these treatments may injure the parathyroid glands and cause hypoparathyroidism. Also ask whether the neck has ever sustained a serious injury in a car crash or by strangulation. Assess whether the patient has any symptoms of hypoparathyroidism, which may range from mild tingling and numbness to muscle tetany. Tingling and numbness around the mouth or in the hands and feet reflect mild to moderate hypocalcemia. Severe muscle cramps, spasms of the hands and feet, and seizures (with no loss of consciousness or incontinence) reflect a more severe hypocalcemia. The patient or family may notice mental changes ranging from irritability to psychosis.

The physical assessment may show excessive or inappropriate muscle contractions that cause finger, hand, and elbow flexion. This can signal an impending attack of tetany. Check for Trousseau and Chvostek signs; positive responses indicate potential tetany (see Figs. 13.11 and 13.12 in Chapter 13). Bands or pits may encircle the teeth, which indicates a loss of tooth calcium and enamel.

The diagnosis of hypoparathyroidism is made by the health care provider based on serum calcium, magnesium, parathyroid hormone, and albumin levels (Table 55.3). Once the diagnosis is confirmed, a 24-hour urine calcium is obtained. Vitamin D levels may also be checked, with the goal of correcting any deficiency.

Take Actions: Interventions

Nonsurgical management of hypoparathyroidism focuses on correcting hypocalcemia and preventing kidney stones. For patients with acute and severe hypocalcemia, calcium is given as IV calcium gluconate. Oral calcitriol and calcium carbonate may also be given depending on the severity of the hypocalcemia and with milder symptoms. Oral Vitamin D supplementation may be given with mild hypocalcemia. Long-term oral therapy for hypocalcemia involves daily intake of calcium (usually calcium carbonate).

Medication dosage is adjusted to keep the patient's calcium level in the low-normal range, enough to prevent symptoms of hypocalcemia. It must also be low enough to prevent increased urine calcium levels, which can lead to kidney stone formation.

Nursing management includes teaching about the drug regimen and interventions. Teach the patient to eat foods high in calcium in moderation, such as milk, yogurt, cheese, and ice cream.

Stress that therapy for hypocalcemia is lifelong. Advise the patient to wear a medical alert bracelet. With adherence to the prescribed drug and diet regimen, the calcium level usually remains high enough to prevent a hypocalcemic crisis.

HYPERPARATHYROIDISM

Pathophysiology Review

Hyperparathyroidism is a disorder in which parathyroid secretion of parathyroid hormone is increased, resulting in *hypercalcemia* and *hypophosphatemia*. In bone, excessive PTH levels increase bone *resorption* by decreasing *osteoblastic* activity and increasing *osteoclastic* activity. This process releases calcium and phosphorus into the blood and reduces bone density. With chronic calcium excess and hypercalcemia, calcium is deposited in soft tissues.

Although the exact trigger is unknown, primary hyperparathyroidism results when one or more parathyroid glands do not respond to the normal feedback of serum calcium levels. Common causes of secondary hyperparathyroidism include vitamin D deficiency and chronic kidney disease (CKD) (El-Hajj et al., 2022). Box 55.7 lists other causes.

BOX 55.7 Causes of Parathyroid Dysfunction

Causes of Hyperparathyroidism
- Calcium absorption difficulties (e.g., as present with celiac disease or in those who have had bariatric surgery)
- Chronic kidney disease with hypocalcemia
- Congenital hyperplasia
- Drug therapy (e.g., diuretics, bisphosphonates)
- Inherited conditions (e.g., multiple endocrine neoplasia type 1 [MEN1])
- Neck trauma or radiation
- Parathyroid hormone–secreting carcinomas of the lung, kidney, or GI tract
- Parathyroid tumor or cancer
- Vitamin D deficiency

Causes of Hypoparathyroidism
- Autoimmune conditions
- Congenital dysgenesis
- Parathyroidectomy
- Thyroid ablation (surgical or radiation-induced)

Interprofessional Collaborative Care

Recognize Cues: Assessment

Symptoms of hyperparathyroidism may be related to either the effects of excessive PTH or the accompanying hypercalcemia.

Ask about any bone fractures, recent weight loss, arthritis, or psychological stress. Ask whether the patient has received radiation treatment to the head or neck. The patient with chronic disease may have a waxy pallor of the skin, and deformities of the bones in the extremities and back.

High levels of PTH cause kidney stones and deposits of calcium in the soft tissue of the kidney. Bone lesions are caused by an increased rate of bone destruction and may result in fractures, bone cysts, and osteoporosis.

GI problems (e.g., anorexia, nausea, vomiting, epigastric pain, constipation, weight loss) are common when serum calcium levels are high. Elevated serum gastrin levels are caused by hypercalcemia and lead to peptic ulcer disease. Fatigue and lethargy may be present and worsen as the serum calcium levels increase. When serum calcium levels are greater than 12 mg/dL (3.0 mmol/L), the patient may have psychosis with confusion, followed by coma and death if left untreated. (See Chapter 13 for more information about hypercalcemia.)

As listed in Table 55.3, serum calcium, magnesium, parathyroid hormone, phosphorus, and vitamin D are laboratory tests used when assessing for hyperparathyroidism. X-rays may show kidney stones, calcium deposits, and bone lesions. Loss of bone density occurs in the patient with chronic hyperparathyroidism. Explain the procedures and care for the patient undergoing diagnostic tests.

Take Actions: Interventions

Surgical management is the treatment of choice for patients with hyperparathyroidism. For asymptomatic patients who wish to delay, drug therapy can help control the problems. Close monitoring of calcium levels, kidney function, and bone density is necessary. Priority nursing interventions focus on monitoring and preventing injury.

Nonsurgical Management. Drug therapy for patients who have more severe symptoms of hyperparathyroidism or who have hypercalcemia related to parathyroid cancer involves the use of cinacalcet, a calcimimetic. When taken orally, the drug binds to calcium-sensitive receptors on parathyroid tissue, reducing PTH production and release. The result is decreased serum calcium levels, stabilization of other minerals, and decreased progression of PTH-induced bone complications. Routine monitoring of calcium levels is required with this therapy.

For patients who have osteoporosis or risk of fracture and cannot or do not want surgery, bisphosphonates are preferred medications.

Patients not undergoing surgery should be counseled on regular exercise, adequate hydration, and avoiding lithium therapy (if taken) if possible (Janicak, 2023), as these can raise calcium levels. Additional teaching points should include avoiding prolonged bed rest and maintaining a diet with moderate amounts of calcium and vitamin D.

Preventing injury is important because the patient with chronic hyperparathyroidism often has significant bone density loss and is at risk for fragile fractures. Teach assistive personnel (AP) to handle the patient carefully and to use a lift sheet to reposition the patient rather than pulling.

Surgical Management. Surgical management of hyperparathyroidism is a parathyroidectomy and is typically curative, meaning that calcium levels return to normal.

The operative procedure can be performed as minimally invasive surgery (especially in the case of a single parathyroid adenoma) or with a traditional transverse incision in the lower neck (if more than one gland needs to be removed). All four parathyroid glands are examined for enlargement during exploration. If a tumor is present on one side but the other side is normal, the surgeon removes the glands containing tumor and leaves the remaining glands on the opposite side intact. If all four glands are diseased, they are all removed. The recurrent laryngeal nerve can be damaged during surgery but is a rare complication. Assess the patient for changes in voice patterns and hoarseness following the procedure.

Nursing care before and after surgical removal of the parathyroid glands is the same as that for thyroidectomy. See the Preoperative Care and Postoperative Care sections under Hyperthyroidism for specific nursing interventions.

NCLEX Examination Challenge 55.3

Health Promotion and Maintenance

A client with hyperparathyroidism is not a surgical candidate. Which of the following instructions would the nurse provide to enhance health maintenance? **Select all that apply.**

A. Regular exercise is important for bone strength.
B. Take bisphosphonates as directed to protect bones.
C. Take lithium as directed to lower calcium level.
D. Ensure proper hydration to help prevent kidney stone formation.
E. Eat a moderate number of foods that contain calcium and vitamin D.

Any remaining glands, which may have atrophied due to PTH overproduction, require several days to several weeks to return to normal function. A hypocalcemic crisis can occur during this critical period, and the serum calcium level must be assessed frequently after surgery. Check serum calcium levels whenever they are drawn until calcium levels stabilize. Monitor for indications of hypocalcemia, such as tingling and twitching in the extremities and face. Check for Trousseau and Chvostek signs, either of which indicates potential tetany (see Figs. 13.11 and 13.12 in Chapter 13). If interventions fail, this means that the resulting hypoparathyroidism is permanent, and the patient will need lifelong treatment with calcium and vitamin D.

GET READY FOR THE NEXT-GENERATION NCLEX® EXAMINATION!

Essential Nursing Care Points

Health Promotion/Disease Prevention

- Teach patients to report signs and symptoms associated with thyroid and parathyroid disorders to their health care provider. Although there is no way to prevent these conditions, early recognition and intervention are important to successful treatment and management.

Chronic Disease Care

- Teach all patients to take antithyroid drugs or thyroid hormone replacement therapy as prescribed. Emphasize which medications are prescribed as lifelong therapy.
- Monitor laboratory results, as well as patient signs and symptoms, as indicators of therapy effectiveness.

Regenerative or Restorative Care

- Keep emergency suctioning and tracheotomy equipment in the room of a patient who has had thyroid or parathyroid surgery.
- When stridor, dyspnea, or other symptoms of obstruction appear after thyroid surgery, notify the Rapid Response Team.
- When caring for a patient with hyperthyroidism, even after a thyroidectomy, immediately report a temperature increase of even 1°F (1.8°C) because it may indicate an impending thyroid crisis.
- Assess the cardiopulmonary status of any patient with hypothyroidism for decreased perfusion or decreased *gas exchange* at least every 8 hours.
- Carefully monitor the hydration status of patients who have hypercalcemia.
- Assess the patient with hypoparathyroidism for manifestations of hypocalcemia, especially numbness or tingling around the mouth and a positive Chvostek sign or Trousseau sign.

Hospice/Palliative/Supportive Care

- Although thyroid cancer is rarely fatal, provide referrals appropriately for patients who may be in need of palliative care or hospice.

Mastery Questions

1. A client has been diagnosed with hypothyroidism. Which instruction would the nurse include about hormone replacement therapy?
   A. Explain that this type of therapy will shrink a goiter.
   B. Take medication before bed with an evening snack.
   C. Report chest discomfort and palpitations to the health care provider.
   D. Hormone replacement therapy is stopped after a euthyroid state is achieved.

2. Which of the following symptoms in a client with untreated hypothyroidism would require the nurse to intervene **immediately? Select all that apply.**
   A. Sodium 149 mEq/L (149 mmol/L) (Reference range: 136–145 mEq/L [136–145 mmol/L])
   B. Blood pressure 130/88 mm Hg
   C. Blood glucose 118 mg/dL (6.6 mmol/L) (Reference range: 74–106 mg/dL [4.1–5.9 mmol/L])
   D. Temperature 97.2°F (36.2°C)
   E. Decreased level of consciousness

3. The nurse hears a client who is scheduled to receive radioactive iodine therapy discussing treatment with the client's partner. Which client statement would require the nurse to provide further teaching?
   A. "We shouldn't share the same toothpaste tube."
   B. "I am going to stay 6 feet away from anyone who is pregnant."
   C. "It will be necessary to work from home for a month after therapy."
   D. "Remind me to flush the toilet two to three times after each use when I am home."

NGN Challenge 55.1

The nurse is caring for a 44-year-old female client who comes to the health care provider reporting progressive symptoms of fatigue, constipation, cold intolerance, and weight gain. She reports no changes in her usual routines or relationships, yet has lost motivation and says she often feels sad.

Complete the diagram by selecting from the choices below to specify what potential condition the client is likely experiencing, **2** nursing actions that are appropriate to take, and **2** parameters the nurse should monitor to determine the effectiveness of nursing actions.

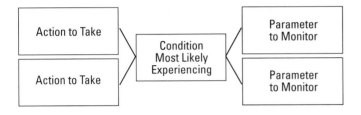

Actions to Take	Potential Conditions	Parameters to Monitor
Increase intake of fiber	Hypoparathyroidism	Urinary changes
Teach to take levo-thyroxine before bed	Hyperparathyroidism	Heart rate
Assess for Chvostek sign	Hypothyroidism	Fever
Teach family signs of myxedema coma	Hyperthyroidism	Development of dysrhythmias
Explain use of bisphosphonate therapy		Calcium levels

NGN Challenge 55.2

The nurse is preparing to care for a 33-year-old female client who has been seeing the primary health care provider for several months. Prior to assessing the client, the nurse reviews select laboratory findings.

Parameters	Results Today	Results Last Month	Results 4 Months Ago
Serum T_3 *Age 20–50 yr.* 70–205 ng/dL (1.2–3.4 nmol/L)	220 ng/dL (3.4 nmol/L)	212 ng/dL (3.3 nmol/L)	200 ng/dL (3.1 nmol/L)
Serum T_4 *Females:* 5–12 mcg/dL (71–142 nmol/L)	14 mcg/dL (180.2 nmol/L)	13 mcg/dL (167.3 nmol/L)	12 mcg/dL (154.5 nmol/L)
Free T_4 0.8–2.8 ng/dL (10–36 pmol/L)	3.4 ng/dL (43.8 pmol/L)	3.1 ng/dL (39.9 pmol/L)	2.9 ng/dL (37.3 pmol/L)
TSH 0.3–5 µU/mL (0.3–5 mU/L)	0.1 µU/mL (0.1 mU/L)	0.2 µU/mL (0.2 mU/L)	0.3 µU/mL (0.3 mU/L)

Complete the following sentences by selecting from the list of word choices below.

Based on the laboratory findings, the nurse expects that the client will have **[Word Choice]** and **[Word Choice]**.

Word Choices
Sleepiness
Exophthalmos
Weight gain
Bradycardia
Constipation
Vision impairment

REFERENCES

African American Wellness Project. (2023). *What Black communities should know about thyroid cancer.* https://aawellnessproject.org/what-black-communities-should-know-about-thyroid-disorders/.

American Cancer Society. (2019). *What is thyroid cancer?* https://www.cancer.org/cancer/thyroid-cancer/about/what-is-thyroid-cancer.html.

American Thyroid Association. (2023). *Older patients and thyroid disease.* https://www.thyroid.org/thyroid-disease-older-patient/.

Burman, K. (2021). Overview of thyroiditis. *UpToDate.* Retrieved June 5, 2023, from https://www.uptodate.com/contents/overview-of-thyroiditis.

Cleveland Clinic. (2023). *Graves' Disease.* https://my.clevelandclinic.org/health/diseases/15244-graves-disease.

Davies, T. (2021). Pathogenesis of Graves' disease. *UpToDate.* Retrieved June 5, 2023, from https://www.uptodate.com/contents/pathogenesis-of-graves-disease.

Davies, T. (2022). Pathogenesis of Hashimoto's thyroiditis (chronic autoimmune thyroiditis). *UpToDate.* Retrieved June 5, 2023, from https://www.uptodate.com/contents/pathogenesis-of-hashimotos-thyroiditis-chronic-autoimmune-thyroiditis.

Davies, T. (2023). Pretibial myxedema (thyroid dermopathy) in autoimmune thyroid disease. *UpToDate.* Retrieved June 5, 2023, from https://www.uptodate.com/contents/pretibial-myxedema-thyroid-dermopathy-in-autoimmune-thyroid-disease.

Duntas, L., & Jonklaas, J. (2021). COVID-19 and thyroid diseases: A bidirectional impact. *Journal of the Endocrine Society, 5*(8), bvab076. https://doi.org/10.1210/jendso/bvab076.

El-Hajj Fuleihan, G., & Silverberg, S. (2022). Primary hyperparathyroidism: diagnosis, differential diagnosis, and evaluation. *UpToDate.* Retrieved June 5, 2023, from https://www.uptodate.com/contents/primary-hyperparathyroidism-diagnosis-differential-diagnosis-and-evaluation.

Ellervik, C., Roselli, C., Christophersen, I., et al. (2019). Assessment of the relationship Between genetic determinants of thyroid function and atrial fibrillation: A Mendelian randomization study. *JAMA Cardiology, 4*(2), 144–152. https://doi.org/10.1001/jamacardio.2018.4635.

Gavryutina, I., Fordjour, L., & Chin, V. (2022). Genetics of thyroid disorders. *Endocrines, 3,* 198–213.

Haymart, M. (2022). Strategies for overcoming barriers to specialty care for thyroid disease and cancer. In *Presented at the ATA 2022 Annual Meeting; October 19-23, 2022; Montreal, QC.*

Janicak, P. (2023). Bipolar disorder in adults and lithium: Pharmacology, administration, and management of adverse effects. *UpToDate.* Retrieved June 5, 2023, from https://www.uptodate.com/contents/bipolar-disorder-in-adults-and-lithium-pharmacology-administration-and-management-of-adverse-effects.

Khalid, N., & Can, A. (2023). Plummer Disease. [Updated 2023 Mar 11]. In *StatPearls [Internet].* Treasure Island (FL): StatPearls Publishing. 2023. Available from: https://www.ncbi.nlm.nih.gov/books/NBK565856/.

Limaiem, F., Rehman, A., Anastasopoulou, C., et al. (2023). Papillary Thyroid Carcinoma. [Updated 2023 Jan 1]. In *StatPearls [Internet].* Treasure Island (FL): StatPearls Publishing. 2023. Available from: https://www.ncbi.nlm.nih.gov/books/NBK536943/.

National Cancer Institute. (2023a). *Differentiated thyroid cancer.* https://www.cancer.gov/publications/dictionaries/cancer-terms/def/differentiated-thyroid-cancer.

National Cancer Institute. (2023b). *Thyroid cancer.* https://www.cancer.gov/types/thyroid#.

Ross, D. (2022a). Diagnosis of and screening for hypothyroidism in nonpregnant adults. *UpToDate.* Retrieved June 5, 2023, from https://www.uptodate.com/contents/diagnosis-of-and-screening-for-hypothyroidism-in-nonpregnant-adults.

Ross, D. (2022b). Graves' hyperthyroidism in nonpregnant adults: overview of treatment. *UpToDate.* Retrieved June 5, 2023, from https://www.uptodate.com/contents/graves-hyperthyroidism-in-nonpregnant-adults-overview-of-treatment.

Ross, D. (2022c). Laboratory assessment of thyroid function. *UpToDate.* Retrieved June 5, 2023, from https://www.uptodate.com/contents/laboratory-assessment-of-thyroid-function.

Ross, D. (2022d). Overview and clinical manifestations of hyperthyroidism in adults. *UpToDate.* Retrieved March 25, 2023, from https://www.uptodate.com/contents/overview-of-the-clinical-manifestations-of-hyperthyroidism-in-adults.

Ross, D. (2023a). Myxedema coma. *UpToDate.* Retrieved June 5, 2023, from https://www.uptodate.com/contents/myxedema-coma.

Ross, D. (2023b). Treatment of primary hypothyroidism. *UpToDate.* Retrieved 3-25-23, from https://www.uptodate.com/contents/treatment-of-primary-hypothyroidism-in-adults.

Tuttle, R. M. (2022). Medullary thyroid cancer: Clinical manifestations, diagnosis, and staging. *UpToDate.* Retrieved June 5, 2023, from https://www.uptodate.com/contents/medullary-thyroid-cancer-clinical-manifestations-diagnosis-and-staging.

Tuttle, R. M., & Sherman, E. (2023). Anaplastic thyroid cancer. *UpToDate.* Retrieved June 5, 2023, from https://www.uptodate.com/contents/anaplastic-thyroid-cancer.

56

Concepts of Care for Patients With Diabetes Mellitus

Michelle L. Litchman and Julia E. Blanchette

http://evolve.elsevier.com/Iggy/

LEARNING OUTCOMES

1. Plan collaborative care with the interprofessional team to promote *glucose regulation* in patients with diabetes mellitus (DM).
2. Teach individuals at risk for impaired *glucose regulation* how to prevent or delay development of type 2 diabetes mellitus (T2DM).
3. Teach the patient and caregiver(s) about common drugs and other management strategies used for DM.
4. Plan patient- and family-centered nursing interventions to decrease the psychosocial impact of living with DM.
5. Apply knowledge of anatomy, physiology, and pathophysiology to provide evidence-based care for patients with DM affecting *glucose regulation.*
6. Analyze assessment and diagnostic findings to generate solutions and prioritize nursing care for patients with DM.
7. Organize care coordination and transition management for patients with DM.
8. Use clinical judgment to plan evidence-based nursing care to promote *glucose regulation* and prevent complications in patients with DM.
9. Incorporate factors that affect health equity into the plan of care for patients with DM.

KEY TERMS

diabetes mellitus (DM) A common, complex, chronic condition in which the ability to produce or utilize the hormone insulin is impaired, resulting in impaired glucose metabolism; can affect many body systems.

diabetic ketoacidosis (DKA) A severe acute complication of diabetes; characterized by uncontrolled hyperglycemia, metabolic acidosis, and increased production of ketones.

diabetic peripheral neuropathy (DPN) Progressive deterioration of nerve function with the loss of sensory perception.

gastroparesis A delay in gastric emptying.

glucagon A hormone produced by the pancreatic alpha cells that stimulates conversion of glycogen stored in the liver into glucose; it is important in glucose regulation and has balancing actions opposite those of insulin and prevents hypoglycemia.

gluconeogenesis Conversion of protein substances into glucose.

glucose regulation (also known as *glucose management)* Process of maintaining blood glucose levels.

glycogenesis Production and storage of glycogen.

glycogenolysis Breakdown of stored glycogen into glucose.

glycosylated hemoglobin (A1C) A standardized test that measures how much glucose attaches to the hemoglobin molecule; it is used to indicate effectiveness of blood glucose control measures.

hyperglycemia Higher-than-normal (or target) blood glucose.

hyperglycemic-hyperosmolar state (HHS) A severe acute hyperosmolar (increased blood osmolarity) state caused by severe dehydration and hyperglycemia.

hyperinsulinemia Chronically high blood insulin levels.

hypoglycemia Lower-than-normal (or target) blood glucose level.

ketogenesis Conversion of fats to acid products.

ketone bodies ("ketones") The acidic by-product formed when there is a lack of insulin and fatty acids are utilized as energy, leading to the acid-base balance problem of metabolic acidosis.

Kussmaul respiration A deep and rapid respiratory pattern triggered by acidosis to reduce blood hydrogen ion concentration by "blowing off" carbon dioxide; can occur in patients with severe DKA.

lipolysis Breakdown of body fats.

metabolic syndrome Simultaneous presence of metabolic factors that increase risk for developing type 2 diabetes mellitus (T2DM) and cardiovascular disease.

proliferative diabetic retinopathy Growth of new fragile retinal blood vessels (neovascularization) that bleed easily and obscure vision.

proteolysis Breakdown of body proteins.

PRIORITY AND INTERRELATED CONCEPTS

The priority concept for this chapter is:
* *Glucose Regulation*
  The *Glucose Regulation* concept exemplar for this chapter is Diabetes Mellitus.

The interrelated concepts for this chapter are:
* *Nutrition*
* *Tissue Integrity*
* *Sensory Perception*
* *Perfusion*
* *Immunity*
* *Fluid and Electrolyte Balance*
* *Acid-Base Balance*

GLUCOSE REGULATION CONCEPT EXEMPLAR: DIABETES MELLITUS

Diabetes mellitus (DM) is a common, complex, chronic condition in which the ability to produce or utilize the hormone insulin is impaired, resulting in impaired glucose metabolism, and can affect the function of all body systems. Although all nutrients are affected, *glucose regulation* is impaired first, which then changes protein and fat metabolism. Glucose regulation is the process of maintaining optimal blood glucose levels (Fig. 56.1). With impaired glucose regulation, many acute and chronic health problems occur as life-shortening complications. In the United States, about 11.3% of the overall population lives with diabetes (Centers for Disease Control and Prevention [CDC], 2022a). Yet, the percentage of hospitalized patients who have DM is over 40%, resulting in a large impact on health care costs and resources (Fingar & Reid, 2021). Therefore a major focus in diabetes care is to identify DM early, help the individual manage diabetes through glucose regulation, and prevent complications or progression of existing complications.

Nurses play a critical role in helping patients and families understand diabetes management. As part of the team, you will help plan, organize, and coordinate care with other team members to promote the patient's health and well-being. These management activities may take place in almost any setting. The desired outcome is to help patients maintain blood glucose levels in the target range *(euglycemia)* while minimizing hyperglycemia (higher than normal [or target] blood glucose levels) and hypoglycemia (lower than target blood glucose level) and maximizing quality of life.

Pathophysiology Review
Classification of Diabetes

Diabetes mellitus (DM) has many subtypes, and all have the main feature of impaired production and/or use of insulin. DM is classified according to the underlying insufficiency in pancreatic beta cell function. Box 56.1 outlines the types of DM. This chapter focuses on the two most common types of DM: type 1 diabetes mellitus (T1DM) and type 2 diabetes mellitus (T2DM). Regardless of the specific type of DM, the organ-damaging consequences and complications of impaired *glucose regulation* are the same.

The Endocrine Pancreas

The pancreas regulates digestion through its exocrine functions and ensures *glucose regulation* through its endocrine functions. The endocrine pancreas has about 1 million small glands, the islets of Langerhans, scattered through the organ. Inside the islets are two types of cells important to glucose regulation. These are the *alpha* cells, which secrete glucagon, and the *beta* cells, which produce insulin and amylin (Fig. 56.2).

Glucagon is a hormone that has balancing actions opposite those of insulin. It prevents *hypoglycemia* by triggering the release of glucose from storage sites in the liver and skeletal muscle. It is sometimes called the "hormone of starvation" because it is secreted when food intake is low to release glucose from the liver to regulate blood glucose levels.

Insulin prevents *hyperglycemia* by allowing body cells to take up, use, and store carbohydrates, fat, and protein. It is sometimes called the "hormone of plenty" because it is secreted when food intake is high and works to move glucose from the blood into cells to keep blood glucose levels in the normal range. Active insulin is a protein made up of 51 amino acids. It is first produced as inactive *proinsulin*, a prohormone that is converted in

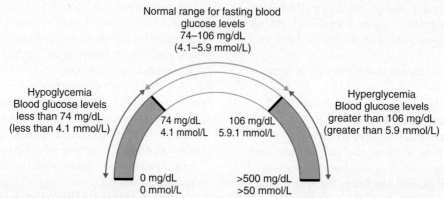

FIG. 56.1 Fasting blood glucose levels. When *glucose regulation* is adequate, fasting levels remain in the normal range. With insufficient insulin usage, hyperglycemia results. Excess insulin or insufficient glucose results in hypoglycemia.

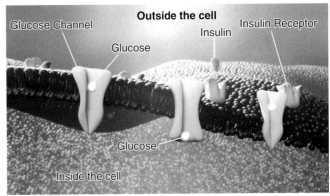

FIG. 56.3 Insulin attaches to receptors on target cells, where it promotes glucose transport into the cells through the cell membranes. (Copyright © Elsevier Animation Collection.)

Glucose Regulation and Homeostasis

Although glucose is a critical nutrient, chronic hyperglycemia contributes to many serious problems, and hypoglycemia can rapidly lead to injury or death. Therefore ***glucose regulation*** that maintains blood glucose levels within target range is important (see Fig. 56.1). Several organs and hormones play a role in maintaining glucose regulation. During fasting, when the stomach is empty, blood glucose is maintained by a balance between glucose uptake by cells and glucose production by the liver. Insulin plays a pivotal role in this process.

Glucose is the main fuel for central nervous system (CNS) cells. Because the brain cannot produce or store much glucose, it needs a continuous supply from the blood to prevent neuron dysfunction and cell death. Other organs can use both glucose and fatty acids to generate energy. Glucose is stored as glycogen in the liver and skeletal muscles, and free fatty acids (FFAs) are stored as triglycerides in fat cells. During a prolonged fast or after illness, proteins are broken down, and some of the amino acids are converted into glucose.

Insulin exerts many effects on metabolism and cellular processes in all tissues and organs. The main metabolic effects of insulin are to stimulate glucose uptake in skeletal muscle and heart muscle and to suppress liver production of glucose and very-low-density lipoprotein (VLDL). In the liver, insulin promotes the production and storage of glycogen (glycogenesis) at the same time that it inhibits glycogen breakdown into glucose (glycogenolysis). It increases protein and lipid (fat) synthesis and inhibits ketogenesis (conversion of fats to acids) and gluconeogenesis (conversion of proteins to glucose). In muscle, insulin promotes protein and glycogen synthesis. In fat cells, it promotes triglyceride storage. Overall, insulin keeps blood glucose levels from becoming too high.

In the *fasting state* (not eating for 8 or more hours), insulin secretion is suppressed, which leads to increased gluconeogenesis in the liver and kidneys, along with increased glucose generation by the breakdown of liver glycogen. In the nonfasting state, insulin released from pancreatic beta cells reverses this process. Instead, glycogen breakdown and gluconeogenesis are inhibited. At the same time, insulin also enhances glucose uptake and use by cells and reduces both body fat breakdown (lipolysis) and body protein breakdown (proteolysis). When

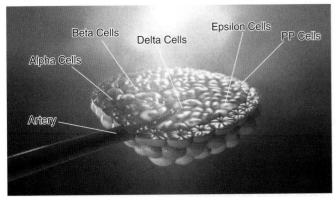

FIG. 56.2 Hormone-secreting cells of the islets of Langerhans in the pancreas. Alpha cells secrete glucagon; beta cells secrete insulin. *PP cells*, Pancreatic polypeptide cells. (Copyright © Elsevier Animation Collection.)

the liver to active insulin. Movement of glucose into most cells requires the presence of specific membrane receptors along with insulin. Insulin is like a "key" that opens "locked" membranes to glucose, allowing blood glucose to move into cells to generate energy. Insulin starts this action by binding to membrane insulin receptors, which changes membrane permeability to glucose (Fig. 56.3).

Insulin is secreted daily in a two-step manner, with low-level secretion during fasting (basal insulin secretion) and a two-phase release after eating *(prandial)*. An early burst of insulin secretion occurs within 10 minutes of eating, followed by an increasing release that lasts until the blood glucose regulates.

more glucose is present in liver cells than can be used for energy or stored as glycogen, insulin causes the excess glucose to be converted to free fatty acids (FFAs). These extra FFAs are deposited in fat cells.

Glucose in the blood after a meal is maintained by the emptying rate of the stomach and delivery of nutrients to the small intestine, where they are absorbed into circulation. *Incretin hormones* (e.g., *glucagon-like peptide 1 [GLP-1]*), secreted in response to food in the stomach, have several actions. They increase insulin secretion, inhibit glucagon secretion, and slow the rate of gastric emptying, thereby preventing hyperglycemia after meals.

Balancing *(counterregulatory)* hormones increase blood glucose by actions opposite those of insulin when more energy is needed. Glucagon is the main balancing hormone. Other hormones that increase blood glucose levels are epinephrine, norepinephrine, growth hormone, and cortisol. The combined actions of insulin and balancing hormones (discussed in the next section) participate in **glucose regulation** and keep blood glucose levels within the target range to support brain function. When blood glucose levels fall, insulin secretion stops and glucagon is released. Glucagon causes glucose release from the liver. Liver glucose is made through breakdown of glycogen to glucose and conversion of amino acids into glucose. When liver glucose is unavailable, the breakdown of body fat and the breakdown of body proteins, especially muscle, provide acids as fuel for energy.

Absence of Insulin

Glucose regulation requires insulin to move glucose into many body tissues. The lack of insulin action in DM, from either a lack of production or a problem with insulin use at its cell receptors, prevents some cells from using glucose for energy. The body then breaks down fat and protein in an attempt to provide energy and increases levels of balancing hormones to make glucose from other sources. Box 56.2 outlines responses to insufficient insulin.

Without insulin, glucose builds up in the blood, causing hyperglycemia, which disturbs **fluid and electrolyte balance,** leading to the classic symptoms of diabetes: polyuria, polydipsia, and polyphagia.

Polyuria is frequent and excessive urination and results from an osmotic diuresis caused by excess glucose in the urine. With diuresis, electrolytes are excreted in the urine, and water loss is severe. Dehydration results and *polydipsia* (excessive thirst) occurs. Because the cells receive no glucose, cell starvation

triggers *polyphagia* (excessive eating). Despite eating, the adult with untreated diabetes remains in metabolic starvation until insulin is available to move glucose into the cells.

With insulin deficiency, the body turns to stored fat for energy, releasing free fatty acids (FFAs). When this stored fat is used for energy, small ketone bodies provide a backup energy source. Ketone bodies ("ketones") are the acidic by-product formed when there is a lack of insulin and fatty acids are utilized as energy, leading to the **acid-base balance** problem of metabolic acidosis.

Dehydration with DM leads to *hemoconcentration* (increased blood concentration); *hypovolemia* (decreased blood volume); poor tissue **perfusion**; and *hypoxia* (poor tissue oxygenation), especially to the brain. Hypoxic cells do not metabolize glucose efficiently, the Krebs cycle is blocked, and lactic acid production increases, causing more acidosis.

The excess acids caused by absence of insulin increase hydrogen ion (H^+) and carbon dioxide (CO_2) levels in the blood, causing anion-gap metabolic acidosis. These products trigger the brain to increase the rate and depth of respiration in an attempt to "blow off" carbon dioxide and acid. This type of breathing is known as Kussmaul respiration. Acetone is exhaled, giving the breath a "citrus fruit" odor. When the lungs can no longer offset acidosis, the blood pH drops. Arterial blood gas studies show a *metabolic acidosis* (decreased pH with decreased arterial bicarbonate [HCO_3^-] levels) and *compensatory respiratory alkalosis* (decreased partial pressure of arterial carbon dioxide [$Paco_2$]).

Lack of insulin causes fluid and electrolyte imbalance, with potassium being most affected. With the increased fluid loss from hyperglycemia, excessive potassium is excreted in the urine, leading to low serum potassium levels. High serum potassium levels may occur in acidosis because of the shift of potassium from inside the cells to the blood in exchange for hydrogen ions. Serum potassium levels in DM, then, may be low *(hypokalemia),* high *(hyperkalemia),* or normal, depending on hydration, the severity of acidosis, and the patient's response to treatment. Chapter 14 discusses **acid-base balance** and acidosis in more detail.

NCLEX Examination Challenge 56.1
Physiological Integrity

The nurse is caring for a healthy adult client who has been NPO for 12 hours. Which of the following physiologic processes work to directly prevent severe hypoglycemia? **Select all that apply.**

A. Gluconeogenesis
B. Glycogenesis
C. Glycogenolysis
D. Ketogenesis
E. Lipogenesis

BOX 56.2   Physiologic Responses to Insufficient Insulin

- Decreased glycogenesis (conversion of glucose to glycogen)
- Increased glycogenolysis (conversion of glycogen to glucose)
- Increased gluconeogenesis (formation of glucose from noncarbohydrate sources such as amino acids and lactate)
- Increased lipolysis (breakdown of triglycerides to glycerol and free fatty acids)
- Increased ketogenesis (formation of ketones from free fatty acids)
- Proteolysis (breakdown of protein with amino acid release in muscles)

Acute Complications of Diabetes

Three glucose-related emergencies can occur in patients with DM:

- Diabetic ketoacidosis (DKA) caused by absence of insulin and generation of ketoacids.

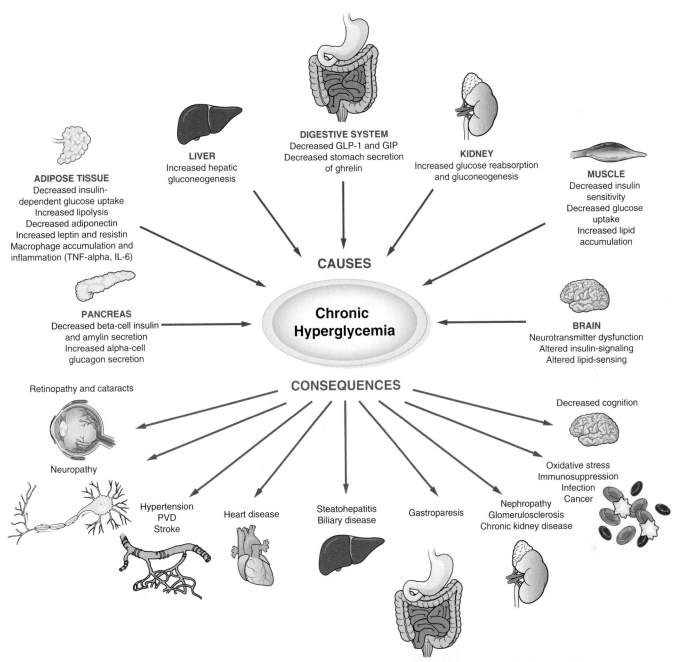

FIG. 56.4 Multiorgan causes and common consequences of chronic hyperglycemia in type 2 diabetes. *GIP, Glucose-dependent insulinotropic polypeptide; GLP-1,* glucagon-like peptide 1; *IL,* interleukin; *PVD,* peripheral vascular disease; *TNF,* tumor necrosis factor. (From Rogers, J. L. (2023). *McCance and Huether's Pathophysiology: The biologic basis for disease in adults and children* [9th ed.]. St. Louis: Elsevier.)

- Hyperglycemic-hyperosmolar state (HHS) caused by severe dehydration and insulin deficiency.
- Hypoglycemia commonly caused by too much insulin, too few carbohydrates, or increased physical activity. Blood glucose <70 mg/dL should be treated quickly to prevent a hypoglycemic emergency.

All three problems require emergency treatment and can be fatal if treatment is delayed or incorrect. These glucose-related emergencies and their management are described later in this chapter.

Chronic Complications of Diabetes

Changes in large blood vessels *(macrovascular)* and small blood vessels *(microvascular)* in tissues and organs result from chronic hyperglycemia and can lead to organ complications and early death (Fig. 56.4). These blood vessel changes lead to complications from poor tissue **perfusion** and tissue ischemia. Macrovascular complications include coronary heart disease, cerebrovascular disease, and peripheral vascular disease, all of which increase the risk of early morbidity and mortality. Microvascular complications of blood vessel structure and function lead to *nephropathy* (kidney dysfunction), *neuropathy* (nerve dysfunction), and *retinopathy* (vision problems). Such problems are responsible for increased morbidity and reduced quality of life. Causes of these diabetic vascular complications include:

- Chronic hyperglycemia thickens basement membranes, which causes organ damage.
- Glucose toxicity directly or indirectly affects functional cell integrity.
- Chronic ischemia in small blood vessels causes tissue hypoxia and microischemia.

Chronic hyperglycemia is the main cause of microvascular complications and allows premature development of macrovascular complications. Additional risk factors contributing to poor health outcomes for adults with DM include smoking, physical inactivity, obesity, hypertension, and hyperlipidemia.

Chronic hyperglycemia from poor **glucose regulation** leads to long-term complications. Intensive therapy to maintain optimal glycemic control can delay the onset and progression of retinopathy, nephropathy, neuropathy, and macrovascular disease. For every percentage point decrease in glycosylated hemoglobin (A1C), a significant reduction in kidney and eye complications can occur.

Macrovascular Complications

Cardiovascular Disease. Patients with diabetes, prediabetes, or metabolic syndrome are at increased risk for cardiovascular disease (CVD) (Rariden, 2019; Rogers, 2023). Because DM is so strongly associated with CVD, it is a target for aggressive CVD risk factor reduction.

Patients with diabetes, especially type 2 diabetes mellitus (T2DM), often have traditional CVD risk factors such as obesity, hyperlipidemia, and hypertension. Cigarette smoking and family history also increase the risk for CVD. Kidney disease, indicated by *albuminuria* (presence of albumin in the urine and elevated albumin-to-creatinine ratio), and retinopathy are associated with increased risk for coronary disease and mortality from coronary artery disease.

Cardiovascular complication rates can be reduced through aggressive management of hypertension, hyperglycemia, and hyperlipidemia. The American Diabetes Association (ADA) recommends that blood pressure be maintained below 140/90 mm Hg, with a target of 120/80 mm Hg in younger adults if that level can be achieved without excessive burden. Lipid profile screening is recommended starting at first diagnosis, every 5 years thereafter if under the age of 40, or every 1 to 2 years thereafter. Patients with DM who do not have overt CVD are recommended to maintain low-density lipoprotein (LDL) cholesterol below 100 mg/dL (2.60 mmol/L), and patients with indications of CVD are recommended to maintain LDL at less than 70 mg/dL (1.8 mmol/L) (ADA, 2022). Increasing intake of omega-3 fatty acids, fiber, and plant sterols; weight loss (if indicated); and increasing physical activity are recommended for all patients living with diabetes (ADA, 2022).

Priority nursing activities focus on interventions to reduce modifiable risk factors associated with CVD. Modifiable risk factors include smoking cessation, stress management, balanced diet, physical activity, blood pressure management, and

maintaining prescribed lipid-lowering drug therapy and aspirin use.

Cerebrovascular Disease. The risk for stroke is two to four times higher in adults with DM compared with those who do not have DM (Rogers, 2023). Diabetes also increases the likelihood of severe carotid atherosclerosis. Hypertension, hyperlipidemia, nephropathy, peripheral vascular disease, and alcohol and tobacco use further increase the risk for stroke in adults with DM.

Reduced Immunity. The combination of vascular changes and hyperglycemia reduces **immunity** by reducing white blood cell activity, inhibiting gas exchange in tissues, and promoting the growth of microorganisms. As a result, any adult who has DM is at an increased risk for developing an infection on exposure to bacteria and other organisms. In addition, infections become serious more quickly and can lead to major complications and sepsis (Rogers, 2023).

Microvascular Complications

Eye and Vision Complications. Blindness is 25 times more common in patients with DM. Diabetic retinopathy (DR) is strongly related to the duration of diabetes. After 20 years of DM, nearly all patients with the disease have some degree of retinopathy (ADA, 2022). Unfortunately, DR has few symptoms until vision loss occurs.

DR is related to problems that block retinal blood vessels and cause them to leak, leading to retinal hypoxia. Nonproliferative diabetic retinopathy causes structural problems in retinal vessels with areas of poor retinal circulation, edema, hard fatty deposits in the eye, and retinal hemorrhages. Fluid and blood leak from the vessels and cause retinal edema and hard exudates. Nonproliferative DR develops slowly and rarely reduces vision to the point of blindness.

Proliferative diabetic retinopathy is the growth of new retinal blood vessels, also known as *neovascularization*. When retinal blood flow is poor and hypoxia develops, retinal cells secrete growth factors that stimulate formation of new blood vessels in the eye. These new vessels are thin and fragile and bleed easily, leading to vision loss.

Visual **sensory perception** loss from DR has several mechanisms. Central vision may be impaired by macular edema with increased blood vessel permeability and deposits of hard exudates at the center of the retina. This problem is the main cause of vision loss in the adult with DM. Vision loss also occurs from macular degeneration, corneal scarring, and changes in lens shape or clarity.

Hyperglycemia may cause blurred vision, even with eyeglasses. Because hyperglycemia can cause temporary vision changes, it is important to wait until blood glucose levels are normal before assessing for refractory changes. Cataracts occur at a younger age and progress faster among patients with DM. Open-angle glaucoma also is more common in patients with DM. The management of cataracts and glaucoma is discussed in Chapter 39.

Keeping blood glucose, blood pressure, and lipid levels within target ranges are important in the prevention of DR. Therefore people with DM should have routine ophthalmic evaluations to detect vision problems early before vision loss occurs.

PATIENT-CENTERED CARE: OLDER ADULT HEALTH

Diabetic Retinopathy

Older patients with diabetic retinopathy also have general age-related vision changes, which may reduce the ability to perform self-care. They may have blurred vision, distorted central vision, fluctuating vision, and loss of color perception. Assess the ability of patients with vision changes to prepare and inject insulin and to monitor blood glucose levels to determine if adaptive devices are needed to assist in self-management (Touhy & Jett, 2023).

Diabetic Peripheral Neuropathy. Diabetic peripheral neuropathy (DPN) is a progressive deterioration of nerve function that results in loss of *sensory perception*. DPN is a common complication of DM and often involves all body areas. Damage to sensory nerve fibers results first in pain, which is eventually followed by loss of sensation. Damage to motor nerve fibers results in muscle weakness. The onset is slow, and the disorder affects both sides of the body, progresses, and is permanent. Late complications include foot ulcers and deformities. Damage to nerve fibers in the autonomic nervous system can cause dysfunction in every organ. The combination of factors leading to the nerve damage in diabetic neuropathy consists of:

- Chronic hyperglycemia, hyperlipidemia
- Damaged blood vessels leading to reduced neuronal oxygen and other nutrients
- Increased genetic susceptibility to nerve damage
- Smoking, nicotine, and alcohol use

Chronic hyperglycemia leads to DPN through blood vessel changes and reduced tissue *perfusion* that cause nerve hypoxia, which leads to poor nerve impulse transmission. Excessive glucose is converted to sorbitol, which collects in nerves and impairs motor nerve conduction (Rogers, 2023). Common diabetic neuropathies are listed in Table 56.1.

Diabetic Autonomic Neuropathy. Cardiovascular autonomic neuropathy (CAN) affects sympathetic and parasympathetic nerves of the heart and blood vessels. This problem is underdiagnosed in diabetes and contributes to left ventricular dysfunction, painless myocardial infarction (MI), and exercise intolerance (Wooton & Melchior, 2020). Most often, CAN leads to *orthostatic* (postural) hypotension and *syncope* (brief loss of consciousness on standing). These problems result from failure of the heart and arteries to respond to position changes by increasing heart rate and vascular tone. As a result, blood flow to the brain is interrupted briefly. Orthostatic hypotension and syncope increase the risk for falls, especially among older adults (Touhy & Jett, 2023).

Autonomic neuropathy can affect the entire GI system. Common GI problems from diabetic neuropathy include gastroesophageal reflex, delayed gastric emptying and gastric retention, early satiety, heartburn, nausea, vomiting, and anorexia (see Table 56.1). Sluggish movement of the small intestine can lead to bacterial overgrowth, which causes bloating, gas, and both diarrhea and constipation. Constipation, the most common GI problem with DM, is intermittent and may alternate with bouts of diarrhea. Gastroparesis (delay in gastric emptying) is a cause of hypoglycemia related to the mismatch of nutrient absorption and insulin action.

Urinary problems from neuropathy cause incomplete bladder emptying and urine retention, which leads to urinary infection and kidney problems. Early symptoms include frequency and urgency. Later symptoms are inability to sense bladder fullness and incontinence.

Diabetic Nephropathy. *Nephropathy* is a pathologic change in the kidney that reduces kidney function and leads to kidney failure. Diabetes is the leading cause of end-stage kidney disease (ESKD) and kidney failure in the United States. Risk factors include chronic hyperglycemia, hypertension, and genetic predisposition. Kidney disease causes progressive albumin excretion and declining glomerular filtration rate (GFR). The onset of diabetic kidney disease may be delayed or prevented by maintaining optimal blood *glucose regulation* (ADA, 2022).

Chronic hyperglycemia can cause hypertension in kidney blood vessels and excess kidney tissue *perfusion.* The blood vessels become leakier, especially in the glomerulus, allowing filtration of albumin and other proteins that deposit in the kidney tissues and blood vessels. Narrowed blood vessels decrease kidney oxygenation, leading to kidney cell hypoxia and cell death, which can progress to chronic kidney disease (see Chapter 60 for a detailed presentation of chronic kidney disease and end-stage kidney disease). Hypertension speeds the progression of diabetic nephropathy.

Sexual Dysfunction. Sexual dysfunction can develop in people with DM as a result of damage to both nerve tissue and vascular tissue. This is made worse by poorly controlled blood glucose levels. Other factors include obesity, hypertension, tobacco use, and some prescribed drugs.

In males, sexual dysfunction manifests with both erectile dysfunction (ED) and retrograde ejaculation. Females may experience decreased vaginal lubrication, uncomfortable or painful sexual intercourse, and decreases in libido and sexual response.

Cognitive Dysfunction. Older adults with DM are at higher risk for developing all types of dementia compared with adults who do not have DM (ADA, 2022). Chronic hyperglycemia with microvascular disease contribute to neuron damage, brain atrophy, and cognitive impairment. These problems are more frequent and more severe in patients with longer-duration DM and increase the complications of neuropathy and retinopathy.

Etiology and Genetic Risk

Type 1 Diabetes. Type 1 diabetes mellitus (T1DM) is an autoimmune disorder in which the pancreatic beta cells are destroyed (Table 56.2). The immune system fails to recognize normal body cells as "self," and immune system cells and antibodies take destructive actions against the insulin-secreting cells in the islets. Viral infections, such as mumps, coxsackievirus infection, and COVID-19, may trigger autoimmune destructive actions.

Type 2 Diabetes and Metabolic Syndrome. Type 2 diabetes mellitus (T2DM) is a progressive disorder in which the person initially has insulin resistance that progresses to decreased

TABLE 56.1	**Features of Diabetic Neuropathy**	
	Complication	**Symptom**
Distal symmetric polyneuropathy	Sensory alterations	Paresthesias: burning/tingling sensations, starting in toes and moving up legs
		Dysesthesias: burning, stinging, or stabbing pain
		Anesthesia: loss of sensation
	Motor alterations in intrinsic muscles of foot	Foot deformities: high arch, claw toes, hammertoes; shift of weight bearing to metatarsal heads and tips of toes
Autonomic neuropathy	Anhidrosis	Drying, cracking of skin
	GI conditions	Gastroparesis: delayed gastric emptying; gastric retention, early satiety, bloating, nausea, vomiting, anorexia, constipation, diarrhea, diffuse sweating while eating, nocturnal diarrhea
	Neurogenic bladder	Atonic bladder, urinary retention
	Sexual dysfunction	Erectile dysfunction
	Cardiovascular autonomic neuropathy (CAN)	Early fatigue, weakness with exercise, orthostatic hypotension
	Defective balancing hormones	Loss of warning signs of hypoglycemia

TABLE 56.2	**Differentiation of Type 1 and Type 2 Diabetes**	
Features	**Type 1**	**Type 2**
Former names	Juvenile-onset diabetes	Adult-onset diabetes
	Ketosis-prone diabetes	Ketosis-resistant diabetes
	Insulin-dependent diabetes mellitus (IDDM)	Non–insulin-dependent diabetes mellitus (NIDDM)
Age at onset	Usually younger than 30 yr	May occur at any age in adults
Symptoms	Abrupt onset, thirst, hunger, increased urine output, weight loss	Frequently none; thirst, fatigue, blurred vision, vascular or neural complications
Etiology	Viral infection, autoimmunity	Not known, genetic predisposition
Pathology	Pancreatic beta cell destruction	Insulin resistance
		Dysfunctional pancreatic beta cells
Inheritance	Complex	Autosomal dominant, multifactorial
Nutritional status	Same obesity prevalence as general adult population	60%–80% obese
Insulin	All dependent on insulin	Required for 20%–30%

PATIENT-CENTERED CARE: GENETICS/GENOMICS

Type 1 Diabetes Mellitus (T1DM)

Inheritance of certain genes and tissue types increases the risk for T1DM (Rogers, 2023). However, inheritance of these genes only *increases the risk,* and most people with these specific tissue types do ***not*** develop T1DM. Development of diabetes is an interactive effect of genetic predisposition and exposure to certain environmental factors. During assessment, always ask whether any family members have been diagnosed with either type 1 or type 2 diabetes or any other autoimmune disorder.

beta cell secretion of insulin. *Insulin resistance* (a reduced cell receptor response to insulin) often develops in a genetically susceptible adult (ADA, 2022). It occurs before the onset of T2DM and often is accompanied by the cardiovascular risk factors of hyperlipidemia, hypertension, and increased clot formation. The specific causes are not known, although insulin resistance and beta cell failure have many genetic and nongenetic causes. Heredity plays a major role in the development of T2DM, although not all gene variations that increase the risk for T2DM are known. Environment, such as neighborhood safety and walkability, food security, air quality, and overall access to health care are also factors in the development of T2DM.

Metabolic syndrome (Fig. 56.5) is the simultaneous presence of metabolic factors that increase risk for developing T2DM and cardiovascular disease. Features of the syndrome include:

- Abdominal obesity: waist circumference of 40 inches (100 cm) or more for men and 35 inches (88 cm) or more for women
- Hyperglycemia: fasting blood glucose (FBG) level of 100 mg/dL or more or on drug treatment for elevated blood glucose levels
- Hypertension: systolic blood pressure of 140 mm Hg or more or diastolic blood pressure of 90 mg Hg or more or on drug treatment for hypertension
- Hyperlipidemia: triglyceride level of 150 mg/dL or more or on drug treatment for elevated triglycerides; high-density lipoprotein (HDL) cholesterol less than 40 mg/dL for men or less than 50 mg/dL for women

Any of these health problems also increase the rate of atherosclerosis and the risk for stroke, CVD, and early death.

Incidence and Prevalence

In the United States, more than 37.3 million people are living with DM, and of those people 23% (8.5 million) are undiagnosed. Another 96 million have prediabetes (CDC, 2022a). *Prediabetes* is defined as impaired fasting glucose (IFG) or an

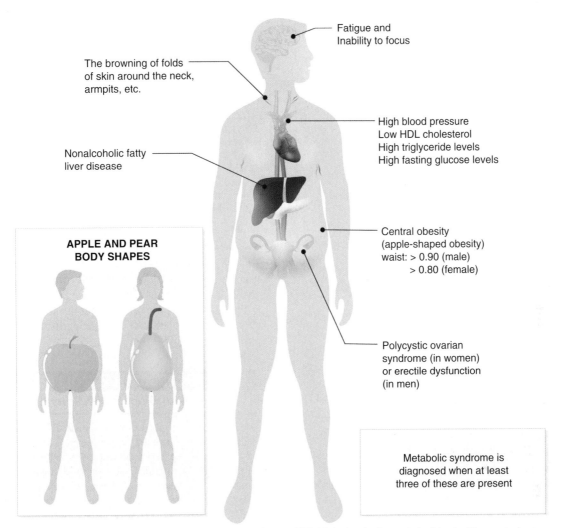

The symptoms of metabolic syndrome

Fatigue and Inability to focus

The browning of folds of skin around the neck, armpits, etc.

Nonalcoholic fatty liver disease

High blood pressure
Low HDL cholesterol
High triglyceride levels
High fasting glucose levels

Central obesity
(apple-shaped obesity)
waist: > 0.90 (male)
      > 0.80 (female)

Polycystic ovarian syndrome (in women) or erectile dysfunction (in men)

APPLE AND PEAR BODY SHAPES

Metabolic syndrome is diagnosed when at least three of these are present

FIG. 56.5 Signs and symptoms of metabolic syndrome. *HDL,* High-density lipoprotein. (Used with permission from istockphoto.com, 2015, ttsz.)

A1C between 5.7 and 6.4, or impaired glucose tolerance (IGT). Over a 3- to 5-year period, adults with prediabetes have a 5-fold to 15-fold higher risk for developing T2DM than do those with in-range blood glucose levels. In Canada, about 5.7 million adults have diabetes (Diabetes Canada, 2022).

About 90% to 95% of adults with diabetes have T2DM (CDC, 2022a). T2DM can be diagnosed even in preadolescents but is more common among middle-age and older adults, affecting about 12.3% of adults over the age of 20 years and 25.9% of adults age 65 years or older (Touhy & Jett, 2023). With the prevalence of obesity rising in North America, diabetes is likely to become even more common (ADA, 2022).

PATIENT-CENTERED CARE: VETERAN HEALTH

Addition Risk for Type 2 Diabetes Mellitus (T2DM)

Diabetes affects almost 25% of the veteran population (U.S. Department of Veterans Affairs, 2019). A possible additional risk factor for T2DM is exposure to the main component of Agent Orange, dioxin, which was used during the military conflicts in Korea and Vietnam. The risk for T2DM appears higher among U.S. military members who were assigned to those geographic areas (U.S. Department of Veterans Affairs, 2016).

Assess veterans who were exposed to Agent Orange at every health care visit for indications of diabetes so that early interventions can be implemented. Encourage veterans to use diabetes prevention strategies of maintaining a healthy weight, eating a balanced diet, and engaging in regular physical activity.

PATIENT-CENTERED CARE: HEALTH EQUITY

Screening for Diabetes Mellitus (DM)

Racially and ethnically diverse populations have a higher prevalence and greater burden of type 2 diabetes mellitus (T2DM). The rate of DM is 14.5% among American Indians and Alaska Natives, 12.1% among non-Hispanic Blacks, 11.8% among those with Hispanic origin, 9.5% among non-Hispanic Asians, and 7.4% among non-Hispanic Whites (CDC, 2022a). Be alert to the risk for DM whenever you are interviewing or assessing adults. The American Diabetes Association (ADA) has identified indications for asymptomatic screening. Be familiar with these screening indications and advocate for early screening to promote early intervention for all adults (Box 56.3).

BOX 56.3 Indications for Screening Asymptomatic Adults

- Testing for diabetes is considered at any age in adults with a BMI greater than 25 kg/m² (or greater than 23 kg/m² in Asian Americans) with one or more of these additional risk factors:
  - First-degree relative with diabetes
  - Physically inactive
  - Member of a high-risk ethnic population (e.g., African American, Latino, Native American, Asian American, or Pacific Islander)
  - Hypertensive (>140/90 mm Hg or on therapy for hypertension)
  - High-density lipoprotein (HDL) cholesterol level less than 35 mg/dL (0.90 mmol/L) and/or a triglyceride level greater than 250 mg/dL (2.82 mmol/L)
  - Polycystic ovary syndrome
  - History of cardiovascular disease
- Patients with prediabetes (A1C ≥5.7% [39 mmol/mol], impaired glucose tolerance, or impaired fasting glucose) should be tested yearly.
- Females diagnosed with GDM should have lifelong testing every 3 years.
- For all other patients, testing should begin at age 35. If results are normal, testing should be repeated at a minimum of 3-year intervals

BMI, Body mass index; *GDM,* gestational diabetes mellitus.
Data from American Diabetes Association (ADA). (2022). Classification and diagnosis of diabetes: Standards of medical care in diabetes—2022. *Diabetes Care, 42*(Suppl. 1): S144–S174.

Health Promotion/Disease Prevention

Diabetes mellitus can contribute to many devastating complications. Managing blood glucose and reducing associated complications are a major focus for health promotion activities. No current interventions or commercially available medications prevent T1DM, but health promotion activities that focus on managing hyperglycemia can reduce the risk of long-term complications.

Adopting a lifestyle that includes a balanced diet, regular physical activity, and weight loss, if applicable, can reduce metabolic and cardiac risk factors and can prevent or delay the onset of T2DM (ADA, 2022). Actions to reduce these risk factors include reducing hypertension, increasing heart rate variability between resting rate and exercise rate, lowering triglyceride levels, increasing high-density lipoprotein (HDL) cholesterol ("healthy" cholesterol) levels, and reducing low-density lipoprotein (LDL) cholesterol ("bad" cholesterol) levels. Smoking cessation and avoidance of excess alcohol consumption also are important in preventing complications of DM.

Teach patients with DM that keeping their blood glucose levels within prescribed target ranges can prevent or delay complications. Encourage them to regularly follow up with their primary health care provider or diabetes health care provider, to have their eyes and vision tested yearly by an ophthalmologist, and to have urine albumin levels assessed yearly. Early detection of changes in the eye or kidney allows adjustments in treatment plans that can slow or halt the progression of retinopathy and nephropathy. Encourage adults to maintain an appropriate weight range for height and body build and to engage in physical activity for at least 150 minutes per week (ADA, 2022). Encourage daily foot inspection and the prompt reporting of ulcers or open areas to the primary health care provider.

PATIENT-CENTERED CARE: HEALTH EQUITY

Increasing Access to Diabetes Prevention

The Centers for Disease Control and Prevention (CDC, 2022b) has launched a national diabetes prevention program that is focused on lifestyle change for people with prediabetes. The goal of this program is to reach communities with fewer resources. The program provides an affordable option to work with a health coach to increase physical activity, make better food choices, and develop stress-reduction strategies. Be aware of resources that are available to promote access and remove barriers to care for patients with prediabetes. This is a critical step in promoting health equity. Visit the CDC website for locations and providers that are part of this national access initiative.

Interprofessional Collaborative Care

Although adults who have DM may be hospitalized for complications of DM, the diagnosis and management generally occur in a clinic or health care provider's office. Much of the essential education about management is performed in the community, as is the overall management. Because DM is a chronic condition and may predispose one to other health problems, you can expect to interact with and care for patients with DM in any health care setting.

INTERPROFESSIONAL COLLABORATION

The Patient With Diabetes Mellitus (DM)

The complicated and chronic nature of DM requires the coordination of an interprofessional team approach for optimal outcomes. The interprofessional team members to help patients achieve desired outcomes include primary health care providers, endocrinologists, diabetes-specialist advanced practice nurses, physician associates, certified diabetes care and education specialists (CDCESs), ophthalmologists, registered nurses, pharmacists, registered dietitian nutritionists (RDNs), podiatrists, physical therapists, and wound care specialists.

Recognize Cues: Assessment

History. Ask about risk factors and symptoms related to DM. Ask females how large their children were at birth, because many females who develop T2DM had gestational diabetes mellitus (GDM) or glucose intolerance during pregnancy (ADA, 2022). Teach females with a history of GDM and those who have prediabetes about lifestyle changes and screening to prevent and detect DM (ADA, 2022).

Assessing weight and weight change is important because excess weight and obesity are risk factors for T2DM. The patient with T1DM often has weight loss with increased appetite during the weeks before diagnosis, but this may also occur in cases of T2DM. For both types of DM, patients usually have fatigue, polyuria, and polydipsia. Ask about recent major or minor infections and assess overall *immunity.* Ask females about frequent vaginal yeast infections. Assess whether they have noticed that small skin injuries become infected more easily or take longer to heal. Also, ask whether they have noticed any changes in vision or in the sense of touch.

TABLE 56.3 Laboratory Profile
Diabetes Mellitus

Test	Normal Range	Prediabetes	Diabetes
Glycosylated hemoglobin (A1C)	4%–5.7% (20–39 mmol/mol)	5.7%–6.4% (39–47 mmol/mol)	≥6.5% (48 mmol/mol)
Fasting blood glucose	74–100 mg/dL (4.1–5.6 mmol/L)	100–125 mg/dL (5.6–6.9 mmol/mol)	≥126 mg/dL (7.0 mmol/mol)
Glucose tolerance (2-hour postprandial glucose [PPG])	<140 mg/dL (<7.8 mmol/L)	140–199 mg/dL (7.8–11.0 mmol/mol)	≥200 mg/dL (11.1 mmol/mol)

Data from American Diabetes Association Standards of Medical Care Abridged for Primary Care Providers (2022) and Pagana, K., Pagana, T. & Pagana, T. (2022). *Mosby's manual of diagnostic and laboratory tests* (7th ed.). St. Louis: Elsevier.

BOX 56.4 Criteria for the Diagnosis of Diabetes

A1C >6.5% (48 mmol/mol). The test should be performed in a laboratory using a method that is NGSP certified and standardized to the DCCT assay.[a]

OR

Fasting blood glucose greater than or equal to 126 mg/dL (7.0 mmol/L). *Fasting* is defined as no caloric intake for at least 8 hours.[a]

OR

Two-hour blood glucose equal to or greater than 200 mg/dL (11.1 mmol/L) during oral glucose tolerance testing. The test should be performed using a glucose load containing the equivalent of 75 g anhydrous glucose dissolved in water.[a]

OR

In a patient with classic symptoms of hyperglycemia or hyperglycemic crisis, a random blood glucose greater than 200 mg/dL (11.1 mmol/L).

[a] In the absence of unequivocal hyperglycemia, diagnosis requires two abnormal tests results from the same sample or in two separate test samples.
DCCT, Diabetes Control and Complications Trial; *NGSP,* National Glycohemoglobin Standardization Program.
Data from American Diabetes Association (ADA). (2022). Classification and diagnosis of diabetes: Standards of medical care in diabetes—2022. *Diabetes Care, 45*(Suppl. 1): 19.

Laboratory Assessment

Diagnosis of Diabetes. Diabetes can be diagnosed by assessing the blood glucose levels listed in Table 56.3. A test result indicating DM should be repeated to rule out laboratory error unless symptoms of hyperglycemia or hyperglycemic crisis are also present. Box 56.4 lists criteria for the diagnosis of DM.

The diagnosis of DM includes elevated glycosylated hemoglobin levels. Glycosylated hemoglobin (A1C) is a standardized test that measures how much glucose attaches to the hemoglobin molecule over the previous 3 months and indicates an average glucose level. Because glucose binds to proteins, including hemoglobin, through a process called *glycosylation,* the higher the blood glucose level is over time, the more glycosylated the hemoglobin becomes.

Fasting plasma glucose (FPG) (fasting blood glucose [FBG]), along with A1C, can be used to diagnose DM in nonpregnant adults. A diagnosis of DM is made with two separate test results greater than 126 mg/dL (7 mmol/L) (ADA, 2022). *Random* or *casual plasma* glucose greater than 200 mg/dL (7.0 mmol/L) is used to diagnose DM in patients with classic hyperglycemia symptoms or hyperglycemic crisis.

The *oral glucose tolerance test (OGTT)* is a sensitive test for the diagnosis of DM. It is often used to diagnose gestational diabetes mellitus (GDM) during pregnancy and is not routinely used for general diagnosis (ADA, 2022).

Screening for Diabetes. Testing to detect prediabetes and T2DM is recommended for patients older than 35 years (ADA, 2022). Testing is recommended for younger adults with risk factors for DM. Screening for DM usually is done with laboratory testing of both A1C levels and fasting plasma glucose levels (ADA, 2022). (See Box 56.3.)

Ongoing Assessment. Glucose levels are assessed through:
- *Glycosylated hemoglobin* (A1C), one indicator of average blood glucose levels
- *Continuous glucose monitoring* (CGM), a diabetes technology system that measures and displays glucose levels on a continual basis
- *Blood glucose monitoring* (BGM), the process of checking a blood glucose level by using a glucose meter

Measurement of A1C shows the average blood glucose level during the previous 120 days—the lifespan of red blood cells. A1C is commonly used to assess long-term glycemic management (or control) and predict the risk for complications. *Unlike the fasting blood glucose test, A1C test results are not altered by the eating habits on the day before the test.* A1C levels are assessed at diagnosis and at specific intervals to evaluate the treatment plan. A1C testing is recommended at least twice yearly in patients who are meeting expected treatment outcomes and have stable blood glucose control. Quarterly assessment is recommended for patients whose therapy has changed or who are not within the glycemic target range (ADA, 2022). An A1C level less than 7% without significant hypoglycemia is the target for nonpregnant adults with DM. Table 56.4 shows the correlation between A1C and mean blood glucose levels.

Continuous glucose monitoring (CGM) can be used for an ongoing time period or for a short assessment time (usually 7–14 days). CGM uses a sensor that is inserted underneath the patient's skin to measure glucose levels on a continual basis. Glucose levels are then displayed on a receiver or mobile phone using a specific application (Fig. 56.6). CGM uses predictive arrows that alert a patient when glucose levels are trending up or down. These predictive arrows can help patients with decision making and overall self-management. CGM data are used to determine for how much time the patient's blood sugar is between 70 and 180 mg/dL. This is called *time-in-range.* The time-in-range goal is 70% for most patients with diabetes. CGM is recommended and often covered by insurance for all patients with T1DM and for patients with T2DM who use insulin.

BGM can help patients understand how their glucose levels are doing on a day-to-day basis when CGM is not available. BGM assesses glucose via capillary plasma using a glucose meter.

TABLE 56.4   Correlation Between A1C Level and Mean Blood Glucose Levels

A1C (%)	MEAN BLOOD GLUCOSE	
	mg/dL	mmol/L
6	126	7.0
7	154	8.6
8	183	10.2
9	212	11.8
10	240	13.4
11	269	14.9
12	298	16.5

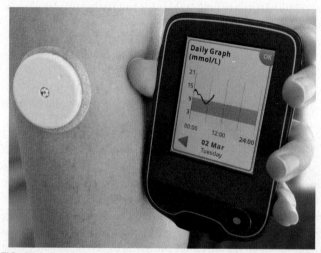

FIG. 56.6 Reading glucose levels by using device for continuous glucose monitoring (CGM) in blood. White sensor is placed on one arm and sends information to the CGM device. (Used with permission from istockphoto.com, 2021, Dragoljub Bankovic.)

Preprandial (before meal) glucose levels are recommended to be 80 to 130 mg/dL (4.4–7.2 mmol/L). Peak postprandial (after meal) glucose levels should be less than 180 mg/dL (10.0 mmol/L). Glucose meter data can also be used to detect time-in-range.

NCLEX Examination Challenge 56.2

Physiological Integrity

The nurse is reviewing preadmission laboratory testing values for a 55-year-old client scheduled for a total knee replacement. The A1C value is 6.2%. How would the nurse interpret this finding? (A1C range: 4%–5.9%)
A. Within normal limits
B. Indicative of type 1 diabetes mellitus
C. Confirmation of type 2 diabetes mellitus
D. Reflects prediabetes mellitus

Analyze Cues and Prioritize Hypotheses: Analysis

The priority collaborative problems for patients with DM include:

1. Potential for injury due to hyperglycemia
2. Potential for surgical complications due to the health complexities with DM
3. Potential for injury due to peripheral neuropathy
4. Potential for kidney disease due to reduced kidney *perfusion*
5. Potential for acute complications associated with glucose-related emergencies

Generate Solutions and Take Actions: Planning and Implementation

Preventing Injury From Hyperglycemia

Planning: Expected Outcomes. The patient is expected to manage DM and prevent disease progression by maintaining blood glucose levels in their target range.

Interventions

Nonsurgical Management. Management of DM involves *nutrition* interventions, glucose monitoring, regular physical activity, stress management and reduction, and, often, drugs to lower blood glucose levels. Nurses, the interprofessional team members, and the patient plan, coordinate, and deliver care.

Drug therapy. Drug therapy is indicated when a patient with T2DM does not achieve target blood glucose levels with a balanced diet, physical activity, and stress management. Several categories of drugs may be used to lower blood glucose levels in those with T2DM. Patients with T1DM require insulin therapy for blood glucose control and may use other antidiabetic drugs, as well.

Drugs are started at the lowest effective dose and increased over time until the desired blood glucose levels or the maximum dosage are reached. Glycemic management may require the use of more than one category of drug. Insulin therapy is indicated for the patient with T2DM when target blood glucose levels cannot be met with the use of two or three different antidiabetic agents, including GLP-1 agonists, or when presenting with an A1C above 10% and symptoms of DM (ADA, 2022).

Antidiabetic drugs should be used in conjunction with balanced eating and regular physical activity. Teach the patient about strategies to maintain balanced eating and the importance of regular physical activity while taking antidiabetic drugs.

💊 NURSING SAFETY PRIORITY

Drug Alert

To avoid drug interactions, teach the patient who is taking an antidiabetic drug to consult with the diabetes health care provider or pharmacist before using *any* over-the-counter drugs, vitamins, or supplements.

Drug selection is based on cost, the patient's ability to manage multiple drug dosages, associated risks for side effects, and response to the drugs. Drugs with once-a-day dosing or once-weekly dosing may be better for adherence. Beta cell function declines over time in T2DM, and some drugs may become less effective. Management of T2DM may eventually require insulin therapy either alone or with other antidiabetic drugs.

Some antidiabetic drugs are oral agents, and other types require subcutaneous injection. See Table 56.5 for common antidiabetic drugs.

Metformin, a *biguanide,* decreases liver glucose production and decreases intestinal absorption of glucose. It also improves insulin sensitivity, which increases peripheral glucose uptake

---

🔖 **TABLE 56.5** **Common Examples of Drug Therapy**

Diabetes Mellitus (DM)

Drug Category	Selected Nursing Implications

For all drugs used in the treatment of DM, teach patient the signs and symptoms of hypoglycemia (hunger, headache, tremors, sweating, confusion) because many antidiabetic drugs lower blood glucose levels even when hyperglycemia is not present.

Biguanides

Lower blood glucose by inhibiting liver glucose production, decreasing intestinal absorption of glucose, and increasing insulin sensitivity.

- Metformin

Instruct patients not to drink alcohol while taking this drug *to reduce the risk for lactic acidosis.*

Remind patients that this drug must be stopped before certain imaging tests using contrast agents *because of the increased risk for kidney damage and lactic acidosis.*

Warn patients that GI problems are common side effects of this drug class. The medication should be taken with food *to lessen GI side effects.*

Incretin Mimetics (GLP-1 Agonists)

Act like natural "gut" hormones that work with insulin to lower blood glucose levels by reducing pancreatic glucagon secretion, reducing liver glucose production, and delaying gastric emptying.

- Dulaglutide
- Exenatide
- Exenatide extended release
- Liraglutide
- Lixisenatide
- Semaglutide

Instruct patients how to inject themselves *because most drugs in this class are only available as subcutaneous formulations.*

Instruct patients to read dosing schedule carefully for exenatide, dulaglutide, and injected semaglutide *because they are injected* **weekly** *rather than daily.*

Teach patients to report persistent abdominal pain and nausea to the health care provider *because these drugs increase the risk for pancreatitis and are contraindicated in gastroparesis.*

Sodium-Glucose Cotransporter 2 (SGLT2) Inhibitors

Lower blood glucose levels by preventing kidney reabsorption of glucose and sodium that was filtered from the blood into the urine. This filtered glucose is excreted in the urine rather than moved back into the blood.

- Canagliflozin
- Dapagliflozin
- Empagliflozin
- Ertugliflozin

Teach the patient the signs and symptoms of dehydration (increased thirst, light-headedness, dry mouth and mucous membranes, orthostatic hypotension) *because these drugs increase urine output and increase dehydration risk.*

Teach patients the signs and symptoms of hyponatremia (muscle weakness, abdominal cramping, rapid heart rate, orthostatic hypotension) *because these drugs increase sodium loss.*

Teach patients the signs and symptoms of urinary tract infection (frequency, pain and burning on urination, foul urine odor) *because the increased glucose in the urinary tract predisposes to infection.*

Instruct to be alert for genital itching and vaginal discharge in females *because these drugs increase the risk for genital yeast infection.*

Teach patients to report any swelling, tenderness, or redness/hyperpigmentation of the genitals or perineal skin *because these drugs increase the risk for Fournier gangrene with perineal fasciitis.*

DPP-4 Inhibitors (Gliptins)

DPP-4 inhibitors are oral agents that prevent the enzyme DPP-4 from breaking down the natural gut hormones (GLP-1 and GIP), which allows these natural substances to work with insulin to lower glucagon secretion from the pancreas, which reduces liver glucose production. These oral drugs also reduce blood glucose levels by delaying gastric emptying and slowing the rate of nutrient absorption into the blood.

- Alogliptin
- Linagliptin
- Saxagliptin
- Sitagliptin

Instruct patients to be alert for rash or other sign of allergic reaction *because this class of drugs is associated with a moderate incidence of drug allergy.*

Teach patients to report persistent abdominal pain and nausea to the health care provider *because these drugs increase the risk for pancreatitis.*

Instruct patients to notify the primary health care provider if shortness of breath, dyspnea on exertion, or cough, especially when lying down, is experienced *because this class of drugs is associated with heart failure.*

Insulin Stimulators (Secretagogues)

Lower blood glucose levels by triggering the release of preformed insulin from beta cells.

Sulfonylureas

- Glipizide
- Glyburide
- Glimepiride

Instruct patients to take these drugs with or just before meals *to prevent hypoglycemia.*

Instruct patients taking a sulfonylurea to check with their health care provider or a pharmacist before taking any over-the-counter drug or supplement *because these drugs interact with many other drugs.*

Meglitinide (Glinides)

- Repaglinide
- Nateglinide

Continued

TABLE 56.5 Common Examples of Drug Therapy—cont'd

Diabetes Mellitus (DM)

Drug Category	Selected Nursing Implications
Insulin Sensitizers	
Lower blood glucose by decreasing liver glucose production and improving the sensitivity of insulin receptors.	
Thiazolidinediones (TZDs or Glitazones) • Pioglitazone • Rosiglitazone	Teach patients with any cardiovascular disease to weigh themselves daily and report a weight gain of more than 2 lb (1 kg) in 1 day or 4 lb (2 kg) in a week to the prescriber *because these drugs increase the risk for heart failure.* Instruct patients to report vision changes immediately *because these drugs increase the risk for macular edema.* Warn patients that weight gain and peripheral edema are *common side effects of these drugs.*
Alpha-Glucosidase Inhibitors	
Act in the intestine to delay the absorption of carbohydrates, preventing after-meal hyperglycemia.	
• Acarbose • Miglitol	Teach patients to take these drugs only with a meal *because the action is in the intestinal tract.* Warn patients that abdominal discomfort and bloating, flatulence, nausea, diarrhea, and indigestion are *common side effects of this drug class.*
Amylin Analogs	
These drugs are similar to amylin, a naturally occurring hormone produced by beta cells in the pancreas that is cosecreted with insulin and lowers blood glucose levels by decreasing endogenous glucagon, delaying gastric emptying, and triggering satiety.	
• Pramlintide	Instruct patients how to inject themselves *because these drugs are available only as subcutaneous formulations.* Warn patients that nausea and vomiting are *common side effects of this drug class.* Do not mix in the same syringe with insulin *because their pH is not compatible.*

DPP-4, Dipeptidyl peptidase 4; *GIP,* glucose-dependent insulinotropic polypeptide; *GLP-1,* glucagon-like peptide 1.

and utilization. Metformin is taken orally and is typically the first-line medication in an adult with T2DM who requires medication therapy.

NURSING SAFETY PRIORITY

Drug Alert

Metformin can cause lactic acidosis in patients with kidney impairment and should not be used by anyone with kidney disease (Burchum & Rosenthal, 2022). To prevent lactic acidosis and acute kidney injury, the drug is withheld 24 hours before using contrast medium or any surgical procedure requiring anesthesia until adequate kidney function is established.

Incretin mimetics work like the natural "gut" hormones, glucagon-like peptide 1 (GLP-1) and glucose-dependent insulinotropic polypeptide (GIP), that are released by the intestine in response to food intake and act with insulin for **glucose regulation.** Drugs in this class include the GLP-1 agonists dulaglutide, exenatide, liraglutide, lixisenatide, and semaglutide. Semaglutide

NURSING SAFETY PRIORITY

Drug Alert

Extended release exenatide, dulaglutide, and semaglutide are injected subcutaneously *once weekly.* Be sure to emphasize this dosing schedule to avoid overdoses.

can be taken orally or subcutaneously. All other GLP-1 drugs are taken subcutaneously on a daily or weekly basis.

Sodium-glucose cotransporter 2 (SGLT2) inhibitors lower blood glucose levels by preventing kidney reabsorption of glucose that was filtered from the blood into the urine. The filtered glucose is excreted in the urine rather than moved back into the blood. These oral drugs include canagliflozin, dapagliflozin, empagliflozin, and ertugliflozin.

Dipeptidyl peptidase 4 (DPP-4) inhibitors (gliptins) work by enhancing the actions of incretin hormones (Burchum & Rosenthal, 2022). Gliptins produce modest glucose reductions and are used as a second-line therapy in T2DM. These drugs include sitagliptin, saxagliptin, linagliptin, and alogliptin.

NURSING SAFETY PRIORITY

Drug Alert

Dipeptidyl peptidase 4 (DPP-4) inhibitors and the incretin mimetics have an increased risk for pancreatitis. Warn patients taking these drugs to immediately report to the diabetes health care provider any signs of jaundice; sudden onset of intense abdominal pain that radiates to the back, left flank, or left shoulder; or gray-blue discoloration of the abdomen or periumbilical area.

Saxagliptin and alogliptin have an increased risk for heart failure. Warn patients to report a sudden weight gain or new-onset shortness of breath.

Insulin stimulators (also known as insulin secretagogues) stimulate insulin release from pancreatic beta cells and are used in patients who are still able to produce insulin. This class includes sulfonylureas and meglitinide analogs.

Sulfonylurea agents lower fasting blood glucose levels by triggering the release of insulin from beta cells. Many drugs interact with sulfonylureas. Be sure to consult a drug reference source or pharmacist when instructing patients who are prescribed a drug from this class. Meglitinides (also known as glinides) are insulin stimulators and have actions and adverse effects similar to those of sulfonylureas. They tend to increase meal-related insulin secretion. Insulin stimulators can cause hypoglycemia and should be used cautiously, especially in combination with insulin.

Insulin sensitizers, also known as thiazolidinediones (TZDs) or glitazones, increase cellular use of glucose, which lowers blood glucose levels. These drugs are associated with an increased risk for heart-related deaths, bone fracture, and macular edema. The U.S. Food and Drug Administration (FDA) has issued a box warning indicating that these drugs are not to be used by patients who have symptomatic heart failure or other specific types of cardiovascular disease.

Alpha-glucosidase inhibitors prevent after-meal hyperglycemia by delaying absorption of carbohydrate (CHO) from the intestine. They inhibit enzymes in the intestinal tract, reducing the rate of starch digestion and glucose absorption. These actions prevent a sudden blood glucose surge after meals. These drugs do not cause hypoglycemia unless given with sulfonylureas or insulin. However, side effects of GI upset and flatulence can deter adherence to the use of these drugs.

Amylin analogs are drugs similar to amylin, a naturally occurring hormone produced by pancreatic beta cells that works with and is secreted with insulin in response to blood glucose elevation. Amylin levels are deficient in patients with T1DM. Pramlintide, an analog of amylin, is approved for patients with DM who are treated with insulin. It works through three mechanisms: delaying gastric emptying, reducing after-meal blood glucose levels, and triggering satiety in the brain. Satiety leads to decreased caloric intake and eventual weight loss.

💊 NURSING SAFETY PRIORITY

Drug Alert

Do not mix pramlintide and insulin in the same syringe because the pH of the two drugs is not compatible.

Combination agents combine drugs with different mechanisms of action. For example, Xigduo XR combines dapagliflozin with metformin extended release. Combining drugs with different mechanisms of action may be highly effective in maintaining desired blood glucose control. Combination medications can also reduce the number of overall prescriptions, reducing costs. Some patients may need a combination of antidiabetic agents and insulin to regulate glucose levels.

Insulin therapy. Insulin therapy is required for patients with T1DM and is used in 20% to 30% of patients with T2DM. The safety of insulin therapy in older patients may be affected by reduced vision, mobility and coordination problems, and decreased memory, increasing the risk for dosage errors. Many types of insulin and regimens are available to achieve normal blood glucose levels. Because insulin is a small protein that is quickly inactivated in the GI tract, it is usually injected.

Types of insulin vary with the source and manufacturing techniques. Insulin analogs are synthetic human insulins in which the structure of the insulin molecule is altered to change the rate of absorption and duration of action within the body (e.g., lispro insulin).

Rapid-, short-, intermediate-, long-, and ultra-long-acting forms of insulin can be injected separately, and some can be mixed in the same syringe. Insulin is available in concentrations of 100 units/mL (U-100), 200 units/mL (U-200), 300 units/mL (U-300), and 500 units/mL (U-500). U-500 insulin concentration is less common and is reserved for when very large doses of insulin are required.

Teach the patient that the insulin types, the injection technique, and the site of injection all affect the absorption, onset, degree, and duration of insulin activity. Reinforce that changing the type of insulin may affect blood glucose control and should be done only under supervision of the diabetes health care provider. Table 56.6 outlines the timed activity of human insulin.

Insulin regimens attempt to replicate the normal insulin release pattern from the pancreas. The pancreas produces a constant *(basal)* amount of insulin that balances liver glucose production with glucose use and maintains normal blood glucose levels between meals. The pancreas also produces additional meal-time *(prandial)* insulin to prevent blood glucose elevation after meals. The insulin dose required for blood glucose control varies among patients. Starting doses may be much lower for older adults or for very thin patients. For multiple-dose regimens or continuous subcutaneous insulin infusion (CSII, also known as an insulin pump), basal insulin makes up about 50% of the total daily dosage, with the remainder divided into premeal doses of rapid-acting insulin analogs or regular insulin. Basal insulin coverage is provided by intermediate-acting insulin (NPH), long, or ultra-long-acting insulin analogs such as insulin glargine, insulin detemir, or insulin degludec. Dosages are adjusted based on the results of blood glucose monitoring.

Single daily injection protocols require insulin injection only once daily. This protocol may include one injection of intermediate-, long-, or ultra-long-acting insulin or an injection of combination short- and intermediate-acting insulin. Some patients with T2DM combine once-daily insulin injection for basal coverage with oral agent therapy or a GLP-1 to stimulate bolus insulin secretion. The effect of basal insulin is assessed by monitoring blood glucose levels before breakfast (fasting).

Multiple-component insulin therapy combines short- (regular) and intermediate-acting (NPH) insulin injected twice daily. Two-thirds of the daily dose is given before breakfast, and one-third before the evening meal. Ratios of intermediate-acting and regular insulin are based on results of blood glucose monitoring. Given the peak of intermediate acting insulin, a bedtime snack may be necessary to avoid nocturnal hypoglycemia.

Intensified regimens, also known as *multiple daily injections (MDIs),* include a basal dose of intermediate-, long-, or ultra-long-acting insulin and a mealtime bolus dose of short- or rapid-acting insulin designed to bring the *next* blood glucose value into the target range. Blood glucose elevations above the target

TABLE 56.6   Timed Activity of Selected Pharmaceutical Insulin Types

Preparation	Onset (min)	Peak (hr)	Duration (hr)
Rapid-Acting Insulin Analogs			
Insulin aspart	10–20	1–3	3–5
Insulin glulisine	10–15	1–1.5	3–5
Insulin lispro (Humalog)	15–30	0.5–2.5	3–6
Short-Acting Insulin			
Regular insulin	30–60	1–5	6–10
Intermediate-Acting Insulin			
NPH insulin	60–120	6–14	16–24
Long-Acting Insulin Analogs			
Insulin glargine U-100	70	None[a]	18–24
Insulin detemir	60–120	None[a]	12–24
Ultra-Long-Acting Insulin			
Insulin degludec	30–90	None	24+

[a]Levels are steady with no discernable peak.
Data from Burchum, J., & Rosenthal, L. (2022). *Lehne's pharmacology for nursing care* (11th ed.). St. Louis: Elsevier.

range are treated with "correction" doses of short- or rapid-acting insulin. The patient's blood glucose patterns determine insulin dosage. Frequency of blood glucose monitoring is based on the timed action of insulin and may occur as often as eight times daily. Blood glucose testing 2 hours after meals and within 10 minutes before the next meal helps determine the adequacy of the previous bolus dose.

Patients on intensified insulin regimens need extensive education to achieve target blood glucose levels. They need to know how to adjust insulin doses and understand **nutrition** therapy for dietary flexibility while meeting target blood glucose levels. Patients must also be able to correctly monitor blood glucose levels using BGM or CGM so that therapy decisions are based on accurate data.

Regardless of the specific insulin regimen, adherence to insulin injection schedules is critical in achieving the glycemic control needed to reduce long-term complications. At times, skipping an occasional insulin dose may be related to an unusual meal pattern for a day or a change in exercise. If a patient is skipping insulin doses often, inquire about barriers, such as cost, fear of hypoglycemia, fear of injections, needing help from others, or embarrassment (Hussein et al., 2019).

Insulin absorption is affected by many factors including injection site; timing, type, or dose of insulin used; and physical activity. Injection site area affects the speed of insulin absorption. Fig. 56.7 shows common insulin injection areas. Absorption is fastest in the abdomen, which is, except for a 2-inch radius around the navel, the preferred injection site. Rotating injection sites allows each injection site to heal completely before the site is used again. Rotation *within* one anatomic site is preferred to rotation from one area to another to prevent day-to-day variability in absorption.

Absorption rate is determined by insulin properties. Longer duration of action makes absorption less reliable. Larger doses

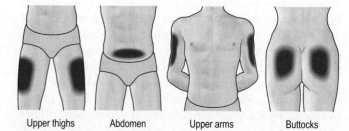

Upper thighs   Abdomen   Upper arms   Buttocks

FIG. 56.7 Common insulin injection areas and sites. (From Peate, I. [2020]. *Alexander's nursing practice: Hospital and home* [5th ed.]. London: Elsevier, Ltd.)

prolong the absorption. Factors that increase blood flow from the injection site, such as applying heat locally, massaging the area, and exercising the injected area, increase insulin absorption. Scarred areas are less sensitive to pain, but these sites usually slow insulin absorption.

Injection depth changes insulin absorption. Usually, injections are made into the subcutaneous tissue. IM injection has a faster absorption and is not used for routine insulin use. Most patients lightly grasp a fold of skin and inject at a 90-degree angle; however, a 45-degree angle is used for frail older adults and those who are very thin. Aspiration for blood is not needed. Patients who are overweight can use 4-mm or 5-mm needles to inject insulin at a 90-degree angle without pinching a skinfold before injection.

Timing of injection affects blood glucose levels. The interval between premeal injections and eating, known as "lag time," affects blood glucose levels after meals. Insulins that have rapid onsets of action are given within 10 minutes before mealtime when blood glucose is in the target range. If hyperglycemia or hypoglycemia is not present, these insulins can be given at any time from 10 minutes before mealtime to just before eating or even immediately after eating. Regular insulin is given at least 20 to 30 minutes before eating when glucose levels are within the target range. When blood glucose levels are *above* the target range, lag time is increased to permit insulin to have a greater glucose-lowering effect before food enters the stomach. When blood glucose levels are *below* the target range, teach patients to inject insulin *immediately* before eating, and to delay rapid-acting insulin injection until sometime *after* eating the meal.

Mixing insulins can change the time of peak action. Mixtures of short- and intermediate-acting insulins produce a more normal blood glucose response in some patients than does a single dose. The patient's response to mixed insulin may differ from the response to the same insulins given separately.

NURSING SAFETY PRIORITY

Drug Alert

Do not mix any other insulin type with insulin glargine, insulin detemir, or any of the premixed insulin formulations such as Humalog Mix 75/25.

Methods of insulin administration vary. These include syringes, insulin pens, smart pens, continuous subcutaneous insulin infusion, and dry powder inhalers.

An insulin pen is an insulin delivery device that is preloaded with insulin and is more convenient than an insulin vial and syringe (Fig. 56.8). A *pen needle* is twisted on the pen for use. The insulin dose is dialed using a twisting motion that has both a tactile and an audible "click." Most insulin pens are disposable after use. However, there are a few reusable ones.

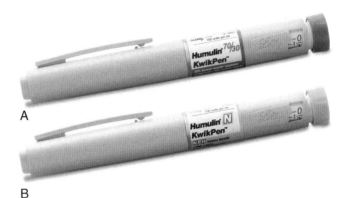

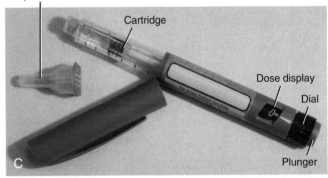

FIG. 56.8 Prefilled insulin pens. (A) Humulin 70/30 short- and intermediate-acting. (B) Humulin N intermediate-acting. (C) Pre-filled pen. (A and B copyright © Eli Lilly and Co. All rights reserved. Used with permission; C from Stein, L. N. M, & Hollen, C. J. [2024]. *Concept-based clinical nursing skills: Fundamental to advanced competencies* [2nd ed.]. St. Louis: Elsevier.)

NCLEX Examination Challenge 56.3

Safe and Effective Care Environment

The nurse is caring for a client who is 5 feet 10 inches tall and weighs 106 lb (48.1 kg). What insulin injection technique would the nurse select?
A. Use a 6-mm needle and inject at a 90-degree angle.
B. Use a 6-mm needle and inject at a 45-degree angle.
C. Use a 12-mm needle and inject at a 90-degree angle.
D. Use a 12-mm needle and inject at a 45-degree angle.

A smart insulin pen is a reusable injector that is connected to a smartphone app. The app helps patients calculate doses of insulin based on programmable settings. These settings include insulin-to-carbohydrate ratio, which delivers a certain amount of insulin based on the number of carbohydrates consumed; a correction factor, which is extra insulin given based on an elevated glucose level; and insulin on board, indicating how much active insulin is circulating in the body. The app can also help patients track their doses, provide reminders, notify when insulin is expired or has reached an unsafe temperature, and provide reports.

Continuous subcutaneous insulin infusion (CSII), also known as an insulin pump, delivers rapid-acting analog insulin (Fig. 56.9) every hour to provide basal insulin coverage with additional insulin at mealtimes. CSII allows flexibility in meal timing, because if a meal is skipped, the additional mealtime dose of insulin is not given. CSII is also programmable to each individual (e.g., insulin-to-carbohydrate ratio, correction factor, insulin on board). CSII consists of an externally worn insulin pump containing a reservoir of rapid-acting insulin that is connected to the patient by an infusion set.

Problems with CSII include skin infections that can occur when the infusion site is not cleaned or the infusion set is not changed every 2 to 3 days. Ketoacidosis may occur more often because of infection, obstruction of the infusion, or mechanical pump problems. Stress the need for ketone testing when blood glucose levels are greater than 300 mg/dL (16.7 mmol/L).

Patients using CSII need intensive and extensive education to operate the pump, adjust the settings, and respond appropriately to alarms. Removing the CSII (insulin pump) for any time can result in hyperglycemia, and some patients may need to administer an insulin bolus after removing the CSII for showering or swimming. Provide supplemental insulin schedules for times when the CSII is not operational.

Automated insulin delivery (AID) is when a CSII (insulin pump) and continuous glucose monitor are combined with an algorithm that takes glucose data from the monitor and sends commands to the pump. Commands might stop the CSII from delivering insulin in response to hypoglycemia or provide extra insulin in response hyperglycemia. The CSII and CGM must be compatible for the AID system to work.

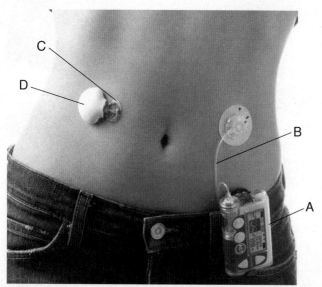

FIG. 56.9 MiniMed Paradigm REAL-Time Insulin Pump and Continuous Glucose Monitoring System. *A*, Pump; *B*, injection cannula; *C*, glucose sensor; *D*, data transmitter. (Courtesy Medtronic Diabetes, Northridge, CA.)

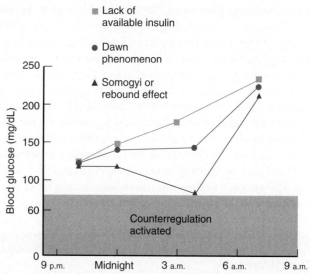

FIG. 56.10 Three blood glucose phenomena in patients with diabetes.

A dry powder inhaler insulin delivery system with single-use cartridges is available for rapid-acting insulin. Its use is limited to adults with T1DM or T2DM who do not have respiratory problems and who are nonsmokers. Pulmonary testing is required before initiating this therapy. Its onset of action is about 12 minutes. Complications of this therapy include new-onset respiratory problems such as bronchospasms.

Hypoglycemia from insulin excess has many causes. Its effects and treatment are discussed in the Interventions for Preventing Hypoglycemia section.

Two conditions of fasting hyperglycemia (in addition to a lack of insulin) can occur (Fig. 56.10). *Dawn phenomenon* results from a nighttime release of adrenal hormones that causes blood glucose elevations at about 5 to 6 a.m. It is managed by providing more insulin for the overnight period (e.g., giving the evening dose of intermediate-acting insulin at 10 p.m. instead of with the evening meal). *Somogyi phenomenon* is morning hyperglycemia from the counterregulatory response to nighttime hypoglycemia. It is managed by ensuring adequate dietary intake at bedtime and evaluating the insulin dose and exercise programs to prevent conditions that lead to hypoglycemia. Both problems are diagnosed by means of blood glucose monitoring during the night. Help identify these problems and teach the patient and family about management.

Patient education: drugs. Provide specific instructions about insulin therapy, new drug therapies, and blood glucose monitoring (BGM).

Insulin storage varies by use. Teach patients to refrigerate insulin that is not in use to maintain potency, prevent exposure to sunlight, and inhibit bacterial growth. Most insulin in use may be kept at room temperature for up to 28 days to reduce injection site irritation from cold insulin.

To prevent loss of drug potency, teach the patient to avoid exposing insulin to temperatures below 36°F (2.2°C) or above 86°F (30°C), to avoid excessive shaking, and to protect insulin from direct heat and light. Insulin should not be allowed to freeze. Teach patients to discard any unused insulin after 28 days.

Teach patients to always have a spare supply of each type of insulin used. Most prefilled syringes are stable for up to 30 days when refrigerated. Store prefilled syringes in the upright position, with the needle pointing upward or flat so insulin particles do not clog it.

Proper dose preparation is critical for insulin effectiveness and safety. Teach patients that the person giving the insulin needs to inspect the vial before each use for changes (e.g., clumping, frosting, precipitation, or change in clarity or color) that may indicate loss in potency. Preparations containing NPH insulin are uniformly cloudy after gently rolling the vial between the hands. Other insulins should be clear. If potency is questionable, another vial or pen of the same insulin type should be used.

Syringes are usually used to inject insulin. Standard insulin syringes are marked in insulin units. They are available in 1-mL (100-U), ½-mL (50-U), and ³⁄₁₀-mL (30-U) sizes. The unit scale on the barrel of the syringe differs with the syringe size and manufacturer. Insulin syringe needles are measured in 28, 29, 30, and 31 gauges and in lengths of 6 mm, 8 mm, and 12.7 mm. To ensure accurate insulin measurement, instruct the patient to always buy the same type of syringe. See Box 56.5 for instructions for drawing up a single insulin injection.

Disposable needles (syringes or pen needles) are used only once. Teach the patient to discard the syringe and needle after one use. Information on needle disposal can be obtained at www.safeneedledisposal.org.

When teaching about insulin pen use, discuss proper storage for prefilled insulin pens or cartridges. Ensure that the product is appropriate for the patient's unique needs. *Insulin pens may be preferred for those who are visually impaired because of the tactile and audible click for each unit.* Ensure that the patient understands the correct use for the selected syringe or cartridge.

! NURSING SAFETY PRIORITY

Action Alert

The Institute for Safe Medication Practices (ISMP) identifies insulin as a *High-Alert* drug. (High-Alert drugs are those that have an increased risk of causing patient harm if given in error.) The ISMP cautions that digital displays on some insulin pens can be misread. If the pen is held upside down, as a left-handed person might do, a dose of 52 units actually appears to be a dose of 25 units, and a dose of 12 units looks like a dose of 21 units.

Patient education: blood glucose monitoring. Blood glucose monitoring (BGM) provides a means to assess effectiveness of the management plan and assists the patient in self-care decisions. Results of BGM are useful in preventing hypoglycemia and hyperglycemia by adjusting drug therapy, diet therapy, and physical activity. Teach patients to assess blood glucose frequently in these situations:

- Symptoms of hypoglycemia or hyperglycemia
- Hypoglycemic unawareness
- Periods of illness
- Before and after exercise
- Gastroparesis
- Adjustment of antidiabetic drugs
- Evaluation of other drug therapies (e.g., steroids)
- Pregnancy

Techniques for BGM follow principles that are the same as for most self-monitoring systems. Blood glucose meter systems now require a very small blood sample, which allows for alternate testing sites (e.g., arm, thigh, hand). The selected site is pricked, a drop of blood is drawn into a testing strip or disk impregnated with chemicals, and the glucose value is displayed or "spoken" (in mg/dL or mmol/L) on a screen.

Data obtained from BGM are evaluated along with other A1C levels or periodic laboratory blood glucose test results. Even when BGM is performed correctly, the results are affected by hematocrit values (anemia falsely elevates glucose values; polycythemia falsely depresses them) and may be unreliable in the hypoglycemic or severely hyperglycemic ranges.

Accuracy of the blood glucose monitor is ensured when the manufacturer's directions are followed. Common user errors involve failing to obtain a sufficient blood drop, poorly storing test strips, using expired strips, not changing the code number on the meter to match the strip bottle code, or using an expired meter. Meter selection is based on cost of the meter and strips, ease of use, and insurance coverage. Provide training, explain and demonstrate procedures, assess visual acuity, and check the patient's ability to perform the procedure using "teach-back" strategies. Newer meters have fewer steps, include error signals for inadequate sample size, and can store hundreds of BGM results that can be downloaded for data reports. Data reports can provide insight regarding the frequency of hypoglycemia or hyperglycemia, and time-in-range.

Accuracy and precision vary widely among capillary blood glucose monitoring devices. If the meter requires calibration, teach patients to properly calibrate the machine. Instruct them to recheck the calibration and retest if they obtain a test result

BOX 56.5 Patient and Family Education

Subcutaneous Insulin Administration

With Vial and Syringe
- Wash your hands.
- Inspect the bottle for the type of insulin and the expiration date.
- Gently roll the bottle of intermediate-acting insulin in the palms of your hands to mix the insulin.
- Clean the rubber stopper with an alcohol swab.
- Remove the needle cover and pull back the plunger to draw air into the syringe. The amount of air should be equal to the insulin dose. Push the needle through the rubber stopper and inject the air into the insulin bottle.
- Turn the bottle upside down and draw the insulin dose into the syringe.
- Remove air bubbles in the syringe by tapping on the syringe or injecting air back into the bottle. Redraw the correct amount.
- Make certain the tip of the plunger is on the line for your dose of insulin. Magnifiers are available to assist in measuring accurate doses of insulin.
- Remove the needle from the bottle. Recap the needle if the insulin is not to be given immediately.
- Select a site within your injection area that has not been used in the past month.
- Clean your skin with an alcohol swab. Lightly grasp an area of skin and insert the needle at a 90-degree angle.
- Push the plunger all the way down. This will push the insulin into your body. Release the pinched skin.
- Pull the needle straight out quickly. Do not rub the place where you gave the shot.
- Dispose of the syringe and needle without recapping in a puncture-proof container.

With a Pen Device
- Wash your hands.
- Check the drug label to be sure it is what was prescribed.
- Remove the cap.
- Look at the insulin to be sure that it is evenly mixed if it contains NPH and that there is no clumping of particles.
- With an alcohol swab, wipe the tip of the pen where the needle will attach.
- Remove the protective pull tab from the needle and screw it onto the pen until snug.
- Remove both the plastic outer cap and the inner needle cap.
- Look at the dose window and turn the dosage knob to the appropriate dose.
- Holding the pen with the needle pointing upward, press the button until at least a drop of insulin appears. This is the "cold shot," "air shot," or "safety shot." Repeat this step if needed until a drop appears.
- Dial the number of units needed.
- Hold the pen perpendicular to and against the intended injection site with your thumb on the dosing knob.
- Press the dosing knob slowly all the way to dispense the dose.
- Hold the pen in place for 6 to 10 seconds, then withdraw from the skin.
- Replace the outer needle cap; unscrew until the needle is removed and dispose of the needle in a hard plastic or metal container.
- Replace the cap on the insulin pen.

that is unusual for them and whenever they are in doubt about test accuracy. Continued retraining of patients performing BGM helps ensure accurate results because performance accuracy deteriorates over time. Laboratory glucose determinations are more accurate than BGM.

Frequency of testing varies with the drug schedules, the patient's prescribed therapy, and expected target outcomes. Patients taking multiple insulin injections or using CSII therapy may need to monitor glucose levels three or more times daily. For patients taking less-frequent injections of insulin or using noninsulin therapy, or for those who are not on antidiabetic medications, daily BGM is useful for evaluation of therapy.

Blood glucose target goals for self-management are set individually for each patient based on the duration of disease, age and life expectancy, other chronic conditions, the severity of cardiovascular disease, and presence of hypoglycemia unawareness (ADA, 2022). The health care team works with the patient to reach target blood glucose levels.

Infection control measures are needed for BGM. The chance of becoming infected from blood glucose monitoring processes is reduced by handwashing before monitoring and by not reusing lancets. *Instruct patients to not share their BGM equipment* because infection can be spread by the lancet holder even when the lancet itself has been changed Regular cleaning of the meter is critical for infection control. Remind staff who perform blood glucose testing and family members who help with testing to wear gloves.

Once the patient learns the technical aspects of meter use, help them to use the results of BGM to achieve glycemic control. Postmeal glucose monitoring provides information about the effects of the size and content of meals. BGM allows the patient to assess effects of exercise on glucose control and provides critical information to help patients who take insulin to exercise safely. Teach patients how to make agreed-on adjustments in the treatment plan when BGM results are consistently out of range for a 3-day period when no change in meal plan, drugs, or activity has occurred.

Alternate site testing uses blood obtained from sites other than the fingertip and is available on many meters and meter-smartphone interfaces. Older meters have wider variation between fingertip and alternate sites, and variation is most evident during times when glucose levels change rapidly. Teach patients about the lag time for blood glucose levels between the fingertip and other sites when blood glucose levels are changing rapidly and that the fingertip reading is the only safe choice at those times.

> **!** **NURSING SAFETY PRIORITY**
>
> *Action Alert*
>
> Teach patients with a history of hypoglycemic unawareness *not* to test at alternative sites.

Continuous blood glucose monitoring systems monitor glucose levels in interstitial fluid to provide real-time glucose information to the user. Many systems consist of three parts: a disposable sensor that measures glucose levels, a transmitter that is attached to the sensor, and a receiver that displays and stores glucose information. The sensor gives glucose values every 1 to 5 minutes that are displayed on a receiver or smartphone app. Most sensors may be used for 6 to 14 days, depending on the manufacturer. Continuous glucose monitoring (CGM) provides information about the current blood glucose level, short-term feedback about results of treatment, and warnings when glucose readings become dangerously high or low. Most available sensors require at least two capillary glucose readings per day for calibration of the sensor. Sensor accuracy depends on these calibrations. There may be a lag time between the capillary glucose measurement and the glucose sensor value. If the blood glucose value is changing rapidly, the time between capillary and interstitial glucose values may be as long as 30 minutes. For this reason, capillary glucose readings need to be checked on all extreme values or if symptoms of hypoglycemia are present before any corrective treatment is given. *With older or less sophisticated systems, give insulin only after confirming the results of any continuous glucose monitoring system.*

Nutrition therapy. Effective self-management of DM requires that **nutrition,** including the meal plan, education, and counseling programs, be individualized for each patient. A registered dietitian nutritionist (RDN) is a member of the interprofessional team. The nurse, RDN, diabetes care team, patient, and family work together on a realistic and flexible meal plan. Plans that consider the patient's cultural background, financial status, access to food, and lifestyle are more likely to be successful. The desired outcomes of nutrition and diet therapy are listed in Box 56.6.

The *principle of medical nutrition* or medical nutrition management (medical nutrition therapy [MNT]) is recommended for use with all adults with DM. For overweight or obese adults with DM, modest weight loss through personalized nutrition plans is beneficial. Blood pressure, blood glucose levels, and lipid profiles are often improved with weight loss (ADA, 2022).

The RDN develops a meal plan based on the patient's usual food intake, weight management goals, and lipid and blood glucose patterns. Consistency in the daily timing and amount of food eaten helps control blood glucose. Patients using insulin therapy need to eat at times that are coordinated with the timed action of insulin. Teach patients using intense insulin therapy to adjust premeal insulin to allow for timing and quantity changes in their meal plan.

No specific percentage of calories from carbohydrates, protein, or fat is ideal for all adults with DM. Recommendations for the distribution of these nutrients is individualized based on food preferences, eating patterns, and metabolic goals (ADA, 2022).

Carbohydrate intake avoids nutrient-deficient sources ("empty calories") and focuses on sources from vegetables, fruits, whole grains, legumes, and dairy products. Adults with DM should eat at least 25 g of fiber daily. Teach patients with DM or prediabetes to avoid sugar-sweetened beverages (including high fructose corn syrup) and sucrose to prevent weight gain and adverse effects on metabolism.

Dietary fat and cholesterol intake for adults with DM focuses on the quality of fat rather than on the quantity of fat. A Mediterranean-style diet rich in monounsaturated fatty acids (MUFAs) is one recommended eating pattern that can lower cardiac risk factors. Such diets include avocados, nuts and seeds, olives, and dark chocolate. Omega-3 fatty acids, including EPA (eicosapentaenoic acid) and DHA (docosahexaenoic acid)

BOX 56.6 Desired Outcomes of Nutrition Therapy for the Patient With Diabetes

- Achieving and maintaining blood glucose levels within target range or as close to target range as possible
- Achieving and maintaining a blood lipid profile that reduces the risk for cardiovascular disease
- Achieving blood pressure levels within the normal range or as close to normal as possible
- Preventing or slowing the development of complications associated with diabetes by modifying nutrient intake and lifestyle
- Addressing **nutrition** needs, taking into account personal and cultural preferences, access to food, and willingness to change
- Meeting the **nutrition** needs during unique times in the life cycle, particularly for pregnant and lactating women and for older adults with diabetes
- Providing self-management training for patients treated with insulin or insulin stimulators for exercising safely, including the prevention and treatment of hypoglycemia, and managing diabetes during acute illness

from fish or fish oil supplements, are recommended as part of a healthy diet to prevent heart disease, as is ALA (alpha-linolenic acid) derived from plant sources. Current recommendations from the ADA to limit *trans* fats, saturated fats, and cholesterol are the same as for the general population (ADA, 2022).

Alcohol consumption affects blood glucose levels, especially with high alcohol use. Teach patients that two alcoholic beverages for males and one for females can be ingested with, and in addition to, the usual meal plan. (One alcoholic beverage equals 12 ounces of beer, 5 ounces of wine, or 1½ ounces of distilled spirits.) The risk for delayed hypoglycemia is increased when drug therapy includes insulin or an insulin stimulator.

! NURSING SAFETY PRIORITY

Action Alert

Because of the potential for alcohol-induced delayed hypoglycemia, instruct the patient with diabetes to ingest alcohol only with or shortly after meals. Even with this precaution, patients must remain alert for delayed hypoglycemia following alcohol ingestion. Patients may want to have someone with them who can provide hypoglycemia support if needed.

Patient education for nutrition is based each patient's **nutrition** recommendations that consider blood glucose monitoring results, total blood lipid levels, and A1C levels. These laboratory values help determine whether current meal and exercise patterns need adjustment or whether present habits need reinforcement. A specific nutrition prescription is developed for each patient.

Reinforce nutrition information provided by the RDN. The patient with DM must understand how to adjust food intake during illness, planned exercise, and social occasions, and when the usual time of eating is delayed. Share dietary information with the person who prepares the meals. The RDN sees each patient yearly to identify changes in lifestyle and make appropriate diet therapy changes. Some patients, such as those with low health literacy, may need more frequent dietary evaluation and counseling. Screening for food insecurity should be done routinely, and appropriate referrals made when present.

Carbohydrate (CHO) counting is one approach to **nutrition** and meal planning that uses label information regarding the nutritional content of packaged food items. Estimation of CHO content when dining out can be taught by the RDN. CHO counting focuses on the nutrient that has the greatest impact on these levels. It uses total grams of CHO, regardless of the food source.

Patients using intensive insulin or CSII therapies can use CHO counting to determine insulin coverage. After the amount of insulin needed to cover the usual meal is determined, insulin may be added or subtracted for changes in CHO intake. An initial formula of 1 unit of rapid-acting insulin for each 15 g of CHO provides flexibility to meal plans and is adjusted based on 2-hour postprandial glucose levels or the next preprandial glucose level. The patient determines the grams of CHO in a specific meal or snack by reading labels or weighing and measuring each item. The total grams of CHO are used to calculate the bolus dose of insulin based on the prescribed insulin-to-carbohydrate ratio.

CHO counting may be challenging for individuals with low health literacy or numeracy skills. In this instance, the MyPlate food plate method is ideal. The MyPlate food plate (see Fig. 52.1)is a visual guide to simplify balanced eating. Half of the plate should be filled with mostly nonstarchy vegetables and an optional small amount of fruit, one-fourth of the plate should be filled with lean protein, and one-fourth of the plate should be filled with whole grains. In addition, the MyPlate food plate is an effective tool to teach anyone with or without DM the principles of balanced eating. Food examples should always be tailored to individual preferences and culture.

Special considerations for patients requiring insulin include developing insulin regimens that conform to the patient's preferred meal routines, food preferences, and exercise patterns. Patients using rapid-acting insulin by injection or CSII must learn to adjust insulin doses based on the CHO content of the meals and snacks. Insulin-to-carbohydrate ratios are developed and are used to provide mealtime insulin doses. Blood glucose monitoring before and 2 hours after meals determines whether the insulin-to-carbohydrate ratio is correct. For patients who are on fixed insulin regimens and do not adjust premeal insulin dosages, consistency in the timing of meals and the amount of CHO eaten at each meal is critical to prevent hypoglycemia.

Exercise can cause hypoglycemia if insulin is not decreased before activity. For planned exercise, hypoglycemia is prevented by a reduction in insulin dosage. For unplanned exercise, intake of additional CHO is usually needed. A 70-kg adult may need 10 to 15 g additional CHO per hour of moderate-intensity activity. More CHO is needed for intense activity.

It is important for patients using insulin to avoid weight gain. Hyperinsulinemia (chronically high blood insulin levels) can occur with intensive management schedules and may result in weight gain. These patients may need to manage hyperglycemia by restricting calories rather than increasing insulin under the guidance of the RDN and diabetes care team. Weight gain can be minimized by following the prescribed meal plan, getting regular exercise, and avoiding overtreatment of hypoglycemia.

Special considerations for overweight and obese patients. A subset of patients with T1DM and T2DM are overweight/obese and insulin resistant. Many patients also have abnormal blood fat levels and hypertension (metabolic syndrome), making reductions of saturated fat, cholesterol, and sodium desirable. A modest reduction in carbohydrates and an increase in physical activity may improve ***glucose regulation*** and weight control. Decreases of 5% to 10% of body weight can significantly improve A1C. Pharmacotherapy for weight loss is also recommended for adults with T2DM who have a body mass index (BMI) of 27 or above, or 25 or above for Asian individuals (ADA, 2022).

PATIENT-CENTERED CARE: OLDER ADULT HEALTH
Nutritional Patterns

Factors that increase the risk for poor **nutrition** in older adults with DM include dental issues, financial stress, changes in appetite, and changes in the ability to obtain and prepare food. Older adults may have reduced awareness of hypoglycemia and hyperglycemia and dehydration, increasing the risk for hyperglycemic-hyperosmolar state (HHS) (Touhy & Jett, 2023). They may eat out or live in situations in which they have little control over meal preparation. Visits by home health nurses can help older adults follow a balanced meal plan.

Changing the eating habits of 60 to 70 years is difficult and requires a realistic approach. The nurse, registered dietitian nutritionist (RDN), and patient assess the patient's usual eating patterns. Teach the older patient taking antidiabetic drugs the importance of eating meals and snacks at the same time every day and eating the same amount of food from day to day.

Physical activity. Regular physical activity is an essential part of DM management and improves carbohydrate metabolism and insulin sensitivity. Increased physical activity and weight loss reduce the risk for T2DM in patients with prediabetes.

Plasma glucose levels remain stable during exercise in adults without DM because of the balance between glucose use by exercising muscles and glucose production by the liver. The patient with T1DM cannot make the hormonal changes needed to maintain stable blood glucose levels during exercise. Without an adequate insulin supply, cells cannot use glucose. Low insulin levels trigger release of glucagon and epinephrine (balancing hormones) to increase liver glucose production, further raising blood glucose levels. Without insulin, FFAs become the source of energy. Exercise in the patient with uncontrolled DM results in hyperglycemia and ketone body formation. Postexercise hyperglycemia can be seen following anaerobic exercise (e.g., powerlifting, bodybuilding) or very vigorous aerobic exercise with intermittent periods of anaerobic exercise (e.g., boxing, mountain biking, mountain climbing).

Exercise also can cause hypoglycemia because of increased muscle glucose uptake and inhibited glucose release from the liver during exercise and for up to 24 hours after exercise. Replacement of muscle and liver glycogen stores, along with increased insulin sensitivity after exercise, causes insulin requirements to drop.

Benefits of exercise include better blood ***glucose regulation*** and reduced insulin requirements. Exercise also increases insulin sensitivity, which enhances cell uptake of glucose and promotes weight loss.

Regular exercise decreases risk for cardiovascular disease. It decreases most blood lipid levels and increases high-density lipoproteins (HDLs, the "good" cholesterol). Exercise decreases blood pressure and improves cardiac function. Regular physical activity prevents or delays T2DM by reducing body weight, insulin resistance, and glucose intolerance.

PATIENT-CENTERED CARE: OLDER ADULT HEALTH
Physical Activity

The ability of the heart and lungs to deliver oxygen to organs declines with age. Muscle strength declines gradually. Range of motion and flexibility decrease, altering gait and increasing the risk for falls. Remaining active can limit loss of muscle mass and function.

Changes in activity levels should be gradual. Formal evaluation by a physical therapist may be needed. Emphasize that the focus for any activity program is on increasing activity levels. Some older adults may need to begin with low-intensity physical activity. Start low-intensity activities in short sessions (less than 5–10 minutes); include warm-up and cool-down components with active stretching. Safe places for physical activity should be assessed to prevent falls or injury. Chair yoga, walking, water aerobics, and resistance band workouts are examples that some older adults might enjoy.

Exercise adjustments are needed when some long-term DM complications are present. Vigorous aerobic or resistance exercise should be avoided in the presence of diabetic retinopathy. Teach the patient with retinopathy about activities that increase blood pressure. Heavy lifting, rapid head motion, or jarring activities can cause vitreous hemorrhage or retinal detachment. Decreased sensation in the extremities increases the risk for skin breakdown and joint damage. Teach patients with peripheral neuropathy to wear proper footwear and examine their feet daily for lesions or injury. Teach anyone with a foot injury or open sore to engage in non–weight-bearing activities such as swimming, bicycling, or arm exercises. Those with autonomic neuropathy are at increased risk for exercise-induced injury from poor temperature control, postural hypotension, and impaired thirst with risk for dehydration. Encourage high-risk patients to start with short periods of low-intensity exercise and to increase the intensity and duration slowly. Patient conditions that often require activity adjustment include:

- Hypertension
- Severe autonomic neuropathy
- Severe peripheral neuropathy or foot lesions
- Unstable proliferative retinopathy

In the absence of contraindications, advise adults with DM to perform at least 150 minutes per week of moderate-intensity aerobic physical activity divided into 5 days (ADA, 2022). Teach patients to avoid going more than 2 consecutive days without aerobic physical activity. Urge patients to perform resistance exercise at least twice weekly, targeting all major muscle groups.

A 5- to 10-minute warm-up period with stretching and low-intensity exercise before exercise prepares the muscles, heart, and lungs for a progressive increase in exercise intensity. After exercising, a cool-down of at least 5 to 10 minutes is performed to gradually bring the heart rate down to preexercise level.

Guidelines for exercise are based on blood glucose levels and ketone levels. Teach patients to check their glucose before exercise, at intervals during exercise, and after exercise to determine if it is safe to exercise, and to evaluate the effects of exercise. The absence of urine ketones indicates that enough insulin is available for glucose transport. *When urine ketones are present, the patient should* **NOT** *exercise.* Ketones indicate that current insulin levels are not adequate and that exercise would elevate blood glucose levels. Carbohydrate foods should be ingested to raise blood glucose levels above 100 mg/dL (5.6 mmol/L) before engaging in exercise. See Box 56.7 for tips to teach about exercise.

❗ NURSING SAFETY PRIORITY

Action Alert

Teach patients with type 1 diabetes mellitus (T1DM) to perform vigorous exercise *only* when blood glucose levels are 100 to 250 mg/dL (5.6–13.8 mmol/L) and no ketones are present in the urine.

BOX 56.7 Patient and Family Education

Physical Activity

- Remember that exercise helps manage blood glucose levels and blood lipid levels and helps reduce complications of diabetes.
- Perform the level of physical activity recommended to you by your diabetes health care provider.
- Wear appropriate footwear designed for physical activity.
- Examine your feet daily and after physical activity.
- Stay hydrated and do not exercise in extreme heat or cold.
- Do not exercise within 1 hour of insulin injection or near time of peak insulin action.
- Prevent hypoglycemia during exercise:
  - Do not exercise unless blood glucose level is at least 100 and less than 250 mg/dL if on insulin.
  - Have a carbohydrate snack before exercising if 1 hour has passed since the last meal or if the planned exercise is of high intensity.
  - Carry a simple sugar to eat during exercise if symptoms of hypoglycemia occur.
- Carry identification information about diabetes during physical activity.
- Check your blood glucose levels more often on days you exercise, and remember that extra carbohydrate and less insulin may be needed during the 24-hour period following exercise.

Blood glucose control in hospitalized patients. Hyperglycemia in hospitalized patients occurs from loss of **glucose regulation** caused by illness; decreased physical activity; withholding of antidiabetic drugs; use of drugs, such as corticosteroids or antipsychotics; and changes in nutrition. Hyperglycemia during hospitalization is associated with poor outcomes, such as higher infection rates, longer hospital stays, increased need for intensive care, and greater mortality. Admission glucose levels greater than 198 mg/dL (10.9 mmol/L) are linked to greater mortality and complications. Hypoglycemia is also a risk factor for mortality.

Current guidelines recommend treatment protocols that maintain blood glucose levels between 140 and 180 mg/dL (7.8 and 10.0 mmol/L) for critically ill patients. For most non–critically ill patients, premeal glucose targets are lower than 140 mg/dL (7.8 mmol/L), with random blood glucose values less than 180 mg/dL (10.0 mmol/L). To prevent hypoglycemia, insulin regimens are reviewed if blood glucose levels fall below 100 mg/dL (5.6 mmol/L) and are modified when blood glucose levels are less than 70 mg/dL (3.9 mmol/L) (ADA, 2022).

Continuous IV insulin solutions (insulin drip) are the most effective method for achieving glycemic targets in the intensive care setting. Scheduled subcutaneous injection with basal, meal, and correction elements is used to maintain glucose control in non–critically ill patients. Use of correction dose to correct premeal hyperglycemia in addition to scheduled prandial and basal insulin is determined by the patient's insulin sensitivity and current blood glucose level.

Prevention of hypoglycemia is also part of managing blood glucose levels. Causes of inpatient hypoglycemia include an inappropriate insulin type, mismatch between insulin type and/or timing of food intake, and altered eating plan without insulin dosage adjustment. Many facilities have protocols for hypoglycemia treatment that direct staff to provide carbohydrate replacement if the patient is alert and able to swallow or to administer concentrated dextrose IV or glucagon by subcutaneous injection if the patient cannot swallow, using the 15-15 rule (see the Nutrition Therapy section under Interventions for Preventing Hypoglycemia later in this chapter for specific 15-15 rule interventions).

There is confusion about whether to give or to hold insulin from a patient who is NPO. Giving rapid-acting or short-acting insulin, as well as amylin and incretin mimetics, will cause hypoglycemia if a patient is not eating. Basal insulin (often at a reduced dose) should be given when the patient is NPO because it controls baseline glucose levels. Insulin mixtures are not given because they contain some short-acting or rapid-acting insulin and will cause hypoglycemia.

Surgical Management. The most common surgical intervention for treating DM is pancreas transplantation. When successful, this procedure eliminates the need for insulin injections, blood glucose monitoring (BGM), and many dietary restrictions. It can eliminate the acute complications related to blood **glucose regulation** but is only partially successful in reversing long-term complications. Pancreas transplant is successful when the patient no longer needs insulin therapy and all blood measures of glucose are normal.

Transplantation requires lifelong drug therapy to prevent graft rejection. These drug regimens have side effects that restrict their use to patients who have serious progressive complications from DM. Some antirejection drugs increase blood glucose levels. A pancreas-alone transplant is most often considered for patients with severe metabolic complications and for those with the inability to prevent acute complications despite intensive insulin use.

Pancreas transplantation is considered in patients with DM and end-stage kidney disease (ESKD) who have had or plan to have a kidney transplant. Pancreas graft survival is better when performed at the time of the kidney transplant. Pancreatic transplantation may be performed as a pancreas transplant alone (PTA), pancreas after kidney transplant (PAK), and simultaneous pancreas and kidney transplant (SPK).

The 1-year survival rate for patients receiving a whole pancreas in North America is above 95%, with most patients remaining free of insulin injection and diet restrictions. The degree of human leukocyte antigen (HLA) tissue-type matching affects the results.

Operative procedures. Most pancreatic transplants involve cadaver donors using a whole pancreas still attached to the exit of the pancreatic duct. The recipient's pancreas is left in place, and the donated pancreas is placed in the pelvis. The insulin released by the pancreas graft is secreted into the bloodstream. The new pancreas also produces about 800 to 1000 mL of fluid daily, which is diverted to either the bladder or the bowel.

Excretion of pancreatic fluids can impair **fluid and electrolyte balance,** and drainage of these fluids into the urinary bladder causes irritation. When the pancreas is attached to the bladder, the loss of fluid rich in bicarbonate may cause acidosis.

Rejection management. Pancreatic transplantation requires a combination of drugs to reverse and prevent rejection. Patients undergoing antirejection therapy first receive drugs to prevent viral, bacterial, and fungal infection because of the risk for opportunistic infections from overall reduced **immunity.** When the regimen includes steroid therapy, the patient will require dosage adjustments in insulin to achieve desired levels of glucose control. Long-term antirejection therapy reduces **immunity** and increases the risk for infection, cancer, and atherosclerosis.

Preventing Surgical Complications

Planning: Expected Outcomes. The patient with DM undergoing a surgical procedure is expected to recover completely without complications.

Interventions. The patient with DM is at higher risk for complications. Anesthesia and surgery cause a stress response with release of counterregulatory hormones that elevate blood glucose by suppressing insulin action and increasing the risk for ketoacidosis. Hyperglycemic-hyperosmolar state (HHS) is a complication of surgery and is associated with increased mortality. Diuresis from hyperglycemia can cause dehydration and increases the risk for acute kidney injury.

Complications of DM increase the risk for surgical problems. Patients with DM are at higher risk for hypertension, ischemic heart disease, cerebrovascular disease, myocardial infarction (MI), and cardiomyopathy. The patient with DM is at risk for acute kidney injury and urinary retention after surgery, especially if they have albumin in the urine (indicator of kidney damage). Nerve function to the intestinal wall and sphincters can be reduced, leading to delayed gastric emptying and reflux of gastric acid, which increases the risk for aspiration with anesthesia. Autonomic neuropathy may cause paralytic ileus after surgery.

Preoperative Care. Before surgery, blood glucose levels are optimized to reduce the risk for complications. Sulfonylureas are discontinued 1 day before surgery. Metformin is stopped at least 24 hours before surgery and restarted only after kidney function is documented as normal. All other oral drugs are stopped the day of surgery. Patients taking long-acting insulin may need to be switched to intermediate-acting insulin forms 1 to 2 days before surgery.

Preoperative blood glucose levels should be less than 200 mg/dL (11.1 mmol/L). Higher levels are associated with increased infection rates and impaired wound healing.

Intraoperative Care. IV infusion of insulin, glucose, and potassium is standard therapy for perioperative management of DM, and infusion rates are based on hourly capillary glucose testing. The object is to keep the glucose level between 140 and 180 mg/dL (7.8 and 10.0 mmol/L) during surgery to prevent hypoglycemia and reduce risks from hyperglycemia. Higher insulin doses may be needed because stress releases glucagon and epinephrine. Patients usually receive about 5 g of glucose per hour during surgery to prevent hypoglycemia, ketosis, and protein breakdown.

Postoperative Care. Hyperglycemia leads to increased mortality after surgical procedures. American Association of Clinical Endocrinology (AACE) and ADA guidelines recommend insulin dosing to maintain blood glucose between 140 and 180 mg/dL (7.8 and 10.0 mmol/L) for critically ill patients (ADA, 2022).

Continue glucose and insulin infusions as ordered until the patient is stable and can tolerate oral feedings. Short-term insulin therapy may be needed after surgery for the patient who usually uses oral agents. For those receiving insulin therapy, dosage adjustments may be required until the stress of surgery subsides.

Opioid analgesics slow GI motility and alter blood glucose levels. The older patient who receives opioids is at risk for confusion, paralytic ileus, hypoventilation, hypotension, and urinary retention. Patient-controlled analgesia (PCA) systems reduce respiratory complications and confusion. (See Chapter 6 for pain interventions and Chapter 9 for general preoperative care.)

Monitoring. Patients with autonomic neuropathy or vascular disease need close monitoring to avoid hypotension or respiratory arrest. Those who take beta blockers for hypertension need close monitoring for hypoglycemia because these drugs mask symptoms of hypoglycemia. Patients with increased blood protein or nitrogen in the blood may have problems with fluid management. Check central venous pressure or pulmonary artery pressure as needed.

Balancing hormones are often activated and cause increased blood glucose levels before patients become febrile. *Hyperglycemia often occurs before a fever.*

! NURSING SAFETY PRIORITY
Action Alert

> When a patient who has had reasonably controlled blood glucose levels in the hospital develops an unexpected rise in blood glucose values, check for infection (e.g., urinary tract infection, pneumonia, cellulitis, wound infection).

Fluid and electrolyte balance is often disrupted by surgery. *Hyperkalemia* (high blood potassium level) is common in patients with mild to moderate kidney failure and can lead to cardiac dysrhythmia. In other patients, *hypokalemia* (low blood potassium level) may occur and be made worse by insulin and glucose given during surgery. Monitor the cardiac rhythm and serum potassium values.

Cardiovascular monitoring by continuous ECG is often used for older patients with DM, those with long-standing T1DM, and those with heart disease. Patients with DM are at higher risk for MI after surgery. Changes in ECG or potassium level may indicate a silent MI.

Kidney monitoring, especially observing fluid balance, helps detect acute kidney injury. Management of infections may require the use of nephrotoxic antibiotics. Ensure adequate hydration when these drugs are used. Check for impending kidney failure by assessing *fluid and electrolyte balance.*

Nutrition. Patients requiring clear or full liquid diets should receive about 200 g of carbohydrate daily in equally divided amounts at meals and snack times. Initial liquids should ***not*** be sugar free. Most patients require 25 to 35 calories per kg of body weight every 24 hours. After surgery, food intake is initiated as quickly as possible, with progression from clear liquids to solid foods occurring as rapidly as tolerated to promote healing and metabolic balance. When oral foods are tolerated, make sure the patient eats at least 150 to 200 g of carbohydrate daily to prevent hypoglycemia.

If total parenteral nutrition (TPN) is used after surgery, severe hyperglycemia may occur. Monitor blood glucose often, usually at least every 6 hours, to determine the need for supplemental insulin.

Preventing Injury From Peripheral Neuropathy

Planning: Expected Outcomes. The patient with DM is expected to identify factors that increase the risk for injury, practice proper foot care, and maintain intact skin on the feet.

Interventions. Patients with DM need intensive education about foot care because foot injury is a common complication. Once a failure of *tissue integrity* has occurred and an ulcer has developed, there is an increased risk for wound progression. Most lower extremity amputations in adults with DM are preceded by foot ulcers, and the 5-year mortality rate after leg or

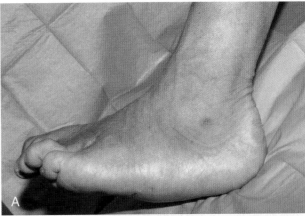
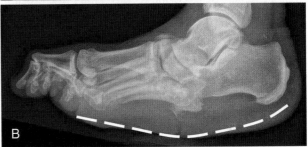

FIG. 56.11 (A) Clinical presentation and (B) lateral radiograph of the rocker-bottom deformity of end-stage Charcot foot. (From Rosskopf, A. B., Loupatatzis, C., Pfirrmann, C. W. A., et al. [2019]. The Charcot foot: a pictorial review. *Insights Imaging, 10* [1].)

foot amputation is high (CDC, 2022a). Neuropathy is the main risk factor for development of a diabetic ulcer, and inadequate ***perfusion*** is the main cause of poor healing.

Motor neuropathy damages the nerves of foot muscles, resulting in foot deformities. These deformities create pressure points that gradually reduce *tissue integrity* with skin breakdown and ulceration. Thinning or shifting of the fat pad under the metatarsal heads decreases cushioning and increases areas of pressure. In claw toe deformity, toes are hyperextended and increase pressure on the metatarsal heads ("ball" of the foot). These changes predispose the patient to callus formation, ulceration, and infection. The *Charcot foot* is a type of diabetic foot deformity with many abnormalities, often including a *hallux valgus* (turning inward of the great toe) (Fig. 56.11). The foot is warm, swollen, and painful. Walking collapses the arch, shortens the foot, and gives the foot a "rocker bottom" shape.

Autonomic neuropathy causes loss of normal sweating and skin temperature regulation, resulting in dry, thinning skin. Skin cracks and fissures increase the infection risk. Sensory neuropathy may cause tingling or burning, but more often it produces numbness and reduced *sensory perception.* Without sensation, the patient does not notice injury and loss of *tissue integrity* in the foot. Peripheral arterial disease reduces blood flow to the foot, increasing the risk for ulcer formation and slowing ulcer healing (Rogers, 2023).

Foot injuries are caused by walking barefoot, wearing ill-fitting shoes, sustaining thermal injuries from heat (e.g., hot water bottles, heating pads, baths), or chemical burns from over-the-counter corn treatments. These injuries lead to loss of *tissue integrity* and often to amputation.

Ulcers result from continued pressure. Ulcers on the sole and ball of the foot are from standing or walking. Those on the top or sides of the foot usually are from shoes. The increased pressure causes calluses. Ulcers usually form over or around the great toe, under the metatarsal heads, and on the tops of claw toes.

Loss of *tissue integrity* with broken skin increases the risk for infection. Skin tends to break in areas of pressure. Infection is common in diabetic foot ulcers and, once present, is difficult to treat. Infection also impairs *glucose regulation,* leading to higher blood glucose levels and reduced *immunity,* which further increases the risk for infection.

Prevention of High-Risk Conditions. Neuropathy of the feet and legs can be delayed by keeping blood glucose levels within the target range. Chronic hyperglycemia increases the risk for neuropathy and amputation. Urge smoking cessation and encourage physical activity to reduce the risk for vascular complications.

The risk for ulcers or amputation increases with the presence of peripheral neuropathy. Other risk factors are male sex; poor glucose control; and cardiovascular, retinal, or kidney complications. Foot-related risks include poor gait and stepping mechanics, peripheral neuropathy, increased pressure (callus, erythema/hyperpigmentation, hemorrhage under a callus, limited joint mobility, foot deformities, or severe nail pathology), peripheral vascular disease, and a history of ulcers or amputation (ADA, 2022).

Peripheral Neuropathy Management. Foot assessment techniques are listed in Box 56.8. A thorough assessment of the feet should be performed by a health care professional at least annually. Table 56.7 lists foot risk categories.

Sensory examination of the foot with Semmes-Weinstein monofilaments is a practical measure of loss of sensation, which increases the risk for foot ulcers. The nylon monofilament is mounted on a holder standardized to exert a 10-g force.

An adult who cannot feel the 10-g pressure at any point is at increased risk for ulcers. A foot exam using a monofilament is recommended at least annually.

Footwear. Patients with any degree of peripheral neuropathy are at risk for loss of *tissue integrity* and need to wear protective shoes fitted by an experienced shoe fitter, such as a certified podiatrist. The shoe should be ½ to ⅝ inch longer than the longest toe. Heels should be less than 2 inches high. Tight shoes

---

BOX 56.8 Assessment of the Diabetic Foot

Assess the patient's risk for diabetic foot problems:
- History of previous ulcer
- History of previous amputation

Assess the foot for abnormal skin and nail conditions:
- Dry, cracked, fissured skin
- Ulcers
- Toenails: thickened, long nails; ingrown nails
- Tinea pedis; onychomycosis (mycotic nails)

Assess the foot for status of circulation:
- Symptoms of claudication
- Presence or absence of dorsalis pedis or posterior tibial pulse
- Prolonged capillary filling time (greater than 25 seconds)
- Presence or absence of hair growth on the top of the foot

Assess the foot for evidence of deformity:
- Calluses, corns
- Prominent metatarsal heads (metatarsal head is easily felt under the skin)
- Toe contractures: clawed toes, hammertoes
- Hallux valgus or bunions
- Charcot foot ("rocker bottom")

Assess the foot for loss of strength:
- Limited ankle joint range of motion
- Limited motion of great toe

Assess the foot for loss of protective sensation:
- Numbness, burning, tingling
- Semmes-Weinstein monofilament testing at 10 points on each foot

Data from American Diabetes Association (ADA). (2022). Standards of medical care in diabetes- 2022. *Diabetes Care, 45* (Suppl. 1). https://diabetesjournals.org/care/issue/45/Supplement_1.

TABLE 56.7 Foot Risk Categories

Risk Categories	Management Categories
Risk Category 0 • Has protective sensation • No evidence of peripheral vascular disease • No evidence of foot deformity or loss of *tissue integrity*	**Management Category 0** • Comprehensive foot examination once a year • Patient education to include advice on appropriate footwear
Risk Category 1 • Does not have protective sensation • May have evidence of foot deformity	**Management Category 1** • Evaluation every 3–6 months • Consider referral to a specialist to assess need for specialized treatment and follow-up • Patient education
Risk Category 2 • Does not have protective sensation • Evidence of peripheral vascular disease	**Management Categories 2 and 3** • Evaluation every 1–3 months • Referral to a specialist • Prescription footwear • Consider vascular consultation for combined follow-up • Patient education
Risk Category 3 • History of ulcer or amputation	

damage tissue. Instruct the patient to change shoes by midday and again in the evening. Socks must fit properly and be appropriate for the planned activity. Socks should feel soft and have no thick seams, creases, or holes. They should pad the foot and absorb excess moisture. White socks are recommended because the presence of blood or drainage is more easily recognized than on colored socks.

Teach patients to avoid tight stockings or those that have constricting bands. Patients with toe deformities need custom shoes with high, wide toe boxes and extra depth. Those with severely deformed feet need specially molded shoes. New shoes need a long break-in period with frequent foot inspection for irritation or blistering.

Foot care. Teach patients about preventive foot care and the need for examination of the feet and legs at each visit to a diabetes health care provider or primary health care provider. A mirror placed on the floor can help the patient visually examine the plantar surface of the foot. Identify patients with high-risk foot conditions. Explain problems caused by loss of protective sensation, the importance of monitoring the feet daily, proper care of the feet (including nail and skin care), and how to select appropriate footwear.

Assess the patient's ability to inspect all areas of the foot and to perform foot care. Teach family members how to inspect and care for the patient's feet using the guidelines in Box 56.9 if the patient is unable to do this independently.

Wound care. The standards of care for diabetic ulcers are a moist wound environment, débridement of necrotic tissue, and elimination of pressure (offloading). Eliminating pressure on an infected area is essential for wound healing. Teach patients with foot ulcers to not wear a shoe on the affected foot while the ulcer is healing. Those with poor **sensory perception** may keep walking on an ulcer because it does not hurt, causing pressure necrosis that delays healing and increases ulcer size. Pressure is reduced by specialized orthotic devices, custom-molded shoe inserts, or shoe adjustments that redistribute weight.

Offloading redistributes force away from ulcer sites and pressure points to wider areas of the foot. Available products include total-contact casting, half shoes, removable cast walkers, wheelchairs, and crutches. Total-contact casts redistribute pressure over the bottom of the foot. Casting material is molded to the foot and leg to spread pressure along the entire surface of contact, reducing vertical force. The almost complete elimination of motion of the total-contact cast reduces plantar shear forces. *Teach the patient that foot ulcers will recur unless weight is permanently redistributed.*

Reducing the Risk for Kidney Disease

Planning: Expected Outcomes. The patient with diabetes is expected to maintain optimum kidney function.

Interventions

Prevention. Diabetic kidney disease is more likely to develop in patients with genetic risk factors, unmanaged hypertension, and chronic hyperglycemia. Progression to end-stage kidney disease can be delayed or prevented by normalizing blood pressure using drugs from either the angiotensin-converting

---

BOX 56.9 Patient and Family Education

Foot Care Instruction

- Inspect your feet daily, especially the area between the toes.
- Wash your feet daily with lukewarm water and soap. Dry thoroughly.
- Apply a moisturizer to your feet (but not between your toes) after bathing.
- Change into clean cotton socks every day.
- Do not wear the same pair of shoes 2 days in a row, and wear only shoes made of breathable materials, such as leather or cloth.
- Check your shoes for foreign objects (pebbles) before putting them on. Check inside the shoes for cracks or tears in the lining.
- Buy shoes that have plenty of room for your toes. Buy shoes later in the day when feet are normally larger. Break in new shoes gradually.
- Wear socks to keep your feet warm.
- Trim your nails straight across with a nail clipper and smooth them with an emery board.
- See your diabetes health care provider immediately if you have blisters, sores, or infections. Protect the area with a dry, sterile dressing. Do not use tape to secure dressing to the skin.
- Do not treat blisters, sores, or infections with home remedies.
- Do not step into the bathtub without checking the temperature of the water with your wrist or thermometer.
- Do not use very hot or cold water. Never use hot-water bottles, heating pads, or portable heaters to warm your feet.
- Do not treat corns, blisters, bunions, calluses, or ingrown toenails yourself.
- Do not go barefooted.
- Do not wear sandals with open toes or straps between the toes.
- Do not cross your legs or wear tight stockings that constrict blood flow.

Data from American Diabetes Association (ADA). (2022). Standards of medical care in diabetes- 2022. *Diabetes Care, 45* (Suppl. 1). https:// diabetesjournals.org/care/issue/45/Supplement_1.

---

enzyme inhibitor (ACEI) class or the angiotensin receptor blocker (ARB) class. Once used to "protect" the kidney, neither class of drug is recommended for patients with DM who have normal blood pressure and normal albumin excretion (ADA, 2022). Hypertension greatly accelerates the progression of diabetic kidney disease.

Stress the need for evaluation of kidney function according to the ADA Standards of Care. An annual test to quantify urine albumin is performed for patients who have had T1DM for over 5 years and in all those with T2DM starting at diagnosis (ADA, 2022). Persistent albuminuria in the range of 30 to 299 mg/24 hours is the earliest stage of nephropathy in T1DM and a marker for the development of nephropathy in T2DM.

Aggressive control of blood glucose, cholesterol levels, and hypertension in patients without albuminuria can prevent nephropathy. Once albuminuria develops, management focuses on controlling blood pressure and blood glucose and avoiding nephrotoxic agents.

Control of blood pressure, cholesterol, and blood glucose levels requires the patient's participation. Prescribed drugs must be taken according to schedules, and dietary restriction must be maintained. Educate patients about the roles of blood pressure and blood glucose levels in kidney disease. Teach them about maintaining normal blood glucose and cholesterol levels and keeping blood pressure levels below 140/80 mm Hg. Stress the need for yearly screening for albuminuria.

Smoking cessation is important in halting the progression of diabetic kidney disease. Teach patients about the risks of smoking and refer them to appropriate resources for assistance in smoking cessation, as described in Chapter 22.

Drugs can affect kidney function through either toxic effects on the kidney or an acute but reversible reduction in function. The most common prescribed nephrotoxic drugs are antifungal agents and aminoglycoside antibiotics. Other common nephrotoxic drugs are NSAIDs such as ibuprofen or naproxen. Teach patients to check with their diabetes health care provider or a pharmacist before taking over-the-counter drugs or herbal remedies.

Radiocontrast media can also affect kidney function, especially in patients with preexisting kidney problems. Monitor IV hydration before and after a contrast agent is used to prevent contrast-induced nephropathy in patients with DM.

Drug Therapy. Use of angiotensin-converting enzyme inhibitors (ACEIs) or angiotensin receptor blockers (ARBs) is recommended for all patients with persistent albuminuria or advanced stages of nephropathy (ADA, 2022). ACEIs reduce the level of albuminuria and the rate of progression of kidney disease, although they do not appear to prevent albuminuria. Monitor serum potassium levels for development of hyperkalemia (ADA, 2022).

Dialysis for patients with DM and kidney failure is the same as for patients without diabetes (see Chapter 60). The dosage of insulin needs to be reduced when dialysis starts, as there is an increased risk of hypoglycemia.

Preventing Complications of Glucose-Related Emergencies

Planning: Expected Outcomes. The patient is expected to maintain optimum blood glucose levels.

Interventions for Preventing Hypoglycemia. Hypoglycemia is a low blood glucose level that induces specific symptoms and resolves when blood glucose concentration is raised. Once plasma glucose levels fall below 70 mg/dL (3.9 mmol/L), a sequence of events begins with release of counterregulatory hormones, stimulation of the autonomic nervous system, and production of *neurogenic* and *neuroglycopenic* symptoms. Peripheral autonomic symptoms, including sweating, irritability, tremors, anxiety, tachycardia, and hunger, serve as an early warning system and occur before the symptoms of confusion, paralysis, seizure, and coma occur from brain glucose deprivation. *Neuroglycopenic symptoms* occur when brain glucose *gradually declines* to a low level. *Neurologic symptoms* result from autonomic nervous activity triggered by a *rapid decline* in blood glucose (Box 56.10).

Central nervous system (CNS) function depends on a continuous supply of glucose in the blood. The brain cannot make glucose and stores only a few minutes' supply as glycogen. This needed supply is not maintained when the blood glucose level falls below critical levels.

BOX 56.10 Symptoms of Hypoglycemia

Neuroglycopenic Symptoms
- Weakness
- Fatigue
- Difficulty thinking
- Confusion
- Behavior changes
- Emotional instability
- Seizures
- Loss of consciousness
- Brain damage
- Death

Neurogenic Symptoms
- Adrenergic:
  - Shaky or tremulous
  - Heart pounding
  - Nervous or anxious
- Cholinergic:
  - Sweaty
  - Hungry
  - Tingling

The first defenses against falling blood glucose levels in the adult without DM are decreased insulin secretion, decreased glucose use, and increased glucose production. Normally, insulin secretion decreases when blood glucose levels drop to about 83 mg/dL (4.5 mmol/L). Balancing (counterregulatory) hormones are activated at about 67 mg/dL (3.7 mmol/L), a level above the threshold for symptoms of hypoglycemia. The main balancing hormone is glucagon. Both glucagon and epinephrine raise blood glucose levels by stimulating liver glycogen breakdown and conversion of protein to glucose. Epinephrine also limits insulin secretion.

A problem with long-standing insulin-dependent T1DM or T2DM is *hypoglycemic unawareness,* in which patients no longer have the warning symptoms of early hypoglycemia that could prompt them to take preventive action. This may occur after years of long-standing history of hypoglycemia.

The blood glucose level at which symptoms of hypoglycemia occur varies among patients. Therefore, clinical criteria used to categorize hypoglycemia are based on symptom severity rather than blood glucose levels. In mild hypoglycemia, the patient remains alert and able to self-manage symptoms. In severe hypoglycemia, neurologic function is so impaired that the patient needs another person's help to increase blood glucose levels.

Blood Glucose Management. Monitor blood glucose levels before giving antidiabetic drugs, before meals, before bedtime, and when the patient is symptomatic. All patients who take insulin, those taking sulfonylureas, and those taking metformin in combination with sulfonylureas are at risk for hypoglycemia. This risk is increased if they are older, have liver or kidney impairment, or are taking drugs that enhance the effects of antidiabetic drugs. In the hospital setting, mealtime insulin *must* be coordinated with timely monitoring and food delivery to avoid episodes of hypoglycemia. In addition, blood glucose should be checked no more than 30 minutes before a meal, and rapid-acting insulin should be given just before the meal to avoid hypoglycemia.

The most common causes of hypoglycemia are:
- Too much insulin relative to food intake and physical activity
- Insulin injected at the wrong time relative to food intake and physical activity

- The wrong type of insulin injected at the wrong time
- Decreased food intake resulting from missed or delayed meals
- Delayed gastric emptying from gastroparesis
- Decreased liver glucose production after alcohol ingestion
- Decreased insulin clearance due to progressive kidney failure

Nutrition Therapy. In hospitalized patients, most protocols for management of hypoglycemia follow the 15-15 rule for hypoglycemia management (Watts et al., 2020). With this rule, 15 g of CHO are given if the blood glucose level is less than 70 mg/dL (3.9 mmol/L) (or 30 g if less than 50 mg/dL [2.8 mmol/L]) or if the patient is experiencing symptoms of hypoglycemia. If the patient can swallow, give a liquid form of CHO, although any fast-acting CHO source can be used (avoid high-potassium options such as orange juice). If the blood glucose recheck within 15 minutes is still low, the same treatment is given again. If at any time the patient is unable to swallow, an IV dose of concentrated dextrose or subcutaneous glucagon is indicated. If the 15-minute recheck is above hypoglycemic range, follow up with a complex carbohydrate such as crackers with nut butter. Specific recommendations are listed in Box 56.11 for management of hypoglycemia at home.

The blood glucose level determines the form and amount of glucose used. Concentrated sweet fluids, such as chocolate, may slow absorption because of the fat content. Initial management of hypoglycemia is most effective with ingestion of glucose or glucose-containing foods rather than foods containing complex carbohydrates. *Ingesting a complex carbohydrate after hypoglycemia resolves helps prevent subsequent hypoglycemia.*

Drug Therapy. Concentrated IV dextrose is often given to patients in the hospital setting who cannot swallow. IM or nasal glucagon is given to patients with severe hypoglycemia who cannot swallow. Glucagon is the main balancing hormone to insulin and is used as first-line therapy for severe hypoglycemia. Glucagon can induce vomiting. To prevent aspiration, be sure to position the patient on the side. Give concentrated dextrose carefully to avoid extravasation because it is hyperosmolar and can damage tissue. The effects of glucagon and dextrose are temporary. Evaluate response by monitoring blood glucose levels every 15 minutes until hypoglycemia resolves, as additional treatment may be needed. Then, monitor for several hours. A target blood glucose level is 70 to 110 mg/dL (3.9–6.2 mmol/L).

✚ NURSING SAFETY PRIORITY

Critical Rescue

Assess patients to recognize the presence and severity of hypoglycemia. For the patient with *severe* hypoglycemia, respond by:
1. Giving the prescribed dose of glucagon
2. Repeating the dose in 10 minutes if the patient remains unconscious
3. Notifying the diabetes health care provider immediately, and following instructions

Prevention Strategies. Teach the patient how to prevent hypoglycemia.

Insulin excess from miscalculating insulin doses can cause hypoglycemia even when insulin is injected correctly.

BOX 56.11 Patient and Family Education

Management of Hypoglycemia at Home

For mild hypoglycemia (hungry, irritable, shaky, weak, headache, fully conscious; blood glucose usually less than 70 mg/dL [3.9 mmol/L]):
- Treat the symptoms of hypoglycemia with 15 g of carbohydrate. You may use one of these:
  - Glucose tablets or glucose gel
  - A half-cup (120 mL) of fruit juice or regular (nondiet) soft drink
  - 5 hard candies
  - 4 cubes of sugar or 4 teaspoons of sugar
  - 1 tablespoon (15 mL) of honey or syrup
- Retest blood glucose in 15 minutes.
- Repeat this treatment if glucose remains less than 70 mg/dL (3.9 mmol/L). Symptoms may persist after blood glucose has normalized.
- Eat a small complex carbohydrate and protein snack.

For moderate hypoglycemia (cold, clammy skin; pale/ash gray skin; rapid pulse; rapid, shallow respirations; marked change in mood; drowsiness; blood glucose usually less than 50 mg/dL [2.2 mmol/L]):
- Treat the symptoms of hypoglycemia with 30 g of rapidly absorbed carbohydrate.
- Glucagon may be indicated.
- Retest glucose in 15 minutes.
- Repeat treatment if glucose is less than 60 mg/dL (3.4 mmol/L).
- Eat a small complex carbohydrate and protein snack once hypoglycemia resolves.

For severe hypoglycemia (unable to swallow; confusion, combativeness, unconsciousness or convulsions):
- Treatment administered by family member:
  - Give prescribed dose of glucagon as IM or subcutaneous injection or nasal powder.
  - Give a second dose in 10 minutes if the person remains unconscious.
  - If still unconscious, call 911 to have the person transported to the emergency department and to receive IV dextrose if needed.
  - Call the diabetes health care provider for insulin instructions.
  - Give a small meal when the person wakes up and is no longer nauseated.

Deficient food intake from inadequate or incorrectly timed meals can result in hypoglycemia. Educate about the importance of regular timing and quantity of food eaten, especially carbohydrates.

Exercise often causes blood glucose levels to fall. Prolonged exercise increases muscle glucose uptake for several hours after exercise. Teach patients about blood glucose monitoring and carbohydrate consumption before and during exercise (if necessary). Also teach them to exercise at times when insulin activity is not peaking.

Alcohol inhibits liver glucose production and can lead to hypoglycemia hours later. It interferes with the hormone response to hypoglycemia and impairs glycogen breakdown. Instruct the patient to ingest alcohol only with or shortly *after* eating a meal with enough carbohydrate to prevent hypoglycemia.

Patient and Family Education. Help each patient develop a personal treatment plan for hypoglycemia. Teach the family the 15-15 rule. Encourage the patient to wear a medical alert bracelet or have a wallet card describing how to manage diabetes emergencies. This information is helpful if the patient becomes hypoglycemic and is unable to perform self-care. Teach the patient to always carry glucagon and blood glucose monitoring supplies.

TABLE 56.8   Differentiation of Hypoglycemia and Hyperglycemia

Feature	Hypoglycemia	Hyperglycemia
Skin	Cool, clammy, "sweaty"	Warm, dry, vasodilated
Dehydration	Absent	Present
Respirations	No particular or consistent change	Rapid, deep[a]; Kussmaul type; acetone odor (rotten "fruity" odor) to breath
Mental status	Anxious, nervous,[a] irritable, mental confusion,[a] seizures, coma	Varies from alert to stuporous, obtunded, or frank coma
Symptoms	Weakness,[a] double vision, blurred vision, hunger, tachycardia, palpitations	None specific for DKA Acidosis; hypercapnia; abdominal cramps, nausea and vomiting Dehydration: decreased neck vein filling, orthostatic hypotension, tachycardia, poor skin turgor
Glucose	<70 mg/dL (3.9 mmol/L)	>180 mg/dL (10.0 mmol/L)
Urine or blood ketones	Negative	Positive

[a]Classic symptoms.
DKA, Diabetic ketoacidosis.

Teach the patient and family about the symptoms of hypoglycemia (see Box 56.10). Stress that delaying a meal for more than 30 minutes raises the risk for hypoglycemia when some insulin regimens are used. Instruct the patient to keep a CHO source nearby at all times. Teach the patient and family how to inject glucagon. The changes in cognition associated with hypoglycemia may cause confusion among family members with those seen in severe hyperglycemia; review the differences in the common signs and symptoms of these two emergencies (Table 56.8).

👤 PATIENT-CENTERED CARE: OLDER ADULT HEALTH

Risk for Hypoglycemia

Older patients are at increased risk for hypoglycemia. Age-related declines in kidney function reduce the elimination of sulfonylureas and insulin, thus potentiating their hypoglycemic effects. Older adults have reduced epinephrine and glucagon release in response to low blood glucose levels and often have hypoglycemic unawareness. Older adults who are living on their own and do not have any caregiver support may need additional support to recognize and treat hypoglycemia.

Instruct the older patient's family to check blood glucose values when symptoms such as unsteadiness, light-headedness, poor concentration, trembling, or sweating occur (Touhy & Jett, 2023). Remind them to make sure that sufficient foods are eaten at appropriate times. Encourage a patient with a poor appetite to eat a small snack at bedtime to prevent hypoglycemia during the night.

Interventions for Preventing Diabetic Ketoacidosis. Diabetic ketoacidosis (DKA) is a complication of diabetes characterized by uncontrolled hyperglycemia, metabolic acidosis, and increased production of ketones. This condition results from the combination of insulin deficiency and the body metabolizing triglycerides and amino acids instead of glucose for energy, and an increase in hormones (Fig. 56.12). Laboratory diagnosis of DKA is shown in Table 56.9. All of these changes increase ketoacid production with resultant ketonemia and metabolic acidosis. The most common precipitating factor for DKA is infection or illness.

Hyperglycemia leads to osmotic diuresis with dehydration and electrolyte loss. Classic symptoms of DKA include polyuria, polydipsia, polyphagia, a fruity odor to the breath, vomiting, abdominal pain, and weakness. If confusion or Kussmaul respirations are present, DKA can quickly lead to shock and coma. Mental status can vary from total alertness to profound coma. As ketones rise, blood pH decreases, and acidosis occurs. Kussmaul respirations cause respiratory alkalosis in an attempt to correct metabolic acidosis by exhaling carbon dioxide. Initial serum sodium levels may be low or normal.

Blood Glucose Management. Monitor for symptoms of DKA (see Table 56.9 and Fig. 56.12). Document and use these findings to determine therapy effectiveness. *First assess the airway, level of consciousness, hydration status, electrolytes, and blood glucose level.* Check the patient's blood pressure, pulse, and respirations every 15 minutes until stable. Record urine output, temperature, and mental status every hour. When a central venous catheter is present, assess central venous pressure every 30 minutes or as ordered. After treatment starts and these values are stable, monitor and record vital signs every 4 hours. Use blood glucose values to assess therapy and determine when to switch from saline to dextrose-containing solutions.

Fluid and Electrolyte Management. **Closely assess the patient's fluid and electrolyte balance.** Assess for acute weight loss, thirst, decreased skin turgor, dry mucous membranes, and oliguria with a high specific gravity. Assess for weak and rapid pulse; flat neck veins; increased temperature; decreased central venous pressure; muscle weakness; postural hypotension; and cool, clammy, and pale/ash gray skin to determine if the patient is at risk for dehydration.

The first outcome of fluid therapy is to restore blood volume and maintain **perfusion** to vital organs. Typically initial infusion rates are 15 to 20 mL/kg/hr during the first hour.

The second outcome of replacing total body fluid losses is achieved more slowly. Usually hypotonic fluids are infused at 4 to 14 mL/kg/hr after the initial fluid bolus. When blood glucose levels reach 250 mg/dL (13.8 mmol/L), give 5% dextrose in 0.45% saline. This solution helps prevent hypoglycemia and cerebral edema, which can occur when serum osmolarity declines too rapidly.

During the first 24 hours of treatment, the patient needs enough fluids to replace the actual volume lost, as well as any ongoing losses, and the total may be as much as 6 to 10 L. Assess cardiac, kidney, and mental status to avoid fluid overload. Watch for symptoms of heart failure and pulmonary edema. Assess the status of fluid replacement by monitoring blood pressure, intake and output, and changes in daily weight.

Drug Therapy. Insulin therapy is used to lower serum glucose by about 50 to 75 mg/dL/hr (2.8–4.2 mmol/L/hr). Unless the episode of DKA is mild, regular insulin by continuous IV

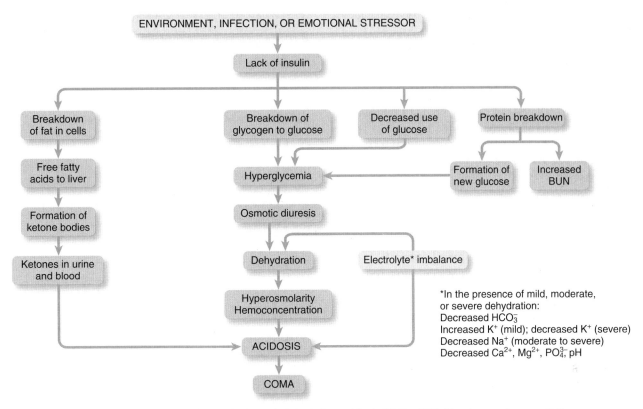

FIG. 56.12 Pathophysiologic mechanism of diabetic ketoacidosis (DKA). *BUN*, Blood urea nitrogen; *Ca²⁺*, calcium; *HCO₃⁻*, bicarbonate; *K⁺*, potassium; *Mg²⁺*, magnesium; *Na⁺*, sodium; *PO₄⁻³*, phosphate.

TABLE 56.9	**Differences Between Diabetic Ketoacidosis and Hyperglycemic-Hyperosmolar State**	
	Diabetic Ketoacidosis (DKA)	**Hyperglycemic-Hyperosmolar State (HHS)**
Onset	Sudden	Gradual
Precipitating factors	Infection Other stressors Inadequate insulin dose	Infection Other stressors Poor fluid intake
Symptoms	Ketosis: Kussmaul respiration, "rotting fruit" breath, nausea, abdominal pain Dehydration or electrolyte loss: polyuria, polydipsia, weight loss, dry skin, sunken eyes, soft eyeballs, lethargy, coma	Altered central nervous system function with neurologic symptoms Dehydration or electrolyte loss: same as for DKA
Laboratory Findings		
Serum glucose	>300 mg/dL (16.7 mmol/L)	>600 mg/dL (33.3 mmol/L)
Osmolarity/osmolality	Variable	>320 mOsm/L (mOsm/kg)
Serum ketones	Positive at 1:2 dilutions	Negative
Serum pH	<7.35	>7.4
Serum HCO₃⁻	<15 mEq/L (mmol/L)	>20 mEq/L (mmol/L)
Serum Na⁺	Low, normal, or high	Normal or low
BUN	>30 mg/dL (10 mmol/L); elevated because of dehydration	Elevated
Creatinine	>1.5 mg/dL (60 mcmol/L); elevated because of dehydration	Elevated
Urine ketones	Positive	Negative

BUN, Blood urea nitrogen; *HCO₃⁻*, bicarbonate; *Na⁺*, sodium.

infusion is the usual management. An initial IV bolus dose is given, followed by an IV continuous infusion. Continuous insulin infusion is used because insulin half-life is short and subcutaneous insulin has a delayed onset of action (Fayfman et al., 2017). Subcutaneous insulin is started when the patient can take oral fluids and ketosis has stopped. DKA is considered resolved when blood glucose is less than 200 mg/mL (11.2 mmol/L) along with a serum bicarbonate level higher than 18 mEq/L (mmol/L), venous pH is higher than 7.30, and a calculated anion gap is less than 12 mEq/L (mmol/L). Assess therapy effectiveness by monitoring blood glucose levels and serial electrolyte levels.

Mild to moderate hyperkalemia is common in patients with hyperglycemia. Insulin therapy, correction of acidosis, and volume expansion decrease serum potassium concentration. To prevent hypokalemia, potassium replacement is initiated after serum levels fall below normal (5.0 mEq/L [mmol/L]). *Assess for signs of hypokalemia, including fatigue, malaise, confusion, muscle weakness, shallow respirations, abdominal distention or paralytic ileus, hypotension, and weak pulse.* An ECG shows conduction changes related to alterations in potassium.

! NURSING SAFETY PRIORITY

Action Alert

Before giving IV potassium-containing solutions, ensure that urine output is at least 30 mL/hr.

Bicarbonate is used only for severe acidosis. Sodium bicarbonate, given by slow IV infusion over several hours, is indicated when the arterial pH is 7.0 or less or the serum bicarbonate level is less than 5 mEq/L (5 mmol/L).

Patient and Family Education. Teach the patient and family to check blood glucose levels every 2 hours as long as symptoms such as anorexia, nausea, and vomiting are present and as long as glucose levels exceed 250 mg/dL (13.8 mmol/L). Teach them to check urine or blood capillary ketone levels when blood glucose levels exceed 250 mg/dL (16.7 mmol/L).

Teach the patient to prevent dehydration by maintaining food and fluid intake. Suggest that the patient drink at least 2 L of fluid daily and increase this amount when infection is present. When nausea is present, instruct the patient to take liquids containing both glucose and electrolytes (e.g., regular sugar-sweetened soda pop, diluted fruit juice, and sports drinks [Gatorade]). Small amounts of fluid may be tolerated even when vomiting is present. When the blood glucose level is normal or elevated, the patient should take 8 to 12 ounces (240–360 mL) of calorie-free and caffeine-free liquids every hour while awake to prevent dehydration.

Liquids containing carbohydrate (CHO) can be taken if the patient cannot eat solid food. Ingesting at least 150 g of CHO daily reduces the risk for starvation ketosis. After consulting the diabetes health care provider, urge the patient to take additional rapid-acting (lispro) or short-acting (regular) insulin based on blood glucose levels.

Instruct the patient and family to consult the diabetes health care provider or primary health care provider when these problems occur:

- Blood glucose exceeds 250 mg/dL (13.8 mmol/L) and does not respond to therapy.

BOX 56.12   Patient and Family Education

Sick-Day Rules

- Notify your primary health care provider or diabetes health care provider that you are ill.
- Monitor your blood glucose at least every 2 to 4 hours.
- Test your urine for ketones even if your blood glucose is in range, particularly if you are vomiting.
- Continue to take insulin or other antidiabetic agents unless instructed otherwise by your diabetes health care provider.
- To prevent dehydration, drink 8 to 12 ounces (240–360 mL) of sugar-free liquids every hour that you are awake. If your blood glucose level is below your target range, drink fluids that contain sugar.
- Continue to eat meals at regular times.
- If unable to tolerate solid food because of nausea, consume more easily tolerated foods or liquids equal to the carbohydrate content of your usual meal.
- Call your diabetes health care provider for any of these problems:
  - Persistent nausea and vomiting
  - Persistent hypoglycemia
  - Moderate or high ketones
  - Blood glucose elevation after two supplemental doses of insulin
  - High (101.5°F [38.6°C]) temperature or increasing fever; fever for more than 24 hours
- Treat diarrhea, nausea, vomiting, and fever as directed by your diabetes health care provider.
- Get plenty of rest.

- Presence of moderate or large ketones.
- The patient cannot take food or fluids or cannot stop vomiting
- Illness lasts more than 1 to 2 days.

Also instruct them to detect hyperglycemia by monitoring blood glucose whenever the patient is ill, as described in Box 56.12 for sick-day rules. Illness can result in dehydration with DKA, hyperglycemic-hyperosmolar state, or both. Insulin therapy should not be omitted during illness.

Interventions for Preventing Hyperglycemic-Hyperosmolar State (HHS). Hyperglycemic-hyperosmolar state (HHS) is a hyperosmolar (increased blood osmolarity) state caused by hyperglycemia. HHS results from a sustained osmotic diuresis leading to extremely high blood glucose levels. The processes of HHS are outlined in Fig. 56.13. Both HHS and diabetic ketoacidosis (DKA) are caused by hyperglycemia and dehydration. HHS differs from DKA in that ketone levels are absent or low and blood glucose levels are much higher. Blood glucose levels may exceed

👤 PATIENT-CENTERED CARE: OLDER ADULT HEALTH

Recognizing Hyperglycemic-Hyperosmolar State (HHS)

HHS occurs most often in older adults with type 2 diabetes mellitus (T2DM), many of whom are unaware they have the disease (Touhy & Jett, 2023). Mortality rates in older patients with HHS have been reported to be as high as 16% (Fayfman et al., 2017). The onset of HHS is slow and may not be recognized. Older patients are at greater risk for dehydration and HHS because of age-related changes in thirst perception, poor urine-concentrating abilities, and use of diuretics. Assess all older adults for dehydration, regardless of whether they are known to have DM.

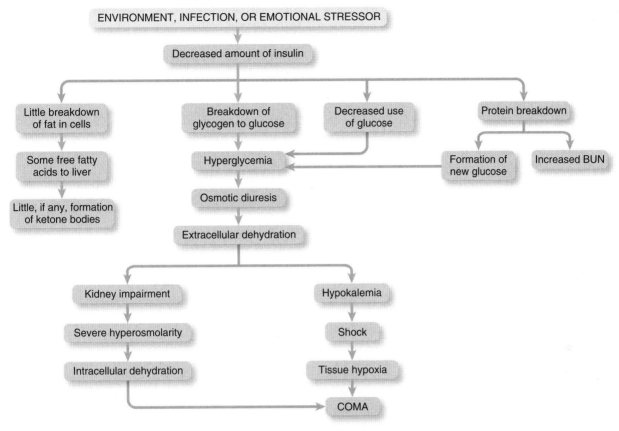

FIG. 56.13 Pathophysiologic mechanism of hyperglycemic-hyperosmolar state (HHS). *BUN,* Blood urea nitrogen.

600 mg/dL (33.3 mmol/L), and blood osmolarity may exceed 320 mOsm/L. Table 56.9 lists the differences between DKA and HHS.

Myocardial infarction, sepsis, pancreatitis, stroke, and some drugs (glucocorticoids, diuretics, phenytoin, beta blockers, and calcium channel blockers) also may cause or contribute to HHS. Central nervous system (CNS) changes range from confusion to complete coma. Patients with HHS may have seizures and reversible paralysis. The degree of neurologic impairment is related to serum osmolarity, with coma occurring once serum osmolarity is greater than 350 mOsm/L (350 mmol/L). Normal serum osmolarity is between 270 mOsm (270 mmol/L) and 300 mOsm/L (300 mmol/L).

The development of HHS rather than DKA is related to residual insulin secretion. In HHS, the patient secretes just enough insulin to prevent ketosis but not enough to prevent hyperglycemia. The hyperglycemia of HHS is usually more severe than that of DKA, greatly increasing blood osmolarity, leading to extreme diuresis with severe dehydration and electrolyte loss.

Fluid Therapy. The expected outcomes of therapy are to rehydrate the patient and restore normal blood glucose levels within 36 to 72 hours. The choice of fluid replacement and the rate of infusion are critical in managing HHS. The severity of the CNS problems is related to the level of blood hyperosmolarity and cellular dehydration. Reestablishing fluid balance in brain cells is a difficult and slow process, and many patients do not

recover baseline CNS function until hours after blood glucose levels have returned to normal.

The *first* priority for fluid replacement in HHS is to increase blood volume. In shock or severe hypotension, normal saline is used. Otherwise half-normal saline is used. Infuse fluids at 1 L/hr until central venous pressure begins to rise or until blood pressure and urine output are adequate. The rate is then reduced to 100 to 200 mL/hr. Half of the estimated fluid deficit is replaced in the first 12 hours, and the rest is given over the next 36 hours. Body weight, urine output, kidney function, and the presence or absence of pulmonary congestion and jugular venous distention determine the rate of fluid infusion. *Assess the patient hourly for signs of cerebral edema (i.e., abrupt changes in mental status, abnormal neurologic signs, and coma).* Lack of improvement in level of consciousness may indicate inadequate rates of fluid replacement or reduction in plasma osmolarity. Regression after initial improvement may indicate a too-rapid reduction in plasma osmolarity. A slow but steady improvement

---

✚ NURSING SAFETY PRIORITY

Critical Rescue

When monitoring the patient being managed for hyperglycemic-hyperosmolar state (HHS), use clinical judgment to recognize status changes and then intervene accordingly. When you notice changes in the level of consciousness; changes in pupil size, shape, or reaction; or seizures, respond by immediately notifying the diabetes health care provider.

in CNS function is the best evidence that fluid management is satisfactory.

Continuing Therapy. IV insulin is administered after adequate fluids have been replaced. Usually an initial bolus dose is given, followed by continuous IV infusion until blood glucose levels fall to 250 mg/dL (13.9 mmol/L). A reduction of blood glucose of 50 to 70 mg/dL (2.8–4.0 mmol/L) per hour is the expected outcome. Monitor the patient closely for hypokalemia because potassium levels drop quickly with insulin therapy. Check serum electrolytes every 1 to 2 hours until stable and monitor cardiac rhythm continuously for signs of hypokalemia or hyperkalemia. Patient education and interventions to minimize dehydration are similar to those for ketoacidosis.

Care Coordination and Transition Management

Self-Management Education. DM is a chronic disease requiring those affected to be actively involved in managing self-care. The interprofessional team of certified diabetes care and education specialists (CDCESs), primary health care providers, nurses, RDNs, pharmacists, social workers, and psychologists all participate in education at every health care encounter (Faminu, 2019; Harris, 2019).

Assessing Learning Needs and Readiness to Learn. First assess the patient's learning needs and readiness to learn to establish what the patient already knows and what they need to know. Assess the needs of both patient and family before teaching as described in Box 56.13.

Provide information that applies directly to the patient. Ask about specific concerns and what the patient wants to learn. Start with what the patient already knows, and build on that

base. Make sure that patients' knowledge is current and applies to their type of DM.

When patients are not ready to learn needed self-management behaviors, ask their permission to teach a family member about DM management. Provide written materials on DM management, as well as telephone numbers for the patient to call when ready to learn.

Assessing Physical, Cognitive, and Emotional Limitations. Assessing the patient's literacy is essential in developing a plan of care and providing self-management education (Watts et al., 2017). It is important to measure the patient's ability to read and understand written materials and perform math calculations. Match the literacy level of materials to the literacy level of the patient.

Assess the patient's ability to read printed information, insulin labels, and markings on syringes and equipment. Many older adult patients have age-related vision problems that are made worse by blurred vision caused by changing blood glucose levels. Also ensure that written materials are provided in the patient's preferred language. Pictographs may be helpful for certain populations.

Assess manual dexterity for any physical limitations that may alter the teaching plan. A hand injury, tremors, or severe arthritis often leads to dosing errors with a standard syringe and may necessitate a change in insulin preparation. Glucometers with a prefilled drum of glucose strips as well as the ability to reapply blood may be preferred when dexterity limitations are present (Fig. 56.14).

Learning styles vary. Successful self-management education provides written or pictograph handouts; discusses steps involved in a procedure, such as insulin administration or self-monitoring of blood glucose (SMBG); and encourages the learner to touch and manipulate equipment. Confirm that the patient understands your instructions by using "teach-back" techniques.

Tailor educational sessions to the time available and to the condition of the patient. Hospitalized adults require only basic education when they are acutely ill. In these situations, it is appropriate to teach basic survival skills or focused problem-solving skills while reserving more detailed education for follow-up sessions.

BOX 56.13 Assessment of Learning Needs for the Patient With Diabetes

- Health and medical history
- Nutrition history and practices
- Physical activity and exercise behaviors
- Prescription and over-the-counter drugs and complementary and integrative therapies and practices
- Factors that influence learning such as education and literacy levels, perceived learning needs, motivation to learn, and health beliefs
- Diabetes self-management behaviors, including experience with self-adjusting the treatment plan
- Previous diabetes self-management training, actual knowledge, and skills
- Physical factors, including age, mobility, visual acuity, hearing, manual dexterity, alertness, attention span, and ability to concentrate or special needs or limitations requiring adaptive support and use of alternative skills
- Psychosocial concerns, factors, or issues, including family and social support
- Current mental health status
- History of substance use, including alcohol, tobacco (especially smoking), and recreational drugs
- Occupation; vocation; education level; financial status; and social, cultural, and religious practices
- Access to and use of health care resources
- Language differences that would require the use of a medically trained interpreter

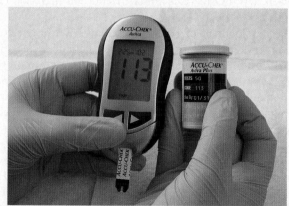

FIG. 56.14 Glucometer with testing strips. (From Sorrentino S, A., & Remmert, L. (2021). *Mosby's textbook for nursing assistants* [10th ed.]. St. Louis: Elsevier.)

Survival Skills Information. The initial phase of education involves teaching just the information necessary for the survival of any adult diagnosed with DM. Survival information includes:

- Simple information on pathophysiology of DM
- Learning how to prepare and inject insulin or how to take other antidiabetic drugs
- Recognition, treatment, and prevention of hypoglycemia and hyperglycemia
- Basic diet information
- Monitoring of blood glucose and urine ketones
- Sick-day management rules
- Where to buy DM supplies and how to store them
- When and how to notify the diabetes health care provider or primary health care provider

In-Depth Education. In-depth education and counseling involve teaching more detailed information about survival skills and actions for avoiding long-term complications. Educational sessions with the patient and family are needed to individualize the DM regimen for their needs and abilities.

The adult with DM must be able to discuss the action of insulin and the effects of insulin deficiency, as well as be able to explain the effects of diet, drugs, and activity on blood glucose. The patient is expected to relate maintaining normal blood glucose levels to preventing complications. This includes relating changes in glucose level to the possible need for a change in insulin dosage.

Provide education about the symptoms of hypoglycemia along with the prescribed treatment options if the patient takes any drugs that will lower blood glucose levels. Educate patients and families about common causes of hypoglycemia described earlier. Review indications of hypoglycemia at each visit. Advise patients to check their blood glucose levels before driving and to make sure they have easy-to-reach snacks and/or fast-acting sugars with them at all times. Remind them to contact their diabetes health care provider if they experience hypoglycemia levels more than twice a week.

Ask patients taking an antidiabetic drug to identify the drug(s) and describe the prescribed schedule. Determine if the patient is able to inject insulin or other injectable antidiabetic drugs accurately by having them demonstrate injection techniques. Ask the patient to discuss the onset, peak, and duration of the insulin used. The patient must be able to state when insulin is to be injected, where it is injected, and how it is stored. Review insulin-to-carbohydrate ratios and correction factors for self-adjustment in insulin (when supported by the diabetes health care provider), and explain blood glucose monitoring requirements needed to evaluate the effects of the insulin dose. Stress the dangers of skipping doses and provide resources if medications are unaffordable. Review drug interactions, especially with older patients taking oral antidiabetic drugs.

Teach patients receiving diet therapy alone, glucose-lowering drugs, or fixed insulin doses to eat consistent amounts of carbohydrate (CHO) at meals and snacks. Patients who adjust mealtime doses of insulin or those on insulin pump therapy can be taught to match their insulin dose to the CHO content of their diet using an insulin-to-carbohydrate ratio. The patient needs to understand balanced eating, including appropriate portion sizes. Stress the importance of eating on time, the dangers of skipping meals, and how to maintain food intake during illness. Ask the patient to describe the meal plan and explain the adjustments needed to meet diabetic diet requirements. Include the family member usually responsible for buying groceries and preparing meals in this teaching.

Teach the patient the skills needed to perform self-monitoring of blood glucose (SMBG), how to interpret results, and when to adjust behaviors and therapy based on the information. In addition, show patients who use insulin how to use SMBG to adjust dosages in order to achieve optimal glucose levels while avoiding episodes of hypoglycemia.

Teach patients sick-day procedures when initially diagnosed with DM. Hyperglycemia often develops before infection symptoms and can serve as a warning sign that infection is developing. Provide guidelines for the frequency of glucose testing, ketone testing, and insulin adjustment for those patients able to self-adjust insulin doses.

The diagnosis of DM may represent a loss of sense of control and flexibility. Although newer diabetes technologies can provide some flexibility, there are still routines that must be followed (e.g., checking blood glucose, taking medications on time). Some events surrounding DM are predictable. Injecting insulin and not eating for several hours causes hypoglycemia. Chronic hyperglycemia can lead to diabetic complications and premature death. Managing blood glucose levels can prevent complications.

Patients are more likely to adhere to disease management activities when the strategies make sense and seem effective. Diabetes education can improve self-efficacy—patients' belief that they can execute behaviors (being active, checking glucose levels, balanced eating, taking medications) to support their diabetes management. SMBG can help the patient understand how different activities affect glucose, and how health behaviors influence glucose levels. Self-efficacy can promote a more positive attitude toward DM. Success in calculating doses (when indicated) and injecting insulin provides concrete evidence that the patient can master the disease. Teach by breaking activities into small tasks that are achievable to ensure mastery. For example, a patient may begin learning how to inject insulin by first obtaining an accurate dose.

Devote as much teaching time as necessary to help the patient understand how to inject insulin and SMBG. Patients with newly diagnosed DM may fear SMBG as well as giving themselves injections. After this technique is mastered, they may be less anxious and more able to attend to other tasks.

Home Care Management. Patients with DM self-manage their disease. Each day they decide what to eat, whether to exercise, and whether to take prescribed drugs. Maintaining blood glucose control depends on the accuracy of self-management skills. The role of the nurse is to provide support and education and to empower the patient to make informed health care decisions.

Self-management education allows patients to identify their problems and provides techniques to help them make decisions, take appropriate actions, and adjust these actions as needed.

BOX 56.14   Home Health Care

The Patient With Diabetes

- Assess overall mental status, wakefulness, and ability to participate in a conversation.
- Take vital signs and weight:
  - Fever could indicate infection.
  - Are blood pressure and weight within target range? If not, why?
- Ask the patient about any change in vision; check current visual acuity.
- Inspect oral mucous membranes, gums, and teeth.
- Ask about injection areas used; inspect areas being used; assess whether the patient is using areas and rotating sites appropriately.
- Inspect skin for intactness; wounds that have not healed; new sores, ulcers, bruises, or burns; assess any previously known wounds for infection, progression of healing.
- Ask patients how often and how they are performing foot care.
- Assess lower extremities and feet for peripheral pulses, lack of or decreased sensation, abnormal sensations, breaks in skin integrity, condition of toes and nails.
- Ask about the color and consistency of stools and frequency of bowel movements; assess abdomen for bowel sounds.
- Review patient's home health diary:
  - Is blood glucose within targeted range? If not, why?
  - Is glucose monitoring being recorded often enough?
  - Is the patient's food intake adequate and appropriate? If not, why?
  - Is exercise occurring regularly? If not, why?
- Assess the patient's ability to perform self-monitoring of blood glucose.
- Assess the patient's procedures for obtaining and storing insulin and syringes, cleaning equipment, and disposing of syringes and needles.
- Assess the patient's insulin preparation and injection technique.
- Assess the patient's knowledge of drug therapy and which side effects to look for.

BOX 56.15   Outcome Criteria for Diabetes Teaching

Before self-management begins at home, the patient with diabetes or the significant other should be able to:

- Tell why insulin or a noninsulin antidiabetic drug is being prescribed
- Name which insulin or noninsulin antidiabetic drug is being prescribed, and name the dosage and frequency of administration
- Discuss the relationship between mealtime and the action of insulin or the other antidiabetic agent
- Discuss plans to follow diabetic diet instructions
- Prepare and inject insulin accurately
- Test blood for glucose or state plans for having blood glucose levels monitored
- Test urine for ketones and state when this test should be done
- Describe how to store insulin
- List symptoms that indicate a hypoglycemic reaction
- Tell which carbohydrate sources are used to treat hypoglycemic reactions
- Tell which symptoms indicate hyperglycemia
- Tell which dietary changes are needed during illness
- State when to call the diabetes health care provider or the nurse (frequent episodes of hypoglycemia, symptoms of hyperglycemia)
- Describe the procedures for proper foot care

Provide information about resources. The patient must know whom to contact in case of emergency. Older adults who live alone need to have daily telephone contact with a friend or neighbor. The patient may also need help shopping and preparing meals. The patient may have limited access to transportation and may not have sufficient supplies of food, particularly in bad weather. Because of the likelihood of vision problems in older patients, they may need help in preparing insulin syringes for injection or in monitoring blood glucose. Make referrals to home care or public health agencies as needed. See Box 56.14.

Evaluate Outcomes: Evaluation

Evaluate the care of the patient with DM based on the identified priority collaborative problems. Outcome success for diabetes education is the ability of the patient to maintain blood glucose levels within the established target range. General outcome criteria are listed here and in Box 56.15. The expected outcomes include that with successful education the patient will be able to:

- Avoid injury by achieving blood glucose control by following the recommended diet, following the prescribed drug regimen, and reaching and maintaining optimum body weight
- Recover from surgery without complications
- Remain free of injury due to peripheral neuropathy including foot lesions, infections, and deformities
- Remain free of kidney disease and maintain optimal urine output
- Avoid acute and chronic complications of diabetes

GET READY FOR THE NEXT-GENERATION NCLEX® EXAMINATION!

Essential Nursing Care Points

Health Promotion/Disease Prevention

- Encourage all patients to maintain weight within an appropriate range.
- Encourage patients with diabetes mellitus (DM) to participate regularly in exercise or physical activity appropriate to their health status.
- Be familiar with screening indications for DM for all adults (see Box 56.3).
- Testing to detect prediabetes and type 2 diabetes mellitus (T2DM) is recommended for patients older than 35 years.
- Adopting a lifestyle that includes a balanced diet, regular physical activity, and weight loss, if applicable, can reduce metabolic and cardiac risk factors and can prevent or delay the onset of T2DM (ADA, 2022).

Chronic Disease Care

- Instruct the patient and family about complications associated with DM and when to seek assistance.
- Urge patients newly diagnosed with DM to attend diabetes education classes to become a fully engaged partner in management of the disease.
- Assess the patient's A1C for indications of adherence to prescribed regimens and their effectiveness.
- Instruct all patients with diabetes to avoid becoming dehydrated and to drink at least 2 L of water each day unless another medical condition requires fluid restriction.
- Teach patients with DM that keeping their blood glucose levels within prescribed target ranges can prevent or delay complications.
- Encourage daily foot inspection and the prompt reporting of ulcers or open areas to the primary health care provider.
- Chronic hyperglycemia increases the risk for neuropathy and amputation.
- In the absence of contraindications, advise adults with DM to perform at least 150 minutes per week of moderate-intensity aerobic physical activity divided into 5 days.

Regenerative or Restorative Care

- Ensure that meals are available with or immediately after the patient receives an antidiabetic drug or insulin.
- Use return demonstration with "teach-back" strategies when teaching the patient about drug regimen, insulin injection, blood glucose monitoring, and foot assessment.
- Immediately report indications of cerebral edema (abrupt changes in mental status; changes in level of consciousness; changes in pupil size, shape, or reaction; seizures) in a patient with hyperglycemic-hyperosmolar state (HHS) to the diabetes health care provider.
- Some antidiabetic drugs are oral agents, and other types require subcutaneous injection. See Table 56.5 for common antidiabetic drugs.
- Insulin therapy is required for patients with type 1 diabetes mellitus (T1DM) and used in 20% to 30% of patients with T2DM.
- For most non–critically ill patients, premeal glucose targets are lower than 140 mg/dL (7.8 mmol/L), with random blood glucose values less than 180 mg/dL (10.0 mmol/L).
- The standards of care for diabetic ulcers are a moist wound environment, débridement of necrotic tissue, and elimination of pressure (offloading).

Hospice/Palliative/Supportive Care

- The complicated and chronic nature of DM requires the coordination of an interprofessional team approach for optimal outcomes. At times, during the course of the disease, patients may need referrals to rehabilitation services such as physical therapy, wound care specialists, or nutritionists.
- The patient with DM is at a higher risk for conditions that are associated with higher mortality, such as diabetic ketoacidosis (DKA) and HHS. Any patient who is critically ill may require a palliative care consultation according to the patient's condition.
- Patients with DM can develop diabetic kidney disease that can progress to end-stage kidney disease (ESKD). Palliative care consultations may be appropriate according to the patient's overall health status.

Mastery Questions

1. The nurse is caring for a client who has a new order for pramlintide. Which teaching would the nurse provide?
   A. Only take this drug once weekly.
   B. Absorption is best if taken at bedtime.
   C. Do not mix in the same syringe with insulin.
   D. Report any genital itching to your primary health care provider.

2. Which of the following instructions would the nurse provide to a client with type 2 diabetes? **Select all that apply.**
   A. "Avoid all dietary carbohydrates and fat."
   B. "Have your eyes and vision assessed by an ophthalmologist every year."
   C. "Reduce your intake of animal fat and increase your intake of plant sterols."
   D. "Be sure to take your antidiabetic drug before you engage in any type of exercise."
   E. "Wearing flip-flops will help to protect your feet when walking long distances."

3. The nurse is preparing to administer a prescribed subcutaneous dose of NPH insulin to a client with diabetes and notes that the solution is cloudy. What action would the nurse take?

A. Roll the vial between the hands until the insulin is clear.

B. Check the expiration date and draw up the insulin dose.

C. Request a new vial of NPH insulin from the pharmacy.

D. Warm the vial in a bowl of warm water until it reaches normal body temperature.

4. While making rounds, the nurse finds a client with type 1 diabetes mellitus pale, sweaty, and slightly confused but able to talk and swallow. The client's blood glucose level is 48 mg/dL (2.7 mmol/L). What would be the appropriate nursing action? (Glucose range: 74–106 mg/dL [4.1–5.9 mmol/L])

A. Call the pharmacy and order a STAT dose of glucagon.

B. Immediately give the client 30 g of glucose orally.

C. Start an IV line and administer a small amount of a concentrated dextrose solution.

D. Recheck the blood glucose level and call the Rapid Response Team.

NGN Challenge 56.1
56.1.1

The nurse is caring for a 64-year-old client who is seeing the primary health care provider for an annual physical examination.

Highlight the findings that require **immediate** follow-up by the nurse.

History and Physical	**Nurses' Notes**	Orders	Laboratory Results

1000: Client here for annual physical examination. Partner present. Last seen 13 months prior. History of hypertension and hypercholesterolemia. Takes amlodipine twice daily and lovastatin once each night. Partner says client is not always adherent to amlodipine therapy when busy in the morning, but usually remembers to take amlodipine and lovastatin at night before bed. Reports two recent urinary tract infections and continued urgency, burning, and frequency today. Reports noticing an increase in thirst over the past few months. Has been feeling somewhat light-headed on occasion and did "not feel right" this morning. During assessment client became somewhat confused; partner verified that client is not confused on baseline. Skin pale and diaphoretic. VS: T 101.9°F (38.8°C); HR 98 beats/min; RR 20 breaths/min; BP 146/98 mm Hg; Spo$_2$ 93% on RA.

56.1.2

During assessment, client became somewhat confused; partner verified that client is not confused on baseline. Skin pale and diaphoretic. Fingerstick glucose is 40 mg/dL. The nurse calls 911.

Complete the following sentence by selecting from the list of word choices below.

Based on analysis of documented assessment findings, the nurse determines that the client is currently at high risk for

[Word Choice].

Word Choices
Atrial fibrillation
Hyperglycemia
Seizure
Hypothyroidism
Sepsis

56.1.3

The client is transported to the local emergency department. The emergency health care provider orders D$_{50}$ IV push × 1 bolus followed by a 5% dextrose drip, hourly blood glucose checks, neurologic checks every 30 minutes or sooner if symptomatic, and oxygen at 2 L per nasal cannula. Laboratory orders include a complete blood count (CBC), complete metabolic profile (CMP), phosphorus, hemoglobin A1C, and urinalysis with urine drug screen (UDS), TSH, and free T$_4$.

Complete the following sentence(s) by selecting from the lists of options below.

When the laboratory values are complete, the nurse will prioritize checking results of the **1 [Select]** and **2 [Select]**.

Options for 1	Options for 2
Hemoglobin A1C	Hematocrit
Casts in urine	TSH
Free T$_4$	White blood cell count

56.1.4

After stabilization in the emergency department, the client is transferred to a medical-surgical unit for monitoring. The admitting health care provider orders ceftriaxone IV every 24 hours in addition to continuing oxygen therapy, performing neurologic checks every 4 hours and blood glucose monitoring before meals and at bedtime. Several hours after admission, the client's partner comes to the nurses' station and reports that the client is not making sense when talking. The nurse assesses that the client is sitting in bed, does not make coherent sentences when speaking, and has pale, cool skin. VS: T 100.9°F (38.3°C); HR 98 beats/min; RR 22 breaths/min; BP 170/100 mm Hg; SpO₂ 91% on RA. Fingerstick glucose is 64 mg/dL. The nurse administers 4 ounces orange juice, which the client consumes, and the client begins to speak more coherently. The nurse contacts the health care provider to request specific orders.

Determine whether each requested order is indicated or unnecessary. Each requested order supports 1 choice.

Requested Order	Indicated	Unnecessary
Place on NPO status		
Prepare for intubation		
Increase oxygen to 4 L per nasal cannula		
Administer bolus of 0.9% normal saline		
Change nasal cannula to facemask		
Administer metformin twice daily		
Increase fingerstick blood glucose order to PRN		

56.1.5

In preparing the client for bed, the nurse changes the client's gown and notes a stage 1 pressure injury on the left heel.

Which 2 actions would the nurse take at this time?

○ Request an order for a wound consultation.
○ Wash the wound gently with alcohol.
○ Obtain a pressure-relieving device.
○ Culture the wound.
○ Apply a wet-to-dry dressing on the wound.
○ Request an order for antibiotic ointment.
○ Review the client's diet for sufficient protein intake.

56.1.6

Several days following discharge, the client follows up with the primary health care provider. The nurse performs an assessment.

Determine whether the following assessment findings indicate that the client's condition has improved, not changed, or declined.

Assessment Finding	Improved	Not Changed	Declined
Blood pressure 130/80 mm Hg			
Respiratory rate 18 breaths/min			
Pulse 90 beats/min			
Heel wound has two small blisters			
Fingerstick glucose 99 mg/dL			

REFERENCES

American Diabetes Association (ADA). (2022). Standards of medical care in diabetes- 2022. *Diabetes Care, 45*(Suppl. 1). https://diabetesjournals.org/care/issue/45/Supplement_1.

Burchum, J., & Rosenthal, L. (2022). *Lehne's pharmacology for nursing care* (11th ed.). St. Louis: Elsevier.

Centers for Disease Control and Prevention (CDC). (2022a). *National diabetes statistics report website.* https://www.cdc.gov/diabetes/data/statistics-report/index.html. Accessed 27 February 2023.

Centers for Disease Control and Prevention (CDC). (2022b). *Increasing access to type 2 diabetes prevention.* https://www.cdc.gov/diabetes/health-equity/increase-type2-prevention.html.

Diabetes Canada. (2022). *Diabetes rates continue to climb in Canada.* https://www.diabetes.ca/media-room/press-releases/diabetes-rates-continue-to-climb-in-canada?.

Faminu, F. (2019). Diabetes: Setting and achieving glycemic goals. *Nursing 2019, 49*(3), 49–54.

Fayfman, M., Pasquel, F., & Umpierrez, G. (2017). Management of hyperglycemic crisis. *Medical Clinics of North America, 101,* 587–606.

Fingar, K., & Reid, L. (2021). *Diabetes-Related Inpatient Stays, 2018. HCUP Statistical Brief #279.* Rockville, MD: Agency for Healthcare Research and Quality. www.hcup-us.ahrq.gov/reports/statbriefs/sb279-Diabetes-Inpatient-Stays-2018.pdf.

Harris, A. (2019). Diabetes self-management education provision by an interprofessional collaborative practice team: A quality improvement project. *Nursing Clinics of North America, 54*(1), 149–158.

Hussein, A., Mostafa, A., Areej, A., et al. (2019). The perceived barriers to insulin therapy among type 2 diabetic patients. *African Health Sciences, 19*(1), 1638–1646.

Pagana, K., Pagana, T., & Pagana, T. (2022). *Mosby's manual of diagnostic and laboratory tests* (7th ed.). St. Louis: Elsevier.

Rariden, C. (2019). Prediabetes: A wake-up call. *Nursing 2019, 49*(4), 38–44.

Rogers, J. L. (2023). *McCance and Huether's Pathophysiology: The biologic basis for disease in adults and children* (9th ed.). St. Louis: Elsevier.

Touhy, T., & Jett, K. (2023). *Ebersole & Hess' toward healthy aging* (11th ed.). St. Louis: Elsevier.

U.S. Department of Veterans Affairs. (2016). *Diabetes type 2 and agent orange.* http://www.publichealth.va.gov/exposures/agentorange/conditions/diabetes.asp.

U.S. Department of Veterans Affairs. (2019). *VA research on diabetes.* https://www.research.va.gov/pubs/docs/va_factsheets/Diabetes.pdf.

Watts, S., Stevenson, C., & Adams, M. (2017). Improving health literacy in patients with diabetes. *Nursing 2017, 47*(1), 25–31.

Watts, S., Nemes, D., Davian, T., & Pensiero, A. (2020). 10 years of inpatient diabetes certification-Lessons learned. *American Nurse Journal, 15*(1), 20–23.

Wooton, A., & Melchior, L. (2020). Diabetes-associated cardiac autonomic neuropathy. *The Nurse Practitioner, 45*(2), 24–31.

57

Assessment of the Renal/Urinary System

Nicole M. Heimgartner

http://evolve.elsevier.com/Iggy/

LEARNING OUTCOMES

1. Use knowledge of anatomy and physiology to perform a focused assessment of the renal/urinary system.
2. Teach evidence-based health promotion activities to help prevent urinary/renal health conditions or trauma.
3. Demonstrate clinical judgment to interpret assessment findings in patients with a renal/urinary system health condition.
4. Identify factors that affect health equity for patients with renal/urinary health conditions.
5. Explain how genetic implications and physiologic aging of the renal/urinary system affects elimination, fluid and electrolyte balance, and acid-base balance.
6. Plan evidence-based care and support for patients undergoing diagnostic testing of the renal/urinary system.

KEY TERMS

bruit An audible swishing sound produced when the volume of blood or the diameter of the blood vessel changes.

calculi Stones.

continence The ability to voluntarily control emptying of the bladder or colon.

cystitis A bladder inflammation, most often with infection.

elimination The excretion of waste from the body by the GI tract (as feces) and kidneys (as urine).

external urethral sphincter Skeletal muscle that surrounds the urethra and helps to control the exit of urine.

incontinence The involuntary loss of urine or stool.

internal urethral sphincter Smooth detrusor muscle of the bladder neck and elastic tissue that helps to control the exit of urine.

microalbuminuria The presence of very small amounts of albumin in the urine that are not measurable with usual urinalysis procedures.

nephron The functional unit of the kidney; forms urine by filtering waste products and water from the blood.

nocturnal polyuria Increased urination at night.

renal threshold The point at which the kidney is overwhelmed with glucose and can no longer reabsorb; also called *transport maximum.*

proteinuria The presence of protein in the urine.

uremia The buildup of nitrogenous waste products in the blood (azotemia).

urethral meatus The opening at the endpoint of the urethra.

urgency A sense of a nearly uncontrollable need to urinate.

✳ PRIORITY AND INTERRELATED CONCEPTS

The priority concept for this chapter is:
• *Elimination*

The interrelated concepts for this chapter are:
• *Fluid and Electrolyte Balance*
• *Acid-Base Balance*

The concept of elimination is the excretion of waste from the body by the GI tract as feces and by the kidneys as urine. See Chapter 3 for an overview of the concept of elimination and how it relates to the concepts of *fluid and electrolyte balance* and *acid-base balance.* In this chapter, the focus is on elimination of waste via the renal system. The kidneys and urinary tract make up the renal system, which is responsible for urine elimination.

The kidneys are responsible for filtering water and wastes from the bloodstream. The filtered-out particles and excess fluid are excreted out of the body into the urinary tract via the ureters, bladder, and ureters ridding the body of these wastes. Structural or functional problems within the renal system may alter **fluid and electrolyte balance** and **acid-base balance.**

The kidneys help maintain health in many ways. *Most important, they maintain body fluid volume and composition and create urine for waste* **elimination.** In addition, the kidneys help regulate blood pressure and **acid-base balance,** produce erythropoietin for red blood cell (RBC) synthesis, and convert vitamin D to an active form.

ANATOMY AND PHYSIOLOGY REVIEW

Kidneys

Structure

The two kidneys are located behind the peritoneum, outside of the abdominal cavity, one on each side of the spine (Fig. 57.1). The adult kidney is 4 to 5 inches (10–13 cm) long, 2 to 3 inches (5–7 cm) wide, and about 1 inch (2.5–3 cm) thick. The left kidney is slightly longer and narrower than the right kidney. Larger than usual kidneys may indicate obstruction or polycystic disease. Smaller than usual kidneys may indicate chronic kidney disease (CKD). A person can be born with only one kidney (renal agenesis), or with two kidneys but only one is functional (kidney dysplasia). In general people with only one working kidney can lead a normal life (National Kidney Foundation, 2022).

Several layers of tissue surround the kidney, providing protection and support. The outer surface of the kidney is a layer of fibrous tissue called the *capsule* (Fig. 57.2). It covers most of the kidney except the *hilum,* which is the indented area where the kidney blood vessels and nerves enter and exit. It is also where

the ureter exits. The capsule is surrounded by layers of fat and connective tissue.

Underneath the capsule fibrous layer are two layers of functional kidney tissue: the cortex and the medulla. The *renal cortex* is the outer tissue layer. The *medulla* is the medullary tissue lying below the cortex in the shape of many fans. Each "fan" is called a pyramid. Pyramids are separated by the *renal columns,* cortical tissue that dips down into the interior of the kidney.

The tip of each pyramid is called a *papilla.* The papillae drain urine into the collecting system. A cuplike structure called a *calyx* collects the urine at the end of each papilla. The calices join together to form the *renal pelvis,* which narrows to become the ureter.

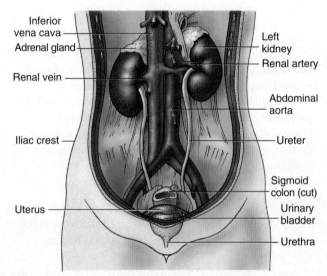

FIG. 57.1 Anatomic location of the kidneys and structures of the urinary system.

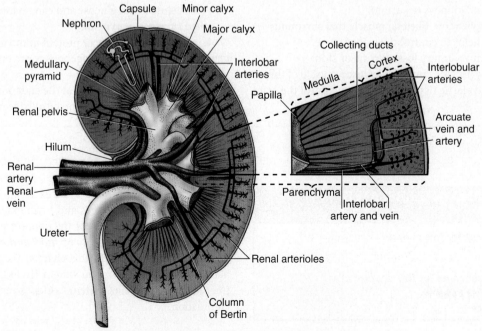

FIG. 57.2 Bisection of the kidney showing its major structures.

The kidneys have a rich blood supply and receive a blood flow from 600 to 1300 mL/min. The blood supply to each kidney comes from the renal artery, which branches off from the abdominal aorta. The renal artery divides into progressively smaller arteries, supplying blood to areas of the kidney tissue and the nephrons. The smallest arteries (*afferent arterioles*) feed the nephrons directly to form urine.

Venous blood from the kidneys starts with the capillaries surrounding each nephron. These capillaries drain into progressively larger veins, with blood eventually returned to the inferior vena cava through the renal vein.

Microscopic Anatomy. The nephron is the functional unit of the kidney and forms urine by filtering waste products and water from the blood. There are about 1 million nephrons per kidney, and each nephron separately performs filtration and makes urine from blood.

There are two types of nephrons: *cortical nephrons* and *juxtamedullary nephrons*. The cortical nephrons are short and lie totally within the renal cortex. The juxtamedullary nephrons (about 20% of all nephrons) are longer, and their tubes and blood vessels dip deeply into the medulla. The purpose of these nephrons is to concentrate urine during times of low fluid intake to allow continued excretion of body waste with less fluid loss (Rogers, 2023).

Blood supply to the nephron is delivered through the *afferent arteriole* (i.e., the smallest, most distal portion of the renal arterial system). From the afferent arteriole, blood flows into the *glomerulus,* which is a series of specialized capillary loops. It is through these capillaries that water and small particles are filtered from the blood to make urine. The remaining blood leaves the glomerulus through the *efferent arteriole,* which is the first vessel in the kidney's venous system. From the efferent arteriole, blood exits into either the *peritubular capillaries* around the tube of the cortical nephrons or the *vasa recta* around the tube of juxtamedullary nephrons.

Each nephron is a tubelike structure with distinct parts (Fig. 57.3). The tube begins with the Bowman capsule, a saclike structure that surrounds the glomerulus. The tubular tissue of the Bowman capsule narrows into the *proximal convoluted tubule (PCT).* The PCT twists and turns, finally straightening into the descending limb of the *loop of Henle.* The descending loop of Henle dips in the direction of the medulla but forms a hairpin loop and comes back up into the cortex as the ascending loop of Henle.

The two segments of the ascending limb of the loop of Henle are the thin segment and the thick segment. The *distal convoluted tubule (DCT)* forms from the thick segment of the ascending limb of the loop of Henle. The DCT ends in one of many collecting ducts located in the kidney tissue. The urine in the collecting ducts passes through the papillae and empties into the renal pelvis.

Special cells in the afferent arteriole, efferent arteriole, and DCT are known as the *juxtaglomerular complex* (Fig. 57.4). These cells produce *renin,* which is a hormone that helps regulate blood flow, glomerular filtration rate (GFR), and blood pressure. Renin is secreted when sensing cells in the DCT (called the *macula densa*) sense changes in blood volume and pressure.

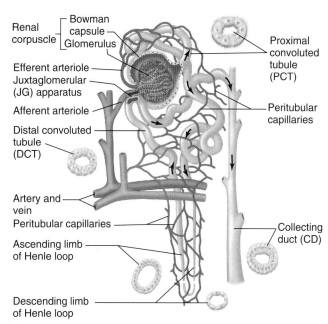

FIG. 57.3 Anatomy of the nephron—the functional unit of the kidney. The differences in appearance in tubular cells seen in a cross section reflect the differing functions of each nephron segment. Note that the particular nephron labeled here is a juxtamedullary nephron. (From Patton, K. T., & Thibodeau, G. A. [2018]. *The human body in health and disease* [7th ed.]. St. Louis: Elsevier.)

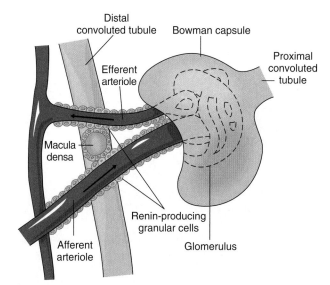

FIG. 57.4 Juxtaglomerular complex showing juxtaglomerular cells and the macula densa.

The macula densa touches the renin-producing cells. Renin is produced when the macula densa cells sense that blood volume, blood pressure, or blood sodium level is low. Renin then converts renin substrate (angiotensinogen) into angiotensin I. This leads to a series of reactions that cause secretion of the hormone aldosterone (Fig. 57.5). Aldosterone increases kidney reabsorption of sodium and water, restoring blood pressure, blood volume, and blood sodium levels (Rogers, 2023). It also promotes excretion of potassium (see Chapter 13).

The glomerular capillary wall has three layers (Fig. 57.6): the endothelium, the basement membrane, and the epithelium. The endothelial and epithelial cells lining these capillaries are

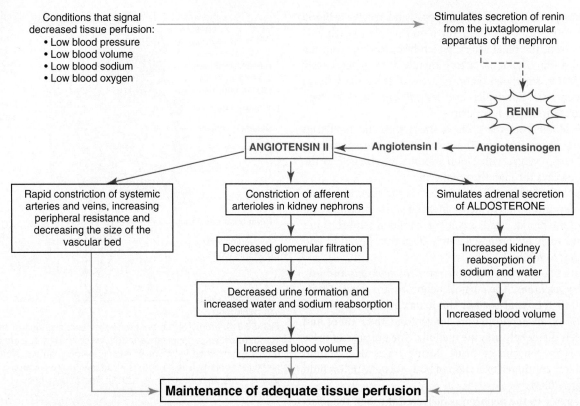

FIG. 57.5 Role of aldosterone, renin substrate (angiotensinogen), angiotensin I, and angiotensin II in the renal regulation of water and sodium.

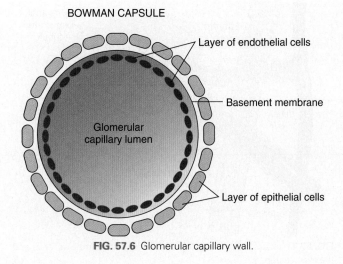

FIG. 57.6 Glomerular capillary wall.

separated by pores that filter water and small particles from the blood into the Bowman capsule. This fluid is called the *filtrate*.

Function

The kidneys have both regulatory and hormonal functions. The regulatory functions control *fluid and electrolyte balance* and *acid-base balance.* The hormonal functions control red blood cell (RBC) formation, blood pressure, and vitamin D activation.

Regulatory Functions. The kidney processes that maintain *fluid and electrolyte balance* and *acid-base balance* through urine *elimination* are glomerular filtration, tubular reabsorption, and tubular secretion. These processes use filtration,

diffusion, active transport, and osmosis. (See Chapter 13 for a review of these actions.) Table 57.1 lists the functions of nephron tubules and blood vessels.

Glomerular filtration is the first process in urine formation. As blood passes from the afferent arteriole into the glomerulus, water, electrolytes, and other small particles (e.g., creatinine, urea nitrogen, glucose) are filtered across the glomerular membrane into the Bowman capsule to form glomerular filtrate. As the filtrate enters the proximal convoluted tubule (PCT), it is called tubular filtrate or early urine.

Large particles, such as blood cells, albumin, and other proteins, are too large to filter through the glomerular capillary walls. These substances are not normally present in the excreted final urine.

Filtration rate is expressed in milliliters per minute. Normal glomerular filtration rate (GFR) averages 125 mL/min, totaling about 180 L daily. If the entire amount of filtrate were excreted as urine, death would occur from dehydration. Actually, only about 1 to 3 L are excreted each day as urine. The rest is reabsorbed back into the blood (Rogers, 2023).

GFR is controlled by blood pressure and blood flow. The kidneys self-regulate their own blood pressure and blood flow, which keeps GFR constant. GFR is controlled by selectively constricting and dilating the afferent and efferent arterioles. When the afferent arteriole is constricted or the efferent arteriole is dilated, pressure in the glomerular capillaries falls and filtration decreases. When the afferent arteriole is dilated or the efferent arteriole is constricted, pressure in the glomerular capillaries rises and filtration increases. This way the kidney

TABLE 57.1   Vascular and Tubular Components of the Nephron

Structure	Anatomic Features	Physiologic Aspects
Vascular Components		
Afferent arteriole	Delivers arterial blood from the branches of the renal artery into the glomerulus	Autoregulation of renal blood flow via vasoconstriction or vasodilation Renin-producing granular cells
Glomerulus	Capillary loops with thin, semipermeable membrane	Site of glomerular filtration Glomerular filtration occurs when hydrostatic pressure (blood pressure) is greater than opposing forces (tubular filtrate and oncotic pressure)
Efferent arteriole	Delivers arterial blood from the glomerulus into the peritubular capillaries or the vasa recta	Autoregulation of renal blood flow via vasoconstriction or vasodilation Renin-producing granular cells
Peritubular capillaries (PTCs) and vasa recta (VR)	PTCs: Surround tubular components of cortical nephrons VR: Surround tubular components of juxtamedullary nephrons	Tubular reabsorption and tubular secretion allow movement of water and solutes to or from the tubules, interstitium, and blood
Tubular Components		
Bowman capsule (BC)	Thin membranous sac surrounding {7/8} of the glomerulus	Collects glomerular filtrate (GF) and funnels it into the tubule
Proximal convoluted tubule (PCT)	Evolves from and is continuous with Bowman capsule Specialized cellular lining facilitates tubular reabsorption	Site for reabsorption of sodium, chloride, water, glucose, amino acids, potassium, calcium, bicarbonate, phosphate, and urea
Loop of Henle	Continues from PCT Juxtamedullary nephrons dip deep into the medulla Permeable to water, urea, and sodium chloride	Regulation of water balance
Descending limb (DL)	Continues from the loop of Henle Permeable to water, urea, and sodium chloride	Regulation of water balance
Ascending limb (AL)	Emerges from DL as it turns and is redirected up toward the renal cortex	Potassium and magnesium reabsorption in the thick segment Thin segment is impermeable to water
Distal convoluted tubule (DCT)	Evolves from AL and twists, so the macula densa cells lie adjacent to the juxtaglomerular cells of afferent arteriole	Site of additional water and electrolyte reabsorption, including bicarbonate Potassium and hydrogen secretion
Collecting ducts	Collect formed urine from several tubules and deliver it into the renal pelvis	Receptor sites for antidiuretic hormone regulation of water balance

maintains a constant GFR, even when systemic blood pressure changes. When systolic pressure drops below 65 to 70 mm Hg, these self-regulation processes do not maintain GFR.

Tubular reabsorption is the second process in urine formation. Tubular reabsorption of most of the filtrate (early urine) keeps normal urine output at 1 to 3 L/day and prevents dehydration. As the filtrate passes through the tubular parts of the nephron, water and electrolytes are reabsorbed from the tubular lumen of the nephron and into the peritubular capillaries. This process returns much of the water, electrolytes, and other particles to the blood.

The tubules return about 99% of filtered water back into the body (Fig. 57.7). Most water reabsorption occurs in the proximal convoluted tubule (PCT). Water reabsorption continues as the filtrate flows down the descending loop of Henle. The thin and thick segments of the ascending loop of Henle are not permeable to water, and no water reabsorption occurs here.

The distal convoluted tubule (DCT) can be permeable to water, and some water reabsorption occurs as the filtrate

continues to flow through the tubule. The membrane of the DCT may be made more permeable to water when vasopressin (antidiuretic hormone [ADH]) and aldosterone are present. Vasopressin increases tubular permeability to water, allowing water to leave the tube and be reabsorbed into the capillaries. Vasopressin also increases arteriole constriction. Arteriole constriction alters blood pressure, which then affects the amounts of fluid and particles that exit glomerular capillaries. Aldosterone promotes the reabsorption of sodium in the DCT. Water reabsorption occurs as a result of the movement of sodium (where sodium goes, water follows).

The ability of the kidneys to vary the volume or concentration of urine helps regulate water balance regardless of fluid intake. In this way, the healthy kidney can prevent dehydration when fluid intake is low and can prevent circulatory overload when fluid intake is high.

In addition to water, electrolytes are reabsorbed as needed to maintain *fluid and electrolyte balance* in the blood. Most sodium, chloride, and water reabsorption occurs in the proximal

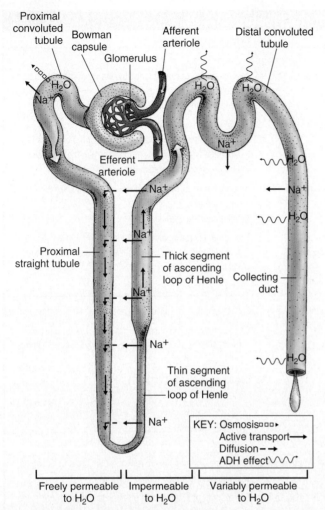

FIG. 57.7 Sodium and water reabsorption by the tubules of a cortical nephron. *ADH,* Antidiuretic hormone; *Na⁺,* sodium.

convoluted tubule (PCT). The collecting ducts are the other site of sodium, chloride, and water reabsorption. Here reabsorption is caused by aldosterone. Potassium is mostly reabsorbed in the PCT and thick segment of the loop of Henle.

Bicarbonate, calcium, and phosphate are mostly reabsorbed in the PCT. Bicarbonate reabsorption helps *acid-base balance* and maintains a normal blood pH. Blood levels of calcitonin and parathyroid hormone (PTH) (see Chapters 13 and 55) control calcium balance.

Some types of particles in the tubular filtrate are also returned to the blood by tubular reabsorption. About 50% of all urea in the filtrate is reabsorbed; creatinine is not reabsorbed.

The kidney reabsorbs some of the glucose filtered from the blood. However, there is a limit to how much glucose the kidney can reabsorb. The point where the kidney is overwhelmed with glucose and can no longer reabsorb is called the renal threshold or *transport maximum* for glucose reabsorption. The renal threshold for glucose is >180 mg/dL (10 mmol/L). This means that at a blood glucose level of 180 mg/dL (10 mmol/L) or less, all glucose is reabsorbed and returned to the blood, with no glucose present in final urine. When blood glucose levels are greater than 180 mg/dL (10 mmol/L), some glucose stays in

the filtrate and is present in the urine (Wald, 2022). Normally, almost all glucose and most proteins are reabsorbed and thus are not present in the urine.

> **! NURSING SAFETY PRIORITY**
> *Action Alert*
>
> Report the presence of glucose or proteins in the urine of a patient undergoing a screening examination to the primary health care provider because this is an abnormal finding and requires further assessment.

Tubular secretion is the third process of urine formation. It allows substances to move from the blood into the urine. During tubular secretion, substances move from the peritubular capillaries in reverse, across capillary membranes, and into the cells that line the tubules. From the cells, these substances are moved into the urine and excreted from the body. Potassium (K⁺) and hydrogen (H⁺) ions are some of the substances moved in this way to maintain *fluid and electrolyte balance* and *acid-base balance* (pH).

Hormonal Functions. The kidneys produce renin, prostaglandins, erythropoietin, and activated vitamin D (Table 57.2). Other kidney products, such as the kinins, change kidney blood flow, regulate blood pressure, and influence capillary permeability. The kidneys also help break down and excrete insulin and many other drugs.

Renin, as discussed in the Microscopic Anatomy section, assists in blood pressure control. It is formed and released when there is a decrease in blood flow, blood volume, or blood pressure through the renal arterioles or when too little sodium is present in kidney blood. These conditions are detected through the receptors of the juxtaglomerular complex.

Renin release causes the production of angiotensin II through a series of steps (see Fig. 57.5). Angiotensin II increases systemic blood pressure with powerful blood vessel constricting effects and triggers the release of aldosterone from the adrenal glands. Aldosterone increases the reabsorption of sodium in the distal tubule of the nephron. Therefore more water is reabsorbed, which increases blood volume and blood pressure. When blood flow to the kidney is reduced, this system also prevents fluid loss and maintains circulating blood volume (see Chapter 13).

Prostaglandins are produced in the kidney and in many other tissues. Those produced specifically in the kidney help regulate glomerular filtration, kidney vascular resistance, and renin production. They also increase sodium and water excretion.

Erythropoietin is produced and released in response to decreased oxygen in the kidney's blood supply. It triggers red blood cell (RBC) production in the bone marrow. When kidney function is poor, erythropoietin production decreases and anemia results.

Vitamin D activation occurs through a series of steps. Some of these steps take place in the skin when it is exposed to sunlight, and then more processing occurs in the liver. From there, vitamin D is converted to its active form in the kidney. Activated vitamin D is needed to absorb calcium in the intestinal tract and regulate calcium balance (Rogers, 2023).

TABLE 57.2 Kidney Hormones and Hormones Influencing Kidney Function

	Site	Action
Kidney Hormones		
Renin	Renin-producing granular cells	Raises blood pressure as result of angiotensin (local vasoconstriction) and aldosterone (volume expansion) secretion
Prostaglandins	Kidney tissues	Regulate intrarenal blood flow by vasodilation or vasoconstriction
Bradykinins	Juxtaglomerular cells of the arterioles	Increase blood flow (vasodilation) and vascular permeability
Erythropoietin	Kidney parenchyma	Stimulates bone marrow to make red blood cells
Activated vitamin D (1,25- dihydroxycholecalciferol)	Kidney parenchyma	Promotes absorption of calcium in the GI tract
Hormones Influencing Kidney Function		
Vasopressin (antidiuretic hormone [ADH])	Released from posterior pituitary	Makes DCT and CD permeable to water to maximize reabsorption and produce a concentrated urine
Aldosterone	Released from adrenal cortex	Promotes sodium reabsorption and potassium secretion in DCT and CD; water and chloride follow sodium movement
Natriuretic hormones	Cardiac atria, cardiac ventricles, brain	Cause tubular secretion of sodium

CD, Collecting duct; *DCT,* distal convoluted tubule.

Ureters

Each kidney usually has a single ureter, which is a hollow tube that connects the renal pelvis with the urinary bladder. The ureter is about ½ inch (1.25 cm) in diameter and about 12 to 18 inches (30–45 cm) in length. The diameter of the ureter narrows in three areas:
- In the upper third of the ureter, at the point where the renal pelvis becomes the ureter, is a narrowing known as the **ureteropelvic junction (UPJ)**.
- The ureter also narrows as it bends toward the abdominal wall (aortoiliac bend).
- Each ureter narrows at the point where it enters the bladder; this point is called the **ureterovesical junction (UVJ)**.

The ureter tunnels through bladder tissue for a short distance and then opens into the bladder at the trigone (Fig. 57.8).

The ureter has three layers: an inner lining of mucous membrane *(urothelium),* a middle layer of smooth muscle fibers, and an outer layer of fibrous tissue. The middle layer of muscle fibers is controlled by several nerve pathways from the lower spinal cord.

Contractions of the smooth muscle in the ureter move urine from the kidney pelvis to the bladder. Stretch receptors in the kidney pelvis regulate this movement. For example, a large volume of urine in the kidney pelvis triggers the stretch receptors, which respond by increasing ureteral contractions and ureter peristalsis.

Urinary Bladder
Structure

The urinary bladder is a muscular sac (see Fig. 57.8) that lies directly behind the pubic bone. In males, the bladder is in front of the rectum. In females, it is in front of the vagina.

The bladder is composed of the *body* (the rounded sac portion) and the *bladder neck* (posterior urethra), which connects to the bladder body. The bladder has three linings: an inner lining of epithelial cells *(urothelium),* middle layers of smooth muscle *(detrusor muscle),* and an outer lining. The *trigone* is an area on the posterior wall between the points of ureteral entry (ureterovesical junctions [UVJs]) and the urethra.

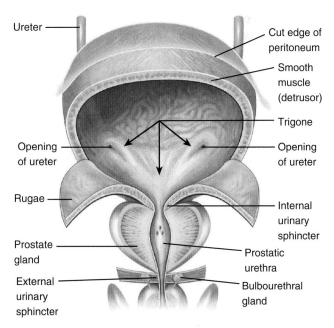

FIG. 57.8 Gross anatomy of the urinary bladder. (Modified from Patton, K. T., & Thibodeau, G. A. [2013]. *Anatomy and physiology* [8th ed.]. St. Louis: Elsevier.)

The **internal urethral sphincter** is the smooth detrusor muscle of the bladder neck and elastic tissue. The **external urethral sphincter** is skeletal muscle that surrounds the urethra. In men, the external sphincter surrounds the urethra at the base of the prostate gland. In women, the external sphincter is at the base of the bladder. The pudendal nerve from the spinal cord controls the external sphincter.

Function

The bladder stores urine, provides continence, and enables voiding. The secretions of the urothelium lining the bladder resist bacteria.

Continence is the ability to voluntarily control bladder emptying. It occurs during bladder filling through the combination of detrusor muscle relaxation, internal sphincter muscle tone, and external sphincter contraction. As the bladder fills with urine, stretch sensations are transmitted to spinal sacral nerves.

Maintaining continence occurs by the interaction of the nerves that control the muscles of the bladder, bladder neck, urethra, and pelvic floor, as well as by factors that close the urethra. In the continent person, the smooth muscle of the detrusor remains relaxed during a period of urine filling and storage. Sympathetic nervous system fibers prevent detrusor muscle contraction. The control centers for voiding are located in the cerebral cortex, the brainstem, and the lower spinal cord. For urethral closure to be adequate for continence, the mucosal surfaces must be in contact and must be adhesive. Contact depends on the presence and proper function of the involved nerves and muscles. Adhesion depends on the secretion of mucuslike substances.

Micturition (voiding, urination) is a reflex of autonomic control that triggers contraction of the detrusor muscle (closing the ureter at the UVJ to prevent backflow) at the same time as relaxation of the external sphincter and the muscles of the pelvic floor. Voluntary urine *elimination* (voiding) occurs as a learned response and is controlled by the cerebral cortex and the brainstem. Contraction of the external sphincter inhibits the micturition reflex and prevents voiding.

Urethra

The urethra is a narrow tube lined with mucous membranes. Its purpose is to allow urine *elimination* from the bladder. The urethral meatus, or opening, is the endpoint of the urethra. In males, the urethra is about 6 to 8 inches (15–20 cm) long, with the meatus located at the tip of the penis. The male urethra has three sections:

- The prostatic urethra, which extends from the bladder through the prostate gland
- The membranous urethra, which extends from the prostate to the wall of the pelvic floor
- The cavernous urethra, which is external and extends through the length of the penis

In females, the urethra is 1 to 1½ inches (2.5–3.75 cm) long and exits through the pelvic floor. The meatus lies slightly below the clitoris and directly in front of the vagina and rectum.

Kidney and Urinary Changes Associated With Aging
Kidney Changes

Changes occur in the kidney as a result of the aging process that can affect urine *elimination* and health (see the Patient-Centered Care: Older Adult Health—Changes in the Renal System Related to Aging box). The kidney loses cortical tissue and nephrons and gets smaller with age as a result of reduced blood flow to the kidney (Touhy & Jett, 2023). The medulla is not affected by aging, and the juxtamedullary nephron functions are preserved. The glomerular and tubular linings thicken. Both the number of glomeruli and their surface areas decrease with aging. Tubule length decreases. The changes reduce the older adult's ability to filter blood and excrete waste products.

👤 PATIENT-CENTERED CARE: OLDER ADULT HEALTH

Changes in the Renal System Related to Aging

Physiologic Change	Nursing Interventions	Rationales
Decreased glomerular filtration rate (GFR)	Monitor hydration status. Ensure adequate fluid intake. Use caution when administering potentially nephrotoxic agents or drugs.	The ability of the kidneys to regulate water balance decreases with age. The kidneys are less able to conserve water when necessary. Dehydration reduces kidney blood flow and increases the nephrotoxic potential of many agents. Acute or chronic kidney failure may result.
Nocturia	Ensure adequate nighttime lighting and a hazard-free environment. Ensure the availability of a bedside toilet, bedpan, or urinal. Discourage excessive fluid intake for 2–4 hr before the patient goes to bed. Evaluate drugs and timing.	Falls and injuries are common among older patients seeking bathroom facilities. Using these items instead of getting up to go the bathroom can help prevent falls. Excessive fluid intake at night may increase nocturia. Some drugs increase urine output and increase the risk for falling when toileting.
Decreased bladder capacity	Encourage the patient to use the toilet, bedpan, or urinal at least every 2 hr. Respond as soon as possible to the patient's indication of the need to void.	Emptying the bladder on a regular basis may avoid overflow urinary incontinence. A quick response may alleviate episodes of urinary stress incontinence.
Weakened urinary sphincters and shortened urethra in women	Provide thorough perineal care after each voiding.	The shortened urethra increases the potential for bladder infections. Good perineal hygiene may prevent skin irritations and urinary tract infection (UTI).
Tendency to retain urine	Observe the patient for urinary retention (e.g., bladder distention) or urinary tract infection (e.g., dysuria, foul odor, confusion). Provide privacy, assistance, and voiding stimulants such as warm water over the perineum as needed. Evaluate drugs for possible contribution to retention.	Urinary stasis may result in a UTI, which may lead to bloodstream infections, urosepsis, or septic shock. Nursing interventions can help initiate voiding. Anticholinergic drugs promote urinary retention.

Blood flow to the kidney declines by about 10% per decade as blood vessels thicken. This means that blood flow to the kidney is not as adaptive in older adults, leaving nephrons more vulnerable to damage during episodes of either hypotension or hypertension.

Glomerular filtration rate (GFR) decreases with age. By age 65 years, the GFR is about 65 mL/min (half the rate of a young adult) and increases the risk for fluid overload. This decline is more rapid in patients with diabetes, hypertension, or heart failure. The combination of reduced kidney mass, reduced blood flow, and decreased GFR contributes to reduced drug clearance and a greater risk for drug reactions and kidney damage from drugs and contrast media in older adults.

Tubular changes with aging decrease the ability to concentrate urine, resulting in urgency (a sense of a nearly uncontrollable need to urinate) and nocturnal polyuria (increased urination at night). The regulation of sodium, acids, and bicarbonate is less efficient. Along with an age-related impairment in the thirst mechanism, these changes increase the risk for disturbances of *fluid and electrolyte balance,* such as dehydration and hypernatremia (increased blood sodium levels) in the older adult. Hormonal changes include a decrease in renin secretion, aldosterone levels, and activation of vitamin D.

Urinary Changes

Changes in detrusor muscle elasticity lead to decreased bladder capacity and reduced ability to retain urine (Touhy & Jett, 2023). The urge to void may cause immediate bladder emptying because the urinary sphincters lose tone and often become weaker with age. In women, weakened muscles in the pelvic floor shorten the urethra and promote incontinence. In men, an enlarged prostate gland makes starting the urine stream difficult and may cause urinary retention.

RECOGNIZE CUES: ASSESSMENT

Patient History

Demographic information, such as age, sex assigned at birth, race, and ethnicity, is important to consider as nonmodifiable risk factors in the patient with any kidney or urinary *elimination* problem. A sudden onset of hypertension in patients older than 50 years suggests possible kidney disease. Clinical changes in polycystic kidney disease typically occur in patients in their 40s or 50s. In men older than 50 years, altered urine patterns accompany prostate disease. Black people are 3 times more likely to have kidney failure, and Latino people are 1.3 times more likely (National Kidney Foundation, 2020). There are many factors that contribute to this risk, including higher rates of hypertension, diabetes mellitus, and heart disease, all of which increase the risk for kidney disease (National Kidney Foundation, 2020).

Anatomic differences according to sex assigned at birth make some disorders worse or more common. For example, males rarely have ascending urinary tract infections. Females have a shorter urethra and more commonly develop cystitis (bladder inflammation, most often with infection) because bacteria pass more readily into the bladder.

Modifiable risk factors, as well as socioeconomic status, level of education, language, and health beliefs, should be considered when assessing renal function. *Socioeconomic status* may influence health care practices. Prevention, early detection, and treatment of kidney or urinary problems may be limited by inability to access health care, lack of transportation, insufficient or no insurance, and/or reduced income. These barriers contribute to inequity in health care and may result in difficulty adhering to a plan of care, having prescriptions filled, following dietary instructions, and keeping follow-up appointments.

Educational level may affect health-seeking practices and the patient's understanding of a disease or its symptoms. Recurring urinary tract infections can result from not completing a course of antibiotic therapy or from not following up to ensure that the infection is cleared.

The language used by patients may be different from that used by the health care professional. When obtaining a history, listen to and explore the terms used by the patient. By using the patient's own terms, you may be able to provide a more complete description of the problem and may decrease the patient's discomfort when discussing bodily functions. The patient's health beliefs affect the approach to health and illness. Cultural background or religious affiliation may influence the belief system, as well as overall comfort when discussing *elimination.*

Ask the patient about previous kidney or urologic problems, including tumors, infections, stones, or urologic surgery. A history of any chronic health problems, especially diabetes mellitus or hypertension, increases the risk for development of kidney disease because these disorders damage kidney blood vessels.

Ask the patient about environmental, food, or medication allergies. Exposure to certain contrast media during imaging can harm the kidneys. Iodinated contrast medium used for CT scans is associated with both acute and chronic kidney injury. High-osmolarity contrast agents can also contribute to kidney function impairment. Exposure to gadolinium-enhanced MRI can result in nephrogenic systemic fibrosis.

Ask the patient about chemical exposures at the workplace or with hobbies. Exposure to hydrocarbons (e.g., gasoline, oil), heavy metals (especially mercury and lead), and some gases (e.g., chlorine, toluene) can impair kidney function. Use this opportunity to teach patients who come into contact with chemicals at work or during leisure-time activities to avoid direct skin or mucous membrane contact with these chemicals. Use of heroin, cocaine, methamphetamine, ecstasy, and volatile solvents (inhalants) has also been associated with kidney damage.

Specifically ask patients whether they have ever been told about the presence of protein or albumin in the urine. The question "Have you ever been told that your blood pressure is high?" may prompt a response different from the one to the question "Do you have high blood pressure?" Ask females about health problems during pregnancy (e.g., proteinuria, high blood pressure, gestational diabetes, urinary tract infections). Obtain information about:

- Chemical or environmental toxin exposure in occupational, diagnostic, or other settings
- Recent travel to geographic regions that pose infectious disease risks
- Recent trauma or injury, particularly to the abdomen or pelvic or genital areas
- A history of altered patterns of urinary *elimination*

Nutrition History

Ask the patient with known or suspected kidney or urologic disorders about diet and any recent dietary changes. Note any excessive intake or omission of certain food categories. Ask about food and fluid intake. Assess how much and which types of fluids the patient drinks daily, especially fluids with a high-calorie or caffeine content. Use this opportunity to teach the patient the importance of drinking sufficient fluid to cause urine to be dilute (clear or very light yellow). If another medical problem does not require fluid restriction, ingestion of about 2 L of fluid daily is recommended. If the patient has followed a diet for weight reduction, the details of the diet plan are important, and collaboration with a registered dietitian nutritionist (RDN) may be needed. A high-protein intake can result in temporary kidney problems. For example, a patient at risk for calculi (stone) formation who ingests large amounts of protein or has a poor fluid intake may form new stones.

Ask about any change in appetite or taste. These symptoms can occur with the buildup of nitrogenous waste products from kidney failure. Changes in thirst or fluid intake may also cause changes in the volume of urine *elimination.* Endocrine disorders may also cause changes in thirst, fluid intake, and urine output. (See Chapter 53 for a discussion of endocrine influences on fluid balance.)

Medication History

Identify all of the patient's prescription drugs because many can impair kidney function. Ask about the duration of drug use and whether there have been any recent changes in prescribed drugs. Drugs for diabetes mellitus, hypertension, cardiac disorders, hormonal disorders, cancer, arthritis, and psychiatric disorders are potential causes of kidney problems. Antibiotics, such as gentamicin, may also cause acute kidney injury. Drug-drug interactions and drug–contrast media interactions also may lead to kidney dysfunction.

Explore the past and current use of over-the-counter (OTC) drugs or agents, including dietary supplements, vitamins and minerals, herbal agents, laxatives, analgesics, acetaminophen, and NSAIDs. Many of these agents affect kidney function and urine *elimination.* For example, dietary supplementation with synthetic creatine, used to increase muscle mass, has been associated with compromised kidney function. High-dose or long-term use of NSAIDs or acetaminophen can seriously reduce kidney function. Some agents are associated with hypertension, hematuria, or proteinuria, which may occur before kidney dysfunction.

Family History and Genetic Risk

The family history of the patient with a suspected kidney or urologic problem is important because some disorders have a familial pattern. Ask whether siblings, parents, or grandparents have had kidney problems. Past terms used for kidney disease include *Bright disease, nephritis,* and *nephrosis.* Although nephritis is a current term for an inflammatory process in the kidney and nephrosis is a current term for a degenerative process in the kidney, these terms have been used by some adults for years to describe any type of kidney problem. Polycystic kidney disease, which is a genetic disorder, can occur in either males or females.

Current Health Problem

The effects of kidney failure are seen in all body systems. Document all of the patient's current health problems. Ask the patient to describe all health concerns, because some kidney disorders cause problems in other body systems. Recent upper respiratory problems, achy muscles or joints, heart disease, or GI conditions may be related to problems of kidney function.

Assess the kidney and urologic system by asking about any changes in the appearance (color, odor, clarity) of the urine, pattern of urine *elimination,* ability to initiate or control voiding, and other unusual symptoms. For example, urine that is reddish, rust-colored, brown or black, greenish, or different from the usual yellowish color may prompt the patient to seek health care assistance. Urine typically has a mild but distinct odor of ammonia. An increase in the intensity of color, a change in odor quality, or a decrease in urine clarity may suggest infection.

Ask about changes in urination patterns, such as incontinence (involuntary bladder emptying), nocturia (urination at night), urgency (nearly uncontrollable urge to urinate), frequency, or an increase or decrease in the amount of urine. The normal urine output for adults is about 1500 to 2000 mL/day or within 500 mL of the volume of fluid ingested daily. Ask about how close the urine output is to the volume of fluid ingested. A bladder diary may be useful. Ask whether:

- Initiating urine flow is difficult
- A burning sensation or other discomfort occurs with urination
- The force of the urine stream is decreased
- Persistent dribbling or leaking of urine is present

The onset of pain in the flank, in the lower abdomen or pelvic region, or in the perineal area triggers concern and usually prompts the patient to seek assistance. Ask about the onset, intensity, and duration of the pain; its location; precipitating and relieving factors; and its association with any activity or event.

Pain associated with kidney or ureteral irritation is often severe and spasmodic. Pain that radiates into the perineal area, groin, scrotum, or labia is described as *renal colic.* This pain occurs with distention or spasm of the ureter, such as in an obstruction or the passing of a stone. Renal colic pain may be intermittent or continuous and may occur with pallor/ash gray skin, diaphoresis, and hypotension. These general symptoms occur because of the location of the nerve tracts near or in the kidneys and ureters.

Because the kidneys are close to the GI organs and the nerve pathways are similar, GI symptoms may occur with kidney problems. These renointestinal reflexes often complicate the description of the kidney problem.

Uremia is the buildup of nitrogenous waste products in the blood from inadequate *elimination* as a result of kidney failure. Symptoms include anorexia, nausea and vomiting, muscle cramps, *pruritus* (itching), fatigue, and lethargy.

Physical Assessment

The physical assessment of the patient with a known or suspected kidney or urologic disorder includes general appearance, a review of body systems, and specific structure and functions of the kidney and urinary system.

Assess the patient's general appearance and check the skin for the presence of any rashes, bruising, or yellowish discoloration. The skin and tissues may show edema associated with kidney disease, especially in the *pedal* (foot), *pretibial* (shin), and sacral tissues and around the eyes. Use a stethoscope to listen to the lungs to determine whether fluid is present. Weigh the patient and measure blood pressure as a baseline for later comparisons.

Assess the levels of consciousness and alertness. Record any deficits in memory, concentration, or thought processes. Family members may report subtle changes. Cognitive changes may be the result of the buildup of waste products when kidney disease is present.

Assessment of the Kidneys, Ureters, and Bladder

Assess the kidneys, ureters, and bladder during an abdominal assessment (Jarvis & Eckhardt, 2024). Auscultate before percussion and palpation because these activities can alter bowel sounds and obscure abdominal vascular sounds.

Inspect the abdomen and the flank regions with the patient in both the supine and sitting positions. Observe the patient for asymmetry (e.g., swelling) or discoloration (e.g., bruising or redness/hyperpigmentation) in the flank region, especially in the area of the costovertebral angle (CVA). The CVA is located between the lower portion of the twelfth rib and the vertebral column.

Listen for a bruit by placing a stethoscope over each renal artery on the midclavicular line. A **bruit** is an audible swishing sound produced when the volume of blood or the diameter of the blood vessel changes. It often occurs with blood flow through a narrowed vessel, as in renal artery stenosis.

Kidney palpation is usually performed by a health care provider. It can help locate masses and areas of tenderness in or around the kidney. The health care provider will lightly palpate the abdomen in all quadrants, ask about areas of tenderness or pain, and examine nontender areas first. The outline of the bladder may be noted as high as the umbilicus in patients with severe bladder distention.

> **! NURSING SAFETY PRIORITY**
>
> **Action Alert**
>
> Performing palpation on a patient with a suspected abdominal tumor or aneurysm may harm the patient.

Because the kidneys are located deep and posterior, palpation is easier in thin patients who have little abdominal musculature. For palpation of the right kidney, the patient is placed in a supine position while the examiner places one hand under the right flank and the other hand over the abdomen below the lower right part of the rib cage. The lower hand is used to raise the flank, and the upper hand depresses the abdomen as the patient takes a deep breath. The left kidney is deeper and often cannot be palpated. A transplanted kidney is readily palpated in either the lower right or left abdominal quadrant. The normal kidney is smooth, firm, and nontender.

A distended bladder sounds dull when percussed. After gently palpating to determine the outline of the distended bladder, begin percussion on the lower abdomen and continue in the direction of the umbilicus until dull sounds are no longer produced. If you suspect bladder distention, use a portable bladder scanner (Fig. 57.9) to determine the amount of retained urine.

If the patient reports flank pain or tenderness, the nontender flank should be percussed first. For percussion, the patient is placed in a sitting, side-lying, or supine position. Percussion, generally performed by the health care provider, is done by forming one hand into a clenched fist while the other hand lies flat over the CVA of the patient. Using the fist, a quick, firm thump is administered to the hand over the CVA area (Jarvis & Eckhardt, 2024). Costovertebral tenderness often occurs with kidney infection or inflammation. Patients with inflammation or infection in the kidney or nearby structures may describe their pain as severe or as a constant, dull ache.

Assessment of the Urethra

Using a good light source and wearing gloves, inspect the urethra by examining the meatus and the tissues around it. Record any unusual discharge such as blood, mucus, or pus. Inspect the skin and mucous membranes of surrounding tissues. Record the presence of lesions, rashes, or other abnormalities of the penis or scrotum or of the labia or vaginal opening. Urethral irritation is suspected when the patient reports discomfort with urination. Use this opportunity to remind females to clean the perineum by wiping from front to back, never from back to front. Teach them that the front-to-back technique keeps organisms in stool from coming close to the urethra and decreases the risk for infection.

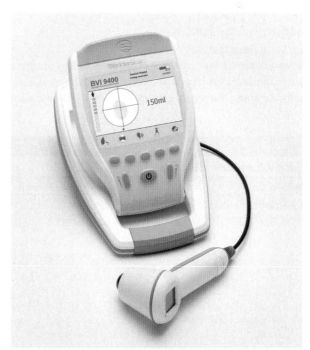

FIG. 57.9 BladderScan BVI 9400, a handheld portable bladder scanner. (Courtesy Verathon Corporation, Bothell, WA.)

PATIENT-CENTERED CARE: CULTURE AND SPIRITUALITY

Female Circumcision

Women from some cultures or religions may have undergone female circumcision. This procedure alters the appearance of the vulvar-perineal area and increases the risk for urinary tract infections. It also makes urethral inspection or catheterization difficult. Document any noted anatomic changes and ask the patient to describe hygiene practices for this area.

Psychosocial Assessment

Concerns about the urologic system may evoke fear, anger, embarrassment, anxiety, guilt, or sadness in the patient. Childhood learning often includes the idea that toileting should take place in private and not be discussed with other people. Urologic disorders may bring up forgotten memories of difficult toilet training and bedwetting or of childhood experiences of exploring one's body. The patient may ignore symptoms or delay seeking health care because of emotional responses or cultural beliefs about the urogenital area.

NCLEX Examination Challenge 57.1

Physiological Integrity

The nurse is completing a health history and physical assessment on a male client who has a history of an enlarged prostate. Which of the following assessment data would the nurse anticipate? **Select all that apply.**

A. Bladder distention
B. Absence of a bruit
C. Frequency of urination
D. Dribbling urine after voiding
E. Chemical exposure in the workplace

Diagnostic Assessment

Laboratory Assessment

Blood Tests. *Serum creatinine* is produced when muscle and other proteins are broken down. Because protein breakdown is usually constant, the serum creatinine level is a good indicator of kidney function. Serum creatinine levels are slightly higher in males than in females because males tend to have a larger muscle mass than females. Similarly, adults with greater muscle mass or muscle mass turnover (e.g., athletes) may have a slightly higher than average serum creatinine level. Muscle mass and the amount of creatinine produced decrease with age. However, because of decreased rates of creatinine clearance, the serum creatinine level remains relatively constant in older adults unless kidney disease is present. See Table 57.3.

No common pathologic condition other than kidney disease increases the serum creatinine level. When the serum creatinine level is doubled, it indicates a 50% reduction in glomerular filtration rate (Pagana et al., 2022); therefore any elevation of serum creatinine values is important and should be assessed further. Creatinine is excreted solely by the kidneys.

! NURSING SAFETY PRIORITY

Action Alert

A serum creatinine of 1.5 mg/dL (110 mcmol/L) or greater places a patient at risk for acute kidney injury (AKI) from iodinated contrast media and some drugs (Lambert et al., 2017). Monitor both baseline and trend values to recognize risk for and actual kidney damage, especially among patients exposed to agents that can cause kidney dysfunction. If indicated, respond by promptly informing the primary health care provider of increases in serum creatinine greater than 1.5 times the baseline and urine output values of less than 0.5 mL/kg/hr for 6 or more hours. Using the baseline and trending creatinine levels is important, especially in older adults and young children, as they have lower creatinine levels than adults due to reduced muscle mass.

Blood urea nitrogen (BUN) measures the effectiveness of kidney excretion of urea nitrogen, a by-product of protein breakdown in the liver. Urea nitrogen is produced mostly from liver metabolism of food sources of protein. The kidneys filter urea nitrogen from the blood and excrete the waste as part of urine *elimination.*

Other factors influence the BUN level, and an elevation does not always mean that kidney disease is present (see Table 57.3). For example, rapid cell destruction from infection, cancer treatment, or steroid therapy may elevate the BUN level. In addition, blood is a protein. Blood in the tissues rather than in the blood

TABLE 57.3 Laboratory Profile

Kidney Function Blood Studies

Test	Normal Range for Adults	Significance of Abnormal Findings
Serum creatinine	*Males:* 0.6–1.2 mg/dL *Females:* 0.5–1.1 mg/dL	An *increased level* indicates kidney impairment. A *decreased level* may be caused by decreased muscle mass.
Blood urea nitrogen (BUN)	10–20 mg/dL (3.6–7.1 mmol/L) *Older adults:* Slightly higher	An *increased level* may indicate liver or kidney disease, dehydration or decreased kidney perfusion, a high-protein diet, infection, stress, steroid use, GI bleeding, or other situations in which blood is in body tissues. A *decreased level* may indicate malnutrition, fluid volume excess, or severe hepatic damage.
BUN/creatinine ratio (BUN divided by creatinine)	6–25 15.5 optimum level for adults	An *increased ratio* may indicate fluid volume deficit, obstructive uropathy, catabolic state, or a high-protein diet. A *decreased ratio* may indicate fluid volume excess.

Data from Pagana, K., Pagana, T., & Pagana, T. (2022). *Mosby's manual of diagnostic and laboratory tests* (7th ed.). St. Louis: Elsevier.

vessels is reabsorbed as if it were a general protein. Reabsorbed blood protein is processed by the liver and increases BUN levels. This means that injured tissues can result in increased BUN levels even when kidney function is normal. In addition, BUN is increased by protein turnover in exercising muscle and is elevated as a result of concentration during dehydration.

The liver must function properly to produce urea nitrogen. When liver and kidney dysfunction are present, urea nitrogen levels are actually *decreased* because the liver failure limits urea production. The BUN level is not always elevated with kidney disease and is not the best indicator of kidney function. However, an elevated BUN level suggests kidney dysfunction.

Blood urea nitrogen to serum creatinine ratio can help determine whether non–kidney-related factors, such as low cardiac output or red blood cell destruction, are causing the elevated BUN level. When blood volume is deficient (e.g., dehydration) or cardiac output is low, the BUN level rises more rapidly than the serum creatinine level. As a result, the ratio of BUN to creatinine is *increased.*

When both the BUN and serum creatinine levels increase at the same rate, the BUN/creatinine ratio remains normal. However, elevations of *both* serum creatinine and BUN levels suggest kidney dysfunction that is not related to dehydration or poor perfusion.

Cystatin-C measures glomerular filtration rate. Cystatin-C is a protein produced by nucleated cells in the body. Because cystatin-C is produced at a constant rate, it can be used as an indicator of glomerular filtration rate. When the glomerular filtration rate is reduced, cystatin-C increases. Increased levels can be considered a predictor of chronic renal disease. Cystatin-C is not influenced by factors that influence BUN and creatinine levels, making it potentially a better indicator of glomerular filtration rate (Pagana et al., 2022).

Blood osmolarity is a measure of the overall concentration of particles in the blood and is a good indicator of hydration status. The kidneys excrete or reabsorb water to keep blood osmolarity in the range of 280 to 300 mOsm/kg (mmol/kg). Osmolarity is slightly higher in older adults. When blood osmolarity is decreased, vasopressin (antidiuretic hormone [ADH]) release is inhibited. Without vasopressin, the distal tubule and collecting ducts are *not* permeable to water. As a result, water is *excreted,* not reabsorbed, and blood osmolarity increases. When blood osmolarity increases, vasopressin is released. Vasopressin increases the permeability of the distal tubule to water. Then water is reabsorbed, and blood osmolarity decreases.

Urine Tests

Urinalysis. Urinalysis is a part of any complete physical examination and is especially useful for patients with suspected kidney or urologic disorders (Table 57.4). Ideally, the urine specimen is collected at the morning's first voiding. Specimens

TABLE 57.4 Laboratory Profile

Urinalysis

Test	Normal Range for Adults	Significance of Abnormal Findings
Color	Yellow	*Dark amber* indicates concentrated urine. *Very pale yellow* indicates dilute urine. *Dark red* or *brown* indicates blood in the urine. Brown may indicate increased bilirubin level. Red also may indicate the presence of myoglobin. *Other color* changes may result from diet or drugs.
Odor	Specific aroma, similar to ammonia	*Foul smell* indicates possible infection, dehydration, or ingestion of certain foods or drugs.
Turbidity	Clear	*Cloudy urine* indicates infection, sediment, or high levels of urine protein.
Specific gravity	1.005–1.030; usually 1.01–1.025 *Older adult:* Decreases with age	*Increased* in decreased kidney perfusion, inappropriate ADH secretion, dehydration, or heart failure. *Decreased* in chronic kidney disease, arginine vasopressin deficiency (AVP-D), arginine vasopressin resistance (AVP-R), hypertensive crisis, diuretic administration, and lithium toxicity.
pH	Average: 6; range: 4.6–8	*Changes* are caused by diet, drugs, infection, age of specimen, acid-base imbalance, and kidney disease.
Glucose	Fresh specimen: Negative 24-hr specimen: 50–300 mg/day (0.3–1.7 mmol/day)	*Presence* reflects hyperglycemia or a decrease in the kidney threshold for glucose.
Ketones	None	*Presence* occurs with diabetic ketoacidosis, prolonged fasting, and anorexia nervosa.
Protein	0–8 mg/dL (50–80 mg in 24-hr specimen at rest; <250 mg in 24-hr specimen with exercise)	*Increased* amounts may indicate stress, infection, recent strenuous exercise, or glomerular disorders.
Bilirubin	None	*Presence* suggests liver or biliary disease or obstruction.
Red blood cells (RBCs)	≤2	*Increased* is normal with catheterization or menses but may reflect tumor, stones, trauma, glomerular disorders, cystitis, or bleeding disorders.

Continued

TABLE 57.4 Laboratory Profile—cont'd

Urinalysis

Test	Normal Range for Adults	Significance of Abnormal Findings
White blood cells (WBCs)	0–4 per low-power field	*Increased* may indicate an infection or inflammation in the kidney and urinary tract, kidney transplant rejection, or exercise.
Casts	None	*Increased* indicates bacteria, protein, or urinary calculi.
Crystals	None	*Presence* may indicate that the specimen has been allowed to stand.
Parasites	None	*Presence* of *Trichomonas vaginalis* indicates infection, usually of the urethra, prostate, or vagina.
Leukocyte esterase	None	*Presence* suggests urinary tract infection.
Nitrites	None	*Presence* suggests urinary *Escherichia coli*.

ADH, Antidiuretic hormone.
Data from Pagana, K., Pagana, T., & Pagana, T. (2022). *Mosby's manual of diagnostic & laboratory tests* (7th ed.). St. Louis: Elsevier.

obtained at other times may be too dilute. The specimen may be collected by several techniques (Table 57.5).

Urine color comes from urochrome pigment. Color variations may result from increased levels of urochrome or other pigments, changes in the concentration or dilution of the urine, and the presence of drug metabolites in the urine. Urine smells faintly like ammonia and is normally clear without turbidity (cloudiness) or haziness.

Specific gravity is the concentration of particles (i.e., electrolytes, wastes) in urine. A high specific gravity indicates concentrated urine from dehydration, decreased kidney blood flow, or excess vasopressin associated with stress, surgery, anesthetic agents, and certain drugs (e.g., morphine, some oral antidiabetic drugs) or syndrome of inappropriate antidiuretic hormone (SIADH) (see Chapter 54). Low specific gravity indicates dilute urine that may occur from high fluid intake, diuretic drugs, or arginine vasopressin deficiency (AVP-D) or arginine vasopressin resistance (AVP-R) (see Chapter 54).

Specific gravity of urine is compared with that of distilled water, which has a specific gravity of 1.000. The normal specific gravity of urine ranges from 1.005 to about 1.030. Kidney disease diminishes the concentrating ability of the kidney, and chronic kidney disease may be associated with a low (dilute) specific gravity.

pH is a measure of urine acidity or alkalinity. A pH value less than 7 is acidic, and a value greater than 7 is alkaline. Urine pH is affected by diet, drugs, systemic disturbances of *acid-base balance,* and kidney tubular function. For example, a high-protein diet produces acidic urine, whereas a high intake of citrus fruit produces alkaline urine. The normal pH of urine ranges from 4.6 to 8 with an average of 6 (Pagana et al., 2022).

Urine specimens become more alkaline when left standing unrefrigerated for more than 1 hour, when bacteria are present, or when a specimen is left uncovered. Alkaline urine increases cell breakdown; thus the presence of red blood cells may be missed on analysis. Ensure that urine specimens are covered and delivered to the laboratory promptly. Urine specimens delayed 2 or more hours require refrigeration or other specific storage and transport precautions to ensure the integrity of the urine specimen (Pagana et al., 2022). During systemic acidosis or alkalosis, the kidneys, along with blood buffers and the lungs, normally respond to keep serum pH normal. Chapter 14 discusses *acid-base balance* and imbalance.

Protein is not normally present in the urine. Protein molecules are too large to pass through intact glomerular membranes. When glomerular membranes are not intact, protein molecules pass through and are excreted with urine *elimination.* Increased membrane permeability is caused by infection, inflammation, or immunologic problems. Some systemic problems cause production of abnormal proteins, such as globulin. Detection of abnormal protein types requires electrophoresis.

A random finding of proteinuria (usually albumin in the urine) followed by a series of negative (normal) findings does not imply kidney disease. If infection is the cause of the proteinuria, urinalyses after resolution of the infection should be negative for protein. Persistent proteinuria needs further investigation.

Microalbuminuria is the presence of albumin in the urine that is not measurable by a urine dipstick or usual urinalysis procedures. Specialized assays are used to quickly analyze a freshly voided urine specimen for microscopic levels of albumin. The normal microalbumin levels in a freshly voided specimen should be less than 2 mg/dL. Higher levels indicate microalbuminuria and could mean mild or early kidney disease, especially in patients with diabetes mellitus. Microalbumin levels greater than 30 mg/24 hr are abnormal (Pagana et al., 2022).

Glucose in the urine may indicate a high level of glucose in the blood. Changes in the renal threshold for glucose may occur temporarily in patients who have infection or severe stress.

Ketone bodies are formed from the incomplete metabolism of fatty acids. Three types of ketone bodies are acetone, acetoacetic acid, and beta-hydroxybutyric acid. *Normally there are no ketones in urine.* Ketone bodies are produced when fat is used instead of glucose for cellular energy. Ketones present in the blood are partially excreted in the urine.

Leukoesterase is an enzyme found in some white blood cells (WBCs), especially neutrophils. When the number of these cells increases in the urine or they are damaged (lysed), the urine then contains leukoesterase. A normal reading is no leukoesterase in the urine. A positive test (+ sign) is an indication of a urinary tract infection.

TABLE 57.5 Collection of Urine Specimens

Nursing Interventions	Rationales
Voided Urine	
Collect the first specimen voided in the morning.	Urine is more concentrated in the early morning.
Send the specimen to the laboratory as soon as possible.	After urine is collected, cellular breakdown results in more alkaline urine.
Refrigerate the specimen if a delay is unavoidable.	Refrigeration delays the alkalinization of urine. Bacteria are more likely to multiply in an alkaline environment.
Catheterized Specimen	
For nonindwelling (straight) catheters:	The one-time passage of a urinary catheter may be necessary to obtain an uncontaminated specimen for analysis or to measure the volume of residual urine.
Use sterile technique and follow facility procedures for urinary catheterization.	These procedures minimize bacterial entry.
For indwelling catheters:	Urine is collected from an indwelling catheter or tubing when patients have catheters for continence or long-term urinary drainage.
• Apply a clamp to the drainage tubing, distal to the injection port for 15–30 minutes	Clamping allows urine to collect in the tubing at the location where the specimen is obtained.
• Clean the injection port cap of the catheter drainage tubing with an appropriate antiseptic and allow to dry. Povidone-iodine solution or alcohol is acceptable.	Surface contamination is prevented by following the cleaning procedures.
• Attach a sterile 5-mL syringe into the port and aspirate the quantity of urine required.	A minimum of 5 mL is needed for culture and sensitivity (C&S) testing.
• Inject the urine sample into a sterile specimen container.	A sterile container is used for C&S specimens.
• Remove the clamp to resume drainage.	
• Properly dispose of the syringe.	
Clean-Catch Specimen	
Instruct the patient to self-clean before voiding:	Surface cleaning is necessary to remove secretions or bacteria from the urethral meatus.
Female patients:	
• Separate the labia and use the wipes provided to clean the urethra with three strokes. The first two wiping strokes are over each side of the urethra; the third wiping stroke is centered over the urethra (from front to back).	
Male patients:	
• Retract the foreskin of the penis and clean the urethra, using three wiping strokes with the wipes provided (from the head of the penis downward).	
Instruct all patients to initiate voiding after cleaning. The patient then stops and resumes voiding into the container.	A midstream collection further removes secretions and bacteria because urine flushes the distal portion of the internal urethra.
Only 1 oz (30 mL) is needed; the remainder of the urine may be discarded into the commode.	
Ensure that the patient understands the procedure.	An improperly collected specimen may result in inappropriate or incomplete treatment.
24-Hour Urine Collection	
Provide written materials to assist in instruction.	Instructional materials for patients, signs, and so on remind patients and staff to ensure that the total collection is completed.
Place signs appropriately.	
Inform all personnel or family caregivers of test in progress.	
Check laboratory or procedure manual on proper technique for maintaining the collection (e.g., on ice, in a refrigerator, or with a preservative).	Proper technique prevents breakdown of elements to be measured.
On initiation of the collection, ask the patient to void, discard the urine, and note the time. If a Foley catheter is in use, empty the tubing and drainage bag at the start time and discard the urine.	Proper techniques ensure that *all* urine formed within the 24-hr period is collected.
Collect all urine of the next 24 hr.	
Twenty-four hours after initiation, ask the patient to empty the bladder and add that urine to the container.	
Do not remove urine from the collection container for other specimens.	Urine in the container is not considered a "fresh" specimen and may be mixed with preservative.

Nitrites are not usually present in urine. Many types of bacteria, when present in the urine, convert nitrates (normally found in urine) into nitrites. A positive nitrites test enhances the sensitivity of the leukoesterase test to detect urinary tract infection (Pagana et al., 2022).

Sediment is precipitated particles in the urine. These particles include cells, casts, crystals, and bacteria. Normally urine contains few, if any, cells. Types of cells abnormally present in the urine include tubular cells (from the tubule of the nephron), epithelial cells (from the lining of the urinary tract), red blood cells (RBCs), and white blood cells (WBCs). WBCs may indicate a urinary tract or kidney infection. RBCs may indicate *glomerulonephritis, acute tubular necrosis, pyelonephritis,* kidney trauma, or kidney cancer.

Casts are clumps of materials or cells. When cells, bacteria, or proteins are present in the urine, minerals and sticky materials clump around them and form a cast of the distal renal tubule and collecting duct. Casts are described by the type of particle they have surrounded (e.g., hyaline [protein based] or cellular [from RBCs, WBCs, or epithelial cells]) or the stage of cast breakdown (whole cell or granular from cell breakdown). Although an isolated urinalysis with sediment from casts may be the result of strenuous exercise, repeated findings with sediment are more likely to be associated with disease.

Urine crystals come from mineral salts as a result of diet, drugs, or disease. Common salt crystals are formed from calcium, oxalate, urea, phosphate, magnesium, or other substances. Some drugs, such as the sulfates, can also form crystals. Crystals can form into calculi.

Bacteria multiply quickly, so the urine specimen must be analyzed promptly to avoid falsely elevated counts of bacterial colonization. Normally urine is sterile, but it can be easily contaminated by perineal bacteria during collection.

Recent advances in technology and molecular biology have led to new diagnostic tests using urine, including identification of biomarkers of disease and profiling for specific proteins. Markers such as cystatin-C are being investigated to identify early-onset kidney dysfunction, target therapy, and predict responsiveness to intervention. Other markers for angiogenesis and kidney cell adhesion, regulation, and apoptosis (i.e., connective tissue growth factor [CTGF], neutrophil gelatinase-associated lipocalin [NGAL]) will likely contribute to clinical diagnostics in the future.

Urine for Culture and Sensitivity. Urine is analyzed for the number and types of organisms present. Symptoms of infection and unexplained bacteria in a urine specimen are indications for urine culture and sensitivity testing. Bacteria from urine are placed in a medium with different antibiotics. In this way, we can know which antibiotics are effective in killing or stopping the growth of the organisms (organisms are "sensitive") and which are not effective (organisms are "resistant"). A clean-catch or catheter-derived specimen is best for culture and sensitivity testing, as these procedures reduce the chance of perineal surface organisms contaminating the specimen.

Composite Urine Collections. Some urine collections are made for a specified number of hours (e.g., 24 hours) for precise analysis of urine levels of substances, such as creatinine or urea nitrogen, sodium, chloride, calcium, catecholamines, or other components. For a composite urine specimen, *all* urine within the designated time frame must be collected. If other urine must be obtained while the collection is in progress, measure and record the amount collected but not added to the timed collection.

The urine collection may need to be refrigerated or stored on ice to prevent changes in the urine during the collection time. Follow the procedure from the laboratory for urine storage, including whether a preservative is to be added. The urine collection must be free from fecal contamination. Menstrual blood and toilet tissue also contaminate the specimen and can invalidate the results.

The collection of all urine for a 24-hour period is often challenging. With hospitalized patients, the cooperation of staff personnel, the patient, family members, and visitors is essential. Placing signs in the bathroom, instructing the patient and family, and emphasizing the need to save the urine are helpful.

Creatinine Clearance. Creatinine clearance is a measure of glomerular filtration rate (GFR) and kidney function. The patient's age, sex assigned at birth, height, weight, diet, and activity level influence the expected amount of excreted creatinine. These factors are considered when interpreting creatinine clearance test results. Decreases in the creatinine clearance rate may require reducing drug doses and often signifies the need to further explore the cause of kidney deterioration.

Commonly, creatinine clearance is calculated from serum creatinine, age, weight, urine creatinine, sex assigned at birth, and race. Creatinine clearance can be based on the excretion of injected inulin or other substances that are not reabsorbed into the blood. Creatinine clearance to estimate GFR can also be based on a 24-hour urine collection, although urine can be collected for shorter periods (e.g., 8 or 12 hours). The analysis compares the urine creatinine level with the blood creatinine level; therefore a blood specimen for creatinine must also be collected. The range for normal creatinine clearance is 107 to 139 mL/min (1.78–2.32 mL/sec) for men and 87 to 107 mL/min (1.45–1.78 mL/sec) for women tested with a 24-hour urine collection (Pagana et al., 2022). Values decrease progressively per decade of life for adults older than 40 years because of age-related decline in GFR.

Current guidelines suggest the use of the 2021 Chronic Kidney Disease Epidemiology Collaboration (CKD-EPI) creatinine equation rather than other estimating equations that include race as a factor in the calculation (Inker & Perrone, 2023). The CKD-EPI uses the patient's age, sex assigned at birth, and serum creatinine level to produce the estimated glomerular filtration rate (eGFR) value. (See the Patient-Centered Care: Healthy Equity box). An eGFR less than or equal to 60 may be indicative of CKD.

PATIENT-CENTERED CARE: HEALTH EQUITY

Estimated Glomerular Filtration Rate (eGFR)

Historically, race has been included in the calculation of eGFR. Currently, the National Kidney Foundation and the American Society of Nephrology have released a new approach to diagnosing kidney disease that removes the variable of race (National Kidney Foundation, 2021). The new equation for estimation is a creatinine-based equation that does not include the social construct of race (Inker & Perrone, 2023). This recommendation is a step forward in promoting health equity (National Kidney Foundation, 2021).

Urine Electrolytes. Urine samples can be analyzed for electrolyte levels (e.g., sodium, chloride). Normally the amount of sodium excreted in the urine is nearly equal to that consumed. Urine sodium levels can vary depending on the amount of water and salt consumed. Normal values for a 24-hour urine sample ranges from 40 to 220 mEq/day (or 40–220 mmol/day). A value greater than 20 mEq/L for a routine urine specimen is considered normal (Pagana et al., 2022).

NCLEX Examination Challenge 57.2
Physiological Integrity

The nurse is caring for a client who is starting a 24-hour urine collection. Which client statement requires further teaching?
A. "I hope I don't have to have a bowel movement in the next 24 hours."
B. "I will make sure that all of my urine is collected over the next 24 hours."
C. "I will throw the toilet paper in the trash, not in the collection container."
D. "I know that the collection container has to be kept on ice."

Urine Osmolarity. Osmolarity measures the concentration of particles in solution. The particles in urine contributing to osmolarity include electrolytes, glucose, urea, and creatinine. Urine osmolarity can vary from 50 to 1200 mOsm/kg or L (mmol/kg or L), depending on the patient's hydration status and kidney function. With average fluid intake, the range for urine osmolarity is 300 to 900 mOsm/kg or L (mmol/kg or L). Electrolytes, acids, and other normal metabolic wastes are continually produced. These particles are the solute load that must be excreted in the urine on a regular basis. This is referred to as *obligatory solute excretion.* If the patient loses excessive fluids, the kidney response is to save water while excreting wastes by excreting small amounts of highly concentrated urine. Diet, drugs, and activity can change urine osmolarity. Urine with an increased osmolarity is concentrated urine with less water and more solutes. Urine with a decreased osmolarity is dilute urine with more water and fewer solutes.

Imaging Assessment

Many imaging procedures are used to diagnose abnormalities within the renal-urinary system (Table 57.6). Explain the procedures, prepare, and provide follow-up care to the patient. Patient education materials for many urologic tests have been developed by organizations, such as the Society of Urologic Nurses and Associates, and are freely available. Encourage the patient to use reliable and credible sources for online information.

Bedside Sonography/Bladder Scanners. The use of portable ultrasound scanners in the hospital and rehabilitation setting by nurses is a noninvasive method of estimating bladder volume (see Fig. 57.9). Bladder scanners are used to screen for postvoid residual volumes and determine the need for intermittent catheterization based on the amount of urine in the bladder rather than the time between catheterizations. There is no discomfort with the scan, and no patient preparation is required beyond an explanation of what to expect.

Explain why the procedure is being done and what sensations the patient might experience during the procedure. For example, "This test will measure the amount of urine in your bladder. I will place a gel pad just above your pubic area and then place the probe, which is a little bigger and heavier than a stethoscope, on the gel."

Before scanning, select the male or female icon on the bladder scanner. Using the female icon allows the scanner software to subtract the volume of the uterus from any measurement. Use the male icon on all men and on women who have undergone a hysterectomy.

Place an ultrasound gel pad right above the pubic bone or moisten the round dome of the scan head area with 5 mL of conducting gel to improve ultrasound conduction. Use gel on the scanner head for obese patients and those with heavy body hair in the area to be scanned. Place the probe midline over the abdomen about 1½ inches (4 cm) above the pubic bone. Aim the scan head so the ultrasound is projected toward the expected location of the bladder, typically toward the patient's coccyx. Press and release the scan button. The scan is complete with the sound of a beep, and a volume is displayed. Two readings are recommended for best accuracy. An aiming icon on the portable bladder scanner indicates whether the bladder image is centered on the crosshairs of the scan head. If the crosshairs on the aiming icon are not centered on the bladder, the measured volume may not be accurate.

Kidney, Ureter, and Bladder X-rays. An x-ray of the kidneys, ureters, and bladder (KUB) is a plain film of the abdomen obtained without any specific patient preparation. The KUB study shows gross anatomic features and obvious stones, strictures, calcifications, or obstructions in the urinary tract. This test identifies the shape, size, and position of the organs in relation to other parts of the urinary tract. Other tests are needed to diagnose functional or structural problems.

There is no discomfort or risk from this procedure. Tell the patient that the x-ray will be taken while in a supine position. No specific follow-up care is needed.

Computed Tomography. Inform the patient that a CT scan provides three-dimensional information about the kidneys, ureters, bladder, and surrounding tissues. The CT scan is performed in a special room, usually in the radiology department. It can provide information about tumors, cysts, abscesses, other masses, and obstruction. CT can also be used to image the kidney's vascular system (i.e., CT angiography). Some hospitals require patients having CT scans to be NPO for some period before the scan, although there is no specific evidence guiding this practice.

Determine whether the scan requires a contrast medium (often called *dye*). The most common contrast agents used for imaging of the kidney are radiopaque, contain iodine, are nonionic, and have varying osmolarity. These include iohexol, iopromide, and iodixanol. Oral or injected contrast medium is usually given before starting the imaging procedure. Dye use may be omitted in patients at risk for contrast-induced acute kidney injury, but the images produced are less distinct.

When a contrast agent is used, ensure that there is sufficient oral or IV intake to dilute and excrete the contrast media. Typically the radiologist will specify a total fluid intake of 1 L

TABLE 57.6 **Radiologic and Special Diagnostic Tests for Patients With Disorders of the Kidney and Urinary System**

Test	Purpose
Radiography of kidneys, ureters, and bladder (KUB) (plain film of abdomen)	To screen for the presence of two kidneys To measure kidney size To detect gross obstruction in kidneys or urinary tract
CT with contrast, CT arteriography or angiography	To measure kidney size To evaluate contour to assess for injury, masses, or obstruction in kidneys or the urinary tract To assess renal blood flow
MRI	Similar to CT Useful for staging of cancers
Ultrasonography (US) Can be used with contrast media	To identify the urine volume in the bladder, size of the kidneys or obstruction (e.g., tumors, stones) in the kidneys or lower urinary tract Assess blood flow to and from the kidney
(Nuclear) renal scan	To evaluate renal perfusion To estimate glomerular filtration rate To provide functional information without exposing the patient to iodinated contrast medium
Cystoscopy	To identify abnormalities of the bladder wall and urethral and ureteral occlusions To treat small obstructions or lesions via fulguration, lithotripsy, or removal with a stone basket
Cystography and cystourethrography With or without retrograde studies With or without contrast medium	To outline bladder's contour when full and examine structure during voiding To examine the structure of the urethra To detect backward urine flow
Metabolic imaging with positron emission tomography (PET)	To evaluate cysts, tumors, and other lesions, eliminating the need for biopsy in some patients

or a variable rate to maintain urine output at 1 to 2 mL/kg/hr for up to 6 hours. When no contrast agent is used, there is no special postprocedural care.

Contrast media are potentially kidney damaging (nephrotoxic). *Contrast-induced acute kidney injury* (previously called *contrast-induced nephropathy*) is the term used for postcontrast kidney injury that is thought to be linked to the administration of the contrast material (Rudnick & Davenport, 2023). The risk for *contrast-induced kidney injury* is greatest in patients who are older or dehydrated, have preexisting chronic kidney disease (CKD), or have comorbidities of diabetes, heart failure, or current hypotension (Pagana et al., 2022). Patients who take nephrotoxic drugs are also at risk. Box 57.1 lists assessment questions to ask before a patient undergoes testing with contrast material.

In addition, patients taking metformin are at risk for lactic acidosis when they receive iodinated contrast media. Metformin should be discontinued at least 24 hours before the time of a procedure and for at least 48 hours after the procedure. Kidney function should be reevaluated before the patient resumes metformin therapy.

⬤ NURSING SAFETY PRIORITY

Drug Alert

Ensure that the patient who is prescribed metformin does not receive the drug after a procedure requiring IV contrast material until adequate kidney function has been determined.

BOX 57.1 **Best Practice for Patient Safety and Quality Care**

Assessing the Patient About to Undergo a Kidney Test or Procedure Using a Contrast Medium

Before the Procedure

Ask the patient:

- Have you ever had a contrast medium? If so, did you have a reaction? If so, describe the reaction (e.g., hives, facial edema, difficulty breathing, bronchospasm). If patients have had a reaction before, they are at higher risk of having another reaction.
- Do you have a history of asthma? Patients with asthma have been shown to be at greater risk for contrast reactions than the general public. When reactions do occur, they are more likely to be severe.
- Do you have hay fever or food or drug allergies? Contrast reactions have been reported to occur in up to 15% of patients with hay fever or food or drug allergies, especially to seafood, eggs, milk, or chocolate.
- Are you taking metformin? Metformin must be discontinued at least 24 hours before any study using contrast media because the life-threatening complication of lactic acidosis, although rare, could occur.
- When did you last eat or drink anything?

Assess for a history of renal impairment and for conditions that have been implicated in increasing the chance of developing kidney injury or impairment after use of contrast media (e.g., diabetic nephropathy, class IV heart failure, dehydration, concomitant use of potentially nephrotoxic drugs such as aminoglycosides or NSAIDs, and cirrhosis).

Assess hydration status by checking blood pressure, heart and respiratory rates, mucous membranes, skin turgor, and urine concentration.

All patients at risk for contrast-induced kidney injury need regular assessment and collaboration with the primary health care provider to maintain hydration and decrease the risk for kidney injury following a CT scan with IV contrast administration. Patients who are at risk of kidney injury are generally prescribed IV saline prior to and during the procedure (Rudnick & Davenport, 2023).

 NURSING SAFETY PRIORITY

Drug Alert

> When a CT scan with contrast is ordered, report the patient's history of immediate hypersensitivity reactions associated with the administration of contrast media to the radiologist and health care provider.

Magnetic Resonance Imaging. MRI provides improved imaging between normal and abnormal tissue in the renal system compared with a CT scan. As with all MRIs, the patient with metal implants (pins, pacemaker, joint replacement, aneurysmal clips, or other cosmetic or medical devices) is not eligible for this test because the magnet can move the metal implant, resulting in harm to the patient. A variation of MRI is magnetic resonance angiography (MRA). This noninvasive procedure is used to detect blockages in large arteries and can determine renal artery stenosis.

Gadolinium-based contrast agents are used with MRI similar to CT scans. The contrast agent is injected intravenously and excreted via the kidneys. These agents have been linked with nephrogenic systemic fibrosis (Pagana et al., 2022) and should not be used in patients with renal impairment, usually defined as a serum creatinine above 1.5 mg/dL (110 mcmol/L) or an estimated GFR less than 30 mL/min. Adults older than 60 years should be carefully evaluated for renal impairment.

Kidney Ultrasonography. Inform the patient that ultrasonography does not cause discomfort and is without risk. This test usually requires a full bladder. Ask the patient to drink 500 to 1000 mL of water, if needed, about 2 to 3 hours before the test to help fill the bladder. The patient should not void after drinking the water until the test is complete. This test applies sound waves to structures of different densities to produce images of the kidneys, ureters, and bladder and surrounding tissues. Ultrasonography allows assessment of kidney size, cortical thickness, and status of the calices. The test can identify obstruction in the urinary tract, tumors, cysts, and other masses without the use of contrast. In addition, it can determine blood flow into and out of the kidney using Doppler color flow imaging.

The patient undergoing kidney ultrasonography is usually placed in the prone position. Sonographic gel is applied to the skin over the back and flank areas to enhance sound wave conduction. A transducer in contact with and moving across the skin delivers sound waves and measures the echoes. Images of the internal structures are produced. Assisting the patient to assume a position of comfort and performing skin care to remove the gel are all that is needed after ultrasonography.

Renal Scan. This imaging test is used to examine the perfusion, function, and structure of the kidneys with the IV administration of a radioisotope. It does not use an iodinated contrast agent and thus may be used in preference to a CT scan when the patient is allergic to iodine or has impaired kidney function that places the patient at risk for kidney injury from IV contrast media.

No fasting or sedation is used. A peripheral IV catheter is inserted to give the radioisotope contrast agent. While the patient lies in a prone or sitting position, a camera is passed over the kidney area and records the isotope uptake on film, minutes after the radioisotope is given. After initial images, the patient may be given furosemide or captopril to better visualize kidney function and blood flow. The isotope is eliminated 6 to 24 hours after the procedure. Encourage the patient to drink fluids to aid in excretion of the isotope. Because only tracer doses of radioisotopes are used, no precautions are needed related to radioactive exposure.

 NURSING SAFETY PRIORITY

Drug Alert

> A renal scan is contraindicated in women who are pregnant unless the benefits outweigh the risks.

Renal Arteriography (Angiography). Renal arteriography allows visualization of the renal arteries using a radiopaque contrast medium that enters the renal blood vessels and generates images to determine blood vessel size and abnormalities. The contrast medium is injected through the femoral or brachial artery as x-ray pictures are taken. This test has largely been replaced by other imaging techniques (e.g., nuclear renal scans, ultrasonography, CT) and is seldom used as a stand-alone diagnostic procedure. The most common use of renal arteriography is at the time of a renal angioplasty or other intervention.

Cystoscopy and Cystourethroscopy

Patient Preparation. Cystoscopy and cystourethroscopy are endoscopic procedures used to evaluate the bladder, urethra, and lower portions of the ureters. An endoscopy scope is inserted through the urethra into the bladder, providing direct visualization. These procedures require completion of a preoperative checklist and a signed informed consent statement. The urologist provides a complete description of and reasons for the procedure, and the nurse reinforces this information. Cystoscopy may be performed for diagnosis or treatment. This test is used to examine for bladder trauma (cystoscopy) or urethral trauma (cystourethroscopy) and to identify causes of urinary tract obstruction. Cystoscopy also may be used to remove bladder tumors or plant radium seeds into a tumor, dilate the urethra and ureters with or without stent placement, stop areas of bleeding, or resect an enlarged prostate gland.

Cystoscopy may be performed with the patient under general anesthesia or under local anesthesia with sedation. The patient's age and general health and the expected duration of the procedure are considered in the decision about anesthesia. A light evening meal may be eaten. Usually the patient is NPO after midnight on the night before the cystoscopy. A bowel preparation with laxatives or enemas is performed the evening before the procedure so that bowel contents do not interfere with the procedure.

Procedure. The cystoscopy is performed in a designated cystoscopic examination room. If the procedure is performed in a surgical suite under general anesthesia, the usual surgical support personnel are present (see Chapter 9). This procedure is often performed in clinics, ambulatory surgery or short-procedure units, or a urologist's office.

Assist the patient onto a table and, after sedation, place the patient in the lithotomy position. After the anesthesia is given and the area cleansed and draped, the urologist inserts a cystoscope through the urethra into the urinary bladder. This examination commonly includes the use of both the cystoscope and urethroscope.

Follow-up Care. After this procedure with general anesthesia, the patient is returned to a postanesthesia care unit (PACU) or area. If local anesthesia and sedation were used, the patient may be returned directly to the hospital room. Patients undergoing cystoscopic examinations as outpatients are transferred to an area for monitoring before discharge to home. Monitor for airway patency and breathing, changes in vital signs (including temperature), and changes in urine output. Also observe for the complications of bladder puncture, excessive bleeding, and infection. Bladder puncture is accompanied by severe pain, including abdominal pain, nausea, and vomiting.

A catheter may or may not be present after cystoscopy. The patient without a catheter has urinary frequency as a result of irritation from the procedure. The urine may be pink tinged, but gross bleeding is not expected. Bleeding or the presence of clots may obstruct the catheter and decrease urine output. Monitor urine output and notify the urologist of obvious blood clots or a decreased or absent urine output. Irrigate the Foley catheter with sterile saline, if ordered. Notify the urologist if the patient has a fever (with or without chills) or an elevated white blood cell (WBC) count, which suggests infection. Urge the patient to take oral fluids to increase urine output (which helps prevent clotting) and reduce the burning sensation on urination.

Cystography and Cystourethrography. These tests are a series of x-rays or a continuous radiographic visualization by fluoroscopy. During the imaging, radiopaque contrast medium fills the bladder and the bladder is emptied. Images show structure and function of the bladder and urethra. Tumors, rupture or perforation of the bladder and urethra, abnormal backflow of urine, and distortion from trauma or other pelvic masses can be seen (Fig. 57.10).

Patient Preparation and Procedure. Explain the procedure to the patient. A urinary catheter is temporarily needed to instill contrast medium directly into the bladder for both procedures. The contrast medium enhances x-ray visibility of the lower urinary tract and is not absorbed into the bloodstream, reducing the risk for contrast-induced kidney injury.

After bladder filling, x-rays are taken from the front, back, and side positions. For the voiding cystourethrogram (VCUG), the patient is requested to void and x-rays are taken during the voiding. A VCUG can determine whether urine refluxes (flows backward) into the ureter. The cystogram is used in cases

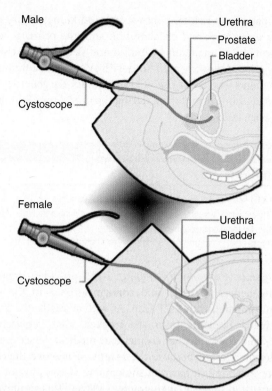

FIG. 57.10 Visualization of cystoscopy in male and female. (From Balas, V. E., Solani, V. K., & Kumar, R. [2020]. Emergence of pharmaceutical industry growth with industrial IoT approach. St. Louis: Elsevier.)

of trauma when urethral or bladder injury is suspected or for patients with recurrent *pyelonephritis* (kidney infection).

Follow-up Care. Monitor for infection as a result of catheter placement. In this test, the contrast medium is not nephrotoxic because it does not enter the bloodstream and does not reach the kidney. Encourage fluid intake to dilute the urine and reduce the burning sensation from catheter irritation after removal. Monitor for changes in urine output because pelvic or urethral trauma may be present.

Retrograde Procedures. *Retrograde* means going against the normal flow of urine. A retrograde examination of the ureters and pelvis *(pyelogram)*, the bladder *(cystogram)*, and the urethra *(urethrogram)* involves instilling radiopaque contrast medium into the lower urinary tract. Because the contrast agent is instilled directly to obtain an outline of the structures desired, the agent does not enter the bloodstream. Therefore the patient is not at risk for contrast-induced kidney injury.

The patient is prepared for retrograde procedures (retrograde pyelography, retrograde cystography, and retrograde urethrography) in the same way as for cystoscopy. Retrograde x-rays are obtained during the cystoscopy. After placement of the cystoscope by the urologist, catheters are placed into each ureter, and contrast material is instilled into each ureter and renal pelvis. The catheters are removed by the urologist, and x-rays are taken to outline these structures as the agent is excreted. The procedure identifies obstruction or structural abnormalities.

For patients undergoing retrograde cystoscopy or urethrography, radiopaque contrast medium is instilled similarly into the bladder or urethra. Cystography and urethrography identify structural problems, such as fistulas, diverticula, and tumors.

After retrograde procedures, monitor the patient for infection caused by placing instruments in the urinary tract. Because these procedures are performed during cystoscopic examination, follow-up care is the same as that for cystoscopy, including monitoring for bladder puncture or perforation.

Other Diagnostic Assessments

Urodynamic Studies. Urodynamic studies examine the processes of voiding and include:
- Tests of bladder capacity, pressure, and tone
- Studies of urethral pressure and urine flow
- Tests of perineal voluntary muscle function

These tests are often used along with voiding urographic or cystoscopic procedures to evaluate problems with urine flow and disorders of the lower urinary tract.

Cystometrography (CMG) can determine how well the bladder wall (detrusor) muscle functions and how sensitive it is to stretching as the bladder fills. This test provides information about bladder capacity, bladder pressure, and voiding reflexes.

Explain the procedure and inform the patient that a urinary catheter will be needed temporarily during the procedure. Ask the patient to void normally. Record the amount and time of voiding. Insert a urinary catheter to measure the residual urine volume. The cystometer is attached to the catheter, and fluid is instilled via the catheter into the bladder. The point at which the patient first notes a feeling of the urge to void and the point at which the patient notes a strong urge to void are recorded. Bladder capacity and bladder pressure readings are recorded graphically. The patient is asked to void when the bladder instillation is complete (about 500 mL). The residual urine after voiding is recorded, and the catheter is removed. Electromyography of the perineal muscles may be performed during this examination.

For any procedure that involves inserting instruments into the urinary tract, monitor for infection. Record the patient's temperature, the character of the urine, and urine output volume.

Urethral pressure profile (also called a *urethral pressure profilometry [UPP]*) can provide information about the nature of urinary incontinence or urinary retention.

Explain the procedure and inform the patient that a urinary catheter will be needed temporarily during the procedure. A special catheter with pressure-sensing capabilities is inserted into the bladder. Variations in the pressure of the smooth muscle of the urethra are recorded as the catheter is slowly withdrawn.

As with any study involving inserting instruments into the urinary tract, monitor the patient for symptoms of infection.

Urine stream testing is used to evaluate pelvic muscle strength and the effectiveness of pelvic muscles in stopping the flow of urine. It is useful in assessing urinary incontinence.

Explain the procedure and reassure the patient that efforts will be made to ensure privacy. The patient is asked to begin urinating. Three to five seconds after urination begins, the examiner gives the patient a signal to stop urine flow. The length of time required to stop the flow of urine is recorded.

Cleaning the perineal area, as after any voiding, is all that is necessary after the urine stream test.

Electromyography (EMG) of the perineal muscles tests the strength of the muscles used in voiding. This information may help identify methods of improving continence. Inform the patient that some mild, temporary discomfort may accompany placement of the electrodes.

In EMG of the perineal muscles, electrodes are placed in either the rectum or the urethra to measure muscle contraction and relaxation. After the completion of EMG, administer analgesics as prescribed to promote the patient's comfort.

Kidney Biopsy

Patient Preparation. Explain that a kidney biopsy can help determine a cause of unexplained kidney problems and help direct or change therapy. Most kidney biopsies are performed percutaneously (through skin and other tissues) using ultrasound or CT guidance. The patient signs an informed consent form. Patients are NPO for 4 to 6 hours before the procedure.

Because of the risk for bleeding after the biopsy, coagulation studies such as platelet count, activated partial thromboplastin time (aPTT), prothrombin time (PT), and bleeding time are performed before surgery. Hypertension is aggressively managed before and after the procedure because high blood pressure can make stopping the bleeding after the biopsy more difficult. Uremia also increases the risk for bleeding, and dialysis may be ordered before a biopsy. A blood transfusion may be needed to correct anemia before biopsy.

Procedure. In a percutaneous biopsy, the nephrologist or radiologist obtains tissue samples without an incision. Patients receive sedation and are monitored throughout the procedure. The patient is placed in the prone position on the procedure table. The entry site is selected after preliminary images are taken. The area is prepared and sterilely draped. A local anesthetic is injected, and the physician then inserts the biopsy device into the tissues toward the kidney. Needle depth and placement are confirmed by ultrasound or CT. While the patient holds the breath, the needle is advanced into the renal cortex. Samples are then taken with a biopsy needle and sent for pathologic study (Pagana et al., 2022).

Follow-up Care. After a percutaneous biopsy, the major risk is bleeding into the kidney or the tissues external from the kidney at the biopsy site. For 24 hours after the biopsy, monitor the dressing site, vital signs (especially fluctuations in blood pressure), urine output, hemoglobin level, and hematocrit. Even if the dressing is dry and there is no hematoma, the patient could be bleeding from the site. An internal bleed is not readily visible but is suspected with flank pain, decreasing blood pressure, decreasing urine output, or other signs of hypovolemia or shock. With severe bleeding, some patients develop bruising along the flank and back accompanied by pain.

The patient follows a plan of strict bed rest, lying in a supine position with a back roll for additional support for 2 to 6 hours after the biopsy. The head of the bed may be elevated, and the patient may resume oral intake of food and fluids. After bed rest, the patient may have limited bathroom privileges if there is no evidence of bleeding.

Monitor for hematuria, the most common complication of kidney biopsy. Hematuria occurs microscopically in most patients, but 5% to 9% have gross hematuria. This problem usually resolves without treatment 48 to 72 hours after the biopsy but can persist for 2 to 3 weeks. In rare cases, transfusions and surgery are required. There should be no obvious blood clots in the urine.

The patient may have some local pain after the biopsy. If aching originates at the biopsy site and begins to radiate to the flank, back, and around the front of the abdomen, bleeding may have started, or a hematoma is forming around the kidney. This pattern of pain with bleeding occurs because blood in the tissues around the kidney increases pressure on local nerve tracts.

If bleeding occurs, IV fluid, packed red blood cells, or both may be needed to prevent shock. In general, a small amount of bleeding creates enough pressure to compress bleeding sites. This is called a *tamponade effect*. If tamponade does not occur and bleeding is extensive, surgery for hemostasis or even nephrectomy may be needed. A hematoma in, on, or around the kidney may become infected, requiring treatment with antibiotics and surgical drainage.

If no bleeding occurs, the patient can resume general activities after 24 hours. Instruct the patient to avoid lifting heavy objects, exercising, or performing other strenuous activities for 1 to 2 weeks after the biopsy procedure. Driving may also be restricted. Refer to Chapter 9 for general postoperative care for the patient who has undergone an open kidney biopsy.

NCLEX Examination Challenge 57.3
Safe and Effective Care Environment

The nurse is conducting an initial assessment on a client who is 1 hour post–kidney biopsy. Which assessment data requires **immediate** intervention?
A. Nausea and vomiting
B. Pink-tinged urine
C. Reports of flank pain
D. The client is ambulating to the bathroom

GET READY FOR THE NEXT-GENERATION NCLEX® EXAMINATION!

Essential Assessment Points

- Wear gloves when handling urine or drainage from the genitourinary tract.
- Evaluate the patient for potential adverse or allergic reactions to radiopaque contrast agents, iodine, or gadolinium.
- Assess the patient for use of drugs that increase risk for kidney dysfunction.
- Assess the patient for bleeding, increased pain, and symptoms of perforation or infection after any invasive test of kidney/urinary function.
- Teach patients to clean the perineal area after voiding, having a bowel movement, and sexual intercourse.
- Urge all patients to maintain an adequate fluid intake (sufficient to dilute urine to a light yellow color) unless another health problem requires fluid restriction.
- Provide privacy for patients undergoing examination or testing of the renal system.
- Use language and terminology that the patient can understand during discussions of kidney/urinary assessment.
- Interpret laboratory data to distinguish between dehydration and kidney impairment.
- Describe how to obtain different types of urine specimens.
- Document renal and urinary system assessment in the patient's electronic health record.
- Assess urine and serum tests of kidney function closely after renal system diagnostic tests.

Mastery Questions

1. Which client admitted to the hospital for dehydration would the nurse consider at greatest risk for reduced kidney function?
   A. 45-year-old female receiving oral and IV fluid therapy
   B. 51-year-old female with a history of urinary incontinence
   C. 62-year-old female with a known allergy to contrast media
   D. 80-year-old male with benign prostatic hyperplasia

2. The nurse is caring for a client during the first 12 hours after a kidney biopsy. Which assessment data indicates a possible complication from the procedure?
   A. The biopsy site is tender to light palpation.
   B. The client experiences nausea and vomiting after drinking juice.
   C. The abdomen is distended, and the client reports abdominal discomfort.
   D. The heart rate is 118 beats/min, blood pressure is 108/50 mm Hg, and peripheral pulses are thready.

REFERENCES

Inker, L., & Perrone, R. (2023). Assessment of kidney function. *UpTo-Date*. Retrieved April 18, 2023, from https://www.uptodate.com/contents/assessment-of-kidney-function.

Jarvis, C., & Eckhardt, A. (2024). *Physical examination & health assessment* (8th ed.). St. Louis: Elsevier.

Lambert, P., Chasson, K., Horton, S., Petrin, C., Marshall, E., Bowdon, S., et al. (2017). Reducing acute kidney injury due to contrast material: How nurses can improve patient safety. *Critical Care Nurse*, *37*(1), 13–26.

National Kidney Foundation. (2020). *Race, ethnicity, and kidney disease*. https://www.kidney.org/atoz/content/minorities-KD.

National Kidney Foundation. (2021). *NKF and ASN release new way to diagnose kidney diseases*. https://www.kidney.org/news/nkf-and-asn-release-new-way-to-diagnose-kidney-diseases.

National Kidney Foundation. (2022). *Living with one kidney*. https://www.kidney.org/atoz/content/onekidney.

Pagana, K., Pagana, T., & Pagana, T. (2022). *Mosby's manual of diagnostic and laboratory test reference* (7th ed.). St. Louis: Elsevier.

Rogers, J. L. (2023). *McCance and Huether's Pathophysiology: The biologic basis for disease in adults and children* (9th ed.). St. Louis: Elsevier.

Rudnick, M., & Davenport, M. (2023). Prevention of contrast-induced acute kidney injury associated with computed tomography. *UpToDate*. Retrieved April 18, 2023, from https://www.uptodate.com/contents/prevention-of-contrast-induced-acute-kidney-injury-associated-with-computed-tomography.

Touhy, T., & Jett, K. (2023). *Ebersole & Hess' toward healthy aging: Human needs & nursing response* (11th ed.). St. Louis: Elsevier.

Wald, R. (2022). Urinalysis in the diagnosis of kidney disease. *UpToDate*. Retrieved April 18, 2023, from https://www.uptodate.com/contents/urinalysis-in-the-diagnosis-of-kidney-disease.

58

Concepts of Care for Patients With Urinary Conditions

Nicole M. Heimgartner

http://evolve.elsevier.com/Iggy/

LEARNING OUTCOMES

1. Plan collaborative care with the interprofessional team to promote *elimination* in patients with urinary conditions.
2. Teach adults how to decrease the risk for urinary conditions.
3. Teach the patient and caregiver(s) about common drugs and other management strategies used for urinary conditions.
4. Plan patient- and family-centered nursing interventions to decrease the psychosocial impact caused by living with urinary conditions.
5. Apply knowledge of anatomy, physiology, and pathophysiology to provide evidence-based care for patients with urinary conditions affecting *elimination*.
6. Analyze assessment and diagnostic findings to generate solutions and prioritize nursing care for patients with urinary conditions.
7. Organize care coordination and transition management for patients with urinary conditions.
8. Use clinical judgment to plan evidence-based nursing care to promote *elimination* and prevent complications in patients with urinary conditions.
9. Incorporate factors that affect health equity into the plan of care for patients with urinary conditions.

KEY TERMS

anuria Absence of urine output.

bacteremia (also called *urosepsis*) Spread of the infection from the urinary tract to the bloodstream.

bacteriuria Presence of bacteria in the urine.

continence Control over the time and place of urine elimination.

cystitis Inflammation of the bladder.

cystocele Herniation of the bladder into the vagina.

dysuria Pain or burning with urination.

frequency Urge to urinate frequently in small amounts.

hydronephrosis Enlargement of the kidney caused by blockage of urine lower in the tract and filling of the kidney with urine.

hydroureter Enlargement of the ureter.

incontinence Involuntary loss of urine.

interstitial cystitis A painful inflammatory bladder condition.

intracorporeal Inside the body.

intravesical Inside the bladder.

lithotripsy Extracorporeal shock wave lithotripsy (ESWL) is the use of sound, laser, or dry shock waves to break stones into small fragments.

nephrolithiasis Formation of stones in the kidney.

oliguria Scant urine output.

pessary Plastic device inserted into the vagina that helps hold internal organs in place.

radical cystectomy Removal of the bladder and surrounding tissue.

renal colic Term used to describe the severe flank pain resulting from stones.

trabeculation Abnormal thickening of the bladder wall caused by urinary retention and obstruction.

ureterolithiasis Formation of stones in the ureter.

urethritis Inflammation of the urethra that can result from infectious and noninfectious conditions.

urgency Feeling that urination will occur immediately.

urolithiasis Presence of calculi (stones) in the urinary tract.

urosepsis (also called *bacteremia*) Spread of the infection from the urinary tract to the bloodstream.

PRIORITY AND INTERRELATED CONCEPTS

The priority concept for this chapter is:
- *Elimination*
  The *Elimination* concept exemplar for this chapter is Urinary Incontinence.

The interrelated concepts for this chapter are:
- *Pain*
- *Immunity*
- *Tissue Integrity*

The urinary tract includes the ureters, bladder, and urethra. Although these structures play no role in the making of urine, their functions are essential for the urine made by the kidneys to be eliminated from the body. Both infectious and noninfectious problems in the urinary tract can disrupt urinary *elimination* and affect control of fluids, electrolytes, nitrogenous wastes, and blood pressure.

Any urinary problem can affect the storage or *elimination* of urine. Both acute and chronic urinary problems are common and costly. Urinary tract infections (UTIs) are the most common type of outpatient infection (Medina & Castillo-Pino, 2019), and it is estimated that 1 million emergency department visits and 100,000 hospitalizations are associated with UTIs (Simmering et al., 2017). In addition, many other people seek treatment for kidney and ureter stones, urinary incontinence (UI), urologic trauma, and cancer involving the urinary system. Although life-threatening complications are rare with urinary problems, patients may have functional, physical, and psychosocial changes that reduce quality of life. Nursing interventions are directed toward prevention, early detection, and early management of urologic disorders.

ELIMINATION CONCEPT EXEMPLAR: URINARY INCONTINENCE

Pathophysiology Review

Continence is the control over the time and place of *elimination*. Urinary continence is specific to control over urinary elimination and is a learned behavior. Efficient bladder emptying (i.e., coordination between bladder contraction and urethral relaxation) is needed for continence. Continence occurs when pressure in the urethra is greater than the pressure in the bladder. For normal voiding to occur, the urethra must relax, and the bladder must contract with enough pressure and duration to empty completely. Voiding normally occurs in a smooth and coordinated manner under conscious control.

Urinary incontinence (UI) is an involuntary loss of urine severe enough to cause social or hygienic problems. It is *not* a normal consequence of aging or childbirth and often is a stigmatizing and an underreported health problem. Many adults suffer in silence, are socially isolated, and may be unaware that treatment is available. In addition, the cost of incontinence can be enormous (Zhang, 2018).

Urinary incontinence has several possible causes (Table 58.1). Except for infection, temporary causes of incontinence

usually do not involve a disorder of the urinary tract. The most common types of adult urinary incontinence are stress incontinence, urge incontinence, overflow incontinence, functional incontinence, and a mixed form of incontinence.

Stress incontinence is the most common type urinary incontinence and will likely affect one in three females at some time in their lives (Cleveland Clinic, 2021). It can occur in males but is much more common in females. Its main feature is the inability to retain urine when laughing, coughing, sneezing, jogging, or lifting. In the continent adult, the urethra can be relaxed and tightened under conscious control because skeletal muscles of the pelvic floor surround it. When an adult feels the urge to urinate, the conscious contraction of the urethra can override a bladder contraction if the urethral contraction is strong enough. Patients with *stress incontinence* cannot tighten the urethra enough to overcome the increased bladder pressure caused by contraction of the detrusor muscle.

Urge incontinence is the loss of urine for no apparent reason after suddenly feeling the need or urge to urinate. Normally when the bladder is full, contraction of the smooth muscle fibers of the bladder detrusor muscle signals the brain that it is time to urinate. Continent adults override that signal and relax the detrusor muscle for the time it takes to locate a toilet. Those who experience urge incontinence cannot suppress the signal and have a sudden strong urge to void and can leak large amounts of urine at this time. Urge incontinence is also known as an *overactive bladder (OAB)* and is more common in older females.

Overflow incontinence occurs when the detrusor muscle fails to contract and the bladder becomes overdistended. This type of incontinence (*reflex incontinence* or *underactive bladder*) occurs when the bladder has reached its maximum capacity and some urine must leak out to prevent bladder rupture. It is important to note that more than one type of incontinence can exist at the same time. This is called *mixed incontinence* and is a combination of stress and urge incontinence.

Functional incontinence occurs as a result of factors other than the abnormal function of the bladder and urethra. A common factor is the loss of cognitive function in patients affected by dementia.

PATIENT-CENTERED CARE: OLDER ADULT HEALTH

Urinary Incontinence

Many factors contribute to urinary incontinence in older adults. An older adult may have decreased mobility from many causes. In inpatient settings, mobility is limited when the older patient is placed on bed rest. Vision and hearing impairments may also prevent the patient from locating a call light to notify the nurse or assistive personnel of the need to void. Assess for these factors and minimize them to prevent urinary incontinence. Getting out of bed to urinate is a common cause of falls among older adults in the home and other settings (Touhy & Jett, 2023).

Etiology

Urinary incontinence may have temporary or permanent causes (see Table 58.1) Evaluation of the patient with urinary

TABLE 58.1   Types of Urinary Incontinence

Type and Description	Causes	Symptoms	Management
Stress Incontinence			
Involuntary loss of urine during activities that increase abdominal and detrusor pressure Inability to tighten the urethra sufficiently to overcome the increased detrusor pressure Leakage of urine	Weakening of bladder neck supports; associated with childbirth Intrinsic sphincter deficiency, such as epispadias (abnormal location of the urethra on the dorsum of the penis) or myelomeningocele Acquired anatomic damage to the urethral sphincter from repeated incontinence surgeries, prostatectomy, radiation therapy, and trauma Vaginal prolapse from vaginal birth or aging	Urine loss with physical exertion, cough, sneeze, or exercise Usually only small amounts of urine are lost with each exertion Normal voiding habits (≤8 times per day, ≤2 times per night) Postvoid residual usually ≤50 mL Pelvic examination shows hypermobility of the urethra or bladder neck with Valsalva maneuvers	Weight reduction for patients who are obese Smoking cessation Pelvic muscle therapy Vaginal cone therapy Bladder training Estrogen therapy for postmenopausal women Electrical stimulation Magnetic resonance therapy Pessary devices Surgery includes slings, bladder suspension, injection of bulking agents, prostatectomy Electrical stimulation device
Urge Incontinence			
Overactive bladder (OAB) Involuntary loss of urine associated with a strong desire to urinate Inability to suppress the signal from the bladder muscle to the brain that it is time to urinate	Idiopathic Neurologic disorders, such as stroke Benign prostatic hypertrophy Bladder inflammation or infection Bladder irritants, such as artificial sweeteners, caffeine, alcohol, citric intake, drugs, nicotine Bladder cancer Medications that cause increased bladder contractility	An abrupt and strong urge to void (urinary urgency) Urinary frequency Nocturia May have loss of large amounts of urine with each occurrence	Bladder training Pelvis muscle therapy Weight reduction for patients who are obese Avoid bladder irritants, such as caffeine and alcohol Smoking cessation Drug therapy if bladder training is not successful: anticholinergics, tricyclic antidepressants with anticholinergic and alpha-adrenergic agonist activity, beta-adrenergic agonist, and onabotulinumtoxinA Electrical stimulation device Surgery includes transurethral resection of the prostate or prostatectomy
Mixed Incontinence			
Combination of stress and urge incontinence	Causes associated with stress and urge incontinence	Symptoms associated with stress and urge incontinence	See management for stress and urge incontinence
Overflow Incontinence (Reflex Incontinence)			
Involuntary loss of urine associated with overdistention of the bladder when the bladder capacity has reached its maximum Detrusor underactivity Bladder outlet obstruction	Urethral obstruction such as benign prostatic hypertrophy or uterine prolapse Diabetic neuropathy Some neurologic disorders, such as multiple sclerosis or spinal cord damage Medication side effects	Bladder distention, Constant dribbling of urine Sense of incomplete emptying of the bladder Pelvic discomfort Palpable bladder	Bladder training Bladder compression (Credé method) Intermittent self-catheterization Drug therapy if bladder training unsuccessful: bethanechol chloride Nonsurgical treatment unless surgery is required to remove the obstruction: i.e., prostatectomy or repair of uterine prolapse
Functional Incontinence			
Leakage of urine caused by factors other than disease of the lower urinary tract	Decreased cognition such as with dementia Impaired mobility, such as paralysis or inability to walk to the toilet; some neurologic disorders	Quantity and timing of urine leakage vary Patterns difficult to discern	Habit training Prompted voiding is used to establish a predictable pattern of bladder emptying to prevent incontinence Applied devices: • Intravaginal pessaries • Penile clamps • Condom catheter Intermittent or long-term catheterization

incontinence means considering all possible causes, beginning with those that are temporary and correctable. Surgical and traumatic causes of urinary incontinence are related to procedures or surgery in the lower pelvic structures, which are areas that contain complex nerve pathways. Radical urologic, prostatic, and gynecologic procedures for treatment of pelvic cancers may result in urinary incontinence. Injury to segments S2–4 of the spinal cord may cause incontinence from impairment of normal nerve pathways.

Inappropriate bladder contraction may result from disorders of the brain and nervous system or from bladder irritation due to chronic infection, stones, chemotherapy, or radiation therapy. Other causes of bladder contraction failure include neuropathies associated with diabetes mellitus, syphilis, and previous treatment with neurotoxic anticancer drugs. Constipation can lead to temporary urinary incontinence. Some drugs or drug-drug interactions from polypharmacy, such as anticholinergics, calcium channel blockers, diuretics, and sedatives, can cause or worsen urinary incontinence.

Incidence and Prevalence

Urinary incontinence is a major health problem. The incidence of UI is increasing, with more than 60% of females in the United States experiencing some form of incontinence (Patel et al., 2022). The incidence also increases with age. Males also experience UI; however, it is less common, and males are much less likely to seek treatment (Clemens, 2022).

Risk for urinary incontinence increases with chronic conditions such as diabetes mellitus, stroke, cognitive impairment, and impaired mobility. Urinary incontinence occurs not only with older age but with a history of vaginal delivery, particularly if the first child was delivered after age 30. Conditions of pelvic prolapse in women, prostate problems in men, diabetes, heart failure, spinal cord or nerve injury, and obesity also increase the risk for urinary incontinence (Lukacz et al., 2017). Both central nervous system diseases (e.g., dementia, multiple sclerosis, Parkinson's disease) and musculoskeletal disorders (e.g., osteoporosis, osteoarthritis, paresthesia, pain, or paralysis) contribute to cognitive and mobility impairment, resulting in the onset and severity of urinary incontinence (Rogers, 2023). Because urinary incontinence is common among older adults, routine screening for incontinence is recommended for all adults 65 years and older.

Interprofessional Collaborative Care

Urinary incontinence can occur in any setting and is very common in the community. Usually the adult with incontinence is treated using self-management strategies. Even when surgical intervention

PATIENT-CENTERED CARE: OLDER ADULT HEALTH
Factors Contributing to Urinary Incontinence

Drugs
- Central nervous system depressants, such as opioid analgesics, decrease the patient's level of consciousness and the urge to void and contribute to constipation.
- Diuretics cause frequent voiding, often of large amounts of urine.
- Multiple drugs can contribute to changes in mental status or mobility, and they can irritate the bladder.
- Anticholinergic drugs or drugs with anticholinergic side effects are especially challenging because they affect both cognition and the ability to void. Monitor patient responses to these drugs early in treatment.

Disease
- Stroke, Parkinson's disease, dementia, and other neurologic disorders decrease mobility, sensation, or cognition.
- Arthritis decreases mobility and causes *pain.*

Depression
- Depression decreases the energy necessary to maintain continence.
- Decreased self-esteem and feelings of self-worth decrease the importance to the patient of maintaining continence.

Inadequate Resources
- Patients who need assistive devices (e.g., eyeglasses, cane, walker) may be afraid to ambulate without them or without personal assistance.
- Products that help patients manage incontinence of urine *elimination* are often costly, and access to these items can be a barrier to successful management of incontinence.
- No one may be available to assist the patient to the bathroom or help with incontinence products.

PATIENT-CENTERED CARE: HEALTH EQUITY
Urinary Incontinence

Evidence indicates that over 50% of females do not seek treatment for urinary incontinence (Agency for Healthcare Research and Quality [AHRQ], 2022). Understanding barriers to treatment for urinary incontinence is a key step in promoting health equity. The existing evidence indicates that barriers to care vary across racial groups, with Latina women experiencing more barriers. A few studies also indicate that access to pelvic floor physical therapy is inconsistent and patients with Medicaid or no insurance were less likely to receive this treatment, which is proven to be beneficial in the treatment of urinary incontinence (Brown & Simon, 2021). It is important for the nurse to assess all patients for urinary health and for signs of incontinence. In addition, teaching patients that most urinary incontinence is very treatable may encourage those who are reluctant to discuss this condition to talk to the provider about treatment options.

PATIENT-CENTERED CARE: OLDER ADULT HEALTH
Underreported Urinary Incontinence

Some age-related changes occur that affect urinary elimination. However, urinary incontinence is not an expected change associated with aging. Urinary incontinence is underreported and undertreated, especially in older adults (Touhy & Jett, 2023). In addition, the associated conditions (or sequalae) associated with urinary incontinence in older adults can be more severe, including the risk for falls, hospitalization, and even the need for long-term care (Touhy & Jett, 2023). It is important for health care providers to recognize that incontinence can be cured in almost 80% of patients (National Association for Continence, 2018). For those patients who cannot be cured, the effects can be minimized with treatment. However, treatment cannot begin without awareness, and that begins with asking about bladder problems with all older adult patients.

is used, hospitalization for incontinence is rare. Because urinary incontinence carries a burden of impaired comfort, activity disruption, shame or embarrassment, and loss of *tissue integrity,* it has a great impact on quality of life for most adults.

Recognize Cues: Assessment

History. Incontinence may be underreported because health care professionals do not ask patients about urine loss. Ask patients about incontinence, as many patients are hesitant to initiate the subject. Only one in five males are likely to seek treatment for UI (Clemens, 2022) Effective screening includes asking patients to respond "always," "sometimes," or "never" to these questions:

- Do you ever leak urine or water when you do not want to?
- Do you ever leak urine or water when you cough, sneeze, laugh, or exercise?
- Do you ever leak urine or water on the way to the toilet?
- Do you ever use pads, tissues, or cloth in your underwear to catch urine?

If any answer is "always" or "sometimes," perform a focused assessment that includes risk factors for UI, signs and symptoms of UI, and potential barriers to toileting. See Box 58.1.

Physical Assessment/Signs and Symptoms. Assess the abdomen to estimate bladder fullness, rule out palpable hard stool, and evaluate bowel sounds. Urinary incontinence is

---

BOX 58.1   The Patient With Urinary Incontinence

Note the presence of risk factors for urinary incontinence:
- Age
- If patient is female, menopausal status
- Central or peripheral neurologic disease with associated impairment in cognition or mobility
- Diabetes mellitus
- History of vaginal delivery; vaginal prolapse
- Urologic procedures
- Prescribed and over-the-counter drugs that affect cognition or mobility
- Bowel patterns; fecal impaction
- Stress/anxiety level

Detail the symptoms of urinary incontinence:
- Leakage
- Frequency
- Urgency
- Nocturia
- Sensation of full bladder before leakage

Obtain a 24-hour intake-and-output record or a voiding diary:
- Time and amount of oral intake and continent voiding
- Time and estimated amount of incontinent leakages
- Activity around the time of leakage

Assess the patient's:
- Mobility
- Self-care ability
- Cognitive ability
- Communication patterns

Assess the environment for barriers to toileting:
- Privacy
- Restrictive clothing
- Access to toilet

---

confirmed by evaluating the force and character of the urine stream during voiding. Ask the patient to cough while wearing a perineal pad to assess for stress incontinence; a wet pad on forceful coughing indicates stress incontinence.

For females, inspect the external genitalia to determine whether there is apparent urethral or uterine prolapse, cysto-cele (herniation of the bladder into the vagina), or rectocele. These conditions occur with pelvic floor muscle weakness. A primary health care provider puts on an examination glove and inserts two fingers into the vagina to assess the strength of these muscles. Strength is described as *weak, adequate,* or *strong* based on the amount of pressure felt by the primary health care provider as the patient tightens vaginal muscles. Describe and document the color, consistency, and odor of any secretions from the genitourinary orifices. The urine stream interruption test (i.e., asking a patient to voluntarily start and stop urine flow during a void at least twice) is another method of determining pelvic muscle strength. For males, inspect the urethral meatus for any discharge.

A digital rectal examination (DRE) is performed by the primary health care provider on both male and female patients. It provides information about the nerve integrity to the bladder. The examiner determines whether there is tactile sensation in the anal area by observing whether the rectal sphincter is relaxed or contracted on digital insertion. Because nerve supply to the bladder is similar to nerve supply to the rectum, the presence of tactile sensation and a rectal sphincter that contracts suggest that the nerve supply to the bladder is intact. Impaction of stool is a cause of transient urinary incontinence and can be detected during a rectal examination. The primary health care provider assesses for prostate enlargement in males as a possible cause of incontinence.

Laboratory Assessment. A urinalysis is useful to rule out urinary tract infection. This test is the first step in the assessment of incontinent patients of any age. The presence of red blood cells (RBCs), white blood cells (WBCs), leukocyte esterase, or nitrites is an indication for culturing the urine. Any infection is treated before further assessment of incontinence.

Imaging Assessment. Determine the amount of postvoid residual urine (urine remaining in the bladder right after voiding) by portable ultrasound (bladder scanner). If ordered, catheterizing the patient immediately after voiding can also be used to assess residual volume. Additional imaging is needed when surgery is being considered. CT is most useful for locating abnormalities in kidneys and ureters. A voiding cystourethrogram (VCUG) or urodynamic testing may be performed to assess the size, shape, support, and function of the urinary tract system. Urodynamic testing (see Chapter 57) may take several hours and more than one visit. Electromyography (EMG) of the pelvic muscles may be a part of the urodynamic studies.

Analyze Cues and Prioritize Hypotheses: Analysis

The priority collaborative problems for patients with urinary incontinence include:
1. Altered urinary elimination due to incontinence
2. Potential for altered tissue integrity due to incontinence

Generate Solutions and Take Actions: Planning and Implementation

The expected outcomes for altered urinary incontinence are to maintain optimal urinary *elimination*, *tissue integrity,* and comfort. Nursing interventions for the management of the different types of urinary incontinence focus on restoring continence, psychosocial comfort, tissue integrity, and patient education.

Promoting Urinary Elimination

Planning: Expected Outcomes. With appropriate therapy, the patient with altered urinary elimination due to incontinence is expected to develop continence of urine *elimination.* Indicators include that the patient consistently or often demonstrates these actions:

- Stress urinary incontinence: No urine leakage between voidings and no urine leakage with increased abdominal pressure (e.g., sneezing, laughing, lifting)
- Urge urinary incontinence: Responds to urge in a timely manner, gets to toilet between urge and passage of urine, and avoids substances that stimulate the bladder (e.g., caffeine, alcohol)
- Overflow urinary incontinence: Recognizes the urge to void, maintains a predictable pattern of voiding, empties bladder completely, and keeps urine volume in the bladder under 300 mL
- Functional urinary incontinence: Uses urine containment or collection measures to ensure dryness and manages clothing independently

Interventions

Nonsurgical Management. Maintaining a diary can be beneficial for patients with stress incontinence to determine patterns of the incontinence events. Collection devices and absorbent pads and undergarments may be used during the often lengthy process of assessment and treatment of urinary incontinence and by patients who elect not to pursue further interventions.

Nutrition therapy. Nutrition therapy plays a role in specific types of urinary incontinence. Nutrition therapy with weight reduction is helpful for patients who are obese because stress incontinence is made worse by increased abdominal pressure from obesity (Lukacz, 2023). Teach the patient to avoid bladder irritants in the diet, such as caffeine and alcohol, that can contribute to urgency and frequency. Stress the importance of maintaining an adequate fluid intake, especially water. Refer the patient to a registered dietitian nutritionist (RDN) as needed.

Drug therapy. Drug therapy with topical estrogen to the perineal and vaginal orifice is used to treat postmenopausal women with stress incontinence. Estrogen may increase the blood flow and tone of the muscles around the vagina and urethra, thus improving the patient's ability to contract those muscles during times of increased intraabdominal stress.

Because the hypertonic bladder contracts involuntarily in patients with urge incontinence, drugs that relax the smooth muscle and increase the bladder's capacity are prescribed (Table 58.2). The most commonly prescribed drugs are anticholinergics (also known as *antimuscarinics* because they target specific receptors in the cholinergic family of receptors), which include darifenacin, fesoterodine, oxybutynin, solifenacin, tolterodine,

and trospium (Burchum & Rosenthal, 2022). This class of drugs has serious side effects, particularly in older adults, and is used along with behavioral interventions. These drugs inhibit the nerve fibers that stimulate bladder contraction. In addition, tricyclic antidepressants with anticholinergic and alpha-adrenergic agonist activity, such as imipramine, have been used successfully in younger patients for enuresis.

A beta-adrenergic agonist, mirabegron, has demonstrated effectiveness in reducing urge incontinence. The evidence comparing different drug categories for effectiveness in managing incontinence is limited, and no single drug or class is recommended over another.

Another drug therapy for urge incontinence is botulinum toxin (Botox). This drug is injected during cystoscopy into multiple areas of the detrusor muscle of the bladder. Usually 10 to 30 different sites are injected during one treatment session. This treatment relaxes the detrusor muscle and relieves the urge to urinate (Hubb et al., 2018). Some patients have relief of incontinence for as long as 6 to 9 months after injection. Side effects may include urinary retention, painful urination, and an increased incidence of urinary tract infections. For most patients who experience urinary retention, the condition is temporary but does require intermittent self-catheterization.

Drugs are prescribed for short-term management of urinary retention seen in overflow incontinence, often after surgery. They are not used in long-term management of overflow incontinence caused by a hypotonic bladder. The most commonly used drug is bethanechol chloride, an agent that increases bladder pressure.

NURSING SAFETY PRIORITY

Drug Alert

Teach patients taking the extended release forms of anticholinergic drugs to swallow the tablet or capsule whole without chewing or crushing. Chewing or crushing the tablet or capsule destroys the extended release feature, allowing the entire dose to be absorbed quickly, which increases adverse drug side effects.

Devices. Devices can be used to assist with continence. A pessary (plastic device, often ring shaped, that helps hold internal organs in place) inserted into the vagina may help with a prolapsed uterus or bladder when this condition is contributing to urinary incontinence. A prolapse occurs when the supportive tissue in the vagina weakens and stretches, allowing pelvic organs to protrude into the vaginal lumen. The pessary presses against the wall of the vagina to reposition pelvic organs. In general, a pessary is removed and cleaned with soap and water on a monthly basis by the patient, but the nurse can do it for adults with cognitive or musculoskeletal impairment.

The Impressa incontinence device is commonly used for activity-induced incontinence in females. The device is like a small tampon that the patient can insert into the vagina and provides support to the urethra to prevent stress incontinence. This device is available over the counter, and a sizing kit can be purchased to determine the best fit for the patient (Clemons, 2022).

TABLE 58.2   Common Examples of Drug Therapy

Urinary Incontinence

Drug Category	Nursing Implications
Hormones	
Thought to enhance nerve conduction to the urinary tract, improve blood flow, and reduce tissue deterioration of the urinary tract	
Estrogen vaginal cream daily or an estrogen-containing ring inserted monthly	Teach patients to use only a thin application of the cream *to minimize excessive absorption and distribution and avoid systemic side effects.* Teach patients that it takes 4–6 weeks to achieve continence benefits and that benefits disappear about 4 weeks after discontinuing regular use *because knowing the drug responses increases the likelihood of its correct use.*
Anticholinergics	
Suppress involuntary bladder contraction and increase bladder capacity	
Darifenacin Fesoterodine Oxybutynin Solifenacin Tolterodine Trospium	Ask whether the patient has glaucoma before starting any drugs from this class *because anticholinergics can increase intraocular pressure and make glaucoma worse.* Suggest that patients increase fluid intake and use hard candy to moisten the mouth *to reduce the dry mouth side effect.* Teach patients to increase fluid intake and the amount of dietary fiber *to prevent constipation associated with this drug category.* Teach patients to monitor urine output and to report an output significantly lower than intake to the primary health care provider *because all of these drugs can cause urinary retention, especially in men with an enlarged prostate.* Instruct patients taking the extended release forms of these drugs not to chew or crush the tablet/capsule *to avoid both ruining the time-release feature and increasing the risk for a bolus dose with more side effects.*
Alpha-Adrenergic Agonists	
Increase contractile force of the urethral sphincter, increasing resistance to urine outflow	
Midodrine[a]	Teach the patient to monitor the blood pressure periodically when starting the drug *because this drug can cause severe supine hypertension and should not be used in patients with severe cardiac disease.*
Beta$_3$ Agonists	
Relax the detrusor smooth muscle to increase bladder capacity and urine storage	
Mirabegron	Teach the patient to periodically obtain a blood pressure and to inform the health care provider if the systolic or diastolic values increase more than 10 mm Hg or above 180/110 mm Hg *because this drug has the potential to increase blood pressure.* If the patient is taking warfarin, avoid this drug or schedule additional blood testing for potential increased risk for bleeding *because this drug uses the same metabolic pathway as warfarin and can potentiate warfarin's effects, leading to a prolonged international normalized ratio (INR) and increasing the risk for bleeding.*
Antidepressants: Tricyclics and Serotonin-Norepinephrine Reuptake Inhibitors (SNRIs)	
Increase norepinephrine and serotonin levels, which are thought to strengthen the urinary sphincters; also have anticholinergic actions	
Tricyclics Imipramine Amitriptyline	Warn patients not to combine these drugs with other antidepressant drugs *to avoid a drug-drug interaction that can lead to a hypertensive crisis.* Instruct patients to inform their primary health care provider if they take drugs to manage hypertension. Teach patients to change positions slowly, especially in the morning, *to avoid dizziness from orthostatic hypotension, which increases the risk for falls.*
SNRI Duloxetine[a]	Teach patients the same interventions as for anticholinergic agents *because these drugs have anticholinergic activity and can produce the same side effects.*

[a]This drug is used off label and do not have U.S. Food and Drug Administration (FDA) approval for use to treat incontinence. However, they are commonly used to manage incontinence syndromes.

The penile clamp is a treatment option for males with stress incontinence. The clamp is applied around the outside of the penis to compress the urethra and prevent urine leakage. Adverse outcomes from pessaries and penile clamps include reduced *tissue integrity* with tissue damage from pressure and infection from colonization of damaged tissues. Both devices require that the patient have either manual dexterity or a caregiver to apply and remove the device. Instruct the patient or caregivers in the use of these devices.

Male patients may use an external collecting device, such as a condom catheter. In acute care settings, the PureWick, a female external collecting device, has demonstrated promise in effectively collecting urine and preventing tissue damage due to urinary leakage (Beeson & Davis, 2018). The PureWick female external catheter is a tube that lies between the labia next to the urethral opening and extends between the buttocks. The tube is secured to the suprapubic area and is attached to low, continuous suction to wick away urine as it leaks from the urethral opening. This external urinary collection device is effective for patients who are lying down or in the sitting position.

Electrical stimulation. Electrical stimulation with either an intravaginal or intrarectal electrical stimulation device is available to treat urge, stress, and mixed incontinence. Treatment consists of stimulating sensory nerves to decrease the sensation of urgency. It is done as an office-based procedure one to three times weekly for 6 to 8 weeks.

Magnetic resonance therapy. Magnetic resonance therapy involves targeted urinary tract nerves and muscles for depolarization. The patient sits on a chair containing a magnetic device that induces depolarization and helps reduce stress-induced incontinence in a manner similar to drug-induced relaxation of muscle and nerves.

Pelvic muscle therapy. Pelvic muscle (Kegel) exercise therapy for women with stress incontinence strengthens the muscles of the pelvic floor (circumvaginal muscles). These muscles become strengthened, as any other skeletal muscle does, by frequent, systematic, and repeated contractions. The most important step in teaching pelvic muscle exercises is to help the patient learn which muscles to exercise. During the pelvic examination in females and the rectal examination in males or females, the patient is instructed to tighten the pelvic muscles around the health care provider's fingers. The health care provider will then provide feedback about the strength of the contraction. Starting and stopping the urine stream or stopping the passage of flatus indicates that the patient has correctly identified the pelvic muscles. Biofeedback devices, such as electromyography or perineometers, measure the strength of contraction. A perineometer is a tampon-shaped instrument inserted into the vagina to measure the strength of pelvic muscle contractions. The graph shows the amplitude of muscle contraction to the patient for biofeedback. Alternatively, retention of a vaginal weight also shows that the patient has identified the proper muscle (see discussion of vaginal cone therapy).

Instructions for pelvic muscle exercises are provided in Box 58.2. Although improvement may take several months, most patients notice a positive change after 6 weeks. Teach patients to continue the exercises 10 times daily to improve and maintain pelvic muscle strength.

Pelvic muscle exercises are also effective for urge incontinence and are taught in the same way as for stress incontinence. Improved urethral resistance helps the patient overcome abnormal detrusor contractions long enough to get to the toilet.

Vaginal cone therapy. *Vaginal cone weight therapy* involves using a set of five small, cone-shaped weights (Touhy & Jett, 2023). They are of equal size but of varying weights and are used together with pelvic muscle exercise. The female patient inserts the lightest cone, labeled 1, into the vagina (Fig. 58.1A), with the string to the outside, for a 1-minute test period. If the patient can hold the first cone in place without its slipping out while walking around, the patient will then proceed to the second cone, labeled 2, and repeat the procedure. The patient begins the treatment with the heaviest cone that can be comfortably held in the vagina for a 1-minute test period. Treatment periods are 15 minutes twice a day. When the patient can comfortably hold the cone in the vagina for 15 minutes, this indicates readiness to progress to the next heaviest weight. Treatment is completed with the cone labeled 5.

Weighted vaginal cones can help strengthen the pelvic muscles and decrease stress incontinence but may not help pelvic prolapse. Vaginal cones do not require a prescription.

Behavioral Interventions. Other interventions for urinary incontinence may include behavior modification or training (i.e., bladder training [Box 58.3]). Bladder training involves a great deal of patient participation and often begins with a thorough

BOX 58.2 **Patient and Family Education**

Pelvic Muscle Exercises

- The pelvic muscles are composed of a sling of muscles that support your bladder, urethra, and vagina. As with any other muscles in your body, you can make your pelvic muscles stronger by alternately contracting (tightening) and relaxing them in regular exercise periods. By strengthening these muscles, you will be able to stop your urine flow more effectively.
- To identify your pelvic muscles, sit on the toilet with your feet flat on the floor about 12 inches apart. Begin to urinate, and then try to stop the urine flow. Do not strain down, lift your bottom off the seat, or squeeze your legs together. When you start and stop your urine stream, you are using your pelvic muscles.
- To perform pelvic muscle exercises, tighten your pelvic muscles for a slow count of 10 and then relax for a slow count of 10. Do this exercise 15 times while you are lying down, sitting up, and standing (a total of 45 exercises). Repeat—and this time rapidly contract and relax the pelvic muscles 10 times. This should take no more than 10 to 12 minutes for all three positions, or 3 to 4 minutes for each set of 15 exercises.
- Begin with 45 exercises a day in three sets of 15 exercises each. You will notice faster improvement if you can do this twice a day, or a total of 20 minutes each day. Remember to exercise in all three positions so your muscles learn to squeeze effectively despite your position. At first, it is helpful to have a designated time and place to do these exercises because you will have to concentrate to do them correctly. After you have been doing them for several weeks, you will notice improvement in your control of urine. However, many people report that improvement may take as long as 3 months.

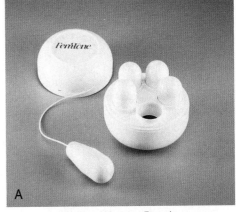

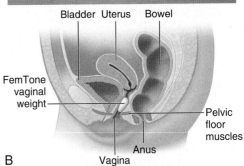

FIG. 58.1 (A) FemTone vaginal weights, or cones. The number on the top of each cone represents increasing weight up to the heaviest cone, number 5. (B) Diagram showing the correct positioning of a vaginal weight, or cone, in place. (A courtesy ConvaTec, A Bristol-Meyers Squibb Company, a Division of E. R. Squibb & Sons, Inc., Princeton, NJ.)

BOX 58.3 Best Practice for Patient Safety and Care

Bladder Training and Habit Training to Reduce Urinary Incontinence

Bladder Training
- Assess the patient's awareness of bladder fullness and ability to cooperate with training regimen.
- Assess the patient's 24-hour urine *elimination* pattern for 2 to 3 consecutive days (bladder diary).
- Base the initial interval of toileting on the voiding pattern (e.g., 45 minutes).
- Teach the patient to void every 45 minutes on the first day and to ignore or suppress the urge to urinate between the 45-minute intervals.
- Take the patient to the toilet or remind the patient to urinate at the 45-minute intervals.
- Provide privacy for toileting and run water in the sink to promote the urge to urinate at this time.
- If the patient is not consistently able to resist the urge to urinate between the intervals, reduce the intervals by 15 minutes.
- Continue this regimen for at least 24 hours or for as many days as it takes for the patient to be comfortable with this schedule and not urinate between the intervals.
- When the patient remains continent between the intervals, increase the intervals by 15 minutes daily until a 3- to 4-hour interval is comfortable for the patient.
- Praise successes. If incontinence occurs, work with the patient to reestablish an acceptable toileting interval.

Habit Training
- Assess the patient's 24-hour voiding pattern for 2 to 3 days.
- Base the initial interval of toileting on the voiding pattern (e.g., 2 hours).
- Help the patient to the toilet or provide a bedpan/urinal every 2 hours (or whatever has been determined to be an appropriate toileting interval for the individual patient).
- During toileting, remind the patient to void and provide cues such as running water.
- If the patient is incontinent between scheduled toiletings, reduce the time interval by 30 minutes until the patient is continent between voidings.
- Help the patient to toilet and prompt to void at prescribed intervals.
- Do not leave the patient on the toilet or bedpan for longer than 5 minutes.
- Ensure that all nursing staff members comply with the established toileting schedule and do not apply briefs or encourage the patient to "just wet the bed."
- Reduce toileting interval by 30 minutes if there are more than two incontinence episodes in 24 hours.
- If the patient remains continent at the toileting interval, attempt to increase the interval by 30 minutes until a 3- to 4-hour continence interval is reached.
- Praise the patient for successes and spend extra time socializing with the patient.
- Discuss daily record of continence with staff to provide reinforcement and encourage compliance with toileting schedule.
- Include assistive personnel in all aspects of the habit training.

explanation of the problem of urge incontinence. Instead of the bladder being in control of the patient, the patient learns to control the bladder. For the program to succeed, the patient must be alert, aware, and able to resist the urge to urinate.

Start a schedule for voiding, beginning with the longest interval that is comfortable for the patient, even if the interval is only 30 minutes. Instruct the patient to void every 30 minutes and to ignore any urge to urinate between the set intervals. Once the patient is comfortable with the starting schedule, increase the interval by 15 to 30 minutes. Instruct the patient to follow the new schedule until achieving success again. As the interval increases, the bladder gradually tolerates more volume. Teach relaxation and distraction techniques to maximize success in the retraining. Provide positive reinforcement for maintaining the prescribed schedule.

Habit training (scheduled toileting) is a type of bladder training that is successful in reducing incontinence in cognitively impaired patients. To use habit training, caregivers help the patient void at specific times (e.g., every 2 hours on the even hours). The goal is to get the patient to the toilet before incontinence occurs. The focus is on reducing incontinence and resulting loss of tissue integrity. When a reduction in incontinence has been achieved, the focus may change to increasing bladder capacity by gradually lengthening the voiding intervals, but this is only secondary.

Prompted voiding, a supplement to habit training, attempts to increase the patient's awareness of the need to void and to prompt the patient to ask for toileting assistance. Habit training otherwise relies completely on a time schedule.

! NURSING SAFETY PRIORITY
Action Alert

Habit training is undermined when absorbent briefs are used in place of timed toileting. Do not tell patients to "just wet the bed." A common cause of falls in health care facilities is related to patient efforts to get out of bed unassisted to use the toilet. Collaborate with all staff members, including assistive personnel (AP), to consistently implement the toileting schedule for habit training.

For overflow incontinence, the most effective common behavioral interventions are bladder compression and intermittent self-catheterization. Bladder compression uses techniques that promote bladder emptying and include the Credé method, the Valsalva maneuver, double-voiding, and splinting.

For the Credé method, teach the patient how to press over the bladder area, increasing the pressure, or to trigger nerve stimulation by tugging at pubic hair or massaging the genital area. These techniques manually help the bladder empty. In the Valsalva maneuver, breathing techniques increase chest and abdominal pressure. This increased pressure is then directed toward the bladder during exhalation. (The Valsalva maneuver is contraindicated in patients who have some cardiac problems because it can trigger a vagal response and cause bradycardia.) With the technique of double-voiding, the patient empties the bladder and then, within a few minutes, attempts a second bladder emptying.

For females who have a large cystocele (prolapse of the bladder into the vagina), a technique called splinting both compresses the bladder and moves it into a better position. The woman inserts her fingers into her vagina, gently lifts the cystocele, and begins to urinate. A pessary, described earlier, can also provide relief from cystocele-related incontinence.

Intermittent self-catheterization is often used to help patients with long-term problems of incomplete bladder emptying. It is effective, can be learned fairly easily, and remains the preferred method of bladder emptying in patients who have incontinence as a result of a neurogenic bladder (Beauchemin et al., 2018). These points are important in teaching the technique:

- Proper handwashing and cleaning of the catheter reduce the risk for infection.
- A small lumen and good lubrication of the catheter prevent urethral trauma.
- A regular schedule for bladder emptying prevents distention and mucosal trauma.

Patients must be able to understand instructions and have the manual dexterity to manipulate the catheter. Caregivers or family members in the home can also be taught to perform intermittent catheterization using clean (rather than sterile) technique with good outcomes (Beauchemin et al., 2018).

Surgical Interventions. Stress incontinence may be treated with a surgical sling or bladder suspension procedure (Table 58.3). A sling procedure creates a sling around the bladder neck and urethra using strips of body tissue or synthetic mesh. Midurethral sling procedures are particularly effective for stress urinary incontinence (Jelovsek & Reddy, 2022). Bladder suspension procedures are more extensive than sling procedures, and the surgeon sutures tissue near the bladder neck to a pubic bone ligament to provide support and prevent sagging. A third surgical procedure is the injection of bulking agents into the urethral wall to provide resistance to urine outflow. Bulking agents include collagen, carbon-coated zirconium beads, and silicone implants. Interventions for the patient with overflow (reflex) incontinence caused by obstruction of the bladder outlet may include surgery to relieve the obstruction. The most common procedures are prostate removal (see Chapter 64) and repair of uterine prolapse (see Chapter 63).

Preoperative care. Teach the patient about the procedure, and clarify the surgeon's explanation of events surrounding the surgery. In contrast to stress urinary incontinence, urge urinary incontinence requires extensive preoperative testing for diagnosis and selection of surgery. The patient may need emotional support during this extensive diagnostic workup. Surgical procedures and preoperative and postoperative management are described in Table 58.3.

Postoperative care. After surgery, assess for and intervene to prevent or detect complications. For prevention of movement or traction on the bladder neck, secure the urethral catheter with tape or a tube holder. If a suprapubic catheter is used instead of a urethral catheter, monitor the dressing for urine leakage and other drainage. Catheters are usually in place until the patient can urinate easily and has residual urine volume of less than 50 mL after voiding. (See Chapter 9 for general care before and after surgery.)

Maintaining Tissue Integrity. A major concern with the use of wearable protective pads is the risk for skin breakdown (loss of *tissue integrity*). Some patients develop incontinence-associated dermatitis (IAD) even when the skin is kept free of contact with urine (McNichol et al., 2018). The wearable pads generate heat and sweat in the area that can cause dermatitis. Materials and costs of protective pads vary. Some are reusable; others are disposable. Avoid use of the word "diaper" when discussing these adult pants because of the association of diapers with a baby. More acceptable terms are "briefs" and "pads." Identifying patients at risk for IAD is important to prevent IAD episodes and maintain tissue integrity. Risk factors may include patients with functional, physical, cognitive, and mobility alterations (Bliss et al., 2017). See Chapter 21 for more information about IAD.

TABLE 58.3	**Surgical Procedures for Stress Incontinence**	
Procedure	**Purpose**	**Nursing Considerations**
Needle bladder neck suspension (Stamey procedure)	Elevates the urethral position and provides longer-lasting results without a long operative time.	The combined vaginal approach with a needle and a small suprapubic skin incision does not allow direct vision of the operative site; however, the high complication rates may be due to the selection of patients who, because of their medical condition, are not good candidates for longer retropubic procedures.
Pubovaginal sling procedures	A sling made of synthetic or fascial material is placed under the ureterovesical junction to elevate the bladder neck.	The operation uses an abdominal, vaginal, or combined approach to treat intrinsic sphincter deficiencies. Temporary or permanent urinary retention is common after surgery.
Midurethral sling procedures	A tensionless vaginal sling is made from polypropylene mesh (or other materials) and placed near the ureterovesical junction to increase the angle, which inhibits movement of urine into the urethra with lower intravesical pressures.	This ambulatory surgical procedure uses a vaginal approach to improve symptoms of stress incontinence. This surgery has become the most common option due to the outcomes as well as shorter recovery times. Temporary or permanent urinary retention can occur after surgery.
Artificial sphincters	A mechanical device to open and close the urethra is placed around the anatomic urethra.	The operation is done more frequently in men. The most common complications include mechanical failure of the device, erosion of tissue, and infection.
Periurethral injection of collagen or Siloxane	Implantation of small amounts of an inert substance through several small injections provides support around the bladder neck.	The procedure can be done in an ambulatory care setting and can be repeated as often as needed. Certain compounds may migrate after injection; an allergy test to bovine collagen must be performed before implantation.

When external devices (condom catheter or female urinary collection device) or containment materials are needed, discuss the possible options and help patients make a selection that is best for their lifestyle and resources. Containment is achieved with absorbent pads and briefs designed to collect urine and keep the patient's skin and clothing dry. Many types and sizes of pads are available:

- Shields or liners inserted inside a panty
- Undergarments that are full-size pads with waist straps
- Plastic-lined protective underpants
- Combination pad and pant systems
- Absorbent bed pads

Correct use of external devices and containment materials is essential to ensure that *tissue integrity* is maintained (Beeson & Davis, 2018).

Catheterization for control of functional incontinence may be intermittent or involve a long-term catheter. Intermittent catheterization is preferred to a long-term catheter because of the reduced risk for infection. A long-term urinary catheter is appropriate for patients with altered *tissue integrity* who need a dry environment for healing, for those who are terminally ill and need comfort, and for those who are critically ill and require precise measurement of urine output.

Care Coordination and Transition Management

Community-based care for the patient with urinary incontinence considers personal, physical, emotional, and social resources. Important personal resources for self-care include mobility and manual dexterity. When planning care, consider who will be the primary caregiver and which factors may influence the effectiveness of the plan. Nonpharmacologic and nonsurgical treatments provide significant clinical benefits with low risk for adverse effects, but these interventions are also associated with poor adherence (Clemens, 2022). Ongoing relationships with primary health care providers may improve adherence.

Home Care Management. Assess the home environment for barriers that limit access to the bathroom. Eliminate hazards that might slow walking or lead to a fall. Such hazards include throw rugs, furniture with legs that extend into the walking area, slippery waxed or polished floors, and poor lighting.

If the patient must climb stairs to reach a bathroom, handrails should be installed and stairs kept free of obstacles. Toilet seat extenders may help provide the right level and height of seating so that maximal abdominal pressure may be applied for voiding.

Portable commodes may be obtained when ambulatory access to toilets is impractical. Physical and occupational therapists are valuable resources for assisting with home care management.

Self-Management Education. Teach the patient and family about the cause of the specific type of incontinence and discuss available treatment options for its management (Box 58.4). The teaching plan should address the prescribed drugs (purpose, dosage, method and route of administration, and expected and potential side effects). Instruct the patient

---

BOX 58.4   Patient and Family Education

Urinary Incontinence

- Maintain a normal body weight to reduce the pressure on your bladder.
- Do not try to control your incontinence by limiting your fluid intake. Adequate fluid intake is necessary for kidney function and health maintenance.
- If you have a catheter in your bladder, follow the instructions given to you about maintaining the sterile drainage system.
- If Kegel exercises are recommended, ask your nurse for specific instructions.
- Following surgical intervention:
  - If you are discharged with a suprapubic catheter in your bladder, inspect the entry site for the tube daily, clean the skin around the opening gently with warm soap and water, and place a sterile gauze dressing on the skin around the tube. Report any redness/hyperpigmentation, swelling, drainage, or fever to your primary health care provider.
  - Do not put anything into your vagina, such as tampons, drugs, hygiene products, or exercise weights, until you check with your primary health care provider at your 6-week checkup after surgery.
  - Do not have sexual intercourse until after your 6-week postoperative checkup.
  - Do not lift or carry anything heavier than 5 lb (2.2 kg) or participate in any strenuous exercise until your primary health care provider gives you postoperative clearance. In some cases, this could be as long as 3 months.
  - Avoid exercises such as running, jogging, step or dance aerobic classes, rowing, cross-country ski or stair-climber machines, and mountain biking. Brisk walking without any additional hand, leg, or body weights is allowed. Swimming is allowed after all drains and catheters have been removed and your incision is completely healed.

---

and family about the importance of weight reduction and dietary modification to help control incontinence of urine *elimination.* Remind the patient who smokes that nicotine can contribute to bladder irritation and that coughing can cause urine leakage.

For urge urinary incontinence, teach the patient to avoid foods that irritate the bladder such as caffeine and alcohol. Spacing fluids at regular intervals throughout the day (e.g., 120 mL every hour or 240 mL every 2 hours) and limiting fluids after the dinner hour (e.g., only 120 mL at bedtime) help avoid fluid overload on the bladder and allow urine to collect at a steady pace. Remind patients that maintaining an ideal body weight helps avoid the pressure that abdominal fat places on pelvic organs, thus reducing incontinence.

For patients who require external devices or containment materials, discuss the options available and work with the patient to determine the best selection. For patients who will use intermittent catheterization or those with artificial urinary sphincters, demonstrate the correct technique to the patient or caregiver. Having the patient return demonstrate correct technique is essential to prevent complications (Beauchemin et al., 2018).

The embarrassment of incontinence can be devastating to self-esteem, body image, and relationships. Sexual intimacy is often adversely affected, and the unpredictable nature of incontinence creates anxiety. Patients may be embarrassed to seek help, and even when resources are identified, they may need help to feel comfortable in using them. Buying supplies at a local store may threaten privacy.

Acknowledge the personal concerns of the patient and caregiver. Never make their concerns seem trivial. As the patient learns the specifics of the plan that will allow control of urinary incontinence, the confidence to resume social interactions should return. Many continence supplies can be purchased online and delivered to the home to maintain privacy.

Health Care Resources. Referral to home care agencies for help with personal care and to continence clinics that specialize in evaluation and treatment may be helpful. In many continence clinics, nurses collaborate with physicians and other health care professionals to evaluate and manage patients. The treatment plan is specific for each patient; supplies and products are custom selected.

Patients may benefit from education and from the support of others who experience similar concerns. The National Association for Continence (NAFC) (www.nafc.org), and the Wound, Ostomy, and Continence Nurses Society (www.wocn.org) publish newsletters and educational materials written with easy-to-understand explanations. The American Urological Association (www.auanet.org) provides information on many areas of urologic dysfunction. Local hospitals often have local NAFC-approved support groups.

Evaluate Outcomes: Evaluation

Evaluate the care of the patient with urinary incontinence based on the identified priority patient problems. The expected outcomes are that the patient will:

- Maintain optimal urinary elimination through a reduction in the number of urinary incontinence episodes
- Maintain tissue integrity of the skin and mucous membranes in the perineal area
- Demonstrate knowledge of proper use of drugs and correct procedures for self-catheterization, use of the artificial sphincter, or care of an indwelling urinary catheter
- Demonstrate effective use of the selected exercise or bladder-training program
- Select and use incontinence interventions, devices, and products

CYSTITIS

Pathophysiology Review

Cystitis is an inflammatory condition of the bladder. Commonly it refers to inflammation from an infection of the bladder. However, cystitis can be caused by inflammation without infection. For example, drugs, chemicals, or local radiation therapy can cause bladder inflammation without an infecting organism. Irritants such as feminine hygiene spray and spermicidal jellies or long-term use of a catheter can cause cystitis without infection. Cystitis may sometimes occur as a complication of other disorders, such as gynecologic cancers, pelvic inflammatory disorders, endometriosis, Crohn's disease, diverticulitis, lupus, or tuberculosis.

An infection can occur in any area of the urinary tract and the kidney. Such infections are known as *urinary tract infections (UTIs).* An acute UTI is the invasion of the urinary tract by an infectious organism. A recurrent UTI is defined as the occurrence of two or more infections in 6 months or three or more infections in 1 year. These distinctions in UTIs are important because they have different approaches to management (Feng et al., 2018). Contributing factors associated with cystitis and other UTIs are listed in Table 58.4.

PATIENT-CENTERED CARE: GENDER HEALTH

Urinary Tract Infections (UTIs)

Women are 30 times more likely to have a UTI than men (U.S. Department of Health and Human Services [USDHHS], 2021). The female urethra is shorter than the male urethra, and this makes it easier for bacteria to get into the bladder. In addition, the female urethra is closer to the anus, which is a source of *Escherichia coli,* a main source of UTIs (USDHHS, 2021).

A UTI is further categorized as *uncomplicated* or *complicated* (Box 58.5). With an uncomplicated UTI, there is no anatomic or functional abnormality of the urinary tract or condition that increases the risk for infection or possibility of treatment failing to resolve the infection (such as the presence of a multidrug-resistant organism or urologic dysfunction). Some factors and conditions that contribute to a diagnosis of complicated UTI are pregnancy, male sex, obstruction, diabetes, neurogenic bladder, chronic kidney disease, and reduced *immunity.* Complicated cystitis or other UTI requires greater vigilance to avoid or detect adverse events from the infection and a longer course of antimicrobial treatment. A diagnosis of complicated UTI may require additional testing to identify and manage other related health problems (comorbidities).

The presence of bacteria in the urine is bacteriuria and may occur with cystitis or any UTI. When the patient has bacteriuria but no symptoms of infection, it is called *colonization* or *asymptomatic bacteriuria (ABU)* and is more common in older adults. This problem may progress to acute infection or renal insufficiency when the patient has other conditions, and only then does it require treatment (Avelluto & Bryman, 2018).

The urinary and genitourinary tracts are normally sterile, apart from the distal urethra. Several host defenses help protect against infection in the urinary tract. Mucin produced by cells lining the bladder helps maintain mucosal integrity and prevents cellular damage. Mucin also prevents bacteria from adhering to urothelial cells. Urine pH also contributes to sustaining sterile urine. White blood cells in the urinary tract are the *immunity* cells that engulf and destroy pathogens. Urine proteins, such as secreted antibodies, also are protective. In men, the prostate gland secretes additional protective proteins. Frequent voiding is another defense against bacterial growth and adherence by preventing urine stasis and flushing out organisms.

Etiology and Genetic Risk

UTIs, like other infections, result from interactions between a pathogen and the host. Usually a high bacterial *virulence*

TABLE 58.4	Factors Contributing to Urinary Tract Infections
Factor	**Mechanism**
Obstruction	Incomplete bladder emptying creates a continuous pool of urine where bacteria can grow, prevents flushing out of bacteria, and allows bacteria to ascend more easily to higher structures.
	Overdistention of the bladder damages the mucosa and allows bacteria to invade the bladder wall.
Stones (calculi)	Large stones can obstruct urine flow.
	The rough surface of a stone irritates mucosal surfaces and creates a spot where bacteria can establish and grow.
	Bacteria can live within stones and cause reinfection.
Vesicoureteral reflux	The urethra is colonized with bacteria. These bacteria are noninfectious until they move to upstream anatomy (bladder, ureters, kidneys) and colonize or form an infection with reflux (backward-flowing urine).
	Reflux of sterile urine can cause kidney scarring, which may promote kidney dysfunction.
Diabetes mellitus	Excess glucose in urine provides a rich medium for bacterial growth.
	Peripheral neuropathy affects bladder innervation and leads to a flaccid bladder and incomplete bladder emptying.
Characteristics of urine	Urine pH can promote different species of bacterial growth.
	Concentrated urine allows bacterial growth and adhesion to urinary tract anatomy.
Sex	**Females:**
	Susceptibility to urethral colonization with coliform or pathogenic bacteria is increased, especially as estrogen levels fall during menopause.
	Use of douches, perfumed pads or toilet tissue, diaphragms, or spermicide can inflame periurethral tissue and contribute to colonization.
	Bladder displacement during pregnancy predisposes to cystitis and the development of pyelonephritis.
	A diaphragm or pessary that is too large can obstruct urine flow or traumatize the urethra.
	Males:
	With increased age, the prostate enlarges and may obstruct the normal flow of urine, producing stasis.
	With increased age, prostatic secretions lose their antibacterial characteristics and predispose to bacterial proliferation in the urine.
	Sexually transmitted infections may cause urethral strictures that obstruct the flow of urine and predispose to urinary stasis.
Age	Urinary stasis may be caused by incomplete bladder emptying as a result of an enlarged prostate in men and cystocele and vaginal prolapse in women.
	Neuromuscular conditions that cause incomplete bladder emptying, such as Parkinson's disease and stroke, affect older adults more frequently.
	The use of drugs with intentional or unintentional anticholinergic properties in older adults contributes to delayed bladder emptying.
	Fecal incontinence contributes to urethral contamination.
	Low estrogen in menopausal females adversely affects the cells of the vagina and urethra, making them more susceptible to infections.
	Overall *immunity* declines with age, increasing the risk for uncomplicated infections to become complicated.
Sexual activity	Sexual intercourse is the strongest risk factor for uncomplicated cystitis, particularly in young females.
	Irritation of the perineum and urethra during intercourse can promote migration of bacteria from the perineal area to the urinary tract in some females.
	Inadequate vaginal lubrication may exacerbate potential urethral irritation.
	Bacteria may be introduced into the male urethra during anal intercourse or during vaginal intercourse with a female who has infectious vaginitis.
Recent use of antibiotics	Antibiotics change *immunity* and normal protective flora, providing opportunity for pathogenic bacterial overgrowth and colonization.
Virulence factors	The more virulent the organism, the more severe the infection.

BOX 58.5	Urinary Tract Infection (UTI) Types
Type	**Description**
Acute uncomplicated cystitis	Acute UTI—bladder involvement only
	No signs/symptoms of upper UTI
	No anatomic or functional abnormality of the urinary tract or condition that increases the risk for infection or possibility of treatment failing to resolve the infection
Acute complicated cystitis	Involves more than the bladder
	Symptoms of upper UTI: fever, flank pain, chills/rigors, malaise, costovertebral angle tenderness, and pelvic and/or perineal pain in men

(ability to invade and infect) is needed to overcome normal host defenses and *immunity*. However, an adult with reduced immunity is more likely to become infected even with bacteria that have low virulence. With UTI, bacteria (and infrequently fungi) move up the urinary tract from the external urethra to the bladder to cause infectious cystitis. Less commonly, spread of infection through the blood and lymph fluid can occur, although this cause of UTI is not common. Invading bacteria with special adhesions are more likely to cause ascending UTIs that start in the urethra or bladder and move up into the ureter and kidney.

Infectious cystitis is typically caused by pathogens from the bowel or, in some cases, the vagina. *Escherichia coli* and *Candida* are the most common causative organisms. Less common organisms include *Enterococcus* and *Klebsiella* (Fekete, 2022). Reflux from the colonized distal urethra can also contribute to UTI in vulnerable patients. Irritation, trauma, or instrumentation of the urinary tract decreases host defenses and contributes to UTIs through the ascending migration of uropathogens.

Urinary tract infections are the fifth most common health care–associated infection; this is related to urinary catheters. The longer a catheter is in place, the greater the risk that a urinary tract infection will develop (Centers for Disease Control and Prevention [CDC], 2022). Within 48 hours of catheter insertion, bacterial colonization along the urethra and the catheter itself begins.

The way that a catheter-associated urinary tract infection (CAUTI) occurs varies between males and females. Bacteria from a female's perineal area are more likely to ascend to the bladder by moving along the urethra. The shorter urethra in women aids in the ascending organisms' migration. In men, bacteria tend to gain access to the bladder from the catheter itself. Any break in the closed urinary drainage system allows bacteria to move through the lumen of the catheter. The external catheter surface also provides route for migration. Best practices to reduce the risk for catheter contamination and CAUTIs are listed in Box 58.6.

Organisms other than bacteria cause cystitis. Fungal infections, such as those caused by *Candida*, can occur during long-term antibiotic therapy because antibiotics change normal protective flora that reduce the adherence and volume of pathogenic bacteria. Patients with reduced *immunity* (those who are severely immunosuppressed, are receiving corticosteroids or other immunosuppressive agents, or have diabetes mellitus or acquired immunodeficiency syndrome [AIDS]) are at higher risk for fungal UTIs.

Viral and parasitic infections are rare and usually transfer to the urinary tract from an infection at another body site. For example, *Trichomonas*, a parasite found in the vagina, can also be found in the urine. Treatment of the vaginal infection also resolves the UTI.

Noninfectious cystitis may result from chemical exposure, such as to drugs (e.g., cyclophosphamide); from radiation therapy; and from *immunity* problems, as with systemic lupus erythematosus (SLE).

Interstitial cystitis/bladder pain syndrome is a chronic inflammation of the entire lower urinary tract (bladder, urethra, and adjacent pelvic muscles) that is related to genetic and *immunity* dysfunction rather than infection. The condition affects females more often than males, and

---

BOX 58.6 Best Practice for Patient Safety and Quality Care

Minimizing Catheter-Associated Urinary Tract Infection (CAUTI)

- Maintain good hand hygiene during insertion and manipulation of the catheter system to avoid contamination.
- Insert urinary catheters for appropriate use only, including:
  - Acute urinary retention or bladder obstruction.
  - Accurate measurement of urine volume in critically ill patients if needed.
  - Perioperative situations only as needed, such as urogenital, gynecologic, laparoscopic, and orthopedic surgeries. Avoid routine use of indwelling catheters in surgical patients.
  - To assist in healing of open sacral or perineal wounds in incontinent patients. Avoid use of indwelling catheters to manage patients who are incontinent.
  - Consider intermittent catheterization or other alternatives to indwelling catheters for patients with spinal cord injuries or conditions.
  - To provide comfort at end of life.
- Ensure that only properly trained personnel insert and maintain catheters.
- Use routine hygiene to clean periurethral area; antiseptic cleaning solutions are *not* recommended.
- Leave catheters in place *only* as long as needed. The strongest predictor of a CAUTI is the length of time the catheter dwells in a patient.
- Assess the need for urinary catheter daily, and document patient needs or indications.
- For example, remove catheters in postanesthesia care unit or as soon as possible after surgery when intraoperative indications have resolved.
- Use aseptic technique and sterile equipment in the acute care setting when inserting a urinary (intermittent or indwelling) catheter.
- Maintain a closed system by ensuring that catheter tubing connections are sealed securely; disconnections can introduce pathogens into the urinary tract.
- Obtain urine samples aseptically.

- If breaks in the system occur, replace the catheter and entire collecting system.
- Maintain unobstructed urine flow:
  - Keep the catheter and collecting tube free from kinking.
  - Keep the urine collection bag below the level of the bladder and do not rest the bag on the floor.
  - Empty the bag regularly, using a separate, clean container for each patient.
  - Ensure that the drainage spigot does not come into contact with nonsterile surfaces.
- Secure the catheter to the patient's thigh (females) or lower abdomen (males); catheter movement can cause urethral friction and irritation.
- Consider the use of antiseptic or antimicrobial catheters for patients requiring urinary catheters for more than 3 to 5 days. These catheters reduce bacterial colonization (i.e., biofilm) along the catheter.
- Consider appropriate alternatives to an indwelling catheter:
  - External (condom) devices in males without obstruction or urinary retention
  - External PureWick collecting device (females)
  - Intermittent catheterization in patients requiring drainage for neurogenic bladder or postoperative urinary retention
- Use portable ultrasound devices to assess urine volume to reduce unnecessary catheterization.
- Implement best practices in quality improvement to ensure that core recommendations for use, insertion, and maintenance are implemented. Examples of projects that improve patient care and reduce CAUTI include:
  - Nurse-initiated protocols for urinary catheter removal
  - Compliance with hand hygiene
  - Impact of educational programs on CAUTI occurrence
  - Compliance with documentation for catheter placement or maintenance
  - Number of CAUTIs per 1000 catheter-days or patient-days on unit
  - Track number of catheters inserted

Adapted from https://www.cdc.gov/nhsn/acute-care-hospital/cauti/.

the diagnosis is difficult to make. Symptoms are pain associated with bladder filling or voiding, usually accompanied by frequency, urgency, and nocturia. Pain occurs in suprapubic or pelvic areas, sometimes radiating to the groin, vulva, or rectum.

Although cystitis is not life-threatening, infection of the urinary tract can lead to life-threatening complications, including pyelonephritis and sepsis. Severe kidney damage from an ascending UTI is a rare complication. Patients with predisposing factors, such as anatomic abnormalities, pregnancy, obstruction, reflux, calculi, or diabetes, are at greater risk for complications.

The urinary tract is often the infection source in severe sepsis or septic shock. The spread of the infection from the urinary tract to the bloodstream is termed bacteremia or urosepsis. Catheter-associated urinary tract infections (CAUTIs) are the leading cause of urosepsis, which has a mortality rate of 10% (Ferguson, 2018). Sepsis, regardless of the source, is a systemic reaction to infection that prolongs hospitalization and can lead to shock, multiple organ failure, and other profound complications (see Chapter 31).

NCLEX Examination Challenge 58.1
Safe and Effective Care Environment

The nurse is caring for a client who has a Foley catheter following gynecologic surgery. Which action by the assistive personnel (AP) requires nursing intervention?

A. Emptying the collection bag into a clean container.
B. Washing hands prior to emptying the Foley catheter.
C. Flushing the urine in the toilet after emptying the collection bag.
D. Placing the collection bag on the floor to prevent kinks in the tubing.

Incidence and Prevalence

Urinary tract infections are very common and are a leading cause of primary care visits. Total costs for UTIs are estimated at $2.8 billion annually. In addition to a high prevalence in primary care, UTIs are one of the most common health care–associated infections (Feng et al., 2018).

Health Promotion/Disease Prevention

Although infectious cystitis is common, in many cases it is preventable. When catheters must be used in institutional settings, strict attention to sterile technique during insertion is essential to reduce the risk for UTIs (see Box 58.6). Long-term placement of urinary catheters requires aseptic technique for insertion. When *intermittent catheterization* was used in home care settings, the use of clean technique resulted in a similar rate of UTI compared with sterile technique. Clean technique, using single-use catheters, for catheter insertion is recommended in home settings where multiple resistant organisms are less likely to be present. Multiuse catheters for home use are no longer recommended. Sterile technique must be used in health care facilities to reduce the risk for infection (Beauchemin et al., 2018).

! NURSING SAFETY PRIORITY
Action Alert

Ensuring that urinary catheters are used appropriately and discontinued as early as possible is required. Do not allow catheters to remain in place for staff convenience.

Certain changes in fluid intake patterns, urinary *elimination* patterns, and hygiene patterns can help prevent or reduce cystitis in the general population. For example, a liberal water intake of 2.2 L for females and 3 L for males can promote general health. Another strategy to promote health is to have sufficient fluid intake to cause 1.5 L of clear or light yellow urine daily. Strategies to prevent cystitis and other UTIs are listed in Box 58.7. Although some of these strategies do not have consistent evidence to support a reduced risk for UTI when followed, they are low risk and reasonable.

NATIONAL PATIENT SAFETY GOALS
Health Care–Associated Infections

The Joint Commission (2022) has implemented a national patient safety goal (NPSG) to prevent infection. Through the use of clear handwashing guidelines, the goal is to reduce infection and prevent hospital-acquired infections such as catheter-associated urinary tract infections (CAUTIs). Improved hand hygiene is associated with a 26% to 45% reduction in health care–associated infections (Joint Commission for Transforming Healthcare, 2022).

Interprofessional Collaborative Care

Cystitis and UTIs can occur in any setting and are very common in the community. Usually the adult with cystitis is treated at home using self-management strategies.

BOX 58.7 Patient and Family Education
Preventing a Urinary Tract Infection

- Drink fluid liberally, as much as 2 to 3 L daily if not contraindicated by health conditions.
- Be sure to get enough sleep, rest, and nutrition daily to maintain immunologic health.
- If spermicides are used, consider changing to another method of contraception.
- Do not routinely delay urination because the flow of urine can help remove bacteria that may be colonizing the urethra or bladder.
- If you experience burning when you urinate, if you have to urinate frequently, or if you find it difficult to begin urinating, notify your primary health care provider right away, especially if you have a chronic medical condition (e.g., diabetes) or are pregnant.
- Females:
  - Clean your perineum (the area between your legs) from front to back.
  - Avoid using or wearing irritating substances such as douches, scented lubricants for intercourse, bubble bath, tight-fitting underwear, and scented toilet tissue. Wear loose-fitting cotton underwear.
  - Empty your bladder before and after intercourse.
- Both males and females:
  - Gently wash the perineal area before intercourse.

BOX 58.8   Key Features

Urinary Tract Infection (UTI)

Common Symptoms
- Frequency
- Urgency
- Dysuria
- Suprapubic pain or tenderness, low back pain
- Nocturia
- Incontinence
- Hematuria
- Pyuria
- Bacteriuria
- Retention
- Suprapubic tenderness or fullness
- Feeling of incomplete bladder emptying

Complicated Cystitis Symptoms
- Fever
- Chills and rigors
- Nausea or vomiting
- Malaise
- Flank pain and costovertebral angle tenderness

Symptoms That May Occur in the Older Adult
- Sudden or worsening: Dysuria, urinary incontinence, nocturia, urgency, and frequency; a general sense of lack of well-being
- **NOTE:** Changes in mental status and falls are not reliable predictors of UTIs. These changes need to be fully assessed to determine the underlying cause.

Recognize Cues: Assessment

Physical Assessment/Signs and Symptoms. The hallmark symptoms of UTI are frequency (an urge to urinate frequently in small amounts), dysuria (pain or burning with urination), and urgency (feeling that urination will occur immediately). See Box 58.8: Key Features—Urinary Tract Infection (UTI).

NURSE WELL-BEING REMINDER!

Remember: The incidence of urinary tract infection (UTI) is higher in those who work in health care, specifically female nurses (Nerbass et al., 2021). This is related to a lack of hydration as well as alterations in voiding patterns while working. Remember that even when working and caring for others, it is important to maintain normal urinary voiding patterns. In addition, be sure to remain hydrated, avoid caffeine, and consume water during breaks.

Urine may be cloudy, foul smelling, or blood tinged. Ask the patient about risk factors for UTI during the assessment (see Table 58.4).

For patients with a urinary catheter, in addition to common signs of UTI (e.g., fever with or without chills; leukocytosis; suprapubic or flank pain; urine with sediment, blood, or foul odor), new onset of hypotension or changes in mental status can indicate a UTI. Diagnostic testing for UTIs in older adults should not be based on mental status changes alone but should be performed when UTI symptoms are present (Gupta, 2022). If a catheter has been in place for more than 2 weeks, it may be necessary to first replace the catheter before obtaining a urine specimen for culture.

Before performing the physical assessment, ask the patient to void so that the urine can be examined and the bladder emptied before palpation. Assess vital signs to help identify the presence of infection (e.g., fever, tachycardia, tachypnea). Inspect the lower abdomen and palpate the bladder. Distention after voiding indicates incomplete bladder emptying.

Using Standard Precautions, record any lesions around the urethral meatus and vaginal opening. To help differentiate between a vaginal and a urinary tract infection, note whether there is any vaginal discharge or irritation. Vaginal discharge and irritation are more indicative of vaginal infection. Females often report burning with urination when urine touches labial tissues that are inflamed or have lost *tissue integrity* with ulcerations by vaginal infections or sexually transmitted infections (STIs). Maintain privacy with drapes during the examination.

The prostate is palpated by digital rectal examination (DRE) by the primary health care provider for size, change in shape or consistency, and tenderness. A large prostate gland can obstruct urine outflow and contribute to urostasis and bacterial colonization of the urinary tract, contributing to the risk for a complicated UTI.

Laboratory Assessment. Laboratory assessment for a UTI begins with a clean-catch urine specimen that is divided into two containers. If the patient cannot produce a clean-catch specimen, you may need to obtain the specimen with a small-diameter (6 Fr) catheter. For a routine urinalysis, 10 mL of urine is needed; smaller quantities are sufficient for culture.

One container is used for a urinalysis. The combination of a positive leukocyte esterase and nitrate from a urinalysis is 68% to 88% sensitive in the diagnosis of a UTI. The presence of white blood cells (WBCs) (pyuria), red blood cells (RBCs) (hematuria), or casts (clumps of material or cells) also may indicate UTI (Pagana et al., 2022).

If the urinalysis suggests a UTI and there are no risk factors or conditions for complicated UTI in a female, treatment can be started. If the UTI is complicated, the second specimen is analyzed as a urine culture. A culture may also be performed when a patient with a UTI does not respond to usual therapy, when the diagnosis is uncertain, to assess for sensitivity, or to determine resolution of UTI (Gupta, 2022). Urinalysis is less specific in diagnosing a UTI in an older adult, especially one who has a urinary catheter.

A urine culture confirms the type of organism and the number of colonies. Urine culture is expensive, and initial results take at least 24 hours. A UTI is confirmed when more than 10^5 colony-forming units per milliliter are in the urine from any patient. In noncatheterized patients who have symptoms of UTI (e.g., fever, dysuria, new-onset frequency or urgency, suprapubic or flank pain, or hematuria), as few as 10^3 colony-forming units/mL in a voided specimen can confirm the infection. For patients with a catheter who are symptomatic, 10^2 colony-forming units per milliliter are diagnostic of a complicated UTI. The presence of many different types of organisms in low colony counts usually indicates that the specimen is contaminated. Sensitivity testing follows culture results when complicating factors are present (e.g., stones or recurrent infection), when the patient is older, or to ensure that appropriate antibiotics are prescribed.

Occasionally the serum WBC count may be elevated, with the differential WBC count showing a "left shift" (see Chapter

16). This shift indicates that the number of immature WBCs is increasing and the number of mature WBCs is decreasing in response to continued infection. Thus the number of "bands," or immature WBCs, is elevated, which indicates reduced *immunity.* Left shift most often occurs with urosepsis and rarely occurs with uncomplicated cystitis, because cystitis is a local rather than a systemic infection.

Other Diagnostic Assessments. The diagnosis of UTI and cystitis is based on history, physical examination, and laboratory data. If urinary retention and obstruction of urine outflow are suspected, pelvic ultrasound or CT may be needed to locate the site of obstruction or the presence of calculi. Voiding cystourethrography (see Chapter 57) is needed when urine reflux is suspected.

Cystoscopy (see Chapter 57) may be performed when the patient has recurrent UTIs (more than three annually). A urine culture is performed first to ensure that no infection is present. If infection is present, the urine is sterilized with antibiotic therapy before the procedure to reduce the risk for sepsis. Cystoscopy identifies abnormalities that increase the risk for cystitis. Such abnormalities include bladder calculi, bladder diverticula, urethral strictures, foreign bodies (e.g., sutures from previous surgery), and trabeculation (an abnormal thickening of the bladder wall caused by urinary retention and obstruction). Retrograde pyelography, along with the cystoscopic examination, shows outlines and images of the drainage tract.

Cystoscopy is needed to accurately diagnose interstitial (noninfectious) cystitis. A urinalysis usually shows WBCs and RBCs but no bacteria. Common findings in interstitial cystitis are a small-capacity bladder, the presence of Hunner ulcers (a type of bladder lesion), and small hemorrhages after bladder distention.

Take Actions: Interventions

Nonsurgical Management. The expected outcome is to maintain an optimal urine *elimination* pattern. Nursing interventions for the management of cystitis focus on *pain* relief and teaching about drug therapy, fluid intake, and prevention measures. In a hospital setting, timely administration of antibiotics can prevent or reduce complications from urosepsis.

Drug Therapy. Drugs used to treat bacteriuria and relieve *pain* include urinary antiseptics or antibiotics, analgesics, and antispasmodics. Cure of a UTI depends on the antimicrobial levels achieved in the urine. Fluconazole is the drug of choice for treatment of *Candida* (fungal) infections. Antispasmodic drugs decrease bladder spasms and promote complete bladder emptying.

Antibiotic therapy is used for bacterial UTIs (Table 58.5). Guidelines for uncomplicated cystitis recommend nitrofurantoin, trimethoprim/sulfamethoxazole, or fosfomycin as first-line therapy for those patients at low risk of resistance to antimicrobials (Gupta, 2022). Longer antibiotic treatment (7–21 days) and sometimes different agents are required for hospitalized patients and those with complicated UTIs (e.g., men, pregnant women, and patients with anatomic, functional or metabolic conditions that affect the urinary tract).

Low-dose antibiotic therapy over 6 to 12 months is sometimes used for chronic, recurring infection caused by structural abnormalities or stones or for long-term management of the older patient with frequent UTIs. For females who have recurrent UTIs after intercourse, antibiotics may be prescribed to be taken after intercourse. The three most common drug treatment regimens are (1) 1 low-dose tablet of trimethoprim, (2) sulfamethoxazole/trimethoprim, or (3) nitrofurantoin.

👤 PATIENT-CENTERED CARE: GENDER HEALTH
Pregnancy and Urinary Tract Infection (UTI)

Pregnant women with a bacterial UTI require prompt and aggressive treatment because a UTI can lead to acute pyelonephritis during pregnancy. Pyelonephritis in pregnancy can cause preterm labor and adversely affect the fetus. Remind patients who are pregnant to contact their health care provider whenever symptoms of UTI are present.

Fluid Intake. Urge patients to drink enough fluid to maintain dilute urine throughout the day and night unless fluid restriction is needed for another health problem. Some urologists recommend sufficient fluid intake to result in at least 1.5 L of urine output or 7 to 12 voidings daily. Food can provide 20% or more of fluid intake, particularly the intake of fruits and vegetables.

Cranberry-containing products appear to decrease the ability of bacteria to adhere to the epithelial cells lining the urinary tract. In some patients, this may result in preventing UTI or decreasing the incidence of recurrent symptomatic UTIs; however, evidence is conflicting (Gupta, 2022). Cranberry juice can be an irritant to the bladder with interstitial cystitis and should be avoided by patients with this condition. Avoiding spices, soy products, and tomato products may decrease bladder irritation and *pain* during cystitis (Feng et al., 2018).

Comfort Measures. A warm sitz bath two or three times a day for 20 minutes may provide *pain* relief and some relief of local symptoms. If burning with urination is severe or urinary retention occurs, teach the patient to sit in the sitz bath and urinate into the warm water. Urinary tract analgesics may also provide comfort (see Table 58.5).

Surgical Management. Surgery for cystitis treats the conditions that increase the risk for recurrent UTIs (e.g., removal of obstructions and repair of vesicoureteral reflux). Procedures may include cystoscopy (see Chapter 57) to identify and remove calculi or obstructions.

TABLE 58.5   Common Examples of Drug Therapy

Urinary Tract Infections

Drug Category	Nursing Implications
Antibiotics	For all antibiotics: • Ask patients about drug allergies prior to administration of any antibiotic drugs *because allergies to antibiotic drugs are common and require changing drug therapy.* • Caution patients to complete the drug regimen even if the symptoms improve or disappear sooner *to prevent bacterial resistance and infection recurrence.* • Remind patients to wear sunscreen and/or avoid direct sun *as most antibiotics can increase sun sensitivity and lead to sunburn.* • Instruct patients to call the primary health care provider if severe or watery diarrhea develops, because *pseudomembranous colitis can occur, which may require discontinuing the drug.*
Common examples of antibiotics:	
• Trimethoprim[a]/sulfamethoxazole	Teach patients to drink a full glass of water with each dose of trimethoprim/sulfamethoxazole and to have an overall fluid intake of 3 L daily *because these drugs can form crystals that precipitate in the kidney tubules. Fluids can prevent this complication.*
• Ciprofloxacin • Levofloxacin • Ofloxacin	Warn patients not to take ciprofloxacin, levofloxacin, or ofloxacin within 2 hours of taking an antacid *to prevent interference with drug absorption.* Teach patients how to take their pulse, to monitor it twice daily while taking ciprofloxacin, levofloxacin, or ofloxacin and to notify the health care provider if new-onset irregular heartbeats occur *to identify serious drug-induced dysrhythmias.*
• Amoxicillin • Amoxicillin/clavulanate	Teach patients to take amoxicillin with food *to reduce the risk for GI upset.*
• Cefdinir • Cefaclor • Cefpodoxime	Remember that cefdinir, cefaclor, and cefpodoxime are structurally similar to penicillin, and anyone with allergies to penicillin may also be allergic to the cephalosporins. Avoid taking cefdinir, cefaclor, and cefpodoxime when also taking metoclopramide or any other drug that increases GI motility *to prevent interference with drug absorption.* Teach patients to drink a full glass of water with each dose of cefdinir, cefaclor, or cefpodoxime and to have an overall fluid intake of at least 3 L daily *to avoid having the drug precipitate in the kidneys and cause kidney damage.*
• Nitrofurantoin	Teach patients to take nitrofurantoin with meals *to reduce the potential for GI disturbance.*
Urinary Analgesic • Phenazopyridine	Remind patients that this drug will not treat an infection, only the symptoms, *because these drugs have no antibacterial activity.* Teach patients to take the drug with or immediately after a meal *to reduce the risk for GI upset.* Warn patients that urine and tears will turn red or orange and may stain clothing and contact lenses.

[a]Trimethoprim can be given alone to patients with a sulfa allergy.

Care Coordination and Transition Management

Assess the patient's level of understanding of the problem. The patient's knowledge about factors that promote the development of cystitis determines the teaching interventions planned.

Teach the patient how to take prescribed drugs. Stress the need for correct spacing of doses throughout the day and the need to complete all of the prescribed antibiotics. If the drug will change the color of the urine, as it does with phenazopyridine, inform the patient to expect this change.

Patients may associate discomfort with sexual activities and have feelings of guilt and embarrassment. Open and sensitive discussions with a female who has recurrences of UTI after sexual intercourse can help in finding techniques to address the problem (see Box 58.7). Explore the factors that contribute to infections in the female, such as sexual penetration when the bladder is full, diaphragm use, and general *immunity* responses against infection. Some positions during intercourse may reduce urethral irritation and subsequent cystitis. Remind the patient that vigorous cleaning of the perineum with harsh soaps and vaginal douching may irritate the perineal tissues and *increase* the risk for UTI.

NCLEX Examination Challenge 58.2

Health Promotion and Maintenance

The nurse is teaching a 45-year-old female client health promotion to avoid recurrent cystitis. Which client statement indicates the need for additional teaching?

A. "I will drink at least 8 glasses of fluid during the daytime."
B. "After toileting, I will wipe from the front to the back."
C. "I will urinate before and after having intercourse."
D. "I will stop the amoxicillin when I have been symptom free for 2 days."

URETHRITIS

Pathophysiology Review

Urethritis is an inflammation of the urethra and can result from infectious and noninfectious conditions. The incidence is highest among adults ages 20 to 24 years. The most common cause of infectious urethritis is sexually transmitted infections (STIs).

Many females with urethritis have symptoms similar to cystitis, vaginitis, or cervicitis. Males with urethritis may report symptoms of cystitis, as well as heaviness in the genitals (*orchalgia*).

Symptoms of urethritis include discharge of mucopurulent or purulent material, dysuria, and itching or discomfort of the area (urethral pruritus). The discharge can be any color, depending on the infecting organism or source of irritation. Additional symptoms may include fever (with or without chills) and urgent or frequent urination.

Interprofessional Collaborative Care

Ask the patient about a history of STI, painful or difficult urination, discharge from the penis or vagina, and discomfort in the lower abdomen. Urinalysis may show pyuria (white blood cells [WBCs] in the urine) without a large number of bacteria. Similarly, a urethral smear may show WBCs. If an STI is suspected, testing for gonorrhea and chlamydia may be performed in addition to a pelvic examination in females.

Urethritis from STIs is treated with antibiotic therapy. More information on STIs can be found in Chapter 65. Noninfectious urethritis symptoms usually resolve spontaneously over time, regardless of treatment.

UROLITHIASIS

Pathophysiology Review

Urolithiasis is the presence of *calculi* (stones) in the urinary tract. (Fig. 58.2) Stones often do not cause symptoms until they

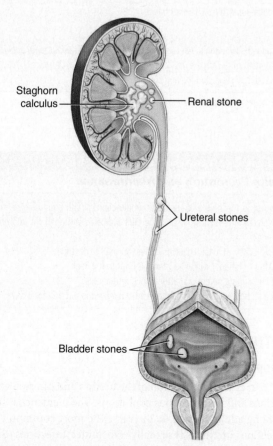

FIG. 58.2 Urolithiasis. (From Shiland, B. J. [2023]. *Mastering healthcare terminology* [7th ed.]. St. Louis: Elsevier.)

pass into the lower urinary tract, where they can cause excruciating pain. Nephrolithiasis is the formation of stones in the kidney; formation of stones in the ureter is ureterolithiasis. Stones are particles in the urine that occur in amounts too high to stay dissolved (become supersaturated) in urine. As a result of supersaturation, the particles precipitate and collect to form calculi.

The most common condition associated with stone formation is dehydration. Everyone excretes crystals in the urine at some time, but less than 10% of adults form stones. Most stones contain calcium as one part of the stone complex. Struvite (15%), uric acid (8%), and cystine (3%) are rarer compositions of stones. Formation of stones involves two conditions:

1. Supersaturation of the urine with the particular element (e.g., calcium, uric acid) that first becomes crystallized and later becomes the stone
2. Formation of a *nidus* (deposit of crystals that can be the point of infection) along the lining of the kidney and urinary tract

In addition, some patients may have decreased amounts of inhibitor substances in the urine that would otherwise prevent supersaturation with crystal aggregation. This type of metabolic risk factor can be inherited.

In addition to low urine volume, high urine acidity (as with uric acid and cystine stones) or alkalinity (as with calcium phosphate and struvite stones), as well as drugs (e.g., topiramate, long-term glucocorticoids, acetazolamide), contribute to stone formation.

One example of a metabolic problem causing stone formation begins when excessive amounts of calcium are absorbed through the intestinal tract, leading to hypercalciuria. As blood circulates through the kidneys, the excess calcium is filtered into the urine, causing supersaturation of calcium in the urine. If fluid intake is poor, such as when a patient is dehydrated, supersaturation is more likely to occur.

Any stone may result in obstruction within the urinary tract, which can threaten both glomerular filtration rate (GFR) and kidney perfusion. When the stone occludes the ureter and blocks the flow of urine, the ureter dilates. Enlargement of the ureter is called hydroureter.

The pain associated with ureteral spasm is excruciating. Hematuria (bloody urine) may result from damage to the urothelial lining. If the obstruction is not removed, urinary stasis can lead to infection and impair kidney function on the side of the blockage. As the blockage persists, hydronephrosis (enlargement of the kidney caused by blockage of urine lower in the tract and filling of the kidney with urine) and permanent kidney damage may develop.

Etiology and Genetic Risk

The vast majority of adults who form stones have a metabolic risk factor. The usual cause of stone formation in a susceptible adult (e.g., one who has a metabolic risk factor) is dehydration. Table 58.6 lists some metabolic problems that cause stone formation. Patients who have a family history of stones, are obese, or have diabetes or gout (hyperuricemia) have increased risk for initial stone formation. Because a metabolic problem is strongly associated with stone formation and is a nonmodifiable risk factor, an adult of any age who develops a stone is always at high risk for future stone development. Diet may be considered a risk for stone formation. Increased sodium intake has been associated with stone formation (Table 58.7).

TABLE 58.6 Metabolic Defects That Commonly Cause Kidney Stones

Metabolic Deficit	Etiology
Hypercalcemia	
Primary	Absorptive: Increased intestinal calcium absorption Renal: Decreased kidney tubular excretion of calcium
Secondary	Resorptive: Hyperparathyroidism, vitamin D intoxication, kidney tubular acidosis, prolonged immobilization
Hyperoxaluria	
Primary	Genetic: Autosomal recessive trait resulting in high oxalate production
Secondary	Dietary: Excess oxalate from foods such as spinach, rhubarb, Swiss chard, cocoa, beets, wheat germ, pecans, peanuts, okra, chocolate, and lime peel
Hyperuricemia	
Primary	Gout is an inherited disorder of purine metabolism (20% of patients with gout have uric acid calculi)
Secondary	Increased production or decreased clearance of purine from myeloproliferative disorders, thiazide diuretics, carcinoma
Struvite	Made of magnesium ammonium phosphate and carbonate apatite; formed by urea splitting by bacteria, most commonly *Proteus mirabilis*; needs an alkaline urine to form
Cystinuria	Autosomal recessive defect of amino acid metabolism that precipitates insoluble cystine crystals in the urine

PATIENT-CENTERED CARE: GENETICS/GENOMICS

Kidney Stone Formation

Family history has a strong association with stone formation and recurrence because of inherited metabolic variations. More than 30 genetic variations are associated with the formation of kidney stones, although single-gene disorders are rare. More commonly, nephrolithiasis is a complex disease, with genetic variation in intestinal calcium absorption, kidney calcium transport, or kidney phosphate transport—all associated with stone formation (Online Mendelian Inheritance in Man [OMIM], 2022). Always ask a patient with a renal stone whether other family members have also experienced this condition.

Incidence and Prevalence

The incidence of stone disease is high and varies with geographic location, race, and family history. It is estimated that 19% of males and 9% of females will develop a renal stone by age 70 (Curhan, 2022). Recurrence rates vary depending on the type of treatment, although any adult who has had a stone is much more likely to have a recurrence.

Interprofessional Collaborative Care

Recognize Cues: Assessment

Ask the patient about a personal or family history of urologic stones. Obtain a diet history, focusing on fluid intake patterns and supplemental vitamin or mineral intake. If the patient has a history of stone formation, ask about past treatment, whether chemical analysis of the stone was performed, and which preventive measures are followed.

The major symptom of stones is severe pain, commonly called renal colic. Flank pain suggests that the stone is in the kidney or upper ureter. Flank pain that extends toward the abdomen or to the scrotum and testes or the vulva suggests that stones are in the ureters or bladder. Pain is most intense when the stone is moving or the ureter is obstructed.

TABLE 58.7 Dietary Treatment for Kidney and Urinary Stones

Stone Type	Dietary Interventions	Rationales
Calcium oxalate	Avoid oxalate sources, such as spinach, black tea, and rhubarb.	Reduction of urinary oxalate content may help prevent these stones from forming. Urinary pH is not a factor.
	Decrease sodium intake.	High sodium intake reduces kidney tubular calcium reabsorption.
Calcium phosphate	Limit intake of foods high in animal protein to 5–7 servings per week and never more than 2 per day.	Reduction of protein intake reduces acidic urine and prevents calcium precipitation.
	Some patients may benefit from a reduced calcium intake (milk, other dairy products).	Reduction of urine calcium concentration may prevent calcium precipitation and crystallization.
	Decrease sodium intake.	High sodium intake reduces kidney tubular calcium reabsorption.
Struvite (magnesium ammonium phosphate)	Limit high-phosphate foods, such as dairy products, organ meats, and whole grains.	Reduction of urinary phosphate content may help prevent these stones from forming.
Uric acid (urate)	Decrease intake of purine sources, such as organ meats, poultry, fish, gravies, red wines, and sardines.	Reduction of urinary purine content may help prevent these stones from forming.
Cystine	Limit sodium and animal protein intake (as above).	It reduces urinary cystine levels.
	Encourage oral fluid intake (500 mL every 4 hours while awake and 750 mL at night).	Increased fluid helps dilute the urine and prevents the cystine crystals from forming.

Renal colic begins suddenly and is often described as "unbearable." Nausea, vomiting, pallor/ash gray skin, and diaphoresis often accompany the pain. However, a large stationary stone in the kidney (staghorn calculus) rarely causes much pain because it is not moving. Frequency and dysuria occur when a stone reaches the bladder. Oliguria (scant urine output) or anuria (absence of urine output) suggests obstruction, possibly at the bladder neck or urethra.

> ! **NURSING SAFETY PRIORITY**
>
> ***Action Alert***
>
> Urinary tract obstruction is an emergency and must be treated immediately to preserve kidney function.

Assess patients for bladder distention. They may appear pale, ashen, and diaphoretic and may have excruciating pain. Vital signs may be elevated with pain; body temperature and pulse are elevated with infection. Blood pressure may decrease if the severe pain causes shock.

Urinalysis is performed in patients with suspected stones. Measurement of urine specific gravity and osmolarity can provide a clue about the adequacy of fluid intake. Urine pH can help in the determination of stone type. High urine acidity (low urine pH) is associated with uric acid and cystine stones; high urine alkalinity (high urine pH) is associated with calcium phosphate and struvite stones. A 24-hour urine analysis can determine whether supersaturation of common stone particles is present. Hematuria during renal colic is common, and blood may make the urine appear smoky or rusty. RBCs are usually caused by stone-induced trauma to the lining of the ureter, bladder, or urethra. WBCs and bacteria may be present as a result of urinary stasis. Increased *turbidity* (cloudiness) and odor indicate that infection may also be present. Microscopic examination of the urine may identify possible stone-forming crystals.

The serum WBC count is elevated with infection. Increases in the serum levels of calcium or phosphate or uric acid levels indicate that excess minerals that may contribute to stone formation are present.

The current standard for confirming urinary stones is an unenhanced helical CT scan of the abdomen and pelvis. Most stones are radiopaque; and the size, location, and surrounding anatomic structures are easily seen. In settings in which CT is not available, a routine abdominal x-ray (x-ray of the of the kidneys, ureters, and bladder [KUB]) is useful (Fig. 58.3). Ultrasonography may be used in pregnant women suspected to have stones, but it is not sensitive for ureteral stones and is not used for general screening.

Take Actions: Interventions

Nursing interventions focus on ***pain*** relief and preventing infection and urinary obstruction. Most patients expel the stone without invasive procedures. Size (i.e., less than 5 mm) is the most important factor for whether a stone will pass on its own; its composition and location are also factors. The larger the stone and the higher up in the urinary tract it is, the less

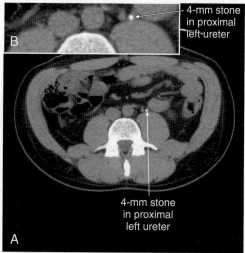

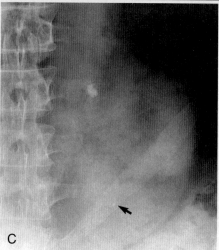

FIG. 58.3 (A and B) Urinary stones on CT scan. (C) Urinary stone *(arrow)* on x-ray of the kidneys, ureters, and bladder (KUB). (A and B from Broder, J. K. [2011]. *Diagnostic imaging for the emergency physician.* Philadelphia: Saunders. C from Pollack, H. M. [2000]. *Clinical urography* [2nd ed.]. Philadelphia: Saunders.)

likely it is to pass. When the stone is passed, it should be captured and sent to the laboratory for analysis. Other interventions are needed when the stone does not pass spontaneously (Fig. 58.4).

Managing Pain. Nonsurgical and surgical approaches are used to help the patient with a kidney stone achieve an acceptable degree of ***pain*** relief.

Nonsurgical Management. Nonsurgical measures to relieve pain include strategies to enhance stone passing, as well as direct pain management.

Drug therapy is needed in the first 24 to 36 hours when pain is most severe. Opioid analgesics are used to control the severe pain caused by stones in the urinary tract and may be given intravenously for rapid pain relief. NSAIDs such as ketorolac in the acute phase are often effective. When NSAIDs are used, there is an increased risk for kidney impairment from reduced perfusion. NSAIDs interfere with renal autoregulation, and the risk for impairment is greater among patients with preexisting kidney dysfunction. Risk for bleeding is also increased from

PROXIMAL URETER
- ESWL
- Retrograde ureteroscopy
- Antegrade nephrostoureterolithotomy
- Stenting alone
- Percutaneous ureterolithotomy or nephrolithotomy

MIDURETER
- Retrograde ureteroscopy
- ESWL
- Antegrade nephrostoureterolithotomy
- Open ureterolithotomy

DISTAL URETER
- ESWL/ureteroscopy
- Antegrade nephrostoureterolithotomy
- Stenting alone
- Open ureterolithotomy

FIG. 58.4 Treatment options for ureteral stones. *ESWL,* Extracorporeal shock wave lithotripsy. (Modified from Singal, R. K., & Denstedt, J. D. [1997]. Contemporary management of ureteral stones. *Urologic Clinics of North America, 24*[1], 59–70.)

platelet inhibition when NSAIDs are used. Bleeding risk is particularly concerning when surgical intervention for stones is needed.

Control of *pain* is more effective when drugs are given at regularly scheduled intervals instead of PRN. Urinary antispasmodic drugs such as oxybutynin are important for control of pain. Administer the drugs as ordered and assess the response by asking the patient to rate the discomfort on a pain-rating scale.

Other management techniques include avoiding overhydration and underhydration in the acute phase to help make the passage of a stone less painful. Strain the urine and teach the patient to monitor for stone passage. If any stone is passed, send it to the laboratory for analysis because preventive therapy is based on stone composition.

Antibiotics may be used to manage struvite stones because these are associated with urinary infections from urease-producing organisms such as *Klebsiella, Enterobacter,* or *Pseudomonas.* When urease-producing bacteria remain in the urine and within the stone, urine becomes alkaline, causing phosphate to precipitate and allowing staghorn-shaped struvite stones to form rapidly.

Several drugs can be used for medical expulsive therapy. The most common is the alpha blocker tamsulosin. This drug is used in patients with ureteral stones that are larger than 5 mm and smaller than 10 mm (Curhan et al., 2023). This medication can shorten the time to stone passage by relaxing the smooth muscle within the ureters.

A stone that has not passed within 1 to 2 months is unlikely to pass spontaneously. Other options for stone intervention are considered when infection occurs, when pain cannot be well managed, or when there is an actual or increased risk for reduced kidney function. An observation period of 1 to 2 weeks may be reasonable if the patient is comfortable or has few symptoms and stones are smaller than 5 mm.

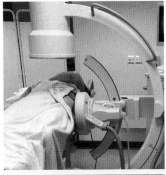
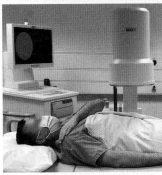

FIG. 58.5 A patient undergoing extracorporeal shock wave lithotripsy (ESWL). (From Strachan, M. W. J., Hobson, R. P., Penman, I. D., et al., eds. [2023]. Davidson's principles and practice of medicine [24th ed.]. St. Louis: Elsevier.)

Lithotripsy or *shock wave lithotripsy (SWL)* is the use of sound, laser, or dry shock waves to break the stone into small fragments (Fig. 58.5). The patient receives moderate sedation and lies on a flat table with the lithotripter aimed at the stone, which is located with fluoroscopy. High-energy shock waves pass through the body until they hit the stone and the waves break the stone into small pieces. Continuous ECG monitoring for dysrhythmia and fluoroscopic observation for stone destruction are maintained.

After lithotripsy, strain the urine to monitor the passage of stone fragments. Bruising may occur on the flank of the affected side. Occasionally a stent is placed in the ureter before SWL to ease passage of the stone fragments.

Surgical Management. Minimally invasive surgical and open surgical procedures are used if urinary obstruction occurs or if the stone is too large to be passed.

Minimally Invasive Surgical Procedures. Minimally invasive surgery (MIS) procedures include stenting, ureteroscopy, percutaneous ureterolithotomy, and percutaneous nephrolithotomy.

Stenting is performed with a small tube (stent) that is placed in the ureter by ureteroscopy. The stent dilates the ureter and enlarges the passageway for the stone or stone fragments. This totally internal procedure prevents the passing stone from coming in contact with the ureteral mucosa, thereby reducing pain, bleeding, and infection risk, all of which could block the ureter. A Foley catheter may facilitate passage of the stone through the urethra.

Ureteroscopy is an endoscopic procedure. The ureteroscope is passed through the urethra and bladder into the ureter. Once the stone is seen, it is removed with grasping baskets, forceps, or loops. Lithotripsy can also be performed through the ureteroscope. A Foley catheter may be placed to facilitate passage of the stone fragments through the urethra.

Percutaneous ureterolithotomy or nephrolithotomy is the removal of a stone in the ureter or kidney through the skin. The patient lies prone or on the side and receives local or general anesthesia. The urologist or radiologist identifies the ideal entry point with fluoroscopy and passes a needle into the collecting system of the kidney. Once a tract has been made in the kidney, other equipment, such as an intracorporeal (inside the body) ultrasonic or laser lithotripter, can be used to break up and remove the stone. An endoscope with a special attachment to grasp and extract the stone can be used. Often a nephrostomy tube is left in place at first to prevent the stone fragments from passing through the urinary tract.

Monitor the patient for complications after the procedure. Complications include bleeding at the site or through the tube, pneumothorax, and infection. Monitor nephrostomy tube drainage for volume and the presence of blood in the urine, which is normal for the first 24 to 48 hours after tube placement. Provide routine nephrostomy tube care, with sterile dressing changes and tube flushing (if ordered).

Open Surgical Procedures. When other stone removal attempts have failed or when risk for a lasting injury to the ureter or kidney is possible, an *open ureterolithotomy* (into the ureter), *pyelolithotomy* (into the kidney pelvis), or *nephrolithotomy* (into the kidney) procedure may be performed. These procedures are used for a large or impacted stone. With the advances in minimally invasive techniques, open surgical procedures are not common and are used only when endoscopic removal has failed or when there are compounding factors such as morbid obesity or anatomic abnormalities in the kidney or ureter.

Preventing Infection. Infection control before invasive procedures is critical for preventing urosepsis. Interventions include giving antibiotics, either to eliminate an existing infection or to prevent new infections, and maintaining nutrition and fluid intake. Because infection occurs with struvite stone formation, the health care team plans for long-term infection prevention.

Drug therapy involves the use of broad-spectrum antibiotics (such as ampicillin). When urine culture and sensitivity (C&S) results are known, more specific antibiotics may be prescribed. C&S studies are often repeated 48 hours after completion of antibiotic therapy to evaluate whether urine sterility has returned.

Urine levels of antibiotics may be measured to ensure that adequate levels have been reached. If the antibiotic is not sufficiently concentrated in urine, organisms may not be completely eliminated. Evidence of a new infection (e.g., chills, fever, altered mental status) warrants the collection of urine sample for new C&S tests.

For the patient with struvite stones, periodic and long-term monitoring of the urine for infection is needed. Urine cultures are checked monthly for up to 6 months. Long-term use of antibiotics, while recommended, makes the development of resistant organisms more likely and can make antibiotic therapy less effective. Review interventions aimed at preventing urinary tract infection (UTI). See Box 58.7.

Nutrition therapy ideally includes adequate calorie intake with a balance of all food groups. Encourage a fluid intake sufficient to dilute urine to a light color throughout the 24-hour day (typically 2–3 L/day) unless another health problem requires fluid restriction.

Preventing Obstruction. Measures to prevent urinary obstruction by stones include a high intake of fluids (3 L/day or more) and accurate measures of intake and output. Fluid intake sufficient to provide diluted urine helps prevent dehydration, promotes urine flow, and decreases the chance of crystals forming a stone. Interventions also depend on the type of stone the patient has formed.

Drug therapy to prevent obstruction depends on what is causing stone formation and the type of stone formed. Teach the patient the reason for the drug and assess for side effects or adverse drug reactions.

Drugs to treat *hypercalciuria* (high levels of calcium in the urine) include thiazide diuretics (e.g., chlorothiazide or hydrochlorothiazide). These drugs promote calcium reabsorption from the renal tubules back into the body, thereby reducing urine calcium loads. For patients with *hyperoxaluria* (high levels of oxalic acid in the urine), vitamin B_6 and thiazide diuretics may be prescribed.

Patients with hyperuricemia or chronic gout have high uric acid levels causing acidic urine and resulting in a higher risk for uric acid stone formation. Acidic urine is more likely to cause uric acid to precipitate, resulting in uric acid stones. Normal urine pH can range from 4.6 to 8.0 with the average at 6.0. Urine pH under 5.0 is considered acidic and over 8.0 is considered alkaline. The desired urine pH range for patients with high uric acid levels and a history of uric acid stone formation is 6.5 to 7.0.

Three measures are commonly used to treat and/or prevent uric stone formation: increasing urine pH, increasing fluid intake, and decreasing uric acid production. To alkalinize the urine, drugs such as potassium citrate and sodium bicarbonate may be prescribed. Drinking 2 to 3 L of water is effective in flushing out excess uric acid and reduces uric acid stone formation. Modifying the diet to restrict purines can be effective in decreasing uric acid production. Foods that contain high levels of purines include organ meats, sardines, and red meats. The use of xanthine oxidase inhibitors such as allopurinol and febuxostat can also be used to decrease the body's production of uric acid.

Cystinuria (high levels of cystine in the urine) can lead to stone formation. Cystinuria is genetic and affects children more than adults. Conservative measures are used to prevent stone formation. Drinking 2 to 3 L of water throughout the day and night is encouraged to reduce high cystine levels in the urine. Moderating sodium and protein consumption has been effective in reducing urine cystine levels. To alkalinize urine, drugs such as potassium citrate are used. However, because moderating sodium has been shown to be effective in reducing urine cystine levels, sodium bicarbonate and sodium citrate are avoided owing to the sodium content in these medications. If conservative measures fail, medications such as tiopronin and D-penicillamine are used to lower urine cystine levels (Goldfarb et al., 2022). *Nutrition therapy* depends on the type of stone formed (see Table 58.7). Collaborate with the registered dietitian nutritionist (RDN) to plan for and teach the appropriate diet to the patient.

Other measures can help the stone pass more quickly. Urge the patient to walk as often as possible. Walking promotes passage of stones and reduces bone calcium resorption. Check the urine pH daily and strain all urine with filter paper or a special urine strainer to collect passed stones and fragments.

Self-management education includes follow-up care to evaluate effects of intervention. The patient often has great anxiety and fear that a stone and its pain may recur. In addition to anxiety about the pain, the risk for repeated surgical interventions or permanent and serious kidney damage may be present. Reassure the patient that preventive and health promotion activities help prevent recurrence. See Box 58.9.

UROTHELIAL CANCER

Pathophysiology Review

Urothelial cancers are malignant tumors of the *urothelium*, which is the lining of transitional cells in the kidney, renal pelvis, ureters, urinary bladder, and urethra. Most urothelial cancers occur in the bladder, and the term *bladder cancer* describes this condition. Urothelial cancer is also known as *transitional cell carcinoma* (TCC).

In North America, most urinary tract cancers are transitional cell carcinomas of the bladder (American Cancer Society [ACS], 2022; Canadian Cancer Society, 2022). The second most common site of urinary tract cancer is the kidney and renal pelvis. Urothelial cancers usually are low grade, have multiple points of origin *(multifocal),* and are recurrent. Once the cancer spreads beyond the transitional cell layer, it is highly invasive and can spread beyond the bladder. Because of the nature of this cancer, patients may have recurrence up to 10 years after being cancer free (ACS, 2022). Less common bladder cancers include squamous cell carcinoma, adenocarcinoma, small cell carcinoma, and sarcoma (ACS, 2022).

BOX 58.9 Patient and Family Education

Urinary Calculi

- Finish your entire prescription of antibiotics to prevent development of a urinary tract infection.
- You may resume your usual daily activities.
- Remember to balance regular exercise with sleep and rest.
- You may return to work 2 days to 6 weeks after surgery, depending on the type of intervention, your personal tolerance, and your primary health care provider's directives.
- Depending on the type of stone you had, you may be advised to take medications or adjust your diet to reduce the risk for further stone formation.
- Remember to drink at least 3 L of fluid a day to dilute potential stone-forming crystals, prevent dehydration, and promote urine flow.
- Monitor urine pH as directed (possibly up to three times per day).
- Expect bruising after lithotripsy. The bruising may take several weeks to resolve.
- Your urine may be bloody for several days after surgery.
- Pain in the region of the kidneys or bladder may signal the beginning of an infection or the formation of another stone. Report any pain, fever, chills, or difficulty with urination immediately to your primary health care provider or nurse.
- Keep follow-up appointments to check on infection and have repeat cultures done.

Tumors confined to the bladder mucosa are treated by simple excision, whereas those that are deeper but not into the muscle layer are treated with excision plus intravesical (inside the bladder) chemotherapy. Cancer that has spread deeper into the bladder muscle layer is treated with more extensive surgery, often a radical cystectomy (removal of the bladder and surrounding tissue) with urinary diversion. Chemotherapy and radiation therapy are used in addition to surgery. If untreated, the tumor invades surrounding tissues; spreads to distant sites (liver, lung, and bone); and ultimately leads to death.

Exposure to toxins such as gasoline and diesel fuel, as well as to chemicals used in hair dyes and in the rubber, paint, electric cable, and textile industries, increases the risk for bladder cancer. The greatest risk factor for bladder cancer is tobacco use.

In the United States and Canada, about 94,000 new cases of bladder cancer are diagnosed each year, and about 19,600 deaths occur each year from the disease (ACS, 2022; Canadian Cancer Society, 2022). This cancer is rare in adults younger than 40 years and is most common after 55 years of age (ACS, 2022).

As with many urologic conditions, sexual health is commonly affected by this diagnosis and treatment. To manage sexual health concerns, encourage patients to discuss sexual health and ensure that the proper interprofessional care team member provides education to patients and their partners about:

- Potential implications of treatment on sexuality
- Treatment options
- Referrals to providers who specialize in sexual dysfunction

Health Promotion/Disease Prevention

Many adults believe that tobacco use is associated with cancers only of organs that come into direct contact with it, such as the lungs. However, many compounds in tobacco enter the bloodstream and affect other organs, such as the bladder. Encourage people who smoke to quit. Just as important, encourage anyone who comes in contact with dry, liquid, or gaseous chemicals to take precautions. Some adults work with chemicals, and others may come into contact with them while engaging in hobbies. Many chemicals and fumes can enter the body through contact with skin and with mucous membranes in the respiratory tract. Use of personal protective equipment, such as gloves and masks, can reduce this contact. Also encourage anyone who works with chemicals to shower or bathe and change clothing as soon as contact is completed.

NCLEX Examination Challenge 58.3

Physiological Integrity

A 68-year-old female client presents to the primary care provider for an annual examination. Which assessment finding would alert the nurse to an increased risk for bladder cancer?

A. A 30-year occupation as a hairdresser
B. A recent colon cancer diagnosis in her sister
C. History of hypertension treated with beta blockers
D. Occasional urine leaking with sneezing or laughing

Interprofessional Collaborative Care

Recognize Cues: Assessment

Physical Assessment/Signs and Symptoms. Ask about patients' perception of their general health. Document the sex and age of the patient. Ask about active and passive exposure to cigarette smoke. To detect exposure to harmful environmental agents, ask patients to describe their occupation and hobbies. Also ask patients to describe any change in the color, frequency, or volume of urine *elimination* and any abdominal discomfort.

Examine the urine for color and clarity. Blood in the urine is often the first indication of bladder cancer. It may be gross or microscopic and is usually painless and intermittent. Dysuria, frequency, and urgency occur when infection or obstruction is also present.

Psychosocial Assessment. Assess the patient's emotions, including the response to a tentative diagnosis of bladder cancer, and note anxiety, fear, sadness, anger, or guilt. Early symptoms are painless, and many patients ignore the blood in the urine because it is intermittent. They also may be reluctant to seek treatment if they suspect a sexually transmitted infection (STI). As a result, they may have guilt or anger about their own delays in seeking medical attention.

Assess the patient's coping methods and available support from family members. Social support may provide motivation and improve coping during recovery from treatment.

Diagnostic Assessment. The only significant finding on a routine urinalysis is gross or microscopic hematuria. Cytologic testing on voided urine specimens is usually not helpful. Bladder-wash specimens and bladder biopsies are the most specific tests for cancer.

Cystoscopy is usually performed to evaluate painless hematuria. A biopsy of a visible bladder tumor can be performed during cystoscopy. This is essential for staging and is usually performed in an ambulatory care surgery center. Cystoureterography may be used to identify obstructions, especially where the ureter joins the bladder. CT scans show tumor invasion of surrounding tissues. Ultrasonography shows masses but is less valuable for tumor staging. MRI may help assess deep, invasive tumors. See Chapter 57 for general care of the patient undergoing diagnostic testing.

Take Actions: Interventions

Therapy for the patient with bladder cancer usually begins with surgical removal of the tumor for diagnosis and staging of disease. For tumors extending beyond the mucosa, surgery is followed by intravesical chemotherapy or immunotherapy. High-grade or recurrent tumors are treated with more radical surgery plus intravesical chemotherapy, radiotherapy, or both. Systemic chemotherapy is reserved for patients with distant metastases. (See Chapter 18 for general care of the patient receiving chemotherapy or radiation therapy.)

Nonsurgical Management. Prophylactic immunotherapy with intravesical instillation of bacille Calmette-Guérin (BCG), a live virus compound, is used to prevent tumor recurrence of superficial cancers. This procedure is more effective than single-agent chemotherapy. Usually the agent is instilled in an outpatient cancer clinic and allowed to dwell in the bladder for a specified length of time, usually 2 hours. When the patient urinates, live virus is excreted with the urine.

Teach patients receiving this treatment to prevent contact of the live virus with other members of the household by not sharing a toilet with others for at least 24 hours after instillation. Instruct males to urinate while sitting down to avoid splashing the urine. After 24 hours, the toilet should be completely cleaned using a solution of 10% liquid bleach. If only one toilet is available in the household, teach the patient to flush the toilet after use and follow this by adding one cup of undiluted bleach to the bowl water. The bowl is then flushed after 15 minutes, and the seat and flat surfaces of the toilet are wiped with a cloth containing a solution of 10% liquid bleach. Instruct the patient to wear gloves during the cleaning and to dispose of the cloth after sealing it in a plastic bag.

Underwear or other clothing that has come in contact with the urine during the immediate 24 hours after instillation should be washed separately from other clothing in a solution of 10% liquid bleach. Sexual intercourse is avoided for 24 hours after the instillation.

Multiagent chemotherapy is successful in prolonging life after distant metastasis has occurred but rarely results in a cure. Radiation therapy is also useful in prolonging life.

Surgical Management. The type of surgery for bladder cancer depends on the type and stage of the cancer and the patient's general health. Complete bladder removal *(cystectomy)* with additional removal of surrounding muscle and tissue offers the best chance of a cure for large, invasive bladder cancers. Four alternatives for urine *elimination* are used after cystectomy: ileal conduit; continent pouch; bladder reconstruction, also known as *neobladder*; and ureterosigmoidostomy.

Preoperative Care. Specific patient education depends on the type and extent of the planned surgical procedure. Coordinate education before surgery with the patient, surgeon, and enterostomal therapist (ET) or wound, ostomy, and continence nurse. Discuss the type of planned urinary diversion and the selection of a site for the stoma. Including the patient in this planning improves the chances for the patient to have a positive attitude about body image and a positive self-image. Use educational counseling to ensure understanding about self-care practices, methods of pouching, control of urine drainage, and management of odor.

The site selected for the stoma should be visible to the patient and avoid folds of skin, bones, and scar tissue. When possible, the waistline or belt area is avoided to reduce the risk for reducing *tissue integrity*. Prepare the patient for the number and type of drains that will be present after surgery. General care before surgery is discussed in Chapter 9.

Operative Procedures. Transurethral resection of the bladder tumor (TURBT) or partial cystectomy is performed for small, early, superficial tumors. In a partial (segmental) cystectomy, a portion of the bladder is removed when there is only a single isolated bladder tumor.

When the entire bladder must be removed (complete cystectomy), the ureters are diverted into a collecting reservoir. Techniques for urinary diversion are shown in Fig. 58.6. With

Ureterostomies divert urine directly to the skin surface through a ureteral skin opening (stoma). After ureterostomy, the patient must wear a pouch.

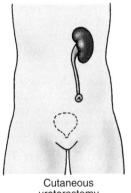

Cutaneous ureterostomy

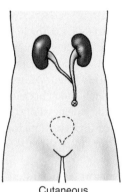

Cutaneous ureteroureterostomy

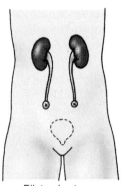

Bilateral cutaneous ureterostomy

Conduits collect urine in a portion of the intestine, which is then opened onto the skin surface as a stoma. After the creation of a conduit, the patient must wear a pouch.

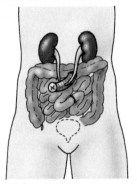

Ileal (Bricker) conduit

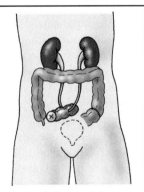

Colon conduit

Ileal reservoirs divert urine into a surgically created pouch, or pocket, that functions as a bladder. The stoma is continent, and the patient removes urine by regular self-catheterization.

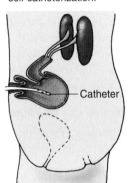

Continent internal ileal reservoir (Kock pouch)

Sigmoidostomies divert urine to the large intestine, so no stoma is required. The patient excretes urine with bowel movements, and bowel incontinence may result.

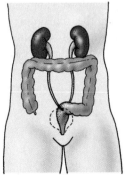

Ureterosigmoidostomy

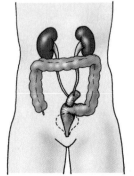

Ureteroiliosigmoidostomy

FIG. 58.6 Urinary diversion procedures used in the treatment of bladder cancer.

an ileal conduit, the ureters are surgically placed in the ileum and urine is collected in a pouch on the skin around the stoma. More often, a continent reservoir known as a "neobladder" is created from an intestinal graft to store urine and replace the surgically removed bladder. With cutaneous ureterostomy or ureteroureterostomy, the ureter opening is brought out onto the skin. The cutaneous ureterostomies may be located on either side of the abdomen or side by side.

Postoperative Care. After cutaneous ureterostomy, an external pouch covers the ostomy to collect urine and maintain *tissue integrity.* Collaborate with the ET to focus care on the wound, the skin, and urinary drainage. (See Chapter 48 for ostomy care.)

The patient with a Kock pouch, a continent reservoir, may have a Penrose drain and a plastic Medena catheter in the stoma. The drain removes lymphatic fluid or other secretions; the catheter ensures urine drainage so incisions can heal. The patient with a neobladder usually requires 2 to 4 days in the ICU and will have a drain at first in the event the neobladder requires irrigation. Later, irrigation can be performed with intermittent catheterization. Irrigation is performed to ensure patency. There is no sensation of bladder fullness with a neobladder because sensory nerves are not attached. As a result, the patient will need to learn new cues to void, such as prescribed times or noticing a feeling of neobladder pressure. General care after surgery is discussed in Chapter 9.

Different types of drains and nephrostomy catheters are used, sometimes on a temporary basis, to drain urine from the kidney. Some are totally internal, with no drainage to the outside. Others may drain exclusively to the outside, and urine is collected in a pouch or bag. For this type of drainage system, urine output remains constant. Decreased or no drainage is cause for concern and must be reported to the surgeon or nephrologist, as is leakage around the catheter. Some nephrostomy tubes are connected both to the new bladder (internal drainage) and to an external drainage system. With this type of system, urine output from the external portion of the catheter varies. With any drainage system, intervention is needed if the external catheter is partially or completely pulled out accidentally. Immediately notify the surgeon or nephrologist. If the catheter remains partially in place, secure it from further movement. This action may result in a reinsertion process rather than a total replacement.

Care Coordination and Transition Management

Self-Management Education. Teach the patient and family about drugs, diet and fluid therapy, the use of external pouching

systems, and the technique for catheterizing a continent reservoir.

With some procedures the patient may need electrolyte replacement to prevent long-term deficits. Teach the patient to avoid foods that are known to produce gas if the urinary diversion uses the intestinal tract. When intestinal production of gas is excessive, flatus can induce incontinence.

Patients who have a neobladder created often have extreme weight loss during the first few weeks after surgery. Collaborate with a dietitian to develop a diet plan specific to the patient to meet caloric needs.

! NURSING SAFETY PRIORITY

Action Alert

Infection is common in patients who have a neobladder. Teach patients and family members the symptoms of infection and the importance of reporting them immediately to the surgeon.

Instruct the patient and family about any changes in self-care activities related to the urinary diversion. In collaboration with the enterostomal therapist, demonstrate external pouch application, local skin care, pouch care, methods of adhesion, and drainage mechanisms. If a Kock pouch has been created, teach the patient how to use a catheter to drain the pouch. For all instruction, observe at least one return demonstration or "teach-back" session by the patient or the caregiver. Ideally the patient assumes responsibility for self-care before discharge.

Help the patient prepare for the impact of urinary diversion on self-image, body image, sexual functioning, and self-esteem. Counseling provides information and support to address the potential impact.

Through discussions with the patient about common social situations, help the patient gain control over new toileting practices. Males with a urinary diversion into the sigmoid colon need to learn the habit of sitting to urinate. For patients of either sex, promote confidence in social situations by encouraging frequent emptying of urinary collection devices before traveling or attending social functions. Resumption of sexual activity is a major concern for many, regardless of age. Address this topic openly and with sensitivity. Cystectomy causes impotence in men, but treatment is available (see Chapter 64).

Health Care Resources. The United Ostomy Association of America (https://www.ostomy.org) and the ACS have educational materials that may be useful to patients. Refer patients and family members to local chapters or units of these organizations. Home care personnel may help with follow-up, easing the transition from hospital to home. The Wound, Ostomy, and Continence Nurses Society has educational programs and a journal for the care of patients with ostomies.

GET READY FOR THE NEXT-GENERATION NCLEX® EXAMINATION!

Essential Nursing Care Points

Health Promotion/Disease Prevention	Chronic Disease Care
• Teach patients to clean the perineal area daily and after voiding, having a bowel movement, and sexual intercourse. • Encourage all patients to maintain an adequate fluid intake. • Teach females who have stress incontinence the proper way to perform pelvic floor–strengthening exercises.	• Use a nonjudgmental approach in caring for patients with urinary incontinence. • Recognize the need for the patient undergoing cystectomy and urinary diversion to grieve about the body image change. • Collaborate with the enterostomal therapist following urinary diversion to teach the patient self-care, including skin and pouch care, as well as external pouch application.
Regenerative or Restorative Care	**Hospice/Palliative/Supportive Care**
• Use sterile technique when inserting a catheter in the acute care environment. • Use Contact Precautions with any drainage from the genitourinary tract. • Identify hospitalized patients at risk for bacteriuria and urosepsis. • Teach patients with urinary tract infection (UTI) to complete all prescribed antibiotic therapy even when symptoms of infection are absent. • Evaluate daily the need for maintaining urinary catheters, and discontinue as soon as possible. • For patients with urolithiasis, nursing interventions focus on pain relief and prevention of infection and obstruction.	• Patients with recurrent or advanced urothelial cancer may benefit from a referral to palliative or hospice care. • Pelvic floor rehabilitation therapy may be beneficial for some patients with certain types of incontinence.

Mastery Questions

1. A 28-year-old female client states, "I don't know why I get cystitis every year. I don't drink much at work so I can avoid using the public toilet." Which of the following teachings by the nurse is most likely to reduce the risk for cystitis? **Select all that apply.**
   A. Reinforce the choice to avoid using a public toilet.
   B. Suggest intake of at least 2 to 3 L of fluid throughout the day.
   C. Instruct to wipe the perineum from front to back after each toilet use.
   D. Reinforce completion of the entire course of antibiotics as prescribed.
   E. Instruct to empty the bladder immediately before intercourse.

2. A client is diagnosed with renal colic. What would the nurse do first?
   A. Prepare the client for lithotripsy.
   B. Encourage oral intake of fluids.
   C. Administer opioids as ordered.
   D. Strain the urine and send for urinalysis.

NGN Challenge 58.1

The nurse is caring for an 82-year-old client admitted to the hospital yesterday with an acute onset of confusion.

History and Physical	Nurses' Notes	Orders	Laboratory Results

1025: The client presents for routine physical. Reports feeling "mostly well" except for a few urinary tract infections recently. The client has a history of seasonal allergies, hypertension, and generalized anxiety. When questioned regarding urination, the client states, "I wet myself sometimes, but that just happens after you have kids." Further assessment reveals involuntary loss of urine when sneezing and occasional "leaking" when exercising. The client reports getting up one time per night to urinate. Bowel sounds are active × 4 and there is no abdominal tenderness or fullness. The client reports regular bowel movements and no incontinence of stool. VS: T 99.2°F (37.3°C); HR 86 beats/min; RR 22 breaths/min; BP 168/88 mm Hg; SpO_2 99% on RA.

Complete the diagram by selecting from the choices below to specify what potential condition the client is likely experiencing, **2** nursing actions that are appropriate to take, and **2** parameters the nurse should monitor to assess the client's progress.

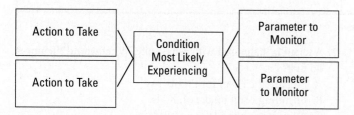

Actions to Take	Potential Conditions	Parameters to Monitor
Insert a Foley catheter	Functional incontinence	Temperature
Obtain a urine sample	Interstitial cystitis	Extremity weakness
Insert a short peripheral IV catheter	Urinary tract infection	Cardiac rhythm
Prepare for lithotripsy	Urolithiasis	SpO_2
Prepare the client for a rectal exam		White blood cell count

NGN Challenge 58.2

The nurse is completing a history and physical on a 52-year-old female who presents to the primary care provider for a routine physical.

History and Physical	Nurses' Notes	Orders	Laboratory Results

1115: Client alert and oriented × 2 (person and place). The client has a history of a left-sided stroke with weakness on the left side of her body. However, visiting family members state that the onset of confusion is new. The night nurse reports that the client was incontinent of urine multiple times last night. On initial assessment, the client stated repeatedly that she needs to urinate; however, when assisted onto the bedside toilet, she is voiding only small amounts. VS: T 101.3°F (38.5°C); HR 122 beats/min; RR 24 breaths/min; BP 144/62 mm Hg; SpO_2 95% on RA. Urine output 20 mL with last void, dark yellow and cloudy in appearance. Bowel sounds × 4. The client reports tenderness over the lower abdominal area. No lesions around the vaginal opening or vaginal discharge noted on assessment.

Complete the diagram by selecting from the choices below to specify what potential condition the client is likely experiencing, **2** nursing actions that are appropriate to take, and **2** parameters the nurse should monitor to assess the client's progress.

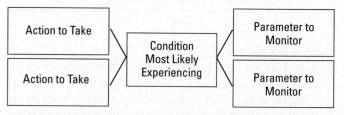

Actions to Take	Potential Conditions	Parameters to Monitor
Teach the use of a pessary	Functional incontinence	Skin integrity
Obtain a urine sample	Stress incontinence	Episodes of incontinence
Insert a short peripheral IV catheter	Urge incontinence	Temperature
Prepare the client for a vaginal exam	Overflow incontinence	White blood cell count
Insert a Foley catheter		Blood pressure

REFERENCES

Agency for Healthcare Research and Quality (AHRQ). (2022). *EvidenceNOW: Managing urinary incontinence.* https://www.ahrq.gov/evidencenow/projects/urinary/index.html.

American Cancer Society (ACS). (2022). *About bladder cancer.* Retrieved from https://www.cancer.org/cancer/bladder/about/what-is-bladder-cancer.

Avelluto, G., & Bryman, P. (2018). Asymptomatic bacteriuria vs. symptomatic urinary tract infection: Identification and treatment challenges in geriatric care. *Urologic Nursing, 38*(3). https://doi.org/10.7257/1053816X.2018.38.3.129.

Beauchemin, L., Newman, D., Danseur, M., Jackson, A., & Ritmiller, M. (2018). Best practices for clean intermittent catheterization. *Nursing 2018, 48*(9). https://doi.org/10.1097/01.NURSE.0000544216.23783.bc.

Beeson, T., & Davis, C. (2018). Urinary management with an external female collection device. *The Journal of Wound, Ostomy and Continence Nursing, 45*(2). https://doi.org/10.1097/WON.0000000000000417.

Bliss, D., Mathiason, M., et al. (2017). Incidence and predictors of incontinence associated skin damage in nursing home residents with new onset incontinence. *The Journal of Wound, Ostomy and Continence Nursing, 44*(2). https://doi.org/10.1097/WON.0000000000000313.

Brown, O., & Simon, M. A. (2021). Applying a Health Equity Lens to Urinary Incontinence. *Clinical obstetrics and gynecology, 64*(2), 266–275. https://doi.org/10.1097/GRF.0000000000000613.

Burchum, J., & Rosenthal, L. (2022). *Lehne's pharmacology for nursing care* (11th ed.). St. Louis: Elsevier.

Canadian Cancer Society. (2022). *Bladder cancer.* https://cancer.ca/en/cancer-information/cancer-types/bladder.

Centers for Disease Control and Prevention (CDC). (2022). *Urinary tract infection (Catheter-associated urinary tract infection [CAUTI] and Non-catheter associated urinary tract infection [UTI]) Events.* National Healthcare Safety Network. https://www.cdc.gov/nhsn/PDFs/pscManual/7pscCAUTIcurrent.pdf.

Clemens, J. Q. (2022). *Urinary incontinence in men. UpToDate.* Retrieved January 29, 2023, from https://www.uptodate.com/contents/urinary-incontinence-in-men.

Clemons, J. (2022). Vaginal pessaries: Indications, devices, and approach to selection. *UpToDate.* Retrieved January 29, 2023, from https://www.uptodate.com/contents/vaginal-pessaries-indications-devices-and-approach-to-selection.

Cleveland Clinic. (2021). *Stress incontinence.* https://my.clevelandclinic.org/health/diseases/22262-stress-incontinence.

Curhan, G. (2022). *Kidney stones in adults: Epidemiology and risk factors. UpToDate.* Retrieved January 29, 2023, from https://www.uptodate.com/contents/kidney-stones-in-adults-epidemiology-and-risk-factors.

Curhan, G., Aronson, M., & Preminger, G. (2023). Kidney stones in adults: Diagnosis and acute management of suspected nephrolithiasis. *UpToDate.* Retrieved January 29, 2023, from https://www.uptodate.com/contents/kidney-stones-in-adults-diagnosis-and-acute-management-of-suspected-nephrolithiasis.

Fekete, T. (2022). *Catheter-associated urinary tract infection in adults. UpToDate.* Retrieved January 29, 2023, from https://www.uptodate.com/contents/catheter-associated-urinary-tract-infection-in-adults.

Feng, F., Hawks, J., Kernen, J., & Kyle, E. (2018). Recurrent urinary tract infection care: Integrating complementary and alternative medicine. *Urologic Nursing, 38*(5). https://doi.org/10.7257/1053-816X.2018.38.5.231.

Ferguson, A. (2018). Implementing a CAUTI prevention program in an acute care setting. *Urologic Nursing, 38*(6). https://doi.org/10.7257/1053816X.2018.38.6.273.

Goldfarb, D., Ferraro, P., Sas, D., & Baum, M. (2022). *Cystinuria and cystine stones. UpToDate.* Retrieved January 29, 2023, from https://www.uptodate.com/contents/cystinuria-and-cystine-stones.

Gupta, K. (2022). *Acute simple cystitis in females. UpToDate.* Retrieved January 29, 2023, from https://www.uptodate.com/contents/acute-simple-cystitis-in-women.

Hubb, A., Stachowicz, A., & Wood, S. (2018). Onabutulinumtoxin A injections for urge incontinence. *American Family Physician, 97*(3) Online.

Jelovsek, E., & Reddy, J. (2022). Female stress urinary incontinence: Choosing a primary surgical procedure. *UpToDate.* Retrieved January 29, 2023, from https://www.uptodate.com/contents/female-stress-urinary-incontinence-choosing-a-primary-surgical-procedure.

Lukacz, E. (2023). *Female urinary incontinence: Treatment. UpToDate.* Retrieved January 29, 2023, from https://www.uptodate.com/contents/female-urinary-incontinence-treatment.

Lukacz, E., Santiago, Y., & Albo, M. (2017). Urinary incontinence in women: A review. *Journal of American Medical Association, 318*(16). https://doi.org/10.1001/jama.2017.12137.

McNichol, L. L., Ayello, E. A., Phearman, L. A., Pezzella, P. A., & Culver, E. A. (2018). Incontinence-Associated Dermatitis: State of the Science and Knowledge Translation. *Advances in skin & wound care, 31*(11), 502–513. https://doi.org/10.1097/01.ASW.0000546234.12260.61.

Medina, M., & Castillo-Pino, E. (2019). An introduction to the epidemiology and burden of urinary tract infections. *Ther Adv Urol.* https://doi.org/10.1177/1756287219832172. 2019 May 2;11:1756287219832172.

National Association for Continence. (2018). *Urinary continence overview.* https://www.nafc.org/urinary-incontinence/.

Nerbass, F., Santo, C., Fialek, E., Calice-Silva, V., & Vieira, M. (2021). Urinary tract infection in different occupations. *Braz. J. Nephrol. 2021, 43*(4), 495–501. https://www.scielo.br/j/jbn/a/Ss6XkJzFY5yRpcK4ZBG3WFJ/?lang=en&format=pdf.

Online Mendelian Inheritance in Man (OMIM). (2022). *Nephrolithiasis, calcium oxalate.* https://www.omim.org/entry/167030.

Pagana, K., Pagana, T., & Pagana, T. (2022). *Mosby's manual of diagnostic and laboratory tests* (7th ed.). St. Louis: Elsevier.

Patel, U. J., Godecker, A. L., Giles, D. L., & Brown, H. W. (2022 Apr 1). Updated Prevalence of Urinary Incontinence in Women: 2015-2018 National Population-Based Survey Data. *Female Pelvic Med Reconstr Surg, 28*(4), 181–187. https://doi.org/10.1097/SPV.0000000000001127. Epub 2022 Jan 12. PMID: 35030139.

Rogers, J. L. (2023). *McCance and Huether's Pathophysiology: The biologic basis for disease in adults and children* (9th ed.). St. Louis: Elsevier.

Simmering, J., Tang, F., Cavannaugh, J., Polgreen, L., & Polgreen, P. (2017). The increase in hospitalizations for urinary tract infections and the associated costs in the United States, 1998-2011. *Open Forum Infectious Diseases, 4*(1). https://doi.org/10.1093/ofid/ofw281.

The Joint Commission. (2022). *Hospital National Patient Safety Goals.* https://www.jointcommission.org/-/media/tjc/documents/standards/national-patient-safety-goals/2022/simple_2022-hap-npsg-goals-101921.pdf.

The Joint Commission for Transforming Healthcare. (2022). *Reduce healthcare-acquired infections*. https://www.centerfortransforminghealthcare.org/products-and-services/targeted-solutions-tool/hand-hygiene-tst.

Touhy, T., & Jett, K. (2023). *Ebersole & Hess' toward healthy aging: Human needs & nursing response* (11th ed.). St. Louis: Elsevier.

U.S. Department of Health and Human Services. (2021). *Urinary tract infections. Office on Women's Health*. https://www.womenshealth.gov/a-z-topics/urinary-tract-infections.

Zhang, N. (2018). An evolutionary concept analysis of urinary incontinence. *Urologic Nursing, 38*(6). https://doi.org/10.7257/1053-816X.2018.38.6.289.

59

Concepts of Care for Patients With Kidney Conditions

Robyn Mitchell

http://evolve.elsevier.com/Iggy/

LEARNING OUTCOMES

1. Plan collaborative care with the interprofessional team to promote urinary elimination in patients with kidney conditions.
2. Teach adults how to decrease the risk for kidney conditions.
3. Teach the patient and caregiver(s) about common drugs and other management strategies used for kidney conditions.
4. Plan patient- and family-centered nursing interventions to decrease the psychosocial impact caused by living with kidney conditions.
5. Apply knowledge of anatomy, physiology, and pathophysiology to provide evidence-based care for patients with kidney conditions affecting elimination, fluid and electrolyte balance, and acid-base balance.
6. Analyze assessment and diagnostic findings to generate solutions and prioritize nursing care for patients with kidney conditions.
7. Organize care coordination and transition management for patients with kidney conditions.
8. Use clinical judgment to plan evidence-based nursing care to promote urinary elimination and prevent complications in patients with kidney conditions.
9. Incorporate factors that affect health equity into the plan of care for patients with kidney conditions.

KEY TERMS

abscess A localized collection of pus caused by an inflammatory response to bacteria in tissues and organs.

acute glomerulonephritis Inflammation of the glomerulus that develops suddenly from an excess immunity response within the kidney tissues.

dysuria Painful urination.

hydronephrosis Abnormal enlargement of the kidney.

hydroureter Abnormal distention of the ureter.

nephrectomy Surgical removal of the kidney.

nephrosclerosis Degenerative kidney disorder resulting from changes in kidney blood vessels.

nephrostomy The surgical creation of an opening directly into the kidney; performed to divert urine externally and prevent further damage to the kidney when a stricture is causing hydronephrosis and cannot be corrected with urologic procedures.

nephrotic syndrome (NS) Immunologic kidney disorder in which glomerular permeability increases so that larger molecules pass through the membrane into the urine and are then excreted; causes massive loss of protein into the urine and decreased plasma albumin levels.

polycystic kidney disease (PKD) Genetic disorder in which fluid-filled cysts develop in the kidneys.

pyelolithotomy Surgical removal of a stone from the kidney.

pyelonephritis A bacterial infection in the kidney and renal pelvis.

stricture Narrowing of the urinary tract.

ureteroplasty Surgical repair of the ureter.

✳ PRIORITY AND INTERRELATED CONCEPTS

The priority concept for this chapter is:

- **Elimination**
  The **Elimination** concept exemplar for this chapter is Pyelonephritis.

The interrelated concepts for this chapter are:

- **Fluid and Electrolyte Balance**
- **Acid-Base Balance**
- **Immunity**
- **Pain**

Healthy kidneys are the major controllers of urinary *elimination*. They perform this function by filtering wastes from the blood and selectively determining which substances remain in the body and which are eliminated. Thus the kidneys maintain homeostasis by contributing to *fluid and electrolyte balance* and *acid-base balance.* Any problem that disrupts kidney function has the potential to impair general homeostasis and all aspects of urinary elimination (Fig. 59.1). Interaction with other organs and systems is necessary for the kidneys to function effectively. In addition, when the kidneys are impaired, the buildup of toxic wastes affects all other body systems and

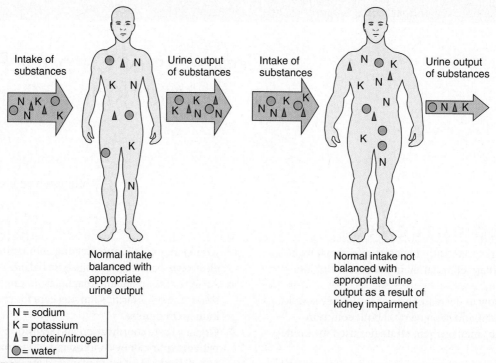

FIG. 59.1 Unbalanced body water, electrolytes, and waste products as a result of kidney problems that prevent adjustments in urinary elimination.

can lead to life-threatening outcomes. This chapter describes a variety of infectious and noninfectious kidney disorders, kidney tumors, and kidney trauma. Acute kidney injury (AKI) and chronic kidney disease (CKD) are discussed in Chapter 60.

✳ ELIMINATION CONCEPT EXEMPLAR: PYELONEPHRITIS

In the healthy adult, urine is normally sterile. Urinary tract infection (UTI) is an infection in any part of this normally sterile system. Pyelonephritis occurs as a complication of an ascending urinary tract infection that spreads from the bladder to the kidneys (Belyayeva & Jeong, 2021). It can be acute or chronic. Pyelonephritis interferes with urinary *elimination,* which is the excretion of waste from the body by the urinary system (as urine). Chapter 3 provides a summary of the concept of elimination in more detail.

Pathophysiology Review

Acute pyelonephritis is an active bacterial infection, whereas *chronic pyelonephritis* results from repeated or continued upper urinary tract infections that occur almost exclusively in patients who have anatomic abnormalities of the urinary tract. Bacterial infection causes local (e.g., kidney) and systemic (e.g., fever, aches, and malaise) inflammatory symptoms.

In pyelonephritis, organisms move up from the urinary tract into the kidney tissue. This is more likely to occur when urine refluxes from the bladder into the ureters and then to the kidney. Reflux is the reverse or upward flow of urine toward the renal pelvis and kidney. Infection also can be transmitted by

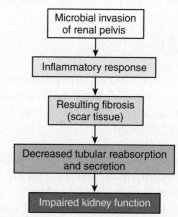

FIG. 59.2 Pathophysiology of pyelonephritis.

organisms in the blood, but this cause of pyelonephritis is rare unless the patient has impaired *immunity.*

Acute pyelonephritis involves acute tissue inflammation, local edema, tubular cell necrosis, and possible abscess formation. Abscesses, which are pockets of infection, can occur anywhere in the kidney. The infection is scattered within the kidney; healthy tissues can lie next to infected areas. Fibrosis and scar tissue develop from chronic inflammation in the kidney glomerular and tubular structures. As a result, filtration, reabsorption, and secretion are impaired, and kidney function is reduced (Fig. 59.2).

Etiology and Genetic Risk

Single episodes of *acute pyelonephritis* result from bacterial infection, with or without obstruction or reflux. *Chronic pyelonephritis* usually occurs with structural deformities, urinary stasis, obstruction, or reflux. Conditions that lead to urinary stasis include prolonged bed rest and paralysis. Obstruction can be caused by stones, kidney cancer, scarring from pelvic radiation or surgery, recurrent infection, or injury. Reflux may occur from scarring or result from anatomic anomalies. Reflux also results from bladder tumors, prostate enlargement, or urinary stones. Reduced bladder tone from diabetic neuropathy, spinal cord injury, and neurodegenerative diseases (e.g., spina bifida, multiple sclerosis) contributes to stasis and reflux.

Pyelonephritis from an ascending infection may follow manipulation of the urinary tract (e.g., placement of a urinary catheter), particularly in patients who have reduced **immunity** or diabetes. In patients with chronic kidney stone disease, stones may retain organisms, resulting in ongoing infection and kidney scarring. Drugs, such as high-dose or prolonged use of NSAIDs, can lead to papillary necrosis and reflux.

The most common pyelonephritis-causing infecting organism among community-dwelling adults is *Escherichia coli*. *Enterococcus faecalis* is common in hospitalized patients. Both organisms are in the intestinal tract. Other organisms that cause pyelonephritis in hospitalized patients include *Proteus mirabilis*, *Klebsiella* species, and *Pseudomonas aeruginosa*. When the infection is bloodborne, common organisms include *Staphylococcus aureus* and *Candida* and *Salmonella* species.

Other causes of kidney scarring contributing to increased risk for pyelonephritis are inflammatory responses resulting from **immunity** excesses with antibody reactions, cell-mediated immunity against the bacterial antigens, or autoimmune reactions.

Incidence and Prevalence

Young females who are sexually active are the most commonly affected by acute pyelonephritis (Belyayeva, & Jeong, 2021). Hormonal changes as well as obstruction caused by the fetus during pregnancy make acute pyelonephritis more common during the second trimester and beginning of the third trimester. Pregnant females are at high risk for premature labor and delivery from acute pyelonephritis (Belyayeva & Jeong, 2021).

Chronic pyelonephritis is rarely characterized by infection alone, so the incidence and prevalence are linked to the underlying condition or conditions that lead to relapsing inflammatory damage of the kidney. These conditions include congenital structural abnormality, neurogenic bladder dysfunction, and primary vesicoureteral reflux (urine flows from the bladder to the kidneys) (Belyayeva & Jeong, 2021).

Interprofessional Collaborative Care

Depending on the severity of the disease, pyelonephritis may be managed in any care setting and in the community. Hospitalization becomes necessary in cases of bacteremia or hemodynamic instability and when oral medication cannot be tolerated. Bacteremia occurs in approximately 10% of cases. Bacteremia is more common in older adult females and females with diabetes (Ayatollahi et al., 2021). The focus of care for patients with chronic pyelonephritis requires continuing attention to managing the structural or functional abnormality that contributes to recurrent infection and inflammatory fibrosis.

Recognize Cues: Assessment

History. Ask about recurrent urinary tract infections (UTIs), diabetes mellitus (DM), stone disease, and known defects of the genitourinary tract. Ask about disease or treatment that results in reduced **immunity**, which also increases the risk for pyelonephritis. Ask about kidney function; knowledgeable patients may be able to describe their stage of chronic kidney disease (CKD) if chronic pyelonephritis has led to permanent kidney damage. Ensure that a woman is not pregnant before radiographic imaging.

Physical Assessment/Signs and Symptoms. Ask about specific symptoms of acute pyelonephritis. See Box 59.1 for key features of acute pyelonephritis. Chronic pyelonephritis has a less dramatic presentation but similar symptoms. Ask the patient to describe any urinary symptoms or abdominal discomfort. Inquire about any history of repeated low-grade fevers. Changes in urine color or odor may accompany bacteriuria. See Box 59.2 for key features of chronic pyelonephritis.

The objective assessment includes inspecting the flanks and gently palpating the costovertebral angle (CVA). Inflammation can be indicated by enlargement, asymmetry, edema, or redness/hyperpigmentation found during the inspection of both CVAs (Fukaguchi, et al., 2021). If there is no tenderness to light palpation in either CVA, the primary health care provider may firmly percuss each area. Tenderness or discomfort may indicate infection or inflammation.

Psychosocial Assessment. Any infection in an older adult can lead to acute confusion. Assess the older adult who has new-onset confusion for signs and symptoms of urinary or renal infection.

The patient with any problem in the genitourinary area may have feelings of anxiety, embarrassment, or guilt. Listen for signs of anxiety or specific fears and prevent embarrassment during assessment. Feelings of guilt, often associated with sexual habits

---

BOX 59.1 Key Features

Acute Pyelonephritis

- Fever
- Chills
- Tachycardia and tachypnea
- Flank, back, or loin pain
- Tenderness at the costovertebral angle (CVA)
- Abdominal, often colicky, discomfort
- Nausea and vomiting
- General malaise or fatigue
- Burning, urgency, or frequency of urination
- Nocturia
- Recent cystitis or treatment for urinary tract infection (UTI)

BOX 59.2 Key Features

Chronic Pyelonephritis

- Hypertension
- Inability to conserve sodium
- Decreased urine-concentrating ability, resulting in nocturia
- Tendency to develop hyperkalemia and acidosis

or practices, may be masked through delay in seeking treatment or through vague, nonspecific responses to specific or direct questions. Encourage patients to tell their own story in familiar, comfortable language.

Laboratory Assessment. Urinalysis shows a positive leukocyte esterase and nitrite dipstick test and the presence of white blood cells (WBCs) and bacteria. Occasional red blood cells (RBCs) and protein may be present. The urine is cultured to determine the specific organisms causing the infection and the susceptibility or resistance of the specific organisms to various antibiotics. The urine sample for culture and sensitivity testing is usually obtained by the clean-catch method. In patients with recurrent pyelonephritis, more specific testing of bacterial antigens and antibodies may help determine whether the same organism is responsible for the recurrent infections.

Blood cultures may be obtained to determine the source and spread of infectious organisms. Other blood tests include the WBC count and differential of the complete blood count, as well as C-reactive protein and erythrocyte sedimentation rate (ESR) to determine *immunity* responses and presence of inflammation. Serum tests of kidney function, such as blood urea nitrogen (BUN) and creatinine, are used as baseline and to trend recovery or deterioration. Estimate of glomerular filtration rate (GFR) also is used to trend kidney function.

Imaging Assessment. An x-ray of the kidneys, ureters, and bladder (KUB) or CT is performed to visualize anatomy, inflammation, fluid accumulation, abscess formation, and defects in kidneys and the urinary tract. These tests also identify stones, kidney tumors or cysts, or prostate enlargement. Urine reflux caused by incompetent bladder-ureter valve closure can be seen with a cystourethrogram. (See Chapter 57 for more information on imaging assessment.)

Other Diagnostic Assessment. Other diagnostic tests include examining antibody-coated bacteria in urine, testing for certain enzymes (e.g., lactate dehydrogenase isoenzyme 5), and performing radionuclide renal scans. Examining urine for antibody-coated bacteria helps identify patients who may need long-term antibiotic therapy. High-molecular-weight enzymes in urine, such as lactate dehydrogenase isoenzyme 5, are present with any kidney tissue deterioration problem and give trend data. The renal scan can identify active pyelonephritis or abscesses in or around the kidney. A kidney biopsy may be performed to rule out less obvious causes of inflammation.

NCLEX Examination Challenge 59.1
Physiological Integrity

The nurse is caring for a newly admitted client. Which of the following assessment data would cause the nurse to suspect acute pyelonephritis? **Select all that apply.**
A. Urinary frequency
B. Dysuria
C. Oliguria
D. Heart rate 120 beats/min
E. Costovertebral angle tenderness

Analyze Cues and Prioritize Hypotheses: Analysis

The priority collaborative problems for the patient with pyelonephritis are:
1. *Pain* (flank and abdominal) due to inflammation and infection
2. Potential for chronic kidney disease (CKD) due to kidney tissue destruction

Generate Solutions and Take Actions: Planning and Implementation

Managing Pain

Planning: Expected Outcomes. With proper intervention, the patient with pyelonephritis is expected to achieve an acceptable state of comfort.

Interventions. Interventions may be nonsurgical or surgical. Interventional radiologic techniques may be used to relieve obstruction or repair a stricture of the urinary tract.

Nonsurgical Management. Interventions include the use of drug therapy, nutrition and fluid therapy, and education to ensure that the patient understands the treatment.

Drug therapy can reduce pain. Acetaminophen is preferred over NSAIDs because it does not interfere with kidney autoregulation of blood flow. Reduction of fever will also reduce *pain.* Some patients may require the use of opioids in the short term for pain control.

Drug therapy with antibiotics is ordered to treat the infection. At first the antibiotics are broad spectrum. After urine and blood culture and sensitivity results are known, more specific antibiotics may be prescribed. Antibiotics are given (usually IV in hospitalized patients; orally in community-dwelling patients) to achieve adequate blood levels or sterile blood culture results. A prophylactic antibiotic is not recommended for patients with impaired voiding or chronic catheter use because it does not limit recurrence or severity of UTI (Belyayeva & Jeong, 2021)

Catheter replacement is supportive for a patient requiring a urinary catheter for 2 or more weeks (e.g., for neurogenic bladder or wound healing). This involves removal and replacement of the catheter and closed drainage system before starting antibiotic therapy. This intervention reduces bioburden by removing a device with a biofilm of concentrated organisms.

Nutritional therapy involves ensuring that the patient's dietary intake has adequate calories from all food groups for healing to occur. A registered dietitian nutritionist should be part of the interprofessional team. Fluid intake is recommended at 2 L/day, sufficient to result in dilute (pale yellow) urine, unless another health problem requires fluid restriction.

Surgical Management. Surgical interventions can correct structural problems causing urine reflux or obstruction of urine outflow or can remove the source of infection. Teach the patient the nature and purpose of the proposed surgery, the expected outcome, and how the patient can participate.

The surgical procedures used may be one of the following: pyelolithotomy (stone removal from the kidney), nephrectomy (removal of the kidney), ureteral diversion, or reimplantation of ureter(s) to restore proper bladder drainage.

A pyelolithotomy is needed for removal of a large stone in the kidney pelvis that blocks urine flow and causes infection.

Nephrectomy is a last resort when all other measures to clear the infection have failed. For patients with poor ureter valve closure or dilated ureters, ureteroplasty (ureter repair or revision) or ureteral reimplantation (through another site in the bladder wall) preserves kidney function and eliminates infections.

Preventing Chronic Kidney Disease

Planning: Expected Outcomes. The patient is expected to conserve existing kidney function. Underlying genitourinary abnormalities must be identified and appropriate interventions taken to manage a current infection and the risk for subsequent infections. The approach by the urologist or nephrologist depends on signs and symptoms, as well as on patient history.

Interventions. Specific antibiotics are ordered to treat the infection. Stress the importance of completing the drug therapy as directed. Discuss with the patient and family the importance of regular follow-up examinations and completing the recommended diagnostic tests.

Blood pressure control slows the progression of kidney dysfunction. Ensure that the patient is able to detect adverse changes in blood pressure using community resources, such as free blood pressure readings at community settings or retail pharmacies. When pyelonephritis causes or worsens CKD, ensure a referral to a nephrologist for additional assessment and management (see CKD in Chapter 60). Encourage the patient to drink sufficient fluid during waking hours to prevent dehydration because dehydration could further reduce kidney function. When dietary protein is restricted, a registered dietitian nutritionist (RDN) can help the family select appropriate food and proportions. Collaborate with the RDN, and reinforce the prescribed interventions.

Care Coordination and Transition Management

Pyelonephritis may cause fear and anxiety in the patient and family. The severity of the acute process and its potential to develop into a chronic process are frightening. The patient and the family need reassurance that treatment and preventive measures can be successful.

If no surgery is performed, the patient may need help with self-care, nutrition, and drug management at home. If surgery is performed, the patient may need help with incision care, self-care, and transportation for follow-up appointments.

Self-Management Education. After assessing the patient's and family's understanding of pyelonephritis and its therapy, explain:

- Drug regimen (purpose, timing, frequency, duration, and possible side effects)
- The role of nutrition and adequate fluid intake
- Best practices for chronic urinary catheter care, if needed
- The need for a balance between rest and activity, including any limitations after surgery
- The signs and symptoms of disease recurrence
- The use of previously successful coping mechanisms and community resources

Advise the patient to complete all prescribed antibiotic regimens and to report any side effects or unusual symptoms to the primary health care provider rather than stopping the drugs.

Ensure that interprofessional care includes nutritional counseling, because many patients have special nutritional requirements, such as those for diabetes or pregnancy.

Evaluate Outcomes: Evaluation

Evaluate the care of the patient with pyelonephritis based on the identified priority patient problems. Expected outcomes may include that the patient will:

- Report that *pain* is controlled
- Be knowledgeable about the disease, its treatment, and interventions to prevent or reduce CKD progression

ACUTE GLOMERULONEPHRITIS

Pathophysiology Review

Glomerulonephritis (GN) is categorized into conditions that primarily involve the kidney (primary glomerular nephritis) and those in which kidney involvement is only part of a systemic disorder (secondary GN). It is a group of diseases that injure and inflame the glomerulus, the part of the kidney that filters blood. Inflamed glomeruli allow passage of protein and blood in the urine. GN is associated with high blood pressure, progressive kidney damage (leading to CKD), and edema. Anemia from reduced production of erythropoietin and high cholesterol often co-occur. GN can cause altered urinary *elimination*.

Acute glomerulonephritis (GN) develops suddenly from an excessive *immunity* response within the kidney tissues. Usually an infection is noticed before kidney symptoms of acute GN are present. The onset of symptoms is about 10 days from the time of infection. Patients usually recover quickly and completely from acute GN.

Many causes of primary GN are infectious (Box 59.3). Secondary GN can be caused by multisystem diseases (Box 59.4) and can manifest as acute or chronic disease. However, the division of primary and secondary GN is complex because diagnostic findings, histologic changes, and other changes are the

---

BOX 59.3 Infectious Agents Associated With Glomerulonephritis

- Group A beta-hemolytic *Streptococcus*
- Staphylococcal or gram-negative bacteremia or sepsis
- Pneumococcal, *Mycoplasma*, or *Klebsiella* pneumonia
- Syphilis
- Dengue
- Hantavirus
- Varicella
- Parvovirus
- Hepatitis B and C
- Cytomegalovirus
- Parvovirus
- Epstein-Barr virus
- Human immunodeficiency virus

Adapted from Patel, N.P. (2018, November 28). Infection-induced kidney diseases. Retrieved from U.S. National Library of Medicine, National Institutes of Health. https://www.ncbi.nlm.nih.gov/pmc/articles/PMC6282040/.

BOX 59.4   Secondary Glomerular Diseases and Syndromes

- Systemic lupus erythematosus (SLE)
- Sustained liver disease (hepatitis B or C, autoimmune hepatitis, and cirrhosis)
- Amyloidosis
- Mesangiocapillary glomerulonephritis (MCGN)
- Alport syndrome
- Vasculitis
- IgA nephropathy
- Wegener granulomatosis
- HIV-associated nephropathy
- Diabetic glomerulopathy

HIV, Human immunodeficiency virus.
Data from Muthu, V.R. (2018, Jan-Feb). *Clinicopathological spectrum of glomerular diseases in adolescents: A single-center experience over 4 years.* Retrieved from U.S. National Library of Medicine, National Institutes of Health. https://www.ncbi.nlm.nih.gov/pmc/articles/PMC5830804/; and Radhakrishnan, J. (2023). Glomerular disease: Evaluation and differential diagnosis in adults. *UpToDate.* Retrieved February 7, 2023, from https://www.uptodate.com/contents/glomerular-disease-evaluation-and-differential-diagnosis-in-adults.

same in both kidney and systemic disease, with both demonstrating altered *immunity.* Drugs and inherited disorders are also implicated in GN with an acute or chronic presentation.

Interprofessional Collaborative Care

Recognize Cues: Assessment

History. Ask about recent infections, particularly of the skin or upper respiratory tract, and about recent travel or other possible exposures to viruses, bacteria, fungi, or parasites. Recent illnesses, surgery, or other invasive procedures may suggest infection. Ask about any systemic diseases that alter *immunity,* such as systemic lupus erythematosus (SLE), which could cause acute GN.

Physical Assessment/Signs and Symptoms. Inspect the patient's skin for lesions or recent incisions, including body piercings, because these may be the source of organisms causing GN. Assess the face, eyelids, hands, and other areas for edema because edema is present in most patients with acute GN. Assess for fluid overload and pulmonary edema that may result from fluid and sodium retention occurring with acute GN. Ask about any difficulty breathing or shortness of breath. Assess for crackles in the lung fields, an S_3 heart sound (gallop rhythm), and neck vein distention.

Ask about changes in urine *elimination* patterns and any change in urine color, volume, clarity, or odor. The patient may describe blood in the urine as smoky, reddish brown, rusty, or cola-colored. Ask about dysuria or oliguria. Weigh the patient to assess for fluid retention.

Take the patient's blood pressure and compare it with the baseline blood pressure. Mild to moderate hypertension occurs with acute GN as a result of impaired *fluid and electrolyte balance* with fluid and sodium retention. The patient may have fatigue, a lack of energy, anorexia, nausea, and/or vomiting if uremia from severe kidney impairment is present.

PATIENT-CENTERED CARE: OLDER ADULT HEALTH

Glomerulonephritis

Glomerulonephritis can lead to chronic kidney disease (CKD), making it essential to prevent and treat in the older adult who is at greater risk for CKD. In the older adult, symptoms of glomerulonephritis can easily be confused with an exacerbation of heart failure. Older adults with immunocompromised backgrounds, such as diabetes mellitus, malignancies, or alcoholism, are reported to be at higher risk for death from glomerulonephritis than younger adults and children, where most cases are resolved without specific treatments (Oda & Yoshizawa, 2021).

Laboratory Assessment. Urinalysis shows red blood cells *(hematuria)* and protein *(proteinuria).* An early morning specimen of urine is preferred for urinalysis because the urine is concentrated, most acidic, and filled with more intact formed elements at that time. Microscopic examination often shows red blood cell casts, as well as casts from other substances.

A 24-hour urine collection for total protein assay is obtained. The protein excretion rate for patients with acute GN may be increased from 500 mg/24 hr to 3 g/24 hr. Serum albumin levels are decreased because this protein is lost in the urine and fluid retention causes dilution.

Serum creatinine and BUN provide information about kidney function and may be elevated, indicating impairment of *elimination.* The glomerular filtration rate (GFR), either estimated from a single serum and urine creatinine value or measured by the 24-hour urine test for creatinine clearance, may be decreased to 50 mL/min. Recall that the older adult has a decline in GFR, which may make GFR results challenging to interpret.

Other Diagnostic Assessment. A kidney biopsy provides a precise diagnosis of the condition, assists in determining the prognosis, and helps in outlining treatment (see Chapter 57). The specific tissue features are determined by light microscopy, immunofluorescent stains, and electron microscopy to identify cell type, the presence of immunoglobulins, or the type of tissue deposits.

Take Actions: Interventions

Interventions focus on managing infection, preventing complications, and providing appropriate patient education.

Managing infection as a cause of acute GN begins with appropriate antibiotic therapy. Penicillin, erythromycin, or azithromycin is prescribed for GN caused by streptococcal infection. Check the patient's known allergies before giving any drug. Stress personal hygiene and basic infection control principles (e.g., handwashing) to prevent spread of the organism. Teach patients the importance of completing the entire course of the prescribed antibiotic.

Modifying *immunity* with drugs can also benefit patients with acute glomerulonephritis (GN) that is not due to acute infection but is related to excessive inflammation. Corticosteroids and cytotoxic drugs (e.g., cyclosporine, cyclophosphamide) to suppress *immunity* responses may be used. Patients receiving immunosuppressants need to take precautions to avoid exposure to new infections.

Preventing complications is an important nursing intervention, especially when *fluid and electrolyte balance* is disrupted. For patients with fluid overload, hypertension, and edema, diuretics and sodium and water restrictions are prescribed. The usual fluid allowance is equal to the 24-hour urine output plus 500 to 600 mL. Patients with oliguria usually have increased serum levels of potassium and blood urea nitrogen (BUN). Potassium and protein intake may be restricted to prevent hyperkalemia and uremia as a result of the elevated BUN. Antihypertensive drugs may be needed to control hypertension (see Chapter 30).

Nausea, vomiting, or anorexia indicates that uremia is present. Dialysis is necessary if uremic symptoms or fluid volume excess cannot be controlled with nutrition therapy and fluid management (see Chapter 60). *Plasmapheresis* (removal and filtering of the plasma to eliminate antibodies) also may be used (see Chapter 34).

Coordinate care to conserve patient energy, and balance activity with rest to maintain function. Relaxation techniques and diversional activities can reduce emotional stress.

Preparing for self-management includes teaching the patient and family members about the purpose of prescribed drugs, the dosage and schedule, and potential adverse effects. Ensure that they understand diet and fluid restrictions. Advise the patient to measure weight and blood pressure daily at the same time each day. Instruct the patient to notify the primary health care provider of any sudden increase in weight or blood pressure.

If short-term dialysis is required to control *fluid and electrolyte balance* or uremic symptoms, explain vascular access care and dialysis schedules and routines (see Chapter 60).

Rapidly progressive glomerulonephritis (RPGN) is a primary GN also called *crescentic glomerulonephritis* because of the presence of crescent-shaped cells in the Bowman capsule. RPGN develops acutely over several weeks or months. Patients become quite ill quickly and have symptoms of kidney impairment (fluid volume excess, hypertension, oliguria, electrolyte imbalances, and uremic symptoms). Regardless of treatment, RPGN often progresses to end-stage kidney disease (ESKD).

CHRONIC GLOMERULONEPHRITIS

Pathophysiology Review

Chronic GN, or *chronic nephritic syndrome*, develops over years to decades. Mild proteinuria and hematuria, hypertension, fatigue, and occasional edema are often the only symptoms.

Although the exact cause is not known, changes in kidney tissue result from infection, hypertension, inflammation from *immunity* excess, or poor kidney blood flow. Kidney tissue atrophies, and functional nephrons are greatly reduced. Biopsy in the late stages of atrophy may show glomerular changes, cell loss, protein and collagen deposits, and fibrosis of the kidney tissue. Microscopic examination shows deposits of immune complexes and inflammation.

The loss of nephrons reduces glomerular filtration. Hypertension and renal arteriole sclerosis are often present. The glomerular damage allows proteins to enter the urine. Chronic GN always leads to end-stage kidney disease (ESKD) (see Chapter 60).

Interprofessional Collaborative Care

Recognize Cues: Assessment

History. Ask about other health problems, including systemic diseases, kidney or urologic disorders, infectious diseases (i.e., streptococcal infections), and recent exposures to infections. Ask about overall health status and whether increasing fatigue and lethargy have occurred.

Identify the patient's urine *elimination* pattern. Ask whether the frequency of voiding has increased or the quantity of urine has decreased. Ask about changes in urine color, odor, or clarity and whether dysuria or incontinence has occurred. Nocturia is a common symptom.

Assess the patient's general comfort, and ask whether new-onset dyspnea has occurred, because fluid overload can occur with decreased urine output. Ask about and observe for changes in cognition (i.e., irritability, an inability to read, or incapacity during job-related functions) or disturbed concentration. Changes in memory and the ability to concentrate occur as waste products collect in the blood.

Physical Assessment/Signs and Symptoms. Assess for systemic circulatory overload. Auscultate lung fields for crackles, observe the respiratory rate and depth, and measure blood pressure and weight. Assess the heart rate, rhythm, and presence of an S_3 heart sound. Inspect the neck veins for venous engorgement and check for edema of the feet and ankles, on the shins, and over the sacrum.

Assess for uremic symptoms, such as slurred speech, ataxia, tremors, or asterixis (flapping tremor of the fingers or the inability to maintain a fixed posture with the arms extended and wrists hyperextended). Inspect the skin for a yellowish color, texture changes, bruises, rashes, or eruptions. Ask about itching, and document areas of dryness or any excoriation from scratching.

Psychosocial Assessment. A diagnosis of chronic GN is associated with psychosocial responses of uncertainty, loss, and fear of the need for lifestyle changes as the disease progresses. While obtaining the history, listen carefully for spoken and unspoken feelings of anger, resentment, sadness, or anxiety, all of which may need further exploration.

Diagnostic Assessment. Urine output decreases and urinalysis shows protein, usually less than 2 g in a 24-hour collection. The specific gravity is fixed at a constant level of dilution (around 1.010) despite variable fluid intake. Red blood cells and casts may be in the urine.

The glomerular filtration rate (GFR) is low. The serum creatinine level is elevated; usually it is greater than 6 mg/dL (500 mcmol/L) but may be as high as 30 mg/dL (2500 mcmol/L) or more because of poor waste *elimination.* The BUN is increased, often as high as 100 to 200 mg/dL (35 to 70 mmol/L).

Decreased kidney function disturbs *fluid and electrolyte balance.* Sodium retention is common, but dilution of the plasma from excess fluid can result in a falsely normal serum sodium level (135 to 145 mEq/L [mmol/L]) or a low sodium level (less than 135 mEq/L [mmol/L]). When oliguria develops, potassium is not excreted, and hyperkalemia occurs when levels exceed 5.4 mEq/L (mmol/L).

Hyperphosphatemia develops with serum levels greater than 4.7 mg/dL (1.73 mmol/L). Serum calcium levels are usually low normal or are slightly below normal.

Disturbances of *acid-base balance* with acidosis develop from hydrogen ion retention and loss of bicarbonate. However, there may be a decrease in serum carbon dioxide (CO_2) levels as patients breathe more rapidly to compensate for the acidosis. If respiratory compensation is present, the pH of arterial blood is between 7.35 and 7.45. A pH of less than 7.35 means that the patient's respiratory system is not completely compensating for the acidosis (see Chapter 14).

The kidneys are abnormally small on x-ray or CT in chronic GN.

Take Actions: Interventions

Interventions focus on slowing the progression of the disease and preventing complications. Management is systemic and consists of diet changes, fluid intake sufficient to prevent reduced blood flow to the kidneys, and drug therapy to control the problems from uremia. Eventually *elimination* is so impaired that the patient requires dialysis or transplantation to prevent death. (Care for the patient requiring dialysis or transplantation is discussed in Chapter 60.)

NEPHROTIC SYNDROME

Pathophysiology Review

Nephrotic syndrome (NS) is an immunologic kidney disorder in which glomerular permeability increases, so larger molecules pass through the membrane into the urine and are then excreted. This process causes massive loss of protein into the urine, edema formation, and decreased plasma albumin levels. Minimal change disease is the most common cause of NS and accounts for 90% of NS in children and 20% in adults. Minimal change disease can be detected using light microscopy and transmission electron microscopy utilizing standard procedures (Yan et al., 2020).

The most common cause of glomerular membrane changes is altered *immunity* with inflammation. Defects in glomerular filtration can also occur as a result of genetic defects of the glomerular filtering system, such as Fabry disease. Altered liver function may occur with NS, resulting in increased lipid production and hyperlipidemia (Mitchell-Brown & Veisze, 2019).

Interprofessional Collaborative Care

The main feature of NS is increased protein *elimination* with severe proteinuria (with more than 3.5 g of protein in a 24-hour urine sample). Patients also have low serum albumin levels of less than 3 g/dL (30 g/L), high serum lipid levels, fats in the urine, edema, and hypertension (Box 59.5). Renal vein thrombosis often occurs at the same time as NS, either as a cause of the problem or as an effect. NS may progress to end-stage kidney disease (ESKD), but treatment can prevent progression.

> ### BOX 59.5 Key Features
> #### *Nephrotic Syndrome*
>
> Key features include sudden onset of these symptoms:
> - Massive proteinuria
> - Hypoalbuminemia
> - Edema (especially facial and periorbital)
> - Lipiduria
> - Hyperlipidemia
> - Delayed clotting or increased bleeding with higher-than-normal values for serum activated partial thromboplastin time (aPTT), coagulation, or international normalized ratio (INR) for prothrombin time (PT)
> - Reduced kidney function with elevated blood urea nitrogen (BUN) and serum creatinine and decreased glomerular filtration rate (GFR)

Management varies, depending on which process is causing the disorder (identified by kidney biopsy). Excess *immunity* may improve with suppressive therapy using steroids and cytotoxic or immunosuppressive agents. Angiotensin-converting enzyme inhibitors (ACEIs) can decrease protein loss in the urine, and cholesterol-lowering drugs can improve blood lipid levels. Heparin may reduce vascular defects and improve kidney function. Diet changes are often prescribed. If the glomerular filtration rate (GFR) is normal, dietary intake of proteins is needed. If the GFR is decreased, protein intake must be decreased. Mild diuretics and sodium restriction may be needed to control edema and hypertension. Assess the patient's hydration status because vascular dehydration is common. If plasma volume is depleted, kidney problems worsen. Acute kidney injury (AKI) may be avoided if adequate blood flow to the kidney is maintained.

NEPHROSCLEROSIS

Pathophysiology Review

Nephrosclerosis is a degenerative disorder resulting from changes in kidney blood vessels. Nephron blood vessels thicken, resulting in narrowed lumens and decreased kidney blood flow. The tissue is chronically hypoxic, with ischemia and fibrosis developing over time.

Nephrosclerosis occurs with all types of hypertension, atherosclerosis, and diabetes mellitus (DM). The more severe the hypertension, the greater the risk for severe kidney damage. Nephrosclerosis is rarely seen when blood pressure is consistently below 160/110 mm Hg. The changes caused by hypertension may be reversible or may progress to end-stage kidney disease (ESKD) within months or years. Hypertension is the second leading cause of ESKD, with many patients requiring kidney replacement therapy (e.g., dialysis or transplantation).

More recent advances in genetic testing have revealed a complex pathogenesis in nephrosclerosis. Patients were often diagnosed with nephrosclerosis thought to be caused by hypertension. However, advanced genetic evidence indicated many as having genetic focal segmental glomerulosclerosis. The apolipoprotein L1 (APOL1) allele is a risk factor for glomerulosclerosis that presents with symptoms such as nephrosclerosis. People with the APOL1 allele are usually of African ancestry. Not all patients with the APOL1 allele will develop kidney disease, suggesting that there may be environmental factors as well. See the Patient-Centered Care: Genetics/Genomics box.

PATIENT-CENTERED CARE: GENETICS/ GENOMICS

APOL1 Gene

About 15% of the general population (37 million people) is affected by chronic kidney disease (Centers for Disease Control and Prevention, 2021). Black Americans, American Indians, and Hispanic Americans are more likely to have chronic kidney disease than White Americans (Deng & Zhang, 2022). About 13% of Black Americans (over 5 million people) have the high-risk *APOL1* gene (Bleyer, 2023). People with this genotype have a 15% to 30% chance of developing ESKD in their lifetime. Patients with this gene should have routine monitoring of kidney function and blood pressure. It is important to provide support to the patient, as well as the clarity that while the risk is increased, two-thirds of those patients who have the *APOL1* gene will not develop ESRD (Bleyer, 2023).

Interprofessional Collaborative Care

Management focuses on controlling high blood pressure and reducing albuminuria to preserve kidney function. Although many antihypertensive drugs may lower blood pressure, the patient's response is important in ensuring long-term adherence to the prescribed therapy. Factors that promote adherence include once-a-day dosing, low cost, and minimal side effects.

Lack of knowledge or misinformation about hypertension poses many challenges to health care professionals working with patients who have hypertension. When kidney disease occurs, adherence to therapy is even more important for preserving health.

Many drugs can control high blood pressure (see Chapter 30), and more than one agent may be needed for best control. Angiotensin-converting enzyme inhibitors (ACEIs) are very useful in reducing hypertension and preserving kidney function. Diuretics can maintain *fluid and electrolyte balance* in the presence of kidney function insufficiency. Hyperkalemia needs to be prevented when potassium-sparing diuretics, alone or in combination with other diuretics, are used to treat hypertensive patients with known kidney disease.

POLYCYSTIC KIDNEY DISEASE

Pathophysiology Review

Polycystic kidney disease (PKD) is a genetic disorder in which fluid-filled cysts develop in the nephrons (Fig. 59.3). Relentless development and growth of cysts from loss of cellular regulation and abnormal cell division result in progressive kidney enlargement. Patients with PKD often experience hypertension, abdominal and flank pain, ruptured cysts, and infections. These complications can lead to kidney failure and reduced quality of life (Ma & Lambert, 2021)

The cysts look like clusters of grapes (see Fig. 59.3). Over time, growing cysts damage the glomerular and tubular membranes. Each cystic kidney enlarges, becoming the size of a football, and may weigh 10 lb or more each. As cysts fill with fluid and become larger, kidney function becomes less effective, and urine formation and waste *elimination* are impaired.

Most patients with PKD have high blood pressure. The cause of hypertension is related to kidney ischemia from the enlarging cysts. As the vessels are compressed and blood flow to the kidneys decreases, the renin-angiotensin system is activated,

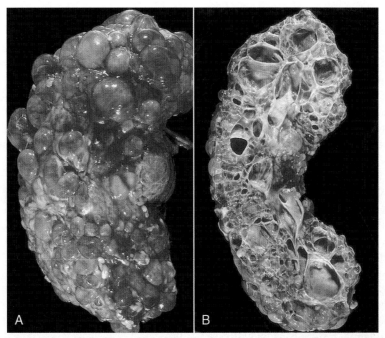

FIG. 59.3 External surface (A) and internal surface (B) of a polycystic kidney. (From Kumar, V., Abbas, A., Fausto, N., & Aster, J. [2010]. *Robbins and Cotran Pathologic basis of disease* [8th ed.]. Philadelphia: Saunders.)

raising blood pressure. Control of hypertension is a top priority because proper treatment can disrupt the process that leads to further kidney damage, as well as avoid complications such as stroke from hypertension.

Cysts may also occur in the liver and blood vessels. The incidence of cerebral *aneurysms* (outpouching and thinning of an artery wall) is higher in patients with PKD. Aneurysms may rupture, causing bleeding and sudden death. For unknown reasons, kidney stones occur in many patients with PKD. Heart valve problems (e.g., mitral valve prolapse), left ventricular hypertrophy, and colonic diverticula also are common in patients with PKD.

Etiology and Genetic Risk

Kidney cysts are genetically and clinically related to many symptoms and problems. PKD can be inherited as either an autosomal dominant trait or, less often, an autosomal recessive trait. Autosomal dominant PKD is the most common inherited kidney disease, occurring in 1 to 1000 live births. Rarely, a new gene mutation can cause PKD in a patient with no family history of the trait. However, the cases of gene mutation tend to be a milder form of PKD. Recent advances have made the genetic forms of cystic disorders of the kidney easier to understand. However, the number of genes influencing PKD is challenging and requires geneticists and genetic counselors to be a part of the interprofessional team caring for patients with or at risk for the disease.

👤 PATIENT-CENTERED CARE: GENETICS/GENOMICS

Autosomal Dominant PKD

Polycystic kidney disease (PKD) is a genetic condition, with the most common form being autosomal dominant. Autosomal dominant PKD is the underlying cause of kidney failure in 5% of patients who begin dialysis annually in the United States (Torres & Bennett, 2023).

There is no way to prevent PKD, although early detection and management of hypertension may slow the progression of kidney damage and impaired *elimination.* Genetic counseling may be useful for adults who have one parent with PKD. Family history analysis is used to help identify people at risk.

Interprofessional Collaborative Care

Recognize Cues: Assessment

Because PKD is a chronic disease with periods of acute problems, most management occurs in the community rather than in an acute care hospital. With acute problems or when surgery is needed, initial care is in a hospital setting, and continuing care can occur in any setting.

History. Explore the family history of a patient with suspected or actual PKD and ask whether either parent was known to have PKD or whether there is any family history of kidney disease. Assess the age at which the problem was diagnosed in the parent and any related complications. Ask about *pain,* abdominal

discomfort, constipation, changes in urine color or frequency, hypertension, headaches, and a family history of stroke or sudden death.

Physical Assessment/Signs and Symptoms. Pain is often the first symptom. Inspect the abdomen. A distended abdomen is common as the cystic kidneys swell and push the abdominal contents forward. Polycystic kidneys are easily palpated because of their increased size. Use *gentle* abdominal palpation because the cystic kidneys and nearby tissues may be tender and palpation is uncomfortable. The patient also may have flank pain as a dull ache or as a sharp and intermittent discomfort. Dull, aching pain is caused by increased kidney size with distention, abnormal stimulation of sensory neurons in the kidney, or infection within the cyst. Sharp, intermittent pain occurs when a cyst ruptures or a stone is present. When a cyst ruptures, the patient may have bright red or cola-colored urine. Infection is suspected if the urine is cloudy or foul smelling or if there is dysuria (pain on urination). See Box 59.6.

Nocturia (the need to urinate excessively at night) is an early symptom and occurs because of decreased urine concentrating ability. Patients with early PKD often have hyperfiltration leading to wasting of sodium and water, which disrupts *fluid and electrolyte balance.* Later, as kidney function declines (i.e., reduced glomerular filtration rate [GFR]), the patient retains water and sodium, which causes hypertension, edema, and uremic symptoms such as anorexia, nausea, vomiting, pruritus, and fatigue (see Chapter 60). Because intracranial aneurysms occur in patients with PKD, a severe headache with or without neurologic or vision changes requires attention.

Psychosocial Assessment. A PKD diagnosis is associated with psychosocial responses of uncertainty, loss, and fear due to the life-threatening complications that can occur (Ma & Lambert, 2021). The patient may have had a parent who died or relatives who required dialysis or transplantation. Listen for spoken and unspoken feelings of anger, resentment, futility, sadness, or anxiety. Such feelings may need further exploration. Feelings of guilt and concern for the patient's children may also complicate the issue.

Diagnostic Assessment. Ultrasound is the primary method for diagnosing PKD. The size of the kidney is measured by ultrasound, as well as cysts within the kidney. MRI or CT may be used in order to confirm ultrasound findings and provide

🔑 BOX 59.6   Key Features

Polycystic Kidney Disease

- Abdominal or flank pain
- Hypertension
- Nocturia
- Frequent urinary tract infections
- Increased abdominal girth
- Constipation
- Hematuria (bloody urine)
- Sodium wasting and inability to concentrate urine in early stage
- Progression to kidney failure with anuria (Nishio et al., 2021)

quantitative data regarding tissue oxygenation, fibrosis, edema, inflammation, and perfusion (Rankin et al., 2021).

Urinalysis may show proteinuria (protein in the urine), which indicates a decline in kidney function and impaired *elimination.* Hematuria may be gross or microscopic. Bacteria in the urine indicate infection, usually in the cysts. Obtain a urine sample for culture and sensitivity testing when there is evidence of infection. As kidney function declines, serum creatinine and blood urea nitrogen (BUN) levels rise. With further decline, creatinine clearance decreases, and the GFR is low. Changes in kidney handling of sodium may cause either sodium losses or sodium retention.

Take Actions: Interventions

Treatment goals are to slow the progression to kidney failure and treat the signs and symptoms supportively (Bennett et al., 2023). This includes management of hypertension and pain, dietary sodium restriction, increased fluid intake, and slowing disease progression.

Blood pressure control and lifestyle and dietary modifications are necessary to reduce cardiovascular complications and slow the progression of kidney dysfunction. Dietary sodium intake of less than 2 g/day is advised. In patients with preserved kidney function, 3 L of fluid daily is recommended to slow cyst growth. Care must be taken to monitor for hypervolemic hyponatremia with excess water intake (Bellos, 2021).

Drug therapy with angiotensin-converting enzyme inhibitors (ACEIs) to reach a blood pressure below 130/80 mm Hg in all patients with PKD or 110/75 mm Hg in young adults with preserved kidney function is recommended (Nishio et al., 2021).

Because PKD-related pain is often persistent and associated with multiple factors, a multidisciplinary *pain* management approach is helpful. Drugs may include opioids along with acetaminophen. NSAIDs are used cautiously because they can reduce kidney blood flow. Aspirin-containing drugs are avoided to reduce bleeding risk. When pain is severe, cysts can be reduced by needle aspiration and drainage; however, they usually refill. When the quality or severity of pain abruptly increases, assess for infection.

Fever, abdominal *pain,* and either leukocytosis or serum markers of inflammation (e.g., elevated erythrocyte sedimentation rate [ESR] or C-reactive protein [CRP]) may be associated with cystic or systemic infection. Blood and urine cultures may or may not be positive with cyst infection. Early infection management can prevent or reduce complications and acute kidney injury.

As the disease progresses, protein intake may be limited to slow the development of ESKD. Help the patient and family understand the diet plan and why it was prescribed. Work closely with the registered dietitian nutritionist (RDN) to foster the patient's understanding.

Strategies for kidney protection include the use of a vasopressin-suppressing agent such as tolvaptan to improve blood flow, slow kidney volume growth, and sustain kidney function. When the disease progresses and the kidneys no longer

function for waste *elimination,* care becomes similar to that needed for the patient with end-stage kidney disease (see Chapter 60).

HYDRONEPHROSIS AND HYDROURETER

Pathophysiology Review

Hydronephrosis and hydroureter are problems of urinary *elimination* with outflow obstruction. Urethral strictures obstruct urine outflow and may contribute to bladder distention, hydroureter, and hydronephrosis. Prompt recognition and treatment are crucial to preventing permanent kidney damage.

In hydronephrosis, the kidney enlarges as urine collects in the renal pelvis and kidney tissue. Because the capacity of the renal pelvis is normally 5 to 8 mL, obstruction in the renal pelvis or at the point where the ureter joins the renal pelvis quickly distends the renal pelvis. Kidney pressure increases as the volume of urine increases. Over time, sometimes in only a matter of hours, the blood vessels and kidney tubules can be damaged extensively (Fig. 59.4).

In patients with hydroureter (enlargement of the ureter), the effects are similar, but the obstruction is in the ureter rather than in the kidney. The ureter is most easily obstructed where the iliac vessels cross or where the ureters enter the bladder. Ureter dilation occurs above the obstruction and enlarges as urine collects (see Fig. 59.4).

Urinary obstruction causes damage when pressure builds up directly on kidney tissue. Tubular filtrate pressure also increases in the nephron as drainage through the collecting system is impaired and glomerular filtration decreases or ceases. Kidney

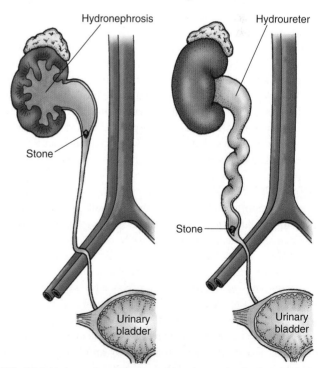

FIG. 59.4 Hydronephrosis is caused by obstruction in the upper part of the ureter. Hydroureter is caused by obstruction in the lower part of the ureter.

necrosis can occur. Nitrogen waste products (urea, creatinine, and uric acid) and electrolytes (sodium, potassium, chloride, and phosphorus) are retained, and **acid-base balance** is impaired.

The cause of hydronephrosis or hydroureter is an obstruction, which can occur at any location between the collecting duct and the urethral meatus. Common causes of urinary obstruction include kidney stones, tumors, fibrosis, structural abnormalities, trauma, abscess, and cysts. With cancer, obstructed ureters may result from tumors pressing on the ureters, pelvic radiation, or surgical treatment. Early treatment of the causes can prevent ureteral problems and permanent kidney damage. The time needed to prevent permanent damage depends on the patient's kidney health. Permanent damage can occur in less than 48 hours in some patients and after several weeks in other patients.

Interprofessional Collaborative Care
Recognize Cues: Assessment

Obtain a history from the patient, focusing on known kidney or urologic disorders. A history of childhood urinary tract problems may indicate previously undiagnosed structural defects. Ask about the usual pattern of urinary **elimination,** especially amount, frequency, color, clarity, and odor. Ask about recent flank or abdominal pain. Chills, fever, and malaise may be present with a urinary tract infection (UTI).

Inspect each flank to identify asymmetry, which may occur with a kidney mass, and *gently* palpate the abdomen to locate areas of tenderness. Palpate the bladder to detect distention, or use a bedside bladder scanner (see Chapter 57). Gentle pressure on the abdomen may cause urine leakage, which reflects a full bladder and possible obstruction.

Urinalysis may show bacteria or white blood cells if infection is present. When urinary tract obstruction is prolonged, microscopic examination may show tubular epithelial cells. Blood chemistries are normal unless glomerular filtration has decreased and waste **elimination** is impaired. Blood creatinine and BUN levels increase with a reduced GFR. Serum electrolyte levels may be altered with elevated blood levels of potassium, phosphorus, and calcium along with a metabolic acidosis (bicarbonate deficit). Urinary outflow obstruction can be seen with ultrasound (US) or CT.

Take Actions: Interventions

Urinary retention and potential for infection are the primary problems. Failure to treat the cause of obstruction leads to infection and acute kidney injury (AKI).

Urologic Interventions. If obstruction is caused by a kidney stone (calculus), it can be located and removed using cystoscopic or retrograde urogram procedures. See Chapter 58 for more information about kidney stone management. After stone removal, a plastic stent is usually left in the ureter for a few weeks to improve urine flow in the area irritated by the stone. The stent is later removed by another cystoscopic procedure.

Radiologic Interventions. When an abnormal narrowing of the urinary tract (stricture) causes hydronephrosis and cannot be corrected with urologic procedures, a nephrostomy is performed. Most nephrostomy drains provide only external drainage (diversion). Other styles of nephrostomy drains enter the kidney and extend to the bladder, draining urine out to a bag or past a ureteral obstruction and into the bladder. With these, there are both internal and external parts to the nephrostomy tubing. Externally, a fully external or an internal/external diversion drain appears the same. The urine output will fluctuate more if all urine goes to the bladder before external drainage.

Patient Preparation. If possible, the patient is kept NPO for 4 to 6 hours before the procedure. Clotting studies (e.g., international normalized ratio [INR], prothrombin time [PT], and partial thromboplastin time [PTT]) should be normal or corrected. Drugs are used to reduce hypertension. The patient receives moderate sedation for the procedure.

Procedure. The patient is placed in the prone position. The kidney is located under ultrasound or fluoroscopic guidance, and a local anesthetic is given. A needle is placed into the kidney, a soft-tipped guidewire is placed through the needle, and then a catheter is placed over the wire. The catheter tip remains in the renal pelvis, and the external end is connected to a drainage bag. The procedure immediately relieves the pressure and prevents further damage. The nephrostomy tube remains in place until the obstruction is resolved.

Follow-up Care. Assess the amount of drainage in the collection bag. The amount of drainage depends on whether a ureteral catheter is also being used (with a separate drainage bag). Patients with ureteral tubes may have all urine pass through to the bladder or may have it drain into the collection bags. The type of urine drainage system placed must be clearly communicated in the chart. If urine is expected to drain into the collection bag, assess the amount of drainage hourly for the first 24 hours. If the amount of drainage decreases and the patient has back pain, the tube may be clogged or dislodged.

Monitor the nephrostomy site for leaking urine or blood. Urine drainage may be bloody for the first 12 to 24 hours after the procedure and should gradually clear. If prescribed, the nephrostomy tube can be irrigated with 5 mL sterile saline to check patency and dislodge clots. It is common for diuresis to occur when a nephrostomy is placed for obstruction. Monitor intake and output hourly for the first several hours, and inform the surgeon if the patient begins to have symptoms of dehydration (i.e., hypotension, poor skin turgor, dry mucous membranes, increased thirst). Assess for indications of infection (i.e., fever, change in urine character).

✚ NURSING SAFETY PRIORITY
Critical Rescue

After nephrostomy, monitor the patient for indications of complications (i.e., decreased or absent drainage, cloudy or foul-smelling drainage, leakage of blood or urine from the nephrostomy site, back pain) (Martin & Baker, 2019). If any indications are present, respond by notifying the surgeon immediately.

RENOVASCULAR DISEASE

Pathophysiology Review

Processes affecting the renal arteries may severely narrow the lumen and greatly reduce blood flow to the kidney tissues. Uncorrected renovascular disease, such as renal vein thrombosis or renal artery stenosis (RAS), atherosclerosis, or thrombosis, causes ischemia and atrophy of kidney tissue, leading to severe impairment of urinary *elimination, fluid and electrolyte balance,* and *acid-base balance* (Fig. 59.5).

Patients with renovascular disease, particularly those older than 50 years, often have a sudden onset of hypertension. Patients with high blood pressure but no family history of hypertension also may potentially have RAS. RAS from atherosclerosis or blood vessel hyperplasia is the main cause of renovascular disease. Other causes include thrombosis and renal vessel aneurysms.

Atherosclerotic changes in the renal artery often occur along with sclerosis in the aorta and in other major vessels. Renal artery changes are often located where the renal artery and aorta meet. Fibrotic changes of the blood vessel wall occur throughout the length of the renal artery.

Interprofessional Collaborative Care

Recognize Cues: Assessment

Hypertension usually first occurs after age 40 to 50, and often the patient does not have a family history of hypertension (Box 59.7). Diagnosis of renovascular disease is made by magnetic resonance angiography (MRA), renal ultrasound, radionuclide imaging, or renal arteriography. MRA provides an excellent image of the renal vasculature and kidney anatomy. Radionuclide imaging is a noninvasive way of evaluating kidney blood flow and excretory function. Combining radionuclide imaging with ingestion of an angiotensin-converting enzyme inhibitor (ACEI) such as lisinopril improves the accuracy of the test. A renal arteriogram makes the features of the renal blood vessels visible.

Take Actions: Interventions

Identifying the type of defect, extent of narrowing, and condition of the surrounding blood vessels is critical for treatment choice, as is the patient's overall health. Many patients with renovascular disease also have cardiovascular disease, and both conditions require treatment.

RAS may be managed by drugs to control high blood pressure and by procedures to restore the blood supply to the kidney. Drugs may control high blood pressure but may not lead to long-term preservation of kidney function. In younger adults, a lifetime of treatment with many drugs for high blood pressure makes treatment difficult and outcomes uncertain.

Endovascular techniques are nonsurgical approaches to repair RAS. Stent placement with or without balloon angioplasty is an example of an endovascular intervention (see Chapter 30). These techniques are less risky and require less time for recovery than does renal artery bypass surgery. After the procedure, the patient usually remains under close observation for 24 hours to monitor for sudden blood pressure fluctuations as the kidneys adjust to increased blood flow.

Renal artery bypass surgery is a major procedure and requires 2 or more months for recovery. A bypass may be performed for either one or both renal arteries. A synthetic blood vessel graft is inserted to redirect blood flow from the abdominal aorta into the renal artery, beyond the area of narrowing. A splenorenal bypass can also restore blood flow to the kidney. The process is similar to other arterial bypass procedures (see Chapter 30).

DIABETIC NEPHROPATHY

Diabetic nephropathy is a vascular complication of diabetes mellitus (DM) and the leading cause of chronic kidney disease in the world. Approximately 40% of patients who are diabetic will develop diabetic kidney disease (Du et al., 2021). It occurs with either type 1 or type 2 DM. Severity of diabetic kidney disease is related to the degree of hyperglycemia the patient generally experiences. With poor control of hyperglycemia, the complicating problems of atherosclerosis, hypertension, and neuropathy (which promotes loss of bladder tone, urinary stasis, and urinary tract infection) are more severe and more likely to cause kidney damage. Chapter 56 discusses diabetic nephropathy. Management of diabetic nephropathy is the same as for chronic kidney disease (see Chapter 60).

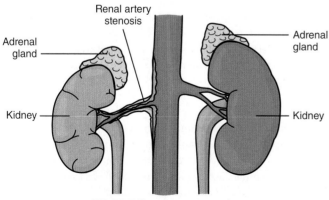

FIG. 59.5 Renal artery stenosis.

> ### BOX 59.7 Key Features
> #### Renovascular Disease
>
> - Significant, difficult-to-control high blood pressure
> - Poorly controlled diabetes or sustained hyperglycemia
> - Elevated serum creatinine
> - Decreased glomerular filtration rate (GFR)

RENAL CELL CARCINOMA

Pathophysiology Review

Renal cell carcinoma (RCC) or adenocarcinoma of the kidney is the most common type of kidney cancer and occurs as a result of impaired cellular regulation. Healthy kidney tissue is damaged and replaced by cancer cells, which impairs urine *elimination* for that kidney.

Systemic effects occurring with this cancer type are called *paraneoplastic syndromes* and include anemia, erythrocytosis, hypercalcemia, and liver dysfunction with elevated liver enzymes, hormonal effects, increased sedimentation rate, and hypertension.

Anemia and erythrocytosis may seem confusing; however, most patients with this cancer have *either* anemia *or* erythrocytosis, not both at the same time. There is some blood loss from hematuria, but the small amount lost does not cause anemia. The cause of the anemia and the erythrocytosis is related to kidney cell production of erythropoietin. At times, the tumor cells produce large amounts of erythropoietin, causing erythrocytosis. At other times, the tumor cells destroy the erythropoietin-producing kidney cells and anemia results.

Parathyroid hormone produced by tumor cells can cause hypercalcemia. Other hormonal changes include increased renin levels (causing hypertension) and increased human chorionic gonadotropin (hCG) levels, which decrease libido and change secondary sex features.

RCC has five distinct carcinoma cell types: clear cell, papillary cell, chromophobe cell, collecting duct carcinoma, and unclassified type (Rogers, 2023).

Kidney tumors are classified into four stages (Box 59.8). Complications include metastasis and urinary tract obstruction. The cancer usually spreads to the adrenal gland, liver, lungs, long bones, or the other kidney. When the cancer surrounds a ureter, hydroureter and obstruction may result.

BOX 59.8 Staging Kidney Tumors

Stage I
Tumors ≤7 cm in largest dimension in the kidney. The renal vein, perinephric fat, and adjacent lymph nodes have no tumor.

Stage II
Tumors are >7 cm in largest dimension in the kidney. However, the tumor remains in the kidney with no lymph node involvement.

Stage III
Tumor has penetrated the major veins or perinephric tissues, yet not beyond Gerota fascia. Tumors extend into the lymph nodes but do have distant metastasis.

Stage IV
Tumors include invasion of adjacent organs beyond Gerota fascia or metastasis to distant tissues.

Adapted from Gallardo, E.A. (2017, November 13). *SEOM clinical guideline for treatment of kidney cancer.* Retrieved from U.S. National Library of Medicine, National Institutes of Health. https://www.ncbi.nlm.nih.gov/pmc/articles/PMC5785618/.

The causes of nonhereditary RCC are unknown, but the risk is slightly higher for adults who use tobacco or are exposed to cadmium and other heavy metals, asbestos, benzene, and trichloroethylene. Males are twice as likely to have kidney cancer as females, and this cancer is more common in Black Americans and American Indians and Alaska Native people (American Cancer Society [ACS], 2022).

There are 79,000 new cases of kidney cancer in the United States each year (American Cancer Society, 2022). About 13,920 people die annually from kidney cancer in the United States. Kidney cancer is among the top 10 most common cancers in men and women, with the average age at diagnosis of 64 years. Kidney cancer is not common in people younger than 45 (ACS, 2022).

Interprofessional Collaborative Care

The most common treatment for RCC is a nephrectomy. When the cancer is local (i.e., only in the kidney), a nephrectomy can provide a cure. For patients with metastasis, nephrectomy is followed by targeted chemotherapy combined with cytokine treatment. Patients with RCC are at risk for CKD and cardiovascular complications. Patients need ongoing, interprofessional care with surveillance for best outcomes. Follow-up therapy is managed on an outpatient basis.

Recognize Cues: Assessment

History. Ask the patient about known risk factors (e.g., smoking or chemical exposures), weight loss, changes in urine color, abdominal or flank discomfort, and fever. Also ask whether any other family member has ever been diagnosed with cancer of the kidney, bladder, ureter, prostate gland, uterus, or ovary.

Physical Assessment/Signs and Symptoms. Some patients with RCC have flank pain, obvious blood in the urine, and a kidney mass that can be palpated. Ask about the nature of the flank or abdominal discomfort. Patients often describe the pain as dull and aching. Pain may be more intense if bleeding into the tumor or kidney occurs. Inspect the flank area, checking for asymmetry or an obvious bulge. An abdominal mass may be felt with *gentle* palpation. A renal bruit may be heard on auscultation.

Bloody urine is a *late* common sign. Blood may be visible as bright red flecks or clots, or the urine may appear smoky or cola colored. Without gross hematuria, microscopic examination may or may not reveal red blood cells (RBCs).

Inspect the skin for pallor/ash gray appearance, darkening of the nipples, and, in men, breast enlargement (*gynecomastia*) caused by changing hormonal levels. Other findings may include muscle wasting, weakness, and weight loss. All tend to occur late in the disease.

Diagnostic Assessment. Urinalysis may show RBCs. Hematologic studies show decreased hemoglobin and hematocrit values, hypercalcemia, increased erythrocyte sedimentation rate, and increased levels of adrenocorticotropic hormone, human chorionic gonadotropin (hCG), cortisol, renin, and parathyroid hormone. Elevated serum creatinine and blood urea nitrogen (BUN) levels indicate impaired kidney function.

Kidney masses may be detected by CT scan or MRI. RCC is often identified incidentally, as a result of another imaging study (Pullen, 2021). This is often when the patient is asymptomatic and when the RCC is in the early stage. Ultrasound is also used to detect masses or for initial screening. Kidney biopsy may be considered to help target therapy.

Take Actions: Interventions

Treatment for kidney cancer focuses on preventing the spread of the cancer and managing complications. Chemotherapy is not as effective when treating advanced kidney cancers. Targeted therapies that block the growth of new blood vessels that nourish cancer and immunotherapies can be effective (ACS, 2021).

Nonsurgical Management. Microwave ablation or cryoablation can slow tumor growth. It is a minimally invasive procedure carried out after MRI has precisely located the tumor. Microwave ablation is used most commonly for patients who have only one kidney or who are not surgical candidates.

Traditional chemotherapy has limited effectiveness against this cancer type (Pullen, 2021). Immunotherapy, such as interleukin-2 and interferon (IFN), and immunomodulating drugs are often used for treatment (Pullen, 2021). See Chapter 18.

Surgical Management. Renal cell carcinoma (RCC) is usually treated surgically by *nephrectomy* (kidney removal). Renal cell tumors are highly vascular, and blood loss during surgery is a major concern. Before surgery, the arteries supplying the kidney may be occluded (embolized) by the interventional radiologist to reduce bleeding during nephrectomy.

Preoperative Care. Instruct the patient about surgical routines (see Chapter 9). Explain the probable site of incision and the presence of dressings, drains, or other equipment after surgery. Reassure the patient about pain relief. Care before surgery may include giving blood and fluids IV to prevent shock.

Operative Procedures. The patient is placed on the nonoperative side, with the kidney to be removed uppermost. The trunk area is flexed to increase exposure of the kidney area. The eleventh or twelfth rib may need to be removed to provide better access to the kidney. The surgeon removes either part or all of the kidney and all visible tumor. The renal artery, renal vein, and fascia also may be removed. A drain may be placed in the wound before closure. The adrenal gland may be removed when the tumor is near this organ.

When a *radical* nephrectomy is performed, local and regional lymph nodes are also removed. The surgical approach may be transthoracic (as discussed in the previous paragraph), lumbar, or through the abdomen, depending on the size and location of the tumor. Radiation therapy may follow a radical nephrectomy.

Postoperative Care. Refer to Chapter 9 for care of the patient after surgery. Nursing priorities are focused on assessing kidney function to determine effectiveness of the remaining kidney, pain management, and preventing complications.

Monitoring includes assessing for hemorrhage and adrenal insufficiency. Inspect the patient's abdomen for distention from bleeding. Check the bed linens under the patient because blood may pool there. Hemorrhage or adrenal insufficiency causes hypotension, decreased urine output, and an altered level of consciousness.

A decrease in blood pressure is an early sign of both hemorrhage and adrenal insufficiency. With hypotension, urine output also decreases immediately. Large water and sodium losses in the urine occur in patients with adrenal insufficiency, leading to impaired *fluid and electrolyte balance.* As a result, a large urine output is followed by hypotension and oliguria (less than 400 mL/24 hr or less than 25 mL/hr). IV replacement of fluids and packed RBCs may be needed.

The second kidney is expected to provide adequate function, but this may take days or weeks. Assess urine output hourly for the first 24 hours after surgery (urine output of 0.5 mL/kg/hr or about 30 to 50 mL/hr is acceptable). A low urine output of less than 25 to 30 mL/hr suggests decreased blood flow to the remaining kidney and potential for acute kidney injury (AKI). The hemoglobin level, hematocrit values, and white blood cell count may be measured every 6 to 12 hours for the first day or two after surgery.

Monitor the patient's temperature, pulse rate, and respiratory rate at least every 4 hours. Accurately measure and record fluid intake and output. Weigh the patient daily.

The patient may be in a special care unit for 24 to 48 hours after surgery for monitoring of bleeding and adrenal insufficiency. A drain placed near the site of incision removes residual fluid. Because of the discomfort of deep breathing, the patient is at risk for atelectasis. Fever, chills, thick sputum, or decreased breath sounds suggest pneumonia.

Managing pain after surgery usually requires opioid analgesics given IV. The incision was made through major muscle groups used with breathing and movement. Liberal use of analgesics is needed for 3 to 5 days after surgery to manage pain. Oral agents may be tried when the patient can eat and drink.

The prevention of complications focuses on infection and management of adrenal insufficiency. Antibiotics may be prescribed during and after surgery to prevent infection. The need for additional antibiotics is based on evidence of infection. Assess the patient at least every 8 hours for indications of systemic infection or local wound infection.

Adrenal insufficiency is possible as a complication of kidney and adrenal gland removal. Although only one adrenal gland may be affected, the remaining gland may not be able to secrete sufficient glucocorticoids immediately after surgery. Steroid replacements may be needed in some patients. Chapter 54 discusses the signs and symptoms of acute adrenal insufficiency in detail, along with specific nursing interventions.

NCLEX Examination Challenge 59.2
Physiological Integrity

The nurse is caring for a male client 8 hours after a nephrectomy. Which assessment finding requires **immediate** nursing intervention?

A. Abdominal distention

B. Urine output 38 mL in the last hour

C. Blood pressure 108/64 mm Hg

D. Hemoglobin 14 g/dL (Reference range: 14–18 g/dL)

KIDNEY TRAUMA

Pathophysiology Review

Trauma to one or both kidneys may occur with penetrating wounds or blunt injuries to the back, flank, or abdomen. Another cause of kidney trauma is urologic procedures. Blunt trauma accounts for most kidney injuries. Traumatic kidney injury is classified into five grades, based on the severity of the injury. Grade 1 consists of low-grade injury in the form of kidney bruising, and grade 5 represents the most severe variety, associated with shattering of the kidney and tearing of its blood supply. Adults of any age can sustain kidney trauma. Strategies to prevent trauma are reviewed in Box 59.9.

Interprofessional Collaborative Care

Recognize Cues: Assessment

Obtain a history of the patient's usual health and the events involved in the trauma from the patient, a witness, or emergency personnel. Document the mechanism of injury to help determine the severity of the injury. For example, blunt trauma of the kidney from car crashes usually results in an injury of low severity. Critical information to acquire is a history of kidney or urologic disease, surgical intervention, or health problems such as diabetes or hypertension.

Ureteral or renal pelvic injury often causes diffuse abdominal pain. Urine outside of the urinary tract may be visible. Ask the patient about pain in the flank or abdomen.

Assess patients with kidney injuries carefully and thoroughly. Take the patient's blood pressure, apical and peripheral pulses, respiratory rate, and temperature. Inspect both flanks for bruising, asymmetry, or penetrating injuries. Also inspect the abdomen, chest, and lower back for bruising or wounds. Percuss the abdomen for distention. Inspect the urethra for blood.

Urinalysis shows hemoglobin or RBCs from tissue damage or kidney blood vessel rupture. Microscopic examination may also show red blood cell casts, which suggest tubular damage. Hemoglobin and hematocrit values decrease with blood loss.

Diagnostic procedures include ultrasound and CT. CT scan shows greater detail about blood vessel and tissue integrity. Hematomas within or through the kidney capsule can be seen, along with the integrity and patency of the urinary tract. If the patient is being taken to the operating room emergently, a high dose of ionic or nonionic IV contrast material can be given, followed by an abdominal x-ray (KUB) to visualize the traumatic injury and any organ damage.

BOX 59.9 **Patient and Family Education**

Preventing Kidney and Genitourinary Trauma

- Wear a seat belt.
- Practice safe walking habits.
- Use caution when riding bicycles and motorcycles.
- Wear appropriate protective clothing when participating in contact sports.
- Avoid all contact sports and high-risk activities if you have only one kidney.

Take Actions: Interventions

Nonsurgical Management. A combination of both drug and fluid therapy may be used to replace blood components and coagulation factors. Drug therapy is used for bleeding prevention or control. Fluid therapy is used to restore circulating blood volume and ensure adequate kidney blood flow. During fluid restoration, give fluids at the prescribed rate and monitor the patient for signs of shock. Take vital signs as often as every 5 to 15 minutes. Measure and record urine output hourly. Output should be greater than 0.5 mL/kg/hr.

The interventional radiologist may use percutaneous or other instrumentation to drain collections of fluid or to embolize (clot) an artery or artery segment or place a stent to repair the urethra or ureters.

! NURSING SAFETY PRIORITY

Action Alert

If the urethral opening is bleeding, consult with the urologist or primary health care provider before attempting urinary catheterization to avoid making the injury worse.

Surgical Management. Most kidney injuries are managed without surgery. Many serious injuries can be treated with minimally invasive techniques such as angiographic embolization, which accesses the arteries of the kidneys through large blood vessels in the groin, similar to a cardiac catheterization. Surgery to explore the injured kidney occurs when the patient is in shock and may be losing a lot of blood from the kidney. Patients who have other significant abdominal injuries, such as injuries to the bowel, spleen, or liver, and require a laparotomy may also undergo inspection and repair of the injured kidney at the same time. The aim of surgical management is to repair the injured kidney and restore its *elimination* function. If the kidney is severely injured (grade 5 injury), a nephrectomy is performed.

Care Coordination and Transition Management

Teach the patient and family how to assess for infection and other complications after kidney trauma. The most common complications are urine leakage and delayed bleeding. Instruct the patient to check the pattern and frequency of urination and to note whether the color, clarity, and amount appear normal. The development of an abscess surrounding the kidney also can occur. Instruct the patient to seek medical attention for worsening hematuria, any worrisome change, or pain with voiding. Chills, fever, lethargy, and cloudy, foul-smelling urine indicate a urinary tract infection or abscess formation. Traumatic kidney injury can also cause hypertension from changes in perfusion and activation of the renin-angiotensin-aldosterone system (see Chapter 57). Advise the patient to seek medical care promptly for all new and concerning signs or symptoms.

GET READY FOR THE NEXT-GENERATION NCLEX® EXAMINATION!

Essential Nursing Care Points

Health Promotion/Disease Prevention	Chronic Disease Care
• Encourage patients with diabetes to achieve tight glycemic control • Encourage patients with hypertension to follow their treatment regimens to maintain proper blood pressure • Refer patients with polycystic kidney disease to a geneticist or a genetic counselor. • Teach patients to match daily urine output with fluid intake, usually at least 2 L for kidney health, unless another health problem requires fluid restriction. • Use language with which the patient is comfortable during assessment of the kidney and urinary system.	• Teach patients with any kidney disorder about strategies to prevent kidney damage from dehydration or trauma. • Instruct patients with any type of kidney problem to weigh daily and to notify the primary health care provider if there is a sudden weight gain. • Be aware of the relationship between kidney disease and hypertension and the associated risk for cardiovascular events. • Use laboratory data and signs and symptoms to determine the effectiveness of therapy for pyelonephritis, polycystic kidney disease, glomerulonephritis (GN), and renal cell carcinoma (RCC).
Regenerative or Restorative Care	**Hospice/Palliative/Supportive Care**
• Report immediately to the primary health care provider sudden decreases of urine output in a patient with kidney disease or trauma. Expected adult urine output is 0.5 to 1 mL/kg/hr. • Check the blood pressure and urine output frequently in patients who have any type of kidney problem. • Teach patients on antibiotic therapy for a UTI (pyelonephritis) to complete the drug regimen. • Teach patients the expected side effects and any adverse reactions to prescribed drugs, especially as they relate to kidney function.	• Allow the patient to express fear or anxiety regarding the potential for chronic kidney disease and end-stage kidney disease. • Some kidney conditions can lead to end-stage kidney disease (ESKD) and may require palliative care consults for support.

Mastery Questions

1. The nurse is teaching a client who experienced kidney trauma 3 days ago and is now being discharged to home. Which teaching would the nurse provide?
   A. Monitor blood pressure carefully for signs of hypotension.
   B. Observe your urine for color and clarity.
   C. Pain can be managed with over-the-counter aspirin.
   D. Lethargy and fever may be present for the next week.

2. The nurse is caring for a client postnephrostomy for treatment of hydronephrosis. Which of the following assessments indicates a possible complication? **Select all that apply.**
   A. Tenderness at the surgical site
   B. Pink-tinged urine draining from the nephrostomy
   C. Urine output of 15 mL for the first hour and then diminishing
   D. A hematocrit value 3% lower than the preoperative value
   E. Sudden onset of abdominal pain that worsens after abdominal palpation

NGN Challenge 59.1

59.1.1

The nurse documents assessment findings for a 48-year-old in the emergency department.

Highlight the findings that would require **immediate** follow-up.

History and Physical	Nurses' Notes	Vital Signs	Laboratory Results

1400: Brought to the emergency department by squad after experiencing pain with urination rated as a 10 on a 0-to-10 scale, severe headache, and flank pain. Health history includes diabetes mellitus, high cholesterol, anxiety, and joint pain. The client takes metformin 500 mg twice daily, simvastatin 20 mg at bedtime, and escitalopram 20 mg at bedtime. The client also reports taking acetaminophen regularly for joint pain. The client works in health care, has two children, and is married. Height: 64.8 in (164.5 cm); weight: 208 lb (94 kg). VS: T 102.8°F (39.3°C); HR 120 beats/min; RR 26 breaths/min; BP 140/90 mm Hg. Spo$_2$ 94% on RA.

59.1.2

The nurse is prioritizing care for this client based on current assessment data.

History and Physical	Nurses' Notes	Vital Signs	Laboratory Results

1405: Client transferred to stretcher and a large-bore IV is inserted into the left forearm. Initial labs drawn per ED protocol. Placed client on cardiac monitor and recurrent blood pressure monitoring. The client is groaning in pain and states, "I feel like I need to urinate, but I cannot. It hurts so bad." A small amount of urine leakage noted with gentle palpation over the bladder area. Bedside blood glucose is 121 mg/dL (range: 74 to 106 mg/dL (4.1 to 5.9 mmol/L).

Complete the following sentence by selecting from the list of word choices below.

Based on the analysis of client findings, the nurse determines that the client is at high risk for **1 [Select]**, as evidenced by **2 [Select]** and **3 [Select]**.

Options for 1	Options for 2	Options for 3
Diabetic ketoacidosis	Glucose 121 mg/dL	Groaning
Pyelonephritis	Urine leakage with bladder palpation	Elevated BMI
Glomerulonephritis	Spo$_2$ 94% on RA	Respirations 26 breaths/min
Hydronephrosis	History of joint pain	History of acetaminophen use

59.1.3

The nurse continues to assess the client and reviews the documentation.

Complete the following sentence(s) by selecting from the list of word choices below.

Based on analysis of documented assessment findings, the nurse determines that the *priority* for the client at this time is to manage [Word Choice] to prevent [Word Choice].

Word Choices
Urinary retention
Kidney injury
Blood sugar
Pain
Anxiety

59.1.4

The client is seen by the health care provider in the ED, and testing reveals a urinary stricture. A urology consult is made, and the client is scheduled for a nephrostomy. The nurse is preparing the client for the nephrostomy procedure and reviews the most recent laboratory values.

Highlight the values that would require follow-up.

Urinalysis Results

Parameter	Result	Reference Range
Appearance	Cloudy	Clear
Color	Yellow	Amber yellow
Odor	Aromatic	Aromatic
White blood cells	6	0–4
Leukocyte esterase	Positive	Negative
Nitrites	Positive	None
Red blood cells	1	≤2

59.1.5

The nurse is caring for the client postnephrostomy. Which of the following actions would the nurse take? **Select all that apply.**

○ Notify the provider if the client reports excessive thirst.
○ Explain that urine will leak from the nephrostomy site.
○ Monitor vital signs hourly or more frequently as needed.
○ Compare current BP results with admission BP.
○ Administer acetaminophen for reports of back pain.
○ Expect pink-tinged urine for the first 12 to 24 hours.
○ Assess patency of the nephrostomy tube by irrigating with saline.

59.1.6

The nurse is preparing the client for discharge 48 hours after the nephrectomy.

For each current client finding, indicate whether the client's condition has improved, not changed, or worsened.

Current Client Finding	Improved	Not Changed	Worsened
Pain level 2 on a 0-to-10 scale			
Temperature 99.2°F (37.3°C)			
Bloody urine			
Bedside glucose 120 mg/dL Range: 74 to 106 mg/dL (4.1 to 5.9 mmol/L)			
Urinalysis WBC 4			

REFERENCES

American Cancer Society. (2021). *Targeted therapies for kidney cancer.* Retrieved from American Cancer Society https://www.cancer.org/cancer/kidney-cancer/treating/targeted-therapy.html.

American Cancer Society. (2022). *Key statistics about kidney cancer.* https://www.cancer.org/cancer/kidney-cancer/about/key-statistics.html.

Ayatollahi, J., Mousavi, S., Hajighasemi, A., & Shahcheraghi, S. (2021). Belya The most common causes of bacteremia and determination of antibiotic sensitivity pattern. *International Medicine,* 117–121.

Bellos, I. (2021). Safety profile of tolvaptan in the treatment of autosomal dominant polycystic kidney disease. *Therapeutics and Clinical Risk Management, 17,* 649–656. https://doi.org/10.2147/TCRM.S286952.

Belyayeva, M., & Jeong, J. M. (2021). Acute Pyelonephritis. In *StatPearls [Internet].* Treasure Island (FL): StatPearls Publishing. 2021 Jan. Available from: https://www.ncbi.nlm.nih.gov/books/NBK519537/.

Bennett, W., Rahbari-Oskoui, F., & Chapman, A. (2023). Patient education: Polycystic kidney disease (Beyond the basics). *UpToDate.* Retrieved February 7, 2023, from https://www.uptodate.com/contents/polycystic-kidney-disease-beyond-the-basics.

Bleyer, A. (2023). Gene test interpretation: APOL1 (chronic kidney disease gene). *UpToDate.* Retrieved February 7, 2023, from https://www.uptodate.com/contents/gene-test-interpretation-apol1-chronic-kidney-disease-gene.

Centers for Disease Control and Prevention. (2021). *Chronic kidney disease in the United States.* 2021 https://www.cdc.gov/kidneydisease/publications-resources/ckd-national-facts.html.

Deng, X., & Zhang, J. (2022). CKD in Minorities: Non-Hispanic Blacks, Hispanics, Asians, and Indian Americans. In J. McCauley, S. M. Hamrahian, & O. H. Maarouf (Eds.), *Approaches to Chronic Kidney Disease.* Cham: Springer. https://doi.org/10.1007/978-3-030-83082-3_19.

Du, X., Liu, J., Xue, Y., et al. (2021). Alteration of gut microbial profile in patients with diabetic nephropathy. *Endocrine, 73,* 71–84(2021). https://doi.org/10.1007/s12020-021-02721-1.

Fukaguchi, K., Yamagami, H., Soeno, S., Liu, K., Nakamura, K., & Goto, T. (2022). The diagnostic accuracy of costovertebral angle tenderness in the emergency department. *Annals of Emergency Medicine, 78*(4), 376–377. https://doi.org/10.1016/j.annemergmed.2021.09.392.

Ma, T., & Lambert, K. (2021). What are the information needs and concerns of individuals with Polycystic Kidney Disease? Results of an online survey using Facebook and social listening analysis. *BMC Nephrology, 22,* 263. https://doi.org/10.1186/s12882-021-02472-1.

Martin, R., & Baker, H. (2019). Nursing care and management of patients with a nephrostomy. *Nursing Times [Online], 115*(11), 40–43.

Mitchell-Brown, F., & Veisze, T. (2019). Minimal change disease: A case report. *Nursing 2019, 49*(1), 33–37.

Nishio, S., Tsuchiya, K., Nakatani, S., et al. (2021). A digest from evidence-based Clinical Practice Guideline for Polycystic Kidney Disease 2020. *Clin Exp Nephrol, 25,* 1292–1302 (2021). Doi: ezproxy.liberty.edu/10.1007/s10157-021-02097-6.

Oda, T., & Yoshizawa, N. (2021). Factors Affecting the Progression of Infection-Related Glomerulonephritis to Chronic Kidney Disease. *International Journal of Molecular Sciences, 2021, 22,* 905. https://doi.org/10.3390/ijms22020905.

Pullen, R. (2021). Renal cell carcinoma, part 2. *Nursing 2021, 51*(8), 25–30.

Rankin, A., Mayne, K., Allwood-Spiers, S., et al. (2021). Will advances in functional renal magnetic resonance imaging translate to the nephrology clinic? *Nephrology,* 1–8. https://doi.org/10.1111/nep.13985.

Rogers, J. L. (2023). *McCance and Huether's Pathophysiology: The biologic basis for disease in adults and children* (9th ed.). St. Louis: Elsevier.

Torres, V., & Bennett, W. (2023). Autosomal dominant polycystic kidney disease (ADPKD) in adults: Epidemiology, clinical presentation, and diagnosis. *UpToDate.* Retrieved February 7, 2023, from https://www.uptodate.com/contents/autosomal-dominant-polycystic-kidney-disease-adpkd-in-adults-epidemiology-clinical-presentation-and-diagnosis. [Accessed 7 February 2023].

Yan, G., Liu, G., Tian, X., et al. (2020). Establishment of a novel nomogram for the clinically diagnostic prediction of minimal change disease, –a common cause of nephrotic syndrome. *BMC Nephrology, 21,* 396. https://doi.org/10.1186/s12882-020-02058-3.

60

Concepts of Care for Patients With Acute Kidney Injury and Chronic Kidney Disease

Robyn Mitchell

http://evolve.elsevier.com/Iggy/

LEARNING OUTCOMES

1. Plan collaborative care with the interprofessional team to promote urinary *elimination* in patients with acute kidney injury or chronic kidney disease.
2. Teach adults how to decrease the risk for acute kidney injury and chronic kidney disease.
3. Teach the patient and caregiver(s) about common drugs and other management strategies used for acute kidney injury and chronic kidney disease.
4. Plan patient- and family-centered nursing interventions to decrease the psychosocial impact caused by living with acute kidney injury and chronic kidney disease.
5. Apply knowledge of anatomy, physiology, and pathophysiology to provide evidence-based care for patients with acute kidney injury and chronic kidney disease

affecting urinary *elimination, fluid and electrolyte balance,* and *acid-base balance.*
6. Analyze assessment and diagnostic findings to generate solutions and prioritize nursing care for patients with acute kidney injury or chronic kidney disease.
7. Organize care coordination and transition management for patients with acute kidney injury or chronic kidney disease.
8. Use clinical judgment to plan evidence-based nursing care to promote urinary function and prevent complications in patients with acute kidney injury and chronic kidney disease.
9. Incorporate factors that affect health equity into the plan of care for patients with acute kidney injury or chronic kidney disease.

KEY TERMS

acute kidney injury (AKI) A rapid reduction in kidney function resulting in a failure to maintain waste *elimination, fluid and electrolyte balance,* and *acid-base balance.*

azotemia An excess of nitrogenous wastes (urea) in the blood.

cardiorenal syndrome Disorders of the kidney or heart that cause dysfunction in the other organ.

dialysate Solution used in dialysis that contains a balanced mix of electrolytes and water and that closely resembles human plasma.

diffusion Movement of molecules from an area of higher concentration to an area of lower concentration.

hyperpnea Abnormal increase in the depth of respiratory movements.

Kussmaul respiration Breathing pattern with respirations that are fast and deep; often associated with metabolic acidosis.

melena Blood in the stool with the appearance of black, tarry stool.

oliguria Urine output less than 400 mL/day.

pruritus Itching.

renal osteodystrophy Bone metabolism and structural damage caused by chronic kidney disease–induced low calcium levels and high phosphorus levels.

uremia The accumulation of nitrogenous wastes in the blood (azotemia); a result of renal failure, with clinical symptoms that include nausea and vomiting.

uremic frost Layer of urea crystals from evaporated sweat; may appear on the face, eyebrows, axillae, and groin in patients with advanced uremic syndrome.

uremic syndrome The systemic clinical and laboratory manifestations of end-stage kidney disease.

⁂ PRIORITY AND INTERRELATED CONCEPTS

The priority concept for this chapter is:

- *Elimination*

  The *Elimination* concept exemplar for this chapter is Chronic Kidney Disease.

The interrelated concepts for this chapter are:

- *Acid-Base Balance*
- *Fluid and Electrolyte Balance*
- *Immunity*
- *Perfusion*

The kidney function of urinary *elimination* includes excretion of waste, *fluid and electrolyte balance,* regulation of *acid-base balance,* and hormone secretion. These processes are greatly impaired with kidney function loss, and every organ system is affected. Acute kidney injury (AKI) is most common in the acute care setting, whereas chronic kidney disease (CKD) is more likely to be seen in community settings or as a coexisting condition in acute care settings. The features of AKI and CKD are described in Table 60.1.

Both types of kidney problems can require kidney replacement therapy (KRT; e.g., dialysis). When kidney function is permanently or persistently impaired, as with end-stage kidney disease (ESKD), dialysis or kidney transplant is a lifesaving approach for urinary *elimination* to maintain homeostasis, *fluid and electrolyte balance,* and *acid-base balance.* ESKD reduces independence, shortens life, and decreases quality of life. Many diseases and conditions are associated with the onset and severity of kidney function loss.

When kidney function declines gradually, it is diagnosed as CKD, formerly termed *chronic renal failure (CRF).* The patient may have many years of abnormal blood urea nitrogen (BUN) and creatinine values, sometimes called *renal insufficiency,* before ESKD develops. When kidney function decline is sudden, acute kidney injury (AKI) is diagnosed. AKI can be a temporary condition that resolves, or it can progress to CKD.

Even when AKI does not progress to CKD, AKI is associated with higher morbidity and mortality, even in young patients without other chronic diseases that increase risks (Fuhrman, 2018). AKI also can occur in a patient with established CKD. When these two conditions co-occur, the loss of kidney function and waste *elimination* is usually more severe and accelerated.

Acute kidney injury affects *many* body systems. Chronic kidney disease affects *every* body system. The problems that occur with kidney function loss are related to disturbances of *fluid and electrolyte balance,* disturbances of *acid-base balance,* buildup of nitrogen-based wastes (uremia), and loss of kidney hormone function.

ACUTE KIDNEY INJURY

Pathophysiology Review

Acute kidney injury (AKI) is a rapid reduction in kidney function resulting in a failure to maintain waste *elimination, fluid and electrolyte balance,* and *acid-base balance.* AKI occurs over a few hours or days. The most current definition of AKI is an increase in serum creatinine by 0.3 mg/dL (26.2 mcmol/L) or more within 48 hours; or an increase in serum creatinine to 1.5 times or more from baseline, which is known or presumed to have occurred in the previous 7 days; or a urine volume of less than 0.5 mL/kg/hr for 6 hours. Criteria for staging the severity of AKI are listed in Table 60.2. The Kidney Disease: Improving Global Outcomes (KDIGO) classification is a universal definition and staging system for AKI.

The creatinine level is most commonly used in the recognition of AKI. However, this value is not ideal because the creatinine level takes time to increase, which can create delays in treatment. A baseline creatinine value is also necessary to evaluate for AKI, as this provides a means for comparison.

Biomarkers that are specific to kidney injury have been approved by the U.S. Food and Drug Administration (FDA) (Gilbert & Weiner, 2023). These biomarkers indicate damage earlier than the creatinine level and do not require a baseline value for comparison. These biomarkers specific to kidney injury can be

TABLE 60.1   Features of Acute Kidney Injury and Chronic Kidney Disease

Characteristic	Acute Kidney Injury	Chronic Kidney Disease
Onset	Sudden (hours to days)	Gradual (months to years)
Percentage of nephron involvement	50%–95%	Varies by stage; generally symptomatic with 75% loss and dialysis with 90%–95% loss
Duration	May not progress; full recovery (return to baseline) possible ESKD occurs in 10%–20% with lifetime reliance on dialysis or kidney transplant	Progressive and permanent Treatment and lifestyle can slow progression and delay onset of ESKD
Prognosis	Good when kidney function is maintained or returns High mortality associated with renal replacement therapy requirements or prolonged illness	Progression of CKD depends on stage of GFR, stage of albuminuria, and specific conditions associated with the onset of the disorder ESKD fatal without renal replacement therapy (dialysis or transplantation) Reduced lifespan and potential for complex medical regimen even with optimal treatment

CKD, Chronic kidney disease; *ESKD,* end-stage kidney disease; *GFR,* glomerular filtration rate.

TABLE 60.2   The KDIGO Classification System for Severity of Acute Kidney Injury

Stage	Serum Creatinine	Urine Output
Stage 1	1.5–1.9 times baseline OR ≥0.3 mg/dL (≥26.5 µmol/L) increase over 48 hr	<0.5 mL/kg/hr for 6–12 hr
Stage 2	2.0–2.9 times baseline	<0.5 mL/kg/hr for ≥12 hr
Stage 3	3.0 times baseline OR Increase in serum creatinine to ≥4.0 mg/dL (≥353.6 µmol/L) OR Initiation of renal replacement therapy OR In patients <18 yr, decrease in eGFR to <35 mL/min/1.73 m²	Anuria lasting for ≥12 hr OR <0.3 mL/kg/hr for ≥24 hr

eGFR, Estimated glomerular filtration rate; *KDIGO,* Kidney Disease: Improving Global Outcomes (2012).
From Kidney Disease Improving Global Outcomes (KDIGO). (2012). Clinical Practice Guideline for Acute Kidney Injury, *Kidney Int Suppl* 2:1–138.

BOX 60.1   Systemic Complications From Acute Kidney Injury

Metabolic
- Metabolic acidosis
- Hyperlipidemia
- Hyperkalemia
- Hyponatremia
- Hypocalcemia
- Hypophosphatemia

Cardiopulmonary
- Peripheral and pulmonary edema
- Heart failure
- Pulmonary embolism
- Pericarditis
- Pericardial effusion
- Hypertension
- Myocardial infarction

Neurologic
- Neuromuscular irritability or weakness
- Asterixis
- Seizures
- Mental status changes

Immune/Infectious
- Pneumonia
- Sepsis

Gastrointestinal
- Nausea
- Vomiting
- Decreased peristalsis
- Enteral nutrition intolerance
- Malnutrition
- Ulcer formation
- Bleeding

Hematologic
- Bleeding
- Thrombosis
- Anemia

Renal
- Chronic kidney disease (CKD)
- End-stage kidney disease (ESKD)

Other
- Hiccups
- Elevated parathyroid hormone
- Low thyroid hormone level

used similarly to biomarkers such as troponin in cardiac injury. These biomarkers can identify patients at high risk for developing AKI during the next 12 to 24 hours and include tissue injury metalloproteinase 2 (TIMP-2) and insulin-like growth factor binding protein 7 (IGFBP-7) (Moore, 2018). Earlier identification of risk allows for earlier intervention. Although these biomarkers show significant promise, they are not yet widely used.

Glomerular filtration rate (GFR) is accepted as the best overall indicator of kidney function, but it is not accurate during acute and critical illness (Gilbert & Weiner, 2023). Estimations of GFR from serum creatinine are affected by metabolic problems and treatments during critical illnesses. Urine output is altered when diuretics or IV fluids are used. AKI also causes systemic effects and complications described in Box 60.1. These complications increase discomfort and risk for death. Duration of oliguria or anuria closely correlates with lack of recovery of kidney function; the longer the duration of oliguria or anuria, the less likely it is that the patient will return to full or baseline kidney function.

Etiology

The causes of AKI are reduced *perfusion* to the kidneys, damage to kidney tissue, and obstruction of urine outflow. Urine outflow obstruction along with tissue damage of the kidneys and reduction of perfusion are causes of AKI. Box 60.2 lists causes of AKI along with the diseases and associated conditions. However, the diseases listed in Box 60.1 are described in greater detail in another section of this text. Risk factors for AKI include shock,

cardiac surgery, hypotension, prolonged mechanical ventilation, and sepsis. Older adults or adults with diabetes, hypertension, peripheral vascular disease, liver disease, or CKD are at higher risk of AKI if hospitalized.

AKI is categorized as prerenal, intrinsic renal (also called intrarenal), and postrenal in order to better understand and treat the disorder. Prerenal AKI is caused by a source outside of the kidney creating conditions that impair renal *perfusion.* Common causes include shock, dehydration, burns, and sepsis. Intrinsic renal injury occurs inside the kidney by disorders that directly affect the renal cortex or medulla. Examples of disorders causing intrinsic renal AKI include allergic disorders, embolism or thrombosis of the renal vessels, and nephrotoxic agents. Postrenal AKI is caused by a urine flow obstruction. The obstruction can be caused by tumors, kidney stones, or strictures (Fig. 60.1) (Rogers, 2023).

With prerenal or postrenal pathology, the kidney compensates with the three responses of constricting kidney blood vessels, activating the renin-angiotensin-aldosterone pathway, and releasing antidiuretic hormone (ADH). These responses increase blood volume and improve kidney *perfusion.* However, these same responses reduce urine *elimination,* resulting in

BOX 60.2 Diseases and Conditions That Contribute to Acute Kidney Injury

Perfusion Reduction (Prerenal Causes)
- Blood or fluid loss
- Blood pressure medications
- Heart attack
- Heart disease
- Infection (e.g., sepsis, septic shock)
- Liver failure
- Use of aspirin, ibuprofen, naproxen, or other related drugs
- Severe allergic reaction (anaphylaxis)
- Severe burns
- Severe dehydration
- Renal artery stenosis
- Bleeding or clotting in the kidney blood vessels (coagulopathy)
- Atherosclerosis or cholesterol deposits that block blood flow in the kidneys

Kidney Damage (Intrinsic or Intrarenal Causes)
- Blood clots in nearby veins and arteries
- Cholesterol deposits that block blood flow in the kidneys
- Glomerulonephritis
- Hemolytic uremic syndrome
- Local infection (pyelonephritis)
- Lupus, an immune system disorder causing glomerulonephritis
- Pharmaceuticals, such as certain chemotherapy agents, antibiotics, iodinated or hyperosmolar contrast media used during imaging tests
- Scleroderma, a group of rare diseases affecting the skin and connective tissues
- Thrombotic thrombocytopenic purpura (TTP), a rare platelet disorder that increases clotting

Urine Flow Obstruction (Postrenal Causes)
- Bladder cancer
- Cervical cancer
- Colon cancer
- Prostate cancer
- Enlarged prostate
- Kidney stones
- Nerve damage involving the nerves that control the bladder
- Blood clots in the urinary tract

oliguria (urine output less than 400 mL/day) and **azotemia** (the retention and buildup of nitrogenous wastes in the blood). Toxins can also cause blood vessel constriction in the kidney, leading to reduced kidney blood flow, oliguria, and azotemia.

Activated *immunity* and damage from kidney toxins (nephrotoxins) (Box 60.3) cause intracellular changes of the tubular system in kidney tissue. Inflammatory proteins and immune-mediated complexes can damage cells and tissues in the kidney. With extensive damage, tubular cells slough and nephrons lose the ability to repair themselves. The presence of tubular debris and sediment in urine from kidney tissue damage (intrarenal failure or *acute tubular necrosis*) is related to systemic ischemia, reduced kidney *perfusion,* or nephrotoxin exposure.

Even with severe AKI (i.e., stage 2 or 3 in Table 60.2), some adults return to baseline kidney function during recovery from illness. It is the responsibility of all health care professionals to be alert to the possibility of AKI and implement prevention strategies when risk factors are present. *Timely interventions to remove the cause of AKI may prevent progression to ESKD and the need for lifelong renal replacement therapy (RRT) or a renal transplant.*

Incidence and Prevalence

Twenty percent of all hospitalized patients and 60% of ICU patients develop AKI. AKI is increasingly recognized as an in-hospital complication that is associated with shock, heart conditions, and surgery (Pavkov et al., 2018). Patients who are older or who have chronic kidney disease or diabetes are at greater risk for AKI.

Health Promotion/Disease Prevention

Keep in mind that dehydration (severe blood volume depletion) reduces **perfusion** and can lead to AKI even in adults who have no known kidney problems. Urge all healthy adults to avoid dehydration by drinking 2 to 3 L of water daily. This is especially important for athletes or anyone who performs strenuous exercise or work and sweats heavily.

Nurses have an essential role in the prevention of AKI in hospitalized patients. Always assess for signs of impending kidney dysfunction including monitoring of laboratory values. Early recognition and correction of problems causing reduced urinary *elimination* may avoid kidney tissue damage. Evaluate the patient's fluid status. Accurately measure intake and output and check body weight to identify changes in fluid balance. Note the characteristics of the urine and report new sediment, hematuria (smoky or red color), foul odor, or other worrisome changes. Report a urine output of less than 30 mL/hr for 2 hours or dark amber urine to the primary health care provider (Jarvis & Eckhardt, 2024). Waiting for 6 hours of oliguria to meet AKI criteria may allow progression of kidney damage—act early!

✚ NURSING SAFETY PRIORITY

Critical Rescue

In any acute care setting, preventing volume depletion and providing intervention early when volume depletion occurs are nursing priorities. Reduced **perfusion** from volume depletion is a common cause of acute kidney injury (AKI). Assess continually to recognize the signs and symptoms of volume depletion (low urine output, decreased systolic blood pressure, decreased pulse pressure, orthostatic hypotension, thirst, rising blood osmolarity). Respond by intervening early with oral fluids or, in the patient who is unable to take or tolerate oral fluid, requesting an increase in IV fluid rate from the primary health care provider to prevent permanent kidney damage.

Monitor laboratory values for any changes that reflect poor kidney function. A significant increase in creatinine, especially when the increase occurs over hours or a few days, is a concern and must be reported urgently to the primary health

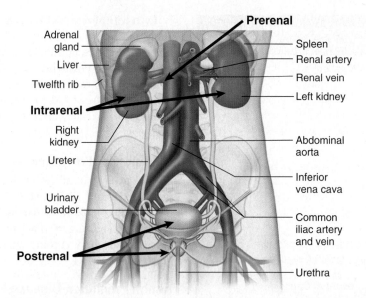

FIG. 60.1 Acute kidney failure categorizations. *Prerenal:* Cause of AKI occurs outside the kidney, impairing perfusion. Examples include extreme hypotension or hypovolemia occurring with conditions such as shock, dehydration, or burns. *Intrarenal:* Cause of AKI occurs inside the kidney. Examples include nephrotoxic agents or embolism or clotting in the renal vessels. *Postrenal:* Cause of AKI occurs due to urinary flow obstruction. Examples include kidney stones or tumors. (Modified from Patton, K. T., & Thibodeau, G. A. [2018]. *The human body in health & disease* [7th ed.]. St. Louis: Elsevier.)

BOX 60.3   Examples of Potentially Nephrotoxic Substances

Drugs

Antibiotics/Antimicrobials
- Amphotericin B
- Colistimethate
- Polymyxin B
- Rifampin
- Sulfonamides
- Tetracycline hydrochloride
- Vancomycin

Aminoglycoside Antibiotics
- Gentamicin
- Neomycin
- Tobramycin

Chemotherapy Agents
- Cisplatin
- Cyclophosphamide
- Methotrexate

NSAIDs
- Celecoxib
- Flurbiprofen
- Ibuprofen
- Indomethacin
- Ketorolac
- Meloxicam
- Nabumetone
- Naproxen
- Oxaprozin
- Tolmetin

Other Drugs
- Acetaminophen
- Captopril
- Cyclosporine
- Fluorinated anesthetics
- Metformin
- Quinine

Other Substances

Organic Solvents
- Carbon tetrachloride
- Ethylene glycol

Nondrug Chemical Agents
- Radiographic contrast media (e.g., iodinated media, hyperosmolar media, and gadolinium)
- Pesticides
- Fungicides
- Myoglobin (from breakdown of skeletal muscle)

Heavy Metals and Ions
- Arsenic
- Bismuth
- Copper sulfate
- Gold salts
- Lead
- Mercuric chloride

care provider. Other laboratory values that help monitor kidney function include serum blood urea nitrogen (BUN); serum potassium, sodium, and osmolarity; and urine specific gravity, albumin-to-creatinine ratio, and electrolytes. Know the baseline (steady-state) GFR because a reduced GFR makes the patient more vulnerable to AKI.

Be aware of nephrotoxic substances that the patient may ingest or be exposed to (see Box 60.3). Question any order for potentially nephrotoxic drugs, and validate the dose before the patient receives the drug. Many antibiotics have nephrotoxic effects. NSAIDs can cause or increase the risk for AKI. Combining two or more nephrotoxic drugs dramatically increases the risk for AKI. If a patient must receive a known nephrotoxic drug, closely monitor laboratory values, including BUN, creatinine, and drug peak and trough levels, for indications of reduced kidney function. When a nephrotoxic agent such as a contrast medium will be used, additional nephrotoxic medications such as metformin should be withheld at least 24 hours before and after the procedure, if possible. IV fluids should be administered before and after exposure to the contrast medium (Moore, 2018).

Interprofessional Collaborative Care

AKI is managed initially in the hospital setting, most commonly in an ICU. During the acute phase of the problem, members of the interprofessional team include the nephrologist, nephrology nurse, registered dietitian nutritionist (RDN), pharmacist, and dialysis technician. The responsibilities of each of these professionals are described within the interventions sections of this chapter. When the patient is discharged before urinary *elimination* returns to normal, continuing management is needed as part of the transition to community care.

Recognize Cues: Assessment

History. The accurate diagnosis of acute kidney injury (AKI), including its cause, depends on a detailed history. Know the risk factors for and criteria of AKI and chronic kidney disease (CKD). Ask about any change in urine appearance, frequency, or volume.

Ask about recent surgery or trauma, transfusions, allergic (hypersensitivity) reactions, or other factors that might lead to reduced kidney *perfusion.* Obtain a drug history, especially use of antibiotics and NSAIDs. Ask about recent imaging procedures requiring injection of a contrast medium. Coexisting conditions of advanced age, chronic kidney disease, diabetes, long-term hypertension, major or systemic infection (sepsis), peripheral vascular disease, chronic liver disease, HIV stage III (AIDS), and prior kidney surgery increase the risk for AKI (Gilbert & Weiner, 2023).

To identify *immunity*-mediated AKI (i.e., acute glomerulonephritis), ask about acute illnesses such as influenza, colds, gastroenteritis, and sore throats. Allergic reactions from a drug or food allergy may result in AKI as late as 10 days after exposure. Ask about rashes, hives, or fever and evaluate the white blood cell (WBC) differential for an increased eosinophil count.

Anticipate AKI following any episode of hypotension or shock. Any problem in which the blood volume is depleted can contribute to AKI by reducing *perfusion.* Such problems include cardiac bypass surgery, extensive bowel preparations, being NPO before surgery, or dehydration from exercise. Recent use of IV vasopressors (e.g., epinephrine or norepinephrine) may contribute to AKI when blood volume is reduced (hypovolemia).

Consider whether there is a history of urinary obstructive problems. Ask the patient about any difficulty in starting the urine stream, changes in the amount or appearance of the urine, narrowing of the urine stream, nocturia, urgency, or symptoms of kidney stones. Also ask about any cancer history that may cause urinary obstruction.

👤 PATIENT-CENTERED CARE: OLDER ADULT HEALTH

Acute Kidney Injury (AKI)

AKI is more common as people age. People ages 80 to 89 years are 55% more likely to develop AKI than people under age 50. As the kidneys age, structural and functional changes occur, including fewer nephrons and sclerosis of glomeruli and the renal arteries. These changes lead to an increased risk for AKI. Older adults also have more comorbid conditions such as diabetes, hypertension, and chronic kidney disease (Johnson et al., 2019).

Further increasing the risk of AKI in the older adult is an increased exposure to nephrotoxic drugs. The use of multiple drugs is associated with drug-induced AKI, particularly in acute and critical care settings. Assess risk and take actions to reduce exposure to nephrotoxic agents, avoid hypotension and hypovolemia, evaluate drug-drug interactions for potential adverse kidney effects, and stop unnecessary drugs to maintain kidney function in older adults.

Physical Assessment/Signs and Symptoms. If a patient has a urinary catheter, assess urine output every hour after surgery until stable, during fluid resuscitation for shock or hypotension, and when the patient has a high risk for AKI following hospital admission. Even a brief period of oliguria, defined as less than 0.5 mL/kg/hr of urine output for 2 or more hours, can signal AKI.

Other symptoms of AKI are related to the buildup of nitrogenous wastes (azotemia) and decreased urine output (oliguria). As AKI progresses in severity, the patient may have symptoms of fluid overload because fluid is not eliminated. Indications of fluid overload include pulmonary crackles, dependent and generalized edema *(anasarca),* decreased oxygenation (low peripheral oxygenation or SpO_2), confusion, increased respiratory rate, and dyspnea. See Chapter 13 for assessment of fluid overload.

Evaluate vital signs to recognize early hypoperfusion and hypoxemia. Symptoms of reduced blood volume such as mean arterial pressure (MAP) below 65 mm Hg, tachycardia, thready peripheral pulses, or decreasing cognition may indicate risk for AKI from poor *perfusion;* an SpO_2 below 88% may indicate potential hypoxemic or ischemic damage to kidney tissue.

Laboratory Assessment. The many changes in laboratory values in the patient with AKI are similar to those occurring in chronic kidney disease (CKD). See Table 60.3. Expect to see rising creatinine and BUN levels and abnormal blood electrolyte values. However, patients with AKI usually do *not* have the anemia associated with CKD unless there is blood loss from another condition (e.g., surgery, trauma) or when BUN levels are high enough to break (lyse) red blood cells (RBCs).

In early AKI, urine tests provide important information. Urine sodium levels may reflect an inability to concentrate urine. Urine may be dilute with a specific gravity near 1.000 or concentrated with a specific gravity greater than 1.030. The presence of urine sediment (e.g., RBCs, casts, and tubular cells), myoglobin, or hemoglobin may lead to nephron damage.

Imaging Assessment. Ultrasonography is useful in the diagnosis of kidney and urinary tract obstruction. Dilation of the renal calyces and collecting ducts, as well as stones, can be detected. Ultrasonography can show kidney size and patency of the ureters. Small kidney size may indicate an underlying CKD with loss of kidney tissue.

CT scans without contrast medium can determine adequacy of kidney *perfusion* and identify obstruction or tumors. Contrast medium is usually avoided to prevent further kidney damage. An MRI may be used in place of a CT scan.

X-rays of the pelvis or kidneys, ureters, and bladder (KUB) may provide an initial view of kidneys and the urinary tract to determine the cause of AKI. Enlarged kidneys with obstruction may show hydronephrosis. X-rays can show stones obstructing the renal pelvis, ureters, or bladder. More commonly, ultrasound is used to screen for hydronephrosis.

A nuclear medicine study called *MAG3* may be used to determine the nature of the kidney failure and measure GFR. A renal scan can determine whether *perfusion* of the kidneys is sufficient. Cystoscopy or retrograde pyelography may be needed to identify obstructions of the lower urinary tract (see Chapter 60).

Other Diagnostic Assessments. Kidney biopsy is performed if the cause of AKI is uncertain and symptoms persist or an immunologic disease is suspected. Prepare the patient before the test, particularly managing both hypotension and hypertension. Hypertension increases the risk for intrarenal hemorrhage following needle biopsy. Provide follow-up care. Be aware of all test results and understand how they might affect the treatment regimen. (See Chapter 57 for a detailed discussion of diagnostic tests related to the kidney.)

TABLE 60.3 Laboratory Profile

Kidney Disease

Test	Normal Range for Adults	Values in Kidney Disease
Serum creatinine	*Male:* 0.6–1.2 mg/dL (53–106 mmol/L) *Female:* 0.5–1.1 mg/dL (44–97 mmol/L) *Older adults:* May be slightly increased	In chronic kidney disease: May increase by 0.5–1.0 mg/dL (50–100 mcmol/L) every 1–2 yr In acute kidney injury: Increase of 1–2 mg/dL (100–200 mmol/L) every 24–48 hr May increase 1–6 mg/dL (100–600 mmol/L) in 1 wk or less
Serum sodium	136–145 mEq/L (136–145 mmol/L)	Normal, increased, or decreased
Serum potassium	3.5–5 mEq/L (3.5–5 mmol/L)	Increased
Serum phosphorus (phosphate)	3–4.5 mg/dL (0.97–1.45 mmol/L) *Older adults:* May be slightly decreased	Increased
Serum calcium	Total calcium: 9–10.5 mg/dL (2.25–2.62 mmol/L) Ionized calcium: 4.5–5.6 mg/dL (1.05–1.3 mmol/L) *Older adults:* Slightly decreased	Decreased
Serum magnesium	1.3–2.1 mEq/L (0.65–1.05 mmol/L)	Increased or decreased
Serum carbon dioxide content	23–30 mEq/L (23–30 mmol/L)	Decreased
Arterial blood pH	7.35–7.45	Decreased (in metabolic acidosis) or normal
Arterial blood bicarbonate (HCO_3^-)	21–28 mEq/L	Decreased
Arterial blood P_{CO_2}	35–45 mm Hg	Decreased
Hemoglobin	*Female:* 12–16 g/dL (7.4–9.9 mmol/L) *Male:* 14–18 g/dL (8.7–11.2 mmol/L) *Older adults:* Slightly decreased	Decreased
Hematocrit	*Female:* 37%–47% (0.37–0.47 volume fraction) *Male:* 42%–52% (0.42–0.52 volume fraction) *Older adults:* May be slightly decreased	Decreased
Blood osmolality	285–295 mOsm/kg (285–295 mmol/kg)	Elevated in volume-depleted states, increasing the risk for acute kidney injury

From Pagana, K., Pagana, T., & Pagana, T. (2022). *Mosby's manual of diagnostic and laboratory tests* (7th ed.). St. Louis: Elsevier.

NCLEX Examination Challenge 60.1

Safe and Effective Care Environment

A 47-year-old male client was admitted yesterday with traumatic injuries and hypovolemic shock. Which lab result would be **most important** for the nurse to report to the health care provider immediately?

A. Serum sodium 132 mEq/L (mmol/L) (Reference range: 136–145 mEq/L [mmol])
B. Serum potassium 6.9 mEq/L (mmol/L) (Reference range: 3.5–4.5 mEq/L [mmol])
C. Blood urea nitrogen 24 mg/dL (8.57 mmol/L) (Reference range: 10–20 mg/dL or 3.6–7.1 mmol)
D. Hematocrit 32% (0.32 volume fraction); hemoglobin 9.2 g/dL (92 g/L) (Reference range: hematocrit 42%–52% [0.42–0.52 volume fraction]; hemoglobin 14–18 g/dL [8.7–11.2 mmol/L])

Take Actions: Interventions

Avoid hypotension and maintain normal fluid balance *(euvolemia)* to prevent and manage AKI. A reduction in kidney **perfusion** may initially not be recognized when there is no associated drop in systemic blood pressure. Autoregulation and the renin-angiotensin-aldosterone system (RAAS) effectively maintain normal kidney perfusion and glomerular filtration rate. Maintaining a mean arterial pressure (MAP) of 80 to 85 mm Hg has been shown to lower rates of AKI in patients with preexisting hypertension. However, there is an increased risk of atrial fibrillation in patients with a mean arterial pressure (MAP) of 80 to 85 mm Hg as opposed to 65 to 70 mm Hg. Accordingly, blood pressure goals are determined based on preexisting conditions and risk versus benefit to the patient (Moore, 2018).

Reduce exposure to nephrotoxic agents and drugs that alter kidney perfusion. When such substances cannot be avoided, monitor drug levels and communicate with the pharmacist to adjust doses to minimize harm. Ensure that kidney function is assessed before an imaging test that includes contrast media. A large volume of contrast agents with high osmolarity (>2000 mOsm/L [mmol/L]), and frequent administration (given twice in 3 months or more often) of agents are more likely to cause contrast-induced nephropathy. Ensure that kidney function is assessed before an imaging test and that both the radiologist and the requesting primary health care provider are aware of reduced kidney function before a contrast medium is given.

Communicate with the radiologist so that the lowest dose of the contrast agent is used in high-risk adults. The patient may receive IV fluids at a rate of 1 mL/kg/hr for 6 to 12 hours before the imaging test or at 3 mL/kg/hr for 1 hour just before the procedure to ensure hydration and dilution of the contrast medium and to speed urinary *elimination* of the agent (Rudnick & Davenport, 2023). A common desired outcome for patients undergoing a procedure with contrast medium is a urine output of 150 mL/hr for the first 6 hours after administration of the contrast agent.

Observations about new-onset or increased peripheral edema, increased daily weight, and reduced urine output can identify patients with a positive fluid balance from AKI who may require treatment with fluid restriction or diuretic therapy. Impairment of *acid-base balance* and electrolyte imbalance can occur and may require treatment, especially in older adults.

Blood sampling of patients at risk for AKI allows early recognition of elevated serum creatinine levels and trend data. Communicate observations about worsening kidney function early and often to the primary health care provider so that interventions can promote kidney health and interrupt the progression of AKI when it occurs.

Not all patients with AKI experience oliguria. **Immunity** and inflammatory causes of AKI may allow proteins to enter the glomerulus, and these proteins can hold fluid in the filtrate, causing a *polyuria* (excess urine output) that disrupts *fluid and electrolyte balance.* During AKI with high-volume urine output, hypovolemia and electrolyte *loss* are the main problems. The patient in the diuretic phase of AKI needs a plan of care that focuses on fluid and electrolyte *replacement* and monitoring. Onset of polyuria can signal the start of recovery from AKI.

Surviving kidney tubule cells possess a remarkable ability to regenerate and proliferate, and early identification can stop progression of AKI, as well as aid in recovery of kidney function. Base the desired outcomes of care on collaboration and communication with interprofessional team members. Update the plan of care for either restriction (when fluid overload from new AKI is present) or liberal administration of fluid (to prevent AKI or promote elimination of contrast medium) based on timely and accurate team communication.

Frequent laboratory value monitoring, close surveillance of intake and output, drug therapy, nutrition, careful administration of fluids and minerals, and renal replacement therapy are commonly used to manage AKI.

Drug Therapy. The interprofessional team consults the inpatient pharmacist for drug adjustment based on kidney function. As kidney function changes, drug dosages are changed. It is important to be knowledgeable about the site of drug metabolism and especially careful when giving drugs. Continuously monitor the patient with AKI for adverse drug events and interactions of the drugs that they are receiving. Diuretics may be used to increase urine output in AKI. Diuretic-induced urine output does not preserve kidney function or stop AKI, but diuretics do rid the body of retained fluid and electrolytes in the patient with AKI that has not progressed to end-stage kidney disease (ESKD).

Fluid challenges are often used to promote kidney *perfusion.* In patients without fluid overload, 500 to 1000 mL of normal saline may be infused over 1 hour. It is important to assess the patient's response to fluid to prevent fluid overload. Fluid overload in critical illness has been shown to increase mortality (Moore, 2018). The term *fluid responsive* is used when identifying patients who have a positive response to fluid. There are many methods to evaluate fluid responsiveness, such as systolic pressure variation, pulse pressure variation, and stroke volume variation, which are obtained from the arterial or pulse oximetry waveforms. In patients with a method of monitoring stroke volume and cardiac output, a passive leg raise can determine if the patient is fluid responsive without the risk of giving fluids. The patient's leg is raised to 45 degrees for 30 to 90 seconds in order to temporarily move fluid by increasing venous return, and if the stroke volume or cardiac output improves, the patient will respond positively to more fluid volume (Brown & Semler, 2019).

Nutrition Therapy. Patients who have AKI often have a high rate of *catabolism* (protein breakdown). Increases in metabolism and protein breakdown may be related to the stress of illness and the increase in blood levels of catecholamines, cortisol, and glucagon. The rate of protein breakdown correlates with the severity of uremia and azotemia. Catabolism causes the breakdown of muscle protein and increases azotemia.

The interprofessional team's registered dietitian nutritionist (RDN) in the ICU setting calculates the patient's protein and caloric needs. A consultation may need to be requested for inpatients outside of the ICU or for those in community settings. Work with the RDN to establish a diet with specified amounts of protein, sodium, and fluids. For the patient who does not require dialysis, 0.6 g/kg of body weight or 40 g of protein per day is usually prescribed. For patients who require dialysis, the protein level needed ranges from 1 to 1.5 g/kg. The dietary sodium ranges from 60 to 90 mEq/kg (mmol/kg). If high blood potassium levels are present, dietary potassium is restricted to 60 to 70 mEq/kg (mmol/kg). The daily amount of fluid permitted is calculated to be equal to the urine volume plus 500 mL. Assess food intake every shift to ensure that caloric intake is adequate.

Many patients with AKI are too ill or their appetite is too poor to meet caloric goals. For these patients, nutrition support

---

NCLEX Examination Challenge 60.2

Safe and Effective Care Environment

The nurse is caring for a 74-year-old client scheduled for a cardiac catheterization with contrast dye. Which of the following nursing actions would be appropriate? **Select all that apply.**

A. Assess creatinine clearance using a 24-hour urine collection test.

B. Assess for coexisting conditions of diabetes, heart failure, and kidney disease.

C. Collaborate with the provider about whether IV fluids should be infused before the test.

D. Notify the provider regarding changes in serum creatinine from 0.2 to 0.4 mg/dL in 24 hours. (Reference range: 0.5–1.1 mg/dL)

E. Alert the provider to a glomerular filtration rate (GFR) below 60 mL/min/1.73 m². (Reference range: >60 mL/min/1.73 m²) with oral supplements, enteral nutrition, or parenteral nutrition (PN, or hyperalimentation) is needed. Nutrition support in AKI aims to provide sufficient nutrients to maintain or improve nutrition status, preserve lean body mass, restore or maintain fluid balance, and preserve kidney function.

There are several kidney-specific formulations of oral supplements and enteral solutions (e.g., Nepro, Suplena, and Novasource Renal). Most specialty formulas for patients with kidney problems are lower in sodium, potassium, and phosphorus and higher in calories than are standard feedings. Enteral nutrition, delivered with a nasogastric or nasojejunal tube (these tubes can also be placed orally), can be used for nutrition support. If PN is used, the IV solutions are mixed to meet the patient's specific needs. Because kidney function is unstable in AKI, continuously monitor intake and output and serum electrolyte levels to determine how the supplementation affects *fluid and electrolyte balance.* IV fat emulsion (Intralipid) infusions can provide a nonprotein source of calories. In uremic patients, fat emulsions are used in place of glucose to avoid the problems of excessive sugars.

Kidney Replacement Therapy. Kidney replacement therapy (KRT), also called *renal replacement therapy (RRT),* is used for patients with loss of kidney function and inadequate waste *elimination.* Indications for KRT include symptomatic uremia (e.g., pericarditis, neuropathy, decline in cognition), persistent or rapidly rising high potassium levels (i.e., greater than 6.5 mEq/L [mmol/L]), severe metabolic acidosis (pH less than 7.1), or fluid overload that inhibits tissue *perfusion.* When AKI occurs with drug or alcohol intoxication, KRT also can remove toxins.

Advancements in KRT over the past 10 years have led to multiple options for patients requiring treatment. Options for KRT include various types of intermittent and continuous hemodialysis (HD) as well as peritoneal dialysis (PD). Despite recent advances, the life expectancy for patients starting KRT ranges from 3 to 5 years. Mortality is highest in the first several months following dialysis (Gilbert & Weiner, 2023).

Immediate vascular access for KRT in patients with AKI is achieved by placement of a catheter specific for dialysis (Fig. 60.2). The temporary catheter is placed in a central vein, most often the internal jugular, using best practices to avoid catheter-associated bloodstream infections (see Chapter 15). Placement of the catheter requires informed consent and a "time-out" similar to that in other surgical procedures (see Chapter 9). This catheter is not used to acquire blood samples, give drugs or fluid, or monitor central venous pressure. Provide site care in accordance with agency policy and best practices to avoid catheter-related bloodstream infection (CRBSI).

A long-term dialysis catheter may be placed in the radiology department using a tunneling technique under moderate sedation. Under ultrasound or fluoroscopic guidance, the health care provider makes a small incision where the internal jugular vein passes behind the clavicle. A 6- to 8-cm tunnel is created away from the site of the incision. A long-term hemodialysis (HD) catheter is inserted through the tunnel and into the jugular vein. Keeping a segment of the catheter within the subcutaneous tissues before entering the jugular vein reduces the risk

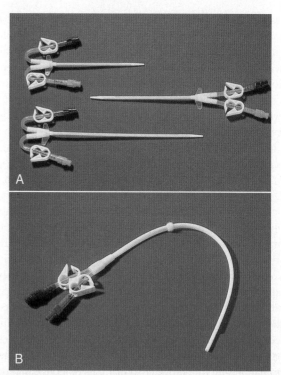

FIG. 60.2 Subclavian dialysis catheters. These catheters are radiopaque tubes that can be used for hemodialysis access. The Y-shaped tubing allows arterial outflow and venous return through a single catheter. (A) Mahurkar catheters, made of polyurethane and used for short-term access. (B) PermCath catheter, made of silicone and used for long-term access. (Courtesy Kendall Company, Bothell, WA.)

for infection. This central catheter is used only for dialysis and requires aseptic dressing changes.

Dialysis catheters have two lumens—one for outflow and one for inflow. This allows the patient's blood to flow out and, once dialyzed, to be returned through the inflow lumen. Some catheters have a third lumen to sample venous blood or give drugs and fluid during dialysis.

Intermittent Versus Continuous Kidney Replacement Therapy. Kidney replacement therapy (KRT) is a supportive strategy to purify blood, substituting for the normal function of the kidney. Particles are separated from blood based on the different ability of particles to pass through (diffuse) a membrane or across the peritoneal lining. KRT can be delivered intermittently, continuously, or as a hybrid of these approaches. Mortality is significant, regardless of modality, among patients who require KRT.

Intermittent KRT, sometimes called *hemodialysis,* is delivered over 3 to 6 hours (see Fig. 60.3). In general, a technician or dialysis nurse brings the dialysis machine to the bedside of a critically ill patient. Patients who do not need intensive care may be transported to an inpatient dialysis unit for the duration of the KRT treatment.

Intermittent KRT uses a dialysis machine to mix and monitor the *dialysate* (the fluid that helps remove the unwanted particles and waste products from blood). Dialysate is prescribed by the nephrology health care provider as an admixture to restore electrolytes and minerals to normal levels in the blood. The machine also monitors the flow of blood while it is outside of the body.

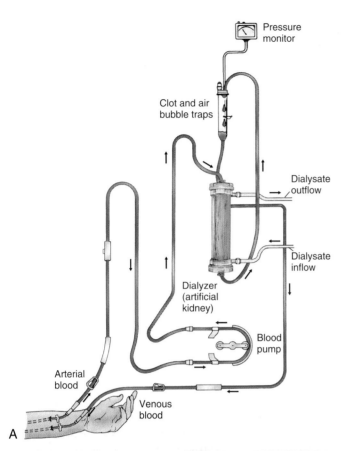

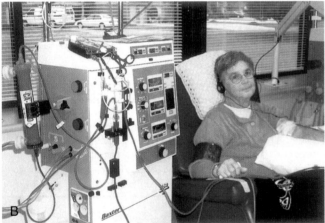

FIG. 60.3 (A) Hemodialysis circuit. Enlarged image to show the process occurring in the hemodialysis machine. (B) Hemodialysis machine. (From Shiland, B. J. [2022]. *Medical assistant: Urinary, blood, lymphatic and immune systems with laboratory procedures—Module E* [2nd ed.]. St. Louis: Elsevier.)

Alarms are set and monitored by the dialysis technician or nurse to ensure safe and effective flow. This type of KRT is delivered three or four times weekly and requires anticoagulation in the dialysis circuit. Dialysis creates shifts of fluid and electrolytes that may not be tolerated in critically ill patients. Another form of intermittent KRT is peritoneal dialysis (PD), which is more commonly used for end-stage kidney disease. This therapy is discussed in detail in the Peritoneal Dialysis section of this chapter.

Continuous kidney replacement therapies (CKRTs), also known as continuous renal replacement therapy (CRRT), are alternative methods for removing wastes and restoring both *acid-base balance* and *fluid and electrolyte balance.* They are used in hospitalized adults who are too unstable to tolerate the changes in blood pressure that occur with intermittent conventional hemodialysis. As with hemodialysis, blood is passed through a filter to remove waste and undesired particles. Although intermittent hemodialysis occurs for 4 hours 3 days a week, CKRTs are typically prescribed for over 24 hours (Ronco et al., 2019). Some CKRT therapies use a different approach to remove particles from the blood. Hemofiltration uses ultrafiltration, whereas diffusion is used in intermittent dialysis to remove toxins and other particles. *Ultrafiltration* is the separation of particles from a suspension by passage through a filter with very fine pores. In ultrafiltration, the separation is performed by convective transport. During intermittent hemodialysis, separation depends on differential diffusion. Some approaches to CKRT combine ultrafiltration with diffusion (combined hemofiltration and hemodialysis).

CKRT occurs only in the ICU, because of the need for frequent monitoring and the specialized skill set of the nurse to maintain safety during extracorporeal circulation (blood flow outside the body). Life-threatening complications can occur if there is an error in the preparation of electrolyte solution or if the conductivity monitors fail (Ronco et al., 2019). The American Nephrology Nurses Association provides resources for intermittent and continuous KRT policies and procedures.

Several strategies can be used to provide CKRT to critically ill patients. The most commonly used CKRTs are continuous venovenous hemofiltration (CVVH) and continuous venovenous hemodialysis (CVVHD). The different CKRT modalities use the same machines, which are set up differently based on the needs of the patient. CVVH uses ultrafiltration, whereas CVVHD uses diffusion to filter the blood. CKRT is powered by a pump that drives blood from the patient catheter into the dialyzer (filter). The ultrafiltrate fluid is then collected into a bag for disposal. There may be a second pump that acts on the ultrafiltrate tubing to create negative pressure and increase fluid removal. Replacement fluid is infused via the inflow circuit in some systems. The pump increases the risk for an air embolus, and KRT systems have alarms that detect air (Ronco et al., 2019).

Another KRT modality is a hybrid of continuous and intermittent approaches. Slow continuous ultrafiltration (SCUF) provides slow removal of fluid over 12 to 24 hours and may be useful when azotemia or uremia is not a concern. Sustained low-efficiency dialysis (SLED) uses the dialysis machine to deliver prolonged dialysis for 12 to 24 hours. Lower blood flow and dialysate flow rates remove both particles and water and may be better tolerated by the unstable or critically ill patient, with fewer episodes of hypotension. A newer type of CKRT is continuous venovenous hemodiafiltration (CVVHDF), which combines the principles of hemodialysis with hemofiltration. Another new type of CKRT is continuous venovenous high-flux hemodialysis (CVVHFD), which uses high-flux membranes in the filter (Ronco et al., 2019).

Continuous KRT is expensive and resource intensive. It requires consultation and collaboration with the nephrologist and close collaboration with a dialysis nurse. Conservative management of *fluid and electrolyte balance, acid-base balance,* and drug therapy is an acceptable and reasonable approach to manage AKI.

Posthospital Care. Patients with AKI may have many outcomes. Some patients recover and return to baseline kidney function and general health. Others have partial recovery with mild or moderate chronic kidney disease (CKD). Still others may require permanent KRT. Some die from the acute illness.

The care for a patient with AKI after discharge from the hospital varies, depending on the status of the kidney function when the patient is discharged. Resolution of kidney injury may occur over several months, and follow-up care may be provided by a nephrologist or by the primary health care provider in consultation with the nephrologist. Frequent medical visits are necessary, as are scheduled laboratory blood and urine tests to monitor kidney function. A registered dietitian nutritionist can plan modifications to the patient's diet according to the degree of kidney function and ongoing nutrition needs. Fluid restrictions and daily weights may be advised to avoid fluid overload while kidneys are recovering.

Recovery of renal function is adversely affected by KRT, putting patients at risk for developing end-stage kidney disease (ESKD). Insult to the kidney by KRT is thought to be related to the loss of autoregulation and inflammation that occurs (Ronco et al., 2019). For patients who require dialysis at discharge following AKI, follow-up care is similar to that needed for patients with ESKD from CKD (see Care Coordination and Transition Management in the Chronic Kidney Disease section). Depending on their level of independence and family support, patients may need home care nursing or social work assistance.

✳ ELIMINATION CONCEPT EXEMPLAR: CHRONIC KIDNEY DISEASE

Pathophysiology Review

Unlike acute kidney injury (AKI), chronic kidney disease (CKD) is a progressive, irreversible disorder lasting longer than 3 months (Ferri, 2022). When kidney function and waste *elimination* are too poor to sustain life, CKD becomes end-stage kidney disease (ESKD). Terms used with CKD include azotemia (buildup of nitrogen-based wastes in the blood), uremia (azotemia with symptoms [Box 60.4]), and uremic syndrome. See Table 60.1 for a comparison of AKI and CKD.

Stages of Chronic Kidney Disease

CKD is classified into five stages based on glomerular filtration rate (GFR) category. Direct measurement of urine creatinine (described in Chapter 57, with a 3-hour or 24-hour urine

🔲 BOX 60.4 **Key Features**
Uremia

- Metallic taste in the mouth
- Anorexia
- Nausea
- Vomiting
- Muscle cramps
- Uremic frost on skin
- Fatigue and lethargy
- Hiccups
- Edema
- Dyspnea
- Paresthesias

collection) is needed for the most accurate GFR estimation. The five stages of CKD are described in Table 60.4. CKD starts with a normal GFR but increased risk for kidney damage. In the first stage, the patient may have a normal GFR (>90 mL/min/1.73 m²) but abnormal urine findings, structural abnormalities, or genetic traits that point to kidney disease. The patient is at increased risk for kidney damage from infection, *immunity* responses with inflammation, pregnancy, dehydration, and hypotension. Careful management of conditions such as diabetes, hypertension, and heart failure (HF) can slow the onset and progression of CKD.

In stage 2 CKD, GFR is reduced, ranging between 60 and 89 mL/min/1.73 m², and albuminuria may be present. Kidney nephron damage has occurred, and there may be slight elevations of metabolic wastes in the blood because of nephron loss. Levels of blood urea nitrogen (BUN), serum creatinine, uric acid, and phosphorus are not sensitive enough to define this stage. Increased output of dilute urine may occur at this stage of CKD and lead to severe dehydration.

❗ NURSING SAFETY PRIORITY
Action Alert

Teach patients with mild chronic kidney disease (CKD) that carefully managing fluid volume, blood pressure, electrolytes, and other kidney-damaging diseases by following prescribed drug and nutrition therapies can slow progression to end-stage kidney disease (ESKD).

In stage 3 CKD, GFR reduction continues and ranges between 30 and 59 mL/min/1.73 m², and albuminuria is usually present. Nephron damage is greater, and azotemia reflecting poor waste *elimination* is present. Ongoing management of the underlying conditions that cause nephron damage is essential, especially diabetes mellitus and blood pressure control. Restriction of fluids, proteins, and electrolytes is needed. Stage 3 is further divided into 3a and 3b to more accurately assess the risk for complications from CKD as GFR decreases below 45 mL/min/1.73 m².

Over time, patients progress to stage 4 CKD and *end-stage kidney disease* (ESKD) (stage 5). Waste *elimination* is poor,

TABLE 60.4 **Stages of Chronic Kidney Disease**		
Stage	**Estimated Glomerular Filtration Rate**	**Intervention**
Stage 1		
At risk; normal kidney function, but urine findings indicate kidney disease	>90 mL/min/1.73 m^2	Screen for risk factors and manage care to reduce risk: • Uncontrolled hypertension • Diabetes with poor glycemic control • Congenital or acquired anatomic or urinary tract abnormalities • Family history of genetic kidney diseases • Exposure to nephrotoxic substances
Stage 2		
Slightly reduced kidney function	60–89 mL/min/1.73 m^2	Focus on reduction of risk factors
Stage 3		
Moderately reduced kidney function	30–59 mL/min/1.73 m^2	Implement strategies to slow disease progression
Stage 4		
Severely reduced kidney function; noticeable jaundice can occur, particularly around the eyes	15–29 mL/min/1.73 m^2	Manage complications Discuss patient preferences and values Educate about options and prepare for renal replacement therapy
Stage 5		
End-stage kidney disease (ESKD)	<15 mL/min/1.73 m^2	Implement renal replacement therapy or kidney transplantation

with excessive amounts of urea and creatinine building up in the blood, and the kidneys cannot maintain homeostasis. Severe impairments of *fluid and electrolyte balance* and *acid-base balance* occur. Without kidney replacement therapy, death results from ESKD.

Three albuminuria stages also are considered in evaluating CKD. These stages are defined by the albumin-to-creatinine ratio in urine. The first stage (A1) is none to mildly increased albumin up to 29 mg/g creatinine (<3 mg/mmol) and is sometimes called *microalbuminuria*. The second (A2) stage has values of 30 to 300 mg/g creatinine (3–30 mg/mmol). The stage of greatest kidney damage (A3) has values >300 mg/g creatinine (>30 mg/mmol). The risk for progression of CKD, ESKD, and mortality is increased when urine albumin increases. Albumin in the urine is a marker of kidney damage, whereas GFR reflects kidney function. The combined values help identify adults at risk for progression of CKD and complications and guide interventions.

Kidney Changes

CKD with greatly reduced GFR causes many problems, including abnormal urine production, severe disruption of *fluid and electrolyte balance,* and metabolic abnormalities. Because healthy nephrons become larger and work harder, urine production and water *elimination* are sufficient to maintain essential homeostasis until about three-fourths of kidney function is lost. As the disease progresses, the ability to produce diluted urine is reduced, resulting in urine with a fixed osmolarity *(isosthenuria)*. As kidney function continues to decline, the BUN increases, and urine output decreases. Extracellular volume overload can occur in CKD because the body loses the capability to excrete sodium (Johnson et al., 2019). At this point, the patient is at risk for fluid overload with edema, pulmonary crackles, shortness of breath, and pleural or pericardial

effusion (with symptoms of a friction rub on auscultation and/or decreased breath sounds or heart sounds).

Metabolic Changes

Urea and creatinine excretion are disrupted by CKD. Creatinine comes from proteins in skeletal muscle. The rate of creatinine excretion depends on muscle mass, physical activity, and diet. Without major changes in diet or physical activity, the serum creatinine level is constant. Creatinine is partially excreted by the kidney tubules, and a decrease in kidney function leads to a buildup of serum creatinine. Urea is made from protein metabolism and is excreted by the kidneys. The BUN level normally varies directly with protein intake.

Sodium excretion changes are common. Early in CKD, the patient is at risk for *hyponatremia* (sodium depletion) because there are fewer healthy nephrons to reabsorb sodium. Thus sodium is lost in the urine. Polyuria of mild to moderate CKD also causes sodium loss.

In the later stages of CKD, kidney excretion of sodium is reduced as urine production decreases. Then sodium retention and high serum sodium levels *(hypernatremia)* occur with only modest increases in dietary sodium intake. This problem leads to severe disruption of *fluid and electrolyte balance* (see Chapter 13). Sodium retention causes hypertension and edema.

Even with sodium retention, the serum sodium level may appear normal because plasma water is retained at the same time. If fluid retention occurs at a greater rate than sodium retention, the serum sodium level is falsely low because of dilution (see Table 60.3).

Potassium excretion occurs mainly through the kidney. Any increase in potassium load during the later stages of CKD can lead to hyperkalemia (high serum potassium levels). Normal serum potassium levels of 3.5 to 5 mEq/L (mmol/L) are maintained until the 24-hour urine output falls below 500 mL. High potassium levels then develop quickly, reaching 7 to 8 mEq/L (mmol/L) or greater. Life-threatening changes in cardiac rate and rhythm result from this elevation because of abnormal depolarization and repolarization. Other factors contribute to high potassium levels in CKD, including the ingestion of potassium in drugs, failure to restrict dietary potassium, tissue breakdown, blood transfusions, and bleeding or hemorrhage. (See Chapter 13 for discussion of potassium imbalance.)

Acid-base balance is affected by CKD. In the early stages, blood pH changes little because the remaining healthy nephrons increase their rate of acid excretion. As more nephrons are lost, acid excretion is reduced and metabolic acidosis results (see Chapter 14).

Many factors lead to acidosis in CKD. First, the kidneys cannot excrete excessive hydrogen ions (acids). Normally, tubular cells move hydrogen ions into the urine for excretion, but ammonium and bicarbonate are needed for this movement to occur (Johnson et al., 2019). In patients with CKD, ammonium production is decreased and reabsorption of bicarbonate does not occur. This process leads to a buildup of hydrogen ions and reduced levels of bicarbonate *(base deficit)*. High potassium levels further reduce kidney ammonium production and excretion.

As CKD worsens and acid retention increases, increased respiratory action is needed to keep blood pH normal. The respiratory system adjusts or compensates for the increased blood hydrogen ion levels (acidosis or decreased pH) by increasing the rate and depth of breathing to excrete carbon dioxide through the lungs. This breathing pattern, called Kussmaul respiration, increases with worsening kidney disease. Serum bicarbonate measures the extent of metabolic acidosis (bicarbonate deficit). Patients usually need alkali replacement to counteract acidosis.

Calcium and phosphorus balance is disrupted by CKD. A complex, balanced normal reciprocal relationship exists between calcium and phosphorus (used interchangeably with phosphate) and is influenced by vitamin D (see Chapter 13). The kidney produces a hormone needed to activate vitamin D, which then enhances intestinal absorption of calcium.

Normally, excess phosphorus is excreted in the urine. In CKD, renal phosphate excretion decreases, which causes elevated phosphate levels. Bone and skeletal changes can occur when the GFR decreases to 25% or less (Rogers, 2023).

Parathyroid hormone (PTH) controls the amount of phosphorus in the blood by causing tubular excretion of phosphorus when there is an excess. An early effect of CKD is reduced phosphorus excretion (Fig. 60.4). As plasma phosphorus levels increase *(hyperphosphatemia),* calcium levels decrease *(hypocalcemia).* Chronic low blood calcium levels stimulate the parathyroid glands to release more PTH. With additional PTH, calcium is released from storage areas in bones *(bone resorption),* which results in bone density loss. The extra calcium from the bone is needed to balance the excess plasma phosphorus level. The problem of low blood calcium levels is made worse with severe CKD because kidney cell damage also reduces production of active vitamin D. Deficiencies in vitamin D lead to even further decreased calcium levels because vitamin D aids in calcium absorption (Rogers, 2023).

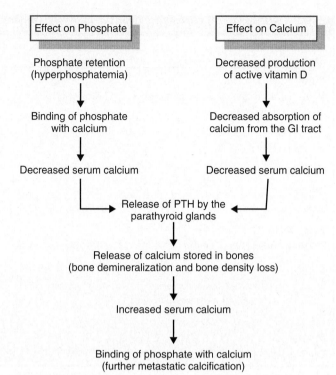

FIG. 60.4 Effects of kidney dysfunction on phosphorus and calcium balance. *PTH,* Parathyroid hormone.

The problems in bone metabolism and structure caused by CKD-induced low calcium levels and high phosphorus levels are called renal osteodystrophy. Bone mineral loss causes bone pain, spinal sclerosis, fractures, bone density loss, osteomalacia, and tooth calcium loss.

Crystals formed from excessive calcium or phosphorus are called *metastatic calcifications* and may precipitate in many body areas. When the plasma level of the calcium-phosphorus product (serum calcium level multiplied by the serum phosphorus level) exceeds 70 mg/dL (6 mmol/L), the crystals may lodge in the kidneys, heart, lungs, blood vessels, joints, eyes (causing conjunctivitis), and brain. Itching increases with calcium-phosphorus imbalances.

Calcium is also deposited in atherosclerotic plaques in the lining of blood vessels. Vascular calcium deposits are a marker of significant risk for cardiovascular disease.

Cardiac Changes

Cardiorenal syndrome refers to disorders of the kidney or heart that cause dysfunction in the other organ. The kidney and the heart have a reciprocal relationship that can make an alteration in one cause an alteration in the other (Ferri, 2022).

Hypertension is common in most patients with CKD. It may be either the cause or the result of CKD. In patients who have other causes of hypertension such as atherosclerosis, the increased blood pressure damages the glomerular capillaries, and eventually ESKD results.

CKD itself elevates blood pressure by causing fluid and sodium overload and dysfunction of the renin-angiotensin-aldosterone system (RAAS). Hypertension alone can damage kidney arterioles, reducing *perfusion.* A decrease in kidney blood flow results in the production and release of a number of signaling chemicals, including renin, to improve blood flow to the kidney. The release of renin triggers the production of angiotensin and aldosterone. Angiotensin causes blood vessel constriction and increases blood pressure. Aldosterone stimulates kidney tubules to reabsorb sodium and water. These actions increase plasma volume and raise blood pressure. However, in the presence of CKD, an increase in blood pressure may not result in increased blood flow, and the production of renin continues, which creates a cycle of vasoconstriction in kidney arterioles and peripheral arterioles. The result is severe hypertension that is difficult to manage and worsens kidney function. Many patients with CKD have heart damage and enlargement from the long-term hypertension that results in coronary artery damage and poor coronary artery perfusion.

Hyperlipidemia occurs in CKD from changes in fat metabolism that increase triglyceride, total cholesterol, and low-density lipoprotein (LDL) levels. These changes increase the patient's risk for coronary artery disease and acute cardiac events. Problems with lipids and atherosclerosis are greatly increased for the patient with both CKD and diabetes mellitus.

Heart failure (HF) may occur in CKD because the workload on the heart is increased as a result of anemia, hypertension, and fluid overload. Left ventricular enlargement and HF are common in ESKD. Uremia may cause *uremic cardiomyopathy,* the uremic toxin effect on the myocardium. HF also may occur in these patients because of hypertension and coronary artery disease. Cardiac disease is a leading cause of death in patients with ESKD.

Pericarditis also occurs in patients with CKD. The pericardial sac becomes inflamed by uremic toxins or infection. If it is not treated, this problem leads to pericardial effusion, cardiac tamponade, and death. Symptoms include shortness of breath from low cardiac output, severe chest pain, tachycardia, narrow *pulse pressure* (close values for systolic and diastolic blood pressure), low-grade fever, and a pericardial friction rub heard with a stethoscope placed over the left sternal border. Dysrhythmias may occur with uremia and uremic pericarditis. Treatment of tamponade, which is a medical emergency, requires immediate removal of pericardial fluid by placement of a needle, catheter, or drainage tube into the pericardium.

Hematologic and Immunity Changes

Anemia is common in patients in the later stages of CKD and worsens CKD symptoms. The causes of anemia include a decreased erythropoietin level with reduced red blood cell (RBC) production, decreased RBC survival time from uremia, and iron and folic acid deficiencies (Norton et al., 2017b). The patient may have increased bleeding or bruising as a result of impaired platelet function.

CKD causes reduced *immunity,* which increases the risk for infection. Uremia disrupts white blood cell (WBC) production and function, decreasing host defenses. Protein, fluid, and electrolyte abnormalities contribute to inflammation and further immunity impairment.

GI Changes

Uremia affects the entire GI system. The flora of the mouth change with uremia. The mouth contains the enzyme *urease,* which breaks down urea into ammonia. The ammonia generated remains and then causes halitosis (uremic fetor) and *stomatitis* (mouth inflammation). Anorexia, nausea, vomiting, and hiccups are common in patients with uremia. The specific cause of these problems is unknown but may be related to high BUN and creatinine levels and acidosis.

Peptic ulcer disease is common in patients with uremia, but the exact cause is unclear. Uremic colitis with watery diarrhea or constipation may also be present with uremia. Ulcers may occur in the stomach or intestine, causing erosion of blood vessels. The blood loss caused by these erosions may lead to hemorrhagic shock from severe GI bleeding.

Cognitive and Functional Changes

Although CKD may be asymptomatic in the early stages, complications include cognitive and physical impairment as CKD progresses. There is also increased risk for systemic drug toxicity and adverse effects from interventions used to prevent or treat CKD.

Etiology and Genetic Risk

The causes of CKD are complex (Box 60.5). More than 100 different disease processes can result in progressive loss of kidney function (see also Chapter 59). Two main causes of

---

BOX 60.5 Selected Causes of Chronic Kidney Disease

Glomerular Disease
- Glomerulonephritis
- Basement membrane disease
- Goodpasture syndrome
- Intercapillary glomerulosclerosis

Tubular Disease
- Chronic hypercalcemia
- Chronic potassium depletion
- Fanconi syndrome
- Heavy metal (lead) poisoning

Vascular Disease of the Kidney
- Ischemic disease of the kidney
- Bilateral renal artery stenosis
- Nephrosclerosis
- Hyperparathyroidism

Inherited or Genetic Conditions
- Hypoplastic kidneys
- Medullary cystic disease
- Polycystic kidney disease

Infection
- Pyelonephritis
- Tuberculosis

Systemic Vascular Disease
- Intrarenal renovascular hypertension
- Extrarenal renovascular hypertension

Metabolic Kidney Disease
- Diabetes
- Amyloidosis
- Gout (hyperuricemic nephropathy)
- Milk-alkali syndrome
- Sarcoidosis

Connective Tissue Disease
- Progressive systemic sclerosis
- Systemic lupus erythematosus
- Polyarteritis

Urinary Tract Disease
- Obstructive uropathy

NOTE: List is not all-inclusive.

CKD leading to dialysis or kidney transplantation are hypertension and diabetes mellitus. Black patients are more likely to develop ESKD and have hypertensive ESKD (National Kidney Foundation [NKF], 2020). In addition, CKD tends to progress to ESKD at a faster rate in Black and Hispanic patients (Chu et al., 2021).

Incidence and Prevalence

The number of patients being treated for CKD is increasing, particularly among older adults. About 15% of adults in the United States (37 million people) are estimated to have CKD (Centers for Disease Control and Prevention [CDC], 2021). Most adults who have CKD (9 out of 10) do not know that they have the disease (CDC, 2021). More than 50,000 Canadians are currently being treated for kidney failure, with 1 in 10 Canadians having CKD, and millions more at risk (Kidney Foundation of Canada, 2020).

Health Promotion/Disease Prevention

Health promotion activities to prevent or delay the onset of CKD focus on controlling the diseases that lead to its development, such as diabetes and hypertension. Educating and encouraging the patient to accept lifestyle modifications and how to implement them are incorporated into the ongoing plan of care. Diet adjustments (e.g., sodium, protein, and cholesterol restriction), weight maintenance (i.e., achieve body mass index of 22–25 kg/m²), smoking cessation, participation in 30 to 60 minutes of moderate-intensity exercise daily, and limitation of alcohol to one or two drinks daily are examples of lifestyle recommendations for the patient with CKD.

Identifying patients who have diabetes or hypertension at an early stage is critical to CKD prevention (Norton et al., 2017a). Teach patients to adhere to drug and diet regimens and to engage in regular physical activity to prevent the blood vessel changes and kidney cell damage d to CKD. Instruct patients with diabetes to keep their blood glucose levels within the prescribed range. Teach patients with hypertension that drug therapy reduces vessel damage. Urge patients with diabetes or hypertension to have yearly testing for urine albumin-to-creatinine ratio (UACR) along with serum creatinine and BUN.

Teach adults treated for an infection anywhere in the kidney/urinary system to take all antibiotics as prescribed. Urge adults to drink at least 2 L of water daily unless a health problem requires fluid restriction. Caution adults who use NSAIDs to use the lowest dose for the briefest time period because these drugs interfere with blood flow to the kidney. High-dose and long-term NSAID use reduces kidney function.

Interprofessional Collaborative Care

Although the patient with CKD may require hospitalization during exacerbation of imbalances or when other health problems require it, the vast majority of care occurs in the community. For best outcomes, the patient with CKD must be engaged in self-management. Because patients with CKD are at risk

---

NCLEX Examination Challenge 60.3
Health Promotion and Maintenance

The nurse is caring for a client with hypertension who reports having frequent urinary tract infections and states, "My kidney function is not the best so I see a kidney doctor every few months." Which nursing assessment query would be **most appropriate** based on the client's history?

A. "What is the color of your urine?"
B. "How much water do you drink daily?"
C. "Have you been urinating more frequently?"
D. "Are you aware of your creatinine or GFR levels?"

for so many adverse outcomes (not just ESKD), the interprofessional care team includes many specialists and health care professionals (e.g., nephrologists, nephrology nurses, pharmacists, registered dietitian nutritionists, mental health therapists, physical therapists, case managers, social workers, clergy or pastoral care workers). The responsibilities of these interprofessional team members are described within the interventions sections for CKD.

Patients with CKD need high levels of coordination between their primary provider, comorbidity management specialists, and renal specialists to achieve the best outcome (see the Systems Thinking/Quality Improvement box). The nurse coordinates the interprofessional team to support and counsel the patient and family, often over many years of treatment. The nurse has the most contact with patients when they are hospitalized or undergoing in-center dialysis treatments.

 SYSTEMS THINKING/QUALITY IMPROVEMENT
Chronic Kidney Disease (CKD) Clinics Improving Patient Outcomes

Himmelfarb, J., & Ikizler, T. A. (2018). *Chronic kidney disease, dialysis and transplantation* (4th ed.). St. Louis: Elsevier.

CKD is a complex disease that affects physical, mental, and social aspects of health. This requires an understanding of available resources in order to improve patient outcomes. CKD clinics use an interprofessional approach, treating all aspects of the patient's health. Hospitals that develop and maintain clinics for patients with chronic diseases such as heart failure and CKD have fewer hospital readmissions and better patient outcomes. CKD clinics are successful because they foster care coordination and promote convenience for the patient.

The following services are recommended at a CKD clinic (Himmelfarb & Ikizler, 2018):

- Scheduling of tests (such as ultrasound and CT scans)
- Scheduling of specialist appointments as necessary
- Providing reminders for appointments and tests
- Following up with test results
- Providing a patient liaison for pharmacy and laboratory tests
- Consulting with interprofessional team members such as registered dietitian nutritionists (RDNs)
- Educating regarding disease processes, transplants, and therapies
- Referring as necessary for dialysis catheter insertion

Recognize Cues: Assessment

History. When taking a history from a patient with risk for or actual CKD, document the patient's age and gender. Accurately measure weight and height and ask about usual weight and recent weight gain or loss. Weight gain may indicate fluid retention from poor kidney function with disrupted *fluid and electrolyte balance.* Weight loss may be the result of anorexia from uremia.

Ask about a history of kidney and urologic disorders, chronic health problems, and drug use. Chronic hypertension, diabetes, inflammatory diseases such as systemic lupus erythematosus or arthritis, cancer, and tuberculosis can cause decreased kidney function. Ask the patient about family members' kidney disease, which might indicate a genetic problem.

Document the use of current and past prescribed and over-the-counter drugs because many drugs are nephrotoxic and drug interactions can cause kidney damage (Burchum & Rosenthal, 2022) (see Box 60.3). Ask whether the patient has had x-rays or CT scans with contrast media.

Examine the patient's dietary habits and discuss any GI problems. A change in the taste of foods often occurs with CKD. Patients may report that sweet foods are not as appealing or that meats have a metallic taste. Ask about the presence of nausea, vomiting, anorexia, hiccups, diarrhea, or constipation. These symptoms may be the result of excess wastes that the body cannot eliminate because of kidney disease.

Ask about the patient's energy level and any recent injuries or bleeding. Explore changes in the daily routine as a possible *result* of fatigue. Fatigue is a common and often profound problem among patients with CKD, particularly among patients receiving dialysis. Weakness, drowsiness, and shortness of breath suggest impending pulmonary edema or neurologic degeneration. Ask about bruising or bleeding caused by hematologic changes from uremia.

Discuss urine *elimination* in detail, including frequency of urination, appearance of the urine, and any difficulty starting or controlling urination. These data can help identify urologic problems that may influence kidney function. See Box 60.6.

Physical Assessment/Signs and Symptoms. CKD causes changes in all body systems (Box 60.7). Most symptoms are related to changes in *fluid and electrolyte balance, acid-base balance,* and buildup of nitrogenous wastes.

Neurologic symptoms of CKD and uremic syndrome vary (see Boxes 60.4 and 60.7). Observe for problems ranging from lethargy to seizures or coma, which may indicate uremic encephalopathy. Fluid overload can cause changes in cognition. Assess for sensory changes that appear in a glove-and-stocking pattern over the hands and feet *(peripheral neuropathy).* Check for weakness in upper and lower extremities *(uremic neuropathy).* Fatigue can result in decreased activity.

If untreated, encephalopathy can lead to seizures and coma. Dialysis is used emergently when neurologic problems result from CKD. The symptoms of encephalopathy may resolve with dialysis. However, improvement in neuropathy can be limited by severe or recurrent episodes of brain dysfunction. Depression may compound cognitive and neurologic problems.

BOX 60.6 Patient and Family Education

Prevention of Kidney and Urinary Problems

- Be alert to the general appearance of your urine. Note any changes in its color, clarity, or odor.
- Changes in the frequency or volume of urine passage occur with changes in fluid intake. More frequent or infrequent voiding not associated with changes in fluid intake may signal health problems.
- Any discomfort or distress with the passage of urine is not normal. Pain, burning, urgency, aching, or difficulty with initiating urine flow or complete bladder emptying is of some concern. Report such symptoms to your primary health care provider.
- The kidneys need 1 to 2 L of fluid a day to flush out your body wastes. Water is the ideal flushing agent.
- Avoid sugary, high-calorie drinks; they provide low-quality calories that contribute to weight gain and sugar-induced urination.
- Changes in kidney function are often silent for many years. Periodically ask your primary health care provider to measure your kidney function with a blood test (serum creatinine) and a urinalysis.
- If you have a history of kidney disease, diabetes mellitus, or hypertension (high blood pressure) or a family history of kidney disease, you should know your serum creatinine level and your glomerular filtration rate (either estimated from serum creatinine or measured with a 24-hour creatinine urine collection). At least one checkup per year that includes laboratory blood and urine testing of kidney function is recommended.
- If you are identified as having decreased kidney function, ask about whether any prescribed drug, diagnostic test, or therapeutic procedure will present a risk to your current kidney function. Evaluate the contribution of diet to risk for kidney disease with your primary health care provider or a registered dietitian nutritionist. Check out all nonprescription drugs with your primary health care provider or pharmacist before using them.

Cardiovascular symptoms of CKD result from fluid overload, hypertension, heart failure (HF), pericarditis, potassium-induced dysrhythmias, and cholesterol/calcium (plaque, atherosclerosis) deposits in blood vessels. Assess for indications of reduced sodium and water excretion. Blood volume overload, if untreated, leads to hypertension, pulmonary edema, peripheral edema, and HF.

Assess heart rate and rhythm, listening for extra sounds (particularly an S_3), irregular patterns, or a pericardial friction rub. Unless a dialysis vascular access has been created, measure blood pressure in each arm. Assess the jugular veins for distention, and assess for edema of the feet, shins, and sacrum and around the eyes. Crackles during lung auscultation and shortness of breath with exertion and at night suggest fluid overload.

Respiratory symptoms of CKD also vary (e.g., breath that smells like urine [*uremic fetor,* or uremic halitosis], deep sighing, yawning, shortness of breath). Observe the rhythm, rate, and depth of breathing. Tachypnea and hyperpnea (increased depth of breathing) occur with metabolic acidosis.

With severe metabolic acidosis, extreme increases in rate and depth of ventilation (Kussmaul respirations) occur. A few patients have pneumonitis, or *uremic lung.* In these patients, assess for thick sputum, reduced coughing, tachypnea, and fever. A pleural friction rub may be heard with a stethoscope. Patients often have pleuritic pain with breathing. Auscultate the lungs for crackles, which indicate fluid overload.

BOX 60.7   Key Features

Severe, Chronic, and End-Stage Kidney Disease

Neurologic Symptoms
- Lethargy and daytime drowsiness
- Inability to concentrate or decreased attention span
- Seizures
- Coma
- Slurred speech
- Asterixis (jerky movements or "flapping" of the hands)
- Tremors, twitching, or jerky movements
- Myoclonus
- Ataxia (alteration in gait)
- Paresthesias from peripheral neuropathy

Cardiovascular Symptoms
- Cardiomyopathy
- Hypertension
- Peripheral edema
- Heart failure
- Uremic pericarditis
- Pericardial effusion
- Pericardial friction rub
- Cardiac tamponade
- Cardiorenal syndrome

Respiratory Symptoms
- Uremic halitosis
- Tachypnea
- Deep sighing, yawning
- Kussmaul respirations
- Uremic pneumonitis
- Shortness of breath
- Pulmonary edema
- Pleural effusion
- Depressed cough reflex
- Crackles

Hematologic Symptoms
- Anemia
- Abnormal bleeding and bruising
- Reduced white blood cell count
- Increased risk for infection

GI Symptoms
- Anorexia
- Nausea
- Vomiting
- Metallic taste in the mouth
- Changes in taste acuity and sensation
- Uremic colitis (diarrhea)
- Constipation
- Uremic gastritis (possible GI bleeding)
- Uremic fetor (breath odor)
- Stomatitis

Urinary Symptoms
- Polyuria, nocturia (early)
- Oliguria, anuria (later)
- Proteinuria
- Hematuria
- Diluted, straw-colored urine appearance (early)
- Concentrated and cloudy urine appearance (later)

Integumentary Symptoms
- Decreased skin turgor
- Yellow-gray pallor/ash gray skin
- Dry skin
- Pruritus
- Ecchymosis
- Purpura
- Soft-tissue calcifications
- Uremic frost (late, premorbid)

Musculoskeletal Symptoms
- Muscle weakness and cramping
- Bone pain
- Fractures
- Renal osteodystrophy

Reproductive Symptoms
- Decreased fertility
- Infrequent or absent menses
- Decreased libido
- Impotence
- Sexual dysfunction

Metabolic Symptoms
- Hyperparathyroidism
- Hyperlipidemia
- Alterations in vitamin D, calcium, and phosphorus adsorption and metabolism
- Metabolic acidosis
- Hyperkalemia

Psychosocial Symptoms
- Depression
- Fatigue
- Sleep disturbances
- Sexual dysfunction
- Cognitive impairment
- Unemployment

Hematologic symptoms of CKD include anemia and abnormal bleeding. Check for indicators of anemia (e.g., fatigue, pallor/ash gray skin, lethargy, weakness, shortness of breath, dizziness). Check for abnormal bleeding by observing for bruising, petechiae, purpura, mucous membrane bleeding in the nose or gums, or intestinal bleeding (black, tarry stools [melena]).

GI symptoms of CKD include foul breath (halitosis) and mouth inflammation or ulceration. Document any abdominal pain, cramping, or vomiting. Test all stools for occult blood.

Skeletal symptoms of CKD are related to osteodystrophy from poor absorption of calcium and continuous bone calcium loss. Adults with osteodystrophy have thin, fragile bones that are at risk for fractures with even slight trauma. Vertebrae become more compact and may bend forward, leading to an overall loss of height. Ask about changes in height and bone pain. Observe for spinal curvatures and any unusual bumps or protrusions in bone areas that may indicate fractures. Handle the patient carefully during examination and care.

Urine symptoms in CKD reflect the kidneys' decreasing function. Urine amount, frequency, and appearance change. Protein, sediment, or blood may be in the urine.

The amount and composition of the urine change as kidney function decreases and waste *elimination* is disrupted. With the onset of mild to moderate CKD, the urine may be more dilute and clearer because tubular reabsorption of water is reduced. The actual urine output in a patient with CKD varies with the amount of remaining kidney function. The patient with severe CKD or ESKD usually has oliguria, but some patients continue to produce 1 L or more daily. Daily urine volume usually changes again after dialysis is started. A long duration of oliguria is an indication that recovery of kidney function is not to be expected.

Skin symptoms of CKD occur as a result of uremia. Pigment is deposited in the skin, causing a yellowish coloration, or darkening when skin is brown or bronze. The anemia of CKD causes sallowness, appearing as a faded suntan on lighter-skinned patients.

Skin oils and turgor are decreased in patients with uremia. A distressing problem of uremia is severe pruritus (itching). Uremic frost, a layer of urea crystals from evaporated sweat, may appear on the face, eyebrows, axillae, and groin in patients with advanced uremic syndrome. Assess for bruises (*ecchymosis*), purple patches (*purpura*), and rashes.

Psychosocial Assessment. CKD and its treatment disrupt many aspects of a patient's life. Psychosocial assessment and support are part of the nurse's role from the time that CKD is first diagnosed. With ongoing issues, a mental health professional is an important member of the care team. Ask about patients' understanding of the diagnosis and what the treatment regimen means to them (e.g., diet, drugs, dialysis). Assess for anxiety and fear and for coping styles used by the patient and family. CKD affects family relations, social activity, work patterns, body image, and sexual activity. The chronic nature of severe CKD and ESKD, the many treatment options, and the uncertainties about the disease and its treatment require ongoing psychosocial assessment, psychosocial interventions, and ongoing support. Support the recommendations of the mental health professional.

Laboratory Assessment. CKD causes extreme changes in many laboratory values (see Table 60.3). Monitor these blood values: creatinine, blood urea nitrogen (BUN), sodium, potassium, calcium, phosphorus, bicarbonate, hemoglobin, and hematocrit. Also monitor GFR for trends.

A urinalysis is performed. In the early stages of CKD, urinalysis may show protein, glucose, red blood cells (RBCs) and white blood cells (WBCs), and decreased or fixed specific gravity. Urine osmolarity is usually decreased. As CKD progresses, urine output decreases dramatically, and osmolarity increases. A urine albumin-to-creatinine ratio (UACR) provides important information about kidney function and damage.

Glomerular filtration rate (GFR) can be estimated from serum creatinine levels, age, gender, race, and body size. But this type of estimation is generally used for screening rather than for staging of CKD. Estimation of GFR based on a formula that includes serum creatinine is also useful to calculate drug dose or drug frequency when reduced kidney function is a concern. To determine stage of CKD, a urine collection of 3 to 24 hours is usually done to assess creatinine clearance. A spot urine albumin-to-creatinine ratio (UACR) also is calculated.

In severe CKD, serum creatinine and BUN levels may be used to determine the presence and degree of uremia. Serum creatinine levels may increase gradually over a period of years, reaching levels of 15 to 30 mg/dL (500–1000 mcmol/L) or more, depending on the patient's muscle mass. BUN levels are directly related to dietary protein intake. Without protein restriction, BUN levels may rise to 10 to 20 times the value of the serum creatinine level. With dietary protein restriction, BUN levels are elevated but less than those of non–protein-restricted patients. Fluid balance also affects BUN.

Imaging Assessment. Few x-ray findings are abnormal with CKD. Bone x-rays of the hand can show renal osteodystrophy. With long-term ESKD, the kidneys shrink (except for ESKD caused by polycystic kidney disease) and may be 8 to 9 cm or smaller. This small size results from atrophy and fibrosis. If CKD progresses suddenly, a kidney ultrasound or CT scan without contrast medium may be used to rule out an obstruction. (See Chapter 57 for a description of kidney function tests.)

Analyze Cues and Prioritize Hypotheses: Analysis

The patient with CKD usually has progressive reduction of kidney function. Management generally occurs in the community setting. In the acute or long-term care setting, the focus of care is to manage problems and prevent complications of CKD. The priority collaborative problems for patients with CKD include:

1. Fluid overload due to the inability of diseased kidneys to maintain body fluid balance
2. Decreased cardiac function due to reduced stroke volume, dysrhythmias, fluid overload, and increased peripheral vascular resistance
3. Weight loss due to inability to ingest, digest, or absorb food and nutrients as a result of physiologic factors
4. Potential for injury due to effects of kidney disease on bone density, blood clotting, and drug elimination
5. Potential for psychosocial compromise due to chronic kidney disease

---

BOX 60.8   Best Practice for Patient Safety and Quality Care

Managing Fluid Volume

- Weigh the patient daily at the same time each day, using the same scale, with the patient wearing the same amount and type of clothing, and graph the results.
- Observe the weight graph for trends (1 L of water weighs 1 kg [2.2 lb]).
- Accurately measure all fluid intake and output.
- Teach the patient and family about the need to keep fluid intake within prescribed restricted amounts and to ensure that the prescribed daily amount is evenly distributed throughout the 24 hours.
- Monitor for these symptoms of fluid overload at least every 4 hours during critical illness:
  - Decreased urine output
  - Rapid, bounding pulse
  - Rapid, shallow respirations
  - Presence of dependent edema
  - Auscultation of crackles or wheezes
  - Presence of distended neck veins in a sitting position
  - Decreased oxygen saturation
  - Elevated blood pressure
  - Narrowed pulse pressure
- Assess level of consciousness and degree of cognition.
- Ask about the presence of headache or blurred vision.

Generate Solutions and Take Actions: Planning and Implementation

Managing Fluid Volume

Planning: Expected Outcomes. The patient with CKD is expected to achieve and maintain an acceptable *fluid and electrolyte balance* and remain free of pulmonary edema.

Interventions. Management of the patient with CKD includes drug therapy, nutrition therapy, fluid restriction, and dialysis (when the patient reaches stage 5). Hemodialysis is performed intermittently for 3 to 4 hours, typically 3 days per week. Alternatively, some patients with ESKD receive peritoneal dialysis (PD). PD uses the peritoneum as the dialyzing membrane. The dialysate is infused through a catheter tunneled into the peritoneum. Dialysis for ESKD is described later in the Kidney Replacement Therapies section.

The purpose of fluid management is to attain fluid balance and prevent complications of fluid overload (see Box 60.8 for best practices to manage fluid volume). Monitor the patient's intake and output and hydration status. Assess for indications of fluid overload (e.g., lung crackles, edema, distended neck veins).

Drug therapy with diuretics is prescribed for patients with mild to severe CKD to increase urinary *elimination* of fluid. The increased urine output with this therapy helps reduce fluid overload and hypertension in patients who still have some urine output. Diuretics are seldom used in ESKD after dialysis is started, because as kidney function is reduced these drugs can accumulate and harm the remaining kidney cells and the patient's hearing. (See Table 60.5 for common examples of drug therapy for chronic kidney disease.

TABLE 60.5   Common Examples of Drug Therapy

Chronic Kidney Disease

Drug	Selected Nursing Implications
Loop Diuretics	
Increase urine output to manage volume overload when urinary elimination is still present.	
• Furosemide • Bumetanide • Dose varies with severity of kidney damage; not effective in ESKD	Monitor intake and output *to assess therapy effectiveness.* In general, the expected outcome is for output to be greater than intake by 500–1000 mL/24 hr. Monitor electrolytes *because these drugs result in loss of potassium;* this can be a desired effect in patients with hyperkalemia.
Vitamins and Minerals	
Used to replace those lost through dialysis or poorly absorbed as a result of dietary restrictions and to lower vitamin or mineral excesses that could lead to more problems.	
Phosphate binders form an insoluble calcium-phosphate complex to inhibit GI absorption to prevent hyperphosphatemia and renal osteodystrophy from hypocalcemia: • Calcium acetate • Calcium carbonate Noncalcium phosphate binders reduce blood phosphate levels without disturbing calcium levels: • Lanthanum carbonate • Sevelamer	Teach patients to take drugs with meals *to increase the effectiveness in slowing or preventing the absorption of dietary phosphorus.* Teach patients not to take these drugs within 2 hours of other scheduled drugs *to prevent the inhibited absorption of other drugs, especially cardiac drugs and antibiotics.* Monitor both serum phosphorus and calcium levels *because these drugs lower phosphorus and can cause hypercalcemia.* Monitor for constipation *because these drugs can cause significant constipation, leading to fecal impaction or ileus.* Teach patients to report muscle weakness, slow or irregular pulse, or confusion to the prescriber *because these are symptoms of hypophosphatemia and indicate that dosage adjustment is required.*
Multivitamins and vitamin B supplements • Folic acid/folate • Cyanocobalamin (B$_{12}$)	Teach patients to take the drugs after dialysis *to prevent the supplement from being removed from the blood during dialysis.* Teach patients to take iron supplements (ferrous sulfate) with meals *to reduce nausea and abdominal discomfort.*
Oral iron salts • Ferrous sulfate • Ferrous fumarate • Ferrous gluconate	Teach patients to take stool softeners daily while taking iron supplements, *which can cause constipation.* Remind patients that iron supplements change the color of the stool *because knowing the expected side effects decreases anxiety when they appear.*
Parenteral iron salts • Iron dextran (IV) • Iron sucrose (IV)	A test dose of iron dextran is recommended before IV administration *because the incidence of allergic reactions is high.* Do not mix with drug with other parenteral drugs *because there are many incompatibilities.*
Vitamin D • Calcitriol • Paricalcitol • Doxercalciferol	Monitor serum levels of calcium *because this active form of vitamin D suppresses parathyroid production and can lead to hypocalcemia.* Monitor serum levels of vitamin D *because this is a lipid-soluble vitamin that can be overingested and lead to toxicity.* Serum calcium levels should stay below 10 mg/dL (Burchum & Rosenthal, 2022).
Erythropoietin-Stimulating Agents (ESAs)	
Used to prevent or correct anemia caused by kidney disease through the stimulation of the bone marrow to increase red blood cell production and maturation.	
• Epoetin alfa • Darbepoetin alfa	Monitor hemoglobin values *because these drugs can overproduce blood cells, which increases blood viscosity and causes hypertension. This problem increases the risk for a myocardial infarction.* Dosage is individualized to produce hemoglobin levels no higher than 10–11 g/dL (Burchum & Rosenthal, 2022). Teach patients to report any of these side effects to the prescriber as soon as possible: chest pain, difficulty breathing, high blood pressure, rapid weight gain, seizures, skin rash or hives, or swelling of feet or ankles, *because these symptoms indicate possible serious cardiac complications.*
Parathyroid Hormone Modulator	
Used to reduce parathyroid gland production of parathyroid hormone by decreasing the gland's sensitivity to calcium. This action helps maintain blood calcium and phosphorus levels closer to normal and can reduce renal osteodystrophy in patients with chronic kidney disease. • Cinacalcet	Monitor blood levels of calcium and phosphorus *to assess drug therapy effectiveness and recognize imbalances of these important electrolytes.* Teach the patient to monitor for and report diarrhea and muscle pain (myalgia), *which are indications of calcium and/or phosphorus imbalance.*

ESKD, End-stage kidney disease.

Assess fluid status by obtaining daily weights and reviewing intake and output. Daily weight gain in these patients indicates fluid retention rather than true body weight gain. Estimate the amount of fluid retained: 1 kg of weight equals about 1 L of fluid retained. Weigh the patient daily at the same time each day, on the same scale, wearing the same amount of clothing, and after voiding (if the patient is not anuric). Monitor weight for changes before and after dialysis.

Fluid restriction is often needed. Consider all forms of fluid intake, including oral, IV, and enteral sources, when calculating fluid intake. Help the patient spread oral fluid intake over a 24-hour period. Monitor the response to fluid restriction, and notify the primary health care provider if symptoms of fluid overload persist or worsen.

Pulmonary edema can result from left-sided heart failure (HF) related to fluid overload or from blood vessel injury. In left-sided HF, the heart is unable to eject blood adequately from the left ventricle, leading to an increased pressure in the left atrium and in the pulmonary blood vessels. The increased pressure causes fluid to cross the capillaries into the pulmonary tissue, forming edema (Rogers, 2023). Pulmonary edema can also occur from injury to the lung blood vessels as a result of uremia. This condition causes inflammation and capillary leak. Fluid then leaks from pulmonary circulation into the lung tissue and alveoli. It may also leak into the pleural space, causing a *pleural effusion.*

Assess the patient for early indicators of pulmonary edema, such as restlessness, anxiety, rapid heart rate, shortness of breath, and crackles that begin at the base of the lungs. As pulmonary edema worsens, the level of fluid in the lungs rises. Auscultation reveals increased crackles and decreased breath sounds. The patient may have frothy, blood-tinged sputum. As cardiac and pulmonary function decrease further, the patient becomes diaphoretic and cyanotic.

The patient with pulmonary edema usually is admitted to the hospital for aggressive treatment and continuous cardiac monitoring. Place the patient in a high-Fowler's position and give oxygen to improve gas exchange. Drug therapy with kidney failure and pulmonary edema is difficult because of potential adverse drug effects on the kidneys (Burchum & Rosenthal, 2022). Loop diuretics such as IV furosemide are used to manage pulmonary edema. Kidney impairment increases the risk for *ototoxicity* (ear damage with hearing loss) with furosemide; IV doses are given cautiously and slowly. Diuresis usually begins within 5 minutes of giving IV furosemide. Measure urine output hourly until the patient is stabilized. Monitor vital signs and assess breath sounds at least every 2 hours to evaluate the patient's response to this treatment.

IV morphine can be prescribed to reduce myocardial oxygen demand by triggering blood vessel dilation and to provide sedation. Dosage adjustments are needed to achieve the desired response and avoid respiratory depression. Monitor the patient's respiratory rate, oxygen saturation, and blood pressure hourly during this therapy. Other drugs that dilate blood vessels, such as nitroglycerin, may be given as a continuous infusion to reduce pulmonary pressure from left-sided HF. Monitor vital signs at least hourly because this drug combination may cause severe hypotension.

Monitor serum electrolyte levels daily and report abnormalities to the primary health care provider so imbalances can be corrected quickly. If using ECG monitoring, identify dysrhythmias as they occur and immediately report changes in rhythm that affect consciousness or blood pressure to the provider. Monitor oxygen saturation levels by pulse oximetry and consult with the respiratory therapist for the optimal method to deliver oxygen (e.g., facemask, nasal cannula, or noninvasive mechanical support [see Chapter 22]). Monitor the patient for worsening of the condition with indications of increasing hypoxemia (decreasing SpO_2 values, restlessness, decreased cognition, or new-onset confusion). Temporary intubation and mechanical ventilation may be needed if respiratory failure occurs.

Patients with CKD who have existing cardiac problems, high blood pressure, or chronic fluid retention are at increased risk for developing pulmonary edema. They are less likely to respond quickly to treatment and are more likely to develop problems related to drug therapy. Kidney replacement therapy with ultrafiltration or dialysis may be used to reduce fluid volume.

Improving Cardiac Function

Planning: Expected Outcomes. The patient with CKD is expected to attain and maintain adequate cardiac function.

Interventions. Many patients with long-standing hypertension are at risk for CKD and accelerated progression of kidney failure once CKD occurs. *Therefore blood pressure control is essential in preserving kidney function* (Norton et al., 2017a). To control blood pressure, diuretics (especially thiazides), calcium channel blockers, angiotensin-converting enzyme inhibitors (ACEIs), alpha-adrenergic and beta-adrenergic blockers, and vasodilators may be prescribed. ACEIs are the most effective drugs to decrease cardiovascular events when patients have CKD and hypertension. Calcium channel blockers can improve the GFR and blood flow within the kidney.

More information on the specific drugs for blood pressure control can be found in Chapter 30. Indications vary, depending on the patient, and these drugs are used carefully to avoid complications. Different dosages and combinations may be tried until blood pressure control is adequate and side effects are minimized. Although there are many blood pressure guidelines available regarding goals of treatment, in CKD (diabetic and nondiabetic) with albumin excretion greater than 30 mg/24 hr, a target blood pressure of 130/80 mm Hg or lower is recommended (Ferri, 2022).

Teach the patient and family to measure blood pressure daily. Evaluate their ability to measure and record blood pressure accurately using their own equipment. Recheck measurement accuracy on a regular basis. Teach the patient and family about the relationship of blood pressure control to diet and drug therapy. Instruct the patient to weigh daily and to bring records of blood pressure measurements and drug administration times and weights for discussion with the health care provider, nurse, or registered dietitian nutritionist.

Assess the patient on an ongoing basis for signs and symptoms of reduced cardiac output, heart failure (HF), and dysrhythmias. These topics are discussed in Chapters 27, 28, and 29.

TABLE 60.6	Dietary Restrictions Needed for Severe Kidney Disease		
Dietary Component	**With Chronic Uremia**	**With Hemodialysis**	**With Peritoneal Dialysis**
Protein	0.55–0.60 g/kg/day	1.0–1.5 g/kg/day	1.2–1.5 g/kg/day
Fluid	Depends on urine output but may be as high as 1500–3000 mL/day	500–700 mL/day plus amount of urine output	Restriction based on fluid weight gain and blood pressure
Potassium	60–70 mEq or mmol daily	70 mEq or mmol daily	Usually no restriction
Sodium	1–3 g/day	2–4 g/day	Restriction based on fluid weight gain and blood pressure
Phosphorus	700 mg/day	700 mg/day	800 mg/day

Enhancing Nutrition

Planning: Expected Outcomes. The patient with CKD is expected to maintain adequate nutrition, demonstrating a protein-caloric intake appropriate for their weight-to-height ratio, muscle tone, and laboratory values (serum albumin, hematocrit, hemoglobin).

Interventions. The nutrition needs and diet restrictions for the patient with CKD vary according to the degree of kidney function and the type of kidney replacement therapy used (Table 60.6). The purpose of nutrition therapy is to provide the food and fluids needed to prevent malnutrition and avoid complications from CKD.

Referral to a registered dietitian nutritionist (RDN) is recommended in patients with a GFR below 50 mL/min/1.73 m^2 and is a Medicare-covered service (Ferri, 2022). Collaborate with the RDN to teach the patient about diet changes that are needed as a result of CKD. Common changes include control of protein intake; fluid intake limitation; restriction of potassium, sodium, and phosphorus intake; taking vitamin and mineral supplements; and eating enough calories to meet metabolic need.

Protein restriction early in the course of the disease prevents some of the problems of CKD and may preserve kidney function. Protein is restricted on the basis of the degree of kidney and waste **elimination** impairment (reduced glomerular filtration rate [GFR]) and the severity of the symptoms. Buildup of waste products from protein breakdown is the main cause of uremia.

The GFR and treatment of CKD are used to guide safe levels of protein intake. In patients with a GFR below 30 mL/min/1.73 m^2, KDIGO has recommended that protein intake should be lowered to 0.8 g/kg/day. Protein intake greater than 1.3 g/kg/day should be avoided in adults with CKD at risk of progression (Ferri, 2022). If protein is lost in the urine, it is added to the diet in amounts equal to that lost. Protein requirements are calculated by the registered dietitian nutritionist based on actual body weight (corrected for edema), not ideal body weight.

The patient with ESKD receiving dialysis needs *more* protein because some protein is lost through dialysis. Protein requirements are tailored according to the patient's postdialysis, or "dry," weight. In general, patients receiving hemodialysis are allowed about 1 to 1.3 g of protein per kilogram per day (Ferri, 2022). Suggested protein-containing foods are meat and eggs. If protein intake is not adequate, muscle wasting can occur. BUN and serum prealbumin levels are used to monitor the adequacy of protein intake. Decreased serum prealbumin levels indicate poor protein intake.

Sodium restriction is needed in patients with little or no urine output to maintain **fluid and electrolyte balance.** Both fluid and sodium retention cause edema, hypertension, and heart failure (HF). Most patients with CKD retain sodium; a few cannot conserve sodium.

Estimate fluid and sodium retention status by monitoring the patient's body weight and blood pressure. In uremic patients not receiving dialysis, sodium is limited to 1 to 3 g daily, and fluid intake depends on urine output. In patients receiving dialysis, the sodium restriction is 2 to 4 g daily, and fluid intake is limited to 500 to 700 mL plus the amount of any urine output. Instruct the patient not to add salt at the table or during cooking. Many foods are significant sources of sodium (e.g., processed food, fast food, potato chips, pretzels, pickles, ham, bacon, sausage) and difficult to moderate or remove from one's diet. Inattention to sodium intake can increase the duration or number of dialysis treatments and contribute to *disequilibrium syndrome* (feeling unsteady or off balance) following dialysis.

Potassium restriction may be needed because high blood potassium levels can cause dangerous cardiac dysrhythmias. Monitor the ECG for tall, peaked T waves caused by hyperkalemia. Instruct patients with ESKD to limit potassium intake to 60 to 70 mEq (mmol) daily. Teach them to read labels of seasoning agents carefully for sodium and potassium content. Foods that are low in potassium and are permitted and foods that are high in potassium should be avoided (see Chapter 13). Instruct patients to avoid salt substitutes composed of potassium chloride. Those receiving peritoneal dialysis (PD) or who are producing urine may not need potassium restriction.

Phosphorus restriction for control of phosphorus levels is started early in CKD to avoid renal osteodystrophy. Monitor serum phosphorus levels. Dietary phosphorus restrictions and drugs to assist with phosphorus control may be prescribed. Phosphate binders must be taken at mealtime. Most patients with CKD already restrict their protein intake; because high-protein foods are also high in phosphorus, this reduces phosphorus intake. Chapter 13 lists foods high in potassium, sodium, and phosphorus. Cinacalcet, a drug to control parathyroid hormone excess, is also used to manage hyperphosphatemia and hypocalcemia.

Vitamin and mineral supplementation is needed daily for most patients with CKD. Low-protein diets are also low in vitamins, and water-soluble vitamins are removed from the blood during dialysis. Anemia also is a problem in patients with CKD because of the limited iron content of low-protein diets and decreased kidney production of erythropoietin. Therefore, supplemental iron is needed. Calcium and vitamin D supplements may be needed, depending on the patient's serum calcium levels and bone status.

Nutrition needs for patients undergoing peritoneal dialysis (PD) are slightly different from those for patients undergoing dialysis. Because protein is lost with the dialysate in PD, protein replacement is needed. Often 1.2 to 1.5 g of protein per kilogram of body weight per day is recommended. Patients may have anorexia and have difficulty eating enough protein. High-calorie oral supplements may also be needed (e.g., Magnacal Renal, Ensure Plus). Sodium restriction varies with fluid weight gain and blood pressure. Dietary potassium usually does not need to be restricted because the dialysate is potassium free, causing excess potassium to be removed from the blood. Any potassium restriction is determined by serum potassium levels.

Collaborate with the RDN to assess each patient's nutrition needs. Teach the patient the dietary regimen and evaluate understanding of and adherence to it. Give the patient and family written examples of the diet to promote adherence. Help patients adapt dietary restrictions to their budget and food preferences.

NCLEX Examination Challenge 60.4

Physiological Integrity

The nurse is teaching a client with end-stage kidney disease who is on hemodialysis regarding dietary selections. Which of the following statements would the nurse include? **Select all that apply.**

A. "A reduction of fluid to 1 to 2 L/day is suggested."
B. "Avoid salty foods and adding salt when cooking."
C. "A dietitian will be consulted to help with food selections at home."
D. "Protein can be lost through hemodialysis, so 1 g/kg per day is suggested."
E. "Foods that are high in potassium are important to replace potential loss."

Preventing Injury

Planning: Expected Outcomes. The patient with CKD is expected to remain free of injury including pathologic fractures, toxic side effects from drug therapy, infection, and bleeding.

Interventions. *Injury prevention strategies* are needed because the patient with long-standing CKD may have brittle, fragile bones that fracture easily and cause little pain. When lifting or moving a patient with fragile bones, use a lift sheet rather than pulling the patient. Teach assistive personnel (AP) the correct use of lift sheets. Observe for normal range of joint motion and for any unusual surface bumps or depressions over bony areas.

Managing drug therapy in patients with CKD is a complex clinical problem. Many over-the-counter drugs contain agents that alter kidney function. Therefore it is important to obtain a detailed drug history. Know the use of each drug, its side effects, and its site of metabolism.

Certain drugs must be avoided, and the dosages of others must be adjusted according to the degree of remaining kidney function. As the patient's kidney function decreases, consult with the nephrologist and pharmacist to determine if further dosage adjustments are necessary. Assess for side effects and indications of drug toxicity and notify the prescriber as appropriate.

⬭ NURSING SAFETY PRIORITY

Drug Alert

Monitor the patient with severe chronic kidney disease (CKD) or end-stage kidney disease (ESKD) closely for drug-related complications, and ensure that dosages are adjusted as needed. Patients with CKD have complex needs due to multiple medications and comorbidities. Consult with the pharmacist to determine safe effective doses.

Drugs to control an excessively high phosphorus level include phosphate-binding agents. These drugs help prevent renal osteodystrophy and related injuries. Stress the importance of taking these agents and all prescribed drugs.

Hypophosphatemia (low serum phosphorus levels) is a complication of phosphate binding, especially in patients who do not eat adequately but continue to take phosphate-binding drugs. *Hypercalcemia* (high serum calcium levels) can occur in patients taking calcium-containing compounds to control phosphorus excess. In patients taking aluminum-based phosphate binders for prolonged periods, aluminum deposits may cause bone disease or neurologic problems. Monitor the patient for muscle weakness, anorexia, malaise, tremors, and bone pain.

Teach patients with kidney disease to avoid antacids containing magnesium. These patients cannot excrete magnesium and thus should avoid additional intake.

Some drugs, in addition to those used to treat kidney failure, require special attention because they either are normally excreted by the kidney or can further damage the kidney. These drugs include antibiotics, opioids, antihypertensives, diuretics, insulin, and heparin.

Monitor carefully for indicators of infection. These indicators include fever, lymph node enlargements, and elevated WBC counts, as well as positive cultures. For patients undergoing dialysis, inspect the vascular access site or PD catheter insertion site every shift for redness/hyperpigmentation, swelling, pain, or drainage. If antibiotics are required, use caution in the patient with CKD. Many antibiotics are safe for patients with CKD, but those excreted by the kidney and those that are nephrotoxic require dose adjustment (Himmelfarb & Ikizler, 2018). To prevent complications of bloodstream infection from mouth bacteria, prophylactic antibiotics are given to patients with CKD before dental procedures.

Give opioid analgesics cautiously in patients with stage 3 or 4 CKD or ESKD because the effects often last longer. Patients with uremia are sensitive to the respiratory depressant effects of these drugs. Because opioids are broken down by the liver and not the kidneys, the dosages are often the same, regardless of the level of kidney function. Monitor the patient's reactions closely after opioids are given to determine whether adjustments are needed.

As CKD progresses, the patient with diabetes often requires reduced doses of insulin or antidiabetic drugs because the failing kidneys do not excrete or metabolize these drugs well. Therefore the drugs are effective longer, increasing the risk for hypoglycemia. Monitor blood glucose levels at least four times daily to assess whether a dosage change is needed.

Poor platelet function and capillary fragility in CKD make anticoagulant therapy risky. Monitor patients receiving heparin, warfarin, or any anticoagulant every shift for bleeding. See Chapter 34 for more information on caring for patients at increased risk for bleeding.

Minimizing Psychosocial Compromise. Due to the chronic nature and impact of CKD, the patient with CKD may experience fatigue and psychosocial impact. These impacts can include anxiety, social isolation, and depression. The patient with CKD often experiences depression (Lotfaliany, 2018). Loss, such as loss of work or family roles, may contribute to depression. Depressive symptoms have been associated with nonadherence to CKD treatments. Sleep disturbances, also interrelated with depression, are common among adults receiving dialysis for ESKD.

Planning: Expected Outcomes. The goal for patients with CKD is to conserve energy by balancing activity and rest, have reduced anxiety and depression, and minimize the overall psychosocial impact of the disease.

Interventions. Perform an ongoing assessment of the patient's level of fatigue as well as reports of anxiety. Ask about sleep patterns and quality. Assess the coping mechanisms and successful methods of dealing with problems. Observe behavior for cues indicating increasing anxiety (e.g., anxious facial expressions, clenching of hands, tapping of feet, withdrawn posture, absence of eye contact) and provide interventions to decrease the anxiety level. Evaluate the support systems and the involvement of family and friends with the patient's care. Provide ongoing supportive interventions throughout therapy. Assess for indicators of depression including despair and loneliness.

Some causes of *fatigue* in the patient with CKD include vitamin deficiency, anemia, and buildup of urea. All patients are given vitamin and mineral supplements because of diet restrictions and vitamin losses from dialysis. Avoid giving these supplements right before hemodialysis (HD) treatment because they will be dialyzed out of the body and the patient will receive no benefit.

The anemic patient with CKD is treated with agents to stimulate red blood cell (RBC) production. The desired outcome of this therapy is to maintain a hemoglobin level around 10 g/dL (100 g/L). This therapy triggers bone marrow production of RBCs if the patient has adequate iron stores. Iron supplements may be needed in patients who are iron deficient. Many who receive these drugs report improved appetite and sexual function along with decreased fatigue. The increased production of all blood cells from this therapy may increase blood pressure. The improved appetite challenges patients in their attempts to maintain protein, potassium, and fluid restrictions and requires additional education.

Unfamiliar settings and lack of knowledge about treatments and tests can increase the patient's anxiety level. Explain all procedures, tests, and treatments. Identify patients' knowledge needs about kidney disease. Provide instruction at a level that they can understand, using a variety of written and visual materials. Provide continuity of care, whenever possible, by using a consistent and trusting nurse-patient relationship to decrease anxiety, and encourage the patient to discuss thoughts and feelings about any current problems or concerns.

Encourage the patient to ask questions and discuss fears about the diagnosis, treatment strategies, and common outcomes. An open atmosphere that allows for discussion can decrease anxiety. Facilitate discussions with family members about the prognosis and the impact on lifestyle.

Identify community resources to maintain independence, including delivered meals, transportation, and financial or health care options.

In the general population, drugs are commonly used to manage depression. However, pharmacologic effects of drugs in adults with CKD or those receiving dialysis are altered, and additional monitoring may be needed with alternative approaches for effective care. Care coordination for patients with CKD is essential because multiple health care professions may be involved in delivering care. Care coordination helps to avoid adverse drug effects (and drug-drug interactions), avoid hospitalizations, and decrease problems related to depression.

Kidney Replacement Therapies

Kidney replacement therapy (KRT) is needed when the pathologic changes of stage 4 and stage 5 CKD are life-threatening or pose continuing discomfort. When the patient can no longer be managed with conservative therapies, such as diet, drugs, and fluid restriction, dialysis is indicated. Transplantation may be discussed at any time.

Hemodialysis. Intermittent hemodialysis (HD) is the most common KRT used with ESKD. Dialysis removes excess fluids and waste products and restores *fluid and electrolyte balance* and *acid-base balance.* HD involves passing the patient's blood through an artificial semipermeable membrane to perform the kidney's filtering and excretion functions. Safe HD therapy requires technicians to provide meticulous care to the machines delivering HD and nurses to implement and supervise direct care. Technical or human error can lead to avoidable complications (e.g., hemolysis, air embolism, dialysate error, contamination, exsanguination).

Patient Selection. Any patient may be considered for intermittent HD therapy. Starting HD depends on symptoms from disruptions of *fluid and electrolyte balance* and waste and toxin accumulation, not the GFR alone. Normally the decision to start dialysis is made by a nephrologist who has been monitoring a patient's decreasing GFR and increasing symptoms. Some indications for emergent dialysis include:

- Pulmonary edema
- Severe uncontrollable hypertension
- Symptomatic hyperkalemia with ECG changes
- Other severe electrolyte or acid-base disturbances
- Some overdoses
- Pericarditis

Most commonly, hemodialysis for CKD is started when uremic symptoms (e.g., intractable nausea and vomiting, confusion, seizures, or severe bleeding from platelet dysfunction) occur.

Many patients survive for years with HD therapy, and others may live only a few months. Length of survival with HD therapy depends on patient's age, the cause of CKD, and the presence of other diseases, such as cardiovascular conditions or diabetes. Selection criteria include:

- Irreversible kidney failure when other therapies are unacceptable or ineffective
- No disorders that would seriously complicate HD
- Patient values and preferences
- Expected ability to continue or resume roles at home, work, or school

Dialysis Settings. Patients with CKD may receive HD treatments in many settings, depending on specific needs. Regardless of the setting of therapy, they need ongoing nursing support to maintain this complex and lifesaving treatment.

Patients may be dialyzed in a hospital-based center if they have recently started treatment or have complicated conditions that require close supervision. Stable patients not requiring intense supervision may be dialyzed in a community or free-standing dialysis center. Selected patients may participate in self-care in an ambulatory care center or with in-home HD.

In-home HD is the least disruptive treatment and allows patients to adapt the regimen to their lifestyle. Newer technologies and HD equipment are making home dialysis an easier process to learn. It is growing in popularity and use. A water-treatment system must be installed in the home to provide a safe, clean water supply for the dialysis process.

Procedure. Dialysis works by using the passive transfer of toxins by diffusion. Diffusion is the movement of molecules from an area of higher concentration to an area of lower concentration. The rate of diffusion during dialysis is most dependent on the difference in the solute concentrations between the patient's blood and the dialysate. Large molecules, such as RBCs and most plasma proteins, cannot pass through the membrane.

When HD is started, blood and dialysate (dialyzing solution) flow in opposite directions across an enclosed semipermeable membrane. The dialysate contains a balanced mix of electrolytes and water that closely resembles human plasma. On the other side of the membrane is the patient's blood, which contains nitrogen waste products, excess water, and excess electrolytes. During HD, the waste products move from the blood into the dialysate because of the difference in their concentrations (diffusion). Some water is also removed from the blood into the dialysate by *osmosis*. Electrolytes can move in either direction, as needed, and take some fluid with them. Potassium and sodium typically move out of the plasma into the dialysate. Bicarbonate and calcium generally move from the dialysate into the plasma. This circulating process continues for a preset length of time, removing nitrogenous wastes, reestablishing ***fluid and electrolyte balance,*** and restoring ***acid-base balance.*** Water volume may be removed from the plasma by applying positive or negative pressure to the system.

The HD system includes a dialyzer, dialysate, vascular access routes, and an HD machine. The artificial kidney, or dialyzer (Fig. 60.5), has four parts: a blood compartment, a dialysate compartment, a semipermeable membrane, and an enclosed support structure.

Dialysate is made from water and chemicals and is free of any waste products or drugs. It is usually dispensed from the

Hemodialysis Process

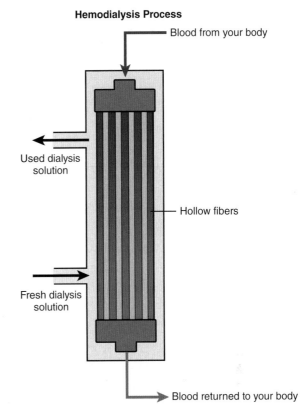

FIG. 60.5 Hollow fiber dialyzer (artificial kidney) used in hemodialysis. (From Feehally, J., Floege, J., & Johnson, R. [2007]. *Comprehensive clinical nephrology* [3rd ed.]. Philadelphia: Mosby.)

pharmacy in an acute care setting. The solution may be mixed in large or small batches by technicians in dialysis centers. Because bacteria and other organisms are too large to pass through the membrane, dialysate is not sterile. Water used in dialysate must meet specific standards and requires special treatment before mixing the dialysate. Dialysate composition may be altered for the patient's needs for management of electrolyte imbalances. During HD, the dialysate is warmed to 100°F (37.8°C) to increase the diffusion rate and prevent hypothermia.

The HD machine has built-in safety features such as the ability to record patient vital signs, blood and dialysate flows, arterial and venous pressures, delivered dialysis dose, plasma volume changes, and temperature changes. If any of these problems are detected, an alarm sounds to protect the patient from life-threatening complications.

All dialyzers function in a similar manner. Fig. 60.6 shows a comparison of fluid and particle movement across the dialyzer membranes, comparing intermittent HD with continuous kidney replacement circuits. For intermittent HD, the number and length of treatments depend on the amount of wastes and fluid to be removed, the clearance capacity of the dialyzer, and the blood flow rate to and from the machine. Fig. 60.7 shows a typical intermittent dialysis machine. Most patients receive three 4-hour treatments over the course of a week. For those with some ongoing urine production, two 5- to 6-hour treatments a week may be adequate. If the patient gains large amounts of fluid, a longer HD treatment time may be needed to remove the fluid without hypotension or other severe side effects.

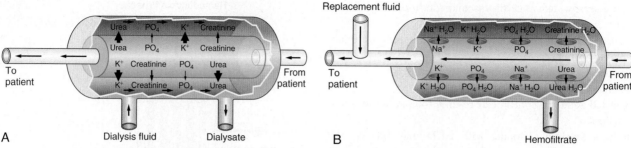

FIG. 60.6 Comparison of hemodialysis and hemofiltration fluid and solute movements across the membrane. Demonstrates this movement in hemodialysis (A) and hemofiltration (B). The *arrows* that cross the membrane indicate the predominant direction of movement of each solute through the membrane; the relative size of the *arrows* indicates the net amounts of the solute transferred. Other *arrows* indicate the direction of flow. (From Feehally, J., Floege, J., & Johnson, R. [2007]. *Comprehensive clinical nephrology* [3rd ed.]. Philadelphia: Mosby.)

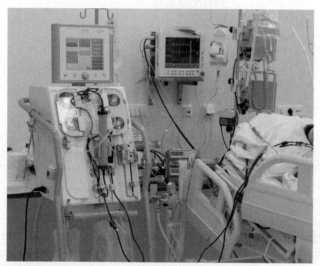

FIG. 60.7 Dialysis machine to which patient is connected in ICU in hospital. (Used with permission from istockphoto.com, 2020, PatrikSlezak.)

Anticoagulation. Blood clotting can occur during dialysis. Anticoagulation, usually with heparin, is delivered into the blood circuit via a pump. In patients with high risk for bleeding, a reduced dose, regional anticoagulation (using citrate rather than heparin for anticoagulation or reversing heparin actions by administering protamine before returning blood to the patient), or no anticoagulation may be used. Patient response to heparin varies, and the dose is adjusted on the basis of each patient's need.

Heparin remains active in the body for 4 to 6 hours after dialysis, increasing the patient's risk for hemorrhage during and immediately after HD treatments. Invasive procedures must be avoided during that time. Monitor the patient closely for any signs of bleeding or hemorrhage. Protamine sulfate is an antidote to heparin and always should be available in the dialysis setting.

Vascular Access. Vascular access is required for hemodialysis (Table 60.7 and Fig. 60.8). The procedure requires the availability of a high blood flow: at least 250 to 300 mL/min, usually for a period of 3 to 4 hours (Norton et al., 2017b). Normal venous cannulation does not provide this high rate of blood flow.

Long-term vascular access is internal for most patients having long-term HD (see Table 60.7). The two common choices are an internal arteriovenous (AV) fistula or an AV graft (see Fig.

60.8). *AV fistulas* are formed by surgically connecting an artery to a vein. The vessels used most often are the radial or brachial artery and the cephalic vein of the nondominant arm. Fistulas increase venous blood flow to the 250 to 400 mL/min needed for effective dialysis.

Time is needed after the surgeon creates the AV fistula for it to develop into a usable access site for HD. As the AV fistula "matures," the increased pressure of the arterial blood flow into the vein causes the vessel walls to thicken. This thickening increases their strength and durability for repeated cannulation. The amount of time needed for the fistula to mature varies. Some fistulas may not be ready for use for as long as 4 months after the surgery, and a temporary vascular access (AV shunt or HD catheter) is used during this time. Fig. 60.9 shows a mature fistula.

To access a fistula, cannulate it by inserting two needles: one toward the venous blood flow and one toward the arterial blood flow. This procedure allows the HD machine to draw the blood out through the arterial needle and return it through the venous needle.

Arteriovenous grafts are used when the AV fistula does not develop or when complications limit its use. The polytetrafluoroethylene (PTFE) graft is a synthetic material (GORE-TEX). This type of graft is commonly used for older patients undergoing HD. Figs. 60.8A and 60.9 show a patient's fistula.

Precautions. Precautions are needed to ensure the functioning of an internal AV fistula or AV graft. First assess for adequate circulation in the fistula or graft and in the lower portion of the arm. Check distal pulses and capillary refill in the arm with the fistula or graft. Then check for a bruit or a thrill by auscultation or palpation over the access site. See Box 60.9 for best practice when caring for a patient with an AV fistula or AV graft.

! NURSING SAFETY PRIORITY

Action Alert

Because repeated compression can result in the loss of the vascular access, avoid taking the blood pressure or performing venipunctures in the arm with the vascular access. Do not use an arteriovenous (AV) fistula or graft for general delivery of IV fluids or drugs.

TABLE 60.7	Types of Vascular Access for Hemodialysis		
Access Type	**Description**	**Location**	**Time to Initial Use**
Permanent			
AV fistula	An internal anastomosis of an artery to a vein	Forearm Upper arm	2–3 mo or longer
AV graft	Looped plastic tubing tunneled beneath the skin, connecting an artery and a vein	Forearm Upper arm Inner thigh	1–3 wk after surgery
Temporary			
Dialysis catheter	A specially designed catheter with separate lumens for blood outflow and inflow	Subclavian, internal jugular, or femoral vein	Immediately after insertion and x-ray confirmation of placement
Subcutaneous catheter	An internal device with two access ports and a cuff or dual-lumen catheter inserted into a large central vein	Subclavian, internal jugular, or femoral vein	Dedicated use; do not access for blood sampling or drug administration

AV, Arteriovenous.

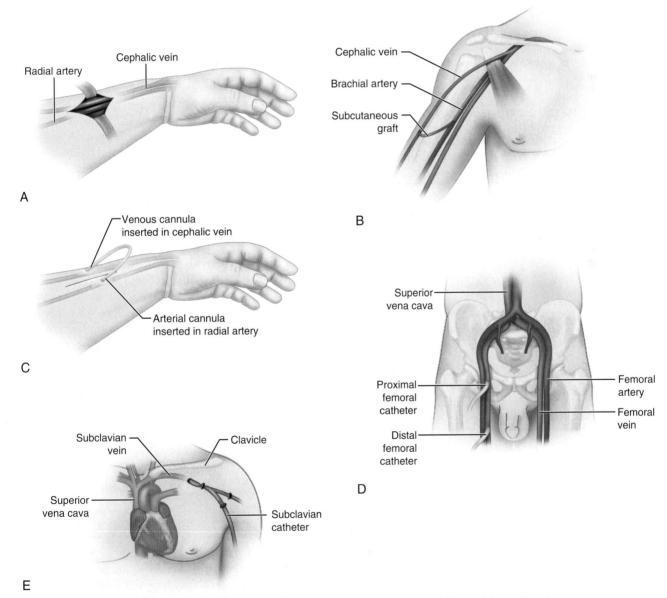

FIG. 60.8 Frequently used means for gaining vascular access for hemodialysis include arteriovenous fistula (A), arteriovenous graft (B), external arteriovenous shunt (C), femoral vein catheterization (D), and subclavian vein catheterization (E). (A) and (B) are options for long-term vascular access for hemodialysis. (C), (D), and (E) are used for short-term access for intermittent hemodialysis or for continuous renal replacement therapy in acute care.

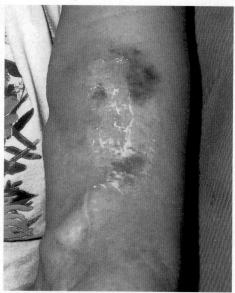

FIG. 60.9 A mature fistula for hemodialysis access. The increased pressure from the anastomosed artery forced blood into the vein. This process caused the vein to dilate enough for fistula needles to be placed for hemodialysis. When the vein is sufficiently dilated, a process that takes 8 to 12 weeks, the fistula is said to be *developed* or *mature*.

BOX 60.9   Best Practice for Patient Safety and Quality Care

Caring for the Patient With an Arteriovenous Fistula or Arteriovenous Graft

- Do not take blood pressure readings using the extremity in which the vascular access is placed.
- Do not perform venipunctures or start an IV line in the extremity in which the vascular access is placed.
- Palpate for thrills and auscultate for bruits over the vascular access site every 4 hours while the patient is awake.
- Assess the patient's distal pulses and circulation in the arm with the access.
- Elevate the affected extremity after surgery.
- Encourage routine range-of-motion exercises.
- Check for bleeding at needle insertion sites.
- Assess for indications of infection at needle sites.
- Instruct the patient not to carry heavy objects or anything that compresses the extremity in which the vascular access is placed.
- Instruct patients not to sleep with their weight on top of the extremity in which the vascular access is placed.

Access Complications. Complications can occur with any type of access. Common problems include thrombosis or stenosis, infection, aneurysm formation, ischemia, and HF (Norton et al., 2017b). Table 60.8 lists strategies to prevent access complications.

Thrombosis, or clotting of the AV access, is the most frequent complication. Most grafts fail because of high-pressure arterial flow entering the venous system. The muscle layers of the veins react to this increased pressure by thickening. The venous thickening reduces or occludes blood flow. An interventional radiologist can reopen failing grafts with the injection of a thrombolytic drug to dissolve the clot. The clot usually dissolves within minutes, and often a stricture is revealed at the point where the graft and the vein connect. The stricture can be corrected by balloon angioplasty.

Most infections of the vascular access are caused by *Staphylococcus aureus* introduced during cannulation. Prepare the skin with an antibacterial agent according to agency policy before cannulation to prevent infection. When using dialysis catheters, be sure to use only the cleansing agent recommended by the catheter manufacturer. Some disinfectants can damage the catheter (Woo, 2019).

Aneurysms can form in the fistula and are caused by repeated needle punctures at the same site. Large aneurysms may cause loss of the fistula's function and require surgical repair.

Ischemia occurs in a few patients with vascular access when the fistula decreases arterial blood flow to areas below the fistula *(steal syndrome)*. Symptoms vary from cold or numb fingers to gangrene. If the collateral circulation is poor, the fistula may need to be surgically tied off and a new one created in another area to preserve extremity circulation.

Shunting of blood directly from the arterial system to the venous system through the fistula can cause HF in patients with limited cardiac function. This complication is rare, but if it does occur, the fistula may need to be revised to reduce arterial blood flow.

Temporary Vascular Access. Temporary access with special catheters can be used for patients requiring immediate HD. A catheter designed for HD may be inserted into the subclavian, internal jugular, or femoral vein. The lumens of these devices are much smaller than the permanent accesses, and more time (4–8 hours) is required to complete a dialysis session.

Subcutaneous devices may also be surgically inserted to provide temporary access for HD. Implanted beneath the skin, these devices are composed of two small metallic ports with attached catheters that are inserted into large central veins. The ports of subcutaneous devices have internal mechanisms that open when needles are inserted and close when needles are removed. Blood from one port flows from the body to the HD machine and returns to the body via the other port.

NCLEX Examination Challenge 60.5
Physiological Integrity

The nurse is preparing a client for discharge after an AV fistula was placed in the left forearm for long-term vascular access. Which client statement indicates that additional teaching is needed?
A. "I will not lay on my left arm while sleeping."
B. "I will not have any IV inserted into my left arm."
C. "I will be able to have the fistula accessed next week for dialysis."
D. "I should be able to feel a pulsation over the site at all times."

Hemodialysis Nursing Care. Many drugs are dialyzable (i.e., can be partially or completely removed from the blood during dialysis). Coordinate with the nephrology health care provider to assess the patient's drug regimen and determine which drugs should be held until after HD treatment. Box 60.10 lists common

TABLE 60.8 Interventions for Preventing Complications in Hemodialysis Vascular Access

Access Type	Bleeding	Infection	Clotting
AV fistula or AV graft	Apply pressure to the needle puncture sites.	Prepare skin using best practices before cannulation. Typically 2% chlorhexidine is used, similar to central line skin preparation. Between hemodialysis sessions, the patient should wash the area with antibacterial soap and rinse with water.	Avoid constrictive devices such as blood pressure cuffs and tourniquets. Rotate needle insertion sites with each hemodialysis treatment. Assess for thrill and bruit.
Hemodialysis catheters (temporary and permanent)	Assess the access site every time you monitor vital signs.	Use aseptic technique to dress site and access catheter. Do not use catheters for blood sampling, IV fluids, or drug administration.	Place a heparin or heparin/saline dwell solution after hemodialysis treatment.

AV, Arteriovenous.

BOX 60.10 Examples of Dialyzable Drugs

Consult the pharmacist, nephrologist, or dialysis nurse to plan the best time to administer a drug based on the dialysis schedule.

Aminoglycosides
- Amikacin
- Gentamicin
- Tobramycin
- Antituberculosis agents
- Ethambutol
- Isoniazid

Antiviral and Antifungal Agents
- Acyclovir
- Ganciclovir
- Fluconazole

Cephalosporins
- Cefaclor
- Cefazolin
- Cefoxitin
- Ceftriaxone
- Cefuroxime
- Cefepime

Anticonvulsants
- Ethosuximide
- Gabapentin
- Phenobarbital

Penicillins
- Amoxicillin
- Ampicillin
- Dicloxacillin
- Penicillin G

Miscellaneous
- Aztreonam
- Cimetidine
- Vitamins
- Clavulanic acid
- Allopurinol
- Enalapril
- Aspirin

dialyzable drugs that should be given *after* rather than before HD. Consult the dialysis nurse or nephrologist to determine if antihypertensive drugs should be given before a scheduled dialysis treatment; some short-acting antihypertensives can contribute to hypotension during dialysis.

The time required to complete an HD treatment usually is at least 4 hours. During this time patients may use various distraction techniques to prevent boredom, such as reading, watching television or videos, visiting with friends or relatives, playing video games, or working puzzles. This time can be used also for brief health teaching opportunities.

Postdialysis Care. Closely monitor the patient immediately and for several hours after dialysis for any side effects from the treatment. Common problems include hypotension, headache, nausea, vomiting, dizziness, and muscle cramps.

Obtain vital signs and weight for comparison with predialysis measurements. Blood pressure and weight are expected to be reduced as a result of fluid removal. Hypotension may necessitate rehydration with IV fluids, such as normal saline. The patient's temperature may also be elevated because the dialysis machine warms the blood slightly. If the patient has a fever, sepsis may be present, and a blood sample is needed for culture and sensitivity testing.

The heparin or citrate required during HD increases the risk for excessive bleeding. All invasive procedures must be avoided for 4 to 6 hours after dialysis. Continually monitor the patient for hemorrhage during and for at least 1 hour after dialysis. See Box 60.11.

Complications of Hemodialysis. Few adverse events occur during a 3- to 4-hour HD treatment under current practice protocols. Improved water treatment, more physiologic solutions, and improvements in HD equipment and procedures have significantly improved safe care for patients receiving this treatment. Complications during HD include hypotension, dialysis disequilibrium syndrome, cardiac events, and reactions to dialyzers (Norton et al., 2017b).

Dialysis disequilibrium syndrome may develop during HD or after HD has been completed. It is characterized by mental status changes and can include seizures or coma, although this severity of disequilibrium syndrome is rare with today's HD practice. A mild form of disequilibrium syndrome includes symptoms of nausea, vomiting, headaches, fatigue, and restlessness. It is thought to be the result of a rapid reduction in electrolytes and other particles. Reducing blood flow at the onset of symptoms can prevent this syndrome.

Cardiac events during HD are associated with underlying cardiovascular disease, especially left ventricular hypertrophy, coronary vascular disease, and a history of cardiac dysrhythmias. These conditions are described in Chapters 28, 29, and 32. Although cardiac arrest is a rare event, the setting should be equipped with an automatic defibrillator, and staff or family should be trained in cardiopulmonary resuscitation. Often cardiac arrest is related to new-onset cardiac ischemia. This problem is managed in an acute care setting in which the presence of myocardial disease can be evaluated and cardiac treatment optimized.

BOX 60.11 Best Practice for Patient Safety and Quality Care

Caring for the Patient Undergoing Hemodialysis

- Weigh the patient before and after dialysis.
- Know the patient's dry weight.
- Discuss with the nephrology health care provider or pharmacist whether any of the patient's drugs should be withheld until after dialysis.
- Be aware of events that occurred during previous dialysis treatments.
- Measure blood pressure, pulse, respirations, and temperature.
- Assess for indications of orthostatic hypotension.
- Assess the vascular access site when taking vital signs and follow agency policy for central line care and dressing changes.
- Observe for bleeding at the vascular access site and other sites where skin integrity is disrupted because anticoagulants given during dialysis and the presence of uremia increase bleeding risk.
- Assess the patient's level of consciousness.
- Assess for headache, nausea, and vomiting.
- Assess serum laboratory tests to evaluate effectiveness of treatment in removing wastes and achieving desired outcomes (e.g., **fluid and electrolyte balance,** reduction of uremia).

✚ NURSING SAFETY PRIORITY

Critical Rescue

Monitor the patient closely during dialysis to recognize hypotension, which is common. Heat transfer from warm solutions can result in vasodilation and a drop in blood pressure. When this occurs, reduce the temperature of the dialysate to 95°F (35°C). Fluid shifts from the plasma volume related to differences in electrolyte concentrations between hemodialysis (HD) solutions and blood also reduce blood pressure. Respond to modest declines in blood pressure by adjusting the rate of dialyzer blood flow and placing the patient in a legs-up (Trendelenburg) position. Respond to sustained or symptomatic hypotension by giving a fluid bolus of 100 to 250 mL of normal saline, albumin, or mannitol (if prescribed). A second bolus may be needed. If hypotension persists, new-onset myocardial injury or pericardial disease may be a contributing factor; respond by applying oxygen, reducing the blood flow, and notifying the primary health care provider urgently. Discontinue HD when hypotension continues despite two bolus infusions.

Pericardial disease is a complication of patients with ESKD. Assess the patient's heart sounds for the presence of a pericardial rub before starting dialysis. Intensification of dialysis may be used to treat this complication. Other treatment might include NSAID use or surgery.

Reactions to dialyzers still occur, although more biocompatible membranes and careful attention to rinsing the dialyzer before use (to eliminate sterilizing agents) have reduced this adverse event during HD. Reactions occur during a "first-time" use of the filter and resemble an anaphylactic episode early during HD, with profound hypotension. (Chapter 17 describes anaphylactic reactions.) With suspected dialyzer reactions, do not return the blood to the patient, and discontinue HD. Corticosteroids may be used to treat the *immunity* reaction.

Other potential complications of HD require the nurse to monitor the level of consciousness and vital signs frequently during treatment and to slow or stop HD when symptoms occur. Hypoglycemia is a rare adverse HD event and is more likely to occur when the patient has diabetes. It is managed by providing glucose and increasing dialysis glucose concentration in subsequent treatments. Hemorrhage can occur when needle dislodgment or circuit connections become loose and is amplified by anticoagulation used to maintain circuit patency. Some hemolysis occurs because of mechanical trauma to RBCs, contributing to anemia in the patient with CKD and, perhaps, to sensations of dyspnea or chest tightness.

Infectious diseases transmitted by blood transfusion are a serious complication of long-term HD. Two of the most serious blood-transmitted infections are hepatitis and HIV infection. *Hepatitis B infection* and *hepatitis C infection* in patients with CKD have decreased because the use of erythropoietin-stimulating agents (ESAs) has reduced the need for blood transfusions to maintain RBC counts. Hepatitis is a problem because of the blood access and the risk for contamination during HD. The viruses can be transmitted through the use of contaminated needles or instruments, by entry of contaminated blood through open wounds in the skin or mucous membranes, or through transfusions with contaminated blood. Monitor all patients receiving HD for indications of hepatitis (see Chapter 50).

The risk for HIV transmission is reduced by the consistent practice of Standard Precautions, routine screening of donated blood for HIV, and decreased need for blood transfusions with CKD and ESKD. Patients who have been undergoing HD or who received frequent transfusions during the early to middle 1980s may have been infected at that time and are at risk for AIDS (HIV-III).

Peritoneal Dialysis. Peritoneal dialysis (PD) allows exchanges of wastes, fluid, and electrolytes to occur in the peritoneal cavity. However, PD is slower than hemodialysis (HD), and more time is needed to achieve the same effect. Other disadvantages of PD are the protein loss in outflow fluid, risk for peritoneal injury, and potential discomfort from indwelling fluid. Advantages and complications are listed in Table 60.9. The use of PD is declining

👤 PATIENT CENTERED CARE: OLDER ADULT HEALTH

Dialysis

Adults over age 75 comprise one of the most rapidly increasing age-groups of dialysis patients. Patients should be educated about all aspects of dialysis care so that they can make an informed decision regarding dialysis initiation. In adults over age 80 with coronary artery disease in addition to other comorbid conditions, dialysis has not been shown to prolong life when compared with patients receiving more conservative treatments. Dialysis patients spend an average of 173 days per year in the hospital or at dialysis; nondialysis, medically treated patients spend an average of 16 days per year in the hospital (Himmelfarb & Ikizler, 2018).

TABLE 60.9	Comparison of Hemodialysis and Peritoneal Dialysis	
Hemodialysis	**Peritoneal Dialysis**
Advantages	
More efficient clearance of wastes	Flexible schedule for exchanges
Short time needed for treatment	Few hemodynamic changes during and following exchanges
	Fewer dietary and fluid restrictions
Complications	
Disequilibrium syndrome	Protein loss
Muscle cramps and back pain	Peritonitis
Headache	Respiratory distress
Itching	Inflammatory bowel disease
Hemodynamic and cardiac adverse events (hypotension, cell lysis	Bowel perforation
contributing to anemia, cardiac dysrhythmias)	Infection
Infection	Weight gain; discomfort from "carrying" 1–2 L in abdomen during dwell time; potential for
Increased risk for subdural and intracranial hemorrhage from	back pain or development of hernia
anticoagulation and changes in blood pressure during dialysis	
Anemia	
Access site complications	
Contraindications	
Hemodynamic instability or severe cardiac disease	Extensive peritoneal adhesions, fibrosis, or active inflammatory GI disease (e.g.,
Severe vascular disease that prevents vascular access	diverticulitis, inflammatory bowel conditions)
Serious bleeding disorders	Ascites or massive central obesity
	Recent abdominal surgery
Access	
Arteriovenous (AV) fistula	Intraabdominal catheter
AV graft	
Central venous catheter	
Procedure	
Complex; requires a second person trained in the technique whether	Simple, easier to complete at home compared with at-home hemodialysis
completed at home or at a dialysis unit/center	Less complex training; typically managed by patient; can be managed by one person
Special training for center personnel and in-home use	

and accounts for less than 10% of the total dialysis population (Johnson et al., 2019).

Patient Selection. Most patients with CKD can select either HD or PD. For those who are unstable and those who cannot tolerate anticoagulation, PD is less hazardous than HD. For some patients, vascular access problems may eliminate HD as an option. At times a patient may use PD until a new arteriovenous (AV) fistula matures. PD is often the treatment of choice for older adults because it offers more flexibility if their status changes frequently.

PD *cannot* be performed if peritoneal adhesions are present or if extensive intraabdominal surgery has been performed (Norton et al., 2017b). In these cases the surface area of the peritoneal membrane is not sufficient for adequate dialysis exchange. Peritoneal membrane fibrosis may occur after repeated infection, which decreases membrane permeability.

Procedure. A siliconized rubber (Silastic) catheter is surgically placed into the abdominal cavity for infusion of dialysate (Fig. 60.10). Usually 1 to 2 L of dialysate is infused by gravity (*fill*) into the peritoneal space over a 10- to 20-minute period, according to the patient's tolerance. The fluid stays *(dwells)* in the cavity for a specified time prescribed for each patient individually by the nephrologist. It then flows out of the body (*drains*) by gravity into a drainage bag. The peritoneal outflow contains the dialysate and the excess water, electrolytes, and nitrogen-based waste products. The dialyzing fluid is called peritoneal *effluent* on outflow. The three phases of the process (infusion, or fill; dwell; and outflow, or drain) make up one PD exchange. The number and frequency of PD exchanges are prescribed by the health care provider, depending on symptoms and laboratory data.

Process. PD occurs through diffusion and osmosis across the semipermeable peritoneal membrane and capillaries. The peritoneal membrane is large and porous. It allows particles and water to move from an area of higher concentration in the blood to an area of lower concentration in the dialyzing fluid (diffusion).

The peritoneal cavity is rich in capillaries and is a ready access to the blood supply. The fluid and waste products dialyzed from the patient move through the blood vessel walls, the interstitial tissues, and the peritoneal membrane and are removed when the dialyzing fluid is drained from the body.

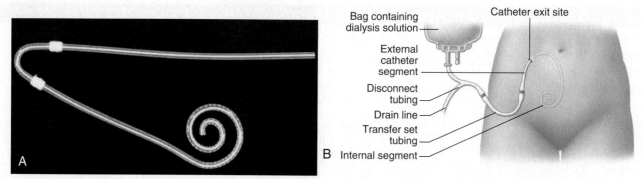

FIG. 60.10 Peritoneal dialysis catheter. (A) The actual Silastic peritoneal dialysis catheter. (B) Positioning of the Silastic catheter within the abdominal cavity. (A From Geary, D. F., & Schaefer, F. [2008]. *Comprehensive pediatric nephrology*. Philadelphia: Mosby.)

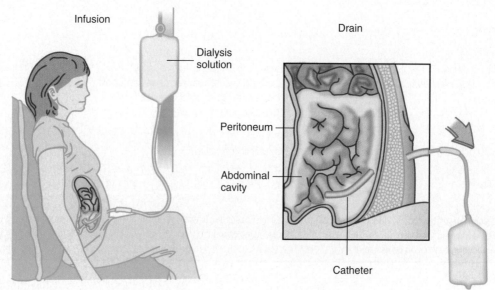

FIG. 60.11 Peritoneal dialysis exchange for control of fluids, electrolytes, nitrogenous wastes, blood pressure, and acid-base balance. The peritoneal membrane acts as the dialyzing membrane.

PD efficiency is affected by many factors. Infection can cause scarring and reduce capillary blood flow. Vascular disease and decreased *perfusion* of the peritoneum reduce PD diffusion. For PD, water removal depends on the concentration of the dialysate. PD efficiency can be altered by the *tonicity* (i.e., number of particles per liter of fluid) of the dialysate. The dialysate concentration is prescribed on the basis of the patient's fluid status (Johnson et al., 2019).

Dialysate Additives. Heparin may be added to the dialysate to prevent clotting of the catheter or tubing. Usually intraperitoneal (IP) heparin is needed only after new catheter placement or if peritonitis occurs. IP heparin is not absorbed systemically and does not affect blood clotting.

Other agents that may be given in the dialysate include potassium and antibiotics. Commercially prepared dialysate does not contain potassium. Some patients need potassium added to the dialysate to prevent hypokalemia. Antibiotics may be given by

the IP route when peritonitis is present or suspected. Potassium and antibiotics are not mixed in the same dialysate bag because interactions may reduce the antibiotic effect.

Types of Peritoneal Dialysis. Many types of PD are available, including continuous ambulatory PD, multiple-bag continuous ambulatory PD, automated peritoneal dialysis (APD), intermittent peritoneal dialysis (IPD), and continuous-cycle PD. The type selected depends on the patient's ability and lifestyle. The two most commonly used types of PD are continuous ambulatory peritoneal dialysis (CAPD) and continuous cycling peritoneal dialysis.

Continuous ambulatory peritoneal dialysis (CAPD) is performed by the patient with the infusion of four 2-L exchanges of dialysate into the peritoneal cavity. Each time, the dialysate remains for 4 to 8 hours, and these exchanges occur 7 days a week (Figs. 60.11 and 60.12). During the dwell period, the patient can use a continuous connect system or disconnect and

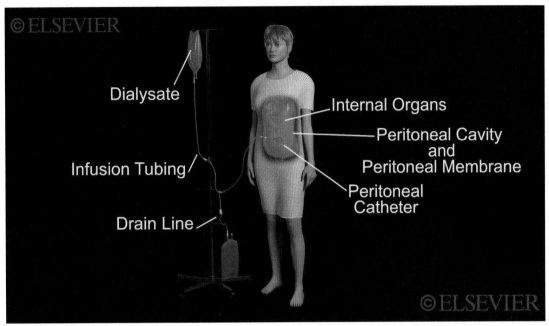

FIG. 60.12 Patient performing continuous ambulatory peritoneal dialysis (CAPD). Note that the patient can walk with this setup.

then reconnect at a later time. Most patients using PD long-term prefer to complete exchanges overnight with an automated cycler (APD).

Automated peritoneal dialysis (APD) may be used in the acute care setting, the ambulatory care dialysis center, or the patient's home. APD uses a cycling machine for dialysate inflow, dwell, and outflow according to preset times and volumes. A warming chamber for dialysate is part of the machine (Fig. 60.13). The functions are programmed for the patient's specific needs. A typical prescription calls for 30-minute exchanges (10/10/10 for inflow, dwell, and outflow) for a period of 8 to 10 hours. The machines have many safety monitors and alarms and are relatively simple to learn to use.

APD has advantages. It permits in-home dialysis during sleep, allowing the patient to be dialysis free during waking hours. The incidence of peritonitis is reduced with APD because fewer connections and disconnections are needed. Also, APD can be used to deliver larger volumes of dialysis solution for patients who need higher clearances.

Intermittent peritoneal dialysis (IPD) combines osmotic pressure gradients with true dialysis. The patient usually requires exchanges of 2 L of dialysate at 30- to 60-minute intervals, allowing 15 to 20 minutes of drain time. For most patients, 30 to 40 exchanges of 2 L three times weekly are needed. IPD treatments can be automated or manual.

Complications. Complications are possible with PD, but many can be prevented with meticulous care and appropriate patient education for self-management. Problems and complications are more common when evidence-based guidelines for catheter care are not followed.

Peritonitis is the major complication of PD, most commonly caused by connection site contamination. To prevent peritonitis, use meticulous sterile technique when caring for the PD catheter and when connecting and disconnecting dialysate bags. See Box 60.12.

Pain during the inflow of dialysate is common when patients are first started on PD therapy. Usually this pain no longer occurs after a week or two of PD. Cold dialysate increases discomfort. Warm the dialysate bags before instillation by using a heating pad to wrap the bag or by using the warming chamber of the automated cycling machine. *Microwave ovens are **not** recommended for warming dialysate.*

Exit-site and tunnel infections are serious complications. The exit site from a PD catheter should be clean, dry, and without pain or inflammation. Exit-site infections (ESIs) can occur with any type of PD catheter. These infections are difficult to treat and can become chronic, leading to peritonitis, catheter failure, and hospitalization. Dialysate leakage and pulling or twisting of the catheter increase the risk for ESIs. A Gram stain and culture should be performed when exit sites have purulent drainage.

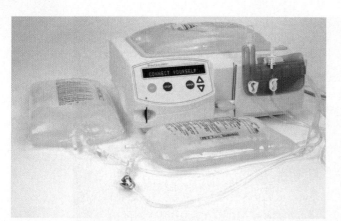

FIG. 60.13 Cycler machine for automated peritoneal dialysis at home. (Courtesy Baxter International, Inc., Deerfield, IL.)

BOX 60.12   Best Practice for Patient Safety and Quality Care

Caring for the Patient With a Peritoneal Dialysis Catheter

- Mask yourself and your patient. Wash your hands.
- Put on sterile gloves. Remove the old dressing. Remove the contaminated gloves.
- Assess the area for signs of infection, such as swelling, redness/hyperpigmentation, or discharge around the catheter site.
- Use aseptic technique:
  - Open the sterile field on a flat surface and place two precut 4 × 4–inch gauze pads on the field.
  - Place three cotton swabs soaked in povidone-iodine or other solution prescribed by the nephrology health care provider on the field. Put on sterile gloves.
  - Use cotton swabs to clean around the catheter site. Use a circular motion starting from the insertion site and moving away toward the abdomen. Repeat with all three swabs.
  - As an alternative (if recommended by the nephrology health care provider or clinic), cleanse the area with sterile gauze pads using soap and water. Use a circular motion starting from the insertion site and moving away toward the abdomen. Rinse thoroughly.
  - Apply precut gauze pads over the catheter site. Tape only the edges of the gauze pads.

Tunnel infections occur in the path of the catheter from the skin to the cuff. Symptoms include redness/hyperpigmentation, tenderness, and pain. ESIs are treated with antimicrobials. Deep cuff infections may necessitate catheter removal.

Poor dialysate flow is often related to constipation. To prevent constipation, a bowel preparation is prescribed before placement of the PD. If prescribed, giving an enema before starting

! NURSING SAFETY PRIORITY

Action Alert

Monitor the patient to recognize indications of peritonitis (e.g., cloudy dialysate outflow (effluent), fever, abdominal tenderness, abdominal pain, general malaise, nausea, and vomiting). *Cloudy or opaque effluent is the earliest indication of peritonitis.* Examine all effluent for color and clarity to detect peritonitis early. When peritonitis is suspected, respond by sending a specimen of the dialysate outflow for culture and sensitivity study, Gram stain, and cell count to identify the infecting organism.

PD may also prevent flow problems. Teach patients to eat a high-fiber diet and to use stool softeners to prevent constipation. Other causes of flow difficulty include kinked or clamped connection tubing, the patient's position, fibrin clot formation, and catheter displacement.

Ensure that the drainage bag is lower than the patient's abdomen to enhance gravity drainage. Inspect the connection tubing and PD system for kinking or twisting. Ensure that clamps are open. If inflow or outflow drainage is still inadequate, reposition the patient to stimulate inflow or outflow. Turning the patient to the other side or ensuring that the patient is in good body alignment may help. Having the patient in a supine low-Fowler's position reduces abdominal pressure. Increased abdominal pressure from sitting or standing or from coughing contributes to leakage at the PD catheter site.

Fibrin clot formation may occur after PD catheter placement or with peritonitis. Milking the tubing may dislodge the fibrin clot and improve flow. An x-ray is needed to identify PD catheter placement. If displacement has occurred, the nephrology health care provider repositions the PD catheter.

Dialysate leakage is seen as clear fluid coming from the catheter exit site. When dialysis is first started, small volumes of dialysate are used. It may take patients 1 to 2 weeks to tolerate a full 2-L exchange without leakage around the catheter site. Leakage occurs more often in obese patients, those with diabetes, older adults, and those on long-term steroid therapy. During periods of catheter leak, patients may require hemodialysis (HD) support.

Other complications of PD include bleeding, which is expected when the catheter is first placed, and bowel perforation, which is serious. When PD is first started, the outflow may be bloody or blood tinged. This condition normally clears within a week or two. After PD is well established, the effluent should be clear and light yellow. Observe for and document any change in the color of the outflow. Brown-colored effluent occurs with a bowel perforation. If the outflow is the same color as urine and has the same glucose level, a bladder perforation is probable. Cloudy or opaque effluent indicates infection.

Nursing Care During in-Hospital Peritoneal Dialysis. In the hospital setting, PD is routinely started and monitored by the nurse. Before the treatment, assess baseline vital signs, including blood pressure, apical and radial pulse rates, temperature, quality of respirations, and breath sounds. Weigh the patient, always on the same scale, before the procedure and at least every 24 hours during treatment. Weight should be checked after a drain and before the next fill to monitor the patient's "dry weight." Baseline laboratory tests, such as electrolyte and glucose levels, are obtained before starting PD and repeated at least daily during the PD treatment.

In the hospital setting, especially with a new access, continually monitor the patient receiving PD fluid exchanges. Take and record vital signs every 15 to 30 minutes. Assess for respiratory distress, pain, and discomfort. Check the dressing around the catheter exit site every 30 minutes for wetness during the procedure. Monitor the prescribed dwell time and initiate outflow. Assess blood glucose levels in patients who absorb glucose.

Observe the outflow pattern (outflow should be a continuous stream after the clamp is completely open). Measure and record the total amount of outflow after each exchange. Maintain accurate inflow and outflow records when hourly PD exchanges are performed. When outflow is less than inflow, the difference is retained by the patient during dialysis and is counted as fluid intake. Weigh the patient daily to monitor fluid status.

Kidney Transplantation. Dialysis and kidney transplant are life-sustaining *treatments* for end-stage kidney disease (ESKD). Kidney transplant is not considered a "cure." Each patient, in consultation with a nephrologist, determines which type of therapy is best suited to the patient's physical condition and lifestyle. About 17,107 kidney transplants take place annually in the United States. Just over 100,000 people are waiting for kidney transplants in the United States (NKF, 2022). The median wait time for a kidney transplant is 4 years (United States Renal Data System, 2019).

Candidate Selection Criteria. Candidates for transplantation have advanced kidney disease, have a reasonable life expectancy, and are medically and surgically fit to undergo the procedure. In the United States, patients can be added to the waiting list once the GFR is less than 20 mL/min/1.73 m². Absolute contraindications to transplant include active cancer, current infection, active psychiatric illness, active substance abuse, and nonadherence with dialysis or medical regimen (Himmelfarb & Ikizler, 2018).

Donors. Kidney donors may be living donors (related or unrelated to the patient), non–heart-beating donors (NHBDs), and cadaveric donors. The available kidneys are matched on the basis of tissue type similarity between the donor and the recipient. NHBDs are patients declared dead by cardiopulmonary criteria. Kidneys from NHBDs are removed (harvested) immediately after death in cases in which patients have previously given consent for organ donation. If immediate removal must be delayed, the organ is preserved by infusing a cool preservation solution into the abdominal aorta after death is declared and until surgery can be performed.

Organs from living donors have the highest rate of graft survival due to healthier donors, shorter cold ischemia times, and less ischemia-reperfusion injury. Patients who are able to find compatible kidney donors have shorter wait times for transplant. Donors must be healthy enough to undergo the procedure and be over the age of 18. Due to the benefits that have been shown, many transplant centers have relaxed their criteria and now accept donors with hypertension, obesity, and glucose intolerance, as well as a glomerular filtration rate (GFR) around the lower limits of the normal range (Himmelfarb & Ikizler, 2018). See Box 60.13 and Fig. 60.14.

Preoperative Care. Many issues related to patient health and the actual transplant procedure must be addressed before surgery.

Immunologic studies are needed because the major barrier to transplant success after a suitable donor kidney is available is the body's ability to reject "foreign" tissue. This immunologic process can attack the transplanted kidney and destroy it. For normal protective **immunity** to be overcome, tissue typing with human leukocyte antigen (HLA) studies and blood typing are performed on all candidates. A donated kidney *must* come from a donor who is the same blood type as the recipient. The HLAs are the main immunologic feature used to match transplant recipients with compatible donors. The more similar the antigens of the donor are to those of the recipient, the more likely the transplant will be successful, and rejection will be avoided (see Chapter 16).

Nursing actions before surgery include teaching about the procedure and care after surgery, in-depth patient assessment, coordination of diagnostic tests, and development of treatment plans. See Chapter 9 for more discussion of standard preoperative nursing care.

BOX 60.13 Never Ending Altruistic Donor (NEAD) Chain

Kidney transplants improve survival rates and lower costs compared with dialysis. The highest survival rates occur in living donor transplants (Himmelfarb & Ikizler, 2018). There are times when a patient needing a transplant has a willing donor who is not compatible and is not able to donate. Previously the patient would have had to wait until another donor was found, and the person who was willing to donate would have been denied. Fig. 60.14 shows an example of a paired exchange kidney donation, which is one option when a recipient has a donor that is not compatible.

Some transplant centers are now using Never Ending Altruistic Donor (NEAD) chains that match donors with recipients. A NEAD chain begins with one nondirected donor. The nondirected donor gives to a person who has a willing but incompatible donor. That willing donor gives to the next person waiting with whom they are compatible, so that each living donor is giving to a stranger. The chain is kept going for as long as possible. For example, if a patient's spouse wanted to donate a kidney but was not compatible, the spouse would be matched with a compatible recipient and the patient would be matched with an acceptable donor. The NEAD chain allows for people to donate to help a specific person without having to be compatible. This simple initiative is improving countless lives (NKF, 2022).

The patient usually requires dialysis within 24 hours of the surgery and often receives a blood transfusion before surgery. Usually blood from the kidney donor is transfused into the recipient. This procedure increases graft survival of organs from living related donors (LRDs).

Operative Procedures. The donor nephrectomy procedure varies depending on whether the donor is a non–heart-beating donor (NHBD), cadaveric donor, or living donor. The NHBD or cadaveric donor nephrectomy is a sterile autopsy procedure performed in the operating room. All arterial and venous vessels and a long piece of ureter are preserved. After removal, the kidneys are preserved until it is time for implantation into the recipient. The technique for kidney removal from living donors is a laparoscopic procedure. Donors need postoperative nursing care and support for the psychological adjustment to loss of a body part.

Transplantation surgery usually takes several hours. The new kidney is placed in the right or left anterior iliac fossa (Fig. 60.15). instead of the usual kidney position. This placement allows easier connection of the ureter and the renal artery and vein. It also allows for easier kidney palpation. The recipient's own failed kidneys are not removed unless chronic kidney infection is present or, as in the case of polycystic kidney disease, the nonfunctioning, enlarged kidneys cause pain. After surgery the patient is taken to the postanesthesia care unit and then, when stable, to a designated unit in the transplant center or to a critical care unit.

Postoperative Care. Care of the recipient after surgery requires nurses to be knowledgeable about the expected responses and potential complications. Nursing care includes ongoing physical assessment, especially evaluation of kidney function. The most common complications occurring in patients after kidney transplant are rejection and infection. Drug therapy used to prevent tissue rejection reduces *immunity,* impairs healing, and increases the risk for infection.

Urologic management is essential to graft success. A urinary catheter is placed for accurate measurements of urine output and decompression of the bladder. Decompression prevents stretch on sutures and ureter attachment sites on the bladder.

Assess urine output at least hourly during the first 48 hours. An abrupt decrease in urine output (see Table 60.2) may indicate complications such as rejection, acute kidney injury (AKI), thrombosis, or obstruction. Examine the urine color. The urine is pink and bloody right after surgery and gradually returns to normal over several days to several weeks, depending on kidney function. Obtain daily urine specimens for urinalysis, glucose

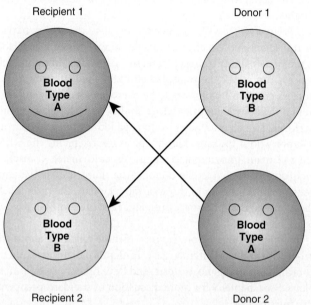

FIG. 60.14 Example of a paired exchange kidney donation. *Donor 1* is related to or acquainted with *recipient 1* and has agreed to donate a kidney but is not a blood type or tissue type match with *recipient 1.* *Donor 1* is compatible with *recipient 2* and agrees to donate a kidney to *recipient 2* if *donor 2* agrees to donate a kidney to *recipient 1* with confirmed compatibility to recipient 1.

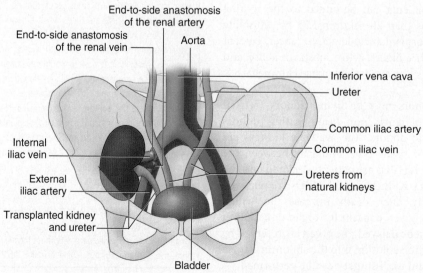

FIG. 60.15 Placement of a transplanted kidney in the right iliac fossa.

measurement, the presence of acetone, specific gravity measurement, and culture (if needed).

Occasionally, continuous bladder irrigation is prescribed to decrease blood clot formation, which could increase pressure in the bladder and endanger the graft. Perform routine catheter care, according to agency policy, to reduce the risk of catheter-associated urinary tract infection (CAUTI). The catheter is removed as soon as possible to avoid infection, usually 3 to 5 days after surgery. After surgery, the function of the transplanted kidney (graft) can result in either oliguria or diuresis. Oliguria may occur as a result of ischemia and acute kidney injury (AKI), rejection, or other complications. To increase urine output, the nephrology health care provider may prescribe diuretics and osmotic agents. Closely monitor the patient's fluid status because fluid overload can cause hypertension, heart failure (HF), and pulmonary edema. Evaluate fluid status by weighing the patient daily, measuring blood pressure every 2 to 4 hours, and measuring intake and output.

Instead of oliguria, the patient may have diuresis, especially with a kidney from a living related donor (LRD). Monitor intake and output and observe for disruptions of *fluid and electrolyte balance,* such as low potassium and sodium levels. Excessive diuresis may cause hypotension.

✚ NURSING SAFETY PRIORITY

Critical Rescue

Monitor the patient to recognize hypotension. If hypotension or excessive diuresis (e.g., unanticipated urine output 500–1000 mL greater than intake over 12–24 hours or other goal for intake and output) is present, respond by notifying the nephrology health care provider because hypotension reduces *perfusion* and oxygen to the new kidney, threatening graft survival.

Complications. Many complications are possible after kidney transplantation. Early detection and intervention improve the chances for graft survival.

Rejection is the most serious complication of transplantation and is the leading cause of graft loss. A reaction occurs between the tissues of the transplanted kidney and the antibodies and cytotoxic T cells in the recipient's blood. These substances treat the new kidney as a foreign invader and cause tissue destruction, thrombosis, and eventual kidney necrosis.

The three types of rejection are hyperacute, acute, and chronic. Acute rejection is the most common type with kidney transplants. It is treated with increased immunosuppressive therapy and often can be reversed. Rejection is diagnosed through symptoms, a CT or renal scan, and kidney biopsy. Table 60.10 lists the features of the three types of rejection. Chapter 16 discusses their causes and treatment.

Ischemia from delayed transplantation following harvesting can contribute to acute kidney injury (AKI). Newly transplanted patients with AKI may need dialysis until adequate urine output returns and the blood urea nitrogen (BUN) and creatinine levels normalize. Biopsy can be used to determine if oliguria is the result of AKI or rejection.

Thrombosis of the major renal blood vessels may occur during the first 2 to 3 days after the transplant. A sudden decrease in urine output may signal impaired *perfusion* resulting from thrombosis. Ultrasound of the kidney may show decreased or absent blood supply. Emergency surgery is required to prevent ischemic damage or graft loss.

Renal artery stenosis may result in hypertension. Other signs include a bruit over the artery anastomosis site and decreased kidney function. A CT or renal scan can quantify the *perfusion* to the kidney. The involved artery may be repaired surgically or with balloon angioplasty in the radiology department. The decision to perform a balloon repair is determined by the amount of healing time after the surgery.

Other vascular problems include vascular leakage or thrombosis, both of which require an emergency transplant nephrectomy.

Other complications may involve the surgical wound or urinary tract. Wound problems, such as hematomas, abscesses, and lymphoceles (cysts containing lymph fluid), increase the risk for infection and exert pressure on the new kidney. Infection from reduced *immunity* is a major cause of death in the transplant recipient. Prevention of infection is essential. Strict aseptic technique and handwashing must be rigorously enforced. Transplant recipients may not have the usual symptoms of infection because of the immunosuppressive therapy. Low-grade fevers, mental status changes, and vague reports of discomfort may be the only symptoms before sepsis. Always consider the possibility of infection with any patient after a kidney transplant. Urinary tract complications include ureteral leakage, fistula, or obstruction; stone formation; bladder neck contracture; and graft rupture. Surgical intervention may be required.

Immunosuppressive Drug Therapy. The success of kidney transplantation depends on changing the patient's *immunity* response so the new kidney is not rejected as a foreign organ. Immunosuppressive drugs protect the transplanted organ. These drugs include corticosteroids, inhibitors of T-cell proliferation and activity (azathioprine, mycophenolic acid, cyclosporine, and tacrolimus), mTOR inhibitors (to disrupt stimulatory T-cell signals), and monoclonal antibodies. Chapter 16 discusses the mechanisms of action of these agents and the associated patient responses. Patients taking these drugs are at an increased risk for death from infection. Usually the patient receives a period of high-dose (induction) therapy followed by lower-dose maintenance immunosuppressive therapy.

Some patients do not follow the maintenance regimen correctly and are at high risk for losing the transplanted kidney. Work with the patient to ensure adherence to the drug regimen.

Despite the complexity of drug regimens following kidney transplantation, 99% of recipients of living kidneys are alive at 1 year and 95% of recipients of kidneys from deceased donors are alive at 1 year. At 4 years, kidney transplant recipients have an average 70% reduction in mortality compared with patients on dialysis (Himmelfarb & Ikizler, 2018)

Although rejection is uncommon with immunosuppressive therapy, kidney transplant recipients are at risk for cardiovascular disease (the most common cause of death among

TABLE 60.10　Comparison of Hyperacute, Acute, and Chronic Posttransplant Rejection

Hyperacute Rejection	Acute Rejection	Chronic Rejection
Onset		
Within 48 hr after surgery	1 wk to any time after surgery; occurs over days to weeks	Occurs gradually during a period of months to years
Signs and Symptoms		
Increased temperature	Oliguria or anuria	Gradual increase in BUN and serum creatinine levels
Increased blood pressure	Temperature over 100°F (37.8°C)	Fluid retention
Pain at transplant site	Increased blood pressure	Changes in serum electrolyte levels
	Enlarged, tender kidney	Fatigue
	Lethargy	
	Elevated serum creatinine, BUN, potassium levels	
	Fluid retention	
Treatment		
Immediate removal of the transplanted kidney	Increased doses of immunosuppressive drugs	Conservative management until dialysis required

BUN, Blood urea nitrogen.

kidney transplant recipients), diabetes, cancer, and infections. Prevention and management of these complications are important to maintaining the health of the transplanted kidney and prolonging patient survival.

! NURSING SAFETY PRIORITY

Action Alert

Teach patients and families about the importance of adhering to the antirejection drug regimen to prevent transplant rejection.

Care Coordination and Transition Management

Home Care Management. Because of the complex nature of CKD, its progressive course, and many treatment options, a case manager is helpful in planning, coordinating, and evaluating care. As kidney disease progresses, the patient is seen by a nephrologist or nephrology nurse practitioner regularly. Together with the registered dietitian nutritionist and social worker, evaluate the home environment and determine equipment needs before discharge. Once the patient is discharged, nephrology home care nurses direct care and monitor progress.

Provide health teaching about the diet in kidney disease and the progression of disease. As CKD approaches end-stage kidney disease (ESKD), treatment with hemodialysis (HD), peritoneal dialysis (PD), or transplantation is selected. For each form of treatment, the patient must learn about the procedures and consider personal lifestyle, support systems, and methods of coping. Decision making about treatment type or even whether to pursue treatment is difficult for patients and families. Provide information and emotional support to help patients with these decisions.

Teach patients who select hemodialysis (HD) about the machine and vascular access care. If in-home HD is selected, preparations are needed for the appropriate equipment, including a water-treatment system. A nephrology nurse is essential for a successful transition to at-home HD to teach the patient

and monitor treatment and care. This nurse performs a home care visit before discharge to coordinate equipment setup. Family members must be available to respond to alarms during treatment. Nocturnal HD is a growing modality, and additional safety considerations must be addressed, including a plan for treatment discontinuation or generator backup during power outages. Regardless of whether the treatment occurs at home or in a center, promote independence through teaching and best practices in self-management.

The patient receiving PD needs extensive training in the procedure and help in obtaining equipment and the many supplies needed. A nephrology nurse assesses patients, monitors vital signs, assesses adherence with drug and diet regimens, and monitors for indications of peritonitis.

The nurse plays a vital role in the long-term care of the patient with a kidney transplant by facilitating acceptance and understanding of the antirejection drug regimen as a part of daily life. Carefully monitor patients for indications of graft rejection and for complications, such as infection.

Self-Management Education. Instruct patients and family members in all aspects of nutrition therapy, drug therapy, and complications. Teach them to report complications, such as fluid overload and infection. When a patient has a specific form of therapy, such as dialysis or transplantation, focus teaching on the chosen type of intervention. Assess the need for immunizations and request a prescription to administer needed ones before transplantation.

Hemodialysis (HD) is the most complex form of therapy for the patient and family to understand. Even if patients receive HD in a dialysis center instead of at home, they are expected to have some knowledge of the process. Teach the patient or a family member to care for the vascular access and to report signs of infection and clotting. Teaching also includes instructing the patient to assess daily for a bruit and thrill in the vascular access. Those who plan to have in-home HD will need a partner. Both the patient and the partner must be taught the entire process of HD and must be able to perform it independently before the patient is discharged.

Peritoneal dialysis (PD) involves extensive health teaching for the patient and family. Emphasize sterile technique because peritonitis is the most common complication of PD. Instruct patients to report any symptoms of peritonitis, especially cloudy effluent and abdominal pain. If peritonitis develops, teach patients how to give themselves antibiotics by the intraperitoneal (IP) route. Stress the importance of completing the antibiotic regimen. Remind patients that repeated episodes of peritonitis can reduce the effectiveness of PD, which may result in the transfer to HD.

The patient receiving a kidney transplant also needs extensive health teaching. Provide instruction about drug regimens, home monitoring, immunosuppression, symptoms of rejection, infection, and prescribed changes in the diet and activity level.

Psychosocial Preparation. In collaboration with the patient's mental health professional or counselor, provide psychosocial support for the patient and family. Help the patient adjust to the diagnosis of kidney failure and eventually accept the treatment regimens.

Many patients view dialysis as a cure instead of lifelong management. For many patients, reduction of uremic symptoms and improved ***elimination*** in the first weeks after starting dialysis treatment create a sense of well-being. They feel better physically, and their mood may be happy and hopeful. At this time they tend to overlook the discomfort and inconvenience of dialysis. Use this time to begin health teaching. Stress that although symptoms are reduced, they should not expect a complete return to the previous state of well-being before ESKD.

Many patients become discouraged during the first year of treatment. This mood state may last a few months to a year or longer. The difficulties of incorporating dialysis into daily life are staggering, and patients may become depressed as problems occur. They may struggle with the idea of having to be permanently dependent on a disruptive therapy. Patients may feel helpless and dependent. Some patients may deny the need for dialysis or may not adhere to drug therapy and diet restrictions. Monitor any behaviors that may contribute to nonadherence and suggest psychiatric referrals. Help the patient and family focus on the positive aspects of the treatments. Continue health education with patients as active participants and decision makers.

Most patients with CKD eventually enter a phase of acceptance or resignation. Each patient reacts differently. To make this long-term adaptation, they must adjust to continuous change. Concerns depend on the patient's health and specific treatment method.

After patients have accepted or become resigned to the chronic aspect of their disease, they usually attempt to return to their previous activities. However, resuming the previous level of activity may not be possible. Help patients develop realistic expectations that allow them to lead active, productive lives.

Health Care Resources. Professionals from many disciplines are resources for the patient with ESKD. Home care nurses monitor the patient's status and evaluate maintenance of the prescribed treatment regimen (HD or PD). Social services are often involved because of the complex process of applying for financial aid to pay for the required medical care. A physical therapist may be beneficial in helping to improve the patient's functional health. A registered dietitian nutritionist can help the patient and family members understand special dietary needs. A psychiatric evaluation may be needed if depressive symptoms are present. Pharmacists provide invaluable insight and teaching about drug therapy and adjustments to meet outcomes. Clergy and pastoral care specialists offer spiritual support.

Patients with CKD are routinely followed by a nephrologist. Organizations such as the National Kidney Foundation (NKF), the American Kidney Fund, and the American Association of Kidney Patients (AAKP) may be helpful to patients and families.

Evaluate Outcomes: Evaluation

Evaluate the care of the patient with CKD based on the identified priority problems. The expected outcomes are that with appropriate management the patient should:

- Achieve and maintain appropriate fluid and electrolyte balance
- Maintain an adequate nutrition status
- Avoid infection at the vascular access site
- Use effective coping strategies
- Prevent or slow systemic complications of CKD, including osteodystrophy
- Report an absence of physical signs of anxiety or depression

GET READY FOR THE NEXT-GENERATION NCLEX® EXAMINATION!

Essential Nursing Care Points

Health Promotion/Disease Prevention

- Urge all healthy adults to avoid dehydration by drinking 2 to 3 L of water daily.
- Teach adults treated for an infection anywhere in the kidney/urinary system to take all antibiotics as prescribed.
- Teach patients the expected side effects, any adverse reactions to prescribed drugs, and when to contact the prescriber.
- Use language and terminology that are understandable for the patient.
- Glomerular filtration rate (GFR) is accepted as the best overall indicator of kidney function. Assess estimated GFR values regularly in patients at risk for kidney disease.

Chronic Disease Care

- Encourage patients with acute kidney injury (AKI), chronic kidney disease (CKD), or end-stage kidney disease (ESKD) to follow fluid and dietary restrictions.
- Teach patients using peritoneal dialysis the early signs and symptoms of peritonitis.
- Teach patients receiving immunosuppressive therapy for kidney transplantation to assess themselves daily for fever, general malaise, and nausea or vomiting, as well as changes in urine output and weight gain that indicate new fluid retention.
- Teach patients in the early stages of CKD the symptoms of dehydration.
- Avoid all invasive procedures in the 4 to 6 hours following hemodialysis.

Regenerative or Restorative Care

- Report a urine output of less than 30 mL/hr for 2 hours or dark amber urine to the primary health care provider.
- Avoid taking blood pressure measurements or drawing blood from an arm with a vascular access.
- Do not use a kidney replacement vascular access device to give IV fluids.
- Collaborate with the registered dietitian nutritionist (RDN) to teach patients about dietary needs.
- Inform the primary health care provider immediately about hemodynamic instability, change in cognition, signs of infection, newly abnormal serum electrolytes, and urine output less than 0.5 mL/kg/hr for more than 2 to 4 hours (unless the patient is oliguric or anuric from ESKD).
- Timely interventions to remove the cause of AKI may prevent progression to ESKD and the need for lifelong renal replacement therapy (RRT) or a renal transplant.

Hospice/Palliative/Supportive Care

- Consider physical therapy referral for patients with CKD osteodystrophy to prevent fractures.
- Allow patients to express concerns about the disruption of lifestyle and considerations for end-of-life care as a result of kidney failure.
- Make appropriate referrals for palliative and/or hospice care based on patient condition and stage of kidney disease.

Mastery Questions

1. The nurse is providing discharge teaching to a client recovering from kidney transplantation. Which client statement indicates understanding?

   A. "I can stop my medications when my kidney function returns to normal."

   B. "If my urine output decreases, I will increase my fluids."

   C. "The antirejection medications will be taken for life."

   D. "I will drink 8 ounces (236 mL) of water with my medications."

2. The nurse is caring for a 38-year-old male with hypertension and stage 1 CKD. The client reports lifestyle changes and feeling "better" and has stopped taking a prescribed diuretic. What is the appropriate nursing response?

   A. "The diuretic will reduce your blood pressure, which may slow or prevent progression of your chronic kidney disease."

   B. "Your primary health care provider prescribed the diuretic because it will reverse the damage caused by kidney disease."

   C. "Taking medications is a personal decision, and you have the right to decline this prescription."

   D. "Since you have implemented lifestyle changes, the diuretic is likely not needed."

3. A client who performs home continuous ambulatory peritoneal dialysis reports that the drainage (effluent) has become cloudy in the past 24 hours. What is the priority nursing action?
   A. Remove the peritoneal catheter.
   B. Notify the nephrology health care provider.
   C. Obtain a sample of effluent for culture and sensitivity.
   D. Teach the client that effluent should be clear or slightly yellow.

NGN Challenge 60.1

The nurse is caring for a 42-year-old client who presents to the primary care provider with reports of nausea and body aches.

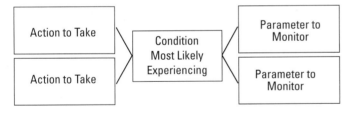

History and Physical	Nurses' Notes	Orders	Laboratory Results

1115: The client has a history of chronic kidney disease requiring dialysis. The client has been doing continuous ambulatory peritoneal dialysis (CAPD) for the last 4 weeks and plans to begin hemodialysis next month. The client reports that the CAPD had been "going well" until yesterday, when he started to feel really achy and noticed that his stomach "looked swollen." The client reports abdominal pain as a 6 on a scale of 0 to 10 and reports that the dialysate outflow is cloudy and flows very slowly. Lung sounds are clear bilaterally. Dressing over peritoneal catheter is clean and dry.
VS: T 100.9°F (38.2°C); HR 80 beats/min; RR 22 breaths/min; BP 140/68 mm Hg; Sp0₂ 98% on RA.

Complete the diagram by selecting from the choices below to specify what potential condition the client is likely experiencing, 2 nursing actions that are appropriate to take, and 2 parameters the nurse should monitor to assess the client's progress.

Actions to Take	Potential Conditions	Parameters to Monitor
Teach use of an enema prior to the instillation	Constipation	Temperature
Culture the dialysis outflow	Peritonitis	Color of effluent
Encourage to warm the dialysate fluid	Catheter displacement	Bowel patterns
Plan for antibiotic therapy	Bowel perforation	Urine output
Plan for diuretic therapy		Blood pressure

NGN Challenge 60.2

The nurse is caring for a 62-year-old male client admitted to the medical unit yesterday after a severe GI viral illness causing prolonged vomiting and diarrhea. The client has a history of diabetes mellitus. To plan the most appropriate care, the nurse reviews relevant client findings recorded on the nursing flow sheet.

NURSING FLOW SHEET

Parameters	Results Today (1000)	Results Yesterday (1030) (Admission)
Temperature	97.6°F (36.4°C)	98°F (36.7°C)
Pulse rate	88 beats/min	84 beats/min
Respiratory rate	24 breaths/min	22 breaths/min
Blood pressure	82/54 mm Hg	90/50 mm Hg
Weight	168 lb (76.2 kg)	165 lb (74.8 kg)
Serum sodium (Reference range 136–145 mEq/L [136–145 mmol/L])	140 mEq/L (128 mmol/L)	138 mEq/L (132 mmol/L)
Serum creatinine (Reference range 0.6–1.2 mg/dL (53–106 mmol/L)	2.6 mg/dL (229.89 mmol/L)	1.4 mg/dL (123.7 mmol/L)
Serum potassium (Reference range 3.5–5 mEq/L or 3.5 mmol/L)	5.4 mEq/L (5.4 mmol/L)	4.9 mEq/L (4.9 mmol/L)
Urine output	120 mL in past 6 hr	400 mL in 24 hr

Complete the following sentence by selecting from the list of Word Choices below.

Based on recent assessment findings and medical history, the nurse determines that the client is currently at high risk for

[Word Choice].

Word Choices
Intrarenal failure
Prerenal failure
Postrenal failure
Chronic kidney failure
Cardiorenal syndrome
Renal osteodystrophy

REFERENCES

Asterisk (*) indicates a classic or definitive work on this subject.

Brown, R. M., & Semler, M. W. (2019). Fluid management in sepsis. *Journal of Intensive Care Medicine, 34*(5), 364–373. https://doi.org/10.1177/0885066618784861.

Burchum, J., & Rosenthal, L. (2022). *Lehne's pharmacology for nursing care* (11th ed.). St. Louis: Elsevier.

Centers for Disease Control and Prevention. (2021). *Chronic kidney disease in the United States, 2021. Centers for Disease Control and Prevention*. Atlanta, GA: US Department of Health and Human Services. https://www.cdc.gov/kidneydisease/publications-resources/ckd-national-facts.html.

Chu, C. D., Powe, N. R., McCulloch, C. E., et al. (2021). Trends in Chronic Kidney Disease Care in the US by Race and Ethnicity, 2012-2019. *JAMA Netw Open, 4*(9), e2127014. https://doi.org/10.1001/jamanetworkopen.2021.27014.

Ferri, F. (2022). *Ferri's clinical advisor 2022, five books in one*. St Louis: Elsevier.

Fuhrman, D. Y. -G. (2018). Acute kidney injury epidemiology, risk factors, and outcomes in critically ill patients 16–25 years of age treated in an adult intensive care unit. *Annals of Intensive Care*, 26–34.

Gilbert, S., & Weiner, D. (2023). *National Kidney Foundation primer on kidney diseases* (8th ed.). St. Louis: Elsevier.

Himmelfarb, J., & Ikizler, T. A. (2018). *Chronic kidney disease, dialysis and transplantation* (4th ed.). St. Louis: Elsevier.

Jarvis, C., & Eckhardt, A. (2024). Physical examinations and health assessment (8th ed.). St. Louis: Elsevier.

Johnson, R., Feehally, J., Floege, J., & Tonelli, M. (2019). *Comprehensive clinical nephrology* (6th ed.). .

Kidney Foundation of Canada. (2020). *Facing the Facts, 2020*. Retrieved from: https://kidney.ca/KFOC/media/images/PDFs/Facing-the-Facts-2020.pdf.

Lotfaliany, M. B. (2018). Depression and chronic diseases: Co-occurrence and communality of risk factors. *Journal of Affective Disorders*, 461–468.

Moore, P. H. (2018). *Management of acute kidney injury: Core Curriculum 2018. American Journal of Kidney Diseases*, 136–148.

National Kidney Foundation (NKF). (2020). *Race, ethnicity, and kidney disease*. Retrieved from https://www.kidney.org/atoz/content/minorities-KD.

National Kidney Foundation (NKF). (2022). *Organ Donation And Transplantation Statistics*. Retrieved from National Kidney Foundation: https://www.kidney.org/news/newsroom/factsheets/Organ-Donation-and-Transplantation-Stats.

Norton, J., Newman, M., Romancito, G., Mahooty, S., Kuracina, T., & Narva, A. (2017a). Improving outcomes for patients with chronic kidney disease: Part 1. *American Journal of Nursing, 117*(2), 22–32.

Norton, J., Newman, M., Romancito, G., Mahooty, S., Kuracina, T., & Narva, A. (2017b). Improving outcomes for patients with chronic kidney disease: Part 2. *American Journal of Nursing, 117*(3), 26–35.

Pavkov, M. E., Harding, J. L., & Burrows, N. R. (2018). Trends in hospitalizations for acute kidney injury — United States, 2000–2014. *MMWR Morb Mortal Wkly Rep, 67*, 289–293. https://doi.org/10.15585/mmwr.mm6710a2external. icon.

Rogers, J. L. (2023). *McCance and Huether's Pathophysiology: The biologic basis for disease in adults and children* (9th ed.). St. Louis: Elsevier.

Ronco, C., Bellomo, R., Kellum, J., & Ricci, Z. (2019). *Critical care nephrology* (3rd ed.). St. Louis: Elsevier.

Rudnick, M., & Davenport, M. (2023). Prevention of contrast-induced acute kidney injury associated with computed tomography. *UpToDate*. Retrieved April 27, 2023, from https://www.uptodate.com/contents/prevention-of-contrast-induced-acute-kidney-injury-associated-with-computed-tomography.

United States Renal Data System. (2019). *USRDS annual data report: Epidemiology of kidney disease in the United States. National Institute of Diabetes and Digestive and Kidney Diseases*. Bethesda, MD: National Institutes of Health. 2019.

Woo, K. (2019). Hemodialysis access: Dialysis catheters. In A. P. Sidawy (Ed.), *Rutherford's vascular surgery and Endovascular therapy* (pp. 2315–2323). Philadelphia: Elsevier.

Assessment of the Reproductive System

Cherie R. Rebar

http://evolve.elsevier.com/Iggy/

LEARNING OUTCOMES

1. Use knowledge of anatomy and physiology to perform a focused assessment of the reproductive system.
2. Teach evidence-based health promotion activities to help prevent reproductive health problems or trauma.
3. Identify factors that affect health equity for patients with reproductive health problems.
4. Explain how genetic implications and physiologic aging of the reproductive system affect *sexuality.*
5. Interpret assessment findings for patients with a suspected or actual reproductive problem.
6. Plan evidence-based care and support for patients undergoing diagnostic testing of the reproductive system.

KEY TERMS

AFAB Assigned female at birth.

AMAB Assigned male at birth.

amenorrhea Absence of menses.

circumcision Surgical removal of the prepuce or foreskin of the penis.

colposcopy Examination of the cervix and vagina using a colposcope, which allows three-dimensional magnification and intense illumination of epithelium with suspected disease. This procedure can locate the exact site of precancerous and malignant lesions for biopsy.

conization Removal of a cone-shaped sample of tissue.

digital 3D mammography (digital breast tomosynthesis) Breast imaging that allows the radiologist to visualize through layers or "slices" of breast tissue, similar to a CT scan.

dilation and curettage (D&C) Procedure in which tissue is removed from inside of the uterus due to abnormal bleeding or to remove pregnancy tissue after an abortion, miscarriage, or childbirth.

human papillomavirus (HPV) test Test that can identify many high-risk types of HPV infection associated with the development of cervical cancer.

hysterosalpingogram An outpatient fluoroscopy procedure that uses an injection of a contrast medium to visualize the cervix, uterus, and fallopian tubes.

hysteroscopy Procedure that uses a fiberoptic camera to visualize the uterus to diagnose and treat causes of abnormal bleeding.

laparoscopy Direct examination of the pelvic cavity through an endoscope.

libido Sex drive or desire.

mammography X-ray of the soft tissue of the breast.

orchitis An acute testicular inflammation resulting from trauma or *infection.*

Papanicolaou test (Pap test or Pap smear) A cytologic study that is effective in detecting precancerous and cancerous cells within the female patient's cervix.

salpingitis Fallopian tube infection.

✴ PRIORITY AND INTERRELATED CONCEPTS

The priority concepts for this chapter are:
- *Infection*
- *Pain*

The interrelated concept for this chapter is:
- *Sexuality*

Reproductive problems affect physical and psychosocial aspects of *sexuality*. They can be difficult for patients to discuss. The nurse can best address patient concerns by showing respect to all people and by creating and maintaining a nonjudgmental environment. It is of critical importance to respect differences in sexual orientation and practices and to respect gender identity when discussing reproductive issues and sexuality. A more detailed discussion of human sexuality is found in Chapter 1.

ANATOMY AND PHYSIOLOGY REVIEW

Structure and Function of the Female Reproductive System

The reproductive system of people assigned female at birth (AFAB) has external and internal components. Estrogen and progesterone are the sex hormones found in these individuals, which include cisgender women, transgender men, and nonbinary people with vaginas (Cleveland Clinic, 2022). Within this chapter, the terms "female," "woman," and "women" apply to all individuals with this type of reproductive system present at birth.

External Genitalia

The female external genitalia, known as the vulva, extend from the mons pubis to the anal opening. The mons pubis is a pad of fat that covers the symphysis pubis and protects it during sexual intercourse (also known as *coitus*).

The labia majora are two vertical folds of adipose tissue that extend posteriorly from the mons pubis to the perineum. The size of the labia majora varies, depending on the amount of fatty tissue present. The skin over the labia majora is usually darker than the surrounding skin and is highly vascular. It protects inner vulval structures and enhances sexual arousal.

The labia majora surround two thinner, vertical folds of reddish epithelium called the *labia minora*. The labia minora are highly vascular and have a rich nerve supply. Emotional or physical stimulation induces marked swelling and sensitivity. Sebaceous glands in the labia minora lubricate the entrance to the vagina. The clitoris is a small, cylindric organ that is composed of erectile tissue with a high concentration of sensory nerve endings. During sexual arousal, the clitoris enlarges and has heightened sensation.

The vestibule is a longitudinal area between the labia minora, the clitoris, and the vagina that contains Bartholin glands, the urethral meatus, the opening of the Skene (paraurethral) glands, the hymen, and the vaginal opening (Jarvis & Eckhardt, 2024). The two Bartholin glands, located deeply toward the back on both sides of the vaginal opening, secrete lubrication fluid during sexual excitement. Their ductal openings are usually not visible.

The perineum is located between the vaginal opening and the anus. The skin of the perineum covers the muscles, fascia, and ligaments that support the pelvic structures.

Internal Genitalia

The internal female genitalia are shown in Fig. 61.1. The *vagina* is a hollow tube that extends from the vestibule to the uterus. Ovarian hormones (primarily *estrogen*) influence the amounts of glycogen and lubricating fluid secreted by the vaginal cells. Normal vaginal bacteria interact with the secretions to produce lactic acid. This process facilitates maintenance of an acidic pH of 4.0 to 4.5 in the vagina, which helps prevent **infection** (Sobel, 2022).

At the upper end of the vagina, the uterine cervix projects into a cup-shaped vault of thin vaginal tissue. The recessed pockets around the cervix permit palpation of the internal pelvic organs. The posterior area provides access into the peritoneal cavity for diagnostic or surgical purposes.

The *uterus* (or "womb") is a thick-walled, pear-shaped muscular organ attached to the upper end of the vagina. This inverted pear-shaped organ is located within the true pelvis,

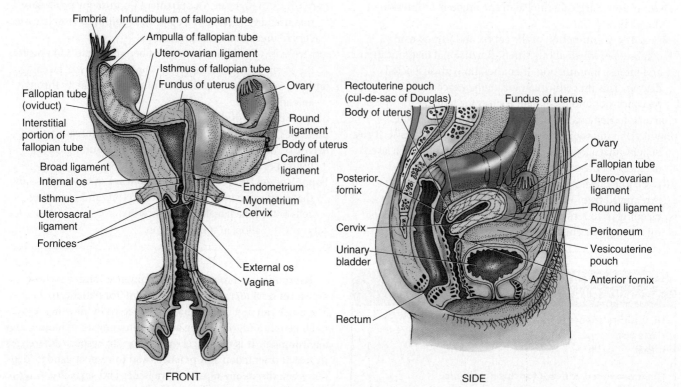

FRONT   SIDE

FIG. 61.1 Internal female genitalia.

between the bladder and the rectum. The uterus is made up of the body and the cervix. The *cervix*, measuring about 1 inch [2.5 cm]), is a narrowed portion of the uterus that extends into the vagina. The surfaces of the cervix and the canal are the sites where Papanicolaou (Pap) testing is performed. (See discussion later in this chapter.)

The *fallopian tubes* insert into the uterine fundus and extend laterally close to the ovaries. They provide a duct between the ovaries and the uterus for the passage of ova and sperm. In most cases, the ovum is fertilized in these tubes up to 72 hours after release.

The *ovaries* are a pair of almond-shaped organs located near the lateral walls of the upper pelvic cavity. These small organs develop and release ova, and produce estrogen and progesterone. Adequate amounts of these hormones are needed for normal female growth and development, and to maintain a pregnancy. Females are born with *oocytes,* germ cells that are involved in reproduction. These are finite in number and do not replenish throughout the life span. After menopause, the ovaries become smaller.

Breasts

The female breasts are a pair of mammary glands that develop in response to secretions from the hypothalamus, pituitary gland, and ovaries and nourish an infant after birth.

Breast tissue is composed of a network of glandular and ductal tissue, fibrous tissue, and fat. The proportion of each component of breast tissue depends on genetic factors, nutrition, age, and obstetric history. The breasts are supported by ligaments that are attached to underlying muscles. They have abundant blood supply and lymph flow that drain from an extensive network toward the axillae (Fig. 61.2).

Structure and Function of the Male Reproductive System

The reproductive system of people assigned male at birth (AMAB) has external and internal components. Testosterone is the primary hormone that is produced by these individuals, which include cisgender men, transgender women, and nonbinary people with penises (New York Presbyterian, n.d.). Within this chapter, the terms "male," "man," and "men" apply to all individuals with this type of reproductive system present at birth.

Testosterone production is predictable in people who are AMAB. After the age of 30, testosterone levels begin to gradually diminish. Low testosterone levels decrease muscle mass, reduce skin elasticity, and lead to changes in sexual performance.

External Genitalia

The reproductive system of people AMAB is comprised of external and internal genitalia. The *penis* is an organ that is used for urination and intercourse. It consists of the body or shaft and the glans penis (the distal end of the penis). The glans is the smooth end of the penis, which contains the opening of the urethral meatus. Urine and semen both exit via the *urethra*. A continuation of skin covers the glans and folds to form the prepuce (foreskin). Circumcision, the surgical removal

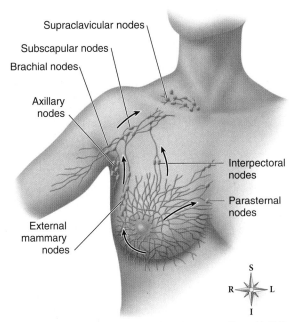

FIG. 61.2 Lymphatic drainage of the female breast. (Found in Wilson, S. F., & Giddens, J. F. [2022]. *Health assessment for nursing practice* [7th ed.]. St. Louis: Elsevier. From Thibodeau, K. T., et. al. [2012]. *Essentials of anatomy and physiology*. St. Louis: Elsevier.)

of the foreskin, is a common procedure performed in various parts of the world for cultural or religious reasons. When chosen, it is often performed very soon after an infant AMAB has been born, or within an established amount of time following the birth.

The scrotum is a thin-walled, fibromuscular pouch that is behind the penis and suspended below the pubic bone. This pouch protects the testes, epididymis, and vas deferens in a space that is slightly cooler than inside the abdominal cavity. The scrotal skin is darkly pigmented and contains sweat glands, sebaceous glands, and few hair follicles. It contracts with cold, exercise, tactile stimulation, and sexual excitement.

Internal Genitalia

The internal male genitalia are shown in Fig. 61.3. The major organs are the *testes* and *prostate gland*. The testes are a pair of oval organs located inside the scrotum that produce sperm and testosterone. Each testis is suspended in the scrotum by the spermatic cord, which provides blood, lymphatic, and nerve supply to the testis. Sympathetic nerve fibers are located on the arteries in the cord, and sympathetic and parasympathetic fibers are on the vas deferens. When the testes are damaged, these autonomic nerve fibers transmit signals of excruciating *pain* and a sensation of nausea.

The *epididymis* is the first portion of a ductal system that transports sperm from the testes to the urethra. It is also the site of sperm maturation. The *vas deferens,* or *ductus deferens*, is a firm, muscular tube that continues from the tail of each epididymis. The end of each vas deferens is a reservoir for sperm and tubular fluids. They merge with ducts from the seminal vesicle to form the ejaculatory ducts at the base of the prostate gland.

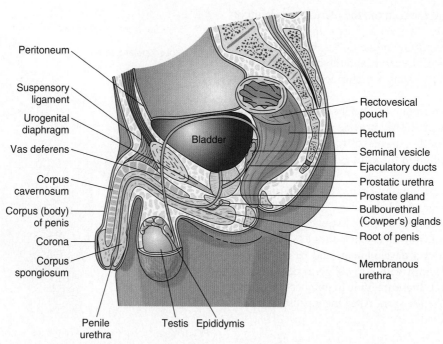

FIG. 61.3 Internal male genitalia.

Sperm from the vas deferens and secretions from the seminal vesicles move through the ejaculatory duct to mix with prostatic fluids in the prostatic urethra.

The *prostate gland* is a large accessory gland of the male reproductive system that can be palpated via the rectum. The gland secretes a milky alkaline fluid that adds bulk to the semen, enhances sperm movement, and neutralizes acidic vaginal secretions. Prostate function depends on adequate levels of testosterone. Men over 50 years of age commonly develop an enlarged prostate (called *benign prostatic hyperplasia* [BPH]),

which can cause problems such as overflow incontinence and nocturia.

Reproductive Changes Associated With Aging

Age brings changes to the function of the male and female reproductive systems (see the Patient-Centered Care: Older Adult Health: Changes in the Reproductive System Related to Aging box). Teach patients the normal and expected signs associated with aging, and remind them to report abnormalities right away to their primary health care provider.

👤 PATIENT-CENTERED CARE: OLDER ADULT HEALTH

Changes in the Reproductive System Related to Aging

Physiologic Change	Nursing Interventions	Rationales
Women		
Graying and thinning of pubic hair Decreased size of labia majora and clitoris	Reassure that these are normal and expected changes.	Education helps patients learn which normal physiologic changes associated with aging to expect and which findings need to be reported to their health care provider. This action can also decrease problems associated with body image by raising awareness that these changes occur in most older adults. (This rationale about education applies when teaching all people about age-related body changes.)
Drying, smoothing, and thinning of vaginal walls	Provide information about vaginal estrogen therapy (if desired and recommended by the health care provider) and water-soluble lubricants to minimize discomfort associated with intercourse.	Education enables the patient to make informed decisions about how or whether to treat vaginal dryness.
Decreased uterine size Atrophy of the endometrium Decreased size and marked convolution of the ovaries Loss of tone and elasticity of the pelvic ligaments and connective tissue	Teach Kegel exercises to strengthen pelvic muscles.	Strengthening exercises can prevent or reduce pelvic relaxation and incidences of urinary incontinence.

Changes in the Reproductive System Related to Aging

Physiologic Change	Nursing Interventions	Rationales
Decreased firmness of the breasts, which allows the breasts to hang lower on the chest wall; decreased erection of the nipples; increased incidence of fibrosis	Teach (1) how to be self-aware of potential breast changes, and (2) the evidence-based recommendations for clinical breast examination and mammography based on the patient's age.	These methods can serve to detect masses or other changes that may indicate the presence of cancer. The sooner a change is noted and examined, the sooner intervention—if the patient desires it—can take place.
Men Graying and thinning of pubic hair	Reassure that this is a normal and expected change.	Education helps patients learn which normal physiologic changes associated with aging to expect and which findings need to be reported to their health care provider. This action can also decrease problems associated with body image by raising awareness that these changes occur in most older adults. (This rationale about education applies when teaching all people about age-related body changes.)
Increased relaxation of the scrotum with loss of rugae	Teach how to be self-aware of potential testicular changes based on evidence-based recommendations for testicular self-examination (TSE).	TSE can serve to detect masses or other changes that may indicate the presence of cancer. The sooner a change is noted and examined, the sooner intervention—if the patient desires it—can take place.
Prostate enlargement, with increased likelihood of urethral obstruction	Teach about symptoms associated with urethral obstruction and the importance of regular prostate cancer screening.	Education helps the patient detect prostate enlargement and/or obstruction, which may indicate the presence of benign prostatic hyperplasia (BPH) or cancer. The sooner a change is noted and examined, the sooner intervention—if the patient desires it—can take place.

Health Promotion/Disease Prevention

Many reproductive system problems can be prevented through health promotion strategies and avoidance of risky lifestyle behaviors. For example, following evidence-based practices for routine preventive screenings, such as mammography and Pap tests, can detect cancer early so that it can be treated with better chance for a cure. The risk for sexually transmitted infections (STIs) and other reproductive infections can be minimized by using safer sex practices such as condoms or practicing abstinence. Teach patients about these health promotion strategies and others that are described under specific reproductive health problems within this unit.

RECOGNIZE CUES: ASSESSMENT

Patients may find it difficult to discuss their reproductive history or concerns about *sexuality*. Establish a trusting relationship with the patient, and provide information about why you are asking these questions. Explain how their answers can help inform the best approach to treatment, and reassure them that their health information is protected via the Health Insurance Portability and Accountability Act (HIPAA). Respect their choice to decline to answer questions if they state that they do not wish to comment.

Patient History

Review the electronic health record. Confirm the history that is present, and ask whether there are any unlisted conditions that need to be added. Disorders that affect a woman's metabolism or nutrition can depress ovarian function and cause amenorrhea, and untreated sexually transmitted infections can lead to

infertility. Ask about childhood conditions that could have an effect on the reproductive system. A history of mumps in men may cause orchitis, which can lead to testicular atrophy and (uncommonly) sterility. A history of undescended testicles can contribute to male infertility.

Assess for chronic illnesses or surgeries that could affect reproductive function. Patients with diabetes mellitus may experience physiologic changes such as vaginal dryness or impotence. Chronic disorders of the nervous system, respiratory system, or cardiovascular system can alter the sexual response, as can psychiatric–mental health disorders.

Ask whether the patient has had infections. Pelvic inflammatory disease or a ruptured appendix followed by peritonitis in females can cause pelvic scarring and strictures or adhesions in the fallopian tubes. Salpingitis, inflammation of the fallopian tubes, is often caused by chlamydia, a sexually transmitted *infection* (STI), and can result in female infertility. A history of infections or prolonged fever in males could have resulted in damaged sperm production or obstruction of the seminal tract, which can cause infertility.

Ask whether the patient has been treated with radiation therapy or had prolonged use of corticosteroids, internal or external estrogen, testosterone, or chemotherapy drugs. These can all lead to reproductive system dysfunction.

Assess general health habits, such as sleep, exercise, and diet, as the amount of body fat a person carries can be related to ovarian dysfunction in females. Determine when patients had their last screening for reproductive concerns. Ask females about the date and result of their most recent Pap test, breast self-examination (if done), and vulvar self-examination (if done). Determine when male patients older than 50 years had their last prostate examination and prostate-specific antigen (PSA) test.

Document any prescribed and over-the-counter drugs the patient is taking, including hormones or hormone replacement therapy, and vitamins or supplements. Certain drugs and supplements can affect libido or the male's ability to obtain and sustain an erection. Adverse effects, including cardiovascular disease and cancer, have been historically associated with the use of menopausal hormone therapy (MHT) (Martin & Barbieri, 2023). Current evidence suggests that cardiovascular risk is dependent upon the timing of exposure to MHT and the type of MHT given (Martin & Rosenson, 2023). Assess all women, particularly those who take combination therapy of estrogen and progesterone, for any signs or symptoms associated with cardiovascular disease and cancer.

PATIENT-CENTERED CARE: GENDER HEALTH
Reproductive Health Assessment

Data about reproductive health are vital parts of the patient's history. Sexual orientation and gender identity should not be assumed. Patients who are lesbian, gay, bisexual, transgender, nonbinary, queer/questioning, intersex, asexual, or two-spirited (LGBTQIA2+) are often not fully assessed by health care professionals due to lack of education on the part of the providers of care. All patients feel more comfortable sharing information about their reproductive health and sexual activity when approached in a caring, nonjudgmental way. Chapter 1 describes interviewing techniques that are appropriate for LGBTQIA2+ patients. Chapter 5 discusses assessment and care of transgender and nonbinary patients in detail.

PATIENT-CENTERED CARE: CULTURE AND SPIRITUALITY
Respecting Patient Beliefs

Cultural, religious, and spiritual beliefs influence lifestyle and *sexuality* practices. These beliefs can influence specific methods of sexual expression, the acceptable number of sexual partners, and philosophy of contraceptive use. Be sensitive to these differences by being nonjudgmental and supportive of each patient and the patient's specific beliefs.

Nutrition History

A nutrition history is important when assessing the reproductive system. Fatigue and low libido may occur because of poor diet and anemia. Consumption of sugar-sweetened beverages and highly processed food is linked to at least 13 types of cancer, including endometrial, breast, and colorectal cancer (Centers for Disease Control and Prevention, 2022). Ask the patient to recall personal dietary intake for a recent 24-hour period to assess general quality of nutrition.

Assess patients' height, weight, and body mass index (BMI). Patients may be hesitant to discuss eating habits such as bingeing, purging, restricting, or excessively exercising. It may also be challenging for them to discuss poor eating habits due to high consumption of fast food or lack of access to nutritious foods if they live in a food desert. Reassure patients that honest assessment information can be used to help connect them with resources to follow a healthier diet.

PATIENT-CENTERED CARE: GENDER HEALTH
Women's Nutrition Needs

Women have special nutrition needs related to reproductive anatomy. Teach that a healthy weight and level of body fat help to maintain regular menstrual cycles and that a decrease in body fat can lead to insufficiency in estrogen levels. Those with heavy menstrual bleeding may require iron supplements. Teach that adequate calcium intake throughout life is needed, especially during and after menopause to help prevent osteoporosis caused by decreased estrogen production (see Chapter 42).

Social History

Assess for alcohol, tobacco, and illicit drug use. In males, libido, sperm production, and the ability to obtain or sustain an erection can be affected by these substances. Women may experience alteration or cessation of the menstrual cycle in response to excessive substance use. Those who have chronically abused drugs and/or alcohol are at higher risk for development of cancer and infectious diseases and may experience fertility concerns as well (American Addiction Centers, 2022).

Family History and Genetic Risk

The family history helps determine the patient's risk for conditions that affect reproductive function. A delayed or early development of secondary sex characteristics may be a familial pattern.

The current age and health status of family members are important. Evidence of diseases or reproductive problems in family members (e.g., diabetes, endometriosis, reproductive cancer) can clarify a patient's current health status or risk for development of certain conditions. For example, daughters of women who were given diethylstilbestrol (DES) (called *DES daughters*) to control bleeding during pregnancy are at increased risk for fertility concerns, adverse pregnancy outcomes, reproductive cancers, and breast cancer (Hatch & Karam, 2022).

Specific *BRCA1* and *BRCA2* gene mutations increase the overall risk for breast or ovarian cancer (American Cancer Society [ACS], 2021b). Men with first-degree relatives (e.g., father, brother) with prostate cancer are at two to three times the risk for development of the disease than are men in the general population (American Society of Clinical Oncology, 2022).

Current Health Problems

Patients often seek medical attention due to pain, bleeding, discharge, or masses. See Box 61.1 for best practices for assessment of these types of concerns (Carusi, 2022). *Pain* related to reproductive system disorders may be confused with GI issues (e.g., abdominal discomfort) or urinary health problems (e.g., urinary frequency), particularly in females.

Menstrual changes may concern the patient. The possibility of pregnancy in any sexually active woman with amenorrhea must be considered. Collaborate with the primary health care provider to obtain a urine pregnancy test. Postmenopausal bleeding needs to be evaluated. Ask the patient to describe the amount and characteristics of any abnormal or unexpected

BOX 61.1 Best Practice for Patient Safety and Quality Care

Assessing the Patient With Reproductive Health Problems

Patient Concern	Nursing Assessment
Pain	• Characteristics (e.g., sharp, stabbing, dull) • Intensity (on a scale of 0 to 10) • Timing (how often it occurs, or if it is constant) • Location (where specifically the pain exists) • Duration (how long the pain has persisted since the onset) • Factors (if any) that exacerbate or relieve pain • Whether pain interferes with sleep and the ability to get adequate rest • Relationship of pain (if any) to menstrual, sexual, urinary, or GI function.
Bleeding and Menstruation	• Presence or absence of bleeding • Characteristics and amount of bleeding • Onset and duration of bleeding (e.g., during or between regular periods, constant) • Presence of associated symptoms, such as **pain** or passing clots • (For females) Relationship of bleeding to events or other factors (e.g., menstrual cycle)
Discharge	• Amount of discharge • Characteristics (e.g., color, thickness, odor) • Frequency of discharge (e.g., 1–2 days a month, all month) • Presence of genital lesions, bleeding, itching, or **pain** • Presence of symptoms or discharge in sexual partner
Masses	• Location and characteristics of mass • Presence of associated symptoms, such as **pain**, discharge • (For females) Relationship of appearance of masses to normal menstrual cycle

BOX 61.2 U.S. Preventive Services Task Force Recommendations for Cervical Cancer Screening

The most current cervical cancer screening recommendations from the *U.S. Preventive Services Task Force Recommendations for Cervical Cancer Screening* were released in 2018. At the time of publication, the Task Force was constructing its final research plan that will contribute to informing an update on these recommendations. Per the 2018 recommendations, the USPSTF recommends:
• Women ages 21 to 29 should have a Pap test every 3 years
• Women ages 30 to 65 should have:
  • A Pap test every 3 years **or**
  • High-risk human papillomavirus testing every 5 years **or**
  • A Pap test <u>and</u> high-risk human papillomavirus (hrHPV) testing every 5 years

The USPSTF recommends against testing for cervical cancer in women who:
• Are younger than age 21 years
• Have had a hysterectomy and haven't had a high-grade precancerous lesion or cervical cancer
• Are older than 65 years, have had adequate screening, and aren't at high risk for cervical cancer

Data from U.S. Preventive Services Task Force. (2018). *Cervical cancer: Screening.* Retrieved from https://www.uspreventiveservicestaskforce.org/uspstf/recommendation/cervical-cancer-screening.

Masses in the breasts, testes, or inguinal area must be evaluated. Ask if the patient can relate the changes in character or size of masses to menstrual cycles, heavy lifting, straining, or trauma. Ask about associated symptoms such as tenderness, heaviness, **pain,** dimpling, and tender lymph nodes.

Physical Assessment
Assessment of the Female Reproductive System

A Papanicolaou test (Pap test or Pap smear) should be scheduled between the patient's menstrual periods so that the menstrual flow does not interfere with laboratory analysis. Teach women not to douche, use vaginal medications, powders, or deodorants, or have sexual intercourse for at least 24 hours before the test, because these may interfere with test results. See Box 61.2 for recommendations from the American Cancer Society (2021a) regarding their Guidelines for the Prevention and Early Detection of Cervical Cancer.

General Canadian recommendations for Pap tests include (Choosing Wisely Canada, 2022):
• Women should begin having an annual Pap test at 21 years of age.
• Women between 21 and 29 years who are sexually active should have a Pap test every 3 years.
• Women between ages 30 and 69 years should have a Pap test every 3 years.
• Women older than 70 years who have had three previous normal Pap tests do not need further Pap testing.
• Women with risk factors such as a history of cancer, precancerous cells in the cervix, or a weakened immune system should speak to their health care provider regarding Pap recommendations.

vaginal bleeding. Assess whether the bleeding occurs in relationship to the usual menstrual cycle or signs of menopause, intercourse, trauma, or strenuous exercise.

For male patients, ask about the presence of penile bleeding. Ask any patient who has abnormal bleeding about associated symptoms, such as **pain,** cramping or abdominal fullness, a change in bowel habits, urinary difficulties, and weight changes.

Discharge from the reproductive tract can cause irritation of the surrounding tissues, itching, **pain,** embarrassment, and anxiety. Ask about the amount, color, consistency, odor, and chronicity of discharge that may be present from orifices used during sexual activity. Certain drugs (e.g., antibiotics) and clothing (e.g., tight clothing, synthetic underwear fabric) may cause or worsen genital discharge. Many types of discharge are caused by STIs or other **infection** (see Chapter 65).

The nurse generalist does not perform the comprehensive reproductive examination. However, the nurse should perform a focused physical assessment related to specific concerns of the patient. The primary health care provider will conduct a detailed reproductive assessment as described in the following paragraphs. You may be asked to assist with preparation for the examination, as well as the examination itself.

The examination should be performed in a room that has adequate lighting for body inspection, has a comfortable temperature, and ensures privacy. Ask patients to empty their bladder before the examination and undress completely. Provide a gown for the patient to wear, and provide draping to provide as much privacy as possible. As needed, assist the primary health care provider in removing drapes only over the region being examined. Replace draping immediately after each area has been assessed. Mirrors can be used to facilitate teaching if the patient desires.

For routine screening examinations, the primary health care provider may begin with assessing the breasts before progressing to the abdomen and pelvic or genital examination. Patients' arms should be at their sides or draped easily over their chest to allow better relaxation of the torso muscles. The primary health care provider will assess for symmetry, shape, skin color and temperature, and presence or absence of lesions or dimpling. Help patients lie on their back during palpation of the breast tissue (and then the abdomen). If patients wish to perform breast self-examinations at home, provide teaching (Chapter 62). Remind them that clinical breast examinations and mammography are still best practices for detecting cancer.

Inspection of the external female genitalia and the pelvic examination are usually performed at the end of a head-to-toe physical assessment, unless the patient has requested to have these done first. Allow the patient to choose when this part of the examination is done. The patient may be apprehensive due to *pain* or a lack of privacy during previous pelvic examinations. Maintain a therapeutic, private environment. Offer reassurance and compassion during this portion of the examination.

Assist patients into the lithotomy position, continuously being mindful of draping for privacy. The health care provider will visualize the mons pubis and vulva. Be aware that removal of pubic hair and/or piercings in this area may compromise tissue integrity and facilitate *infection*. In preparation for the internal genitalia examination, obtain a Graves speculum for most adult patients or a Pederson speculum (which is narrower and flatter) for patients who are younger or postmenopausal;

run warm water over it and apply a dime-sized amount of water-soluble gel lubricant (Jarvis & Eckhardt, 2024). Teach that a plastic speculum makes a loud clicking sound when it locks and unlocks so that this noise does not startle the patient (Jarvis & Eckhardt, 2024). This portion of the examination can help to determine pregnancy or reasons for infertility, as well as assess for:

- Menstrual irregularities
- Unexplained abdominal or vaginal *pain*
- Vaginal discharge, itching, sores, or *infection*
- Physical changes in the vagina, cervix, and uterus
- Rape trauma or other pelvic injury

During the speculum examination, the health care provider palpates for symptomatic and asymptomatic abdominopelvic masses. These can be of reproductive, intestinal, or urinary tract origin. Gynecologic masses, such as ovarian masses, may be further differentiated from lesions on the body of the uterus during the bimanual portion of the pelvic examination.

Several samples of cells from the cervix are obtained with a small brush or spatula during the Pap test, placed on a glass slide, and sent to the laboratory for examination. Nucleic acid amplification tests (NAATs) are collected to test for sexually transmitted infections, and samples for HPV testing are also obtained at this time.

A bimanual examination will be performed by the health care provider to palpate the internal genitalia for location, size, mobility, and the presence of masses or tenderness (Jarvis & Eckhardt, 2024). The health care provider may also perform a rectal examination, which can demonstrate external or internal hemorrhoids, fissures, or masses.

When the examination is complete, provide the patient with a towel to remove any residual water-soluble gel. If needed, assist the patient to a sitting position, and then provide privacy for redressing.

PATIENT-CENTERED CARE: CULTURE AND SPIRITUALITY
Influences on Sexuality

A patient's personal experiences, culture, and/or spiritual beliefs may influence thoughts about **sexuality**, which can affect the patient's ability to enjoy a satisfactory sex life. Influences may include:

- Sexual trauma or abuse experienced during childhood or adulthood
- Childhood punishment for masturbation
- Childhood or adult psychological trauma
- Cultural, religious, or spiritual beliefs
- Concerns about sexual partners or sexual practices
- Use of alcohol, prescribed drugs, and/or other substances

Assessment of the Male Reproductive System

Unless a male patient seeks care for a specific reproductive problem, the health care provider may not perform this type of assessment. That decision depends on the setting where the patient is being seen, the patient's age, and the presenting concern.

Men may be embarrassed and anxious when the reproductive system is assessed. The patient may be concerned about *pain,* genitalia development, or the possibility of experiencing an erection during assessment. If the patient does experience an erection, remind the patient that this is a natural response to stimulus. It is appropriate to nonjudgmentally continue the examination unless the patient requests to stop the assessment.

Explain each step of the assessment procedure before it is performed. Provide privacy within a well-lit environment and have the patient undress. Use appropriate draping to achieve as much privacy as possible throughout the examination. Remove drapes only as needed for the examination, and replace them after that area has been assessed. Reassure the patient that the health care provider will stop and change the assessment approach if requested.

The health care provider will examine the pubis, penis, and scrotum, looking for lesions or compromised skin integrity. If a sexually transmitted *infection* is suspected, swabs may be obtained at this time by the provider. Provide nonjudgmental support, and teach relaxation techniques that can be helpful to relieve discomfort, especially if the provider performs a digital rectal examination (DRE) to palpate the prostate gland to assess for masses or *pain*. This type of examination will not be performed for all patients; the health care provider will discuss with each individual patient whether this evaluation is recommended.

The health care provider may also conduct a breast examination that is similar to what is performed for women. Although men are less likely to have breast cancer than women, it is important to assess for this possibility, especially if the patient has been exposed to radiation, has a high level of estrogen, or has a family history of breast cancer (National Breast Cancer Foundation, 2022).

When the examination is complete, provide the patient with a towel for cleaning (if needed) and privacy for redressing.

Psychosocial Assessment

Ask about sources of support, strengths, and coping reactions to illness or dysfunction. It is not uncommon for people with reproductive concerns to feel anxiety or fear. For patients who have few support systems in place, consider referral to community groups or social services that can be of assistance. Collaborate with the health care provider for appropriate referral of the patient with fertility concerns.

Diagnostic Assessment
Laboratory Assessment

As noted earlier, the Pap test is a cytologic study performed during a female reproductive examination that is effective in detecting precancerous and cancerous cells within the cervix. The human papillomavirus (HPV) test performed on cervical cells can identify many high-risk types of HPV *infection* associated with development of cervical cancer. The HPV test can be done at the same time as the Pap test for women between the ages of 25 and 65, or as a follow-up for those who have had an abnormal Pap test result. The HPV test does not replace the Pap test, as each test is used for assessment of unique concerns. Women with normal Pap test results and no HPV infection are at a low risk for developing cervical cancer. Conversely, those with an abnormal Pap test and a positive HPV test result are at higher risk if not treated.

Table 61.1 summarizes important laboratory tests associated with reproductive function, normal ranges, and the significance of abnormal findings. Serum levels of follicle-stimulating

TABLE 61.1 Laboratory Profile
Reproductive Assessment

Serum Test	Normal Range for Adults	Significance of Abnormal Findings
Follicle-stimulating hormone (FSH)	*Men:* 1.42–15.4 IU/L *Women:* • Follicular phase, 1.37–9.9 IU/L • Ovulatory peak, 6.17–17.2 IU/L • Luteal phase, 1.09–9.2 IU/L • Postmenopause, 19.3–100.6 IU/L ***Canadian:*** *Men:* 1.0–10.0 IU/L *Women:* • Follicular phase, 1.37–9.9 IU/L • Ovulatory peak, 6.17–17.2 IU/L • Luteal phase, 1.09–9.2 IU/L • Postmenopausal, 40–250 IU/L	Increased levels may indicate polycystic ovaries (in women), complete testicular feminization syndrome (in men), or pituitary adenoma. Decreased levels may indicate pituitary or hypothalamic failure, stress, anorexia nervosa, or malnutrition.
Luteinizing hormone (LH)	*Men:* 1.24–7.8 IU/L *Women:* • Follicular phase, 1.68–15 IU/L • Ovulatory peak, 21.9–56.6 IU/L • Luteal phase, 0.61–16.3 IU/L • Postmenopausal, 14.2–52.3 IU/L ***Canadian:*** *Men:* 1.0–9.0 IU/L *Women:* • Follicular phase, 2.0–10.0 IU/L • Ovulatory peak, 15.0–65.0 IU/L • Luteal phase, 1.0–12.0 IU/L • Postmenopausal, 12–65 IU/L	Same significance as FSH above.

Continued

TABLE 61.1   Laboratory Profile—cont'd

Reproductive Assessment

Serum Test	Normal Range for Adults	Significance of Abnormal Findings
Prolactin	*Men:* 3–13 ng/mL *Women:* 3–27 ng/mL **Canadian:** *Men:* 1–20 ng/mL *Women:* 1–25 ng/mL	Increased levels may indicate galactorrhea, amenorrhea (in women), prolactin-secreting pituitary tumor, metastatic cancer of the pituitary gland, hypothyroidism, stress, renal failure, or polycystic ovary syndrome (in women). Decreased levels may indicate possible pituitary apoplexy (in women) or pituitary destruction from tumor.
Estradiol	*Men:* 10–50 pg/mL *Women:* • Follicular phase, 20–350 pg/mL • Midcycle, 150–750 pg/mL • Luteal phase, 30–450 pg/mL • Postmenopausal, ≤20 pg/mL **Canadian:** *Men:* 36.7–183.5 pmol/L *Women:* • Follicular phase, 73.4–1284.8 pmol/L • Midcycle, 550.6–2753.3 pmol/L • Luteal phase, 110.1–1651.9 pmol/L • Postmenopausal, ≤73.4 pmol/L	Increased levels may indicate possible adrenal tumor, ovarian tumor (in women), or testicular tumor (in men), normal pregnancy development (in women), or feminization syndromes (in men). Decreased levels may indicate possible pregnancy concerns or menopause (in women), hypopituitarism, primary and secondary hypogonadism (in men), or anorexia nervosa.
Progesterone	*Men:* 10–50 ng/dL *Women:* • Follicular phase, <50 ng/dL • Luteal phase, 300–2500 ng/dL • Postmenopausal, <40 ng/dL **Canadian:** *Men:* 0–1.3 nmol/L *Women:* • Follicular phase, 0.3–4.8 nmol/L • Luteal phase, 8.0–89.0 nmol/L • Postmenopausal, <1.27 nmol/L	Increased levels in women may indicate ovulation, pregnancy, molar pregnancy, luteal cysts of the ovary, hyperadrenocorticalism, adrenocortical hyperplasia, or choriocarcinoma of the ovary. Decreased levels in women may indicate preeclampsia, toxemia of pregnancy, threatened abortion, placental failure, fetal death, ovarian neoplasm, ovarian hypofunction, or amenorrhea.
Testosterone (Total Testosterone)	*Men:* 280–1080 ng/dL *Women:* <70 ng/dL **Canadian:** *Men:* 275–875 ng/dL *Women:* 23–875 ng/dL	Increased levels in women may indicate possible adrenal or ovarian tumor, polycystic ovaries, or idiopathic hirsutism. Increased levels in men may indicate possible testicular, extragonadal, or adrenocortical tumor; pinealoma; testosterone resistance syndrome; or hyperthyroidism. Decreased levels in men may indicate possible cryptorchidism, hypogonadism, trisomy 21, or orchidectomy.
Prostate-specific antigen	*Men:* • 0–2.5 ng/mL = low • 2.6–10 ng/mL = slightly to moderately elevated • 10–19.9 ng/mL = moderately elevated • 20 ng/mL or more = significantly elevated **Canadian:** *Men:* 0–4 ng/mL	Increased levels in men may indicate prostatitis, benign prostatic hyperplasia, or prostate cancer.

Data from Pagana, K. D., Pagana, T. J., & Pagana, T. N. (2022). *Mosby's manual of diagnostic and laboratory tests* (7th ed.). St. Louis: Elsevier.

hormone (FSH), luteinizing hormone (LH), and prolactin are helpful in the diagnosis of reproductive tract disorders. Serum testing can detect estrogen, progesterone, and testosterone levels. Teach the patient that no dietary restrictions are necessary before having these tests performed.

Other types of laboratory testing include cytologic vaginal *cultures,* which can detect bacterial, viral, fungal, and parasitic disorders. Examination of cells from the vaginal walls can evaluate estrogen balance in female patients.

Serologic studies detect antigen-antibody reactions that occur in response to foreign organisms. This form of diagnostic testing is helpful only after an *infection* has become well established. Serologic testing can be used in the evaluation of exposure to organisms causing syphilis, rubella, and herpes simplex virus type 2 (HSV2). Results may be read as *nonreactive* or *reactive.* A single titer is not as revealing as serial titers, which can detect the rise in antibody reactions as the body continues to fight the infection.

The *prostate-specific antigen (PSA)* test is used to screen for prostate cancer in men, and to monitor the disease during and after treatment (if elected). Although elevated PSA levels may be associated with prostate cancer, there is variance among health care providers regarding interpretation of results. Levels of 0 to 4.0 ng/mL may be considered normal, depending on the resource used (Hoffman & Preston, 2023; Pagana et al., 2022). Certain factors such as prostatitis, acute urinary retention, recent prostate biopsy, or transurethral resection of the prostate (TURP) can cause transient rises in PSA (Hoffman & Preston, 2023). The health care provider will collaborate with the patient to determine the individual's specific risk level and recommend diagnostic evaluation accordingly.

PATIENT-CENTERED CARE: HEALTH EQUITY

Prostate Cancer in African-American Men

African-American men are 1.6 times as likely to develop prostate cancer and twice as likely to die from it than are White men (Research on Prostate Cancer in Men of African Ancestry, 2019). To address this concern related to health equity, diligently advocate for African-American male patients to begin prostate cancer screening at age 40. Early detection facilitates early intervention.

Imaging Assessment

Mammography. Mammography is an x-ray of the soft tissue of the breast. Mammograms assess differences in breast tissue density. They are especially helpful in evaluating poorly defined masses, multiple masses or nodules, nipple changes or discharge, skin changes, and factors that may cause *pain.* Mammography can detect many cancers that are not palpable by physical examination. However, false-positive and false-negative readings can occur (ACS, 2022b).

In breasts of younger female patient, there is little difference in the density between normal glandular tissue and malignant tumors. Cancer and cysts may have the same density. This makes the mammogram less useful for evaluation of breast masses in this population. For this reason, annual screening mammograms are not recommended for women younger than 40 years. In older women, it is not uncommon to have a high amount of fatty tissue present and for this tissue to appear lighter than cancers.

Organizations such as the U.S. Preventive Services Task Force, the American Cancer Society (ACS), the American College of Obstetricians and Gynecologists (ACOG), and others have different guidelines on screening for breast cancer. Teach all patients to collaborate with their health care provider to determine the timing that is right for a mammogram based on age and risk factors.

No dietary restrictions are necessary before having a mammogram. Remind the patient to refrain from using creams, lotions, powders, or deodorant on the breasts or underarms before the study. These products may be visible on the mammogram and contribute to misdiagnosis. If someone has come to their appointment and used one of these products, provide washcloths and premoistened wipes to remove the residue. If there is any possibility that the patient is pregnant, the test should be rescheduled.

Explain the purpose of the study and its anticipated discomforts. The mammographer provides a gown and privacy for the patient to undress above the waist. The patient will be asked about the presence of any lumps or recent breast changes.

In some places, digital 3D mammography—also called digital breast tomosynthesis, *digital tomosynthesis,* or

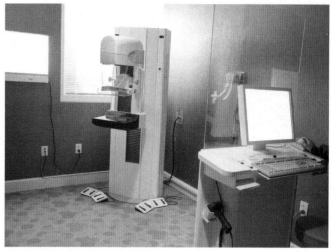

FIG. 61.4 System for digital 3D mammography, also known as digital breast tomosynthesis. (Copyright ©iStock/JodiJacobson.)

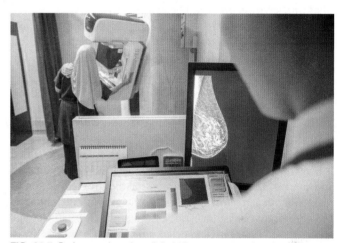

FIG. 61.5 Patient undergoing digital 3D mammography, also known as digital breast tomosynthesis. (Copyright ©iStock/JohnnyGreig.)

tomosynthesis—is used regularly (Figs. 61.4 and 61.5); in other places, 2D mammography is performed. In select locations, the patient may be able to choose which kind to have. A benefit of 3D mammography is that a three-dimensional image of each breast is created, using multiple images from different angles around the breast (Breastcancer.org, 2023). In 2D mammography, a two-dimensional image of each breast is created, using two x-rays of each breast (Breastcancer.org, 2023). Compared with conventional digital mammography, digital 3D mammography has been shown to increase cancer detection rates, although it does increase the radiation dose to the patient (Venkataraman et al., 2021).

To capture 3D mammography, the mammographer positions the patient next to the machine and exposes one breast. The breast tissue is laid across the mechanism and secured into place with mild compression by the machine (initiated by the mammographer). The patient's hand and arm on the side of the examined breast will be positioned by the mammographer so that they are out of the viewing area, allowing the machine to capture as much of the breast tissue as possible. Once the breast, arm, and hand are properly positioned, the mammographer may continue to manually compress the breast just a bit further.

Patients are then asked to hold their breath for a few seconds, and to exhale as soon as the image is properly captured. It is not unusual for patients to feel some temporary discomfort while the breast is imaged. The process lasts about 15—20 seconds for each of two positions for each breast. The patient is usually asked to wait while the mammographer reviews the images to make sure that everything is visualized properly.

Remind patients of when to expect the report of the results. Because this is a time when anxiety may be high, allow patients to express their concerns. Provide follow-up information as needed.

CT Scans. CT scans for reproductive system disorders are often done of the abdomen and pelvis. Primary health care providers can detect and evaluate masses and identify lymphatic enlargement from metastasis. This scan can differentiate solid tissue masses from cystic or hemorrhagic structures.

Magnetic Resonance Imaging. MRI uses a magnetic field and radiofrequency energy to distinguish between normal and malignant tissues, and to detect pelvic tumors. MRI is used in addition to mammograms to assess for breast cancer in women who are at high risk, or for further diagnostic purposes for those who have already been diagnosed with breast cancer (ACS, 2022a). The use of MRI in evaluating patients with dense breast tissue may reduce the need for biopsy.

Ultrasonography. Ultrasonography (US) is a technique that is used to assess females for fibroids, cysts, ectopic pregnancy, and masses. It can be used to monitor the progress of tumor regression after treatment. US is also helpful in differentiating solid tumors from cysts in breast examinations. Prostate, scrotal, and rectal US can be used to detect abnormalities in these areas, such as prostate or testicular masses, varicoceles, or problems of the ejaculatory ducts, seminal vesicles and vas deferens (Pagana et al., 2022).

For an external US of the abdomen, breast, or scrotum, the technician exposes the area and applies gel to the area to be scanned, which provides better transmission of sound waves from the transducer through the patient's skin. The transducer is moved in a linear pattern across the area being tested to outline and define soft-tissue masses and to differentiate tumor type, ascites, and encapsulated fluid.

Prior to an internal *transvaginal scan*, ask women to empty their bladder. Patients having an internal transvaginal or transrectal ultrasound should be informed that they might feel some mild *pain* associated with pressure of the *transducer* (also called a *probe*). Prior to insertion, the transducer is covered with a condomlike sac. Teach the patient to report any allergies to latex, as the condomlike sac is often made of this substance (Pagana et al., 2022). Also, ask about food allergies, as certain foods such as avocado, banana, kiwi, and chestnuts (among others) are "latex cross-reactive foods" (Allergy & Asthma Network, 2023). Once the sac is in place, transducer gel is applied to the transducer, and it is inserted into the vagina or rectum as indicated.

NCLEX Examination Challenge 61.2
Physiological Integrity

The nurse is scheduling a transrectal ultrasound for a client. When reviewing the electronic health record, which of the following food allergies would the nurse identify to **immediately** discuss with the client? **Select all that apply.**

A. Eggs
B. Corn
C. Wheat
D. Banana
E. Avocado

Hysterosalpingography. A hysterosalpingogram is an outpatient fluoroscopy procedure that uses an injection of a contrast medium to visualize a female's cervix, uterus, and fallopian tubes. This test is used to evaluate tubal anatomy and patency and is commonly done as part of an infertility evaluation, after placement of an internal contraception device, or after tubal ligation or tubal reversal (Lee & Kilcoyne, 2023). It can also be useful in the assessment of uterine problems such as fibroids, tumors, and fistulas. Assess the patient for pregnancy, vaginal bleeding, pelvic *infection* (even if taking antibiotics), and history of reaction to iodine, as these are all contraindications to this procedure.

The examination is best performed on days 6 to 11 from the patient's last menstrual cycle, which reduces the chance that the patient may be pregnant and helps to avoid menstruation (Lee & Kilcoyne, 2023). Teach that the procedure may cause some mild and self-limited *pain*, as well as a small amount of postprocedure bleeding; if cramping continues after the procedure, an NSAID can be used to alleviate discomfort (Lee & Kilcoyne, 2023).

On the day of the examination, confirm the date of the patient's last menstrual period. Again, ask about allergies to iodine dye. The health care provider communicates benefits and risks of the procedure with the patient. As the nurse, you may witness the signed informed consent. Be aware that the patient may experience some nausea and vomiting, abdominal cramping, or faintness during the procedure. Communicate this possibility to the patient, and provide support and assistance with relaxation techniques as needed.

After the patient is placed in lithotomy position, the health care provider will insert a speculum to view the cervix. Dye is injected through the cervix to fill and highlight the interior of the cervix, uterus, and fallopian tubes. If the fallopian tubes are patent, the contrast material spills into the peritoneal cavity. Usually only two or three views are obtained to show the path and distribution of the contrast medium.

As noted earlier, the patient may experience a small amount of vaginal bleeding and pelvic *pain* after the study. If ordered, administer analgesic medications. Inform the female that it is not uncommon to experience referred pain to the shoulder because of irritation of the phrenic nerve. Provide a perineal pad after the test to prevent soiling of clothes as the dye drains from the cervix. Instruct the patient to contact the health care provider if bloody discharge continues for 4 days or longer and to immediately report any signs of **infection,** such as lower quadrant pain, fever, chills, malodorous discharge, or tachycardia.

NCLEX Examination Challenge 61.3
Physiological Integrity

A client who underwent a hysterosalpingogram 5 days ago calls the telehealth nurse to report a heart rate of 110 beats/minute, LLQ discomfort, scant bleeding, and intermittent chills. Which of the following responses would the nurse provide? **Select all that apply.**

A. Seek emergency care immediately.
B. Take aspirin to alleviate the pain.
C. These findings are expected.
D. Record your temperature for the next 2 days.
E. Notify your primary health care provider in the morning.

Endoscopic Studies

Colposcopy. A colposcope allows three-dimensional magnification and intense illumination of tissue of the female's cervix, vagina, or vulva (Feltmate & Feldman, 2023). Because it provides accurate site selection, this procedure can locate the exact site of precancerous and cancerous lesions for biopsy in preparation for early treatment. Colposcopy can also be used for further diagnosis after a woman has an abnormal Pap test result or has been diagnosed with HPV (Feltmate & Feldman, 2023).

This nearly painless procedure is better tolerated if it is explained in advance and if a picture of a colposcope is shown to the patient. Explain that the health care provider may take a biopsy specimen while performing colposcopy. Teach the patient to refrain from douching or using vaginal preparations for 24 to 48 hours before the test.

The day of the procedure, the provider will obtain informed consent, and you, as the nurse, may witness this. Provide the patient with a gown and privacy, and ask the patient to undress from the waist down. Help the patient to assume the lithotomy position.

The health care provider locates the cervix or vaginal site through a speculum, and a visual examination is performed. After 30 to 60 seconds, acetic acid is applied to the cervix to draw moisture from the tissue, which allows large or dense nuclei (e.g., metaplastic or dysplastic cells, or cells infected with HPV) to be visualized more easily. If no abnormalities are noted, other solutions composed of iodine, potassium iodine, and distilled water are applied to the cervix (Feltmate & Feldman, 2023), and cells with glycogen turn dark brown. The health care provider may use a green or blue filter to visualize differences between the abnormal vascularities and epithelium. During the procedure, a biopsy specimen can be taken if abnormal cells are seen. (See Cervical Biopsy section later in this chapter.)

After the procedure, allow the patient to rest for a few minutes, especially if a biopsy has been performed. Provide privacy and supplies to clean the perineum and a perineal pad to absorb dye or discharge. Inform the patient that a menstrual pad can be worn because mild cramping, spotting, or dark or black-colored discharge (from medication applied to the cervix to reduce

bleeding) may occur for several days. Remind the patient to take pain relievers as recommended by the health care provider but to avoid aspirin to decrease the chance of bleeding. The patient should be instructed to refrain from douching, using tampons, and having sexual intercourse for 1 week (or as instructed by the health care provider).

Dilation and Curettage. A dilation and curettage (D&C) is a procedure in which tissue is removed from inside the uterus because of abnormal bleeding or to remove pregnancy tissue after an abortion, miscarriage, or childbirth. Done through a hysteroscope (see Hysteroscopy section later in this chapter), a type of endoscope, this procedure is done under anesthesia and takes about 10 to 15 minutes although the patient is kept longer for monitoring (ACOG, 2022).

Prior to the procedure, teach patients about the anesthesia that will be used, and assess for any prior adverse reactions to sedation. If prescribed, teach the patient about techniques or medication that is used before the procedure to begin dilating, or softening, the cervix. Ensure that patients have someone to drive them home after the procedure concludes, and teach that mild spotting, light bleeding, and/or mild **pain** may occur.

On the day of the procedure, the health care provider will obtain informed consent, and you may witness the patient signing this. Remind the patient to report heavy bleeding, fever, abdominal pain, or foul-smelling discharge to the health care provider right away. Also, explain that the next menstrual cycle may occur earlier or later than its normally anticipated date.

Laparoscopy. Laparoscopy is a direct examination of the pelvic cavity through an endoscope. This procedure can be used to rule out an ectopic pregnancy, evaluate ovarian disorders and pelvic masses, and aid in the diagnosis of infertility and unexplained pelvic **pain.** Laparoscopy is also used during surgical procedures such as:

- Tubal sterilization
- Ovarian biopsy
- Cyst aspiration
- Removal of endometriosis tissue or fibroids
- Lysis of adhesions around the fallopian tubes
- Retrieval of intrauterine devices that the patient cannot self-retrieve

A laparoscopy is often preferred over laparotomy for minor surgical procedures because it is less costly, sometimes requires a shorter operative time, produces smaller scars, and lends itself to a faster recovery time without formation of adhesions (Sharp, 2023).

On the day of the procedure, the surgeon describes benefits and risks to the patient. Risks include complications associated with the use of anesthesia, postoperative shoulder pain from irritation of the phrenic nerve, effects of carbon dioxide gas and/or peritoneal stretching, irritation at the incision site, and the rare occurrence of **infection** or electrical burns. As the nurse, you may witness the patient signing the informed consent form. A laparoscopy can be performed with use of a regional or general anesthetic, depending on the patient's risk factors related to sedation, the type of position the patient will be placed in during the procedure, and the anticipated length of procedural time (Joshi, 2022).

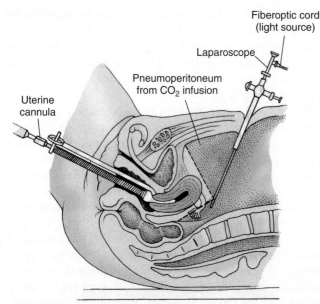

FIG. 61.6 Laparoscopy. (*CO_2,* Carbon dioxide.)

After the patient is anesthetized and placed in supine or dorsal lithotomy position, a urinary catheter is inserted to drain the bladder. The operating table is placed in slight Trendelenburg position to allow the intestines to fall away from the pelvis so that the pelvic viscera can be better visualized (Sharp, 2023). The cervix is held with a cannula to allow movement of the uterus during laparoscopy (Fig. 61.6). The surgeon inserts a needle below the umbilicus to infuse carbon dioxide (CO_2) into the pelvic cavity, which distends the abdomen and permits better visualization of the organs. After the trocar and cannula are in place in the abdominal cavity, the surgeon removes the trocar and inserts the laparoscope. The surgeon can then visualize the pelvic cavity and reproductive organs. Further instrumentation is possible through one or more small incisions. The laparoscope is removed at the end of the procedure, and the abdomen is deflated. The small incision is closed with absorbable sutures and dressed with an adhesive bandage.

The patient is usually discharged on the day of the procedure. Incisional *pain* is managed by oral analgesics. The greatest discomfort is usually caused by referred shoulder pain. Most of these sensations disappear within 48 hours, depending on the extent of the procedure. Instruct the patient to change the small adhesive bandage as needed and to observe the incision for signs of *infection* or hematoma. Teach about the importance of avoiding strenuous activity for the first week after the procedure.

Hysteroscopy. Hysteroscopy is a procedure that uses a fiberoptic telescope to visualize the uterus to diagnose and treat causes of abnormal bleeding. The hysteroscope includes a fiberoptic camera that is inserted into the vagina to examine the cervix and uterus. Diagnostic hysteroscopy is used to diagnose new problems with the uterus or to confirm results from other tests. Hysteroscopy can also be used before or during other procedures (e.g., laparoscopy) for infertility and unexplained bleeding. The procedure is best performed in the proliferative stage to best visualize the uterine cavity (Bradley, 2023).

The health care provider informs the patient of benefits and risks associated with the procedure and obtains consent. You, as the nurse, may witness the patient signing the informed consent form. The preparation is the same as for a pelvic examination. After the patient is placed in lithotomy position, anesthesia with a paracervical block may be given before the cervix is dilated if the procedure will involve uterine biopsy (Bradley, 2023).

The health care provider inserts the hysteroscope through the cervix. Because this distends the uterus, cells can be pushed through the fallopian tubes and into the pelvic cavity. Therefore, hysteroscopy is contraindicated in patients with suspected cervical or endometrial cancer, in those with *infection* of the reproductive tract, and in patients who are pregnant. Postprocedure care is the same as that given following a pelvic examination. Analgesics may be prescribed if the patient has cramping or shoulder pain.

Biopsy Studies

Cervical Biopsy. In a cervical biopsy, cervical tissue is removed for cytologic study. A biopsy is indicated for an identifiable cervical lesion, regardless of the cytologic findings. The health care provider usually performs a biopsy in conjunction with colposcopy as a follow-up to a suspicious Pap test finding. The procedure may be performed in the health care provider's office setting.

The biopsy is usually scheduled when the patient is in the early proliferative phase of the menstrual cycle, when the cervix is least vascular. Because a biopsy evaluates potentially cancerous cells, the patient may be anxious and need time to discuss feelings and fears. Provide a supportive presence, and encourage the use of relaxation techniques as appropriate. Assist the patient into the lithotomy position, recognizing that further preparation depends on the type of procedure to be performed.

The health care provider may anesthetize the patient according to the needs of the chosen procedure. The type of anesthetic used determines the type of immediate care that is needed after the procedure.

Several techniques can be used for a cervical biopsy. If a lesion is clearly visible, endocervical curettage can be performed as an ambulatory care procedure and with little or no anesthetic. This tissue sample is immediately placed into a formalin solution. Conization (removal of a cone-shaped sample of tissue) and loop electrosurgical excision procedures (LEEPs) can be done later if there is a discrepancy between the Pap test and biopsy findings (Cooper et al., 2022). Conization can be done as a cold-knife procedure, a laser excision, or an electrosurgical incision. Discharge instructions can be found in Box 61.3.

Endometrial Biopsy. Endometrial biopsy and aspiration are used to obtain cells directly from the lining of the uterus to assess for cancer of the endometrium. Biopsy also helps assess menstrual disturbances (especially heavy bleeding) and infertility (corpus luteum dysfunction).

When menstrual disturbances are being evaluated, the biopsy is generally done in the immediate premenstrual period to provide an index of progesterone influence and ovulation. A biopsy performed in the second half of the menstrual cycle (about days 21 and 22) evaluates corpus luteum function and

BOX 61.3 **Patient and Family Education**

Recovering From Cervical Biopsy

- Do not lift any heavy objects until the site is healed (about 2 weeks).
- Rest for 24 hours after the procedure.
- Report any excessive bleeding (more than that of a normal menstrual period) to your health care provider.
- Report signs of *infection* (fever, increased *pain*, foul-smelling drainage) to your health care provider right away.
- Do not douche, use tampons, or have vaginal intercourse until the site is healed (about 2 weeks).
- Keep the perineum clean and dry by using antiseptic solution rinses (as directed by your health care provider) and changing pads frequently.

the presence or absence of a persistent secretory endometrium. Postmenopausal women may undergo biopsies at any time.

An endometrial biopsy is usually done as an office procedure with or without anesthesia. Menstrual data—if the patient still has periods—should be obtained from the patient and are included on the specimen request for the pathologist. Confirm that the patient is not pregnant, as this is an absolute contraindication for this procedure.

Prepare the patient in the same way as you would for a pelvic examination. Explain that some cramping may occur when the cervix is dilated. Analgesia before the procedure and relaxation and breathing techniques during the procedure may be helpful to make her more comfortable. Some providers will prescribe an NSAID 30 to 60 minutes prior to the procedure to decrease cramping; others may administer a paracervical block or administer local anesthetic via intrauterine instillation (Del Priore, 2022).

After the uterus is measured and the cervix dilated, the health care provider inserts the curette or intrauterine cannula into the uterus. A portion of the endometrium is withdrawn, using either the cuplike end of the curette or suction equipment. The sample is placed into a formalin solution to be sent for histologic examination. This is the most likely time that the patient could experience moderate cramping.

Allow the patient to rest on the examining table until the cramping has subsided. Provide a perineal pad and a wipe to clean the perineum. Explain that spotting may be present for 1 to 2 days but that any signs of *infection* or excessive bleeding should be reported to the health care provider right away. Instruct the patient to avoid intercourse or douching until all discharge has stopped.

Breast Biopsy. All breast masses should be evaluated for the possibility of cancer. It is important to recognize that breast cancer can occur in men and women; less than 1% of breast cancers occur in men (National Cancer Institute at the National Institutes of Health, 2022). About 2800 men are diagnosed with breast cancer annually in the United States, and approximately 530 die from this condition yearly (ACS, 2023).

Fibrocystic lesions, fibroadenomas, and intraductal papillomas can be differentiated by biopsy. Any discharge from the breasts is examined histologically. Prior to the procedure, provide instructions to the patient based on the type of biopsy performed and the type of anesthesia that is to be used. The patient

usually will receive a local anesthetic, and the tissue will either be aspirated through a large-bore needle (core-needle biopsy) or removed using a small incision to extract multiple samples of tissue.

Aspirated fluid from benign cysts may appear clear to dark green or brown. Bloody fluid suggests cancer. These specimens undergo histologic evaluation. If cancer is found, the tissue is evaluated for estrogen receptor analysis. Chapter 62 discusses types of breast cancer and their relationship to estrogen receptors.

Teach that discomfort after the procedure is usually mild and can be controlled with analgesics or the use of ice or heat, depending on the type and extent of the biopsy. Educate the patient about how to assess the area or incision for bleeding and edema. Teach the patient that the surgeon may recommend that a supportive bra be worn continuously for 1 week after procedure. Remind the patient that numbness around the biopsy site may last several weeks. If cancer is identified, provide emotional support and reinforce information about follow-up treatment options as suggested by the surgeon.

Prostate Biopsy. When prostate cancer is suspected, a biopsy must be performed. This can be done by transurethral biopsy, by inserting a needle through the area of skin between the anus and scrotum, or, most commonly, by transrectal biopsy. Preparation for the procedure depends on the technique used to puncture the gland. A urinalysis should be performed before the procedure; if the patient has a urinary tract infection (UTI), the procedure will need to be rescheduled after the *infection* has been successfully treated (Benway & Andriole, 2021).

Because the purpose of this procedure is to evaluate prostate cells for cancer, allow the patient to discuss fears. Some health care providers will prescribe an anxiolytic to address the patient's anxiety about the procedure (Benway & Andriole, 2021). Prophylactic antibiotics are usually prescribed to lower the incidence of postbiopsy bacteriuria (Benway & Andriole, 2021). Patients taking aspirin, warfarin, or other anticoagulants should talk with the health care provider about whether to continue taking these or to withhold them before the procedure. The health care provider will discuss benefits and risks to the procedure; you may witness the patient signing the informed consent form.

Explain to the patient that some discomfort may be experienced. Provide information about breathing and relaxation techniques that may be helpful to use during the procedure. Assist the patient who is undergoing transrectal biopsy into the side-lying position with the knees pulled up toward the chest. The health care provider will cleanse the area, apply gel, and then insert a thin ultrasound probe into the patient's rectum to anesthetize (if needed) and guide the biopsy needle into place. The biopsy specimen is collected over a 5- to 10-minute period. The patient may experience a brief, uncomfortable feeling each time the needle collects a sample.

Following the biopsy, remind the patient that slight soreness, a small amount of bright red rectal bleeding, and moderate hematuria are common. These should resolve over the coming few days after the procedure (Benway & Andriole, 2021). Explain that semen may be red or rust colored for several weeks. Pain can be treated with over-the-counter acetaminophen. NSAIDs should be avoided due to the risk for bleeding. Teach the patient to contact the health care provider if fever, prolonged or heavy bleeding, worsening *pain,* fever, penile discharge, swelling in the biopsy area, and/or difficulty with urination occur. Rarely, sepsis can develop after a prostate biopsy, usually in patients who did not adhere to taking prophylactic antibiotics.

GET READY FOR THE NEXT-GENERATION NCLEX® EXAMINATION!

Essential Assessment Points

- Provide a safe, professional environment for the discussion of issues related to reproductive health and *sexuality.*
- Encourage all adults to follow recommended guidelines for screening and early detection of reproductive cancers.
- Determine which reproductive changes are age-related versus abnormal.
- Explain diagnostic procedures, restrictions, and follow-up care associated with reproductive system testing and treatment.
- Teach women to report symptoms of *infection* or bleeding to their health care provider after endoscopic procedures and biopsies of the breast, cervix, and endometrium.
- Instruct men to report symptoms of *infection* to their health care provider after a transrectal biopsy of the prostate.
- Teach patients with *pain,* bleeding, discharge, masses, or changes in reproductive function to see their primary health care provider right away.
- Provide thorough pre- and postprocedure teaching for patients having diagnostic testing associated with reproductive system concerns.

Mastery Questions

1. A client who had a prostate biopsy contacts the telehealth nurse. Which symptom would the nurse report to the primary health care provider?
   A. Semen discoloration 1 week after biopsy
   B. Scrotal pain the evening after the procedure
   C. Swelling at the biopsy site 2 days postbiopsy
   D. Hematuria on the morning following the procedure

2. A client having a Pap smear today reports having had sexual intercourse and douching right before coming to this morning appointment. Which nursing action is appropriate?
   A. Reschedule the Pap smear for next month.
   B. Prepare the client for the examination now.
   C. Delay the procedure until the last appointment today.
   D. Make an appointment that falls during the next menstrual cycle.

REFERENCES

Allergy & Asthma Network. (2023). *Latex allergy and foods.* https://allergyasthmanetwork.org/allergies/latex-allergy/latex-allergy-foods/.

American Addiction Centers. (2022). *Effects of drugs and alcohol on the reproductive system.* Retrieved from https://americanaddictioncenters.org/health-complications-addiction/reproductive-system.

American Cancer Society (ACS). (2021a). *Guidelines for the Prevention and Early Detection of Cervical Cancer.* https://www.cancer.org/cancer/cervical-cancer/detection-diagnosis-staging/cervical-cancer-screening-guidelines.html.

American Cancer Society (ACS). (2021b). *Testing for BRCA gene mutation.* Retrieved from https://www.cancer.org/cancer/breast-cancer/risk-and-prevention/genetic-testing.html.

American Cancer Society (ACS). (2022a). *Breast MRI scans.* Retrieved from https://www.cancer.org/cancer/breast-cancer/screening-tests-and-early-detection/breast-mri-scans.html.

American Cancer Society (ACS). (2022b). *Limitations of mammograms.* Retrieved from https://www.cancer.org/cancer/breast-cancer/screening-tests-and-early-detection/mammograms/limitations-of-mammograms.html.

American Cancer Society (ACS). (2023). *Key statistics for breast cancer in men.* Retrieved from https://www.cancer.org/cancer/breast-cancer-in-men/about/key-statistics.html.

American College of Obstetricians and Gynecologists (ACOG). (2022). *Dilation and curettage.* Retrieved from https://www.acog.org/patient-resources/faqs/special-procedures/dilation-and-curettage.

American Society of Clinical Oncology. (2022). *Prostate cancer: Risk factors and prevention.* Retrieved from https://www.cancer.net/cancer-types/prostate-cancer/risk-factors-and-prevention.

Benway, B., & Andriole, G. (2021). Prostate biopsy. *UpToDate.* Retrieved May 26, 2023, from https://www.uptodate.com/contents/prostate-biopsy.

Bradley, L. (2023). Overview of hysteroscopy. *UpToDate.* Retrieved May 26, 2023, from https://www.uptodate.com/contents/overview-of-hysteroscopy.

Breastcancer.org. (2023). *Mammography technique and types.* https://www.breastcancer.org/screening-testing/mammograms/types.

Carusi, D. (2022). The gynecologic history and pelvic examination. In R. Barbieri (Ed.), *UpToDate.* Retrieved May 26, 2023, from https://www.uptodate.com/contents/the-gynecologic-history-and-pelvic-examination.

Centers for Disease Control and Prevention. (2022). *Poor nutrition.* https://www.cdc.gov/chronicdisease/resources/publications/fact-sheets/nutrition.htm.

Choosing Wisely Canada. (2022). *Pap tests: When you need them and when you don't.* Retrieved from https://choosingwiselycanada.org/pap-tests/.

Cleveland Clinic. (2022). Estrogen. https://my.clevelandclinic.org/health/body/22353-estrogen.

Cooper, D., Carugno, J., & Menefee, G. (2022). Conization of cervix. [Updated 2022 Sep 12]. In: *StatPearls* [Internet]. Treasure Island, FL. StatPearls Publishing; 2023 Jan-. Available from: https://www.ncbi.nlm.nih.gov/books/NBK441845/.

Del Priore, G. (2022). Endometrial sampling procedures. *UpToDate.* Retrieved May 27, 2023, from https://www.uptodate.com/contents/endometrial-sampling-procedures.

Feltmate, C., & Feldman, S. (2023). Colposcopy. *UpToDate.* Retrieved May 27, 2023, from https://www.uptodate.com/contents/colposcopy.

Hatch, E., & Karam, A. (2022). Outcome and follow-up of diethylstilbestrol (DES) exposed individuals. *UpToDate.* Retrieved May 27,

2023, from https://www.uptodate.com/contents/outcome-and-fol-low-up-of-diethylstilbestrol-des-exposed-individuals.

Hoffman, R., & Preston, M. (2023). Screening for prostate cancer. *UpToDate*. Retrieved May 27, 2023, from https://www.uptodate.com/contents/screening-for-prostate-cancer.

Jarvis, C., & Eckhart, A. (2024). *Physical examination & health assessment* (9th ed.). St. Louis: Elsevier.

Joshi, G. (2022). Anesthesia for laparoscopic and abdominal robotic surgery in adults. *UpToDate*. Retrieved May 27, 2023, from https://www.uptodate.com/contents/anesthesia-for-laparoscopic-and-abdominal-robotic-surgery-in-adults.

Lee, S., & Kilcoyne, A. (2023). Hysterosalpingography. *UpToDate*. Retrieved May 27, 2023, from https://www.uptodate.com/contents/hysterosalpingography.

Martin, K., & Barbieri, R. (2022). Menopausal hormone therapy: Benefits and risks. *UpToDate*. Retrieved May 27, 2023, from https://www.uptodate.com/contents/menopausal-hormone-therapy-benefits-and-risks.

Martin, K., & Rosenson, R. (2023). Menopausal hormone therapy and cardiovascular risk. *UpToDate*. Retrieved May 27, 2023, from https://www.uptodate.com/contents/menopausal-hormone-therapy-and-cardiovascular-risk.

National Breast Cancer Foundation. (2022). *Male breast cancer*. Retrieved from https://www.nationalbreastcancer.org/male-breast-cancer.

National Cancer Institute at the National Institutes of Health. (2022). *General information about male breast cancer*. www.cancer.gov/cancertopics/pdq/treatment/malebreast/Patient/page1#Keypoint3.

New York Presbyterian. (n.d.). *LGBTQ+ Terminology / Vocabulary Primer*. https://www.nyp.org/documents/pps/cultural-competency/Understanding%20Disparities%20-%20LGBTQ%-20Terminology.pdf.

Pagana, K. D., Pagana, T. J., & Pagana, T. N. (2022). *Mosby's manual of diagnostic and laboratory tests* (7th ed.). St. Louis: Elsevier.

Research on Prostate Cancer in Men of African Ancestry: Defining the Roles of Genetics, Tumor Markers and Social Stress. (2019). *Respond: African American prostate cancer study*. Retrieved from http://respondstudy.org/Default.aspx.

Sharp, H. (2023). Overview of gynecologic laparoscopic surgery and non-umbilical entry sites. *UpToDate*. Retrieved May 27, 2023, from https://www.uptodate.com/contents/overview-of-gynecologic-laparoscopic-surgery-and-non-umbilical-entry-sites.

Sobel, J. (2022). Vaginal discharge: Vaginitis (initial evaluation). *UpToDate*. Retrieved May 27, 2023, from https://www.uptodate.com/contents/vaginal-discharge-vaginitis-initial-evaluation.

Venkataraman, S., Slanetz, P., & Lee, C. (2021). Breast imaging for cancer screening: Mammography and ultrasonography. *UpToDate*. Retrieved May 27, 2023, from https://www.uptodate.com/contents/breast-imaging-for-cancer-screening-mammography-and-ultrasonography.

62

Concepts of Care for Patients With Breast Conditions

Hannah M. Lopez

http://evolve.elsevier.com/Iggy/

LEARNING OUTCOMES

1. Plan collaborative care with the interprofessional team to promote tissue integrity in patients with breast disorders.
2. Teach adults how to decrease the risk for breast disorders.
3. Teach the patient and caregiver(s) about common drugs and other management strategies used for breast disorders.
4. Plan patient- and family-centered nursing interventions to decrease the psychosocial impact caused by living with breast disorders.
5. Apply knowledge of anatomy, physiology, and pathophysiology to provide evidence-based care for patients with breast disorders.
6. Analyze assessment and diagnostic findings to generate solutions and prioritize nursing care for patients with breast disorders.
7. Organize care coordination and transition management for patients with breast disorders.
8. Use clinical judgment to plan evidence-based nursing care to promote favorable *cellular regulation* and prevent *infection* and *pain* in patients with breast conditions.
9. Incorporate factors that affect health equity into the plan of care for patients with breast disorders.

KEY TERMS

adjuvant therapy Additional treatment following an initial surgical procedure; performed to help keep cancer from recurring.

atypical hyperplasia (AH) A proliferative breast disorder that is a change in the cellular structure of a cell but is not considered cancerous.

breast augmentation Surgery to increase or improve the size, shape, or symmetry of the breasts.

breast-conserving surgery (also known as lumpectomy or partial mastectom*y*) Procedure in which the surgeon removes part of the breast that contains cancer and some normal tissue around it.

cysts Spaces filled with fluid lined by breast glandular cells.

ductal carcinoma in situ (DCIS) An early noninvasive form of breast cancer; in DCIS, cancer cells are located within the duct and have not invaded the surrounding fatty breast tissue.

fibroadenoma A well-defined solid mass of connective tissue that is unattached to the surrounding breast tissue and is usually discovered by the woman herself or during mammography.

fibrocystic changes (FCCs) A range of changes involving the lobules, ducts, and stromal tissues of the breast.

fibrosis Replacement of normal cells with connective tissue and collagen.

gynecomastia A benign ridge of glandular tissue within the male breast.

inflammatory breast cancer (IBC) Aggressive type of breast cancer characterized by diffuse erythema/hyperpigmentation and edema (peau d'orange).

invasive ductal carcinoma The most common type of invasive breast cancer, in which the disease originates in the mammary ducts and breaks through the walls of the ducts into the surrounding breast tissue.

lobular carcinoma in situ (LCIS) A noninvasive disease in which the cells look like cancer cells and are contained within the lobules (milk-producing glands) of the breast; LCIS is less common than DCIS and is not thought to be a precursor of invasive cancer.

prophylactic mastectomy Preventive surgical removal of one or both breasts.

prophylactic oophorectomy Preventive removal of the ovaries.

reduction mammoplasty Breast reduction surgery in which the surgeon removes excess breast tissue and then repositions the nipple and remaining skin flaps to produce the best cosmetic effect.

triple-negative breast cancer (TNBC) A type of breast cancer that lacks expression of the estrogen receptor (ER), progesterone receptor (PR), and human epidermal growth factor receptor 2 (HER2).

PRIORITY AND INTERRELATED CONCEPTS

The priority concepts for this chapter are:
- *Cellular Regulation*
- *Infection*
- *Pain*

The **Cellular Regulation** concept exemplar for this chapter is Breast Cancer.

The interrelated concept for this chapter is:
- *Sexuality*

Improper *cellular regulation* (see Chapter 1) can cause breast tissue changes that create a great deal of anxiety for patients. Although many breast disorders are benign rather than malignant, it is important to encourage all patients to have clinical breast examinations (CBEs) regularly and to speak to their primary health care provider about any changes as soon as they are noticed. Early detection of breast cancer is critical in the treatment and management of this condition.

Breast cancer is often associated with women. However, it can occur in male patients as well. Within this chapter, the terms "female," "woman," and "women" apply to all individuals who were *assigned female at birth (AFAB)*, including cisgender women, transgender men, and nonbinary people with vaginas (Cleveland Clinic, 2023). The terms "male," "man," and "men" apply to all individuals who were *assigned male at birth (AMAB)*, including cisgender men, transgender women, and nonbinary people with penises.

BENIGN BREAST DISORDERS

Benign breast disorders (BBDs)—also known as benign breast disease—are very common and represent a spectrum of conditions (Sabel, 2023). They are more prevalent in women but can occur in men as well. BBDs include noncancerous breast-related changes such as irregular cysts or lumps, breast pain, infections, nipple discharge, and skin changes (American College of Obstetricians and Gynecologists [ACOG], 2023b), as well as simple cysts, lipomas, or fat necrosis (Sabel, 2023). Table 62.1 highlights select, common BBDs and the age at which these are likely to occur. BBDs are classified as nonproliferative, proliferative without atypia, or proliferative with atypia.

PROLIFERATIVE BREAST LESIONS WITH ATYPIA

Lesions classified as proliferative with atypia are considered high risk for development of breast cancer. They are further distinguished as *atypical ductal hyperplasia (ADH), atypical lobular hyperplasia (ALH), or lobular carcinoma in situ (LCIS)* (Sabel & Collins, 2022). The term atypical hyperplasia (AH), which includes ADH and ALH, represents a proliferative breast disorder involving growth of breast cells that are abnormal. LCIS involves the highest risk factor for later development of invasive breast cancer (Sabel & Collins, 2022). The younger the woman is when diagnosed with AH, the higher the lifetime risk of developing cancer. The patient should be managed by a surgical oncologist or breast surgeon and taught to undergo yearly mammography and twice-yearly clinical breast examinations (Sabel, 2023). Women with AH should be taught to stop taking oral contraceptives (under the supervision of their primary health care provider) and to avoid hormone replacement therapy (HRT) (Sabel, 2023). Surgical excision and tamoxifen can also be considered as a treatment for AH.

PROLIFERATIVE BREAST LESION WITHOUT ATYPIA: FIBROADENOMA

Fibroadenomas are common benign tumors that occur in women in their 20s and 30s, although they can occur at any age (American Cancer Society [ACS], 2022c). A fibroadenoma is a well-defined solid mass of connective tissue that is unattached to the surrounding breast tissue and is usually discovered personally by the patient or during mammography. Although the immediate fear is that of breast cancer, these changes are generally not associated with an increased risk for such. On clinical examination, these various-sized tumors are oval, freely mobile, and rubbery.

Fibroadenomas may occur anywhere in the breast. The health care provider may request a breast ultrasound examination or may perform a needle aspiration to establish whether the lump is cystic (filled with fluid) or solid.

NONPROLIFERATIVE BREAST LESIONS: FIBROCYSTIC CHANGES (FCCs) AND CYSTS

Pathophysiology Review

Fibrocystic changes of the breast include a range of changes involving the lobules, ducts, and stromal tissues of the breast.

TABLE 62.1 Typical Presentation of Select Benign Breast Disorders

Breast Disorder	Description	Incidence
Fibroadenoma	Most common benign lesion; solid mass of connective tissue that is unattached to the surrounding tissue	During teenage years into the 30s (most commonly)
Fibrocystic changes (FCCs)	Breast **pain** and tender lumps; the lumps are rubbery, ill defined, and commonly found in the upper outer quadrant of the breast	Onset late teens and 20s; usually subsides after menopause
Ductal ectasia	Hard, irregular mass or masses with nipple discharge, enlarged axillary nodes, redness/hyperpigmentation, and edema; difficult to distinguish from cancer	Women approaching menopause
Intraductal papilloma	Mass in duct that results in bloody nipple discharge; mass is usually not palpable	Women 40–55 years of age

Because these alterations affect at least half of women over the life span, they are referred to as fibrocystic changes (FCCs) rather than *fibrocystic disease*. See Fig. 62.1, which demonstrates normal breast tissue, versus Fig. 62.2, which shows FCCs. This condition most often occurs in premenopausal women between 20 and 50 years of age and is thought to be caused by an imbalance in the normal estrogen-to-progesterone ratio. Areas of fibrosis are made up of fibrous connective tissue. Typical symptoms include breast *pain* and firm, hard, tender lumps or swelling in the breasts, particularly before the onset of a menstrual period. Having FCCs does not increase the chance of developing breast cancer (Huether & McCance, 2020).

Cysts are spaces filled with fluid lined by breast glandular cells. They often enlarge in response to monthly hormonal changes, stretch the surrounding breast tissue, and become painful. Symptoms usually resolve after menstruation and then recur before the next menstrual period in a cyclic fashion. In postmenopausal women, symptoms often resolve completely because estrogen decreases. However, postmenopausal patients using hormone replacement therapy (HRT) may not have a significant reduction in symptoms.

Breast ultrasonography is used to confirm the presence of a cyst. If a lump is very firm or has other features raising a concern for cancer, mammography is indicated. A *needle biopsy* (aspiration) may also be ordered if a mammogram shows suspicious findings. A *surgical biopsy* may be performed if no fluid can be aspirated, the mass remains palpable after aspiration, or the aspirated fluid reveals cancer cells.

Interprofessional Collaborative Care

Management of FCCs focuses on the symptoms of the condition. Teach supportive measures such as the use of analgesics to address discomfort. Teach patients that wearing a supportive bra, even to bed, can reduce *pain* by decreasing tension on the ligaments. Local application of ice or heat may provide temporary relief. For some patients, draining the cysts via needle aspiration relieves painful symptoms.

Limiting salt intake before menses can help decrease swelling. Some patients find relief by reducing dietary caffeine and other stimulants. Hormonal drugs such as oral contraceptives or selective estrogen receptor modulators (SERMs) may be prescribed for some women with severe symptoms of FCCs to suppress oversecretion of estrogen. Diuretics may be prescribed to decrease premenstrual breast engorgement.

Encourage the patient to continue prescribed drug therapy and monitor the effectiveness of these interventions. Teach the patient to become familiar with the normal feel and texture of the breasts so that she is aware of any ongoing changes.

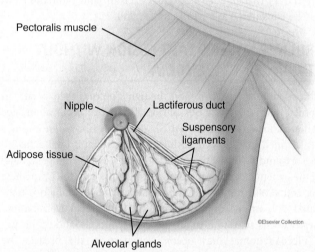

FIG. 62.1 Normal breast. (Copyright © Elsevier Collection.)

> ### 💊 NURSING SAFETY PRIORITY
> #### *Drug Alert*
>
> Explain the benefits and risks associated with hormonal drug therapy for fibrocystic changes (FCCs). Risks include increased chance of thrombotic events (e.g., stroke or blood clots) and development of uterine cancer. Teach patients to seek medical attention immediately if any signs or symptoms of these complications occur.

LARGE BREASTS

In Men

In men, a benign ridge of glandular tissue within the breast, caused by an increase in ratio of estrogen to androgen activity, is referred to as gynecomastia (Braunstein & Anawalt, 2021). It may be bilateral or unilateral, with a palpable mass of tissue at least 0.5 cm in diameter. Most men are asymptomatic, although some may report tenderness or sensitivity when clothing touches the nipple or the affected area.

Drugs such as spironolactone can cause gynecomastia. Because of that, the first line of treatment is to discontinue any drug(s) that may exacerbate or cause this condition. If a condition such as hyperthyroidism or hypogonadism contributes to the condition, treatment of the underlying issue often helps

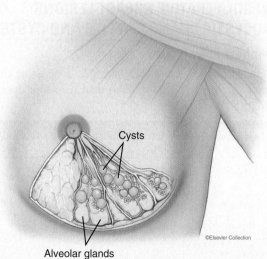

FIG. 62.2 Breast with fibrocystic changes. (Copyright © Elsevier Collection.)

to resolve gynecomastia. Selective estrogen receptor modulators (SERMs) such as tamoxifen, aromatase inhibitors (AIs), and androgens may also be used for treatment. Surgery can be considered for men who have unresolved gynecomastia when nonsurgical management does not resolve the condition.

In Women

Women with excessive breast tissue often have back *pain* and shoulder indentations from bra straps. They may also have recurrent fungal infections under the breasts during hot or humid conditions due to the difficulty in keeping skin in this area dry. The breast size of some individuals declines during weight loss; however, large breasts can and do occur in people who do not have obesity.

Larger bras are expensive and may need to be specially ordered. If well-fitting bras do not help, or weight loss does not alter the condition for the individual whose weight has reduced, reduction mammoplasty may be an appropriate intervention. This procedure, also called *breast reduction surgery,* can be accomplished in several ways, depending on the breast position and shape prior to surgery. Sometimes the nipples can be left intact during surgery, and in other cases they may need to be moved for cosmetic reasons (Figs. 62.3, 62.4, and 62.5). Insurance usually covers the cost of reduction mammoplasty if health detriments are well documented by the health care provider prior to surgery.

The decision to have the procedure is usually made after years of living with the discomfort of excess breast tissue. Provide

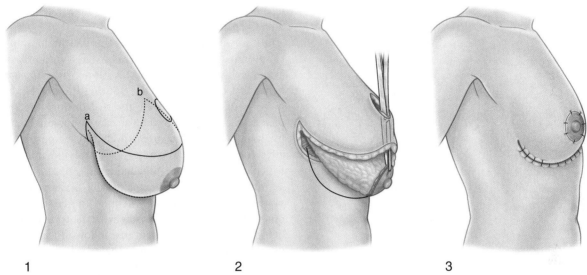

FIG. 62.3 Reduction mammoplasty: Passot technique of nipple transposition. (From Neligan, P. C., & Buck, D. W. [2020]. *Core procedures in plastic surgery* [2nd ed.]. Philadelphia: Elsevier.)

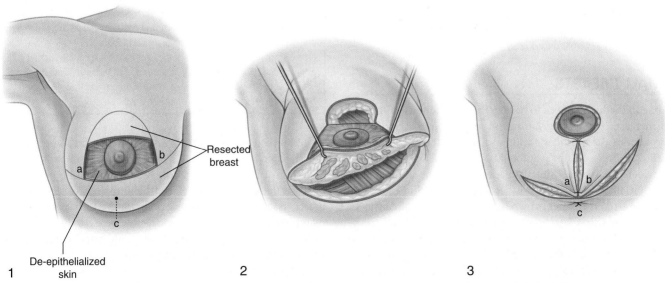

FIG. 62.4 Reduction mammoplasty: Strombeck horizontal bipedicle technique. (From Neligan, P. C., & Buck D. W. [2020]. *Core procedures in plastic surgery* [2nd ed.]. Philadelphia: Elsevier.)

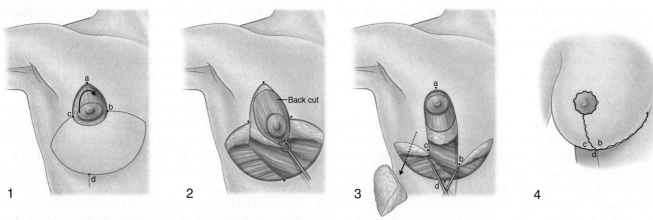

1   2   Back cut   3   4

FIG. 62.5 Reduction mammoplasty: Superomedial pedicle with Wise-pattern skin closure. (From Neligan, P. C., & Buck, D. W. [2020]. *Core procedures in plastic surgery* [2nd ed.]. Philadelphia: Elsevier.)

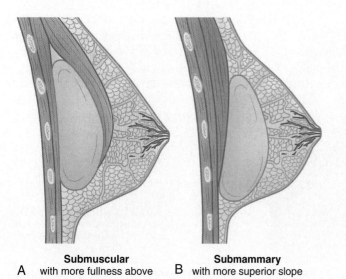

A **Submuscular**
with more fullness above

B **Submammary**
with more superior slope

FIG. 62.6 Augmentation mammaplasty. (A) Submuscular implant placement. (B) Submammary implant placement. (Used with permission of Mayo Foundation for Medical Education and Research, all rights reserved.)

appropriate preoperative teaching (see Chapter 9). Nursing care after surgery is similar to that for the individual having reconstructive surgery, discussed later in this chapter.

SMALL BREASTS

Some individuals choose to have breast augmentation surgery to increase or improve the size, shape, or symmetry of their breasts, or to create breasts within a naturally flatter chest. Most health insurers do not pay for this procedure, as it is usually considered cosmetic. Most surgeries involve the implantation of saline-filled or silicone prostheses (Fig. 62.6). Some are constructed from the patient's own tissue in much the same way as for reconstruction after mastectomy. *Saline* implants are commonly used. These are filled with sterile saline to achieve the shape and firmness the patient wants. If the implanted shell leaks, the saline is safely absorbed by the body. *Silicone* implants are filled with a silicone gel, which can leak into the breast and will not be absorbed. The plastic surgeon reviews the advantages

and disadvantages of each type of implant or surgical option with the patient.

Before breast surgery, teach the patient to stop smoking (to promote healing and decrease overall cardiovascular risk); avoid aspirin and other NSAIDs; and avoid supplements and herbs that can cause bleeding during the procedure. One or more wound drains will be inserted during surgery, and the patient will need to know how to care for these at home. Provide teaching on incisional care as well. Review possible postoperative complications, including *infection* and implant leakage, which can cause severe *pain* and fever.

After surgery, the patient is usually discharged home on the same or the following day. Remind the family or significant other that someone should stay with the patient for at least 24 hours after surgery. Confirm that follow-up care that is scheduled, and answer any questions the patient or family may have.

❗ NURSING SAFETY PRIORITY
Action Alert

Remind the patient who has undergone breast augmentation to expect soreness in the chest and arms for the first few postoperative days and breast swelling for 3 to 4 weeks. The breasts will feel tight and sensitive, and the skin over the breasts may feel warm or may itch. Teach patients that they will have difficulty raising the arms over the head and should not lift, push, or pull anything until the surgeon clears them to do so. Teach to avoid strenuous activity or twisting above the waist. Remind the patient to walk every few hours to prevent venous thromboembolism (VTE).

Teach patients who have breast augmentation surgery about breast cancer surveillance. Breast self-examination (BSE) and clinical breast examination (CBE) can still be performed because the prosthesis is placed behind the woman's normal breast tissue, actually pushing it forward. However, screening mammography may not be as sensitive because the amount of visualized breast tissue is decreased. Additional x-rays, called *implant displacement views,* may be used to examine the breast tissue more completely.

Although there is no conclusive evidence that breast augmentation increases breast cancer risk, women must be informed that there is an increased risk for development of a rare form of non-Hodgkin lymphoma called breast implant–associated anaplastic large cell lymphoma (BIA-ALCL) (U.S. Food and Drug Administration, 2019).

BREAST INFLAMMATION AND INFECTION

Breast Abscess

Nonlactational breast abscesses can occur peripherally from the nipple, or in the vicinity of the areola. Recurrent infections are often found in patients 18 to 50 years old who have diabetes, smoke, have obesity, and/or have nipple piercings (American Society of Breast Surgeons Foundation, 2023). Risk factors that increase the chance for nonlactational breast abscesses include clogged sweat glands, acne, or trauma to the area. Common signs and symptoms include pain and swelling in the affected region. Treatment includes broad-spectrum antibiotics, ultrasound-guided aspiration, and/or incision and drainage (American Society of Breast Surgeons Foundation, 2023).

Mastitis

Mastitis—inflammation of the breast that may be accompanied by *infection* and *pain* (Dixon & Pariser, 2022)—is often associated with lactating and breast-feeding women; however, it can occur in women who are not lactating or breast-feeding. This condition is more common in women who smoke and in women who have nipple piercings where bacteria can enter through a milk duct. Treatment options, including antibiotic therapy, steroid therapy, or watchful waiting, are dependent on the type of specific presentation of mastitis (Dixon & Pariser, 2022). Mastitis does not increase the risk for the woman to develop breast cancer in the future (ACS, 2022e).

✴ CELLULAR REGULATION CONCEPT EXEMPLAR: BREAST CANCER

Pathophysiology Review

Cancer is a common problem of impaired *cellular regulation.* Cancer of the breast begins as a single transformed cell that grows and multiplies in the epithelial cells lining one or more of the mammary ducts or lobules. It is a heterogeneous disease, having many forms with different clinical signs and symptoms, and varying responses to therapy. Some breast cancers present as a palpable lump in the breast, whereas others show up only on a mammogram.

There are two broad categories of breast cancer: noninvasive and invasive. As long as the cancer remains within the mammary duct, it is referred to as *noninvasive.* The more common type of breast cancer is classified as *invasive*; this type grows into surrounding breast tissue. *Metastasis* occurs when cancer cells spread beyond the breast tissue and lymph nodes, via the blood and lymph systems, to distant sites. The most common sites of metastasis are brain, bones, liver, and lung, but breast cancer

can spread to any organ. The course and treatment of metastatic breast cancer is related to the site affected and the level of functional impairment. The processes involved in cancer development are described in Chapter 18.

Breast cancer is often considered a disorder that affects women. Although uncommonly, men can also develop breast cancer, accounting for less than 1% of all breast cancer cases (Breastcancer.org, 2023a). Risk factors for male breast cancer include a family history of breast cancer, *BRCA1* and/or *BRCA2* mutation, age (over 50), history of radiation or hormone therapy, liver disease, testicular conditions (injury, swelling, or surgery), and overweight or obesity (Centers for Disease Control and Prevention, 2022).

Men present with a hard, painless, subareolar mass; gynecomastia may also be present. Other symptoms include nipple discharge (often containing blood), rash around the nipple, inverted nipple, ulceration or swelling of the chest, and possibly swollen lymph nodes. Because men usually do not suspect breast cancer, they often ignore the symptoms and postpone seeing their primary health care provider. As a result, many men are diagnosed at later stages than women. Treatment of breast cancer in men is the same as in women at a similar stage of disease.

Noninvasive (In Situ) Breast Cancers

Ductal carcinoma in situ (DCIS) is an early *noninvasive* form of breast cancer. In DCIS, cancer cells are located within the duct and have not invaded the surrounding fatty breast tissue. Because of more precise mammography screening and earlier detection, the number of women diagnosed with DCIS has increased. Almost all women with this type of condition can be cured (ACS, 2021a).

Another type of noninvasive disease is lobular carcinoma in situ (LCIS). The cells look like cancer cells and are contained within the lobules (milk-producing glands) of the breast. LCIS is not considered cancer but does increase the patient's risk for developing invasive breast cancer (ACS, 2022d). It is usually diagnosed before menopause in women 40 to 60 years of age. LCIS may be treated by maintaining close observation, or by removal via a needle biopsy.

Invasive Breast Cancers

The most common type of invasive breast cancer is invasive ductal carcinoma. As the name implies, the disease originates in the mammary ducts and breaks through the walls of the ducts into the surrounding breast tissue. Once invasive, the cancer grows into the tissue around it in an irregular pattern. If a lump is present, it is felt as an irregular, poorly defined mass. As the tumor continues to grow, fibrosis (replacement of normal cells with connective tissue and collagen) develops around the cancer. This fibrosis may cause shortening of the Cooper ligaments and the resulting typical skin dimpling that is seen with more advanced disease (Fig. 62.7). Another sign, sometimes indicating late-stage breast cancer, is an edematous thickening and pitting of breast skin called *peau d'orange* (orange peel skin) (Fig. 62.8).

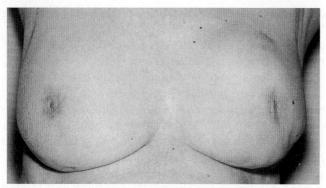

FIG. 62.7 Skin dimpling on a breast as a result of fibrosis or breast cancer. (From Mansel, R., & Bundred, N. [1995]. *Color atlas of breast disease.* St. Louis: Mosby.)

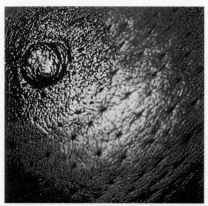

FIG. 62.8 Breast edema giving the skin an "orange peel" *(peau d'orange)* appearance. (From Gallager, H. S., Leis, H. P. Jr., Snyderman, R. K., et al. [1978]. *The breast.* St. Louis: Mosby.)

A rare but highly aggressive form of invasive breast cancer is **inflammatory breast cancer (IBC)**. It is characterized by diffuse erythema/hyperpigmentation and edema (peau d'orange). Patients typically report breast ***pain*** or a rapidly growing breast lump. Other common symptoms include a tender, firm, enlarged breast and breast itching. Because of its aggressive nature, IBC is usually diagnosed at a later stage than other types of breast cancer and is often harder to treat successfully (ACS, 2022f).

Other Types of Breast Cancer

Paget Disease. Paget disease is a rare breast cancer that occurs in or around the nipple (Breastcancer.org, 2023b). Although more common in women, it can also occur in men. It usually affects the nipple ducts, followed by the nipple surface, and then the areola, leaving the area scaly, red, and irritated (Breastcancer.org, 2023b). It is critical to teach patients to see their health care provider if they have these symptoms, as people with Paget disease often have other types of breast cancer.

Triple-Negative Breast Cancer. **Triple-negative breast cancer (TNBC)** lacks expression of the estrogen receptor (ER), progesterone receptor (PR), and human epidermal growth factor receptor 2 (HER2) (Anders & Carey, 2023). This type of breast cancer grows rapidly and is often found in women with *BRCA* mutation who are premenopausal (Anders & Carey, 2023).

PATIENT-CENTERED CARE: GENDER HEALTH
Genetics and Younger Women

Genetic predisposition is a stronger risk factor for development of breast cancer in younger women than older women. Younger women frequently present with more aggressive forms of the disease; they are usually diagnosed at a later stage, have triple-negative breast cancer, and must receive more aggressive treatment. Screening tools can be less effective for this group because the breasts tend to be denser and mammographic recognition of breast cancer may be impaired in areas of dense tissue. Nurses should encourage women who have symptoms to seek evaluation and not watch and wait.

PATIENT-CENTERED CARE: HEALTH EQUITY
Disparities in Mortality Associated With Breast Cancer

The rate of mortality associated with breast cancer in Black women is higher than that for White women (Breast Cancer Research Foundation, 2023). Black women are also 40% more likely to die from breast cancer than White women (Breast Cancer Research Foundation, 2023). Black women have a higher risk for triple-negative breast cancer (Anders & Carey, 2023). Nurses must recognize these differences in health equity and create targeted interventions that are appropriate for each specific patient. Advocate for Black women, especially those younger than 50 years, to receive breast screenings so that cancer, if detected, can be identified in its earliest stage.

Incidence and Prevalence

One of every eight women in the United States will develop breast cancer in her lifetime (ACS, 2023a). It is the most common cancer diagnosis in women. Breast cancer is the second leading cause of cancer death in women, after lung cancer (ACS, 2023a). Similar statistics can be found in Canada (Canadian Cancer Society [CCS], 2022). Early detection is the key to effective treatment and survival. The 5-year relative survival rate for localized breast cancer is 99%, whereas the rate drops to 86% for regional breast cancer (spread to nearby structures or lymph nodes), and 30% for metastatic breast cancer (ACS, 2023b; ACS, 2022b). Metastatic cancer is not considered curable, but rather is treated as a chronic disease.

Etiology and Genetic Risk

Increased age is the primary risk factor for developing breast cancer in both women and men. Examples of other factors that are known to increase the risk of developing breast cancer include family and genetic history, early menarche, nulliparity or older age at the first full-term pregnancy, and late menopause. These factors are not modifiable. Modifiable factors include but are not limited to increased weight and body fat (especially in postmenopausal women), physical inactivity,

NCLEX Examination Challenge 62.1
Health Promotion and Maintenance

The nurse is assessing people at a community health fair. Which person would the nurse identify as being at the **highest** risk for development of breast cancer?

A. 38-year-old male with gynecomastia and obesity
B. 47-year-old female whose mother and aunt had breast cancer
C. 63-year-old male whose father died from lymphoma at age 83
D. 70-year-old female who has a history of fibrocystic breast changes

TABLE 62.2   Risk Factors for Breast Cancer

Factors	Comments
Nonmodifiable Risk Factors	
Female gender	Most breast cancer occurs in women.
Age >55 years	Risk increases with aging, especially after the age of 55.
Genetic factors	Inherited mutations of *BRCA1* and/or *BRCA2* increase risk.
Race	Overall, White women are more likely to develop breast cancer than Black women; however, in women <40 years old, breast cancer is more common in Black women.
Jewish heritage	Women of Ashkenazi Jewish heritage have higher incidences of *BRCA1* and *BRCA2* genetic mutations, which raises the risk.
Being taller	Although the reason for this factor is unknown, research shows that taller women have a higher risk for developing breast cancer compared with shorter women.
Personal history of previous breast cancer	The risk for developing a cancer in the opposite breast is higher than in the average population at risk.
Personal history of certain benign breast conditions	Benign breast conditions that slightly raise the risk for breast cancer: • Fibroadenoma • Papillomatosis • Radial scar • Sclerosing adenosis • Unusual ductal hyperplasia (without atypia) Benign breast conditions that significantly raise the risk for breast cancer: • Atypical ductal hyperplasia (ADH) • Atypical lobular hyperplasia (ALH) • Lobular carcinoma in situ (LCIS)
Breast density	Dense breasts contain more glandular and connective tissue, which increases the risk for developing breast cancer.
Family history of breast cancer	Having a first-degree relative with breast or ovarian cancer increases risk.
Ionizing radiation	Receiving frequent radiation therapy to the chest increases risk, especially if the exposure occurred during periods of rapid breast formation when the woman was a teen or young adult.
High postmenopausal bone density	High estrogen levels over time both strengthen bone and increase breast cancer risk.
Menstrual history: early menstruation (younger than 12 years) *or* late menopause (at or older than 55 years) *or* both	The risk for breast cancer rises as the interval between menarche and menopause increases.
Exposure to diethylstilbestrol (DES)	Women who took DES, and women whose mothers took DES, have a slightly higher risk of developing breast cancer.
Other Risk Factors	
Alcohol consumption	Risk is dependent on drinking patterns: • Consumption of 1 alcoholic drink daily increases risk by 7% to 10%. • Consumption of 2–3 drinks per day is associated with a 20% increased risk • The risk increases with increased consumption.
Hormone replacement therapy (HRT) use	Use of HRT containing both estrogen and progesterone for 4 or more years increases risk; risk diminishes 5 years after discontinuation.
Lack of physical activity	Lack of physical activity has been associated with an elevated risk for developing breast cancer.
Overweight or obesity after menopause	Postmenopausal obesity (especially increased abdominal fat), increased body mass, insulin resistance, and hyperglycemia have been reported to be associated with an increased risk for breast cancer.
Oral contraceptive use	There is a slight increase in breast cancer risk in women taking oral contraceptives. The risk returns to normal 10 years after stopping the pill.
Reproductive factors: • Nulliparity *or* first child born after age 30 years • Not breastfeeding	• Having no children or the first child after the age of 30 slightly raises risk. • Not breastfeeding appears to slightly raise the risk for developing breast cancer.

Data from American Cancer Society (ACS). (2021). *Breast cancer risk factors you cannot change.* https://www.cancer.org/cancer/breast-cancer/risk-and-prevention/breast-cancer-risk-factors-you-cannot-change.html; American Cancer Society (ACS). (2022). *Lifestyle-related breast cancer risk factors.* https://www.cancer.org/cancer/breast-cancer/risk-and-prevention/lifestyle-related-breast-cancer-risk-factors.html; Breastcancer.org. (2023). *Ashkenazi Jewish women who know they have* BRCA *mutation have better breast cancer outcomes.* https://www.breastcancer.org/research-news/ashkenazi-brca-status-and-bc-outcomes.

PATIENT-CENTERED CARE: GENETICS/ GENOMICS

Hereditary Breast Cancer

> Mutations in several genes, such as *BRCA1* and *BRCA2,* are related to hereditary breast cancer. People who have specific mutations in either one of these genes are at an increased risk for developing breast cancer and ovarian cancer. Encourage women to talk with a genetics counselor to carefully consider the benefits and potential consequences of genetic testing before these tests are performed.

use of combined estrogen and progestin postmenopausal hormone replacement therapy (HRT), smoking, and alcohol consumption (Chlebowski, 2023). Having several risk factors increases one's risk more than having a single risk factor. Table 62.2 provides major risk factors for breast cancer.

Health Promotion/Disease Prevention

The American Cancer Society (ACS) and the Canadian Cancer Society (CCS) establish evidence-based guidelines for breast cancer screening in women (ACS, 2022a; CCS, 2023). Guidelines have not been recommended for screening men in the general population because breast cancer in men is so rare. Encourage men with a strong family history or known genetic mutations to discuss screening with their primary health care provider or request referral to a genetics counselor.

In addition to other screening and assessment methods, the National Cancer Institute (n.d.) offers a Breast Cancer Risk Assessment Tool that can be used by a health care professional to estimate risk. Teach women that no single method for early detection of breast cancer is effective when used alone. The evidence-based approach for average-risk women is a screening mammogram, clinical breast examination (CBE), and breast self-awareness.

Mammography

The American Cancer Society (ACS, 2022a) breast cancer screening guidelines recommend that women:

- Ages 40 to 44 have the choice to start annual mammograms after the risks and potential benefits have been explained by their health care provider
- At average risk of breast cancer begin annual screening mammography at age 45 up to age 54
- Age 55 and older may switch to mammograms every 2 years, or continue annual screening mammograms if they choose to do so
- Age 55 and over continue with screening while in good health and with a life expectancy of at least 10 years

Canadian guidelines for mammography differ from those of the United States, recommending that women (CCS, 2023):

- Ages 40 to 49 speak with their health care provider about whether screening is recommended for them based on risk factors
- Ages 50 to 74 have a mammogram every 2 years until age 74
- Age 75 and over speak with their health care provider about whether they should have mammography

Breast Self-Awareness

Evidence does not show a clear benefit of breast self-examination (BSE) (ACS, 2022a). Most breast cancer is detected via mammogram or when a women discovers a symptom (e.g., a breast lump) during ADLs such as bathing or dressing (ACS, 2022a). Recommend that women become familiar with how their breasts normally look and feel, and to report any changes to their primary health care provider immediately after discovery.

Clinical Breast Examination

Clinical breast examination (CBE) is performed by advanced practice nurses and other health care providers. It is recommended that the CBE be part of a periodic health assessment at least every 1 to 3 years for asymptomatic women of average risk between the ages of 25 to 39 and every year for asymptomatic women 40 years of age and older (ACOG, 2023a). Although CBE is not a stand-alone assessment tool, providers may notice changes that the patient does not (National Breast Cancer Foundation, 2022b).

Teach patients what to expect during this examination. First, they will be asked to undress from the waist up. The health care provider inspects the breasts for abnormalities in size and shape and for skin and nipple changes. Then, using the pads of the fingers, the provider palpates the breasts for any lumps and, if present, whether such lumps are attached to the skin or deeper tissues. The area under both arms is also examined. Remind patients to report any breast changes they may have noted to the health care provider performing the clinical breast examination.

NCLEX Examination Challenge 62.2

Physiological Integrity

A 28-year-old client is seeing the health care provider for an annual wellness visit. Which assessment finding would the nurse report to the provider?
A. Breast tenderness prior to menses
B. Nipple irritation following piercing
C. Firm and moveable lump in left breast
D. Left breast slightly larger than right breast

👤 **PATIENT-CENTERED CARE: OLDER ADULT HEALTH**

Breast Changes in Older Women

> As women age, the breast tissue becomes flattened and elongated and is suspended loosely from the chest wall. On palpation, the breast tissue of the older woman has a finer, more granular feel than the lobular feel in a younger woman. The inframammary ridge may be more prominent as a result of atrophy of the breast tissue. Breast examination in older adults may be easier because of tissue atrophy and relaxation of the suspensory ligaments.

Options for High-Risk Women

Those with a personal history of breast cancer are at risk for developing a recurrence or a new breast cancer. It is estimated that 55% to 65% of women with a *BRCA1* mutation and 45% of women with a *BRCA2* mutation will develop breast cancer by the age of 70 (National Breast Cancer Foundation, 2020).

These women usually practice *close surveillance* as a prevention option. It is a method of *secondary prevention* and is used to detect cancer early in the initial stages. In addition to annual mammography and clinical breast examination, high-risk women are recommended to have an annual breast MRI screening (ACS, 2022a). Close surveillance may begin as early as age 30 years. Encourage high-risk women to discuss their personal preferences for close surveillance with their primary health care provider.

PATIENT-CENTERED CARE: VETERAN HEALTH

The Million Veteran Program

U.S. Department of Veterans Affairs (VA) researchers are using data generated through the Million Veteran Program (MVP) initiative to study how military experience and race may affect the risk for developing breast cancer (U.S. Department of Veterans Affairs, 2021). Encourage all veterans to talk to their health care provider about screening based on their individual risk factors.

Other options currently available for reducing a woman's breast cancer risk are prophylactic mastectomy (preventive surgical removal of one or both breasts), prophylactic oophorectomy (preventive removal of the ovaries), and chemopreventive drugs. Although each option significantly reduces the risk for breast cancer, no option eliminates it. Each option has its own risks and potentially serious complications.

Even though a woman may decide to have a prophylactic mastectomy, there is a small risk that breast cancer will develop in residual breast glandular tissue because no mastectomy reliably removes all mammary tissue. Women must also understand that breast reconstruction after a prophylactic mastectomy is very different from breast augmentation. It is a more complex surgical procedure with a greater potential for complications. The decision to have this type of surgery can be a very difficult one to make. Women may find it helpful to reach out to a breast cancer support organization and talk to someone who has been through a prophylactic mastectomy.

Women undergoing prophylactic oophorectomy will likely experience menopausal symptoms, although some estrogen remains in body fat tissue. Chemoprevention drugs, such as tamoxifen, reduce breast cancer recurrence but carry other risks such as blood clots and endometrial cancer. Encourage women to carefully consider the benefits and risks of breast cancer risk–reducing options and discuss them with their health care provider.

Interprofessional Collaborative Care

Recognize Cues: Assessment

History. Early breast cancer often has no symptoms (ACS, 2022a). At other times, the history is taken after a mass has been discovered but before a diagnosis has been made. For some patients the history may be obtained when they are seen for treatment of an identified cancer. The interview should focus on three major areas: risk factors, the breast mass, and health maintenance practices.

PATIENT-CENTERED CARE: CULTURE AND SPIRITUALITY

Culturally Sensitive Care

Some cultures do not allow men to be part of a woman's care and allow only women to care for a woman. Other cultures are male predominant, and all decisions about care for a female are made by the significant man in her life, who may be a father, spouse, older brother, or oldest son. It is important for the health care provider and nurse to provide culturally sensitive care and to respect the beliefs and practices of the patient.

Ask specific information about personal and family histories of breast cancer. In addition to increasing the woman's own risk, these factors also affect any sisters' or daughters' risk and should be part of later counseling.

Ask about the woman's gynecologic and obstetric (if any) history, including:
- Age at menarche
- Age at menopause
- Symptoms of menopause
- Age at first child's birth (or nulliparity—having no children)
- Number of children and pregnancies, including miscarriages or terminations
  Recognize that increased risk factors include:
- Prolonged hormonal stimulation (e.g., early menses, late menopause)
- Use of contraceptives
- Birth of the first child after 30 years of age

A history of the breast mass or lump can reveal the course of the disease and information related to health care–seeking practices and health-promoting behaviors. Ask the patient about how, when, and by whom the mass was discovered and the time between discovery and seeking care. The answer to this question reveals the need for discussion and teaching about health promotion practices, regardless of whether the mass proves to be cancerous. If there was a delay between discovery and seeing the health care provider, inquire what caused the delay. These questions are linked to the psychosocial assessment but also reveal the length of time that the mass has been untreated. Review with the patient which procedures have been performed to diagnose the problem and if they have noticed any other changes in their body within the past year. This information can help determine if there will be the likelihood of metastasis. Ask especially about the presence of joint and bone *pain* or cognitive changes.

Assess the use of alcohol intake because this is a factor that may increase breast cancer risk. Perform an in-depth medication review, including prescribed and over-the-counter (OTC) drugs that are used. Specifically ask about hormonal supplements, such as estrogen and natural or herbal substances that stimulate hormones, and birth control use. Estrogen can be taken orally, intravaginally, or via a transdermal patch. Document the type and form of hormones (birth control pills or patches, supplements) and length of use.

Physical Assessment/Signs and Symptoms. Document any abnormal findings from the clinical breast examination. Describe specific information about a breast mass (as described in Box 62.1), such as location, using the "face of the clock" method; shape; size; consistency; and whether the mass is mobile or fixed to the surrounding tissue. Note any skin change, such as *peau d'orange*, redness/hyperpigmentation and warmth, nipple retraction, or ulceration, which can indicate advanced disease. Document the location of any enlargements of axillary and supraclavicular lymph nodes. Evaluate for the presence of *pain* or tenderness in the affected breast.

Psychosocial Assessment. A breast cancer diagnosis is usually an unanticipated event in the life of a woman who feels physically well. It initiates a sudden and distressing transition into a potentially life-threatening illness. Feelings of fear, shock, and disbelief are predominant as a woman learns about the disease

BOX 62.1   Best Practice for Patient Safety and Quality Care

Assessing a Breast Mass

- Identify the location of the mass by using the "face of the clock" method.
- Describe the shape, size, and consistency of the mass.
- Assess whether the mass is fixed or movable.
- Note any skin changes around the mass, such as dimpling of the skin, increased vascularity, nipple retraction, nipple inversion, or skin ulceration.
- Assess the adjacent lymph nodes, both axillary and supraclavicular nodes.
- Ask patients if they experience **pain** or soreness in the area around the mass.

and faces numerous treatment decisions. Psychological distress is common at cancer diagnosis and at the various transitions of treatment. A previous history of mental illness, age, and life circumstances can contribute to increased psychological distress. Encourage expression of feelings, focusing on the human component of care, and determine if a referral to a counselor would be helpful. There are also multiple community resources available for the person diagnosed with breast cancer. Talking with someone who has been through the experience is particularly helpful in dealing with the emotional aspects of the disease.

Assess the patient for concerns related to **sexuality.** Sexual dysfunction affects most breast cancer survivors in some way. Sometimes it is related to the loss of a breast and the threat to one's femininity, the self-image, or how the patient perceives the significant other's response. Lack of libido related to hormonal changes, psychological distress, and anxiety are commonly experienced by women with breast cancer. If the patient does not discuss sexual concerns voluntarily, open the conversation in a nonthreatening, nonjudgmental way. Use resources that provide education about alternative expressions of intimacy and a focus on pleasure rather than performance. Refer the patient and significant other to counseling if appropriate. See the Interprofessional Collaboration: The Patient With Psychosocial Concerns Related to Breast Cancer box.

INTERPROFESSIONAL COLLABORATION

The Patient With Psychosocial Concerns Related to Breast Cancer

The patient with psychosocial concerns related to breast cancer may benefit from referral to a licensed oncology social worker (Association of Oncology Social Work, 2023). These individuals provide psychosocial care for patients with cancer, utilizing a special skill set and knowledge base related to oncology. Family and caregivers can be included in this support at the discretion of the patient (Board of Oncology Social Work, 2022).

These members of the interprofessional team are masters-prepared professionals who provide individualized support to patients with breast cancer, survivors of breast cancer, institutions and agencies that provide oncology services, and the community.

According to the Interprofessional Education Collaborative (IPEC) Expert Panel's Competency of Roles and Responsibilities, using the unique and complementary abilities of other team members optimizes health and patient care (IPEC, 2016; Slusser et al., 2019).

Laboratory Assessment. The diagnosis of breast cancer relies on pathologic examination of tissue from the breast mass. After the diagnosis of cancer has been established, laboratory tests, including pathologic study of the lymph nodes, help detect possible metastases. Elevated liver enzyme levels indicate possible liver metastases, and increased serum calcium and alkaline phosphatase levels could suggest bone metastases.

PATIENT-CENTERED CARE: GENDER HEALTH

Lesbian Women and Breast Cancer

Research about breast cancer risk and lesbian women is ongoing, as previous research has been contradictory (National LGBT Cancer Network, 2023). Four common risk factors for breast cancer—cigarette smoking, alcohol use, overweight or obesity, and not having children before the age of 30—apply to women of all sexual orientations. Lesbian women may not seek care due to fear and distrust of health care providers. Nurses' awareness of and sensitivity to these issues help establish trust. Continue to educate yourself to deliver the best care possible to all populations. Resources such as the National LGBT Cancer Network (2023) can be helpful.

Imaging Assessment. *Mammography* is a sensitive screening tool for breast cancer. The uniqueness of this test results from its ability to reveal preclinical lesions (masses too small to be palpated manually). Most breast centers now use *digital mammography,* a system that is able to read, file, and transmit mammograms electronically. Patient preparation and the procedure for mammography are discussed in Chapter 61. Some women may voice concern about radiation exposure with mammograms. Reassure them that the dose is very small and the risk for harm from radiation is minimal.

The American College of Radiology created the Breast Imaging-Reporting and Data System, known as BI-RADS, as a risk assessment and quality assurance tool that standardizes mammography reporting (Niknejad, 2022). Some people receive a numeric BI-RAD score printed on their results. Teach women to follow up with their health care provider regarding specific findings, as BI-RAD terminology is used by providers to describe mammography findings.

Digital breast tomosynthesis (3D mammography, digital tomosynthesis, or tomosynthesis) is technology that is similar to mammography but uses three-dimensional images (Fig. 62.9). It is useful in evaluating dense breasts and is more accurate in women younger than 50. In the United States, currently it is covered by Medicare and most other major health insurances. This advanced technology is also available in Canada.

Ultrasonography of the breast is an additional diagnostic tool used to clarify findings on mammography. If the mammogram reveals a lesion, ultrasonography is helpful in differentiating a fluid-filled cyst from a solid mass. Mammography screening combined with ultrasound may be effective for detecting cancers in women with dense breasts, but currently it is not recommended for routine breast cancer screening as a stand-alone imaging tool.

MRI is used for screening high-risk women and better examination of suspicious areas found on a mammogram (ACS, 2022a). Although higher-quality images are produced, there is concern about high costs and access to high-quality breast MRI services for high-risk women. It is more expensive than mammography.

If the patient has an invasive breast cancer, other imaging tests may be done to rule out metastases. Positron emission tomography (PET) scan, brain MRI, and CT scans of the chest, abdomen, and pelvis can reveal distant metastases.

Imaging Technology

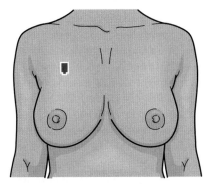
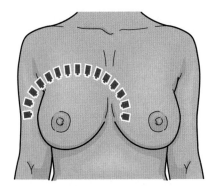

Takes one mammogram image of the breast from the top and one from the side, which may create images with overlapping tissue.

Takes 15 images of the breast in an arc from the top and from the side, which are then transformed into multiple nonoverlapping thin slices through the breast tissue.

FIG. 62.9 2D versus 3D mammography. (Adapted from UCLA Health, 2023. https://www.uclahealth.org/medi-cal-services/radiology/breast-imaging/diagnostic-exams/breast-imaging-3d-mammography-tomosynthesis.)

Other Diagnostic Assessment. Although imaging techniques serve as tools for screening and more precise visualization of potential breast cancers, *breast biopsy (pathologic examination of the breast tissue) is the only definitive way to diagnose breast cancer.* Tissue samples are analyzed by a pathologist to determine the presence of breast cancer. If breast cancer is identified, it is classified according to the size and type of breast cancer, the histologic grade, and the type of receptors on the cells. These characteristics are used to guide treatment. For example, a small, noninvasive breast cancer may be treated with only lumpectomy and radiation, whereas a larger, aggressive tumor (one with a high histologic grade) may be treated with a mastectomy and chemotherapy, followed by radiation.

Cancer cells that contain estrogen receptors *(ER positive)* or progesterone receptors *(PR positive)* have a better prognosis and usually respond to hormonal therapy. If the type of breast cancer is *HER2 positive,* it may be treated with trastuzumab, which is a HER2-positive breast cancer–specific *targeted therapy.*

Most women, even those with very small tumors, receive some sort of treatment in addition to surgery for breast cancer. Research has focused on ways to predict clinical outcomes so that low-risk women may avoid unnecessary treatments. Genomic tests, such as Oncotype DX and MammaPrint, have been developed to help predict clinical outcomes by analyzing genes in breast cancer tissue. Some health care providers use this information in addition to the pathologic analysis for guiding treatment decisions. These multigene tests have been shown to be accurate predictors of patient prognosis and response to therapy in breast cancer (Bou Zerdan et al., 2021).

Analyze Cues and Prioritize Hypotheses: Analysis

The priority collaborative problems for patients with breast cancer include:

1. Potential for cancer metastasis due to lack of, or inadequate, treatment
2. Potential for impaired coping due to breast cancer diagnosis and treatment

Generate Solutions and Take Actions: Planning and Implementation

Decreasing the Risk for Metastasis

Planning: Expected Outcomes. The goal for the patient who is treated for breast cancer is to remain free of metastases or recurrence of disease, if possible. If cancer recurs, the patient will experience optimal health outcomes, including potential palliation and end-of-life care.

Interventions. Although patients are living longer with metastatic disease, the 5-year survival rate remains low. Once cancer is diagnosed, the extent and location of breast cancer and metastases (if applicable) determine the overall treatment strategy. The emphasis of breast cancer treatment is on preventing or stopping the spread of tumor cells that lead to distant metastasis. Treatment is tailored specifically to each patient, considering other health problems and the patient's ability to tolerate a particular therapy.

Nonsurgical Management. For patients with breast cancer at a stage for which surgery is the main treatment, follow-up with adjuvant (in addition to surgery) radiation, chemotherapy, hormone therapy, or targeted therapy is commonly prescribed. For those who cannot have surgery or whose cancer is too advanced, these therapies may be used to promote comfort (palliation). End-of-life care is discussed in Chapter 8.

Palbociclib is a new drug that is a targeted therapy. It is used in the treatment of hormone receptor-positive (HR+), human epidermal growth factor receptor 2-negative (HER2−) metastatic breast cancer (mBC), or HR+/HER2− mBC (Pfizer, Inc., 2023).

Complementary and integrative health. Women with breast cancer often cope with distressing symptoms related to the disease itself or the side effects of treatment. Common symptoms associated with these treatments include *pain,* nausea and vomiting, hot flashes, anxiety, depression, and fatigue. Physical and emotional symptoms associated with breast cancer may be eased with the use of complementary and integrative therapy. Prayer is also widely used. Other types of therapies include guided imagery and massage. The most frequently used strategies are

TABLE 62.3 Common Complementary and Integrative Therapies Used by Patients With Breast Cancer

Symptom	Complementary and Integrative Therapy
Physical	
Pain	Acupuncture, chiropractic therapy, hypnosis, massage, music, reiki, shiatsu
Nausea/vomiting	Acupuncture, aromatherapy, ginger, hypnosis, progressive muscle relaxation, shiatsu
Fatigue	Acupuncture, massage, meditation, reiki, tai chi, yoga
Hot flashes	Acupuncture, flaxseed, black cohosh (Use caution with all herbal and ingested supplements; there are no substantial data to support one treatment over others.)
Muscle tension	Aromatherapy, massage, shiatsu
Emotional	
Anxiety, stress, fear	Aromatherapy, guided imagery, hypnosis, journaling, massage, meditation, music therapy, progressive muscle relaxation, prayer, support groups, tai chi, yoga
Depression	Aromatherapy, yoga, journaling, progressive muscle relaxation

biologically based therapies such as vitamins, special cancer diets, and herbal therapy. Teach the patient that all ingested complementary agents potentially risk interaction with conventional drugs.

Encourage women to seek a practitioner with a certification or license for the specific type of integrative therapy intervention. In some states, a certification or license is required for acupuncture, chiropractic therapy, massage, and shiatsu. Some types of complementary and integrative therapy can be self-taught or done alone after a few sessions of instruction. Table 62.3 lists complementary and integrative therapies for specific symptoms associated with breast cancer and its treatments.

Although the use of complementary and integrative therapy can improve quality of life, its use does not alter the outcome of breast cancer, and it should not be used in place of standard treatment. Encourage patients who are interested in trying these therapies to check with their health care provider before using them. The website https://www.breastcancer.org/treatment/comp_med provides accurate information about complementary therapies and the extent to which they have been researched in breast cancer patients. Cost may be a factor in decision making because not all insurances provide coverage for complementary and integrative therapies. Remind the patient that it is important to disclose to the health care provider all treatments and supplements taken.

Surgical Management. The management of early-stage breast cancer is surgery. A large tumor is sometimes treated with chemotherapy, called *neoadjuvant therapy,* to shrink the tumor before it is surgically removed. An advantage of this therapy is that cancer can be removed by means of lumpectomy rather than mastectomy. This may provide less invasive surgery and a better cosmetic outcome for the patient.

Axillary lymph nodes are analyzed for the presence of cancer and staging purposes. Axillary lymph node dissection (ALND) is usually done when there are clinically positive nodes. Sentinel lymph node biopsy (SLNB) is a much less invasive approach and is recommended by guidelines for analyzing lymph nodes in early-stage breast cancers with low to moderate risk for lymph node involvement. In this method, the sentinel lymph node is identified during breast surgery by injecting the breast with radioisotope and/or dye that travels via lymphatic pathways to the sentinel lymph node. The nodes that take up the dye are removed and examined for the presence of cancer cells. It is believed that if cancer cells have traveled through the lymph channels, the cells will lodge in the sentinel nodes. Travel beyond these nodes to higher-level nodes may occur as a secondary event. Therefore the absence of cancer cells in the sentinel nodes is an indicator that no other nodes in the regional area are involved.

Preoperative care. Care of the patient facing surgery for breast cancer focuses on psychological preparation and preoperative teaching. Priority nursing interventions are directed toward relieving anxiety and providing information to increase patient knowledge. Include the spouse, significant other, or other family member who may be experiencing similar stress and confusion in health teaching unless the patient does not desire this or the patient's culture does not permit this approach.

Review the type of procedure planned. Use open-ended questions (e.g., "What type of surgery are you having? Can you explain what will happen?") to assess the patient's current level of knowledge. Provide postoperative information, including:

- The need for a drainage tube
- The location of the incision
- Mobility restrictions
- The length of the hospital stay
- General preoperative and postoperative information needed by any surgical patient (see Chapter 9)

Supplement teaching with written or digital materials for the patient and family. This information should include whom to call in case there are any complications or questions. Address body image issues and expectations before surgery to avoid misconceptions about appearance after surgery. If available, suggest that patients and their caregivers attend classes before surgery in an ambulatory care setting, such as a breast cancer center, to promote successful early discharge from the hospital. Programs that provide emotional support, information, and opportunities for discussion related to **sexuality,** body image, and preoperative and postoperative care enhance the recovery of the short-stay mastectomy patient.

Operative procedures. Types of breast surgeries are shown in Fig. 62.10. During breast-conserving surgery, also known as *lumpectomy* or *partial mastectomy,* the surgeon removes part of the breast that contains cancer and some normal tissue around it. The term *margins* refers to the distance between the tumor and the edge of the surrounding tissue. The desired outcome of breast-conserving surgery is to obtain *negative margins* in which no cancer cells extend to the edge of the tissue. Patients undergoing breast-conserving surgery may have drainage tubes

Breast-conserving Surgery

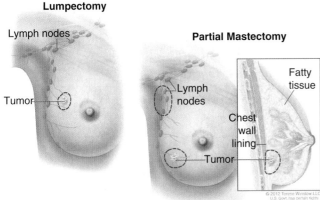

Breast-conserving surgery. Dotted lines show the area containing the tumor that is removed and some of the lymph nodes that may be removed.

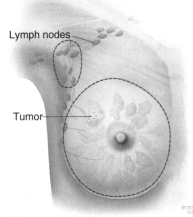

Total (simple) mastectomy. The dotted line shows where the entire breast is removed. Some lymph nodes under the arm may also be removed.

Modified radical mastectomy. The dotted line shows where the entire breast and some lymph nodes are removed. Part of the chest wall muscle may also be removed.

FIG. 62.10 Surgical treatment for breast cancer. (Copyright ©2010 Terese Winslow. U.S. Govt. has certain rights.)

placed if the lump is large or if axillary node dissection is performed. Typically, radiation therapy follows to kill any residual tumor cells.

Breast-conserving procedures are usually performed in same-day surgical settings. The cosmetic results of these surgeries are good to excellent, and the psychological benefits of avoiding breast removal are significant for patients who choose this option.

Indications for a mastectomy include multicentric disease (tumor is present in different quadrants of the breast), inability to have radiation therapy, presence of a large tumor in a small breast, genetic testing results, and patient preference. Mastectomy does not conserve the breast; the affected breast is completely removed. A total (simple) mastectomy is surgery to remove the whole breast that has cancer. A *modified radical mastectomy* removes the breast tissue, lymph nodes, and sometimes part of the underlying chest wall muscle. During this procedure, the surgeon places one or two drainage tubes, usually Jackson-Pratt (JP) drains, under the skin flaps and attaches the tubes to a small collection chamber. These collect any fluid that accumulates under the surgical area. Reconstruction can be performed at the same time as the mastectomy. Skin flaps or expanders may be used to create a breast mound at the time of the original procedure.

Postoperative care. The hospital stay after breast surgery is short, often same day or just overnight, and recovery is usually not complicated. After surgery, avoid using the affected arm for measuring blood pressure, giving injections, or drawing blood. If lymph nodes are removed, it is critical to prevent trauma to the affected arm. The patient returns from the postanesthesia care unit (PACU) as soon as vital signs return to baseline levels and if no complications have occurred. Assess vital signs on a schedule of decreasing frequency, such as every 30 minutes for two times, every hour for two times, and then every 4 hours (or as ordered). During these checks, assess the dressing for bleeding.

When taking vital signs, monitor for the amount and color of drainage if drains are present. Document this in the intake and output section of the electronic health record.

> **!** **NURSING SAFETY PRIORITY**
>
> ***Action Alert***
>
> To decrease the chance of surgical site ***infection,*** carefully observe the surgical wound after breast surgery for signs of swelling and infection throughout recovery. Assess the incision and flap of the postmastectomy patient for signs of bleeding, infection, and poor tissue perfusion. Drainage tubes are usually removed about 1 to 3 weeks after hospital discharge when the patient returns for an office visit. The drainage amount should be less than 30 mL in a 24-hour period. Inform the patient that tube removal may cause temporary ***pain.*** Provide or suggest analgesia before tubes are removed. Document all findings and report any abnormalities to the surgeon immediately.

Assess the patient's position to ensure that the drainage tubes or collection device is not pulled or kinked. The patient should have the head of the bed elevated at least 30 degrees, with the affected arm elevated on a pillow while awake. Keeping the affected arm elevated promotes lymphatic fluid return after removal of lymph nodes and channels. Provide other basic comfort measures, such as repositioning and analgesics as pre-scribed, on a regular basis until *pain* ceases. Patient-controlled analgesia may be used for some patients for a short time, depending on the type of surgery that was performed.

Ambulation and a regular diet are resumed by the day after surgery. While the patient is walking, the arm on the affected side may need to be supported at first. Gradually the arm should be allowed to hang straight by the side. Encourage the patient to use good posture to prevent mobility issues. Beginning exercises that do not stress the incision can usually be started on the first day after surgery. These exercises include squeezing the affected hand around a soft, round object (a ball or rolled washcloth) and flexion/extension of the elbow. The progression to more strenuous exercises depends on the subsequent procedures planned (e.g., reconstruction) and the surgeon's directions. The patient can be discharged to home after safely ambulating and when surgical *pain* is under con-trol. Common instructions for exercises after mastectomy are listed in Box 62.2.

Breast reconstruction. Breast reconstruction after or during mastectomy for women is common with few complications. Patients consult with the plastic surgeon to discuss the type of reconstruction, timing of the procedure, and technique desired. Many women prefer reconstruction immediately after mas-tectomy, using their own tissue (autogenous reconstruction).

BOX 62.2   Patient and Family Education

Postmastectomy Exercises

The surgeon or physical therapist can provide additional stretches and exer-cises. Hold each stretch until you feel a gentle pulling. Exercises can be done standing, sitting, or lying down.

Hand Wall Climbing
- Face the wall and put the palms of your hands flat against the wall at shoul-der level.
- Flex your fingers so your hands slowly "walk" up the wall.
- Stop when your arms are fully extended.
- Slowly "walk" your hands back down the wall until they return to shoulder level.

Wand Exercise
- Lie down on your back. Bend knees for comfort.
- Position your hands so your thumbs are pointing to each other. With both hands, hold a wand-shaped object, such as a broom handle or a cane. Your hands should be about shoulder width apart on the object.
- Start with the object resting across your hips. Slowly lift the wand toward the ceiling.

Side Bends
- Sit in a chair.
- Clasp your hands together.
- Slowly raise your arms over your head and then gently bend to each side.

Shoulder Blade Squeeze
- Sit in chair. Do not rest your back against the chair.
- Place arms at side, elbows bent.
- Squeeze your shoulder blades together behind you. Do not lift your shoul-ders up toward your ears.

Breast reconstruction at the time of mastectomy, both autoge-nous and prosthetic, may lessen the psychological strain associ-ated with undergoing a mastectomy.

NCLEX Examination Challenge 62.3
Physiological Integrity

The nurse is caring for a client with breast cancer who just underwent a radi-cal left mastectomy. Which intervention is appropriate postoperatively?
A. Maintain NPO status
B. Obtain blood pressure in left arm
C. Remove sutures to facilitate healing
D. Administer analgesics for reported pain level

Although reconstruction is not appropriate for some women and others may not be interested in it, the surgeon should discuss the indications and contraindications, advantages and disadvan-tages, and typical recovery. If immediate reconstruction is cho-sen, the breast surgeon should be aware of this before surgery so plans can be coordinated with those of the plastic surgeon.

Several procedures are available for restoring the appearance of the breast (Table 62.4). Reconstruction may begin during the original operative procedure or later in one to several stages. Common types of breast reconstruction are:
- Breast expanders (saline or silicone)
- Autologous reconstruction using the patient's own skin, fat, and muscle

Breast expanders are the most common method of breast reconstruction used in the United States. A tissue expander is a balloonlike device with a resealable metal port that is placed under the pectoralis muscle. A small amount of normal saline is injected intraoperatively into the expander to partially inflate it. The patient then receives additional weekly saline injections for about 6 to 8 weeks until the expander is fully inflated. When full expansion is achieved, the tissue expander is then exchanged for a permanent implant during surgery in an ambulatory care center. The permanent implant is filled with either saline or silicone.

Autologous reconstruction using the patient's own skin, fat, and muscle is advantageous because the donor site tissue is similar in consistency to that of the natural breast. This option provides results that more closely resemble a real breast compared with implant reconstruction. Flap donor sites include the latissimus dorsi flap (back muscle); transverse rectus abdominis myocuta-neous flap, known as the *TRAM flap* (abdominal muscle); and the gluteal flap (buttock muscle). Reconstruction of the nipple-areola complex is the last stage in the reconstruction of the breast.

Women who have had a mastectomy and breast reconstruc-tion in one breast should have close-surveillance breast can-cer screening in the contralateral (opposite) breast, including imaging with mammography or mammography and MRI. Mammography and MRI are not recommended to be done rou-tinely in reconstructed breasts because most local recurrences of breast cancer in the residual tissue are palpable during clin-ical breast examination. Nursing care of the woman who has undergone breast reconstruction is outlined in Box 62.3.

Refer the patient to the American Cancer Society's *Reach to Recovery* program. This program has trained breast can-cer

TABLE 62.4 Examples of Breast Reconstruction Procedures

Procedure	Description
Implantation	An implant matching the size of the other breast is placed under the muscle on the operative side to create a breast mound.
Flaps	A flap of skin, fat, and muscle is transferred from the donor site to the operative area. The flap contains an appropriate amount of fat to match the other breast and is similar in appearance to breast tissue. A blood supply is established by reanastomosis of vessels from the operative area to those with the flap when possible. A new nipple may be created with tissue from areas such as the labia or upper, inner thigh. Nipples can also be created by tattooing.

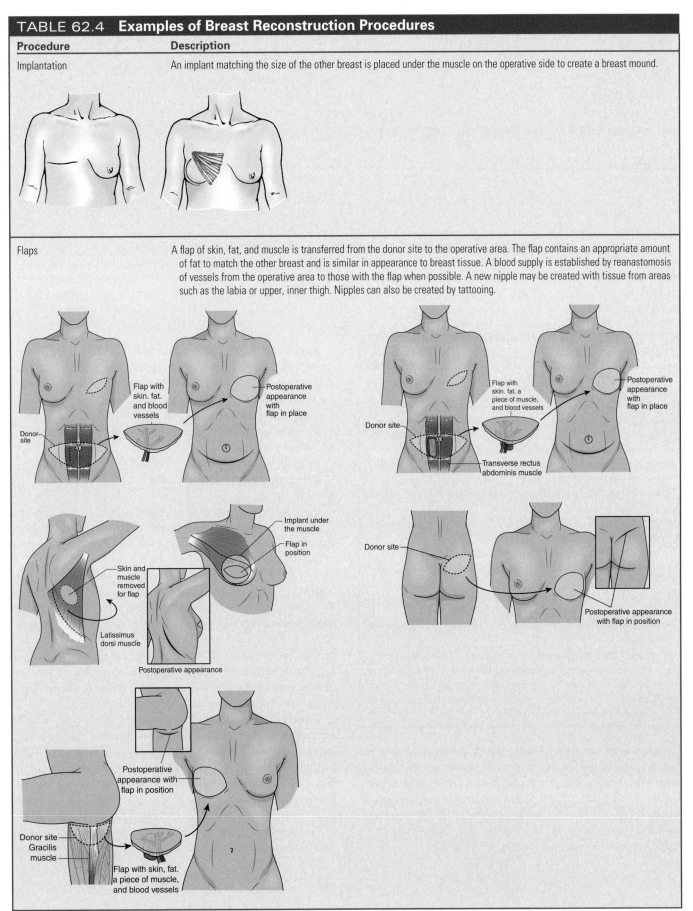

Continued

TABLE 62.4   Examples of Breast Reconstruction Procedures—cont'd

Procedure	Description
Tissue expansion DIEP reconstruction (deep inferior epigastric perforator flap)	A tissue expander is placed under the muscle and gradually expanded with saline to stretch the overlying skin and create a pocket. After several weeks, the tissue expander is exchanged for an implant.

Flap figures adapted from American Cancer Society (ACS), 2023. https://www.cancer.org/cancer/breast-cancer/reconstruction-surgery/breast-reconstruction-options/breast-reconstruction-using-your-own-tissues-flap-procedures.html.

BOX 62.3   Best Practice for Patient Safety and Quality Care

Postoperative Care of the Patient After Breast Reconstruction

- Assess the incision and flap for signs of *infection* (excessive redness/hyperpigmentation, drainage, odor) and poor tissue perfusion (duskiness, decreased capillary refill) during dressing changes.
- Avoid pressure on the flap and suture lines by positioning on the nonoperative side and avoiding tight clothing.
- Monitor and measure drainage in collection devices (e.g., Jackson-Pratt [JP] drains).
- Teach to return to usual activity level gradually (per the surgeon's orders) and to avoid heavy lifting.
- Remind to avoid sleeping in the prone position.
- Teach to avoid participation in contact sports or other activities that could cause trauma to the chest.
- Teach to minimize pressure on the breast during sexual activity.
- Remind to refrain from driving until advised by the surgeon.
- Remind to ask at the 6-week postoperative visit when full activity can be resumed.
- Reassure that optimal appearance may not occur for 3 to 6 months after surgery.
- If implants have been inserted, teach the proper method of breast massage to enhance expansion and prevent capsule formation (consult with the surgeon).
- Remind about the importance of clinical breast examination and follow-up surveillance by the health care provider.

survivors who can help navigate the decisions needed when facing breast cancer. In this program, a volunteer who has had breast cancer visits the woman, offering information on breast forms, clothing, coping with breast cancer, and possible reconstructive options. For this intervention to be as helpful as possible, the volunteer should be about the same age as the patient and have experienced the same surgical procedure.

Adjuvant therapy. The decision to follow the original surgical procedure with additional treatment to help keep the cancer from recurring is known as adjuvant therapy. This decision is based on several factors:

- Stage of the disease
- Patient's age and menopausal and functional status
- Patient preferences
- Pathologic examination
- Hormone receptor (ER/PR) status
- HER2 status
- Presence of a known genetic predisposition

Adjuvant therapy for breast cancer consists of systemic chemotherapy, radiation therapy, or a combination of both. The purpose of radiation therapy is to reduce the risk for local recurrence of breast cancer. The goal of systemic therapy (with chemotherapy, hormone therapy, and targeted therapy) is to reduce the risk of recurrence (locally or at distant sites) and prevent cancer-related death. These drugs destroy breast cancer cells that may be present anywhere in the body. They are typically delivered after surgery for breast cancer, although neoadjuvant chemotherapy may be given to reduce the size of a tumor before surgery. Endocrine therapy may also be used as a chemoprevention option for high-risk women with a personal history of breast cancer.

RADIATION THERAPY. Radiation therapy is usually administered after surgery to destroy breast cancer cells that may remain near the site of the original tumor (Fig. 62.11). This therapy can be delivered to the whole breast or to only part of the breast. Whole-breast irradiation is delivered through external beam radiation over a period of 5 to 6 weeks. Partial breast irradiation (PBI) is an option for some women (Forster, 2020). PBI is a convenient alternative to whole-breast irradiation. Less time is needed for completion, and outcomes are comparable

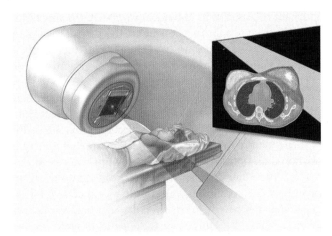

FIG. 62.11 Radiation therapy. (Used with permission of Mayo Foundation for Medical Education and Research, all rights reserved.)

to those of whole-breast irradiation. The advantage of this type of radiation is that it is delivered over a much shorter time interval, eliminating the need for weeks of treatment. The types of methods available for delivering PBI include the following:

- Brachytherapy is a form of treatment in which an external catheter is inserted at the lumpectomy cavity and surrounding margin, and radioactive seeds are inserted into a multicatheter or balloon catheter device. Radiation is given over a period of 5 days. Ten treatments are given in total, with at least 6 hours between treatments.
- Intraoperative radiation therapy is the most accelerated form of PBI. It uses a high single dose of radiation delivered during the lumpectomy surgery.

Nursing care for the patient undergoing radiation therapy includes patient education and side effect management. Skin changes are a major side effect during this therapy. If brachytherapy is planned, instruct patients about the procedure. Assure them that they will be radioactive only while the radiation source is dwelling inside the breast tissue.

> ### ! NURSING SAFETY PRIORITY
> #### *Action Alert*
>
> Teach women undergoing brachytherapy for breast cancer that radiation is contained in the temporary catheter and then removed before the patient goes home. The risk for others to be exposed to radiation is very small. Body fluids and items contacted by patients with brachytherapy are not radioactive. However, during the time that radiation is delivered, the patient will be alone in the room.

DRUG THERAPY. The National Comprehensive Cancer Network (NCCN, 2023) provides a database of evidence-based practice and treatments for various cancers. *Chemotherapy* for breast cancer is a systemic treatment used to kill undetected breast cancer cells that may have left the original tumor and moved to more distant sites. Generalist nurses do not administer chemotherapy; consult your agency policies regarding the specific training and education that is needed to demonstrate and maintain competence in chemotherapy administration (Oncology Nursing Society, 2019).

Chemotherapy is recommended for treatment of invasive breast cancer after surgery (adjuvant chemotherapy). It may also be given before surgery to reduce the size of the tumor (neoadjuvant chemotherapy) and is most effective when combinations of more than one drug are used. Sometimes a patient needs to have a surgically implanted IV catheter before chemotherapy administration. Chemotherapy drugs are usually delivered in four to six cycles, with each period of treatment followed by a rest period to give the body time to recover from the adverse effects of the drugs. Each cycle is 2 to 3 weeks long. The total treatment time is 3 to 6 months, although treatment may be longer for advanced or HER2-positive breast cancer.

A common chemotherapy regimen for breast cancer treatment is doxorubicin, cyclophosphamide, and paclitaxel, which in the United States is also known as AC-T. If the patient is HER2 positive, a trastuzumab-based regimen will be used. In early-stage breast cancer, chemotherapy regimens lower the risk for breast cancer recurrence and death. In metastatic breast cancer, chemotherapy regimens reduce cancer size and slow the progression of disease.

Nurses who are qualified to give chemotherapy must be very proficient in the preparation and administration of these drugs and knowledgeable about various venous access devices. They must also be able to manage the distressing symptoms associated with side effects of these drugs. Chapter 18 discusses chemotherapy in more detail and general nursing management of alopecia, nausea and vomiting, mucositis, and bone marrow suppression.

Chemotherapy can be unpleasant and expensive and can have life-threatening short-term and long-term side effects. Because more women are living longer with breast cancer, more long-term effects are emerging. For example, ovarian suppression from chemotherapy drugs can result in infertility, which can be devastating for some women of childbearing age.

> ### ! NURSING SAFETY PRIORITY
> #### *Action Alert*
>
> Teach patients undergoing chemotherapy with doxorubicin and trastuzumab to be aware of cardiotoxic effects. Patients will have routine testing of their cardiac function and ejection fraction (EF) because these side effect are often asymptomatic (Morgan, 2022). Instruct them to report excessive fatigue, shortness of breath, chronic cough, and edema to the health care provider. These side effects can manifest years after treatment.

Targeted cancer therapies are drugs that target specific characteristics of cancer cells, such as a protein, an enzyme, or the formation of new blood vessels. The advantage of targeted therapy over traditional chemotherapy is that targeted therapy is less likely to harm normal, healthy cells, and therefore it has fewer side effects. One of the first targeted therapies developed for breast cancer is the monoclonal antibody *trastuzumab*. This drug targets the *HER2 protein* overexpression in breast cancer cells. Other targeted therapies are available.

Drugs that alter hormone levels may also be used in breast cancer prevention and treatment. The purpose of endocrine therapy is to reduce the estrogen available to breast tumors to stop or prevent their growth. *Premenopausal* women whose main estrogen source is the ovaries may benefit from drugs that inhibit estrogen synthesis. These drugs include leuprolide and goserelin, which suppress the hypothalamus from making luteinizing hormone–releasing hormone (LHRH). When LHRH is inhibited, the ovaries do not produce estrogen. Although the suppression of ovarian function decreases breast cancer risk, the drastic drop in estrogen causes significant menopausal symptoms. The decision to use these drugs is not made lightly and patients should discuss this with their health care provider.

Selective estrogen receptor modulators (SERMs), on the other hand, do not affect ovarian function. Rather, they block the effect of estrogen in women who have estrogen receptor (ER)–positive breast cancer (Burchum & Rosenthal, 2022). SERMs are also used as chemoprevention in women at high risk for breast cancer and in women with advanced breast cancer. For women with hormone receptor–positive breast cancer, tamoxifen reduces the chances of the cancer coming back by about 40% (ACS, 2021b). This drug is usually prescribed for 5 to 10 years following a diagnosis of breast cancer. Common side effects of SERMs include hot flashes and weight gain. Rare but serious side effects of these drugs include endometrial cancer and thromboembolic events.

Aromatase inhibitors (AIs), such as letrozole and anastrozole, are used in *postmenopausal* women whose main source of estrogen is not the ovaries but, rather, body fat (Burchum & Rosenthal, 2022). AIs reduce estrogen levels by inhibiting the conversion of androgen to estrogen through the action of the enzyme *aromatase.* They are beneficial when given to postmenopausal women for up to 10 years to prevent recurrence (NCCN, 2023). A side effect of AIs, not seen with tamoxifen, is loss of bone density. Women taking AIs are candidates for bone-strengthening drugs and must be closely monitored for osteoporosis. Weight-bearing exercises and supplementation should be implemented into the daily routine.

Enhancing Coping Strategies

Planning: Expected Outcomes. The patient who is treated for breast cancer will verbalize enhanced coping ability related to the diagnosis and treatment of the condition.

Interventions. The patient with breast cancer may have difficulty coping and experience anxiety related to the disease or treatment. The fear and uncertainty for the patient with breast cancer begin the moment a lump is discovered or when a mammogram reveals an abnormality. These feelings may be related to past experiences and personal associations with the disease. Assess the patient's situational perceptions. Allow the expression of feelings even if a diagnosis has not been established.

Assess the patient's need for knowledge. Some may want to read and discuss any available information. Provide accurate information and clarify any misinformation the patient may have received through the media, on the Internet, or from family and friends. If the mass has been diagnosed as cancer, people may feel a partial sense of relief to be dealing with a known entity. A feeling of shock or disbelief usually occurs. It is difficult to accept a diagnosis of cancer. Patients and their families or significant others deal in individual ways with the mix of feelings. Adjust your approach to care as the patient's emotional state changes. The goal is to have the patient, and significant other and family (as desired by the patient), be active participants in management of the disease.

An integral part of the plan to meet these emotional needs is the use of outside resources. For example, the patient who is worried in particular about the side effects of radiation therapy may benefit more from talking to someone who has undergone radiation than from talking to the nurse or primary health care provider. The American Cancer Society Reach to Recovery program is just one community resource that connects breast cancer patients to a peer who has lived through the treatment the patient is facing. Be sure to assess the patient's preference and make appropriate referrals.

Another helpful resource for patients who desire to receive care at one location is a full-service cancer center. Some agencies have all cancer services offered comprehensively in one location, including surgeon and provider services, counseling, nursing care, social services, nutrition services, rehabilitation, various therapies (including chemotherapy), and spiritual ministry. Obtaining all services in one familiar location can decrease the stress that the patient feels.

Concerns about appearance after surgery are common and are often a threat to the patient's self-concept as a woman. Before breast surgery, the woman and significant other can benefit from an explanation of the expected postoperative appearance. After a modified radical mastectomy, the chest wall is fairly smooth and has a horizontal incision from the axilla to the mid-chest area. After breast-conserving surgery, scars vary according to the amount of breast tissue removed. Emphasize that scars will fade and edema will lessen with time. Scars may be red and raised at first, but these features lessen in the first few months. After surgery, encourage the woman to look at the incision when ready. Do not push the patient to accept this body image change immediately.

Much of one's body image reflects how others respond. The response of the patient's significant other or family members to the surgery affects self-esteem. These people may also need the support of the nurse. They may have concerns about their ability to accept the changes and need to discuss these feelings with an objective listener. They may also need help with communicating their feelings to their loved one. Involving them in teaching, if the patient desires, may also help reinforce learning and increase retention.

Discuss sexual concerns before discharge. Most surgeons recommend avoiding sexual intercourse for 4 to 6 weeks. Patients may prefer to lay a pillow over the surgical site or to wear a bra, camisole, or T-shirt to prevent contact with the surgical site during intercourse. Patients or significant others may be embarrassed to discuss the topic of *sexuality.* Be sensitive to possible concerns and approach the subject first.

For young women, issues related to childbearing may be a concern. Chemotherapy and radiation are considered serious teratogenic (birth defect–causing) agents. Advise sexually active patients receiving chemotherapy or radiotherapy to use birth control during therapy. The method and length of birth control should be discussed with the health care provider. Patients with hormone ER/PR–positive breast cancer need to avoid estrogen, including contraceptives, HRT, and vaginal creams.

Care Coordination and Transition Management

Home Care Management. In collaboration with the case manager and members of the interprofessional health care team, make the appropriate referrals for care after discharge. Preoperative teaching and arrangements for home care management and referrals can be started before surgery or other treatment.

The patient who has undergone breast surgery can be discharged to the home setting unless other physical disabilities exist. Some are discharged the day after surgery with drains in place; some are discharged to home on the day of surgery. Patients should not be sent home without a family member or friend who can stay with them for 1 to 2 days. They may need assistance at home with drain care, dressings, and ADLs because of *pain* and impaired range of motion of the affected arm. See Box 62.4.

Teach patients that activities involving stretching or reaching for heavy objects should be avoided temporarily. This restriction

can be discussed with a family member or significant other who can perform these tasks or place the objects within easy reach.

Self-Management Education. The education plan for the patient after surgery includes:
- Teaching how to care for the incision and drainage device
- Showing exercises that will help reestablish full range of motion
- Explaining measures to avoid lymphedema
- Sharing measures to improve body image, coping, and self-esteem
- Providing information about interpersonal relationships and roles
- Encouraging avoidance of large crowds and ill people to decrease the risk for *infection*
- Reminding about immunizations to prevent illnesses, including the vaccine for COVID-19 (Breast Cancer Research Foundation, 2022)

See Box 62.5 for additional important patient teaching.

Postoperative Mastectomy Teaching. Teach incisional care to the patient, family, and/or other caregiver. The patient may wear a light dressing to prevent irritation. Although swelling and redness/hyperpigmentation of the scar itself are normal

---

🏠 BOX 62.4 Home Health Care
Patients Recovering From Breast Cancer Surgery

Assess cardiovascular, respiratory, and urinary status:
- Vital signs
- Lung sounds
- Urine output patterns

Assess for *pain* and effectiveness of analgesics.

Assess dressing and incision site:
- Excess drainage
- Symptoms of *infection*
- Wound healing
- Intact staples, sutures

Assess drain and site:
- Drainage around site and within drain reservoir
- Color and amount of drainage
- Symptoms of *infection*
- Review patient's recordings of drainage.
- Evaluate patient's ability to care for and empty drain reservoir.

Assess status of affected extremity:
- Range of motion
- Ability to perform exercise regimen
- Lymphedema

Assess nutritional status:
- Food and fluid intake
- Presence of nausea and vomiting
- Bowel sounds

Assess functional ability:
- ADLs
- Mobility and ambulation

Assess home environment:
- Safety
- Structural barriers

Assess patient's compliance and knowledge of illness and treatment plan:
- Follow-up appointment with surgeon
- Symptoms to report to health care provider
- Hand and arm care guidelines

BOX 62.5 Patient and Family Education
Recovery From Breast Cancer Surgery

- There may be a dry gauze dressing over the incision when you leave the hospital. You may change this dressing if it becomes soiled.
- A small, dry dressing will be around the site where a drain is placed. Often there is some leakage of fluid around the drain. Check the gauze dressing for drainage and change it if it becomes soiled. Some leakage is normal, but if the dressing becomes soaked more than once a day, call your health care provider.
- You have been taught how to empty the reservoir from your drain and how to measure the volume of drainage. You should empty the reservoir twice a day and record the measurements.
- Drains are generally removed when drainage is less than 30 mL/day for 3 consecutive days.
- You may take sponge baths or tub baths, making certain that the area of the drain and incision stays dry. You may shower after the stitches, staples, and drains are removed.
- You can begin using your arm for normal activities, such as eating or combing your hair. Exercises involving the wrist, hand, and elbow, such as flexing your fingers, circular wrist motions, and touching your hand to your shoulder, are very good. You can usually resume more strenuous exercises after the drains have been removed and your surgeon has cleared you to do so.
- You can expect mild *pain* after surgery; but within 4 to 5 days, most patients have no need for pain medication or require medication only at bedtime. If serious pain persists, contact your surgeon.
- Numbness in the area of the surgery and along the inner side of the arm from the armpit to the elbow occurs in almost all patients owing to injury to the nerves. Patients have described sensations of burning, and "pins and needles." This is neuropathic pain, and short-acting analgesics may be given. These sensations may change over the next several months, becoming less and less noticeable, and may resolve entirely by the end of the first year following surgery.
- Pamphlets on exercises, hand and arm care, and general facts about breast cancer are available from your hospital or from a volunteer visitor of the local or national office on cancer or breast cancer.

for the first few weeks, swelling, redness/hyperpigmentation, increased heat, and tenderness of the surrounding area indicate *infection* and should be reported to the surgeon immediately. If a lymph node dissection was performed, instruct the patient to elevate the affected arm on a pillow and to use interventions to decrease risk of lymphedema. Encourage the patient to dress in comfortable street clothes at home, not pajamas, to further enhance a positive self-image.

Teach the patient to continue performing the exercises that were begun in the hospital. Active range-of-motion exercises should begin 1 week after surgery and should be continued after sutures and drains are removed. Emphasize that reaching and stretching exercises should continue only to the point of *pain* or pulling, never beyond that.

Patients should be screened for mobility and provided education on exercises to perform after surgery. In addition, if the patient is unable to raise the arm over the head, positioning for radiation therapy will be difficult. Referral to physical therapy prior to surgery allows for education and assessment to be done in an unrushed environment. Attempt to choose resources and providers who are well educated in breast cancer rehabilitation, as people with this training have specific awareness of surgical interventions, and chemotherapy, radiation, and medication implications that may affect the patient's recovery from surgery for breast cancer (Physiological Oncology Rehabilitation Institute, 2022).

Lymphedema (Fig. 62.12), an abnormal accumulation of protein fluid in the subcutaneous tissue of the affected limb after a mastectomy, is a commonly overlooked topic in health teaching. Risk factors include injury or *infection* of the extremity, obesity, presence of extensive axillary disease, and radiation treatment. Once lymphedema develops, it can be very difficult to manage, and *lifelong measures must be taken to prevent it.* In some cases

infection causes lymphedema, and in other situations lymphedema leads to infection.

Nurses play a vital role in educating patients about this complication. Teach patients, especially those who have had axillary lymph nodes removed, that measures to prevent lymphedema are lifelong and include avoiding trauma to the arm on the side of the mastectomy. Teach your patient to immediately report symptoms of lymphedema such as sensations of heaviness, aching, fatigue, numbness, tingling, restricted range of motion (beyond what is expected after surgery) and/or swelling in the affected arm, and swelling in the upper chest (Mehrara, 2022).

Nurses should not assume that women with lymphedema are disabled; they are able to live full lives within this condition. A referral to a lymphedema specialist may be necessary for the patient to be fitted for a compression sleeve and/or glove, to be taught exercises and manual lymph drainage, and to discuss ways to modify daily activities to avoid worsening the problem. Management is directed toward measures that promote drainage of the affected arm.

! NURSING SAFETY PRIORITY
Action Alert

Teach the patient how to avoid lymphedema and *infection* of the affected arm after the mastectomy. Teach the importance of avoiding having blood pressure measurements taken on, injections in, or blood drawn from the arm on the side of the mastectomy, especially if lymph node dissection has occurred. Instruct the patient to wear a mitt when using the oven, wear gloves when gardening, and treat cuts and scrapes appropriately. If lymphedema occurs, early intervention provides the best chance for control.

Health Care Resources. Resources available to the patient after discharge include personal support and community programs. After discharge, the significant other may need help in planning support for home responsibilities. This caregiver may be assuming additional duties at home and work and may feel stressed. Discussing the need for ongoing emotional support is also beneficial to both the patient and caregiver.

The American Cancer Society (ACS) is a comprehensive resource for information and support in the United States. Breastcancer.org (2023c) provides evidence-based information in language a layperson can understand.

The Canadian Cancer Society (CCS) offers information, resources, and support services for breast cancer patients and their families. The Breast Cancer Society of Canada conducts research on breast cancer in Canada.

Numerous support and educational resources are available to those diagnosed with breast cancer. Nurses must provide accurate and current information to patients who may have obtained inaccurate or outdated information from various sources. There are over 3.8 million breast cancer survivors in the United States (National Breast Cancer Foundation, 2022a), and many people are active in breast cancer support and advocacy organizations. National breast cancer organizations are accessible online, and many of them have local affiliates. Examples of such organizations are Susan G. Komen for the Cure, the

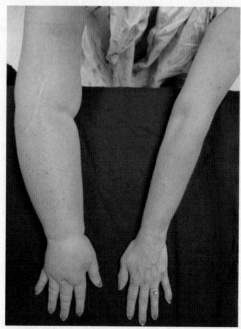

FIG. 62.12 Lymphedema of the arm. (From Song, D. H., & Neligan, P. C. [2018]. Plastic surgery. Volume 4. *Lower extremity, trunk, and burns* [4th ed.]. Philadelphia: Elsevier.)

National Breast Cancer Coalition, Sisters Network, and Young Survival Coalition. Local support organizations can be found and accessed through the health care provider, the local hospital, wellness centers, or home care agencies; by word of mouth; or by Internet search.

Recognize that some women may choose to forego or discontinue treatment for breast cancer for a variety of reasons. Honor the patient's decision, and collaborate with hospice and palliative care resources to provide the patient with support.

Helping patients diagnosed with breast cancer to be active participants in their care, to find resources to help them cope, and to gain support with physical and emotional changes are priorities for the nurse and members of the interprofessional team.

Evaluate Outcomes: Evaluation

Evaluate the care of the patient with breast cancer based on the identified priority patient problems. The expected outcomes include that the patient:

- Has no recurrence or metastasis of breast cancer after completion of treatment; if metastasis occurs, have optimal palliative and end-of-life care
- Reports adequately coping with breast cancer and the chosen plan of care.

▌GET READY FOR THE NEXT-GENERATION NCLEX® EXAMINATION!

Essential Nursing Care Points

Health Promotion/Disease Prevention	Chronic Disease Care
• Identify and educate patients about the importance of mammograms and clinical breast examinations for women according to national guidelines and risk factors. • Teach women factors that place them at a higher risk for developing breast cancer. • Discuss ways to change modifiable risk factors to decrease the chance for developing breast cancer. • Teach women and men the signs of breast cancer that should be reported immediately to their primary health care provider.	• Provide support, education, and community referrals to the patient with breast cancer and their significant others. • Recognize that treatment for breast cancer may take months to years; refer patients who need psychosocial support to social services or mental health professionals who can provide long-term assistance. • Teach patients prescribed tamoxifen to prevent breast cancer recurrence that this therapy is taken for 5 to 10 years following a diagnosis of breast cancer.
Regenerative or Restorative Care	**Hospice/Palliative/Supportive Care**
• Notify the interprofessional health care team that the arm on the surgical mastectomy side should not be used for blood pressures, blood drawing, IV therapy, or injections. • Following surgery, elevate the head of the bed to at least 30 degrees; elevate the affected arm on a pillow to promote lymphatic fluid return. • Assess dressings and drains following surgery for breast cancer; drainage amount should be less than 30 mL in a 24-hour period. • Teach postmastectomy exercises that will help the patient to regain function following surgery.	• Refer patients who will undergo surgery for breast cancer to physical and occupational therapists with breast cancer rehabilitation expertise. • Refer patients at end of life to hospice, palliative care, and support groups as appropriate.

Mastery Questions

1. The nurse is caring for a young client with breast cancer who will start chemotherapy soon. Which of the following nursing interventions are appropriate? **Select all that apply.**
   A. Explain that few side effects are expected.
   B. Refer to support groups for people with breast cancer.
   C. Provide self-care resources before chemotherapy begins.
   D. Teach client about birth control options that are available.
   E. Ask if there are sexuality concerns the client wishes to discuss.

2. Which assessment finding in a client who underwent a left mastectomy yesterday would the nurse communicate to the health care provider?
   A. Numbness in the left arm
   B. Temperature of 99.9°F (37.7°C)
   C. Drainage of 26 mL collected over 24 hours
   D. Scant fluid noted around the drain insertion

NGN Challenge 62.1

62.1.1

The oncoming nurse reviews the documentation of the previous nurse for a 58-year-old client who had a left mastectomy 2 days ago following a breast cancer diagnosis.

Highlight the findings that would require **immediate** follow-up.

History and Physical	Nurses' Notes	Vital Signs	Laboratory Results

0602: Dressing clean and dry. Drain emptied of 24 mL serosanguineous fluid. Reports feeling very tired. Pain rated at 6 on a 0-to-10 scale. Height: 68 inches (173 cm); weight: 184 lb (83.5 kg). VS: T 99.6°F (37.6°C); HR 72 beats/min; RR 18 breaths/min; BP 118/78 mm Hg; Spo$_2$ 98% on RA. IV line in right forearm infusing 0.9% NS at 100 mL/hr. Site clean, dry, cool to touch. No redness noted.

62.1.2

The nurse performs an assessment and adds the following information to the electronic health record.

History and Physical	Nurses' Notes	Vital Signs	Laboratory Results

0602: Postoperative day 1 following left mastectomy. Dressing clean and dry. Drain emptied of 24 mL serosanguineous fluid. Reports feeling very tired. Pain rated at 6 on a 0-to-10 scale. Oxycodone administered per orders in medical administration record (MAR). Height: 68 inches (173 cm); weight: 184 lb (83.5 kg). VS: T 99.6°F (37.6°C); HR 72 beats/min; RR 18 breaths/min; BP 118/78 mm Hg; Spo$_2$ 98% on RA. IV line in right forearm infusing 0.9% NS at 100 mL/hr. Site clean, dry, cool to touch. No redness noted.

0730: Patient resting in bed; sleepy but easily aroused. States generalized pain persists at 6 on a 0-to-10 scale and that her left arm feels "heavy" and "kind of like it is numb." Left arm with mild swelling, difficulty with shoulder movement, and difficulty bending at the elbow.

The nurse analyzes the findings to determine the client's condition. Complete the following sentence by selecting from the lists of options below.

The client is at high risk for **1 [Select]** as evidenced by **2 [Select]** and **3 [Select]** .

Options for 1	Options for 2	Options for 3
Osteomyelitis	Generalized pain of 6 on 0-to-10 scale	24 mL serosanguineous drainage
Lymphedema	BMI indicating overweight	Left arm numbness
Sepsis	Tiredness	Temperature 99.6°F (37.6°C)
Cellulitis	Left arm heaviness	Sleepiness

62.1.3

The nurse determines the priority for the plan of care.

History and Physical	Nurses' Notes	Vital Signs	Laboratory Results

0602: Postoperative day 1 following left mastectomy. Dressing clean and dry. Drain emptied of 24 mL serosanguineous fluid. Reports feeling very tired. Pain rated at 6 on a 0-to-10 scale. Oxycodone administered per orders in medical administration record (MAR). Height: 68 inches (173 cm); weight: 184 lb (83.5 kg). VS: T 99.6°F (37.6°C); HR 72 beats/min; RR 18 breaths/min; BP 118/78 mm Hg; Spo$_2$ 98% on RA. IV line in right forearm infusing 0.9% NS at 100 mL/hr. Site clean, dry, cool to touch. No redness noted.

0730: Patient resting in bed; sleepy but easily aroused. States generalized pain persists at 6 on a 0-to-10 scale and that her left arm feels "heavy" and "kind of like it is numb." Left arm with mild swelling, difficulty with shoulder movement, and difficulty bending at the elbow.

Complete the following sentence by selecting from the list of word choices below.

The **priority** for the client at this time is to manage __[Word Choice]__ to prevent __[Word Choice]__ .

Options
Recurrence of breast cancer
Pain
Lymphedema
Arm impairment
Increased weight

62.1.4

The nurse enters the client room to provide care.

History and Physical	Nurses' Notes	Vital Signs	Laboratory Results

0602: Postoperative day 1 following left mastectomy. Dressing clean and dry. Drain emptied of 24 mL serosanguineous fluid. Reports feeling very tired. Pain rated at 6 on a 0-to-10 scale. Oxycodone administered per orders in medical administration record (MAR). Height: 68 inches (173 cm); weight: 184 lb (83.5 kg). VS: T 99.6°F (37.6°C); HR 72 beats/min; RR 18 breaths/min; BP 118/78 mm Hg; Spo$_2$ 98% on RA. IV line in right forearm infusing 0.9% NS at 100 mL/hr. Site clean, dry, cool to touch. No redness noted.

0730: Patient resting in bed; sleepy but easily aroused. States generalized pain persists at 6 on a 0-to-10 scale and that her left arm feels "heavy" and "kind of like it is numb." Left arm with mild swelling, difficulty with shoulder movement, and difficulty bending at the elbow.

Based on the client's findings, select the **4** nursing interventions that are appropriate to meet the client's priority need.

○ Place ice pack on swelling in left arm.
○ Assist with gentle range-of-motion exercises.
○ Administer antibiotics as prescribed.
○ Encourage regular ambulation as tolerated.
○ Position right arm over the head when resting.
○ Monitor temperature every 4 hours.
○ Apply tourniquet below site of swelling.

62.1.5

In addition to interventions that promote lymphatic drainage, the nurse collaborates with the surgeon regarding the client's pain management. The surgeon increases the dose of oxycodone every 4 to 6 hours as needed. After administering this dose, which of the following nursing actions would the nurse take? **Select all that apply.**

○ Monitor respiratory status.
○ Request that family monitor the client.
○ Evaluate pain intensity 30 minutes later.
○ Facilitate ambulation an hour after this dose.
○ Remind the client to use the call light if the bathroom is needed.
○ Teach about how to properly care for the incision and drain at home.

62.1.6

A week later following discharge from the hospital, the client follows up with the surgeon on an outpatient basis. The nurse performs an assessment. For each client finding, determine whether the interventions instituted by the hospital nurses were effective (helped to meet expected outcomes) or not effective (did not help to meet expected outcomes).

Previous Client Finding	Current Client Finding	Effective	Not Effective
Left arm with mild swelling	Left arm with mild swelling		
Temperature immediately following surgery: 99.6°F (37.6°C)	Current temperature: 98°F (36.7°C)		
Limited range of motion in left elbow	Full range of motion in left elbow		
Limited range of motion in left shoulder	Limited range of motion in left shoulder		
Numbness in left arm	Sensation in left arm		

REFERENCES

American Cancer Society (ACS). (2021a). *Ductal carcinoma in situ (DCIS)*. https://www.cancer.org/cancer/breast-cancer/understanding-a-breast-cancer-diagnosis/types-of-breast-cancer/dcis.html.

American Cancer Society (ACS). (2021b). *Tamoxifen and raloxifene for lowering breast cancer risk*. https://www.cancer.org/cancer/breast-cancer/risk-and-prevention/tamoxifen-and-raloxifene-for-breast-cancer-prevention.html.

American Cancer Society (ACS). (2022a). *American Cancer Society recommendations for the early detection of breast cancer*. https://www.cancer.org/cancer/breast-cancer/screening-tests-and-early-detection/american-cancer-society-recommendations-for-the-early-detection-of-breast-cancer.html.

American Cancer Society (ACS). (2022b). *Breast cancer facts and figures 2022*. https://www.cancer.org/content/dam/cancer-org/research/cancer-facts-and-statistics/annual-cancer-facts-and-figures/2022/2022-cancer-facts-and-figures.pdf.

American Cancer Society (ACS). (2022c). *Fibroadenomas of the breast*. https://www.cancer.org/cancer/breast-cancer/non-cancerous-breast-conditions/fibroadenomas-of-the-breast.html.

American Cancer Society (ACS). (2022d). *Lobular carcinoma in situ (LCIS)*. https://www.cancer.org/cancer/breast-cancer/non-cancerous-breast-conditions/lobular-carcinoma-in-situ.html.

American Cancer Society (ACS). (2022e). *Mastitis*. https://www.cancer.org/cancer/breast-cancer/non-cancerous-breast-conditions/mastitis.html.

American Cancer Society (ACS). (2022f). *Treatment of inflammatory breast cancer*. https://www.cancer.org/cancer/breast-cancer/treatment/treatment-of-inflammatory-breast-cancer.html.

American Cancer Society (ACS). (2023a). Key statistics for breast cancer: How common is breast cancer? https://www.cancer.org/cancer/breast-cancer/about/how-common-is-breast-cancer.html.

American Cancer Society (ACS). (2023b). *Survival rates for breast cancer*. https://www.cancer.org/cancer/breast-cancer/understanding-a-breast-cancer-diagnosis/breast-cancer-survival-rates.html.

American College of Obstetricians and Gynecologists (ACOG). (2023a). *Benign breast conditions*. https://www.acog.org/womens-health/faqs/benign-breast-problems-and-conditions.

American College of Obstetricians and Gynecologists (ACOG). (2023b). Breast cancer risk assessment and screening in average-risk women. *Practice Bulletin, 179*. (2011, 2017, 2021). https://www.acog.org/clinical/clinical-guidance/practice-bulletin/articles/2017/07/breast-cancer-risk-assessment-and-screening-in-average-risk-women.

American Society of Breast Surgeons Foundation. (2023). *Breast abscess*. Retrieved from https://breast360.org/topic/2017/01/01/breast-abscess/.

Anders, C., & Carey, L. (2023). ER/PR negative, HER2-negative (triple-negative) breast cancer. *UpToDate*. Retrieved June 7, 2023, from https://www.uptodate.com/contents/er-pr-negative-her2-negative-triple-negative-breast-cancer.

Association of Oncology Social Work. (2023). *Oncology social work certification*. https://aosw.org/publications-media/oncology-social-work-specialty-certification/.

Board of Oncology Social Work. (2022). *Our mission*. https://oswcert.org/.

Bou Zerdan, M., et al. (2021). Genomic assays in node positive breast cancer patients: A review. *Frontiers in Oncology*, 10:609100. https://doi.org/10.3389/fonc.2020.609100.

Braunstein, G., & Anawalt, B. (2023). Clinical features, diagnosis, and evaluation of gynecomastia in adults. *UpToDate*. Retrieved June 7, 2023, from https://www.uptodate.com/contents/clinical-features-diagnosis-and-evaluation-of-gynecomastia-in-adults.

Breast Cancer Research Foundation. (2022). *COVID-19 and breast cancer: What patients need to know*. https://www.bcrf.org/blog/coronavirus-covid-19-and-breast-cancer-common-questions-and-answers/.

Breast Cancer Research Foundation. (2023). *Black women and breast cancer: Why disparities persist and how to end them*. https://www.bcrf.org/blog/black-women-and-breast-cancer-why-disparities-persist-and-how-end-them/.

Breastcancer.org. (2023a). *Male breast cancer*. https://www.breastcancer.org/symptoms/types/male_bc.

Breastcancer.org. (2023b). *Paget's disease of the nipple*. https://www.breastcancer.org/symptoms/types/pagets.

Breastcancer.org. (2023c). *Trusted guidance when you need us most. Because no one should face breast cancer alone*. https://www.breastcancer.org/.

Burchum, J. L. R., & Rosenthal, L. D. (2022). *Lehne's pharmacology for nursing care* (11th ed.). St. Louis: Elsevier.

Canadian Cancer Society. (2022). *Breast cancer statistics*. Retrieved from https://www.cancer.ca/en/cancer-information/cancer-type/breast/statistics/?region=on.

Canadian Cancer Society. (2023). *Screening for breast cancer*. https://cancer.ca/en/cancer-information/cancer-types/breast/screening.

Centers for Disease Control and Prevention. (2022). *Breast cancer in men*. https://www.cdc.gov/cancer/breast/men/index.htm.

Chlebowski, R. (2023). Factors that modify breast cancer risk in women. *UpToDate*. Retrieved June 7, 2023, from https://www.uptodate.com/contents/factors-that-modify-breast-cancer-risk-in-women.

Cleveland Clinic. (2023). *Estrogen*. https://my.clevelandclinic.org/health/body/22353-estrogen.

Dixon, J., & Pariser, K. (2022). Nonlactational mastitis in adults. *UpToDate*. Retrieved June 7, 2023, from https://www.uptodate.com/contents/nonlactational-mastitis-in-adults.

Forster, T. (2020). Accelerated partial breast irradiation: A new standard of care? *Breast Care, 15*, 136–137.

Huether, S., & McCance, K. (2020). *Understanding Pathophysiology* (7th ed.). St. Louis: Elsevier.

Interprofessional Education Collaborative (IPEC). (2016). *Core competencies for interprofessional collaborative practice: 2016 update*. https://ipec.memberclicks.net/assets/2016-Update.pdf.

Mehrara, B. (2022). Breast cancer-associated lymphedema. *UpToDate*. Retrieved June 7, 2023, from https://www.uptodate.com/contents/breast-cancer-associated-lymphedema.

Morgan, J. (2022). Cardiotoxicity of trastuzumab and other HER-2 targeted agents. *UpToDate*. Retrieved June 7, 2023, from https://www.uptodate.com/contents/cardiotoxicity-of-trastuzumab-and-other-her2-targeted-agents.

National Breast Cancer Foundation. (2020). *BRCA: The breast cancer gene*. Retrieved from https://www.nationalbreastcancer.org/what-is-brca.

National Breast Cancer Foundation. (2022a). *Breast cancer facts*. https://www.nationalbreastcancer.org/breast-cancer-facts.

National Breast Cancer Foundation. (2022b). *Clinical breast exam*. https://www.nationalbreastcancer.org/clinical-breast-exam.

National Cancer Institute. (n.d). *Breast Cancer Risk Assessment Tool*. Bethesda, MD. Retrieved from: https://bcrisktool.cancer.gov/calculator.html.

National Comprehensive Cancer Network (NCCN). (2023). *NCCN clinical practice guidelines in Oncology (NCCN Guidelines®). [v.4.2023]*. Retrieved from https://www.nccn.org/professionals/physician_gls/default.aspx.

National LGBT Cancer Network. (2023). *Lesbians and breast cancer risk*. https://cancer-network.org/cancer-information/lesbians-and-cancer/lesbians-and-breast-cancer-risk/.

Niknejad, M. (2022). Breast imaging - reporting and data system (BI-RADS). https://radiopaedia.org/articles/breast-imaging-reporting-and-data-system-bi-rads.

Oncology Nursing Society. (2019). *Chemotherapy and Immunotherapy Guidelines and Recommendations for Practice* (4th ed.). Pittsburgh, PA: Author.

Pfizer, Inc. (2023). A scientific advancement in the treatment Of HR+, HER2- metastatic breast cancer. https://www.ibrance.com/about-ibrance.

Physiological Oncology Rehabilitation Institute. (2022). *Breast cancer rehabilitation*. https://www.pori.org/breast-cancer-rehabilitation.html.

Sabel, M., & Collins, L. (2022). Atypia and lobular carcinoma in situ: High-risk lesions of the breast. *UpToDate*. Retrieved June 7, 2023, from https://www.uptodate.com/contents/atypia-and-lobular-carcinoma-in-situ-high-risk-lesions-of-the-breast.

Sabel, M. (2023). Overview of benign breast disease. *UpToDate*. Retrieved June 7, 2023, from https://www.uptodate.com/contents/overview-of-benign-breast-diseases.

Slusser, M., Garcia, L., Reed, C., & McGinnis, P. (2019). *Foundations of interprofessional collaborative practice in health care*. St. Louis: Elsevier.

Susan G. Komen. (2023). *Hyperplasia and other benign breast conditions*. https://www.komen.org/breast-cancer/risk-factor/hyperplasia-and-other-benign-breast-conditions/.

U.S. Department of Veterans Affairs. (2021). *Women veterans in research*. https://www.research.va.gov/pubs/docs/va_factsheets/MVP_womens_factsheet.pdf.

U.S. Food and Drug Administration. (2019). Questions and answers about breast implant-associated anaplastic large cell lymphoma (BIA-ALCL). https://www.fda.gov/medical-devices/breast-implants/questions-and-answers-about-breast-implant-associated-anaplastic-large-cell-lymphoma-bia-alcl.

63

Concepts of Care for Patients With Gynecologic Conditions

Cherie R. Rebar

http://evolve.elsevier.com/Iggy/

LEARNING OUTCOMES

1. Plan collaborative care with the interprofessional team to promote gynecologic health in patients with gynecologic disorders.
2. Teach adults how to decrease the risk for gynecologic disorders.
3. Teach the patient and caregiver(s) about common drugs and other management strategies used for gynecologic disorders.
4. Plan patient- and family-centered nursing interventions to decrease the psychosocial impact caused by living with a gynecologic disorder.
5. Apply knowledge of anatomy, physiology, and pathophysiology to provide evidence-based care for patients with a gynecologic disorder affecting *sexuality* and *reproduction.*
6. Analyze assessment and diagnostic findings to generate solutions and prioritize nursing care for patients with a gynecologic disorder.
7. Organize care coordination and transition management for patients with a gynecologic disorder.
8. Use clinical judgment to plan evidence-based nursing care to promote *sexuality* and *reproduction* and prevent *pain* and complications in patients with a gynecologic disorder.
9. Incorporate factors that affect health equity into the plan of care for patients with gynecologic disorders.

KEY TERMS

anterior colporrhaphy Surgery for severe symptoms of cystocele in which the pelvic muscles are tightened for better bladder support.

bilateral salpingo-oophorectomy (BSO) Surgical removal of both fallopian tubes and both ovaries.

colposcopy Examination of the cervix and vagina using a colposcope, which allows three-dimensional magnification and intense illumination of epithelium with suspected disease. This procedure can locate the exact site of precancerous and malignant lesions for biopsy.

concurrent chemoradiation The use of chemotherapy and radiation together at the same time.

cystocele Protrusion of the bladder through the vaginal wall (urinary bladder prolapse).

dyspareunia Painful intercourse.

endometrial cancer Cancer of the inner uterine lining.

fibroid See *leiomyoma.*

leiomyoma Benign, slow-growing solid tumor of the uterine myometrium.

loop electrosurgical excision procedure (LEEP) Diagnostic procedure or treatment in which a thin loop-wire electrode that transmits a painless electrical current is used to cut away affected cervical cancer tissue.

myoma See *leiomyoma.*

myomectomy Removal of leiomyomas from the uterus.

pelvic organ prolapse (POP) Condition in which the sling of muscles and tendons that support the pelvic organs becomes weak and is no longer able to hold them in place.

posterior colporrhaphy Surgery to repair a rectocele by strengthening pelvic supports and reducing the bulging.

rectocele Protrusion of the rectum through a weakened vaginal wall (rectal prolapse).

stress urinary incontinence (SUI) Loss of urine during activities that increase intraabdominal pressure, such as laughing, coughing, sneezing, or lifting heavy objects.

total hysterectomy Removal of the uterus and cervix; the procedure may be vaginal or abdominal.

uterine artery embolization Use of a percutaneous catheter by a radiologist, inserted through the femoral artery to inject sandlike pellets into the uterine artery. The resulting blockage starves the tumor of circulation, allowing it (or them) to shrink.

uterine prolapse The most common kind of pelvic organ prolapse (POP); the downward displacement of the uterus into the vagina.

vulvovaginitis Inflammation of the lower genital tract resulting from a disturbance of the balance of hormones and flora in the vagina and vulva.

✳ PRIORITY AND INTERRELATED CONCEPTS

The priority concepts for this chapter are:
- *Sexuality*
- *Infection*
- *Pain*

The **Sexuality** concept exemplar for this chapter is Uterine Leiomyoma.

The interrelated concepts for this chapter are:
- *Elimination*
- *Reproduction*

Gynecologic concerns can range in complexity from mild to life-threatening. *Pain*, vaginal discharge, abnormal bleeding, and urinary *elimination* problems are commonly experienced symptoms. These problems can affect *sexuality* and the patient's feelings about intimacy with others, as well as *reproduction* capability.

Because of the private nature of these concerns, it can be challenging for some people to seek medical care or to talk about symptoms. Create an open, nonjudgmental, and therapeutic environment in which the patient can feel comfortable expressing concerns.

Within this chapter, the terms "female," "woman," or "women" and the pronouns "she" and "her" apply to all individuals who were *assigned female at birth (AFAB)*, which includes cisgender women, transgender men, and nonbinary people with vaginas (Cleveland Clinic, 2023).

✳ SEXUALITY CONCEPT EXEMPLAR: UTERINE LEIOMYOMA

Pathophysiology Review

Leiomyomas, also called fibroids or myomas, are commonly found in women. These are benign, slow-growing solid tumors of the uterine myometrium (muscle layer) that develop from excessive local growth of smooth muscle cells. The growth of leiomyomas may be related to stimulation by estrogen, progesterone, and growth hormone. They are classified according to their position in the layers of the uterus (Fig. 63.1) (Stewart & Laughlin-Tommaso, 2023):

- *Intramural* leiomyomas are contained in the uterine wall within the myometrium.
- *Submucosal* leiomyomas protrude into the uterine cavity and can cause bleeding and disrupt pregnancy.
- *Subserosal* leiomyomas protrude through the outer surface of the uterine wall and may extend to the broad ligament, pressing other organs. These may have a broad or pedunculated base.

Although most fibroids develop within the uterine wall, a few may appear in the cervix, called cervical leiomyomas. Pedunculated leiomyomas are attached by a pedicle (stalk) to the outside of the uterus and occasionally break off and attach to other tissues (parasitic fibroids).

Etiology and Genetic Risk

The etiology of leiomyomas is not fully understood. Researchers continue to search for answers, recognizing that leiomyomas are

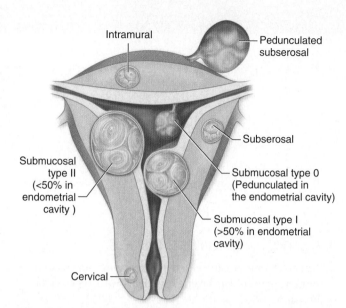

FIG. 63.1 Classification of uterine leiomyomas. (From Fielding, J.R., Brow, D.L., & Thrumond, A.S. [2011]. *Gynecologic Imaging*. Philadelphia: Elsevier.)

diagnosed primarily during the reproductive years (Stewart & Laughlin-Tommaso, 2023).

There is a genetic component associated with the risk for development of leiomyomas. Risk factors for the development of leiomyomas include (Stewart & Laughlin-Tommaso, 2023):

- Nulliparity
- Menarche before the age of 10 years
- In utero exposure to diethylstilbestrol (DES)
- Significant consumption of beef and red meats or ham
- Vitamin D insufficiency
- Alcohol consumption (especially beer)
- Hypertension
- Smoking

🔸 PATIENT-CENTERED CARE: HEALTH EQUITY

Vitamin D Deficiency and Leiomyomas

Evidence confirms that a low serum level of vitamin D is correlated with the presence and size of leiomyomas (Mohammadi et al., 2020; Szydlowska et al., 2022). Vitamin D intake can be consumed via dairy products; however, Black, American Indian, Asian American, and Hispanic/Latino people commonly experience lactose malabsorption (National Institute of Diabetes and Digestive and Kidney Disorders, 2018). Thoroughly assess all women at risk for leiomyomas for signs and symptoms of vitamin D deficiency. Collaborate with the primary health care provider to determine whether an over-the-counter vitamin D supplement is recommended or if further evaluation for vitamin D deficiency should be performed.

Incidence and Prevalence

Although leiomyomas are the most diagnosed pelvic tumor, incidence is difficult to determine based on the lack of longitudinal studies (Stewart & Laughlin-Tommaso, 2023). Up to 70%

of White women and up to 80% of women of African ancestry will develop fibroids in their lifetime (Giuliani et al., 2020).

Health Promotion/Disease Prevention

There is no way to fully prevent formation of leiomyomas. Encourage all women to eat a healthy diet, participate in regular exercise, and maintain a normal vitamin D level.

Interprofessional Collaborative Care

Recognize Cues: Assessment

History. Many women with leiomyomas report ongoing abnormal uterine bleeding and pelvic pain or pressure (Stewart & Laughlin-Tommaso, 2023). These symptoms are often what prompt the patient to seek health care. Establish whether the patient has a predictable menstrual pattern, experiences bleeding between periods, or whether she has prolonged bleeding (periods that exceed the normal 5 to 6 days). Ask about how many tampons or menstrual pads she uses in a day, if she must change tampons or pads overnight, if clots are passed, and if she has ever been diagnosed with anemia.

Determine whether she has a feeling of pelvic pressure or altered **elimination** patterns, including constipation and urinary frequency or retention. These symptoms result when the enlarged fibroid presses on other organs. Ask whether she experiences dyspareunia. Depending on the location of the leiomyoma, it can make intercourse uncomfortable. Acute discomfort may also occur with twisting of the fibroid on its stalk.

Physical Assessment/Signs and Symptoms. The patient may notice or feel that her abdomen has increased in size. Assess for distention or enlargement. Abdominal, vaginal, and rectal examinations performed by the health care provider usually reveal the presence of a uterine enlargement. Further diagnostic procedures are needed to differentiate benign tumors from malignant ones.

Psychosocial Assessment. Symptoms such as dyspareunia may significantly impact the patient's quality of life. A woman may fear that she has cancer, experience anxiety about abnormal bleeding, or fear the possibility of being unable to conceive. She may also be concerned if surgery is recommended, particularly if she desires to become pregnant in the future. Assess the woman's feelings and concerns. If hysterectomy is recommended, explore the significance of the loss of the uterus for the woman and her partner, including its effects on **sexuality** and potential plans for **reproduction**.

Diagnostic Assessment. Laboratory testing is usually limited to a hemoglobin/hematocrit (in the case of heavy bleeding) and a human chorionic gonadotropin (hCG) test to determine whether pregnancy is the cause of the uterine enlargement. An endometrial biopsy may be performed to evaluate for endometrial cancer.

Transvaginal ultrasound (US), a procedure in which the ultrasound probe is placed into the vagina for visualization, is the diagnostic study of choice (Stewart & Laughlin-Tommaso, 2023). Saline infusion sonography, hysteroscopy, and MRI (which can differentiate between benign and malignant tumors) may also be ordered if the results from the transvaginal ultrasound are inconclusive.

Analyze Cues and Prioritize Hypothesis: Analysis

The priority collaborative problem for patients with uterine leiomyoma is:

- Potential for prolonged or heavy bleeding due to abnormal uterine growth

Generate Solutions and Take Actions: Planning and Implementation

Managing Bleeding

Planning: Expected Outcomes. The expected outcome for the patient with a uterine leiomyoma is to have resolution of abnormal uterine bleeding after treatment.

Interventions. Asymptomatic leiomyomas may not require treatment. Leiomyomas in menopausal women usually shrink, so surgery may be unnecessary. Management depends on the size and location of the tumor, as well as the woman's desire for future pregnancy. Women who want to become pregnant may be prescribed drug therapy or have a myomectomy performed to remove the tumor. Hysterectomy may be recommended for women who no longer desire pregnancy.

Nonsurgical Management. If the woman has few symptoms or desires future pregnancy, the health care provider may recommend intermittent observation and monitoring. Mild leiomyoma symptoms can be managed with hormonal therapies. Combined estrogen-progestin drugs are most frequently used (Stewart, 2023), especially in premenopausal women. These can be delivered in oral form, as a vaginal ring, or as a transdermal patch. A progestin-releasing intrauterine device (IUD) is another alternative for women who do not want to take contraceptives with estrogen (Stewart, 2023).

Uterine artery embolization (UAE) is a procedure performed under local anesthesia, or with sedation if the patient requests it (van der Kooij & Hehenkamp, 2022). UAE is usually not performed if the patient desires future pregnancy. The interventional radiologist uses a percutaneous catheter inserted through the femoral artery to inject sandlike particles into the uterine artery. The uterine artery then carries these materials into the blood vessels that feed the leiomyoma. The resulting blockage starves the tumor of circulation, allowing it (or them) to shrink.

Common concerns reported following uterine artery embolization include pelvic pain, which is most severe in the first 24 hours, and nonpurulent vaginal discharge (without fever), which is self-limiting and can last for months (van der Kooij & Hehenkamp, 2022). Teach the patient to resume usual activities slowly and avoid strenuous activity until the surgeon recommends it. Most patients can return to work or their daily routine within a week.

Surgical Management. When possible, minimally invasive surgery (MIS) techniques are performed, such as a myomectomy, to prevent removal of the uterus. If not, a hysterectomy is the procedure of choice.

Uterus-sparing surgeries. If the woman desires children, the surgeon usually performs a hysteroscopic myomectomy. This procedure is used to remove submucosal leiomyomas and certain intramural leiomyomas where the fibroid protrudes into the uterine cavity (Bradley, 2021). When possible, this MIS procedure is performed very soon after the completion of a menstrual period to minimize blood loss and avoid the possibility of interrupting an unsuspected pregnancy. About 20% of leiomyomas recur after surgery, and about 20% of those who undergo this procedure still experience subsequent abnormal uterine bleeding (Bradley, 2022).

Normal activities can resume as quickly as the woman is comfortable after the laparoscopic procedure. She can return to work, daily activities, and sexual activity whenever she is ready. Other nursing care is similar to that for a woman undergoing a hysterectomy.

➕ **NURSING SAFETY PRIORITY**

Critical Rescue

Monitor the client who had hysteroscopic myomectomy. The fluid used to distend the uterine cavity during the procedure can be absorbed, resulting in fluid overload (Bradley, 2021). Although this potential complication is rare, assess carefully for signs and symptoms of pulmonary edema or heart failure, such as dyspnea, cough with frothy sputum, subjective report of "suffocating" or "smothering," and palpitations. *Report this information to the surgeon immediately.*

Hysterectomy. Leiomyomas may require removal via hysterectomy, which can be performed abdominally, vaginally, or with laparoscopic or robotic assistance (Fig. 63.2) based on the patient's clinical reason for hysterectomy and the surgeon's area of technical expertise. It can be performed as a partial, total or radical hysterectomy (Fig. 63.3), based on the patient's presentation and risk factors. Box 63.1 defines common terminology associated with common gynecologic surgeries.

PREOPERATIVE CARE. Preoperative teaching begins at the time the patient considers having a hysterectomy. Explain procedures that routinely take place before surgery, including laboratory tests and whether prophylactic antibiotics will be ordered. Depending on the type of surgical technique planned, teach about the need for turning, coughing, and deep-breathing exercises; incentive spirometry; early ambulation; and how *pain* will be controlled. (See Chapter 9 for a discussion

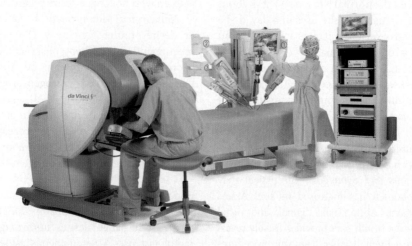

FIG. 63.2 Operating room layout for robotic surgery with da Vinci Robotic Surgery System. (Copyright ©2016 Intuitive Surgical, Inc.)

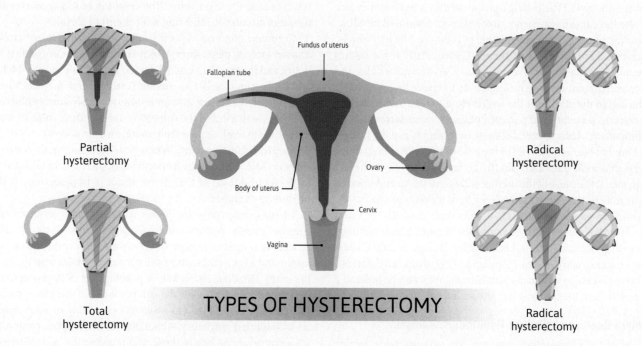

FIG. 63.3 Types of hysterectomy. (Used with permission from istockphoto.com, 2020, Anastasiia Krasavina.)

EVIDENCE-BASED PRACTICE

Effectively Discussing Sexuality and Sexual Health with Patients

Åling, M., et al. (2021). A scoping review to identify barriers and enabling factors for nurse–patient discussions on sexuality and sexual health. *Nursing Reports, 11*, 253-266.

The authors conducted a systematic review of research regarding therapeutic discussions between nurses and patients regarding sexuality and sexual health. Although it is well-researched that sexual health is an important part of overall well-being, health care providers continue to report that having open conversations about this with patients is difficult. Using the Preferred Reporting Items for Systematic Reviews and Meta-Analyses (PRISMA) checklist, 438 initial articles were identified for review; a final set of 19 articles (11 quantitative, 8 qualitative) met the selection criteria for this review and were used.

One factor associated with enabling successful conversations about sexuality and sexual health with patients included having a professional approach and core care values. Strategies such as having environmental privacy, connecting implications of physical problems to *sexuality* and sexual health, and having a favorable care relationship with the patient fostered helpful discussions between nurses and patients. It was also noted that having available education, policies, and checklists helped to foster meaningful conversation.

Barriers to discussion on sexuality and sexual health included nurses' perceived difficulty in addressing these topics with older adults, preconceived notions about who is or is not sexually active, and personal comfort level. Other barriers included nurses' fear of making patients feel uncomfortable or insulted, nurses' inability to place personal convictions about sexuality and sexual health aside, and the comfort level between nurses and patients of different ethnicities, cultural backgrounds, and religious beliefs. A common theme in one study noted that nurses avoided discussions about sexuality and sexual health to avoid offending patients or creating misunderstanding.

The review demonstrated that nurses agree that conversations about sexuality and sexual health influence overall patient well-being and that this type of information has significance to physical and psychological patient health. However, nurses overwhelmingly still felt it was difficult to have these conversations for the reasons noted above, which can create a disconnect in the provision of holistic care.

Level of Evidence: 1

The study was a systematic review, which is a strong source of evidence.

Implications for Research and Practice

The authors recommend that a professional approach be taken to equip nurses with what they need to professionally discuss sexuality and sexual health with patients. This approach includes providing nurses with training and access to vital tools and resources, and application of trust within the nurse-patient relationship, to foster professional discussions and collection of a sexual history.

Having training and tools provides the nurse with readiness and the ability to initiate and continue conversations about these topics that influence overall patient health.

BOX 63.1 Common Gynecologic Surgeries

Total Hysterectomy
- The entire uterus and cervix are removed. The procedure may be performed via the vagina or abdominally, with laparoscopic or robotic assistance.

Radical Hysterectomy
- The uterus, cervix, adjacent lymph nodes, upper third or half of the vagina, and surrounding tissues (parametrium) are removed.

Supracervical Hysterectomy (Also Called "Subtotal" or "Partial" Hysterectomy)
- The upper part of the uterus is removed; however, the cervix is left in place. This procedure is performed laparoscopically or abdominally.

Salpingo-Oophorectomy
- Removal of the fallopian tube(s) and ovary/ovaries. This can be done on one side of the body or both (termed *bilateral salpingo-oophorectomy*, or *BSO*).
- If only one or both fallopian tubes are removed, it is known as a *salpingectomy*.
- If only one or both ovaries are removed, it is known as an *oophorectomy*.
- For patients at risk of ovarian or breast cancer who choose to have both ovaries removed (even if healthy) in order to decrease their risk of developing cancer, it is known as a *risk-reducing bilateral salpingo-oophorectomy*.

Data from American College of Obstetricians and Gynecologists. (2021). *Hysterectomy.* https://www.acog.org/Patients/FAQs/Hysterectomy; Mann, W. (2023). Radical hysterectomy. *UpToDate.* Retrieved June 5, 2023, from https://www.uptodate.com/contents/radical-hysterectomy.

of general patient care before surgery.) Correct any misperceptions about the effects of hysterectomy, such as association with weight gain.

Psychological assessment is essential. Maintain an environment where it is safe for the patient to discuss feelings about sexual health. Provide reassurance that it is normal to have feelings and questions about the significance of a hysterectomy to *sexuality* and any potential desire for *reproduction*. Some women relate their uterus to self-image, femininity, and/or sexuality. Although surgically induced menopause can contribute to a loss of libido and vaginal changes if the ovaries are also removed, teach that vaginal estrogen cream, lubricants, and gentle dilation can help with these issues.

Remain nonjudgmental, building on a trusting nurse-patient relationship to provide the patient with the best evidence-based care and information based on her individual needs. See the Evidence-Based Practice box regarding the importance of fostering unbiased, open discussions about sexuality and sexual health with patients.

Assess the patient's support system. Ask whether she would like to include the partner in teaching sessions, and respect her decision.

OPERATIVE PROCEDURES. Hysterectomy can be performed vaginally, abdominally, laparoscopically, or via robotic-assisted laparoscopy. The choice of route is based on (Walters & Ferrando, 2022):
- Risk for injury
- Total operating time
- Feasibility of removal
- Hospitalization duration after surgery
- Time from surgery to resuming normal activity

POSTOPERATIVE CARE. Nursing care of the woman who has undergone a total abdominal hysterectomy is similar to that of any patient who has had laparoscopic or traditional open abdominal surgery. Chapter 9 contains information on general postoperative care. Also see Box 63.2 for additional information on caring for the patient who has had an open total abdominal hysterectomy.

BOX 63.2   Postoperative Nursing Care of the Patient After Open Total Abdominal Hysterectomy

Following hysterectomy, assess and monitor:

- Vital signs, including pain level
- Activity tolerance level
- Temperature and color of the skin
- Heart, lung, and bowel sounds
- Incision characteristics
  - Presence or absence of bleeding at the site (a small amount is normal)
  - Intactness of incision
  - Pain at site of incision
- Dressing and drains for color and amount of drainage
- Fluid intake (via IV until peristalsis returns and oral intake is tolerated)
- Urine output
  - Provide catheter care (catheter will be removed in about 24 hours)
- Red blood cell, hemoglobin, and hematocrit levels
- Vaginal discharge and/or bleeding
  - Provide perineal care
  - Assess perineal pads for vaginal bleeding and clots (should be less than one saturated perineal pad in 4 hours)

NCLEX Examination Challenge 63.1

Physiological Integrity

Following a laparoscopic total abdominal hysterectomy, which assessment finding would the nurse report to the surgeon as the **priority**?

A. Pain level of 5 on a 0-to-10 scale
B. Temperature of 99.2°F (37.3°C)
C. Saturation of one perineal pad in an hour
D. Decreased bowel sounds in all quadrants

Care Coordination and Transition Management

Self-Management Education. Discharge teaching following hysterectomy depends on the type of surgical procedure performed. General teaching points include expected physical changes, any activity restrictions, diet, wound care (if any), complications, and the need for follow-up care.

Some women experience abdominal or shoulder discomfort because of the introduction of carbon dioxide gas during a laparoscopic procedure. Teach patients who had a vaginal hysterectomy to promptly report excessive or increasing bleeding to their surgeon.

Driving should be avoided until the patient no longer takes opioid drugs (if prescribed). Showers can be taken, yet baths, hot tubs, and swimming should be avoided until cleared by the surgeon. Sexual activity and the use of tampons and douches should be avoided until up to 6 weeks after surgery; the surgeon will determine the time frame in which these are again permissible. Remind the patient that it may take from 2 to 6 weeks to return to work and normal function, depending on the type of procedure that was done.

See Box 63.3 for more specific health teaching, and see Chapter 9 for additional information about the postoperative period.

BOX 63.3   Patient and Family Education

Care After a Hysterectomy

Expected Physical Changes

- You will no longer have a period, although you may have some vaginal discharge or spotting for several weeks after you go home. Wear a perineal pad until the discharge or spotting stops.
- Although birth control methods are no longer needed to prevent pregnancy, condoms should still be used to decrease the chance of getting a sexually transmitted infection (STI).
- If your ovaries were removed, you may experience menopausal symptoms such as hot flushes, night sweats, and vaginal dryness. If these are become bothersome, discuss treatment options with your primary health care provider.
- It is normal to tire more easily and require more sleep and rest during the first few weeks after surgery.

Activity (Typically for Vaginal and Traditional Open Surgeries)

- Limit stair climbing; follow your surgeon's recommendations for this activity if you have stairs in your home.
- Do not lift anything heavier than you can pick up with one hand.
- Gradually increase walking as exercise, but stop before you become fatigued.
- Avoid the sitting position for extended periods. When you sit, do not cross your legs at the knees.
- Avoid strenuous activity and exercise for 2 to 6 weeks, depending on which type of surgical procedure was performed.
- Do not drive until your surgeon has cleared you and opioid medications have been discontinued.

Sexual Activity

- Do not engage in sexual intercourse for 6 weeks or as prescribed by your surgeon.
- If you had a vaginal "repair" as part of your surgery, you may experience some tenderness or *pain* the first time you have intercourse because the vaginal walls are tighter. This sensation usually diminishes with time. Careful intercourse and the use of water-based lubricants can help reduce this discomfort.

Complications

- Take your temperature twice each day for the first 3 days after surgery. Report fevers of over 100°F (38°C).
- Check any incisions daily for signs of infection (increasing redness/hyperpigmentation, open areas, drainage that is thick or foul smelling, incision *pain*).

Symptoms to Report to Your Surgeon

- Increased vaginal drainage or a change in drainage (bloodier, thicker, foul-smelling)
- Signs of infection at an incision site
- Temperature over 100°F (38°C)
- **Pain**, tenderness, redness/hyperpigmentation, or swelling in your calves
- **Pain** or burning on urination

Health Care Resources. Loss of female reproductive organs causes many women to experience a grieving process. Psychological reactions can occur months to years after surgery, particularly if sexual functioning and libido are diminished. Intermittent sadness is normal, but continued feelings of low self-esteem or loss of interest or pleasure in usual activities is not expected and should be evaluated. As appropriate, refer the patient with persistent grieving or depressive feelings to a mental health professional who can provide long-term follow-up. Community groups can also be of benefit for women who are experiencing similar circumstances to support each other.

Evaluate Outcomes: Evaluation

Evaluate the care of the patient with leiomyomas on the basis of the identified priority problem. The expected outcomes are that she:

- Has relief of bleeding after effective management

PELVIC ORGAN PROLAPSE

Pathophysiology Review

The pelvic organs are supported by a sling of muscles and tendons, which sometimes become weak and no longer able to hold an organ in place. Uterine prolapse, the most common type of pelvic organ prolapse (POP), can be caused by neuromuscular damage of childbirth; increased intraabdominal pressure related to pregnancy, obesity, or physical exertion; or weakening of pelvic support caused by decreased estrogen. The stages of uterine prolapse are described by the degree of descent of the uterus through the pelvic floor.

Whenever the uterus is displaced, other structures such as the bladder, rectum, and small intestine can protrude through the vaginal walls (Fig. 63.4). A cystocele is a protrusion of the bladder through the vaginal wall (urinary bladder prolapse), which can lead to stress urinary incontinence (SUI) and urinary tract infections (UTIs). A rectocele is a protrusion of the rectum through a weakened vaginal wall (rectal prolapse).

Interprofessional Collaborative Care

Recognize Cues: Assessment

Patients with suspected uterine prolapse may report a feeling of "something falling out," dyspareunia, backache, and/or heaviness or pressure in the pelvis.

Ask the patient whether she has urinary **elimination** problems, such as difficulty emptying her bladder, urinary frequency and urgency, a urinary tract **infection** (UTI), or stress urinary incontinence (SUI) (loss of urine during activities that increase intraabdominal pressure, such as laughing, coughing, sneezing, or lifting heavy objects). These symptoms may be associated with a *cystocele* (bladder prolapse).

Diagnostic assessment methods performed by the health care provider may include (Fashokun & Rogers, 2023):

- Visual, speculum, bimanual, rectovaginal, and neuromuscular examinations
- Imaging studies to demonstrate the anatomic characteristics of the prolapse
- Urinary tract and urinary retention evaluation (done because many cases of prolapse also involve incontinence)
- Perineal ultrasound and/or postvoid residual urine volume (PRUV) test
- Bowel function evaluation (if bowel incontinence accompanies pelvic organ prolapse)

During the pelvic examination, the health care provider may be able to visualize protrusion of the cervix or anterior vaginal wall when the woman is asked to bear down.

Take Actions: Interventions

Interventions are based on the severity of the POP. Conservative management is preferred over surgical treatment when possible.

Nonsurgical Management. Teach women to improve pelvic support and tone by doing pelvic floor muscle exercises (PFMEs, or Kegel exercises) (see Chapter 58). Space-filling devices such as a vaginal pessary can be worn to elevate the uterine prolapse. Women with bladder symptoms may benefit from bladder training and attention to complete emptying. Management of a rectocele focuses on promoting bowel **elimination.** The primary health care provider usually orders a high-fiber diet, stool softeners, and laxatives to facilitate bowel elimination that will not further aggravate the rectocele.

Surgical Management. Various surgical approaches may be considered for severe symptoms of POP, with preference given to the least invasive approach. Most women with symptomatic POP are treated with a reconstructive procedure, which may or may not include hysterectomy (Jelovsek, 2023). Synthetic mesh is often used in *transabdominal* POP repair; mesh intended for *transvaginal* surgical repair was discontinued in the United

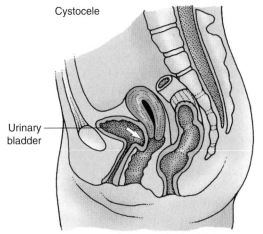
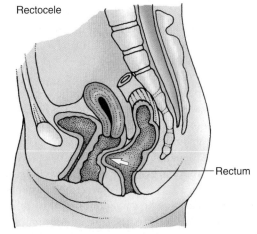

FIG. 63.4 In cystocele, the urinary bladder is displaced downward, causing bulging of the anterior vaginal wall. In rectocele, the rectum is displaced, causing bulging of the posterior vaginal wall.

States in 2019 because of complications associated with this procedure (U.S. Food and Drug Administration [FDA], 2021a). Follow preoperative assessment processes as in Chapter 9.

> **! NURSING SAFETY PRIORITY**
>
> **Action Alert**
>
> If a patient is recommended to have transabdominal surgical mesh used for pelvic organ prolapse, provide information for her to review. The surgeon will explain information about mesh and obtain informed consent after communicating benefits and risks, specifically about complications that may arise when using synthetic mesh, such as erosion through the vagina (U.S. Food and Drug Administration, 2021b). Reinforce information about possible adverse events, signs and symptoms of **infection,** and when the patient should contact the surgeon.

Teach patients who have just had the mesh procedure to avoid strenuous exercise, heavy lifting, and sexual intercourse for 6 weeks. After 6 weeks, the patient may gradually begin to return to regular activities but must be educated about prevention of increasing intra-abdominal pressure (e.g., constipation, weight lifting, cigarette smoking) for a minimum of 3 months to allow proper healing and prevent POP recurrence.

If caring for a patient who previously underwent a transvaginal mesh procedure prior to discontinuation of this product, advise her to see her health care provider if she has any concerns or complications. No additional action is needed unless complications have arisen since the time of implantation (U.S. Food and Drug Administration, 2021b).

Alternatives to minimally invasive surgery (MIS) are open surgical techniques. An anterior colporrhaphy (anterior repair) tightens the pelvic muscles for better *bladder* support, and is usually performed only after the patient has unsuccessfully tried conservative management and continues to have bothersome symptoms. This procedure is usually deferred until the woman no longer wishes to have children. Teach the patient to adhere to preoperative teaching (as in Chapter 9) and to consult her surgeon about the possible use of transvaginal estrogen prior to the procedure, which helps to maximize vaginal mucosal thickening (Mahajan, 2021).

A vaginal surgical approach is used and may be done as a laparoscopic-assisted procedure. Nursing care for a woman undergoing an anterior repair is similar to that for a woman undergoing a vaginal hysterectomy.

After surgery, the woman will have a urinary catheter in place for about 24 hours. Provide appropriate catheter care, and follow other postoperative care recommendations as in Chapter 9. Instruct the patient in how to splint her abdomen to protect sutures, and teach her to limit activities. She should *avoid* lifting anything heavier than 5 pounds (2.27 kg), strenuous exercises, straining with bowel movements, and sexual intercourse for up to 6 weeks (Mahajan, 2021). If she is prescribed postoperative vaginal estrogen, teach her how to administer this. Tell the woman to notify her surgeon if she has signs of **infection,** such as fever, persistent **pain,** or purulent, foul-smelling discharge, and to be sure to keep her follow-up appointment after surgery.

Although there are numerous approaches to managing posterior vaginal defects, traditional posterior colporrhaphy, which reduces *rectal* bulging, is used most commonly. If both a cystocele and a rectocele are present, an *anterior and posterior colporrhaphy* (A&P repair) is performed. In this case, the woman may return from surgery with a urinary catheter in place to keep the surgical area clean and dry.

The nursing care after a posterior repair is similar to that after any rectal surgery. After surgery, a low-residue (low-fiber) diet is usually ordered to decrease bowel movements and allow time for the incision to heal. Instruct the patient to avoid straining when she does have a bowel movement so that she does not put pressure on the suture line. Bowel movements are often painful, and she may need pain medication before having a stool. Provide sitz baths or delegate this activity to assistive personnel (AP) to relieve the woman's **pain**; this is a task that the AP can easily perform and then report outcomes back to you. Health teaching for the patient undergoing a posterior repair is similar to that for the patient undergoing an anterior repair.

> **NCLEX Examination Challenge 63.2**
>
> **Physiological Integrity**
>
> A client who had surgery for pelvic organ prolapse is being discharged today. Which of the following client statements require further teaching by the nurse? **Select all that apply.**
> A. "I plan to eat more high-fiber cereal."
> B. "Sitz baths can help relieve discomfort."
> C. "Intercourse should be postponed for at least 6 weeks."
> D. "My partner is going to bring our groceries in from the car."
> E. "Some discharge that smells bad is normal after this procedure."

ENDOMETRIAL CANCER

Pathophysiology Review

Cancer can affect any organ in the reproductive tract. This chapter covers very common gynecologic cancers. Endometrial cancer (cancer of the uterine lining) is the most common gynecologic malignancy; its incidence continues to rise in the United States, with an estimated 65,950 new cases diagnosed annually (American Cancer Society [ACS], 2022).

Endometrial cancer grows slowly in most cases, and early symptoms of vaginal bleeding generally lead to prompt evaluation and treatment. As a result, this type of cancer has a generally favorable prognosis. *Adenocarcinoma* of the endometrium is the most common type of uterine cancer. Abnormal uterine bleeding (AUB) is the most common symptom, resulting from estrogen exposure that leads to endometrial hyperplasia (Rogers, 2023).

The initial growth of the cancer is within the uterine cavity, followed by extension into the myometrium and the cervix. Staging reflects the location of the cancer and whether it has spread. Categorized by histology, type I uterine tumors (the most common) result from endometrial hyperplasia (described above). Type II, which reflect 10% to 20% of endometrial cancers, are likely to invade the uterine muscle and metastasize (Plaxe & Mundt, 2022).

Endometrial cancer is strongly associated with conditions causing prolonged exposure to estrogen without the protective effects of progesterone. Although most cases of endometrial cancer do not involve a genetic predisposition, it is more common in families that have gene mutations for hereditary nonpolyposis colon cancer (HNPCC) (Plaxe & Mundt, 2022). Other risk factors are listed in Box 63.4.

Interprofessional Collaborative Care

Recognize Cues: Assessment

The main symptom of endometrial cancer is abnormal uterine bleeding [AUB], especially postmenopausal bleeding. Ask the patient how many tampons or menstrual pads she uses each day. Some women also have a watery, bloody vaginal discharge or low back, low pelvis, or abdominal **pain** (caused by pressure of the enlarged uterus). Ask the patient to describe the exact location and intensity of discomfort. A pelvic examination performed by the health care provider may reveal the presence of a palpable uterine mass or uterine polyp. The uterus is enlarged if the cancer is advanced.

Several laboratory tests are used to determine the health status of the woman with possible or confirmed endometrial cancer. A complete blood count may show anemia due to heavy bleeding. Serum tumor markers to assess for metastasis include CA 125 (cancer antigen 125) and alpha fetoprotein (AFP), both of which may be elevated when ovarian cancer is present (Pagana et al., 2022). A human chorionic gonadotropin (hCG) level may be obtained to rule out pregnancy before treatment for cancer begins.

Transvaginal ultrasound (TVUS) and *endometrial biopsy* are the gold standard diagnostic tests to determine the presence of endometrial thickening and cancer. A saline infusion sonography can be performed subsequently to detect small lesions that the TVUS or endometrial biopsy may have missed (Feldman & Levine, 2023).

Other diagnostic tests to determine the patient's overall health status and the presence of metastasis include (Plaxe & Mundt, 2022; Feldman & Levine, 2023):

> ### BOX 63.4 Risk Factors for Endometrial Cancer
>
> Women at higher risk for endometrial cancer include those who:
> - Are middle-aged or older
> - Consume a high-fat diet
> - Experienced early menarche or late menopause
> - Use (or used) estrogen (without progesterone) after menopause
> - Have undergone radiation therapy for treatment of the pelvis
> - Have a personal history of type 2 diabetes, ovarian tumors, polycystic ovarian syndrome (PCOS) (Fig. 63.5), breast or ovarian cancer, or endometrial hyperplasia
> - Have a family history of colon cancer or Lynch syndrome
> - Have obesity
> - Have never been pregnant, especially if this was due to infertility
> - Take (or took) tamoxifen
>
> Data from American Cancer Society. (2019). *Endometrial cancer risk factors.* https://www.cancer.org/cancer/endometrial-cancer/causes-risks-prevention/risk-factors.html; Katz, A. (2019). Obesity-related cancer in women: A clinical review. *American Journal of Nursing, 119*(8), 34-40; and Rogers, J. L. (2023). *McCance and Huether's Pathophysiology: The biologic basis for disease in adults and children* (9th ed.). St. Louis: Elsevier.

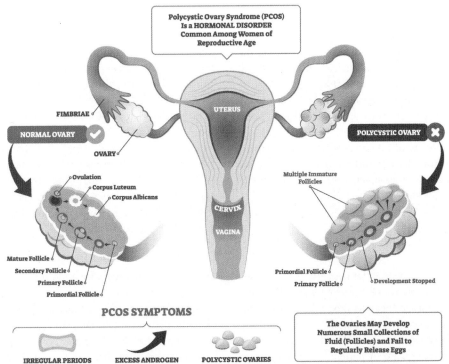

FIG. 63.5 Polycystic ovarian syndrome (PCOS). (Used with permission from istockphoto.com, 2019, VectorMine.)

- Dilation and curettage (when the patient cannot tolerate an endometrial biopsy)
- Hysteroscopy after dilation and curettage (for better visualization of the endometrial cavity)
- Chest x-ray
- Whole-body imaging of chest, abdomen, and pelvis (CT, MRI, positron emission tomography [PET], or combined PET/CT can be used)
- Liver and bone scans to assess for distant metastasis

Take Actions: Interventions

Surgical removal and cancer staging of the tumor with adjacent lymph nodes are the most important interventions for endometrial cancer. Cancer staging is often done using minimally invasive techniques, such as laparoscopic or robotic-assisted procedures.

Nonsurgical Management. Nonsurgical interventions (radiation therapy and chemotherapy) are typically used after surgery and depend on the surgical staging.

Radiation Therapy. The oncologist may prescribe radiation therapy to be delivered by external beam and/or brachytherapy, depending on stage and grade.

External beam radiation therapy can be used in combination with surgery, brachytherapy, and/or chemotherapy. It is given on an ambulatory basis in 30-minute increments, 5 days a week for 4 to 6 weeks (ACS, 2019). While the patient lies still, an external radiation beam is directed toward the radiation field. Teach the patient to monitor for signs of skin breakdown, especially in the perineal area; to avoid sunbathing; and to avoid washing the markings outlining the treatment site.

Brachytherapy is used to prevent disease recurrence. This procedure is used for women who have had their uterus and cervix removed (ACS, 2019). The upper part of the vagina is treated when a cylinder is placed inside it by the radiologist. In high-dose-rate (HDR) brachytherapy, each treatment takes about 10 to 20 minutes, and is given 3 to 5 times. While the radioactive implant is in place, radiation is emitted that can affect other people, so others will not be in the room.

Inform the patient that she is restricted to bed rest during the treatment session to prevent dislodgment of the radioactive source. At the completion of treatment, the patient may go home the same day. There are no restrictions to avoid family or the public between treatments. Depending on the oncologist's determination, treatments may be given weekly or daily for at least three doses (ACS, 2019).

Box 63.5 lists additional health teaching for the patient having brachytherapy for gynecologic cancer.

Reactions to radiation therapy vary. Some women report feeling "radioactive" after treatments and may exhibit withdrawal behaviors. Some patients may be concerned about how radiation affects ***sexuality***. Reassure them by correcting any misconceptions and encourage them to talk with their health care provider to receive specific recommendations regarding intimacy while receiving radiation treatment (ACS, 2020a). Chapter 18 discusses nursing care of patients receiving radiation therapy in more detail.

BOX 63.5 Best Practice for Patient Safety and Quality Care

Health Teaching for the Patient Having Brachytherapy for Gynecologic Cancer

Teach the patient that these short-term side effects are expected:
- Fatigue
- Urinary discomfort
- Urinary frequency (which may persist even beyond treatment)
- Loss of pubic hair, which is temporary
- Loose stools

Teach the patient to report any of these signs and symptoms to the health care provider immediately:
- Heavy vaginal bleeding
- Urethral burning for more than 24 hours
- Hematuria
- Extreme fatigue
- Severe diarrhea
- Fever over 100°F (38°C)
- Abdominal *pain*

Drug Therapy. Multiagent *chemotherapy* is used as palliative treatment in advanced and recurrent disease when it has spread to distant parts of the body, but it is not always effective (Campos & Cohn, 2022). For that reason, it is important to also consider other methods of palliative care, as discussed in Chapter 8. Chapter 18 describes chemotherapy and general nursing care during treatment.

Complementary and Integrative Health. Certain complementary and integrative therapies have been shown to decrease side effects of drug therapy, improve pain management, and support the patient's mental health (e.g., art therapy). Provide your patient with information that will help her make informed, evidence-based decisions. Remind her to check with her oncologist and/or pharmacist because some integrative therapies can be harmful or interfere with cancer treatment. Current evidence-based information is available at the American Cancer Society (www.cancer.org) and Canadian Cancer Society (www.cancer.ca) websites about various therapies available.

Surgical Management. The most common surgical procedure to treat endometrial cancer involves the removal of the uterus, fallopian tubes, and ovaries (total hysterectomy and bilateral salpingo-oophorectomy [BSO]) (Chen & Berek, 2022). Laparoscopy or robotic-assisted surgery is preferred when the disease is confined to the uterus (Cohn, 2022), as these surgeries are usually less expensive and have fewer complications and shorter hospital stays. If minimally invasive surgery is not possible, laparotomy can be considered. Vaginal or abdominal hysterectomies are also options.

Care Coordination and Transition Management

Home care after surgery for endometrial cancer is the same as that after a hysterectomy. Patients who are receiving chemotherapy or radiation therapy may be surprised by the fatigue that occurs. Help the patient and family plan daily activities around treatment requirements so that the patient can effectively conserve energy.

Every woman experiences cancer differently. It is not uncommon for the patient to express disbelief, anger, depression, anxiety, or withdrawal after a diagnosis of cancer. Assess these emotional reactions, and encourage the patient to discuss her feelings. Assess her support systems, and provide referrals as appropriate. In the United States, local American Cancer Society chapters provide written materials about endometrial cancer and information about local support groups. Each province in Canada also has a division of the Canadian Cancer Society.

Death can occur with or without treatment. The goal is for the patient to meet and exceed the 5-year survival mark without a recurrence of disease. If the tumor recurs and cure is unlikely, the woman and her family can consider hospice care and whether she can be cared for in the home. If nursing care is needed at home, assist with coordination of care with a home health care agency. A referral to a social services agency may be needed if the patient needs financial assistance for treatment and long-term follow-up.

OVARIAN CANCER

Pathophysiology Review

Ovarian cancer is the leading cause of gynecologic cancer death and the second most common type of gynecologic cancer in the United States (Chen & Berek, 2023). One of the most common types of ovarian cancer begins with precursor lesions, small groups of abnormal cells in a fallopian tube (Begun, 2022). Most ovarian cancers are epithelial tumors that grow on the surface of the ovaries. These tumors grow rapidly as a result of disordered cellular regulation. They spread quickly, and are often bilateral in nature. Tumor cells spread by direct extension into nearby organs and through blood and lymph circulation to distant sites. Free-floating cancer cells also spread through the abdomen to seed new sites, usually accompanied by ascites (abdominal fluid).

Risk factors include older age, being overweight or having obesity, nulliparity or having children later in life, use of estrogen with or without progesterone after menopause, and a family history of ovarian, breast, or colorectal cancer (ACS, 2021; Centers for Disease Control and Prevention [CDC], 2022b). Women with genetic mutations of *BRCA1* or *BRCA2* are at higher risk (National Ovarian Cancer Coalition [NOCC], 2022a). Of these, some choose to have a *risk-reducing bilateral salpingo-oophorectomy* (BSO) (see Box 63.1) to prevent ovarian cancer.

For many years, the use of talcum powder has been associated with the development of ovarian cancer. This myth continues to be perpetrated. However, the most current research shows that this correlation is not statistically significant (National Cancer Institute, 2022). Box 63.6 lists known and suspected risk factors for ovarian cancer.

Formerly, it was thought that ovarian cancer was a "silent" disease where symptoms did not present until the late stages of the disease. Evidence now shows that common symptoms of bloating; urinary urgency or frequency; difficulty eating, anorexia, or feeling full after a few bites of food; and abdominal or pelvic pain are often experienced very early in the disease process (Chen & Berek, 2023). Caught early, ovarian cancer is curable in 90% of women (Begun, 2022). However, many women do not seek care because they associate vague symptoms (weight gain, constipation, bloating) with menopause (Bohnenkamp et al., 2019)

BOX 63.6   Risk Factors for Ovarian Cancer

Women at higher risk for ovarian cancer include those who:
- Are middle-aged or older
- Are of Eastern European or Ashkenazi Jewish ethnicity
- Have close maternal or paternal family members with ovarian cancer
- Have a genetic mutation of the *BRCA1* or *BRCA2* gene or the gene associated with Lynch syndrome
- Have a personal history of breast, uterine, or colon cancer
- Have endometriosis
- Have never given birth or who have a history of trouble getting pregnant

Data from Centers for Disease Control and Prevention (CDC). (2022). What are the risk factors for ovarian cancer? https://www.cdc.gov/cancer/ovarian/basic_info/risk_factors.htm; Hall, M., & Neumann, C. (2022). Lynch syndrome (Hereditary nonpolyposis colorectal cancer): Cancer screening and management. Retrieved June 5, 2023, from https://www.uptodate.com/contents/lynch-syndrome-hereditary-nonpolyposis-colorectal-cancer-cancer-screening-and-management; Centers for Disease Control and Prevention. (2022). Obesity and cancer. https://www.cdc.gov/cancer/obesity/.

---

or an acute illness. Survival rates are much lower when this type of cancer is discovered in its later stages.

Interprofessional Collaborative Care
Recognize Cues: Assessment

As a matter of prevention, teach women to *"think ovarian"* even at the onset of vague abdominal and GI symptoms, such as **pain**, swelling, indigestion, or gas. Many women with ovarian cancer have experienced mild symptoms for several months but have associated them with perimenopausal changes, acute illness, or stress. Ask the patient whether she has had urinary frequency or incontinence, unexpected weight loss, and/or vaginal bleeding.

In some instances, patients present acutely and require urgent evaluation due to ascites, pleural effusion, bowel obstruction, or venous thromboembolism (Chen & Berek, 2023). These conditions are associated with advanced disease.

On pelvic examination, an abdominal mass may not be palpable until it reaches a size of 4 to 6 inches (10 to 15 cm). Any enlarged ovary found after menopause should be evaluated as though it were malignant.

A cancer antigen test, *CA 125,* measures the presence of damaged endometrial and uterine tissue in the blood. It may be elevated if ovarian cancer is present, but it can also be elevated in patients with endometriosis, fibroids, pelvic inflammatory disease, pregnancy, and even menses (Pagana et al., 2022). It can still be useful for monitoring a patient's progress during and after treatment.

A chest x-ray can be obtained to assess for metastasis, while CT scans can assess for ascites, pleural effusion, and mediastinal lymphadenopathy (Chen & Berek, 2023).

NCLEX Examination Challenge 63.3
Psychosocial Integrity

A client with ovarian cancer tells the nurse, "I don't know why I need surgery; I'm going to die from cancer anyway." Which nursing response is appropriate?
A. "Ovarian cancer is not always fatal."
B. "I can help you to arrange for hospice services."
C. "What if your family wants you to still have surgery?"
D. "It sounds as if you are concerned about your diagnosis."

Take Actions: Interventions

Nursing care of the patient with ovarian cancer is similar to that for the patient with endometrial or cervical cancer. The options for treatment depend on the extent of the cancer and usually include surgery first, followed by chemotherapy. External beam radiation therapy may be used for treatment of recurrent ovarian cancer (National Ovarian Cancer Coalition, 2022b).

A total abdominal hysterectomy, bilateral salpingo-oophorectomy (BSO; removal of the ovaries and fallopian tubes), and pelvic and paraaortic lymph node dissection are usually performed. Tumors are staged during surgery. Very large tumors that cannot be removed are debulked (reduced). These procedures can be performed via laparoscopic technique or robotic-assisted laparoscopy to decrease recovery time, minimize *pain,* and reduce postoperative complications.

A once-daily oral pill, Zejula (niraparib), is approved for maintenance therapy of newly diagnosed or recurrent germline BRCA-mutated (gBRCAm) ovarian cancer. This drug is used after complete or partial response to the most recent chemotherapy (GSK, 2022).

Nursing care of the patient is similar to that for any patient having abdominal surgery (see Chapter 9). As for any patient after abdominal surgery, assess vital signs and *pain* and maintain catheters and drains. Teach her the importance of antiembolism stockings, incentive spirometry, and early ambulation. Evaluate for respiratory or urinary *infection.* Assess vital signs, and monitor the quantity and quality of urine output.

After removing and staging ovarian cancer, *chemotherapy* is used often. See Chapter 18 for care of the patient with cancer for more information. Chemotherapeutic agents may be given IV and/or intraperitoneally.

Care Coordination and Transition Management

Teach patients discharged to home to avoid tampons, douches, and sexual intercourse for at least 6 weeks or as instructed by the surgeon. Remind them to keep their follow-up surgical appointment and to follow the surgeon's other recommendations about resuming usual activities.

Refer patients and their families to Gilda's Club within their local demographic (known as Red Door Community in New York City), and the National Ovarian Cancer Coalition (NOCC) (www.ovarian.org) for more information and support groups. In Canada, Ovarian Cancer Canada (www.ovariancanada.org) is available for the same purpose.

Ovarian cancer has a high recurrence rate. After recurrence, the cancer is considered treatable but no longer curable. If the patient refuses maintenance therapy, or if maintenance therapy is unsuccessful, the patient may deny symptoms at first or express feelings of anger and grief. The patient and family are often fearful of the outcome. Provide encouragement and support during this difficult time, and refer to grief counseling, spiritual leaders (if desired), and community support groups. For patients with advanced metastatic disease, collaborate with members of the interprofessional team for possible referral to hospice. Refer to Chapter 8 for more information on end-of-life care.

CERVICAL CANCER

Pathophysiology Review

The uterine cervix is covered with squamous cells on the outer cervix and columnar (glandular) cells that line the endocervical canal. Papanicolaou (Pap) tests sample cells from both areas as a screening test for cervical cancer. The squamocolumnar junction is the *transformation zone* where most cell abnormalities occur. The adolescent woman has more columnar cells exposed on the outer cervix, which may be one reason that she is more vulnerable to sexually transmitted infections (STIs) and human immunodeficiency virus (HIV). In contrast, in the menopausal woman the squamocolumnar junction may be higher up in the endocervical canal, making it difficult to sample for a Pap test.

Premalignant changes are classified on a continuum from cervical intraepithelial neoplasia (dysplasia) to cervical carcinoma in situ (where the full epithelial thickness of the cervix is involved) to invasive carcinoma (Rogers, 2023).

Most cervical cancers arise from the squamous cells on the outside of the cervix. The other cancers arise from the mucus-secreting glandular cells (adenocarcinoma) in the endocervical canal. The disease spreads by direct extension to the vaginal mucosa, lower uterine segment, parametrium, pelvic wall, bladder, and bowel. Metastasis is usually confined to the pelvis, but distant spread can occur through lymphatic spread and the circulation to the liver, lungs, or bones.

Human papillomavirus (HPV) *infection* is the most common type of sexually transmitted infection (STI) in the United States (CDC, 2022a). Almost all women will have HPV at some time in their lives, but not all types lead to cancer. Most cases of cervical cancer are caused by certain types of HPV. The high-risk HPV types 16 and 18 are responsible for 50% of cervical cancers (World Health Organization [WHO], 2022). They impair the tumor-suppressor gene and cause most of the cervical cancers. The unrestricted tissue growth can spread, becoming invasive and metastatic (Rogers, 2023). Risk factors for cervical cancer are listed in Box 63.7. Teach patients how to reduce their risk of sexual exposure to HPV by being immunized with an HPV vaccine, and using condoms during sexual intimacy.

Health Promotion/Disease Prevention

Girls and young women should be immunized with one of the HPV vaccines:

- *Gardasil* (available in Canada)—available for ages 9 through 26
- *Gardasil 9* (available in the United States and Canada)—available for ages 9 to 26; can be administered until age 45
- *Cervarix* (available in Canada)—available for ages 9 through 25

See Chapter 65 for a thorough discussion of the importance of HPV vaccination; Pap and HPV testing recommendations; and associated patient teaching. In addition to being immunized, women should be taught to follow the U.S. Preventive Services Task Force recommendations on Papanicolaou (Pap)

BOX 63.7 Risk Factors for Cervical Cancer

Women at higher risk for cervical cancer include those who:

- Are immunocompromised (e.g., have HIV or are taking immunosuppressant drugs for an autoimmune condition)
- Are daughters of women who took diethylstilbestrol (DES; a hormone to prevent miscarriage) between 1940 and 1971
- Became sexually active at a young age
- Do not eat a diet high in fruits and vegetables
- Smoke tobacco
- Have a family history of cervical cancer
- Have infection with human papillomavirus (HPV) and/or chlamydia
- Have obesity
- Have many sexual partners or one partner who is high risk
- Have used oral contraceptives (OCs) for a long length of time (risk diminishes when OCs are discontinued)
- Have had multiple full-term pregnancies
- Had a first full-term pregnancy earlier than age 20

Data from American Cancer Society. (2020). *Risk factors for cervical cancer.* https://www.cancer.org/cancer/cervical-cancer/causes-risks-prevention/risk-factors.html; Katz, A. (2019). Obesity-related cancer in women: A clinical review. *American Journal of Nursing, 119*(8), 34-40; Centers for Disease Control and Prevention. (2022). *Obesity and cancer.* https://www.cdc.gov/cancer/obesity/.

tests and HPV testing (U.S. Preventive Services Task Force, 2018).

Teach women to follow the U.S. Preventive Services Task Force (2018) recommendations on Pap and HPV testing:

A. If 21 to 29 years old, get a Pap test every 3 years.

B. If 30 to 65 years old, get:
  - A Pap test every 3 years, or
  - An HPV test every 5 years, or
  - A Pap test and HPV test together (called cotesting) every 5 years

C. If older than 65, ask the health care provider whether Pap tests and HPV tests can be stopped.

The Canadian Cancer Society (2023) recommends beginning Pap smears by the age of 21 if sexually active, and continuing every 1 to 3 years thereafter even if not sexually active. Patients in Canada are encouraged to talk to their health care provider for specific recommendations based on their own history and risk factors.

Interprofessional Collaborative Care

Recognize Cues: Assessment

The patient who has preinvasive cervical cancer is often asymptomatic. The classic symptoms of invasive cancer include painless vaginal bleeding, which may be irregular or heavy, and bleeding after sexual intercourse. As the cancer grows, bleeding increases in frequency, duration, and amount and may become continuous. As the disease advances, other symptoms may include pelvic or back pain, hematuria, hematochezia, or vaginal passage of stool or urine (Frumovitz, 2023). A physical examination may not reveal any abnormalities; however, the internal pelvic examination may identify late-stage disease.

An HPV-typing DNA test of the cervical sample taken alone or during the Pap test (ACS, 2020c) can determine the presence of one or more high-risk types of HPV (CDC, 2022a; Emory Winship Cancer Institute, 2023). The health care provider may perform a colposcopic examination to view the transformation zone. Colposcopy is a procedure in which application of an acetic acid solution is applied to the cervix. The cervix is then examined under magnification with a bright filter light that enhances the visualization of the characteristics of dysplasia or cancer. If abnormal tissue is recognized, multiple biopsies of the cervical tissue are performed.

If atypical glandular cells are suspected, the health care provider may perform a cervical biopsy in the form of a punch biopsy, a cone biopsy, or *endocervical curettage* (scraping of the endocervix wall) as well. Inform the patient that a small amount of bleeding is expected for several days after this procedure and that she should not douche, use tampons, or have sexual intercourse for at least a week.

Take Actions: Interventions

Interventions for the woman with cervical cancer are similar to those for endometrial cancer: surgery, which can be followed by radiation and chemotherapy for late-stage disease.

Nonsurgical Management. Radiation therapy, including brachytherapy and external beam radiation therapy (EBRT), can be used to treat certain stages of cervical cancer, or cervical cancer that has spread to other organs. A combination of chemotherapy and radiation, referred to as concurrent chemoradiation, may also be used. This treatment modality has been shown to be effective because the chemotherapy enhances the effect of the radiation. See Chapter 18 for more information about general nursing care for the patient on chemotherapy and radiation.

Surgical Management. Choice of surgical management approach is dependent on the patient's overall health, desire for future childbearing, tumor size and stage, cancer cell type, degree of lymph node involvement, and patient preference.

The loop electrosurgical excision procedure (LEEP) is short (10 to 30 minutes) and is performed in a health care provider's office or an ambulatory care setting with a local anesthetic injected into the cervix. A thin loop-wire electrode that transmits a painless electrical current is used to cut away affected tissue. LEEP (Fig. 63.6) is a diagnostic procedure as well as a treatment because it provides a specimen that can be examined by a pathologist to ensure that the lesion was completely removed. Spotting (very scant bleeding) and slight *pain* after the procedure is common. Teach patients to adhere to the restrictions listed in Box 63.8 for 3 weeks, or for the time frame recommended by the health care provider.

Laser surgery is also an office procedure done under local anesthesia to address early cancers. A laser beam is directed through the vagina to burn off abnormal cells. The procedure takes about 10 to 15 minutes. A small amount of bleeding occurs with the procedure, and the woman may have a slight vaginal discharge for several weeks. She can usually return to work in 2 to 3 days, yet be cautioned to avoid tampons and vaginal sexual activity for at least 2 to 3 weeks. A disadvantage of this procedure is that no specimen is available for study.

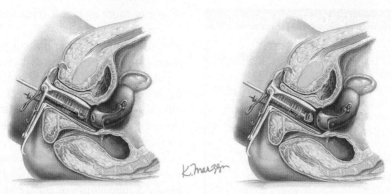

FIG. 63.6 Loop electrosurgical excision procedure (LEEP). (From Smith, R.P. [2018]. *Netter's Obstetrics and Gynecology* [3rd ed.]. Philadelphia: Elsevier.)

> ### BOX 63.8 Patient and Family Education
> #### Care After Local Cervical Ablation Therapies
>
> - Refrain from sexual intercourse.
> - Do not use tampons.
> - Do not douche.
> - Take showers rather than tub baths.
> - Avoid lifting heavy objects.
> - Report any heavy vaginal bleeding, foul-smelling drainage, or fever.

Cryosurgery involves freezing of the cancer, causing subsequent necrosis. The procedure is usually painless, although some women have slight cramping after it. Teach the patient that she will have heavy, watery brown discharge for several weeks after the procedure. Instruct her to follow the restrictions in Box 63.8.

In cases of microinvasive cancer, a *conization* can remove the affected tissue while still preserving fertility. This procedure is done when the lesion cannot be visualized by colposcopic examination. A cone-shaped area of cervix is removed surgically and sent to the laboratory to determine the extent of the cancer. Potential complications from this procedure include hemorrhage and uterine perforation. Long-term follow-up care is needed because new cancers can develop.

For women who may wish to become pregnant in the future, a *radical trachelectomy* can be done. This procedure does not guarantee the ability to carry a pregnancy to term, but it does provide a chance for that, although the risk for miscarriage is raised (ACS, 2020b). Going through the vagina or abdomen (sometimes laparoscopically), the cervix and upper part of the vagina are removed, leaving the body of the uterus intact (ACS, 2020b). A "purse-string" stitch is made to hold the opening of the uterus closed.

A hysterectomy may be performed as treatment of microinvasive cancer if the woman does not wish to become pregnant in the future. Care for patients undergoing hysterectomy is discussed earlier in this chapter in the Sexuality Concept Exemplar: Uterine Leiomyoma section.

Care Coordination and Transition Management

As with all patients who have undergone treatment, provide discharge teaching that is congruent with the procedure used.

Refer to psychosocial support as needed, and encourage the patient to keep all follow-up appointments.

VULVOVAGINITIS

Pathophysiology Review

Vaginal discharge and itching are two common problems experienced by most women at some time in their lives. Vaginal infections may be transmitted sexually or nonsexually. Gonorrhea, syphilis, chlamydia, and herpes simplex virus infections are sexually transmitted infections (STIs) discussed in Chapter 65.

Vulvovaginitis is inflammation of the lower genital tract resulting from a disturbance of the balance of hormones and flora in the vagina and vulva. It may be characterized by itching, change in vaginal discharge, odor, or lesions. Pediculosis pubis, known as crab lice, or "crabs," and scabies are parasitic infections of the vulvar skin that are *sexually* transmitted. The most common causes of *nonsexually* transmitted infections causing vulvovaginitis include (U.S. National Library of Medicine, 2022):

- Infections
  - Yeast infections related to *Candida albicans*
- Chemicals
  - Spermicide
  - Vaginal sponges
  - Feminine hygiene sprays
  - Bubble baths and soaps
  - Body lotion
- Other causes
  - Low levels of estrogen
  - Wearing tight-fitting or nonabsorbent clothing
  - Wiping from back to front, introducing bacteria from the stool into the vagina

Some women may develop an *itch-scratch-itch cycle*, in which the itching leads to scratching, which causes excoriation that then must heal. As healing takes place, itching occurs again. If the cycle is not interrupted, the chronic scratching may lead to the white, thickened skin of lichen planus. This dry, leathery skin cracks easily, increasing the risk for **infection.**

Interprofessional Collaborative Care

Assess for vulvovaginitis by asking questions about the symptoms, collecting information about whether the condition may

Prevention and Treatment of Vulvovaginitis

- Wear cotton underwear; nylon and other fabrics retain heat and moisture, which increases the risk for infection.
- Avoid wearing tight clothing because it can cause chafing. You can also get hot and sweaty, which can increase the risk for **infection.**
- Always wipe front to back after having a bowel movement or urinating.
- Use fragrance-free laundry detergent.
- During a bath or shower, cleanse the inner labial mucosa with water, not soap.
- Do not douche or use feminine hygiene sprays.
- Choose other methods of contraception instead of spermicide or vaginal sponges, which can irritate the condition.
- If your sexual partner has an **infection** of the sex organs, do not have intercourse with that partner until you both have been treated.
- You are more likely to get an **infection** if you are pregnant, have diabetes, take oral contraceptive drugs, or are menopausal. Make sure your primary health care provider is aware of any preexisting health conditions.
- If irritation is due to a yeast or parasitic infection, take or apply the prescribed drug treatment as ordered by the primary health care provider.
- Applying cool compresses several times a day can be helpful to minimize itching.

Prevention of Toxic Shock Syndrome

- Wash your hands before inserting a tampon.
- Do not use superabsorbent tampons.
- Do not use a tampon if it is dirty.
- Insert the tampon carefully to avoid injuring the delicate tissue in your vagina.
- Change your tampon every 3 to 6 hours.
- Use perineal pads ("sanitary napkins") instead of tampons at night.
- Avoid the use of insertable contraceptive devices.
- Regularly change tampons, cervical caps, and menstrual cups.
- Contact your primary health care provider if you experience a sudden onset of high temperature, vomiting, or diarrhea.
- Do not use tampons at all if you have had toxic shock syndrome.

have been transmitted sexually, assisting with a pelvic examination, and obtaining vaginal smears for laboratory testing. Ask whether the patient is experiencing an itching or burning sensation, erythema or erosions, edema, and/or superficial skin ulcers.

Interventions for vulvovaginitis depend on the specific cause. Sometimes treatment is as easy as removing the offending agent (e.g., avoiding bubble baths), whereas other treatment may be required if the condition is precipitated by a fungal or parasitic **infection**. Topical drugs such as estrogens and lidocaine may also be prescribed to relieve itching. Treatment of pediculosis and scabies is used if needed and includes:

- Applying a topical pediculicide to the affected area as prescribed
- Cleaning affected clothes, bedding, and towels
- Disinfecting the home environment (Lice cannot live for more than 24 hours away from the body.)

Remind patients that healthy habits such as good personal hygiene can benefit treatment. Teach patients how to manage the condition and prevent further infections per the instructions in Box 63.9.

TOXIC SHOCK SYNDROME

Pathophysiology Review

Toxic shock syndrome (TSS) can result from leaving a tampon, contraceptive sponge, diaphragm, menstrual cup, cervical cap, or other device in the vagina. The highest risk is associated with women who have preexisting staphylococcal colonization of the vagina and leave a device in place (Bush & Vazquez-Pertejo, 2023).

Risk factors for TSS, usually of streptococcal origin, include surgical wound **infection,** minor trauma, viral infection (e.g., varicella), diabetes, alcohol use, and the use of nonsteroidal antiinflammatory medications (NSAIDs) (Bush & Vazquez-Pertejo, 2023). *TSS can be fatal.*

Menstrual blood provides a growth medium for *Staphylococcus aureus* (or, less frequently, group A beta-hemolytic *Streptococcus* [GABHS], also known as *Streptococcus pyogenes*). Exotoxins produced from the bacteria cross the vaginal mucosa to the bloodstream via a mucosal break or via the uterus (Bush & Vazquez-Pertejo, 2023).

TSS usually develops within 5 days after the onset of menstruation. Its most common symptoms include:

- Fever of 102.2° to 104.9°F (39° to 45.5°C) that remains elevated despite treatment
- Diffuse macular rash, which often looks like a sunburn and begins 3 to 7 days after onset
- Hypotension
- Involvement of at least two other organ systems.

TSS due to *Staphylococcus aureus* also causes vomiting, diarrhea, confusion, thrombocytopenia, and elevated creatinine kinase; TSS due to streptococcal infection can cause acute respiratory distress syndrome (ARDS), coagulopathy, and hepatic damage (Bush & Vazquez-Pertejo, 2023). Renal impairment can occur in TSS caused by either organism.

Interprofessional Collaborative Care

Educate all women on prevention of TSS as covered in Box 63.10.

Treatment includes removal of the **infection** source, such as a tampon or other device; restoring fluid and electrolyte balance; administering drugs to manage hypotension; and infusion of IV antibiotics. Other measures may include transfusions to reverse low platelet counts, corticosteroids to treat skin changes, and hemodialysis and ventilatory support for patients in critical condition.

GET READY FOR THE NEXT-GENERATION NCLEX® EXAMINATION!

Essential Nursing Care Points

Health Promotion/Disease Prevention	Chronic Disease Care
• Identify and educate patients about the importance of screening for gynecologic cancers according to national guidelines and risk factors. • Teach women factors that place them at a higher risk for developing gynecologic cancer. • Discuss ways to change modifiable risk factors to decrease the chance for developing gynecologic cancers and conditions, pelvic organ prolapse, leiomyomas, and toxic shock syndrome. • Teach women to always use condoms during sexual intimacy to decrease the risk for *infection*.	• Provide support, education, and community referrals to patients with gynecologic cancer and their significant others. • Recognize that a diagnosis of gynecologic cancer can greatly impact a patient's life; refer those who need psychosocial support to social services or mental health professionals who can provide long-term assistance. • Remind patients desiring complementary and integrative therapies to discuss these with their health care provider.
Regenerative or Restorative Care	**Hospice/Palliative/Supportive Care**
• Monitor patients closely for bleeding after gynecologic surgery. • Use best practices when caring for a patient with a radioactive implant. • Ensure that the patient who is prescribed drug therapy understands the route of administration and how to properly take or administer the medication.	• Refer patients with terminal gynecologic cancer to hospice, palliative care, and support groups as appropriate.

Mastery Questions

1. The nurse is caring for a 26-year-old female client who reports becoming sexually active recently. Which of the following statements would the nurse provide? **Select all that apply.**
   A. "Use condoms at all times when sexually active."
   B. "The Gardasil-9 immunization is highly recommended."
   C. "Yellow or green vaginal discharge following intercourse is expected."
   D. "Plan on having a Pap test every 1 to 3 years to screen for cervical cancer."
   E. "Birth control pills can lower your chance of pelvic inflammatory disease."

2. The nurse has provided teaching to a client with a new diagnosis of vulvovaginitis. Which of the following client statements indicate that teaching has been effective? **Select all that apply.**
   A. "It is important to wear nylon underwear at all times."
   B. "My partner and I will use spermicide to prevent pregnancy."
   C. "I will wipe from the front to the back after I go to the bathroom."
   D. "It is time for me to get rid of some of my pants that fit too tightly."
   E. "Fragranced soap or body wash can help to prevent gynecologic odor."

NGN Challenge 63.1
63.1.1

The nurse documents assessment findings for a 52-year-old client who has come to the primary health care provider today for an annual visit.

Highlight the findings that would require **immediate** follow-up.

History and Physical	Nurses' Notes	Vital Signs	Laboratory Results

0900: Here today for annual visit; pelvic examination and Pap smear requested. Denies health problems within the past 12 months with the exception of irregular menstrual periods, which sometimes last more than a week, and "gaining weight in the abdomen." Reports that sometimes the bleeding is scant, whereas other times she has to get up two to three times at night to replace a perineal pad. Weight one year ago was 164 lb (74.4 kg) and today is 163 lb (73.9 kg). Denies passing clots, urinary symptoms, or bowel changes. Health history positive for hypertension for 10 years for which she takes amlodipine 5 mg twice daily. Works from home as a business consultant. Height: 67 in (170 cm); weight: 163 lb (73.9 kg). VS: T 98.4°F (36.9°C), HR 82 beats/min, RR 18 breaths/min, BP 132/80 mm Hg. Spo$_2$ 98% on RA.

63.1.2

The nurse documents the assessments performed.

| History and Physical | **Nurses' Notes** | Vital Signs | Laboratory Results |

0900: Here today for annual visit; pelvic examination and Pap smear requested. Denies health problems within the past 12 months with the exception of irregular menstrual periods, which sometimes last more than a week, and "gaining weight in the abdomen." Reports that sometimes the bleeding is scant, whereas other times she has to get up two to three times at night to replace a perineal pad. Weight one year ago was 164 pounds (74.4 kg) and today is 163 lb (73.9 kg). Denies passing clots, urinary symptoms, or bowel changes. Health history positive for hypertension for 10 years for which she takes amlodipine 5 mg twice daily. Works from home as a business consultant. Height: 67 in (170 cm); weight: 163 lb (73.9 kg). VS: T 98.4°F (36.9°C), HR 82 beats/min, RR 18 breaths/min, BP 132/80 mm Hg. Spo$_2$ 98% on RA.
0910: Abdominal assessment by nurse reveals no visible anomalies. Abdomen is soft and nontender with bowel sounds in all quadrants.
0920: Health care provider in to perform pelvic examination. Assisted with obtaining specimens for laboratory testing. Upon manual examination, provider states uterus feels enlarged. Ultrasounds ordered.

The nurse analyzes the findings to determine the client's condition. Complete the following sentence(s) by selecting from the lists of options below.

The client is at high risk for **1 [Select]**, as evidenced by **2 [Select]** and **3 [Select]**.

Options for 1	Options for 2	Options for 3
Toxic shock syndrome	History of hypertension	Taking amlodipine
Uterine leiomyoma	Bleeding that exceeds a week	Weight reduction of 1 lb in a year
Cystocele	Sitting often when working from home	Changing perineal pads at night
Vulvovaginitis	Not seeing the primary health care provider for a year	BMI overweight

63.1.3

The nurse considers the client data to determine the priority for the plan of care.

| Health History | **Nurses' Notes** | Vital Signs | Laboratory Results |

0900: Here today for annual visit; pelvic examination and Pap smear requested. Denies health problems within the past 12 months with the exception of irregular menstrual periods, which sometimes last more than a week, and "gaining weight in the abdomen." Reports that sometimes the bleeding is scant, whereas other times she has to get up two to three times at night to replace a perineal pad. Weight one year ago was 164 pounds (74.4 kg) and today is 163 lb (73.9 kg). Denies passing clots, urinary symptoms, or bowel changes.
Health history positive for hypertension for 10 years for which she takes amlodipine 5 mg twice daily. Works from home as a business consultant. Height: 67 in (170 cm); weight: 163 lb (73.9 kg). VS: T 98.4°F (36.9°C), HR 82 beats/min, RR 18 breaths/min, BP 132/80 mm Hg. Spo$_2$ 98% on RA.
0910: Abdominal assessment by nurse reveals no visible anomalies. Abdomen is soft and nontender with bowel sounds in all quadrants.
0920: Health care provider in to perform pelvic examination. Assisted with obtaining specimens for laboratory testing. Upon manual examination, provider states uterus feels enlarged. Ultrasounds ordered.

Complete the following sentence(s) by selecting from the list of word choices below.

The *priority* for the client at this time is to manage **[Word Choice]** to prevent **[Word Choice]**.

Word Choices
Hypertension
Weight concerns
Abnormal uterine bleeding
Pelvic organ prolapse
Anemia

63.1.4

Several days later, the client's ultrasound results are available and confirm the presence of a 14-cm leiomyoma. The primary health care provider refers care to a gynecologic surgeon, who recommends a hysterectomy.

Which of the following information would the nurse plan to include as a part of preoperative teaching? **Select all that apply.**

○ How pain will be controlled
○ Periods will be lighter after procedure
○ Need for early ambulation after surgery
○ Expectation that weight gain will occur
○ Birth control is not needed after hysterectomy
○ Hysterectomy helps to avoid menopausal symptoms

63.1.5

Twelve hours after surgery, the nurse is monitoring the client on a medical-surgical floor. Select the **2** assessment findings the nurse would report to the surgeon.

○ Hematocrit 32% (0.32 volume fraction) (Reference range: 37%–47% [0.37–0.47 volume fraction])
○ WBC 6500/mm^3 (6.5 x 10^9/L) (Reference range: 5000–10,000/mm^3 [5–10 × 10^9/L])
○ Hemoglobin 9.6 g/dL (5.6 mmol/L) (Reference range: 12–16 g/dL [7.4–9.9 mmol/L])
○ Temperature 99.4°F (37.4°C)
○ Saturated one perineal pad in 6 hours
○ Pain level 4 out of 10 on 0-to-10 scale
○ Used incentive spirometer once hourly

63.1.6

Twenty-four hours later, the nurse assesses the client again. For each current client finding, indicate if the interventions were effective (helped to meet expected outcomes) or not effective (did not help to meet expected outcomes).

Previous Client Finding	Current Client Finding	Effective	Not Effective
Hematocrit 32% (0.32 volume fraction) (Reference range: 37%–47% [0.37–0.47 volume fraction])	Hematocrit 33% (0.33 volume fraction)		
WBC 6500/mm^3 (6.5 x 10^9/L) (Reference range: 5000–10,000/mm^3 [5–10 × 10^9/L])	WBC 14,500/mm^3 (14.5 x 10^9/L)		
Hemoglobin 9.6 g/dL (5.6 mmol/L) (Reference range: 12–16 g/dL [7.4–9.9 mmol/L])	Hemoglobin 10.8 g/dL (6.7 mmol/L)		
Saturated one perineal pad in 6 hours	Saturated one perineal pad in 8 hours		
Pain level of 4 on a 0-to-10 scale	Pain level of 2 on a 0-to-10 scale		

REFERENCES

Asterisk (*) indicates a classic or definitive work on this subject.

American Cancer Society (ACS). (2018). *About ovarian cancer.* Retrieved from https://www.cancer.org/cancer/ovarian-cancer/about/what-is-ovarian-cancer.html.

American Cancer Society (ACS). (2019). *Radiation therapy for endometrial cancer.* Retrieved from https://www.cancer.org/cancer/endometrial-cancer/treating/radiation.html.

American Cancer Society (ACS). (2020a). *Radiation therapy can affect the sex life of females with cancer.* Retrieved from http://www.cancer.org/treatment/treatments-and-side-effects/physical-side-effects/fertility-and-sexual-side-effects/sexuality-for-women-with-cancer/pelvic-radiation.html.

American Cancer Society (ACS). (2020b). *Surgery for cervical cancer.* Retrieved from https://www.cancer.org/cancer/cervical-cancer/treating/surgery.html.

American Cancer Society (ACS). (2020c). *The HPV DNA test.* Retrieved from https://www.cancer.org/cancer/cervical-cancer/prevention-and-early-detection/hpv-test.html.

American Cancer Society (ACS). (2021). Ovarian cancer risk factors. https://www.cancer.org/cancer/ovarian-cancer/causes-risks-prevention/risk-factors.html.

American Cancer Society (ACS). (2022). *Key statistics for endometrial cancer.* Retrieved from https://www.cancer.org/cancer/endometrial-cancer/about/key-statistics.html.

Begun, C. (2022). *Key to detecting ovarian cancer early may be in the fallopian tubes.* https://www.pennmedicine.org/news/news-blog/2022/march/key-to-detecting-ovarian-cancer-early-may-be-in-the-fallopian-tubes.

Bohnenkamp, S., McClurg, E., & Bohnenkamp, Z. (2019). What medical-surgical nurses need to know about caring for patients with epithelial ovarian cancer: Part I. *Medsurg Nursing, 28*(5), 334–338.

Bradley, L. (2021). Hysteroscopy: Managing fluid and gas distending media. *UpToDate.* Retrieved June 6, 2023, from https://www.uptodate.com/contents/hysteroscopy-managing-fluid-and-gas-distending-media.

Bradley, L. (2022). Uterine fibroids (leiomyomas): Hysteroscopic myomectomy. *UpToDate.* Retrieved June 6, 2023, from https://www.uptodate.com/contents/uterine-fibroids-leiomyomas-hysteroscopic-myomectomy.

Bush, L., & Vazquez-Pertejo, M. (2023). *Toxic shock syndrome.* https://www.merckmanuals.com/professional/infectious-diseases/gram-positive-cocci/toxic-shock-syndrome-tss.

Campos, S., & Cohn, D. (2023). Treatment of metastatic endometrial cancer. *UpToDate.* Retrieved June 6, 2023, from https://www.uptodate.com/contents/treatment-of-metastatic-endometrial-cancer.

Canadian Cancer Society. (2023). *When should I be screened for cervical cancer?* https://cancer.ca/en/cancer-information/find-cancer-early/get-screened-for-cervical-cancer/when-should-i-be-screened-for-cervical-cancer.

Centers for Disease Control and Prevention (CDC). (2022a). *Genital HPV infection: Basic fact sheet.* www.cdc.gov/std/hpv/stdfact-hpv.htm.

Centers for Disease Control and Prevention (CDC). (2022b). *What are the risk factors for ovarian cancer?* Retrieved from https://www.cdc.gov/cancer/ovarian/basic_info/risk_factors.htm.

Chen, L., & Berek, J. (2022). Patient education: Endometrial cancer treatment after surgery (Beyond the basics). *UpToDate.* Retrieved June 6, 2023, from https://www.uptodate.com/contents/endometrial-cancer-diagnosis-staging-and-surgical-treatment-beyond-the-basics.

Chen, L., & Berek, J. (2023). Epithelial carcinoma of the ovary, fallopian tube, and peritoneum: Clinical features and diagnosis. *UpToDate*. Retrieved June 6, 2023, from https://www.uptodate.com/contents/epithelial-carcinoma-of-the-ovary-fallopian-tube-and-peritoneum-clinical-features-and-diagnosis.

Cleveland Clinic. (2023). Estrogen. https://my.clevelandclinic.org/health/body/22353-estrogen.

Cohn, D. (2022). Endometrial carcinoma: Staging and surgical treatment. *UpToDate*. Retrieved June 6, 2023, from https://www.uptodate.com/contents/endometrial-carcinoma-staging-and-surgical-treatment.

Emory Winship Cancer Institute. (2023). *HPV DNA test*. https://www.cancerquest.org/patients/detection-and-diagnosis/hpv-dna-test.

Fashokun, T., & Rogers, R. (2023). Pelvic organ prolapse in women: Diagnostic evaluation. *UpToDate*. Retrieved June 6, 2023, from https://www.uptodate.com/contents/pelvic-organ-prolapse-in-women-diagnostic-evaluation.

Feldman, S., & Levine, D. (2023). Overview of evaluation of the endometrium for malignant or premalignant disease. *UpToDate*. Retrieved June 6, 2023, from https://www.uptodate.com/contents/overview-of-the-evaluation-of-the-endometrium-for-malignant-or-premalignant-disease.

Frumovitz, M. (2023). Invasive cervical cancer: Epidemiology, risk factors, clinical manifestations, and diagnosis. *UpToDate*. Retrieved June 6, 2023, from https://www.uptodate.com/contents/invasive-cervical-cancer-epidemiology-risk-factors-clinical-manifestations-and-diagnosis.

Giuliani, E., As-Sanie, S., & Marsh, E. (2020). Epidemiology and management of uterine fibroids. *International Journal of Gynecology & Obstetrics*, 149(1), 3–9.

GSK. (2022). *Why Zejula (niraparib)?* https://zejula.com/about/why-zejula/.

Jelovsek, J. (2023). Pelvic organ prolapse in women: Choosing a primary surgical procedure. *UpToDate*. Retrieved June 22, 2023, from https://www.uptodate.com/contents/pelvic-organ-prolapse-in-women-choosing-a-primary-surgical-procedure.

Mahajan, S. (2021). Pelvic organ prolapse in women: Surgical repair of anterior vaginal wall prolapse. *UpToDate*. Retrieved June 22, 2023, from https://www.uptodate.com/contents/pelvic-organ-prolapse-in-women-surgical-repair-of-anterior-vaginal-wall-prolapse.

Mohammadi, R., Tabrizi, R., Hessami, K., et al. (2020). Correlation of low serum vitamin-D with uterine leiomyoma: A systematic review and meta-analysis. *Reproductive Biology & Endocrinology*, 18, 85. https://doi.org/10.1186/s12958-020-00644-6.

National Cancer Institute. (2022). *Ovarian, fallopian tube, and primary peritoneal cancer prevention (PDQ®)–Health professional version*. https://www.cancer.gov/types/ovarian/hp/ovarian-prevention-pdq#cit/section_3.51.

National Institute of Diabetes and Digestive and Kidney Disorders. (2018). *Definition and facts for lactose intolerance*. https://www.niddk.nih.gov/health-information/digestive-diseases/lactose-intolerance/definition-facts.

National Ovarian Cancer Coalition (NOCC). (2022a). Information for every woman: Ovarian cancer risk factors. https://ovarian.org/about-ovarian-cancer/whos-at-risk/.

National Ovarian Cancer Coalition (NOCC). (2022b). *Overview: External beam radiation therapy*. https://ovarian.org/treatment-options/radiation/.

Pagana, K. D., Pagana, T. J., & Pagana, T. N. (2022). *Mosby's manual of diagnostic and laboratory tests* (7th ed.). St. Louis: Elsevier.

Plaxe, S., & Mundt, A. (2022). Overview of endometrial carcinoma. *UpToDate*. Retrieved June 6, 2023, from https://www.uptodate.com/contents/overview-of-endometrial-carcinoma?search=overview%20of%20endometrial%20carcinoma%20plaxe&source=search_result&selectedTitle=2~150&usage_type=default&display_rank=2.

Rogers, J. L. (2023). *McCance and Huether's Pathophysiology: The biologic basis for disease in adults and children* (9th ed.). St. Louis: Elsevier.

Stewart, E. (2023). Uterine fibroids (leiomyomas): Treatment overview. *UpToDate*. Retrieved June 5, 2023, from https://www.uptodate.com/contents/uterine-fibroids-leiomyomas-treatment-overview.

Stewart, E., & Laughlin-Tommaso, S. (2023). Uterine Fibroids: Epidemiology, clinical features, diagnosis, and natural history. *UpToDate*. Retrieved June 6, 2023, from https://www.uptodate.com/contents/uterine-fibroids-leiomyomas-epidemiology-clinical-features-diagnosis-and-natural-history.

Szydłowska, I., Nawrocka-Rutkowska, J., Brodowska, A., Marciniak, A., Starczewski, A., & Szczuko, M. (2022). Dietary natural compounds and vitamins as potential cofactors in uterine fibroids growth and development. *Nutrients*, 14(4), 734. https://doi.org/10.3390/nu14040734.

U.S. Food and Drug Administration (FDA). (2021a). *Pelvic organ prolapse: Surgical mesh considerations and recommendations*. https://www.fda.gov/medical-devices/urogynecologic-surgical-mesh-implants/pelvic-organ-prolapse-pop-surgical-mesh-considerations-and-recommendations.

U.S. Food and Drug Administration (FDA). (2021b). *Urogynecologic surgical mesh implants*. Retrieved from https://www.fda.gov/medical-devices/implants-and-prosthetics/urogynecologic-surgical-mesh-implants.

U.S. National Library of Medicine. (2022). *Vulvovaginitis*. Retrieved from https://medlineplus.gov/ency/article/000897.htm.

U.S. Preventive Services Task Force. (2018). *Cervical cancer: Screening*. Retrieved from https://www.uspreventiveservicestaskforce.org/uspstf/recommendation/cervical-cancer-screening.

van der Kooij, S., & Hehenkamp, W. (2022). Uterine leiomyomas (fibroids): Treatment with uterine artery embolization. *UpToDate*. Retrieved June 7, 2023, from https://www.uptodate.com/contents/uterine-fibroids-leiomyomas-treatment-with-uterine-artery-embolization.

Walters, M., & Ferrando, C. (2022). Hysterectomy for benign indications: Selection of surgical route. *UpToDate*. Retrieved June 6, 2023, from https://www.uptodate.com/contents/hysterectomy-benign-indications-selection-of-surgical-route.

World Health Organization (WHO). (2022). *Human papillomavirus (HPV) and cervical cancer*. Retrieved from https://www.who.int/news-room/fact-sheets/detail/human-papillomavirus-(hpv)-and-cervical-cancer.

64

Concepts of Care for Patients With Male Reproductive Conditions

Cherie R. Rebar

http://evolve.elsevier.com/Iggy/

LEARNING OUTCOMES

1. Plan collaborative care with the interprofessional team to promote *elimination* and *cellular regulation* in patients with male reproductive disorders.
2. Teach adults how to decrease the risk for male reproductive disorders.
3. Teach the patient and caregiver(s) about common drugs and other management strategies used for male reproductive disorders.
4. Plan patient- and family-centered nursing interventions to decrease the psychosocial impact caused by living with a male reproductive disorder.
5. Apply knowledge of anatomy, physiology, and pathophysiology to provide evidence-based care for patients with a male reproductive disorder affecting *elimination* or *cellular regulation.*
6. Analyze assessment and diagnostic findings to generate solutions and prioritize nursing care for patients with a male reproductive disorder.
7. Organize care coordination and transition management for patients with a male reproductive disorder.
8. Use clinical judgment to plan evidence-based nursing care to promote *elimination* and *cellular regulation* and prevent complications in patients with a male reproductive disorder.
9. Incorporate factors that affect health equity into the plan of care for patients with male reproductive disorders.

KEY TERMS

active surveillance (AS) Observation for cancer without immediate active treatment.

azoospermia The absence of living sperm in the semen.

brachytherapy Procedure in which small pellets are inserted internally into tissue; also known as *seed implantation* or *interstitial radiation therapy.*

cryptorchidism Failure of the testes to descend into the scrotum.

erectile dysfunction (ED) The inability to achieve or maintain a penile erection sufficient for sexual intercourse.

external beam radiation therapy (EBRT) Radiation focused on a target area from a machine outside the body.

gynecomastia Abnormal enlargement of the breasts in men.

hydronephrosis Abnormal enlargement of the kidney caused by a blockage of urine lower in the tract and filling of the kidney with urine.

hydroureter Abnormal distention of the ureter.

hyperplasia Growth that causes tissue to increase in size by increasing the number of cells; abnormal overgrowth of tissue.

lower urinary tract symptoms (LUTS) Symptoms that occur because of prostatic hyperplasia, such as urinary retention and overflow incontinence, or urinary leaking.

oligospermia Low sperm count.

orchiectomy The surgical removal of one or both testes.

prostate artery embolization A procedure in which the interventional radiologist threads a small vascular catheter into the prostate's arteries and injects particles blocking some of the blood flow to shrink the prostate gland.

prostate-specific antigen (PSA) A glycoprotein produced solely by the prostate.

prostatitis Inflammation and possible infection of the prostate.

retrograde ejaculation A condition in which semen flows backward into the bladder so that only a small amount will be ejaculated from the penis; usually is a result of nerve damage during surgery.

transurethral resection of the prostate (TURP) The traditional "closed" surgical procedure for removal of the prostate.

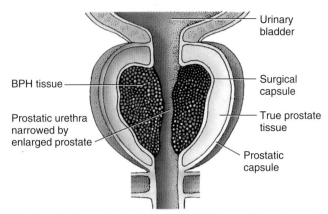

FIG. 64.1 Benign prostatic hyperplasia (BPH) grows inward, causing narrowing of the urethra.

Within this chapter, the terms "male," "man," or "men" and the pronouns "he" and "him" apply to all individuals who were assigned male at birth (AMAB), which includes cisgender men, transgender women, and nonbinary people with penises (New York Presbyterian, n.d.).

The nurse's role in caring for men with reproductive problems is to be open, supportive, and nonjudgmental. Male reproductive problems are very personal and can range from short-term infections to long-term health care problems that require end-of-life care. These conditions can affect the human needs for *sexuality, elimination,* and *reproduction,* all of which can affect the patient's physiologic and psychosocial sense of well-bring. See Chapter 1 for a review of the nursing concepts applied in this chapter.

ELIMINATION CONCEPT EXEMPLAR: BENIGN PROSTATIC HYPERPLASIA

Pathophysiology Review

With aging and increased dihydrotestosterone (DHT) levels, the glandular units in the prostate undergo nodular tissue hyperplasia (an increase in the number of cells; an abnormal overgrowth of tissue). This altered tissue promotes local inflammation by attracting cytokines and other substances (Rogers, 2023).

As the prostate gland enlarges, it extends upward into the bladder and inward, causing bladder outlet obstruction (BOO) (Fig. 64.1). In response, urinary *elimination* is affected in several ways, causing lower urinary tract symptoms (LUTS)—an umbrella term that includes problems such as urinary retention, urinary leaking, or incontinence.

First, the detrusor (bladder) muscle thickens to help urine push past the enlarged prostate gland (Rogers, 2023). Despite the bladder muscle change, the patient experiences increased residual urine (stasis) and chronic urinary retention. The increased volume of residual urine often causes overflow urinary incontinence, in which the urine "leaks" around the enlarged prostate, causing dribbling. Urinary stasis can also result in urinary tract infections and bladder calculi (stones).

In some instances, the prostate becomes very large and results in *acute urinary retention* (AUR). The patient with this problem requires *emergent* care. In other patients, *chronic* *urinary retention* may result in a backup of urine and cause a gradual, abnormal distention of the ureters (hydroureter) and enlargement of the kidneys (hydronephrosis) if benign prostatic hyperplasia (BPH) is not treated. These urinary *elimination* problems can lead to chronic kidney disease, as described in Chapter 60.

Etiology and Genetic Risk

BPH is a very common male health problem, but the exact cause is unclear. Its relationship to aging is the only known factor (Rogers, 2023). Other nonmodifiable risk factors include (McVary, 2023b):
- Race
  - Black men younger than 65 need treatment more often than White men.
  - LUTS is more common in Black men than White men.
  - Asian men have BPH less often than Black and White men.
  - Asian men are less likely to need surgery for BPH than White men.
- Genetic susceptibility—Variants in the *GATA3* gene have been associated with development of BPH/LUTS.
- Family history of cancer—Men with a family history of bladder cancer (*not* prostate cancer) are at higher risk to develop BPH.

Modifiable risk factors include (McVary, 2023a; McVary, 2023b):
- Obesity and metabolic syndrome—Obesity, glucose intolerance, dyslipidemia, and hypertension are associated with a higher risk for development of BPH.
- Beverage consumption—Coffee and caffeine intake have been associated with an increase in risk for progression of existing LUTS/BPH.
- Physical activity—Lower levels of activity are associated with development of LUTS.

Incidence and Prevalence

Benign prostatic hyperplasia (BPH) affects 50% of men between the ages of 51 and 60 and over 80% of men older than 70 years (Yale Medicine, 2023). BPH is one of the common reasons that men seek urology care (Yale Medicine, 2023).

Health Promotion/Disease Prevention

Teach men that BPH occurs commonly and that sexual frequency does not cause this condition. Current evidence does not show that there are absolute specific actions that prevent the development of BPH; however, teach men that addressing modifiable risk factors can improve their overall health.

Interprofessional Collaborative Care

Recognize Cues: Assessment

History. When taking a history, several standardized assessment tools are used to help the health care provider determine the severity of lower urinary tract symptoms (LUTS) associated with prostatic enlargement. One of the most commonly used assessments is the International Prostate Symptom Score (I-PSS) (Fig. 64.2). This tool incorporates the American Urological Association Symptom Index (AUA-SI) as questions 1 through 7 and asks an eighth question about the implication of the patient's urinary symptoms on quality of life. Most patients complete the questions as a self-administered tool because it is available in many languages. If the patient cannot read, or does not wish to read, the nurse or health care provider can ask the questions to complete the assessment.

Physical Assessment/Signs and Symptoms. Ask about the patient's current urinary *elimination* pattern, and ask whether it has changed recently. Assess for urinary frequency and urgency. Determine the number of times the patient awakens during sleep to void. Also assess for:

- Difficulty in starting (hesitancy) and continuing urination
- Reduced force and size of the urinary stream ("weak" stream)
- Sensation of incomplete bladder emptying
- Straining to begin urination
- Postvoid dribbling or leaking

The patient is also at risk to develop an *infection* or other bladder problem. Ask whether the patient has noticed blood in the urine, as BPH is a common cause of hematuria in older men due to *infection.*

Remind the patient to void before the physical examination. Inspect and palpate the abdomen. If the patient has a sense of urgency when gentle pressure is applied, the bladder may be distended. Patients with obesity are best assessed by percussion (done by the health care provider) or bedside ultrasound bladder scanner rather than by inspection or palpation.

Prepare the patient for the prostate gland examination, which will be conducted by the health care provider. Tell him that he may feel the urge to urinate as the prostate is palpated. Because the prostate is close to the rectal wall, it is easily examined by *digital rectal examination* (DRE). If needed, help the patient bend over the examination table or assume a side-lying fetal position, whichever is the easiest position for him. The health care provider assesses for size and consistency of the prostate. BPH presents as a uniform, elastic, nontender enlargement, whereas cancer of the prostate gland feels like a stony-hard nodule. Advise the patient that after the prostate gland is palpated, it may be massaged to obtain a fluid sample for examination to rule out prostatitis (inflammation and possible *infection* of the prostate), a common problem that can occur with BPH. If the patient has bacterial prostatitis, he is treated with broad-spectrum antibiotic therapy to prevent the spread of infection (Rogers, 2023).

Psychosocial Assessment. Patients who have nocturia and other LUTS may be frustrated or depressed as a result of interrupted sleep and ongoing visits to the bathroom. Assess the effect of sleep interruptions on the patient's mood and mental status. Ask him about the impact of symptoms on *sexuality* and libido.

Postvoid dribbling and overflow incontinence may cause embarrassment and prevent the patient from socializing or leaving the home. For some patients, social isolation can affect quality of life and lead to clinical depression and/or severe anxiety. Provide time for the patient to express his feelings about these concerns.

Laboratory Assessment. A *urinalysis* and a urine *culture* are typically obtained to diagnose urinary tract infection and microscopic hematuria. If *infection* is present, the urinalysis measures the number of white blood cells (WBCs).

Other laboratory studies that may be performed include:

- A *complete blood count* (CBC) to evaluate any evidence of systemic infection (elevated WBCs) or anemia (decreased red blood cells [RBCs]) from hematuria.
- *Blood urea nitrogen* (BUN) and *serum creatinine* levels to evaluate renal function (both are usually elevated with kidney disease).
- A *prostate-specific antigen* (PSA) test for screening purposes
- A *serum acid phosphatase* level if metastatic prostate cancer is suspected (this is typically elevated in patients who have prostate cancer that has metastasized).
- A biopsy, which may be performed if life expectancy is greater than 5 to 10 years and if needed to confirm a histologic diagnosis (Taplin & Smith, 2023).

Other Diagnostic Assessment. Imaging studies that are typically performed are transrectal ultrasound (TRUS) and MRI (Taplin & Smith, 2023). The patient having a TRUS lies on his side while the transducer is inserted into the rectum for viewing the prostate and surrounding structures. A tissue biopsy may also be done during this procedure. Prostate-specific membrane antigen (PSMA) positron emission tomography (PET) scanning can be used to detect soft tissue and distant metastases (Taplin & Smith, 2023).

In some cases, cystoscopy may be ordered to view the interior of the bladder, the bladder neck, and the urethra. This procedure is used to study the presence and effect of bladder neck obstruction and is usually done in an ambulatory care setting. Residual urine can also be measured when the cystoscope is inserted. See Chapter 57 for a detailed description of *cystoscopy* and the nursing care needed for patients having this procedure.

Residual urine may be determined by *bladder ultrasound* immediately after the patient voids. *Urodynamic pressure-flow studies* can be helpful in determining whether there is urine blockage or weakness of the detrusor muscle.

Analyze Cues and Prioritize Hypotheses: Analysis

The priority collaborative problem for the patient with benign prostatic hyperplasia (BPH) is:

1. Urinary retention due to bladder outlet obstruction (BOO)

International Prostate Symptom Score (I-PSS)

Patient Name:_____ Date of Birth:_____ Date Completed_____

In the past month:	Not at All	Less Than 1 in 5 Times	Less Than Half the Time	About Half the Time	More Than Half the Time	Almost Always	Your Score
1. Incomplete Emptying How often have you had the sensation of not emptying your bladder?	0	1	2	3	4	5	
2. Frequency How often have you had to urinate less than every 2 hours?	0	1	2	3	4	5	
3. Intermittency How often have you found you stopped and started again several times when you urinated?	0	1	2	3	4	5	
4. Urgency How often have you found it difficult to postpone urination?	0	1	2	3	4	5	
5. Weak Stream How often have you had a weak urinary stream?	0	1	2	3	4	5	
6. Straining How often have you had to strain to start urination?	0	1	2	3	4	5	
	None	**1 Time**	**2 Times**	**3 Times**	**4 Times**	**5 Times**	
7. Nocturia How many times do you typically get up at night to urinate?	0	1	2	3	4	5	
Total I-PSS Score							

Score: 1-7: Mild   8-19: Moderate   20-35: Severe

Quality of Life Due to Urinary Symptoms	Delighted	Pleased	Mostly Satisfied	Mixed	Mostly Dissatisfied	Unhappy	Terrible
If you were to spend the rest of your life with your urinary condition just the way it is now, how would you feel about that?	0	1	2	3	4	5	6

FIG. 64.2 The International Prostate Symptom Score (I-PSS). (Adapted from the American Urological Association Practice Guidelines Committee. [2003]. Guideline on the management of benign prostatic hyperplasia [BPH]. *Journal of Urology, 170*[2 Pt 1], 530–547.)

About the I-PSS

The International Prostate Symptom Score (I-PSS) is based on the answers to seven questions concerning urinary symptoms and one question concerning quality of life. Each question concerning urinary symptoms allows the patient to choose one out of six answers indicating increasing severity of the particular symptom. The answers are assigned points from 0 to 5. The total score can therefore range from 0 to 35 (asymptomatic to very symptomatic).

The questions refer to the following urinary symptoms:

Questions	Symptom
1	Incomplete emptying
2	Frequency
3	Intermittency
4	Urgency
5	Weak stream
6	Straining
7	Nocturia

Question 8 refers to the patient's perceived quality of life.

The first seven questions of the I-PSS are identical to the questions appearing on the American Urological Association (AUA) Symptom Index, which currently categorizes symptoms as follows:

Mild (symptom score less than or equal to 7)

Moderate (symptom score range 8 to 19)

Severe (symptom score range 20 to 35)

The International Scientific Committee (SCI), under the patronage of the World Health Organization (WHO) and the International Union Against Cancer (UICC), recommends the use of only a single question to assess the quality of life. The answers to this question range from "delighted" to "terrible," or 0 to 6. Although this single question may or may not capture the global impact of benign prostatic hyperplasia (BPH) symptoms or quality of life, it may serve as a valuable starting point for a doctor-patient conversation.

The SCI has agreed to use the symptom index for BPH, which has been developed by the AUA Measurement Committee, as the official worldwide symptoms assessment tool for patients suffering from prostatism.

The SCI recommends that physicians consider the following components for a basic diagnostic workup: history; physical examination; appropriate labs such as U/A, creatinine, etc.; and DRE or other evaluation to rule out prostate cancer.

Fig. 64.2, cont'd

Generate Solutions and Take Actions: Planning and Implementation

Improving Urinary Elimination

Planning: Expected Outcomes. The patient with BPH is expected to have a normal urinary *elimination* pattern without lower urinary tract symptoms (LUTS) or *infection.*

Interventions. Treatment for BPH ranges from careful monitoring to surgery, depending on the degree of impairment the patient is experiencing. If the patient is not experiencing complications or discomfort, behavioral modification may be recommended. Patients with symptomatic BPH are usually first treated with nonsurgical interventions, such as drug therapy.

Nonsurgical Management

Behavioral modification. Teach patients with BPH to avoid drinking large amounts of fluid in a short time, especially before going out or at bedtime (McVary, 2023b). Caffeine and alcohol consumption should be limited, as these have a diuretic effect. Caution patients to talk with their primary health care provider about drugs that can cause urinary retention, especially anticholinergics, antihistamines, antipsychotics, and muscle

TABLE 64.1 Common Examples of Drug Therapy

Drug Therapy Used to Treat Benign Prostatic Hyperplasia (BPH)

Drug Category	Selected Nursing Implications
5-Alpha-Reductase Inhibitors	
Common examples of 5-alpha-reductase inhibitors: • Dutasteride • Finasteride	Monitor blood pressure, and teach to move slowly from sitting to standing; *orthostatic hypotension can occur.* Teach about possible side effect of gynecomastia; *men taking a 5-alpha-reductase inhibitor are three times more likely to develop this condition.* Teach about the increased risk for development of prostate cancer; *men taking these drugs are at higher risk for development of prostate cancer.* Teach to keep medications stored away from anyone who is pregnant or who may become pregnant; *these drugs are teratogenic and can be absorbed through the skin.* Teach patients taking dutasteride to take the capsule with a full glass of water and to refrain from opening the capsule to sprinkle on food; *dutasteride irritates oropharyngeal mucosa.*
Alpha₁ₐ-Blocker/5-Alpha-Reductaste Inhibitor	
• Tadalafil	Monitor blood pressure, and teach to move slowly from sitting to standing; *orthostatic hypotension can occur.* Teach that this drug is usually given to treat erectile dysfunction (ED) but is also used to improve lower urinary tract symptoms (LUTS); *the patient needs to know the mechanism of action as it relates to treatment of BPH and LUTS.* Teach to refrain from taking this drug with grapefruit juice or grapefruit. *Drinking grapefruit juice while taking tadalafil can increase the amount of drug in the body.*
Alpha₁-Adrenergic Antagonists	
Common examples of alpha₁-adrenergic antagonists: • Alfuzosin • Doxazosin • Silodosin • Tamsulosin • Terazosin	Monitor blood pressure, and teach to move slowly from sitting to standing; *orthostatic hypotension can occur.* Monitor for side effects such as ongoing dizziness, headache, and weakness; *these side effects may require dose reduction or discontinuation of the drug.* Teach patients taking alfuzosin or tamsulosin to take it 30 minutes after meals at the same time daily. *This increases absorption of the drug.* Teach patient to report taking this type of drug to all health care providers; *alpha₁-adrenergic antagonists can increase or decrease the side effects of other drugs such as beta-blockers, calcium channel blockers, or medications used to treat ED.*

Data from Burchum, J.R., & Rosenthal, L.D. (2022). *Lehne's Pharmacology for nursing care* (11th ed.). St. Louis: Elsevier.

relaxants (McVary, 2023b). *Emphasize the importance of telling any health care provider about the diagnosis of BPH so that these drugs are not prescribed.*

Drug therapy. *Alpha₁-adrenergic antagonists* (also known as *alpha blockers*), which act to relax smooth muscle in the bladder neck, and *5-alpha-reductase inhibitors* (5-ARIs), which act to reduce prostate size, are often prescribed in combination, as evidence shows that they work better in combination (Burchum & Rosenthal, 2022). See Table 64.1 for an overview of drug therapy used to treat BPH.

NURSING SAFETY PRIORITY

Drug Alert

If giving alpha-blockers in an inpatient setting, assess for orthostatic (postural) hypotension, tachycardia, and syncope, especially after the first dose is given to older men. If the patient is taking the drug at home, *teach about being careful when changing position and to report any weakness, light-headedness, or dizziness to the primary health care provider immediately.* Bedtime dosing may decrease the risk for problems related to hypotension.

The most effective drug therapy approach used for many patients is a combination of a 5-ARI drug and an alpha₁-adrenergic antagonist. Commonly prescribed drug regimens include finasteride and doxazosin, dutasteride and tamsulosin, and the newly released finasteride and tadalafil (Veru Inc., 2021).

NURSING SAFETY PRIORITY

Drug Alert

Teach patients taking a 5-ARI to keep these drugs stored away from pregnant women or women who may become pregnant. These drugs are absorbed through the skin and are teratogenic.

NURSING SAFETY PRIORITY

Drug Alert

Remind patients taking a 5-ARI for BPH that they may need to take it for as long as 6 months before improvement is noticed. Teach about possible side effects, including erectile dysfunction (ED), decreased libido, and dizziness due to orthostatic hypotension. *Remind them to change positions carefully and slowly!*

Other drugs may be helpful in managing specific urinary symptoms. For example, low-dose oral desmopressin, a synthetic antidiuretic analog, has been used successfully for nocturia (Wang et al., 2022).

Complementary and integrative health. Saw palmetto *(Serenoa repens)* has long been associated with usefulness in treating BPH. However, studies continue to show no data supporting its use in treatment (Saper, 2022). Remind patients who are interested in taking saw palmetto to talk with their primary health care provider before taking this herb because of potential interactions with drug therapy.

Other nonsurgical interventions. Frequent sexual intercourse can reduce obstructive symptoms because it causes the release of prostatic fluid. This approach is helpful for the man whose obstructive symptoms result from an enlarged prostate with a large amount of retained prostatic fluid.

Surgical Management. If drug therapy or other measures are not helpful in relieving urinary symptoms, several minimally invasive techniques are available to shrink or destroy excess prostate tissue. The minimally invasive prostate artery embolization is performed by an interventional radiologist (IR), who threads a small vascular catheter into an artery in the wrist or groin. An arteriogram (dye injected in the blood vessels) allows the IR to see the vessels that feed the prostate, into which particles are injected to reduce some of the blood flow. In turn, this shrinks the prostate gland. This procedure has a low side effect profile for development of incontinence or erectile dysfunction (ED), so it is preferred by many patients. Local anesthesia or procedural sedation is used rather than general anesthesia, which allows a typical discharge from the hospital in as little as 3 hours after the procedure.

Other select procedures are described in Table 64.2. All of these minimally invasive treatments use local or regional anesthesia, or procedural sedation. Some, but not all, require an indwelling urinary catheter for a short period after the procedure. They are also associated with less risk for complications such as intraoperative bleeding and erectile dysfunction when compared with traditional surgical approaches. Patients can return to their usual activities in a short time as prescribed by their provider.

For patients who are not candidates for, or are not interested in, medication therapy or other less invasive options, more complex surgery may be performed. Some or all of these criteria indicate the need for surgery:

- Acute urinary retention (AUR) due to obstruction
- Chronic urinary tract infections secondary to residual urine in the bladder
- Hematuria
- Hydronephrosis
- Persistent pain with decrease in urine flow

If a lesser invasive procedure is not indicated or desired, for years the historical gold standard surgery was a transurethral resection of the prostate (TURP), in which the enlarged part of the prostate is removed through an endoscopic instrument. More recently, the growing popularity of the holmium laser enucleation of the prostate (HoLEP) procedure has become the new gold standard for the surgical treatment of BPH (Shvero et al., 2021; University of Wisconsin Hospitals and Clinics Authority, 2023).

A procedure similar to the TURP is the transurethral incision of the prostate (TUIP), in which small cuts are made into the prostate to relieve pressure on the urethra. This alternate technique is used for smaller prostates.

The HoLEP procedure usually requires 1 to 2 days of hospitalization; the TURP and TUIP procedures usually require 1 to 3 days, depending on complexity.

Preoperative care. When planning surgical interventions, the patient's general physical condition, the size of the prostate gland, and the patient's preferences are considered. The patient may have fears and misconceptions about prostate surgery, such as believing that automatic loss of sexual functioning or permanent incontinence will occur. Assess for anxiety, correct any misconceptions about the surgery, and provide accurate information to the patient and his family.

Regardless of the type of surgery to be performed, reinforce information about anesthesia (see Chapter 9). Help patients taking anticoagulants or antiplatelet therapy to coordinate with their surgeon. Sometimes these drugs are stopped briefly before the procedure, and other times they are continued, dependent upon multiple risk factors, risk for bleeding, and the specific drug(s) being taken.

The patient may have other medical problems that increase the risk for complications of general anesthesia and may be advised to have spinal anesthesia. Because the patient is conscious during spinal anesthesia, it is easier to assess for hyponatremia (low serum sodium), fluid overload, and water intoxication, which can result from large-volume bladder irrigations.

Teach that after a HoLEP or TURP, patients will have an indwelling urethral catheter; however, select patients who undergo a HoLEP procedure may have the catheter removed later during the day of surgery (Agarwal et al., 2020). If it is not removed the same day, it usually stays in for 1 to 2 days before removal. Patients who undergo a TURP generally have their catheter removed within 1 to 2 days.

Be sure that all patients who have a catheter in place know that they will feel the urge to void while the catheter is in place. Tell the patient that he will probably have traction on the catheter that may cause discomfort, and reassure him that analgesics will be prescribed to relieve pain. Explain that it is normal for the urine to be blood-tinged after surgery. Small blood clots and tissue debris may pass while the catheter is in place and immediately after it is removed. Some patients also have continuous bladder irrigation (CBI), depending on the procedure performed Other general preoperative care is described in Chapter 9.

Operative procedures. The HoLEP surgery is minimally invasive, while the traditional TURP is a "closed" surgery. To perform the HoLEP, a laser and scope are inserted through the urethra to remove tissue that is blocking urinary flow. A benefit of this procedure is that the entire amount of prostate tissue can be removed, leaving only the prostate capsule (The University of Utah, 2023). The patient usually goes home the same day as surgery; he may or may not have the catheter removed prior to discharge.

To perform the TURP procedure, the surgeon inserts a resectoscope (an instrument similar to a cystoscope, but with a cutting and cauterizing loop) through the urethra. The enlarged portion of

TABLE 64.2 Other Procedures Used to Treat Benign Prostatic Hyperplasia (BPH)

Procedure	Description	Nursing Implications
Aquablation	A robotic heat-free waterjet is used, in combination with a cystoscope with ultrasound imaging, to remove the prostate tissue.	Teach: • This is a surgical procedure that requires an overnight stay in the hospital. • A catheter will be in place following the procedure and removed in a day. • Minor burning upon urination may occur for 1 to 2 weeks after the procedure.
Photoselective vaporization (PVP)—(e.g., GreenLight ™ Laser Therapy)	Laser energy is used to vaporize the prostate tissue.	Teach: • This is a same-day surgical procedure; usually relief is noted within 24 hours. • A catheter will be in place following the procedure and removed in a day. • Retrograde ejaculation may occur.
Transurethral needle ablation (TUNA)	Low radiofrequency energy is used to shrink the prostate.	Teach: • This is a same-day surgical procedure; usually relief is noted in 2 to 6 weeks, with full improvement in 2 to 3 months. • A urinary catheter will be needed for 2 to 3 days after the procedure. • Minor burning upon urination may occur for 1 to 2 weeks after the procedure.
Transurethral microwave thermotherapy (TUMT)	An antenna is inserted through the penis toward the prostate to deliver electromagnetic waves (EMs) that heat and destroy prostate tissue.	Teach: • This is a same-day surgical procedure. • A urinary catheter will be needed after the procedure for about 1 week. • Burning at the tip of the penis is expected for about a week after the procedure. • It may take up to several months to experience the best procedural benefit, as this is dependent on how long the body needs to absorb the overgrown prostate that has been destroyed. • Have continued digital rectal examinations (DREs) and screenings for prostate cancer annually, even after the procedure.
Transurethral electro-vaporization of the prostate (TUEVAP or TUVP)	A heated ball or wire loop is inserted through the urethra to heat the prostate tissue, reducing it to vapor.	Teach: • Avoid heavy lifting; avoid straining when having a bowel movement. • Drink 8 cups of water daily. • It may take several months before fully normal urination occurs, although the stream will likely be stronger right after the procedure.
Transurethral water vapor therapy (e.g., Rezum™)	Sterile heated water is transformed from liquid to vapor; vapor is delivered by needle to targeted tissue at slightly above interstitial pressure as ablative therapy (Boston Scientific Corporation, 2023).	Teach: • This is a same-day surgical procedure; improvement is usually noted within 2 weeks, with full benefits at around 3 months postoperative. • A catheter may be placed for a few days. • Dysuria, hematuria, frequency, and urgency may occur postprocedure.
Urolift	A delivery device is placed through the obstructed urethra; small implants are placed to lift and hold the enlarged prostate tissue, which increases the urethral opening (Neotract, 2023).	Teach: • This is a same-day surgical procedure; improvement is usually noted within 2 weeks. • Dysuria, hematuria, pelvic pain, and urgency may be experienced postprocedure; these usually resolve in 2 to 4 weeks.

Data from Boston Scientific Corporation. (2023). Rezum™ water vapor therapy. https://www.bostonscientific.com/en-US/products/lithotripsy/rezum-water-vapor-therapy/science-of-rezum.html; Mayo Clinic. (2023). Transurethral microwave thermotherapy (TUMT). https://www.mayoclinic.org/tests-procedures/tumt/about/pac-20384886; McVary, K. (2022). Surgical treatment of benign prostatic hyperplasia (BPH). *UpToDate*. Retrieved June 9, 2023, from https://www.uptodate.com/contents/surgical-treatment-of-benign-prostatic-hyperplasia-bph; Neotract. (2023). The UroLift® system treatment. https://www.urolift.com/what-is-urolift?; PROCEPT BioRobotics Corporation. (2023). Aquablation®. https://aquablation.com/aquablation-therapy/; Ziętek, R. J., & Ziętek, Z. M. (2023). Transurethral Microwave Thermotherapy (TUMT) in the treatment of benign prostatic hyperplasia: A preliminary report. Medical science Monitor: *International Medical Journal of Experimental and Clinical Research, 27*, e931597. https://doi.org/10.12659/MSM.931597.

the prostate gland is then removed in small pieces (prostate chips). The estimated blood loss during TURP is less than 500 mL.

The disadvantage of a TURP is that only small pieces of the gland are removed. Remaining prostate tissue may continue to grow and cause urinary obstruction, requiring additional TURPs. Urethral trauma from the resectoscope with resulting urethral strictures is also possible.

Postoperative care. During any surgical procedure for BPH, a urinary catheter is placed into the bladder. Traction is often applied on the catheter by pulling it taut and taping it to the patient's abdomen or thigh. If the catheter is taped to the patient's thigh, instruct him to keep his leg straight.

The patient who undergoes the HoLEP procedure may have the catheter removed the same day as surgery. The patient who

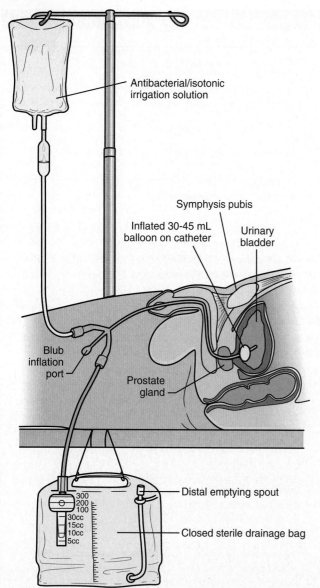

Antibacterial/isotonic irrigation solution

Symphysis pubis

Inflated 30-45 mL balloon on catheter

Urinary bladder

Blub inflation port

Prostate gland

300
200
100
30cc
15cc
10cc
5cc

Distal emptying spout

Closed sterile drainage bag

FIG. 64.3 Continuous bladder irrigation system after a TURP. *TURP,* Transurethral resection of the prostate.

undergoes a TURP may have a catheter and continuous bladder irrigation (CBI) in place for 1 to 2 days. For the CBI, a three-way urinary catheter is used to allow drainage of urine and inflow of a bladder irrigating solution (Fig. 64.3). Be sure to maintain the flow of the irrigant to keep the urine clear. When measuring the fluid in the urinary drainage bag, subtract the amount of irrigating solution that was used, to determine actual urine output.

NCLEX Examination Challenge 64.1
Physiological Integrity

A client has continuous bladder irrigation after surgery yesterday. The amount of bladder irrigating solution that has infused over the past 12 hours is 1200 mL. The amount of fluid in the urinary drainage bag is 2050 mL. The nurse records that the client had _____ mL of urine output in the past 12 hours. **Fill in the blank.**

BOX 64.1 Best Practice for Patient Safety and Quality Care

Care of the Patient After Transurethral Resection of the Prostate

- Monitor the patient closely for signs of *infection.* Older men undergoing prostate surgery often also have underlying chronic diseases (e.g., cardiovascular disease, chronic lung disease, diabetes).
- Help the patient out of the bed to a chair as soon as permitted to prevent complications of immobility. Provide assistance, especially for patients with underlying changes in the musculoskeletal system (e.g., decreased range of motion, stiffness in joints). These patients are at *high risk* for falls.
- Assess the patient's pain every 2 to 4 hours, and intervene as needed to control pain.
- Provide a safe environment for the patient.
  - Anticipate a temporary change in mental status for the older patient related to anesthesia and unfamiliar surroundings.
  - Reorient frequently.
  - Keep catheter tubes secure.
- Maintain the rate of the continuous bladder irrigation to ensure clear urine without clots and bleeding.
- Use normal saline solution (which is isotonic) for the intermittent bladder irrigant unless otherwise prescribed.
- Monitor and document the color, consistency, and amount of urine output.
- Check the drainage tubing frequently for external obstructions (e.g., kinks) and internal obstructions (e.g., blood clots, decreased output).
- Assess the patient for reports of severe bladder spasms with decreased urine output, which may indicate obstruction.
- If the urinary catheter is obstructed, irrigate it per agency or surgeon protocol.
- Notify the surgeon immediately if the obstruction does not resolve by hand irrigation or if the urinary return looks like ketchup.

Remind the patient who had a TURP that because of the urinary catheter's large diameter and the pressure of the retention balloon on the internal sphincter of the bladder, he will feel the urge to void continuously. This is a normal sensation, not a surgical complication. Advise him not to try to void around the catheter, as this causes the bladder muscles to contract and may result in painful spasms. Box 64.1 summarizes the nursing care for patients after a TURP.

PATIENT-CENTERED CARE: OLDER ADULT HEALTH
Reorientation After Surgery

When caring for older patients who become confused after surgery, reorient them frequently and remind them not to pull on the catheter. If the patient pulls tubes, provide a familiar object such as a family picture for him to hold for distraction and a feeling of security. Do not restrain the patient unless all other alternatives have failed.

NURSING SAFETY PRIORITY
Critical Rescue

Monitor the patient for the rare, yet critical, complication of post-TURP syndrome characterized by dilutional hyponatremia related to excessive absorption of hyperosmolar fluids (Emmett et al., 2022). This degree of absorption places stress on the heart. Signs and symptoms include headache, dizziness, hypoxemia, hypertension, bradycardia, and an altered level of consciousness. Notify the surgeon immediately, as the patient is likely to need intensive care during diuresis.

✚ NURSING SAFETY PRIORITY

Critical Rescue

After a TURP, monitor the patient's urine output every 2 to 4 hours and vital signs (including pain assessment) every 4 hours for the first postoperative day or according to agency or surgeon protocol. Assess for postoperative bleeding. *Patients who undergo a TURP are at risk for severe bleeding or hemorrhage after surgery. Although rare, bleeding is most likely within the first 24 hours.* Bladder spasms or movement may trigger fresh bleeding from previously controlled vessels. This bleeding may be arterial or venous, but venous bleeding is more common.

✚ NURSING SAFETY PRIORITY

Critical Rescue

If arterial bleeding occurs, the urinary drainage is bright red or ketchup-like with numerous clots. *Notify the surgeon immediately, and irrigate the catheter with normal saline solution per surgeon or hospital protocol.* Surgical intervention may be needed to clear the bladder of clots and stop bleeding.

If the bleeding is *venous,* the urine output is burgundy, with or without any change in vital signs. *Inform the surgeon of any bleeding.* Closely monitor the patient's hemoglobin (Hgb) and hematocrit (Hct) levels for anemia as a result of blood loss.

Observe for other possible but uncommon complications of TURP, such as *infection* and incontinence. Explain that temporary incontinence immediately following surgery is not unusual, but that fever, swelling, purulent drainage, and swelling must be reported to the surgeon right away.

Teach the patient that sexual function should not be affected after surgery but that retrograde ejaculation is possible, wherein semen flows backward into the bladder so that only a small amount will be ejaculated from the penis. Also remind the patient that *reproduction* ability should not be affected by surgery. Encourage the patient to express feelings and concerns about sexual dysfunction that may occur or persist following treatment. Provide objective information, and refer to supportive resources as needed.

NCLEX Examination Challenge 64.2

Physiological Integrity

The nurse is caring for a client on continuous bladder irrigation who had a transurethral resection of the prostate (TURP) yesterday. When bright red urinary drainage is noted, which **primary** action would the nurse take?

A. Calculate intake and output.
B. Monitor hemoglobin and hematocrit.
C. Increase the rate of the bladder irrigation.
D. Document findings in the electronic health record.

Care Coordination and Transition Management

The patient with benign prostatic hyperplasia (BPH) is typically managed at home. Patients who have surgery are also discharged to their home or other setting from where they were admitted.

Home Care Management. Depending on the procedure performed, some patients may be discharged with a urinary catheter in place for a short period of time. Older men may benefit from one or two visits from a home health care agency to ensure that they are not experiencing postsurgical complications and can provide safe self-care.

Self-Management Education. Teach patients not to take a bath or swim, and ways to prevent a urinary tract *infection* while the catheter is in place. When the urinary catheter is removed, the patient may experience burning on urination and some urinary frequency, dribbling, and leakage. Reassure the patient that these symptoms are normal and will decrease. Teach the patient to keep the penis and perineal area clean and dry to prevent skin breakdown. Remind him to toilet when he feels the urge and, if needed, to wear a small absorbent pad to prevent undergarment soiling.

If not contraindicated by another health condition, instruct the patient to increase fluid intake to at least 2000 to 2500 mL daily, which helps decrease dysuria and keeps the urine clear. *Be aware that a patient with renal disease or who is at risk for heart failure may not be able to tolerate this much fluid.*

Instruct the patient to contract and relax his sphincter frequently to reestablish urinary *elimination* control (Kegel exercises). External urinary (condom) catheters are not used except in extreme cases because they may give the patient a false sense of security and delay urinary control.

Teach patients to have follow-up care as recommended by their primary health care provider and surgeon (if surgery was performed).

Health Care Resources. Patients being managed for BPH usually do not require extensive health care resources.

After surgery, some men experience a return of LUTS and/or erectile dysfunction, which can decrease their quality of life. Encourage them to talk with their primary health care provider if symptoms are present.

Evaluate Outcomes: Evaluation

Evaluate the care of the patient with BPH based on the identified priority patient problem. The primary expected outcome is that the patient will:

• Have improved urinary *elimination* following appropriate and effective interprofessional management

✳ CELLULAR REGULATION CONCEPT EXEMPLAR: PROSTATE CANCER

Pathophysiology Review

Testosterone and dihydrotestosterone (DHT) are the major androgens (male hormones) in the adult male. Testosterone is produced by the testis and circulates in the blood. DHT is a testosterone derivative in the prostate gland. In some patients, the prostate grows very rapidly, leading to noncancerous high-grade prostatic intraepithelial neoplasia (PIN). This impairment of *cellular regulation* causes men to be at a higher risk

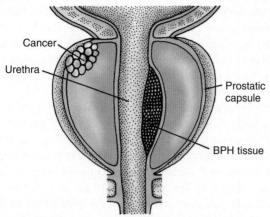

FIG. 64.4 Prostate gland with cancer and benign prostatic hyperplasia (BPH). Note that cancer normally arises in the periphery of the gland, whereas BPH occurs in the center of the gland.

for developing prostate cancer than men who do not have that growth pattern.

Many prostate tumors are androgen sensitive (Rogers, 2023). Most are adenocarcinomas and arise from epithelial cells located in the posterior lobe or outer portion of the gland (Fig. 64.4).

Of all malignancies, prostate cancer is one of the slowest growing, and it metastasizes in a predictable pattern. Common sites of metastasis are bones and nearby lymph nodes (Rogers, 2023), although the cancer can also metastasize to the lungs or liver. The bones of the pelvis, sacrum, and lumbar spine are most often affected. Chapter 18 describes staging categories of localized and advanced cancers.

Etiology and Genetic Risk

Advanced age is the leading risk factor for development of prostate cancer (Centers for Disease Control and Prevention [CDC], 2023). The risk increases for men with a first-degree relative (father, brother, son) with the disease, men who had prostate cancer at or before the age of 55, and for those with family members who have had breast, ovarian, or pancreatic cancer (CDC, 2023).

> ### 👤 PATIENT-CENTERED CARE: HEALTH EQUITY
>
> #### *Prostate Cancer*
>
> Prostate cancer affects African Americans more often than other ethnic/racial groups (Centers for Disease Control and Prevention [CDC], 2023). Males of African descent who live in the Caribbean have the highest mortality rates in the world (Rogers, 2023). Mortality is increasing in Asia as well as in Central and Eastern European countries, whereas it has decreased in Australia, Canada, Italy, Norway, the United Kingdom, and the United States (Rogers, 2023). Be aware of epidemiologic factors, and advocate for all men to talk with their primary health care providers about screening for prostate cancer.

> ### 👤 PATIENT-CENTERED CARE: GENETICS/GENOMICS
>
> #### *Genes and Prostate Cancer*
>
> Many gene mutations play a role in various types of prostate cancer. Some men with the most aggressive prostate cancers have *BRCA2* mutations similar to those women who have *BRCA2*-associated breast and ovarian cancers. The most common genetic factor that increases the risk for prostate cancer is a mutation in the glutathione *S*-transferase *(GSTP1)* gene. This gene is normally part of the pathway that helps to protect against carcinogen damage (Rogers, 2023).

Incidence and Prevalence

Prostate cancer is the most diagnosed nonskin cancer in men in the United States (Rogers, 2023). If found and treated early, it has a nearly 100% cure rate. Men older than 65 years have the greatest risk for the disease (Rogers, 2023), with the average age at diagnosis being 66 (American Cancer Society, 2023b). In the United States, one man in eight will receive a prostate cancer diagnosis in his lifetime; about 1 in 41 men will die from this disorder (American Cancer Society, 2023b).

Health Promotion/Disease Prevention

Teach men about the most current evidence-based guidelines for prostate cancer screening and early detection. The current recommendations from the U.S. Preventive Services Task Force (2018) states that men aged 55 to 69 should talk with their primary health care provider and make an informed decision about whether to have prostate cancer screening. This same agency recommends against PSA screening for men who are 70 years old and older.

Other organizations, such as the American Urological Association, the American College of Physicians, and the American Cancer Society, have varying guidelines. It is important to note that:

- Men at a high risk for prostate cancer, including African Americans or men whose father or brother had prostate cancer before the age of 65 years, should discuss screening with their health care provider at the age of 45 (American Cancer Society, 2023a).
- Men with multiple first-degree relatives with prostate cancer at an early age should discuss screening with their primary health care provider at age 40 (American Cancer Society, 2023a).

Although a family history of prostate cancer cannot be changed, certain nutritional habits can be modified to possibly decrease the risk for the disease. First, teach men to eat a healthy, balanced diet, including decreases in the intake of animal fat (e.g., red meat) and dairy products (Sartor, 2022). Also reinforce the need to increase fruits and vegetables—especially tomatoes, which are high in lycopene (Sartor, 2022).

Interprofessional Collaborative Care
Recognize Cues: Assessment

History. Assess the patient's age, ethnicity, and family history of prostate cancer. Ask about his nutritional habits, especially focusing on the intake of red meat and dairy products as a source of concern.

Recognize that in early prostate cancer, there are often no signs or symptoms experienced by the patient. Assess whether the patient has existing or new problems with urinary *elimination.* Ask about medications that are being taken to determine whether any could affect voiding. The first symptoms that the man may report are related to bladder outlet obstruction (BOO), such as difficulty in starting urination, frequent bladder infections, and urinary retention. Ask about urinary frequency, hematuria, and nocturia. Inquire whether he has had or currently has any other pain (particularly bone pain in the hips and legs), a symptom associated with advanced prostate cancer. Ask whether there has been recent unexpected weight loss.

Take a sexual history for recent changes in *sexuality,* including libido or function. Ask about current or previous sexually transmitted infections, penile discharge, or scrotal pain or swelling. Ask whether he has had any pain during intercourse, especially when ejaculating.

Physical Assessment/Signs and Symptoms. Most *early* cancers are diagnosed while the patient is having a routine physical examination or is being treated for benign prostatic hyperplasia (BPH). Gross blood in the urine is a common sign of *late* prostate cancer. Pain in the pelvis, hips, spine, or ribs, and swollen nodes indicate advanced disease that has spread. Take and record the patient's weight because unexpected weight loss is also common when the disease is advanced.

Prepare the patient for a digital rectal examination (DRE) by the primary health care provider. A prostate that is stony hard with palpable irregularities or indurations is suspected to be malignant.

Psychosocial Assessment. A diagnosis of any type of cancer causes fear and anxiety for most people. Some men develop the disease earlier in life, when they are putting their children through school, looking toward retirement in the coming years, or enjoying their middle years. Assess the reaction of the patient and family to the diagnosis. Men may describe their feelings as shock, fear, or anger, or a combination of these. Expect that patients usually go through the grieving process and may be in denial or depressed. Determine what support systems they have, such as family, friends, spiritual leaders, or community group support, to help them through diagnosis, treatment, and recovery.

A concern the patient may have following treatment is his ability for sexual function. Tell him that function will depend on the type of treatment he has. Common surgical techniques used today do not involve cutting the perineal nerves that are needed for an erection. A dry climax may occur if the prostate is removed because it produces most of the fluid in the ejaculate. Refer the patient to his surgeon (urologist), sex therapist, or intimacy counselor as needed.

Laboratory Assessment. Prostate-specific antigen (PSA) is a glycoprotein produced by the prostate. If the patient and health care provider have agreed to screening, PSA analysis can be used as a screening test for prostate cancer. *Because other prostate problems also increase the PSA level, it is not specifically diagnostic for cancer.* Up to 80% of PSA screenings demonstrate a false-positive result (Burchum & Rosenthal, 2022). This test can be used alone or in combination with a digital rectal examination; most guidelines do not recommend DRE as a standard screening tool (Hoffman, 2023). If the test is performed, the specimen should be drawn before the DRE because the examination can cause an increase in PSA as a result of prostate irritation.

It is ideal that men younger than 50 years have a PSA of less than 2.4 ng/mL. PSA levels increase to as high as 6.5 ng/mL when men reach their 70s (Pagana et al., 2022). African Americans aged 50 and 59 have a slighter higher normal value than men who are White or Japanese, but the reason for this difference is not known (Pagana et al., 2022). Levels greater than 4 ng/mL have been noted in more than 80% of men with prostate cancer (Pagana et al., 2022).

An elevated PSA level should decrease a few days after a prostatectomy for cancer. An increase in the PSA level several weeks after surgery may indicate that the disease has recurred (Pagana et al., 2022).

Other laboratory testing includes evaluation for prostate-specific proteins, PSA isoforms, and prostate cancer specific biomarkers (Burchum & Rosenthal, 2022). These are much more accurate tests than the traditional PSA.

Other Diagnostic Assessment. After assessments by PSA with or without DRE, most patients have a *transrectal ultrasound (TRUS)* of the prostate in an ambulatory care or imaging setting. Before the procedure, the health care provider uses lidocaine jelly on the ultrasound probe and/or injects lidocaine into the prostate gland to promote patient comfort. The provider inserts a small probe into the rectum and obtains a view of the prostate using sound waves. If prostate cancer is suspected, a *biopsy* is usually performed at that time to obtain an accurate diagnosis.

> **! NURSING SAFETY PRIORITY**
>
> *Action Alert*
>
> After a transrectal ultrasound with biopsy, instruct the patient about possible complications, although rare, including hematuria with clots, signs of *infection,* and perineal pain. Teach the patient to report fever, chills, bloody urine, and any difficulty voiding. Advise him to avoid strenuous physical activity and to drink plenty of fluids, especially in the first 24 hours after the procedure. Teach him that a small amount of bleeding turning the urine pink is expected during this time. However, bright red bleeding should be reported to the health care provider immediately.

After prostate cancer is diagnosed, the patient has additional imaging and blood studies to determine the extent of the disease. Common tests include lymph node biopsy, CT of the pelvis and abdomen, and MRI to assess the status of the pelvic and para-aortic lymph nodes. A radionuclide bone scan may be performed to detect metastatic bone disease. An enlarged liver or abnormal liver function study results indicate possible liver metastasis.

Patients with advanced prostate cancer often have *elevated serum acid phosphatase.* Most men with bone metastasis have *elevated serum alkaline phosphatase* levels and severe pain.

As with any cancer, accurate staging and grading of prostate tumors guide monitoring and treatment plans during the

TABLE 64.3 Prostate Cancer Staging

Stage	Description	Grade Group (Likelihood of Cancer Growing and Spreading)	Metastasis
I	Tumor not detectable by digital rectal examination (DRE); cannot be seen on imaging studies (was found during TURP or via needle biopsy); PSA <10; *or* Tumor can be detected by DRE or seen with imaging, and is in one-half or less of only one side of the prostate, and PSA <10; *or* Prostate has been surgically removed (tumor was only in the prostate), and PSA <10	1	No
IIA	Tumor not detectable by DRE; cannot be seen on imaging studies (was found during TURP or via needle biopsy); PSA is at least 10 but less than 20; *or* Tumor can be detected by DRE or seen with imaging, and is in one-half or less of only one side of the prostate; PSA is at least 10 but less than 20	1	No
IIB	Tumor can be detected by DRE or seen with imaging, and is in more than one-half of one side of the prostate, or in both sides; PSA <20; *or* Tumor may or may not be felt by DRE or seen with imaging; PSA <20	2	No
IIC	Tumor can be detected by DRE or seen with imaging; PSA <20	3 or 4	No
IIIA	Tumor may or may not be felt by DRE or seen with imaging; cancer has not grown outside the prostate; PSA at least 20	1 to 4	No
IIIB	Cancer has grown outside the prostate and may have spread to seminal vesicles, or spread to other tissues near the prostate (e.g., urethral sphincter, rectum, bladder, pelvis); PSA can be any value	1 to 4	No (although has spread locally beyond prostate)
IIIC	Cancer may or may not be growing outside prostate and into nearby tissues; PSA can be any value	5	No (although has spread locally beyond prostate)
IVA	Tumor may or may not be growing into tissues near the prostate; cancer **has** spread to local lymph nodes; PSA can be any value	Any grade	No (although has spread to nearby lymph nodes)
IVB	Cancer may or may not be growing into tissues near prostate and may or may not have spread to local lymph nodes; **has** spread to other parts of body (e.g., distant lymph nodes, bones, other organs); PSA can be any value.	Any grade	Yes

Adapted from American Cancer Association. (2021). https://www.cancer.org/cancer/prostate-cancer/detection-diagnosis-staging/staging.html.

course of the disease. Based on diagnostic assessment results, the cancer is staged, which can help to guide treatment choices. Table 64.3 shows how prostate cancer is staged.

Analyze Cues and Prioritize Hypotheses: Analysis

The priority collaborative problem for the patient with prostate cancer is:

1. Potential for cancer metastasis due to lack of, or inadequate, treatment

Generate Solutions and Take Actions: Planning and Implementation

Preventing Metastasis

Planning: Expected Outcomes. The patient with prostate cancer is expected to remain free of metastases or recurrence of disease, if possible. If cancer recurs, the patient will experience optimal health outcomes, including potential palliation and end-of-life care.

Interventions. Patients are faced with several treatment options. A urologist and an oncologist usually collaborate to help patients make the best decisions about treatment options.

Active Surveillance. Because prostate cancer is slow growing with late metastasis, older men who are asymptomatic and have other illnesses may choose observation without immediate active treatment, especially if the cancer is at an early stage. This option is known as active surveillance (AS). Factors that are considered in choosing AS include potential side effects of treatment (e.g., urinary incontinence, erectile dysfunction), estimated life expectancy, the presence of comorbid medical conditions, and the risk for increased morbidity and mortality from not seeking active treatment.

This form of treatment involves a predefined follow-up schedule at regular intervals for DRE and PSA testing. The intent of AS is to implement curative treatment if subclinical progression is detected (Punnen et al., 2022). The average time from diagnosis to start of treatment is up to 10 years.

Patients with prostate cancer at a very early stage who choose AS require close follow-up by their primary health care provider. If obstruction occurs, a transurethral resection of the prostate (TURP) may be done. The care of patients having this procedure is described in the discussion of Surgical Management under the section titled Elimination Concept Exemplar: Benign Prostatic Hyperplasia, earlier in this chapter.

Specific management is based on the extent of the disease and the patient's physical condition. The patient may undergo surgery for a biopsy (if not previously done), staging and removal of the tumor, or palliation to control the spread of disease or relieve distressing symptoms. As with AS, the health care provider and patient must weigh the benefits of treatment against potential adverse effects, such as incontinence and erectile dysfunction (ED).

Nonsurgical Management. Nonsurgical management may be an adjunct to surgery or alternative intervention if the cancer is widespread or the patient's condition or age prevents surgery. Available modalities include radiation therapy, hormone therapy, and chemotherapy (less often).

Radiation therapy. External or internal radiation therapy may be used in the treatment of prostate cancer or as salvage treatments when cancer recurs. It may also be done for palliation of the patient's symptoms.

EXTERNAL BEAM RADIATION THERAPY. External beam radiation therapy (EBRT) comes from a source outside the body. Patients are usually treated 5 days a week for a minimum of several weeks. EBRT can also be used to relieve pain from bone metastasis. Three types of EBRT include three-dimensional conformal radiation therapy (3D-CRT), intensity-modulated radiation therapy (IMRT), and stereotactic body radiation therapy.

Three-dimensional conformal radiation therapy (3D-CRT) can accurately target prostate tissue and reduce damage to nearby organs and tissue.

An advanced type of 3D-CRT radiation is *intensity-modulated radiation therapy* (IMRT), which provides very high doses to the prostate. It is the most commonly used type of external beam radiation therapy for prostate cancer (American Cancer Society, 2023c).

Stereotactic body radiation therapy (SBRT), also known as Gamma Knife, X-Knife, CyberKnife, and Clinac, involves the delivery of large doses of radiation to the prostate over a period of a few days (American Cancer Society, 2023c). This treatment takes less time than IMRT but usually has more prominent side effects.

Teach patients that external beam radiation causes ED in many men well after the treatment is completed. Remind the patient that other complications from EBRT include urinary frequency, diarrhea, and acute *radiation cystitis,* which causes persistent pain and hematuria (American Cancer Society, 2023c). Symptoms are usually mild to moderate and subside after treatment is discontinued, although there is a rare chance that this will not go away. Teach the patient to avoid caffeine and continue drinking plenty of water and other fluids.

Radiation proctitis, irritation of the rectum, may also develop but is less likely with 3D-CRT. In some instances, a device or gel is placed between the rectum and prostate before treatment to lessen the amount of radiation to which the rectum is exposed (American Cancer Society, 2023c). Radiation that has irritated the rectum can cause urgency and cramping, diarrhea that is sometimes blood, and rectal leakage (American Cancer Society, 2023c). Teach the patient to report these symptoms to the primary health care provider. Like cystitis, this problem usually resolves following treatment, although in rare cases it is permanent. If proctitis occurs, teach patients to limit spicy or fatty foods, caffeine, and dairy products.

BRACHYTHERAPY. Low-dose brachytherapy is a type of internal radiation (Fig. 64.5) that is delivered by implanting low-dose radiation "seeds" (the size of a grain of rice) directly into the prostate gland (American Cancer Society, 2023c). This treatment involves transrectal ultrasound, CT scans, or MRI, which are used to guide implantation of the seeds. These procedures

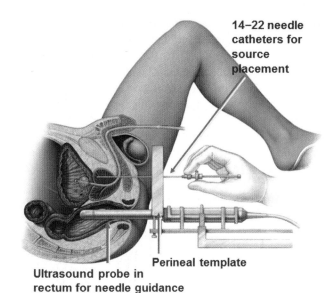

FIG. 64.5 Patient position and vital components of prostate brachytherapy with transrectal ultrasound guidance. (From Stish, B. J., Davis, B. J., Mynderse, L. A., Deufel, C. L., & Choo, R. [2017]. Brachytherapy in the management of prostate cancer. *Surgical Oncology Clinics of North America, 26*[3], 491–513. https://doi.org/10.1016/j.soc.2017.01.008.)

are usually done on an ambulatory care basis under spinal or general anesthesia and are the most cost-effective treatment for early-stage prostate cancer.

Reassure the patient that the dose of radiation is low and that the radiation will not pose a hazard to him or others. Teach him that ED, urinary incontinence, and rectal problems do occur in a small percentage of cases. Fatigue is also common and may last for several months after the treatment stops. Chapter 18 describes general nursing care for patients having radiation therapy.

Radiation proctitis can develop as a side effect of brachytherapy; this usually resolves, and long-term concerns are uncommon. Urinary and erection problems are not commonly associated with brachytherapy (American Cancer Society, 2023c).

RADIOPHARMACEUTICALS. Radiopharmaceutical treatment is usually used to treat prostate cancer that has spread and that has been previously treated with hormone therapy and chemotherapy, or to treat prostate cancer that has spread to the bones (American Cancer Society, 2023c). Depending on the agent, these drugs are given intravenously in specific cycles. Each agent has specific recommendations for whether the patient needs to avoid contact with other people for a period of time; provide information according to the treatment that has been prescribed.

Side effects of radiopharmaceutical agents include low blood counts of RBCs, platelets, and WBCs. The agents that treat nonmetastasized prostate cancer also can contribute to kidney damage (American Cancer Society, 2023c). Teach patients to protect themselves from infection and to drink plenty of fluids to flush the drug from their system.

Drug therapy. Drug therapy may consist of hormone therapy or chemotherapy. Because most prostate tumors are hormone dependent, patients with extensive tumors or those with metastatic disease may be managed by androgen deprivation. *Luteinizing hormone–releasing hormone (LHRH) agonists* or antiandrogens can be used.

LHRH agonists available in the United States include leuprolide, goserelin, histrelin, and triptorelin. These drugs first stimulate the pituitary gland to release luteinizing hormone (LH). After about 3 weeks, the pituitary gland is depleted of LH, which reduces testosterone production by the testes (Burchum & Rosenthal, 2022). Leuprolide is used most for advanced prostate cancer with the goal of palliation (Burchum & Rosenthal, 2022).

🖊 NURSING SAFETY PRIORITY

Drug Alert

Teach patients taking LHRH agonists that side effects include "hot flashes," which usually decrease as treatment continues. The subsequent reduction in testosterone may contribute to erectile dysfunction and decreased libido. Some men also develop **gynecomastia** (abnormal enlargement of the breasts in men). These drugs can also increase the patient's risk for osteoporosis and fractures. Teach the patient to take calcium and vitamin D and to engage in regular weight-bearing exercise. Bisphosphonates can be prescribed to prevent bone fractures.

Gonadotropin-releasing hormone antagonists such as degarelix and relugolix suppress the testes' ability to produce androgens. Degarelix, an injection, is used for palliative therapy in advanced prostate cancer (Burchum & Rosenthal, 2022). Relugolix, a oral medication, is used for the treatment of advanced prostate cancer.

Androgen receptor blockers (also known as *antiandrogens*) work differently in that they block the body's ability to use the available androgens (Burchum & Rosenthal, 2022). Antiandrogens may be used alone or in combination with LHRH agonists for total or maximal androgen blockade (hormone ablation). These drugs are the major treatment for metastatic disease in addition to surgical or chemical castration with a gonadotropin-releasing hormone antagonist. Examples include flutamide, bicalutamide, and nilutamide. They inhibit tumor progression by blocking the uptake of testicular and adrenal androgens at the prostate tumor site.

Patients should be taught to follow up closely with their health care provider and to undergo all laboratory testing as prescribed. These medications increase the risk for liver toxicity. Regular liver function tests will be ordered at baseline, monthly during the first 4 months, and periodically thereafter (Burchum & Rosenthal, 2022).

Systemic *chemotherapy* may be an option for patients whose cancer has spread and for whom other therapies have not worked. For example, small cell prostate cancer is rare and is more responsive to chemotherapy than to hormone therapy. The goal of therapy is not curative; it is to slow the cancer's growth so that the patient experiences a better quality of life. Chapter 18 describes general nursing care for patients receiving chemotherapy.

Surgical Management. Surgery is the most common intervention for a cure. Minimally invasive surgery (MIS) or, less commonly, an open surgical technique for radical prostatectomy (prostate removal) can be performed. A bilateral orchiectomy (removal of both testicles) is another palliative surgery that slows the spread of cancer by removing the main source of testosterone.

Preoperative care. Preoperative care depends on the type of surgery that will be done. Minimally invasive surgery (MIS) is most appropriate for localized prostate cancer and is used as a curative intervention.

The most common procedure is the *laparoscopic radical prostatectomy (LRP),* often done with robotic assistance. In this procedure, the entire prostate gland, its surrounding tissues, and seminal vesicles are removed.

The transurethral resection of the prostate procedure (TURP) for BPH can also be used to relieve symptoms in men with advanced prostate cancer, yet it is not curative in nature (American Cancer Society, 2019).

Patients who qualify for LRP must have a PSA of less than 10 ng/mL and have had no previous hormone therapy or abdominal surgeries. Remind the patient that the advantages of this procedure over open surgery include:

- Decreased hospital stay (1 to 2 days)
- Minimal bleeding
- Smaller or no incisions and less scarring
- Less postoperative discomfort
- Decreased time for urinary catheter placement (usually removed on third postoperative day)
- Fewer complications
- Faster recovery and return to usual activities
- Nerve-sparing advantages

For the patient undergoing an *open* radical prostatectomy, provide preoperative care as for any patient having surgery (see Chapter 9).

Operative procedures. For the *LRP procedure,* the patient is placed in lithotomy positioning with steep Trendelenburg. The urologist makes one or more small punctures or incisions into the abdomen. A laparoscope with a camera on the end is inserted through one of the incisions while other instruments are inserted into the other incisions. The robotic system may be used to control the movement of the instruments by a remote device. The prostate is removed along with nearby lymph nodes, but perineal nerves are not affected.

The *open* radical prostatectomy can be performed via several surgical approaches, depending on the patient's desired outcomes and the staging of the disease. The perineal and retropubic (nerve-sparing) approaches are most used.

The surgeon removes the entire prostate gland along with the prostatic capsule, the cuff at the bladder neck, the seminal vesicles, and the regional lymph nodes. The remaining urethra is connected to the bladder neck. The removal of tissue at the bladder neck allows the seminal fluid to travel upward into the bladder rather than down the urethral tract, resulting in retrograde ejaculation. A catheter will remain in place following a radial retropubic or perineal prostatectomy for 1 to 2 weeks.

Postoperative care. Provide postoperative care of the patient after a radical prostatectomy as summarized in Box 64.2. Nursing interventions include typical care for any patient undergoing major surgery. Maintaining hydration, caring for

BOX 64.2 Best Practice for Patient Safety and Quality Care

Care of the Patient After a Radical Prostatectomy

- Encourage use of patient-controlled analgesia (PCA) as needed.
- Assist with moving from the bed into a chair on the night of surgery, and ambulate by the next day.
- Maintain the sequential compression device until the patient begins to ambulate.
- Monitor for venous thromboembolism and pulmonary embolus.
- Keep an accurate record of intake and output, including drainage from a Jackson-Pratt or other drainage device.
- Keep the urinary meatus clean using soap and water.
- Avoid rectal procedures or treatments.
- Emphasize the importance of not straining during a bowel movement, yet to avoid suppositories or enemas.
- Remind about the importance of follow-up appointments with the surgeon and oncologist to monitor progress.
- For patients who had an open procedure, teach how to care for the urinary catheter at home, which will be in place for 1 to 2 weeks.

wound drains (open procedure), managing pain, and preventing pulmonary complications are important aspects of nursing care. (See general postoperative care in Chapter 9.)

Assess the patient's pain level and monitor the effectiveness of pain management with opioids given as patient-controlled analgesia (PCA), a common method of delivery during the first 24 hours after surgery. Administer a stool softener if needed to prevent possible constipation from the drugs.

The patient has an indwelling urinary catheter to straight drainage to promote urinary *elimination*. Monitor intake and output every shift and record or delegate this activity to assistive personnel (AP), as this is a task that is within an AP's scope that can effectively and quickly be reported back to the nurse. An antispasmodic may be prescribed to decrease bladder spasm induced by the indwelling urinary catheter that will be in place 3 days if laparoscopic surgery was done, or 1 to 2 weeks if an open surgery was done.

Ambulation should begin no later than the day after surgery. Provide assistance in walking the patient when he first gets out of bed. Assess for scrotal or penile swelling from the disrupted pelvic lymph flow. If this occurs, elevate the scrotum and penis, and apply ice to the area intermittently for the first 24 to 48 hours.

Many patients who have the minimally invasive techniques are discharged 1 to 2 days after surgery and can resume usual activities in about a week or two. Those who have open procedures are discharged in 2 to 3 days or longer, depending on their progress.

Remind patients that common potential long-term complications of open radical prostatectomy are erectile dysfunction (ED) and urinary incontinence. For ED, drugs such as sildenafil may be effective.

Urge incontinence may occur because the internal and external sphincters of the bladder lie close to the prostate gland and are often damaged during the surgery. Kegel perineal exercises may reduce the severity of urinary incontinence after radical

prostatectomy. Teach the patient to contract and relax the perineal and gluteal muscles in several ways. For one of the exercises, teach him to:

1. Tighten the perineal muscles for 3 to 5 seconds as if to prevent voiding, and then relax
2. Bear down (but not to strain) as if having a bowel movement
3. Relax and repeat the exercise

Explain how to inhale through pursed lips while tightening the perineal muscles and how to exhale when he relaxes. He may also sit on the toilet with the knees apart while voiding and practice starting and stopping the stream several times.

Care Coordination and Transition Management

Interprofessional collaborative care of the patient with prostate cancer should include his partner, if the patient desires. The diagnosis and treatment of cancer greatly affect couples who experience the disease. Recognize that the patient and partner have specific physical and psychosocial needs that should be addressed before hospital discharge, and management should continue in the community setting.

Patients with prostate cancer may require care in a wide variety of settings at any stage of the disease process: at the hospital, the radiation therapy department, the oncologist's office, or home. Specific interventions depend on which treatment or combinations of treatment the patient had. Regardless of treatment, coordination to effectively manage transitions in care is essential. This section focuses on the needs of those who had a *radical prostatectomy*.

Home Care Management. Discharge planning and health teaching start early, even before surgery. A patient can better plan home care management when he knows what to expect. Collaborate with the case manager to coordinate the efforts of various health care providers, surgical unit nursing staff, and possibly a home nurse.

Self-Management Education. An important area of teaching for the patient going home with a urinary catheter is appropriate care. An indwelling urinary catheter may be in place for 3 days for the patient who had an LRP, or up to several weeks for the patient who underwent an open radical prostatectomy. Teach how to care for the catheter, use a leg bag, and identify signs and symptoms of *infection* and other potential complications. See Box 64.3.

Remind the patient to shower but to avoid tub baths, swimming pools, and hot tubs while the catheter is in place. Those whose catheter has been removed can shower, yet they still should not immerse themselves in water until cleared by the surgeon.

Teach patients who underwent a laparoscopic procedure to leave the wound closure tape in place and allow it to fall off naturally in about a week. Show patients how to inspect the incision or puncture site(s) daily for signs of *infection.*

Encourage the patient to walk short distances at a reasonable pace. Vigorous exercise such as running or jumping should be avoided for at least 6 weeks and then gradually introduced. Patients should not drive for about a week following surgery.

BOX 64.3   Patient and Family Education

Urinary Catheter Care at Home

- Once a day, gently wash the first few inches of the catheter, starting at the penis and washing outward with mild soap and water.
- Rinse and dry the catheter well.
- If you have not been circumcised, push the foreskin back to clean the catheter site; when finished, push the foreskin forward.
- Change the drainage bag at least once a week as needed:
  - Hold the catheter with one hand and the tubing with the other hand and twist in opposite directions to disconnect.
  - Place the end of the catheter in a clean container to catch leakage of urine.
  - Remove the rubber cap from the tubing of the leg bag or clean drainage bag.
  - Clean the end of the new tubing with alcohol swabs.
  - Insert the end of the new tubing into the catheter and twist to connect securely.
  - Clean the drainage bag just removed by pouring a solution of one part vinegar to two parts water through the tubing and bag. Rinse well with warm water and allow the bag to dry.

BOX 64.4   Patient and Family Education

Testicular Self-Examination

- Examine your testicles monthly immediately after a bath or a shower, when your scrotal skin is relaxed.
- Examine each testicle by gently rolling it between your thumbs and fingers. Testicular tumors tend to appear deep in the center of the testicle.
- Look and feel for any lumps; smooth, rounded masses; or any change in the size, shape, or consistency of the testes.
- Report any lump or swelling to your primary health care provider as soon as possible.

PATIENT-CENTERED CARE: HEALTH EQUITY

The ZERO® Initiative

The ZERO® (2023) initiative exists to advance health equity to "help bridge the gap between racial and health disparities in prostate cancer among Black men" (¶ 3). This organization provides men and their families with educational resources geared toward early detection of prostate cancer in an effort to ZERO the disease permanently. In 2021, they merged with Us TOO, the first prostate cancer support group in the United States, creating a dynamic resource with the aim to "create Generation ZERO—the first generation of men free from prostate cancer" (ZERO®, 2023).

Again, depending on the procedure that was done and the patient's occupation, the patient can return to work in 1 to 3 weeks at the surgeon's recommendation. Lifting may be restricted based on the type of procedure that was done.

Teach the patient not to strain to defecate. A stool softener may be prescribed to reduce the need for straining. If an opioid is prescribed for pain management, encourage the patient to drink adequate water to prevent constipation.

Remind all patients to keep all follow-up appointments. PSA blood tests are usually performed 6 weeks after surgery and then every 4 to 6 months to monitor progress.

Health Care Resources. Refer the patient (and partner, if the patient desires) to agencies or support groups such as the American Cancer Society's Cancer Survivors Network. This program provides discussion boards where people can engage in open and candid discussions.

Further information can be obtained from the Prostate Cancer Foundation (www.prostatecancerfoundation.org) or the National Alliance of State Prostate Cancer Coalitions (www.naspcc.org). In Canada, the Canadian Cancer Society (www.prostatecancer.ca) is dedicated to research and support for this disease. Other personal and community support services such as spiritual leaders or churches, synagogues, or mosques are also important to many patients.

For all LGBT patients surviving prostate cancer, *Malecare* (http://malecare.org) is an excellent resource. This nonprofit organization organized the first cancer survivorship program for gay and bisexual men in 1988, and the first cancer survivorship program to serve all LGBT people in 2005.

Some men have erectile dysfunction (ED) for the first 3 to 18 months after a prostatectomy. Refer them to a specialist who can help with this problem. (ED is discussed later in this chapter.) Refer patients with urinary incontinence to a urologist who specializes in this area. Chapter 58 discusses incontinence management in detail.

For the patient with terminal prostate cancer, refer to hospice and palliative care as appropriate.

Evaluate Outcomes: Evaluation

Evaluate the care of the patient with prostate cancer based on the identified priority patient problem. The primary expected outcome is that the patient with prostate cancer is expected to remain free of metastases or recurrence of disease, if possible. If cancer recurs, the patient will experience optimal health outcomes, including potential palliation and end-of-life care.

TESTICULAR CANCER

Pathophysiology Review

Testicular cancer is a rare cancer that most often affects young men but can affect men of any age. Although it can present bilaterally, it is usually confined to one testicle. The average age of diagnosis is 33 (American Society of Clinical Oncology, 2023). It usually strikes men at a productive time of life and thus has significant economic, social, and psychological impact on the patient and his family and/or partner. With early detection by testicular self-examination (TSE) (Box 64.4 and Fig. 64.6) and with treatment, testicular cancer has a greater than 95% cure rate (Rogers, 2023).

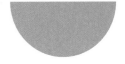

Monthly Self-Exam

HOW TO PERFORM A MONTHLY SELF EXAM.

Always perform monthly self-exams and ask your doctor for a testicular exam at your annual appointment, or sports physical.

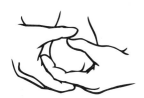

One.
Cup one testicle at a time using both hands.
This is best performed during or after a warm shower.

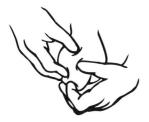

Two.
Examine by rolling the testicle between thumb and fingers.
Use slight pressure.

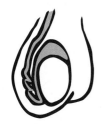

Three.
Familiarize yourself with the spermatic cord and epididymis.
The tube like structures connected on the back side of each testicle.

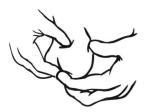

Four.
Feel for lumps, changes in size, or irregularities.
It is normal for one testis to be slightly larger than the other.

KNOW THE FACTS ABOUT TESTICULAR CANCER
- *Leading cancer in men 15-44*
- *Early detection is key*
- *Every hour a male is diagnosed*
- *Every day a life is lost*

RISK FACTORS
- *Undescended testicles (cryptorchidism)*
- *Family history*
- *Personal history of TC*
- *Intratubular germ cell neoplasia*

SIGNS & SYMPTOMS
- *A painless lump, change in size or any irregularity*
- *Pain or discomfort in the scrotum or testicle*
- *A dull ache or sense of pressure in the lower abdomen, back or groin*

ADVANCED SIGNS
- *Significant weight loss*
- *Back and/or abdominal pain*
- *Chest pain, coughing or difficulty breathing*
- *Headaches*
- *Enlarged lymph nodes in abdomen and/or neck*

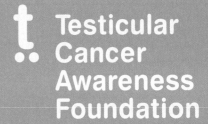

Testicular Cancer Awareness Foundation

Awareness •• Support •• Survivorship

FIG. 64.6 Monthly self-examination of testicles. (Courtesy of Testicular Cancer Awareness Foundation.)

BOX 64.5 Classification of Testicular Tumors

Germ Cell Tumors (GCTs)
- Seminomas
  - Classic
  - Spermatocytic
- Nonseminomas
  - Embryonal carcinoma
  - Yolk sac carcinoma
  - Choriocarcinoma
  - Teratoma

Non–Germ Cell Tumors
- Leydig cell
- Sertoli cell
- Granulosa cell
- Thecal cell

Mixed Tumors
- Teratocarcinoma
- Other

Data from Rogers, J. L. (2023). McCance and Huether's *Pathophysiology: The biologic basis for disease in adults and children* (9th ed.). St. Louis: Elsevier; Johns Hopkins Medicine. (2023). *Types of testicular cancer.* https://www.hopkinsmedicine.org/health/conditions-and-diseases/testicular-cancer/types-of-testicular-cancer; Steele, G., Richie, J., & Michaelson, M. (2023). Clinical manifestations, diagnosis, and staging of testicular germ cell tumors. *UpToDate.* Retrieved June 9, 2023, from https://www.uptodate.com/contents/clinical-manifestations-diagnosis-and-staging-of-testicular-germ-cell-tumors.

Primary testicular cancers fall into two major groups:
- Germ cell tumors (GCTs) arising from the sperm-producing cells (account for most testicular cancers)
- Non–germ cell tumors arising from the stromal, interstitial, or Leydig cells that produce testosterone (account for a very small percentage of testicular cancers)

Testicular germ cell tumors are classified into two broad categories: germ cell tumors (GCTs) and others (Box 64.5). The most common type of testicular tumor is *seminoma*. Patients with seminomas have the most favorable prognoses because the tumors are usually localized, metastasize late, and respond to treatment. They often are diagnosed when they are still confined to the testicles and retroperitoneal lymph nodes.

The risk for testicular tumors is higher in males who have an undescended testis (cryptorchidism); human immunodeficiency virus (HIV) infection; infertility; high intake of dietary fat, cholesterol, and dairy; engage in frequent use of marijuana; or history of hypospadias or testicular cancer (Michaelson & Oh, 2023).

PATIENT-CENTERED CARE: GENETICS/GENOMICS

Testicular Cancer Risk

Men are at a higher risk for testicular cancer if they have a family history of the disease (Michaelson & Oh, 2023). The incidence is higher among brothers and sons. White men are at a higher risk for testicular cancer than men of other ethnicities (Michaelson & Oh, 2023).

Interprofessional Collaborative Care

Recognize Cues: Assessment

History. When taking a history from a patient with a suspected testicular tumor, assess for risk factors, including a history or presence of an undescended testis, or a family history of testicular cancer.

The most common report is a painless, hard swelling or enlargement of the testicle, although a small portion of patients do report pain. Patients with testicular pain, lymph node swelling, bone pain, abdominal masses or aching, sudden hydrocele (fluid in the scrotum), or gynecomastia may have metastatic disease. Determine and document how long any signs and symptoms have been present.

Questions about *sexuality* and *reproduction* are important. If the patient undergoes a retroperitoneal lymph node dissection (RPLND) or chemotherapy, he may become sterile because of treatment effects on the sperm-producing cells or surgical trauma to the sympathetic nervous system, resulting in retrograde ejaculation. Therefore, collect information regarding whether the patient is sexually active, whether he wishes to have children in the future, and if so, whether he would be interested in learning about sperm storage in a sperm bank.

Physical Assessment/Signs and Symptoms. The testes, lymph nodes, and abdomen should be examined thoroughly. Patients may feel embarrassed about having this examination. Provide privacy and explain the procedure to the patient. Inspect the testicles for swelling or a lump that the patient reports is painless. A health care provider will palpate the testes for lumps and swelling that are not visible.

Psychosocial Assessment. Because testicular cancer and its treatment can lead to sexual dysfunction, be aware of the psychosocial aspects of the disease. *Sexuality* is likely to be a prime concern for any patient, yet it may be even more concerning for younger men, who may have a fear of being unable to perform sexually or father children. Assess the man's support systems, and refer to community support resources as necessary.

Diagnostic Assessment. Common serum tumor markers and other diagnostic methods that are used when formulating a diagnosis of testicular cancer are:
- Alpha fetoprotein (AFP)
- Beta human chorionic gonadotropin (hCG)
- Lactate dehydrogenase (LDH)
- Scrotal ultrasound
- Bone scan (to determine whether there is metastasis to the bones)
- Chest x-ray (to assess for metastasis)
- CT of the chest (if metastasis is suspected)
- CT scan of the abdomen and pelvis (if metastasis is suspected)
- MRI of the brain (if metastasis is suspected)

Take Actions: Interventions

The incidence of oligospermia (low sperm count) and azoospermia (absence of living sperm) is common in patients diagnosed with testicular cancer. In the pretreatment phase, review the normal reproductive function, as well as possible effects of cancer and its treatment on reproductive function. Explore various reproductive options if the patient desires (Box 64.6). A sperm bank facility provides comprehensive information on semen collection, storage of semen, the storage contract, costs, and the insemination process.

Sperm Banking

- You may want to investigate sperm storage (called "cryopreservation") in a sperm bank to preserve your sperm for future use.
- Studies confirm that intrauterine insemination is just as effective when using sperm that has been frozen as when using freshly ejaculated sperm (Cherouveim et al., 2022).
- Frozen sperm appears to be viable indefinitely. For example, sperm frozen for 27.5 years prior was used to successfully create a twin pregnancy (Guinness World Records Limited, 2023).
- Check with the sperm bank to see how much it charges to process and store your sperm and whether you must pay when the service is provided.
- Investigate whether your health insurance company will reimburse you for sperm collection and storage.

Data from Cherouveim, P., Vagios, S., Hammer, K., et al. (2022). The impact of cryopreserved sperm on intrauterine insemination (IUI) outcomes: Is frozen as good as fresh? *Human Reproduction, 37*(Supplement_1), deac105-098; Guinness World Records Limited. (2023); Oldest sperm used in successful IVF treatment. https://www.guinnessworldrecords.com/world-records/oldest-sperm-used-in-successful-ivf-treatment.

Nonsurgical Management. Chemotherapy or radiation therapy may be used, depending on the tumor staging, whether surgery is performed, and based on the degree of adherence to treatment that is anticipated (Oh, 2023). The specific treatment, including frequency, cycling, and duration, will vary from patient to patient, depending on the extent of the disease and the protocol being followed. Chapter 18 discusses the general nursing care for the patient receiving chemotherapy.

Surgical Management. Surgery is the main treatment for testicular cancer. For localized disease, the surgeon performs a unilateral orchiectomy to remove the affected testicle, which is usually curative (Oh, 2023).

Preoperative Care. Like most patients with cancer, men with testicular cancer may be very apprehensive. Offer support and reinforce the teaching provided by the surgeon. Teach the patient and caregivers what to expect after surgery.

Operative Procedures. Most patients with seminoma have only one surgery, an orchiectomy, to remove the diseased testicle through the groin (inguinal) for a cure. A frozen section of the tumor is examined to confirm the type and stage of the cancer. A saline-filled silicone prosthesis may be surgically implanted into the scrotum at the time of the orchiectomy or later if the patient desires. This type of reconstructive surgery gives the appearance of having two testes. With one functioning testicle, the man is still able to achieve an erection for sexual intercourse.

Some men have lymph nodes that are affected around the aorta and inferior vena cava (American Cancer Society, 2018). The preferred method to address this is laparoscopic retroperitoneal lymph node dissection (RPLND). This technique can be done at the same time as an orchiectomy or in a separate surgery. As an open procedure, this surgery is long and complex (up to 5 hours in length), with the torso being incised

for abdominal removal of lymph nodes (American Cancer Society, 2018).

In laparoscopic RPLND, very small skin incisions in the abdomen are made by a laparoscope, through which the nodes are dissected for examination. Bleeding, postoperative pain, and postoperative complications are minimized. The patient who has had laparoscopic RPLND can still achieve an erection, yet if there has been nerve damage during surgery, he may experience retrograde ejaculation. Newer nerve-sparing surgeries have shown to be very successful when performed by experienced surgeons (American Cancer Society, 2018).

Postoperative Care. Nursing care for the patient after surgery depends on the type of surgical procedure that was performed and the extent of the disease process. The patient is usually hospitalized for multiple days after an *open* radical retroperitoneal lymph node dissection. The patient having the laparoscopic procedure may have a urinary catheter in place following the procedure, which is removed before discharge 1 to 2 days later. Refer to Chapter 9 for general postoperative care.

Physiological Integrity

The nurse is caring for a client who had an orchiectomy and laparoscopic radical retroperitoneal lymph node dissection yesterday. Which assessment finding would the nurse report to the health care provider?

A. Total urine output in 24 hours of 1314 mL
B. BP 130/90 mm Hg, T 99.0°F (37.2°C), RR 18, P 90
C. Reports pain of 7 on a 0-to-10 scale after receiving opioid medication
D. Expresses uncertainty about ability to obtain an erection in the future

Care Coordination and Transition Management

After an open *orchiectomy,* the patient is discharged without a dressing on the inguinal incision (if there is no wound complication). A scrotal support may be needed for several days. The patient may want to wear a dry dressing to prevent clothing from rubbing on the sutures and causing irritation. Tell him that the sutures will be removed in the health care provider's office 7 to 10 days after surgery.

Patients who also had an *open* RPLND recover more slowly. They should avoid lifting, stair climbing, and driving for several weeks. Be sure that bathroom facilities are on the first floor of the house, where he can easily access them. It may take 3 to 6 weeks to be able to return to work that is not physically demanding, or up to 3 months if the patient performs heavy lifting or physical labor (Memorial Sloan Kettering Cancer Center, 2022).

Teach the patient who had a laparoscopic procedure that he will be able to resume most of his usual activities within 1 week after discharge. He can take a shower 1 or 2 days after surgery, but should not remove the wound closure tape. These strips of tape will loosen and fall off about a week after surgery.

⚠ NURSING SAFETY PRIORITY
Action Alert

For the patient who has undergone testicular surgery, emphasize the importance of keeping the follow-up visit with the surgeon to examine the incision for proper healing. Instruct him to notify the surgeon immediately if chills, fever, vomiting, increasing incisional pain, drainage, or dehiscence of the incision occurs. These signs and symptoms may indicate **infection** for which antibiotics are needed.

Explain the importance of performing monthly testicular self-examination (TSE) on the remaining testis and scheduling follow-up examinations with the health care provider. The patient who has had testicular cancer should be seen regularly by his health care provider for follow-up care and testing.

For the patient with *reproduction* concerns, refer to the American Society for Reproductive Medicine (www.reproductivefacts.org) or RESOLVE: The National Infertility Association (www.resolve.org). For the patient with terminal testicular cancer, refer to hospice and palliative care as appropriate.

ERECTILE DYSFUNCTION

Pathophysiology Review

Erectile dysfunction (ED), also known as *impotence,* is the inability to achieve or maintain an erection for sexual intercourse. It affects millions of men throughout the world. There are two major types of ED: organic and psychogenic.

Organic ED is a gradual deterioration of function. The man may first notice diminishing firmness and a decrease in frequency of erections. Causes include (Schreiber, 2019; Rogers, 2023):

- Vascular, endocrine, or neurologic disease
- Chronic disease (e.g., diabetes mellitus, renal failure)
- Penile disease or trauma
- Surgery or pharmaceutical therapies
- Obesity

If the patient has episodes of ED, it usually has a *psychogenic* cause that may be related to anxiety, depression, trauma, stress, relationship concerns, or other psychological factors (Khera, 2020). Men with this type of ED usually still have normal nocturnal (nighttime) and morning erections. Onset is usually sudden and follows a period of high stress.

Interprofessional Collaborative Care

The health care provider will attempt to determine the cause of the ED through a variety of diagnostic tests. These may include evaluating glycated hemoglobin, a lipid panel for cardiac risk factors, thyroid-stimulating hormone (TSH) to rule out thyroid disease, and serum total testosterone (Khera, 2020). Doppler ultrasonography can be used to determine blood flow to the penis. Treatment depends on the underlying cause, and may include (Khera, 2023):

- Lifestyle modifications (e.g., smoking cessation, weight loss, management of hypertension)
- Management of medications that may cause ED (e.g., antidepressants)
- Penile self-injection with prostaglandin E1
- Phosphodiesterase-5 (PDE5) drug therapy
- Psychotherapy
- Testosterone and PDE5 drug therapy (for men with hypogonadism)
- Surgery (prosthesis)
- Vacuum-assisted erection devices

See Table 64.4 for select treatment options for ED.

💊 NURSING SAFETY PRIORITY
Drug Alert

Instruct patients taking PDE5 inhibitors to abstain from alcohol before sexual intercourse because it could impair the ability to have an erection. Common side effects of these drugs include dyspepsia (heartburn), headaches, facial flushing, and stuffy nose. If more than one pill a day is being taken, leg and back cramps, nausea, and vomiting also may occur. *Teach men who take nitrates to avoid PDE5 inhibitors because the vasodilation effects can cause profound hypotension and reduce blood flow to vital organs* (Burchum & Rosenthal, 2022).

VASECTOMY

Vasectomy is the most effective mode of male contraception. It involves interruption or occlusion of each vas deferens (Viera, 2023). The preferred procedure is the "no-scalpel" vasectomy in the United States, performed with local anesthetic (without epinephrine) in an outpatient setting.

Teach the patient to leave the dressing and scroll support in place for at least 48 hours postprocedure, and to apply an ice pack intermittently to the scrotum for 24 to 48 hours to minimize pain and swelling. Confirm that mild pain, swelling, and bruising are normal for the first few days. Teach the patient to rest for the first 24 hours after the procedure and to report increasing pain, incisional bleeding, increased swelling, or fever to the health care provider (Viera, 2023).

In 2 days, the patient can return to light work. Heavy lifting, sports, and sexual intercourse should be avoided for at least 1 week. A barrier method of contraception should still be used to prevent pregnancy until a semen analysis has confirmed sterility. This is usually performed 3 months postoperatively.

Although this procedure is performed with the intention of permanent sterilization, vasectomy can be reversed microsurgically in about 50% to 70% of cases (Viera, 2023).

OTHER CONDITIONS AFFECTING THE MALE REPRODUCTIVE SYSTEM

Other conditions that can affect the male reproductive system include inflammation, infection, swelling, trauma, and torsion (Fig. 64.7). Table 64.5 lists select examples of these common conditions with their nursing implications.

TABLE 64.4   Select Treatment Options for Erectile Dysfunction

Procedure	Description	Nursing Implications
Phosphodiesterase-5 (PDE5) inhibitors (drug therapy including avanafil, sildenafil, tadalafil, vardenafil)	Relaxes the smooth muscles in the corpora cavernosa so that blood flow to the penis is increased. The veins exiting the corpora are compressed, limiting outward blood flow and resulting in penile swelling.	Teach: • Notify the primary health care provider if taking or prescribed a nitrate drug or alpha-adrenergic blocker; *use of these with a PDE5 inhibitor can induce hypotension*. • Any PDE5 drug can lower blood pressure; *take safety precautions before use*. • When taking any PDE5 drug, refrain from eating grapefruit or drinking grapefruit juice; *these can interfere with action of the drug*. • Avanafil: Sexual stimulation is needed within 15 to 30 minutes to promote an erection, depending on prescribed dose. • Sildenafil: Sexual stimulation is needed within ½ to 1 hour to promote the erection. Take pill about 1 hour before intercourse on an empty stomach. • Tadalafil: Low-dose daily therapy may be prescribed. • Vardenafil: Sexual stimulation is needed within 15 to 30 minutes to promote an erection, depending on prescribed dose. A high-fat diet may lower effectiveness.
Intraurethral alprostadil injections	Self-administered pellet is placed into urethra immediately after urination; penis is rolled between hands for 10 seconds to complete administration.	Teach: • Cost of this type of drug therapy may be prohibitive. • Penile pain and/or bleeding can occur. • This type of drug therapy should not be used in men with sickle cell anemia, sickle cell trait, leukemia, and other health conditions that may be accompanied by priapism.
Penile injections	Self-injection into the shaft of the penis. Patient uses an insulin syringe with prostaglandin E1.	Teach: • Erection occurs within a few minutes of injection. • Use a condom due to increased risk for infection created at the injection site. • Ibuprofen can be used to treat penile pain. • Priapism is a *urologic emergency* that can occur when using penile injection therapy; seek emergency care immediately.
Penile prostheses	Semirigid or inflatable options. • Semirigid option results in permanent erection. • Inflatable option involves placement of two hollow cylinders in the corpora cavernosa and a saline reservoir. Use of a pump moves the saline from the reservoir to the penile cylinders, causing an erection.	Teach: • Report any signs of infection immediately to the health care provider.
Vacuum-assisted erection device	A cylinder is placed over the penis, sitting firmly against the body. Using a pump, a vacuum is created to draw blood into the penis to maintain an erection. A rubber ring (tension band) is placed around the base of the penis to maintain the erection, and the cylinder is removed.	Teach: • Do not apply vacuum for more than 30 minutes. • Device can be used in tandem with PDE5 inhibitors.

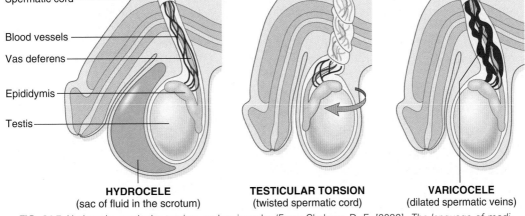

Spermatic cord

Blood vessels

Vas deferens

Epididymis

Testis

HYDROCELE
(sac of fluid in the scrotum)

TESTICULAR TORSION
(twisted spermatic cord)

VARICOCELE
(dilated spermatic veins)

FIG. 64.7 Hydrocele, testicular torsion, and varicocele. (From Chabner, D. E. [2020]. *The language of medicine* [12th ed.]. St. Louis: Elsevier.)

TABLE 64.5 Select Conditions Affecting the Male Reproductive System

Condition Examples of Type	Condition	Description	Signs and Symptoms	Nursing Considerations
Emergent	Paraphimosis	The foreskin (of an uncircumcised male) cannot be returned back over the penis tip, resulting in the foreskin becoming stuck, impeding blood flow to the penile tip and lymphatic drainage	Enlargement and congestion of glans and foreskin, with a band of constrictive tissue that prevents moving the foreskin forward over the penile tip (glans)	Recognize: • Treatment may be manual or surgical in nature. Teach: • Paraphimosis is a *urologic emergency;* seek emergency care immediately. • Topical antibiotic ointment may be prescribed following reduction of the paraphimosis; apply as directed. • Do not retract the foreskin for at least a week following reduction.
	Phimosis	Tightness that results in the inability to retract the foreskin	Swelling and pain at the head of the penis, causing difficulty in retraction of the foreskin Is often associated with hygienic concerns (neglecting to replace the foreskin after cleaning, intercourse, or urination), or body piercing of the glans or foreskin.	Teach: • Proper hygiene is important to avoid this problem in the future. • Topical corticosteroids may be prescribed; use as directed. • Circumcision may be recommended by the health care provider.
	Priapism	Persistent, painful erection (usually >4 hours initially) not associated with sexual stimulation; is common in patients with sickle cell disease, and can be associated with use of certain drugs	Painful erection unrelated to sexual stimulation that lasts >2 to 4 hours (patients with recurrent priapism may have shorter duration of erection)	Recognize: • Priapism *can become a urologic emergency;* seek emergency care immediately. • Treatment varies depending on underlying cause; medical therapy involves intracavernosal injection of a sympathomimetic drug (e.g., phenylephrine) into the penis. After 4 hours duration, aspiration may be required in addition to sympathomimetic drug therapy. Surgical intervention includes placement of a shunt. • Patients with sickle cell disease may require additional treatment, including automated red blood cell exchange transfusions. Intervene: • Administer venous thromboembolism prophylaxis, correction of dehydration (or other sickle cell–related manifestations), and adequate pain control for patients with sickle cell disease and priapism. • See Chapter 9 for postoperative procedures.
	Testicular torsion	Twisting of the spermatic cord that results in ischemia from decreased arterial inflow and venous outflow obstruction; can occur spontaneously or as a result of trauma	Nausea Vomiting Lower abdominal pain Tender mass or knot above the testis	Intervene: • Immediately prepare patient for surgery. • See Chapter 9 for postoperative procedures. Teach: • This is a *urologic emergency;* seek emergency care immediately. Damage may be irreversible after 8 hours. • Surgery is usually performed urgently; manual detorsion is attempted if surgery is not available immediately.

Continued

TABLE 64.5 Select Conditions Affecting the Male Reproductive System—cont'd

Condition Type	Examples of Condition	Description	Signs and Symptoms	Nursing Considerations
"Cele"	Hydrocele	Swelling in the scrotum where fluid has collected around one or both testicles	Painless testicle swelling; often the sensation is described as "heaviness" of the scrotum	Teach: • Confirm that treatment is usually not needed unless the condition becomes painful or too large for comfort; at that time, surgery may be recommended. • If pain does occur, acetaminophen or ibuprofen can be taken. • Report any changes involving pain, fever, redness/hyperpigmentation, or swelling.
	Spermatocele	A cyst that develops in the epididymis; usually is painless	Usually asymptomatic; sometimes pain and/or heaviness occurs in the affected testicle	Teach: • Confirm that treatment is usually not needed unless the condition becomes painful or too large for comfort; at that time, surgery may be recommended. • If pain does occur, acetaminophen or ibuprofen can be taken.
	Varicocele	Vein enlargement inside the scrotum (usually on the left side), which can cause low sperm production	Can be asymptomatic; pain, if experienced, may be dull or sharp, worsening with activity and throughout the day	Teach: • Confirm that treatment is usually not needed unless the condition becomes painful or too large for comfort; at that time, surgery may be recommended, particularly if the patient wishes to maintain fertility.
Infection	Epididymitis	Inflammation or infection of the epididymis; often caused by *Neisseria gonorrhoeae* or *Chlamydia trachomatis* in men under 35 years of age; in older men, it often occurs in association with obstructive uropathy from benign prostatic hyperplasia (BPH). For men of any age who practice insertive anal intercourse, this condition is often associated with exposure to rectal coliform bacteria.	Localized testicular pain Tenderness and swelling on palpation of the epididymis May have scrotal erythema/hyperpigmentation Advanced cases may include testicular swelling	Intervene: • Administer antibiotics and NSAIDs as prescribed. Teach: • Take the full course of antibiotics, even if feeling better. • Ibuprofen can be used for pain. • Elevate the scrotum and apply ice intermittently. • Refrain from sexual intercourse until treatment is completed. • Always use a condom when engaging in sexual intercourse. • Report development of fever, chills, and/or lower urinary tract symptoms (LUTS) to the health care provider right away.

Data from Bragg, B., Kong, E., & Leslie, S. (2023). *Paraphimosis*. [Updated 2023 May 30]. In: StatPearls [Internet]. Treasure Island (FL): StatPearls Publishing; 2023 Jan-. Available from https://www.ncbi.nlm.nih.gov/books/NBK459233/; Deveci, S. (2022). Priapism. *UpToDate*. Retrieved June 9, 2023, from https://www.uptodate.com/contents/priapism; Eyre, R. (2023). Acute scrotal pain in adults. *UpToDate*. Retrieved June 9, 2023, from https://www.uptodate.com/contents/acute-scrotal-pain-in-adults; Eyre, R. (2021). Nonacute scrotal conditions in adults. *UpToDate*. Retrieved June 9, 2023, from https://www.uptodate.com/contents/nonacute-scrotal-conditions-in-adults; DeBaun, M., Burnett, A., & Idris, I. (2023). Priapism and erectile dysfunction in sickle cell disease. *UpToDate*. Retrieved June 9, 2023, from https://www.uptodate.com/contents/priapism-and-erectile-dysfunction-in-sickle-cell-disease; Silberman, M., Stormont, G., Leslie, S., Hu, E. (2023). *Priapism*. [Updated 30 May 2023]. In: StatPearls [Internet]. Treasure Island (FL): StatPearls Publishing; 2023 Jan-. Available from https://www.ncbi.nlm.nih.gov-/books/NBK459178/.

GET READY FOR THE NEXT-GENERATION NCLEX® EXAMINATION!

Essential Nursing Care Points

Health Promotion/Disease Prevention

- Educate patients about the importance of screening for male reproductive cancers according to national guidelines and risk factors.
- Teach men how to perform testicular self-examination.
- Teach men factors that place them at a higher risk for developing male reproductive cancers.
- Discuss ways to change modifiable risk factors to decrease the chance for developing male reproductive cancers and conditions.
- Assess the patient's understanding regarding the fact that some procedures and drugs related to reproductive problems cause temporary or permanent erectile dysfunction and/or incontinence.

Chronic Disease Care

- Teach patients with male reproductive cancer about resources available to provide support.
- Remind patients wanting to use complementary and integrative therapies to check with their health care provider first.

Regenerative or Restorative Care

- Monitor closely for bleeding in patients who have had surgery for a male reproductive problem.
- Use best practices when caring for a patient with a radioactive implant.
- Ensure that the patient who is prescribed drug therapy understands the route of administration and how to properly take or administer the medication.
- Maintain traction on the urinary catheter and continuous bladder irrigation after a TURP.
- Observe for and report complications after surgery, including **infection,** severe pain, urinary infection, **elimination** problems, bloody urine with clots, and/or erectile dysfunction.

Hospice/Palliative/Supportive Care

- Refer patients with terminal male reproductive cancer to hospice, palliative care, and support groups as appropriate.
- Teach patients with a urinary catheter how to properly care for it at home.

Mastery Questions

1. The nurse has provided teaching to a client with erectile dysfunction who was prescribed sildenafil. Which client statement demonstrates an understanding of this drug?
   A. "I might get a headache or stuffy nose when this drug is used."
   B. "After I take this drug, I can have intercourse up to 4 hours later."
   C. "Taking this drug with a drink of alcohol will enhance my performance."
   D. "If one pill doesn't work, I can take another pill to achieve an erection."

2. A client with a history of BPH contacts the telehealth nurse, reporting the sudden onset of testicular pain after moving heavy furniture. Which nursing response is appropriate?
   A. "Taking acetaminophen will help alleviate the pain intensity."
   B. "The BPH is probably increasing because you were moving furniture."
   C. "Please call 911 to take you to the closest emergency department right away."
   D. "The pain will go away soon, as this is a common reaction when performing labor."

NGN Challenge 64.1

The nurse is conducting a history for a 67-year-old male client who has come to the primary care provider reporting difficulty starting a urinary stream. He says that once the urinary stream begins, it feels weak, and then he feels as if his bladder is not empty after urinating. This issue has worsened over the past few months. He denies blood in the urine, burning upon urination, or change in bowel habits.

Complete the diagram by selecting from the choices below to specify what potential condition the client is likely experiencing, **2** nursing actions that are appropriate to take, and **2** parameters the nurse should monitor to assess the client's progress.

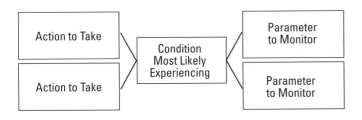

Actions to Take	Potential Conditions	Parameters to Monitor
Administer IV antibiotic therapy	Epididymitis	Biopsy results
Elevate scrotum	Testicular cancer	Increase in pain
Discourage use of caffeine and alcohol	Spermatocele	Results following brachytherapy
Prepare for CT of abdomen and pelvis	Benign prostatic hyperplasia	Decrease in symptom severity
Explain alpha₁-adrenergic antagonists and 5-ARI therapy		Adherence to drug therapy

NGN Challenge 64.2

A client has come to the emergency department. He reports a painful erection that has lasted several hours yet denies being engaged in sexual activity. Rates pain at 8 on a 0-to-10 scale. Electronic health record shows a history of sickle cell disease.

Complete the diagram by selecting from the choices below to specify what potential condition the client is likely experiencing, **2** nursing actions that are appropriate to take, and **2** parameters the nurse should monitor to assess the client's progress.

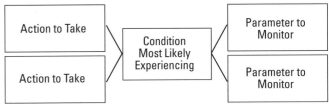

Actions to Take	Potential Conditions	Parameters to Monitor
Refer for circumcision	Hydrocele	Adherence to topical steroid therapy
Administer IV opioids	Phimosis	Congestion of the glans
Watchful waiting for symptom resolution	Priapism	Response to sympathomimetic drug injection
Contact the health care provider	Testicular torsion	Reduction in pain rating
Prepare for emergent surgery		Ability to replace foreskin

REFERENCES

Agarwal, D. K., Rivera, M. E., Nottingham, C. U., Large, T., & Krambeck, A. E. (2020). Catheter removal on the same day of Holmium laser enucleation of the prostate: Outcomes of a pilot study. *Urology, 146,* 225–229. https://doi.org/10.1016/j.urology.2020.09.038.

American Cancer Society (ACS). (2018). *Surgery for testicular cancer.* https://www.cancer.org/cancer/testicular-cancer/treating/surgery.html.

American Cancer Society (ACS). (2019). *Surgery for prostate cancer.* https://www.cancer.org/cancer/prostate-cancer/treating/surgery.html.

American Cancer Society (ACS). (2021). *About prostate cancer.* Retrieved from https://www.cancer.org/content/dam/CRC/PDF/Public/8793.00.pdf.

American Cancer Society (ACS). (2023a). *American Cancer Society recommendations for prostate cancer early detection.* https://www.cancer.org/cancer/prostate-cancer/detection-diagnosis-staging/acs-recommendations.html.

American Cancer Society (ACS). (2023b). *Key statistics for prostate cancer.* Retrieved from https://www.cancer.org/cancer/prostate-cancer/about/key-statistics.html.

American Cancer Society (ACS). (2023c). *Radiation therapy for prostate cancer*. Retrieved from https://www.cancer.org/cancer/prostate-cancer/treating/radiation-therapy.html.

American Society of Clinical Oncology. (2023). *Testicular cancer: Statistics*. https://www.cancer.net/cancer-types/testicular-cancer/statistics.

Boston Scientific Corporation. (2023). *Rezum™ water vapor therapy*. https://www.bostonscientific.com/en-US/products/lithotripsy/rezum-water-vapor-therapy/science-of-rezum.html.

Burchum, J. L. R., & Rosenthal, L. D. (2022). *Lehne's pharmacology for nursing care* (10th ed.). St. Louis: Elsevier.

Centers for Disease Control and Prevention. (2023). *Who is at risk for prostate cancer?* Retrieved from https://www.cdc.gov/cancer/prostate/basic_info/risk_factors.htm.

Emmett, M., Istre, O., & Hahn, R. (2022). Hyponatremia following transurethral resection, hysteroscopy, or other procedures involving electrolyte-free irrigation. *UpToDate*. Retrieved June 9, 2023, from https://www.uptodate.com/contents/hyponatremia-following-transurethral-resection-hysteroscopy-or-other-procedures-involving-electrolyte-free-irrigation.

Guinness World Records Limited. (2023). *Oldest sperm used in successful IVF treatment*. https://www.guinnessworldrecords.com/world-records/oldest-sperm-used-in-successful-ivf-treatment.

Hoffman, R., & Preston, M. (2023). Screening for prostate cancer. *UpToDate*. Retrieved June 9, 2023, from https://www.uptodate.com/contents/screening-for-prostate-cancer.

Khera, M. (2020). Evaluation of male sexual dysfunction. *UpToDate*. Retrieved June 9, 2023, from https://www.uptodate.com/contents/evaluation-of-male-sexual-dysfunction.

Khera, M. (2023). Treatment of male sexual dysfunction. *UpToDate*. Retrieved June 9, 2023, from https://www.uptodate.com/contents/treatment-of-male-sexual-dysfunction.

McVary, K. (2023a). Epidemiology and pathophysiology of benign prostatic hyperplasia. *UpToDate*. Retrieved June 9, 2023, from https://www.uptodate.com/contents/epidemiology-and-pathophysiology-of-benign-prostatic-hyperplasia.

McVary, K. (2023b). Medical treatment of benign prostatic hyperplasia. *UpToDate*. Retrieved June 9, 2023, from https://www.uptodate.com/contents/medical-treatment-of-benign-prostatic-hyperplasia.

McVary, K. (2023c). Surgical treatment of benign prostatic hyperplasia. *UpToDate*. Retrieved June 9, 2023, from https://www.uptodate.com/contents/surgical-treatment-of-benign-prostatic-hyperplasia-bph.

Memorial Sloan Kettering Cancer Center. (2022). *About your retroperitoneal lymph node dissection*. https://www.mskcc.org/cancer-care/patient-education/about-your-retroperitoneal-lymph-node-dissection.

Michaelson, M., & Oh, W. (2023). Epidemiology of and risk factors for testicular germ cell tumors. *UpToDate*. Retrieved June 9, 2023, from https://www.uptodate.com/contents/epidemiology-of-and-risk-factors-for-testicular-germ-cell-tumors.

Neotract. (2023). *The UroLift® system treatment*. https://www.urolift.com/what-is-urolift?.

New York Presbyterian. (n.d.). *LGBTQ+ Terminology / Vocabulary Primer*. https://www.nyp.org/documents/pps/cultural-competency/Understanding%20Disparities%20-%20LGBTQ%20Terminology.pdf

Oh, W. (2023). Overview of the treatment of testicular germ cell tumors. *UpToDate*. Retrieved June 9, 2023, from https://www.uptodate.com/contents/overview-of-the-treatment-of-testicular-germ-cell-tumors.

Pagana, K. D., Pagana, T. J., & Pagana, T. N. (2022). *Mosby's manual of diagnostic and laboratory tests* (7th ed.). St. Louis: Elsevier.

Punnen, S., Carroll, P., & Washington, S., III. (2022). Active surveillance for men with clinically localized prostate cancer. *UpToDate*. Retrieved June 9, 2023, from https://www.uptodate.com/contents/active-surveillance-for-males-with-clinically-localized-prostate-cancer.

Rogers, J. L. (2023). *McCance and Huether's Pathophysiology: The biologic basis for disease in adults and children* (9th ed.). St. Louis: Elsevier.

Saper, R. (2022). Clinical use of saw palmetto. *UpToDate*. Retrieved June 9, 2023, from https://www.uptodate.com/contents/clinical-use-of-saw-palmetto.

Sartor, A. (2022). Risk factors for prostate cancer. *UpToDate*. Retrieved June 5, 2023, from https://www.uptodate.com/contents/risk-factors-for-prostate-cancer.

Schreiber, M. (2019). Erectile dysfunction. *MedSurg Nursing, 28*(5), 327–330. https://doi.org/10.1155/2018/2146080.

Shvero, A., Calio, B., Humphreys, M. R., & Das, A. K. (2021). HoLEP: The new gold standard for surgical treatment of benign prostatic hyperplasia. *The Canadian Journal of Urology, 28*(5), 6–10.

Taplin, M., & Smith, J. (2023). Clinical presentation and diagnosis of prostate cancer. *UpToDate*. Retrieved June 9, 2023, from https://www.uptodate.com/contents/clinical-presentation-and-diagnosis-of-prostate-cancer.

The University of Utah. (2023). *HoLEP: Holmium laser enucleation of the prostate*. https://healthcare.utah.edu/urology/conditions/enlarged-prostate/surgery/holep.php.

University of Wisconsin Hospitals and Clinics Authority. (2023). *A gold standard for BPH treatment*. https://www.uwhealth.org/treatments/holep-holmium-laser-enucleation-of-the-prostate.

U.S. Preventive Services Task Force. (2018). *Final recommendation statement: Prostate cancer: Screening*. Retrieved from https://www.uspreventiveservicestaskforce.org/Page/Document/RecommendationStatementFinal/prostate-cancer-screening.

Veru Inc. (2021). *Entadfi™*. https://www.accessdata.fda.gov/drugsatfda_docs/label/2021/215423s000lbl.pdf.

Viera, A. (2023). Vasectomy. *UpToDate*. Retrieved March 19, 2023, from https://www.uptodate.com/contents/vasectomy.

Wang, Q., Alshayyah, R., & Yang, B. (2022). The efficacy and safety of desmopressin acetate applied for nocturia in benign prostatic hyperplasia patients: A systematic review and meta-analysis. *Lower Urinary Tract Symptoms, 14*(3), 155–162.

Yale Medicine. (2023). *Enlarged prostate (benign prostatic hyperplasia)*. https://www.yalemedicine.org/conditions/enlarged-prostate-benign-prostatic-hyperplasia-bph.

ZERO®. (2023). *Our story*. https://zerocancer.org/why-zero/our-mission-impact/our-story/.

65

Concepts of Care for Patients With Sexually Transmitted Infections

Cherie R. Rebar

http://evolve.elsevier.com/Iggy/

LEARNING OUTCOMES

1. Plan collaborative care with the interprofessional team to promote health in patients with a sexually transmitted infection.
2. Teach adults how to decrease the risk for sexually transmitted infections.
3. Teach the patient and caregiver(s) about common drugs and other management strategies used for sexually transmitted infections.
4. Plan patient- and family-centered nursing interventions to decrease the psychosocial impact caused by living with a sexually transmitted infection.
5. Apply knowledge of anatomy, physiology, and pathophysiology to provide evidence-based care for patients with a sexually transmitted infection.
6. Analyze assessment and diagnostic findings to generate solutions and prioritize nursing care for patients with a sexually transmitted infection.
7. Organize care coordination and transition management for patients with a sexually transmitted infection.
8. Use clinical judgment to plan evidence-based nursing care to promote health and prevent complications in patients with a sexually transmitted infection.
9. Incorporate factors that affect **health equity** into the plan of care for patients with a sexually transmitted infection.

KEY TERMS

chancre The ulcer that is the first sign of syphilis. It develops at the site of entry (inoculation) of the organism, usually 3 weeks after exposure. The lesion may be found on any area of the skin or mucous membranes but occurs most often on the genitalia, lips, nipples, and hands and in the oral cavity, anus, and rectum.

dyspareunia Painful sexual intercourse.

dysuria Painful urination.

expedited partner therapy (EPT) The practice of treating sexual partners of patients diagnosed with chlamydia infection or gonorrhea by providing prescriptions or medication to the patient, which they can take to their partner(s), without the primary health care provider examining the partner(s). Also called *patient-delivered partner therapy*.

genital herpes (GH) An acute, recurring incurable viral disease of the genitalia caused by the herpes simplex virus and transmitted through contact with an infected person.

pelvic inflammatory disease (PID) An acute syndrome resulting in tenderness in the fallopian tubes and ovaries (adnexa) and, typically, dull pelvic pain.

safer sex practices Interventions that reduce the risk of nonintact skin or mucous membranes coming in contact with infected body fluids and blood, such as using a condom.

salpingitis Fallopian tube infection.

sexually transmitted disease (STD) Term used in some instances by the Centers for Disease Control and Prevention for sexually transmitted infection.

sexually transmitted infection (STI) Infectious organisms that have been passed from one person to another through intimate contact.

syphilis A complex sexually transmitted disease that can become systemic and cause serious complications and even death.

INTRODUCTION TO SEXUALLY TRANSMITTED INFECTIONS

Sexually transmitted infections (STIs) are infectious conditions that have been passed from one person to another through intimate contact—usually oral, vaginal, or anal intercourse. STIs can also be passed by parenteral exposure to infected blood, via fecal-oral transmission, by intrauterine transmission to the fetus, and by perinatal transmission from mother to neonate.

In some instances, the term sexually transmitted disease (STD) is used by the Centers for Disease Control and Prevention (CDC, 2023c). The CDC provides best practice guidelines for the treatment of STIs (Workowski et al., 2021). This includes information, treatment standards, and counseling recommendations to help decrease the spread of these diseases and their complications.

The reported numbers of cases of STIs are influenced by improved diagnostic techniques, increased knowledge about organisms that can be sexually transmitted, and changes in *sexuality* (see Chapter 1) and sexual practices. Other factors, such as an increasing population, cultural practices, political and economic policies, sexual abuse, human trafficking, and international travel and migration, also affect the prevalence of STIs.

The prevalence of STIs is a major public health concern worldwide. People at greatest risk for acquiring an STI include those who (American College of Obstetricians and Gynecologists, 2023; World Health Organization, 2022a):

- Have more than one sexual partner currently (especially anonymous partners)
- Have had more than one sexual partner in the past
- Engage in sexual activity with someone who has an STI
- Have a history of having an STI
- Use intravenous drugs
- Have or had a partner who uses (used) intravenous drugs
- Engage in anal, vaginal, or oral sex without a condom
- Have sex while using drugs or alcohol

While some populations are more affected by STIs than others, it is important to not assume that certain groups are less vulnerable than others, as sexual practices and knowledge about self-protection vary greatly. A key nursing role is to ensure that *all* people are equally assessed for, and educated about, STIs. Within this chapter, the terms "female," "woman," and "women"

and the pronouns "she" and "her" apply to all individuals who were *assigned female at birth (AFAB),* which includes cisgender women, transgender men, and nonbinary people with vaginas (Cleveland Clinic, 2023). The terms "male," "man," and "men" and the pronouns "he" and "him" apply to all individuals who were *assigned male at birth (AMAB),* which includes cisgender men, transgender women, and nonbinary people with penises.

👤 **PATIENT-CENTERED CARE: OLDER ADULT HEALTH**

Older Adults and STIs

Older adults may not realize that they are at risk for STIs or feel comfortable discussing *sexuality* with health care providers. Provide a safe and private environment to teach older adults who are sexually active about their risk for developing STIs and how to protect themselves.

One of the greatest factors associated with STI prevalence is the interest in *sexuality*, sexual behaviors, and intimacy in the American culture. The stigma of STIs in the United States has been associated with higher rates of these infections compared with rates in other developed countries. The prevalence of STIs is also affected by changing human physiology patterns, such as earlier onset of menarche, comorbidities associated with human immunodeficiency virus (HIV) and diabetes, and imbalances in *health equity* (see Chapter 1). Misuse of substances has also been identified as a significant risk factor because of the effects that drugs have on decision making and risk-taking behavior.

STIs can cause complications that contribute to severe physical and emotional pain, including ectopic pregnancy; cancer; infertility, which can affect future plans for *reproduction;* and death. Some of the most common complications that can result from sexually transmitted organisms are listed in Table 65.1.

Certain types of STIs must be reported to local health authorities. Check requirements in your state, and communicate reportable STIs accordingly (see the Legal/Ethical Considerations box).

❓ **LEGAL/ETHICAL CONSIDERATIONS**

Reporting Sexually Transmitted Infections (STIs)

Certain conditions such as chlamydia, gonorrhea, syphilis, chancroid, and HIV *infection* (through HIV Stage III—acquired immunodeficiency syndrome [AIDS]) are notifiable nationally (CDC, 2022a). Other STIs such as genital herpes (GH) may or may not be reported, depending on state and local legal requirements. Professional nursing implications include reporting positive results to the appropriate authorities, recognizing that reports are kept strictly confidential by the receiving authority.

Nurses in all environments of care have a responsibility to recognize patients who are at risk for or who have STIs, possibly while being treated for another unrelated health problem. Sexual issues, particularly those involving suspected or actual STIs, are sensitive, personal, and sometimes controversial. As a patient advocate, demonstrate a nonjudgmental attitude when caring for people who have concerns related to *sexuality.* Providing confidentiality and privacy is essential for patients

TABLE 65.1 Complications That Can Result From Sexually Transmitted Organisms

Causative Organism	Complication
Candida albicans	Female: • Increased localized inflammation and pain Male: • Balanitis (inflammation of the penile head)
Chlamydia trachomatis	Female: • Pelvic inflammatory disease • Premature labor/birth, low-birth-weight neonate (in pregnant women) • Scarring in, or obstruction of, fallopian tubes • Sexually acquired reactive arthritis Male: • Epididymitis or epididymo-orchitis • Sexually acquired reactive arthritis
Condylomata acuminata (Genital warts caused by HPV)	Female: • Cellular changes resulting in cancer • Transmission of infection to neonate born vaginally Male: • Cellular changes resulting in cancer
Herpes simplex virus-1 (HSV-1) Herpes simplex virus-2 (HSV-2)	Female and Male: • Meningoencephalitis
Neisseria gonorrhoeae	Female: • Ectopic pregnancy • Infertility • Miscarriage, premature labor/birth, neonate eye infection (in pregnant women) • Pelvic inflammatory disease • Pelvic pain (long term) • Sepsis (if left untreated) Male: • Fertility reduction • Proctitis • Sepsis (if left untreated)
Treponema pallidum (Causative agent of syphilis)	Female and Male: • Progression to secondary or tertiary stage of syphilis • Neurosyphilis • Ocular syphilis • Otosyphilis
Trichomonas vaginalis	Female: • Increased risk for HIV infection • Premature labor/birth, low-birth-weight neonate (in pregnant women) Male: • Infertility • Prostatitis • Epididymitis • Urethral stricture

to receive correct information, make informed decisions, and obtain evidence-based care.

Recognize that 70% of victims of human trafficking have had to seek medical care at some point (Pourmand & Marcinkowski, 2022). In any clinical setting, you are in a key position to identify and assist victims (Rapoza, 2022). Signs of trafficking can be found in Chapter 10. Best practices for identifying and caring for people who may need assistance include:

- Interviewing the patient without the presence of a partner or other person who accompanies them
- Providing professional interpreters, if needed; never rely on the partner or others to speak for the patient
- Collaborating with social workers, sexual assault nurse examiners (SANEs), and other members of the interprofessional team, as indicated
- Ensuring that documentation is consistent if there are concerns regarding trafficking.

👤 PATIENT-CENTERED CARE: GENDER HEALTH

Screening for STIs

Because of the very vascular and large surface area of the mucous membranes of the vagina, women are more easily infected with STIs and are vulnerable to infections because of the exposure of cervical basal epithelium cells. Men who have sex with men (MSM) are disproportionately affected by STIs (Indiana Department of Health, 2021). Screen all people for STIs, recognizing that some of these conditions do not have symptoms that prompt people to seek health care.

Changing social relationships later in life affects the risk for exposure to STIs. Women who are no longer concerned with pregnancy may be at risk for STIs if they do not use barrier methods. Physiologic changes experienced by postmenopausal women such as mucosal tears from vaginal atrophy increase risk.

Women have more asymptomatic infections, which may delay diagnosis and treatment. Many infectious organisms reside in the cervical os and cause little change in vaginal discharge or vulvar tissue, so women are unaware that they are infected. This delay increases the risk for complications, including ascending infections, which may cause reproductive organ damage and illness. Embarrassment, denial, or fear about STIs may further delay treatment, increasing the potential for serious complications.

Health Promotion/Disease Prevention

Select examples of *Healthy People 2030* objectives related to sexually transmitted infections include (U.S. Department of Health and Human Services, Office of Disease Prevention and Health Promotion, 2023):

- Reduction of the syphilis rate in men who have sex with men, and in females
- Increase in the proportion of sexually active female adolescents and young women who get screened for chlamydia
- Reduction of deaths associated with hepatitis B or C

See Box 65.1 for more *Healthy People 2030* objectives related to sexually transmitted infections.

One of the primary tools for prevention of sexually transmitted infections (STIs) is education. All people, regardless of age, sex assigned at birth, gender identity, ethnicity, socioeconomic status, education level, or sexual orientation, are susceptible to these diseases. Health literacy, motivation, and perceived risk can affect the health status of any patient. Do not assume that a person is not sexually active because of age, education, marital status, profession, culture, or religion.

Use a variety of venues for teaching people about methods of prevention, including available technology platforms, mobile applications, and professional social media presences such as the CDC's Twitter account (Curry et al., 2022). These forums can be used to provide education about vaccination, safer sex practices, available health resources, and expedited partner therapy.

STIs are largely preventable through safer sex practices—actions that that reduce the risk for nonintact skin or mucous membranes coming in contact with infected body fluids and blood. Discuss prevention methods, including safer sex, with all patients who are or may become sexually active. These practices include:

- Using a latex or polyurethane condom for genital and anal intercourse
- Using a condom or latex barrier (dental dam) over the genitals or anus during oral-genital or oral-anal sexual contact
- Wearing gloves for finger or hand contact with the vagina or rectum
- Practicing abstinence
- Practicing mutual monogamy
- Decreasing the number of sexual partners

GENITAL HERPES

Pathophysiology Review

Genital herpes (GH) is an acute, recurring common viral disease. More than half a million new infections are diagnosed in the United States annually (CDC, 2021a). Two serotypes of herpes simplex virus (HSV) affect the genitalia: type 1 (HSV-1) and type 2 (HSV-2) (Rogers, 2023). In the United States, about 12% of people between the ages of 14 and 49 have HSV-2 (CDC, 2021a).

Most *nongenital* lesions such as cold sores are caused by HSV-1, transmitted via oral-oral contact. Historically, HSV-2 caused most of the genital lesions. However, either type can produce oral or genital lesions through oral-genital or genital-genital contact with an infected person. HSV-2 recurs and sheds asymptomatically more often than HSV-1. Many people with GH have not been diagnosed because they have mild symptoms and shed the virus intermittently.

The incubation period of genital herpes is 2 to 20 days (average is 1 week). Many people do not have symptoms during the primary outbreak. The virus remains dormant and recurs periodically, even if the patient is asymptomatic. Recurrences are not caused by reinfection; they are related to *viral shedding, and the patient is infectious.*

Long-term complications of GH include the risk for neonatal transmission and an increased risk for acquiring HIV *infection* (Rogers, 2023). GH is still considered incurable (American Sexual Health Association, 2023) although vaccine clinical trials continue.

Interprofessional Collaborative Care
Recognize Cues: Assessment

The diagnosis of GH is based on the patient's history and physical examination (Box 65.2).

Ask the patient if they experience itching or a tingling sensation in the skin 1 to 2 days before the outbreak, known as the *prodrome.* These sensations are usually followed by the appearance of vesicles (blisters) in a typical cluster on the vulva (Fig. 65.1), vagina, cervix, scrotum, penis (Fig. 65.2), or perianal region at the site of inoculation. The blisters rupture spontaneously in a day or two and leave ulcerations that can become extensive and cause *pain.*

Assess for other symptoms such as headaches, fever, general malaise, and swelling of inguinal lymph nodes. Ask whether urination is painful. External dysuria is a painful symptom when urine passes over the eroded areas. Patients with urinary retention may need to be catheterized. Lesions resolve within 2 to 6 weeks. After the lesions heal, the virus remains in a dormant state in the sacral nerve ganglia.

Periodically the virus activates, and symptoms recur. These recurrences can be triggered by stress, fever, sunburn, poor nutrition, menses, and sexual activity. Provide anticipatory guidance regarding stressor management to prevent outbreaks.

GH is usually confirmed through laboratory testing, which may include a viral culture, polymerase chain reaction (PCR), direct fluorescent antibody, and type-specific serologic

BOX 65.2 Assessing the Patient With a Suspected Sexually Transmitted Infection

Assess history of present illness:
- Chief concern
- Time of onset
- Symptoms by quality and quantity, precipitating and palliative factors
- Any treatments taken (self-prescribed or over-the-counter products) and whether they have been helpful

Assess past medical history:
- Major health problems, including any history of STIs, PID, or immunosuppression
- Surgeries: obstetric and gynecologic; circumcision

Assess current health status:
- Menstrual history for irregularities
- Sexual history:
  - Type and frequency of sexual activity
  - Number of sexual contacts/partners (lifetime and past 6 months); or monogamous
  - Sexual orientation
  - Contraception history
- Medications
- Allergies
- Lifestyle risks: drugs, alcohol, tobacco

Assess preventive health care practices:
- Papanicolaou (Pap) tests
- Regular STI screening
- Use of barrier contraceptives to prevent STIs and/or pregnancy

Assess physical examination findings:
- Vital signs
- Oropharyngeal findings
- Abdominal findings
- Genital or pelvic findings
- Anorectal findings

Assess laboratory data:
- Urinalysis
- Hematology
- ESR or CRP if PID is being considered
- Cervical, urethral, oral, rectal specimens
- Lesion samples for microbiology and virology
- Pregnancy testing

CRP, C-reactive protein; *ESR*, erythrocyte sedimentation rate; *PID*, pelvic inflammatory disease; *STI*, sexually transmitted infection.

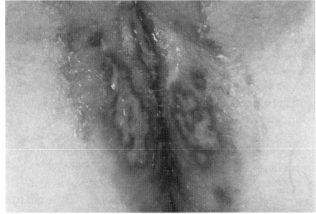

FIG. 65.1 Herpes simplex virus type 2 (HSV-2) infection; blisters on the vulva. (From Jarvis, C, & Eckhardt, A. [2024]. *Physical examination and health assessment* [9th ed.]. St. Louis: Elsevier.)

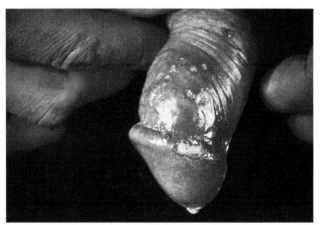

FIG. 65.2 Herpes simplex virus type 2 (HSV-2) infection; blisters on the penis. (From Jarvis, C, & Eckhardt, A. [2024]. *Physical examination and health assessment* [9th ed.]. St. Louis: Elsevier.)

tests (Albrecht, 2022a). Fluid from inside the blister obtained within 48 hours of the first outbreak will yield the most reliable results because accuracy decreases as the blisters begin to heal. Serology testing, which is glycoprotein G antibody–based, can identify the HSV type, either 1 or 2. Antibodies may not be present soon after the initial infection, so false-negative results are possible (Albrecht, 2022a).

Take Actions: Interventions

The desired outcomes of treatment for patients infected with GH are to decrease **pain** from ulcerations, promote healing without secondary infection, decrease viral shedding, and prevent **infection** transmission.

Drug Therapy. Antiviral drugs are used to treat GH. The drugs decrease the severity, promote healing, and decrease the frequency of recurrent outbreaks but do not cure the **infection.**

Drug therapy should be offered to anyone with an initial outbreak of GH regardless of the severity of the symptoms. The CDC (2021a) recommends treatment with acyclovir, famciclovir, or valacyclovir. Intravenous acyclovir and hospitalization may be indicated for patients with HSV and more severe symptoms, including aseptic meningitis, encephalitis, end-organ disease, or disseminated (systemic) disease (Albrecht, 2022b).

Dosage and length of treatment differ and can be discussed between the patient and health care provider. *Episodic therapy*, taking an antiviral drug at the first sign of a recurrent outbreak, is most beneficial if it is started within 1 day of the appearance of lesions or when itching or tingling occur before lesions appear. *Suppressive therapy*, taking a prescribed antiviral drug daily, can also be offered to patients (Albrecht, 2022b). Suppression reduces recurrences in most patients, but it does not prevent viral shedding, even when symptoms are absent. Encourage patients on chronic suppressive therapy to follow up annually with their provider (or more frequently as needed) to continue to determine which type of drug therapy is most beneficial.

Self-Management Education. Nursing interventions focus on **pain** control by treatment of the underlying problem and on patient education. Teach about the **infection,** modes of sexual transmission, potential for recurrent episodes, and correct use

---

BOX 65.3   Patient and Family Education

Teaching the Patient With Genital Herpes (GH)

- Take oral analgesics and antiviral medication as prescribed.
- Apply local anesthetic sprays or ointments as prescribed.
- Apply ice packs or warm compresses to lesions.
- Take sitz baths three or four times a day.
- Increase fluid intake to replace fluid lost through open lesions.
- Practice frequent urination.
- Pour water over genitalia while voiding or while standing in a shower.
- Maintain genital hygiene, keeping the skin clean and dry.
- Wear gloves when applying ointments or making any direct contact with lesions.
- Wash hands thoroughly after contact with lesions
- Launder towels that have had direct contact with lesions.
- Avoid sexual activity when lesions are present.
- Use latex or polyurethane condoms during all sexual exposures.
- Discuss the diagnosis of GH with former, current, and new partners so that effective treatment or prevention of transmission takes place.

---

and possible side effects of antiviral therapy. Clear discussion about sexual activity, including whether the patient has new or multiple partners, is an essential component of the nurse's intervention. Box 65.3 contains important information to teach the patient for effective self-management.

! NURSING SAFETY PRIORITY

Action Alert

Remind patients to abstain from sexual activity while GH lesions are present. Sexual activity can cause *pain* and the likelihood of viral transmission is higher. Urge condom use during all sexual encounters because of the increased risk for HSV transmission from viral shedding, which can occur even when lesions are not present. Teach the patient how to properly use condoms (Box 65.4).

Assess the patient's and partner's emotional responses to the diagnosis of GH. Many people are initially shocked and need reassurance that they can manage the disease. Patients who are infected may have feelings of disbelief, anger, guilt, isolation, or loneliness. They may be angry at their partner(s) for transmitting the *infection* or fear rejection because they have it. Help patients cope with the diagnosis by being nonjudgmental, sensitive, and supportive during assessments and interventions. Encourage social support and refer patients to support groups (e.g., local support groups of the Herpes Resource Center [http://www.ashasexualhealth.org/stdsstis/herpes/]) and therapists.

SYPHILIS

Pathophysiology Review

Syphilis is a complex sexually transmitted **infection** (STI) that can become systemic and cause serious complications, including death. Rates of syphilis in the United States have continued to rise annually (CDC, 2023d). The causative organism is a spirochete called *Treponema pallidum*. The infection is usually transmitted by sexual contact and blood exposure, but transmission

---

BOX 65.4   Patient and Family Education

Proper Use of Condoms

- Use external latex or polyurethane condoms; avoid natural membrane condoms as they provide much less protection against STIs.
- Use a new condom with each sexual encounter (including oral, vaginal, and anal), even with the same person.
- Internal condoms ("female condoms")—polyurethane or nitrile sheaths placed in the vagina or anus—have not been studied as closely as traditional male condoms (Hoke et al., 2022).
- Do not use an external condom with an internal condom; this causes friction and can cause a condom to break.
- Condoms can break during sexual intercourse. If a condom breaks, replace it immediately.
- Keep condoms (especially latex) in a cool, dry place, out of direct sunlight.
- Do not use condoms that are in damaged packages or that are brittle or discolored.
- Always handle a condom with care to avoid damaging it with fingernails, teeth, or other sharp objects.
- Put condoms on before any genital contact. Hold the condom by the tip, and unroll it on the penis. Leave a space at the tip to collect semen.
- Ensure that lubricant, if used, is water based and washes away with water. Oil-based products damage latex condoms.
- Recognize that nonoxynol-9 does not protect against GH and can irritate tissues; this may increase the risk for transmission of HIV in women during vaginal and anal intercourse (Bartz, 2023).
- After ejaculation, withdraw the erect penis carefully, holding the condom at the base of the penis to prevent the condom from slipping off.
- Never use a condom more than once.

Data from Centers for Disease Control and Prevention. (2022). *How to use condoms and other barriers.* https://www.cdc.gov/condomeffectiveness/index.html; Workowski, K., et al. (2021). Sexually transmitted infections treatment guidelines. *Morbidity and Mortality Weekly Report Recommendations and Reports, 70*(No. RR-4), 1–192.

---

can occur through close body contact such as touching or kissing where there are open lesions (e.g., on the breast, genitals, or lips, or in the oral cavity) (Hicks & Clement, 2022a).

Untreated syphilis is divided into two categories—early and late—and progresses through four stages: primary (localized chancre), secondary (systemic illness), early latent (seropositive yet without symptoms), and tertiary (symptomatic infection). Neurosyphilis can occur at any time in any stage; patients with this form of the disease may experience meningitis, vision or hearing loss, and brain and spinal cord dysfunction.

The appearance of an ulcer called a chancre is the first sign of *primary* syphilis (Fig. 65.3). It develops at the site of entry (inoculation) of the organism from 12 days to 12 weeks after exposure (3 weeks is average) (Rogers, 2023). Chancres may be found on any area of the skin or mucous membranes but occur most often on the genitalia (Hicks & Clement, 2022a).

During this highly infectious stage, the chancre begins as a small papule, about 1 to 2 cm in diameter with a raised, indurated margin (Hicks & Clement, 2022a). Within 3 to 7 days, it breaks down into its typical appearance: a painless, indurated, smooth, weeping lesion. Regional lymph nodes enlarge, feel firm, and are not painful. Without treatment, the chancre usually disappears within 3 to 6 weeks (Hicks & Clement, 2022a). However, the organism spreads throughout the body, and the patient is still infectious.

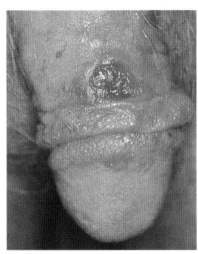

FIG. 65.3 Syphilitic chancre on the penis. (From Jarvis, C., & Eckhardt, A. [2024]. *Physical examination and health assessment* [9th ed.]. St. Louis: Elsevier.)

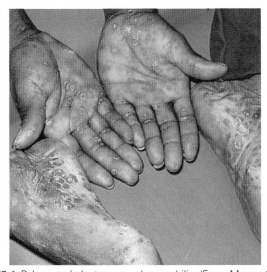

FIG. 65.4 Palmar and plantar secondary syphilis. (From Morse, S., Ballard, R., Holmes, K., & Moreland, A. [2003]. *Atlas of sexually transmitted diseases and AIDS* [3rd ed.]. Edinburgh: Mosby.)

Secondary syphilis develops in about 25% of untreated infected persons within a few months (Hicks & Clement, 2022a). During this stage, syphilis is a systemic disease because the spirochetes circulate throughout the bloodstream. Commonly mistaken for influenza, signs and symptoms include malaise, low-grade fever, headache, sore throat, hoarseness, generalized adenopathy, joint pain, and skin or mucous membrane leisons or rash (Rogers, 2023). There is no typical appearance of this rash, but it usually appears on the palms, soles, trunk, and mucous membranes. It can appear as diffuse macules (reddish brown), papules (usually less than 5 mm) or pustules, scaly psoriasis-like lesions (Fig. 65.4), or gray-white wartlike lesions (condylomata lata). *All of these lesions are highly contagious and should not be touched without gloves.* Patchy alopecia on the scalp or facial hair (missing part of the eyebrow, "moth-eaten" appearance) is another symptom. The rash subsides without treatment

in 2 to 10 weeks (Rogers, 2023), and the patient enters the early latent stage, during which the patient is seropositive but asymptomatic. The stage may last as little as a year, or as long as a lifetime (Rogers, 2023).

Tertiary, or late, syphilis is uncommon because of the widespread availability of antibiotics (Rogers, 2023). If experienced, this occurs after a highly variable period, from 4 to 20 years. This stage develops in untreated cases and can mimic other conditions because any organ system can be affected. Signs and symptoms of late syphilis include (Rogers, 2023):

- Cardiovascular lesions
- Neurosyphilis, including tabes dorsalis and general paresis
- Gummatous syphilis lesions (granulomatous lesions) on the skin, bones, or internal organs

PATIENT-CENTERED CARE: HEALTH EQUITY

Patients With Syphilis

Advocate for ***health equity*** when caring for patients with syphilis. Disparities exist between racial and ethnic groups in the incidence of primary and secondary syphilis. In recent reports from the CDC (2022h), the rates of syphilis increased in most racial/Hispanic ethnicity groups. The greatest increases were noted among non-Hispanic American Indian/Alaska Native individuals and in non-Hispanic people of multiple races (CDC, 2022h). Access to high-quality care is critical to the health of all people.

PATIENT-CENTERED CARE: HEALTH EQUITY

Equitable Health Assessment

Identify unique needs regarding sexual health and prevention and treatment of STIs for lesbian, gay, bisexual, transgender, and questioning (LGBTQ) patients. Discrimination, ***health equity*** imbalances**,** and lack of understanding by health care providers can greatly affect the health status of this population. People who are LGBTQIA2+ may have difficulty finding health care providers who ask about and address their specific needs, risks, and concerns. Taking a health history that provides an opportunity for the patient to share their sexual orientation, gender identity, and sexual activity is crucial.

Especially among transgender and nonbinary people, opportunities for health assessment may be avoided by the patient or missed by the provider because of fears of being misunderstood or inadequately prepared to give or receive appropriate care. Chapter 5 discusses the special health care needs of these patients.

PATIENT-CENTERED CARE: GENDER HEALTH

Syphilis in MSM

Men who have sex with men (MSM) are at high risk for contracting primary and secondary syphilis (CDC, 2023d). Do not assume that people have only had sexual experiences congruent with their noted sexual orientation, as this limits the accuracy of the nurse's risk assessment. Collect an appropriate sexual history for all patients, and design a plan of care based on that specific information.

Interprofessional Collaborative Care

Recognize Cues: Assessment

Assessment of the patient with signs and symptoms of syphilis begins with gathering a history about ulcers or rash. Take a sexual history and conduct a risk assessment to include whether previous testing or treatment for syphilis or other STDs has ever been done (see Box 65.2). Ask about an allergy to penicillin, as this is the treatment of choice for syphilis.

Ask whether there is a history of a chancre. A woman may report inguinal lymph node enlargement resulting from a chancre in the vagina or cervix that is not easily visible to her. Men usually discover the chancre on the penis or scrotum.

Conduct a physical assessment, including inspection and palpation. *Wear gloves while palpating any lesions because of the highly contagious treponemes that are present.* Observe for and document rashes of any type because of the variable presentation of secondary syphilis.

The health care provider will obtain a specimen of the chancre for examination under a darkfield microscope. Diagnosis of primary or secondary syphilis is confirmed if *T. pallidum* is present.

Nontreponemal blood tests include the *Venereal Disease Research Laboratory (VDRL)* serum test, the more sensitive *rapid plasma reagin (RPR)* test. These tests are based on an antibody-antigen reaction that determines the presence and amount of antibodies produced by the body in response to an **infection** by *T. pallidum*. False-positive and false-negative results are a downfall of these types of tests.

Treponemal tests detect antibodies directed against treponemal antigens; they are more reliable than nontreponemal tests (Hicks & Clement, 2022b). These include:

- Fluorescent treponemal antibody absorption (FTA-ABS) test
- Microhemagglutination test for antibodies to *T. pallidum* (MHA-TP)
- *T. pallidum* particle agglutination assay (TPPA)
- *T. pallidum* enzyme immunoassay (TP-EIA)
- Chemiluminescence immunoassay (CIA)

Most patients who are shown to be reactive to one of these nontreponemal tests will have this positive result for their entire lives, even after treatment. This may be surprising news for a patient who denies a history of or does not know of a personal history of syphilis. Use therapeutic communication skills and a nonjudgmental attitude to objectively discuss this finding.

Patients with neurosyphilis symptoms may have a cerebrospinal fluid evaluation performed, particularly if cranial nerve dysfunction is present (Workowski et al., 2021). The health care provider will use the findings from this test in aggregate with other diagnostic results to formulate a firm diagnosis.

Take Actions: Interventions

Drug Therapy. Interprofessional collaborative care includes drug therapy and health teaching to resolve the **infection** and prevent transmission to others. Benzathine penicillin G given IM as a single dose at the time of the initial visit with the health care provider is the evidence-based treatment for primary, secondary, and early latent syphilis (Workowski et al., 2021). Patients in the late latent stage and tertiary stage have a longer duration of drug therapy (Workowski et al, 2021).

NURSING SAFETY PRIORITY

Drug Alert

Allergic reactions to benzathine penicillin G can occur. Monitor for allergic signs and symptoms (e.g., rash, edema, shortness of breath, chest tightness, anxiety). Penicillin desensitization is recommended for penicillin-allergic patients. *Keep all patients at the health care agency for at least 30 minutes after they have received the antibiotic so that signs and symptoms of an allergic reaction can be detected and treated. The most severe reaction is anaphylaxis. Treatment should be available and implemented immediately if symptoms occur.* Chapter 17 describes the management of drug allergies in detail.

The *Jarisch-Herxheimer reaction* may also follow antibiotic therapy for syphilis. This febrile reaction is caused by the rapid release of products from the disruption of the cells of the organism. Additional symptoms include generalized aches, rigors, vasodilation, diaphoresis, hypotension, and worsening of any rash that was present. These symptoms are usually benign and begin within 24 hours after therapy, and are treated symptomatically with analgesics and antipyretics (Workowski et al., 2021). Teach the patient the difference between this possible reaction and an allergic reaction to penicillin.

Self-Management Education. To provide teaching, choose a setting that offers privacy and encourages open discussion. Discuss the importance of partner notification and treatment, including the risk for reinfection if the partner goes untreated. All sexual partners must be prophylactically treated as soon as possible, preferably within 90 days of the syphilis diagnosis.

Inform the patient that the disease will be reported to the local health authority and that all information will be held in strict confidence. Urge the patient to keep follow-up appointments. For primary and secondary syphilis, drug therapy is provided at the first visit, which may suggest to the patient that no further visits are indicated or important. Remind the patient that follow-up for self and partner(s) is critical and that sexual abstinence is recommended until full treatment is complete. After the initial antibiotic, the CDC recommends follow-up evaluation, including blood tests at 6, 12, and 24 months. Repeat treatment may be needed if the patient does not respond to the initial antibiotic.

The emotional responses to syphilis vary and may include feelings of fear, depression, guilt, and anxiety. Patients may experience guilt if they have infected others or anger if a partner has infected them. If further psychosocial interventions are needed, encourage the patient to discuss these feelings or refer the patient to other resources, such as psychotherapy, self-help support groups, or STI/STD clinics.

NCLEX Examination Challenge 65.1

Physiological Integrity

The nurse is caring for a client in an outpatient clinic who has been diagnosed with primary syphilis. Which of the following client statements requires further teaching by the nurse? **Select all that apply.**

A. "I will get an antibiotic injection today."

B. "I am going to tell my partner about my diagnosis."

C. "I will need to continue taking oral antibiotics at home."

D. "I do not need any further follow-up appointments after today."

E. "I am staying here for at least 30 minutes after you give me a shot."

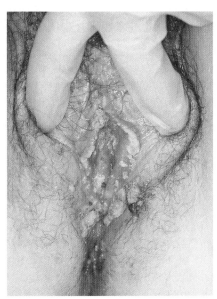

FIG. 65.5 Genital warts on the vulva. (From Jarvis, C., & Eckhardt, A. [2024]. *Physical examination and health assessment* [9th ed.]. St. Louis: Elsevier.)

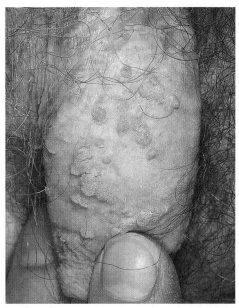

FIG. 65.6 Genital warts on the penis. (From Jarvis, C., & Eckhardt, A. [2024]. *Physical examination and health assessment* [9th ed.]. St. Louis: Elsevier.)

CONDYLOMATA ACUMINATA (GENITAL WARTS)

Pathophysiology Review

Condylomata acuminata (genital warts) are caused by certain types of *human papillomavirus (HPV)*. Genital warts are a very common viral disease that is sexually transmitted and often coexists with other infections. Most of these infections originate from HPV types 6 and 11, which cause 90% of genital warts (Palefsky, 2022). There are 14 to 15 HPV types that are associated with precancerous or dysplastic lesions, as well as cervical, vulvar, vaginal, and anal cancers, with types 16 and 18 being responsible for most HPV-related cancers (National Cancer Institute, 2023; Palefsky, 2022). HPV infection has been established as the primary risk factor for development of cervical cancer. Evidence shows that HPV can also cause cancer of the vulva, vagina, penis, anus, and oropharynx (throat, tongue, and tonsils) (CDC, 2022c). High-risk HPV (strains that cause cancer) *infection* may coexist with low-risk HPV (strains that cause warts). The presence of one strain increases the risk for acquiring other strains.

Interprofessional Collaborative Care

Recognize Cues: Assessment

The diagnosis of condylomata acuminata is made by examination of the lesions. They are initially small, papillary growths that are white or resemble the color of the patient's skin (Figs. 65.5 and 65.6) and may grow into large cauliflower-like masses (Fig. 65.7). Multiple warts usually occur in the same area. Bleeding may occur if the wart is disturbed. Warts may disappear or resolve on their own without treatment. They may occur once or recur at the original site. Warts can occur on the external or internal surfaces of the genitalia,

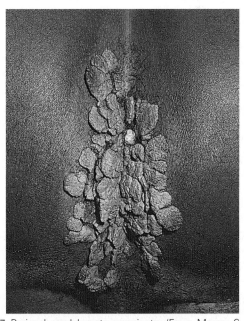

FIG. 65.7 Perianal condylomata acuminata. (From Morse, S., Ballard, R., Holmes, K., & Moreland, A. [2003]. *Atlas of sexually transmitted diseases and AIDS* [3rd ed.]. Edinburgh: Mosby.)

including the mucosal surfaces of the vagina and urethra. Screening for HPV and dysplasia of the cervix is done by obtaining cervical specimens for Papanicolaou (Pap) and HPV DNA testing.

The health care provider will also consider condyloma lata (which occurs in secondary syphilis) as a coexisting diagnosis because STIs frequently coexist. Blood tests, an HIV test, and cultures for chlamydia and gonorrhea infections are done. If a wart-like lesion bleeds easily, appears infected, is atypical, or persists, a biopsy of the lesion is performed to rule out other pathologic problems such as cancer. A biopsy of warts that are seen on the cervix should be performed before any treatment to eradicate them.

Take Actions: Interventions

The outcome of treatment is to remove the warts. No current therapy eliminates the HPV *infection,* and recurrences after treatment are likely. It is not known whether removal of visible warts decreases the risk for disease transmission.

Nonsurgical Management. Patients may be prescribed cryo-destructive therapies such as podophyllotoxin, podophyllum resin, or trichloroacetic acid (TCA) as applied topical applications for treatment of warts (Carusi, 2023). TCA must be applied by a health care provider.

Immune-mediated therapies include imiquimod (topical), sinecatechins (topical), and interferons (available as a topical treatment, as well as through IM and subcutaneous injections). Patients taking imiquimod should be taught that this medication is applied at bedtime and washed off upon awakening (Burchum & Rosenthal, 2022). These treatments are less expensive than those performed in the health care provider's office but take longer for healing. *Teach patients that over-the-counter (OTC) wart treatments should not be used on genital tissue.*

Topical treatment of perianal warts in men with bacillus Calmette-Guérin is another therapy that is starting to be used more frequently (Carusi, 2023).

Surgical Management. Surgical excision, cryoablation, laser ablation, electrocautery, and ultrasonic aspiration are treatment options that the health care provider can perform (Carusi, 2023). The choice of treatment is based on the patient's individualized presentation, including number, size, and location of warts; preference of the patient; cost; adverse effects; the skills of the clinician; and treatment availability.

Care Coordination and Transition Management

Self-Management Education. The priority nursing intervention is patient and partner education about the mode of transmission, incubation period, treatment, and complications, especially the association with various types of cancer. Teach about local care

---

💊 NURSING SAFETY PRIORITY
Drug Alert

Teach patients that after treatment with podophyllotoxin, podophyllum resin, or trichloroacetic acid (TCA) they may experience **pain,** bleeding, or discharge from the site or sloughing of parts of warts. Teach to keep the area clean and dry and to be alert for any signs or symptoms of further **infection** or side effects of the treatment.

---

for postsurgical lesions or patient-applied treatment for self-management.

Inform patients that recurrence is likely, especially in the first 3 months, and that repeated treatments may be needed. Urge all patients to have complete STI testing, since exposure to one STI increases the risk for contracting another. Sexual partners should also be evaluated and offered treatment if warts are present. Teach patients to avoid intimate sexual contact until external lesions are healed, and to use condoms to help reduce transmission even after warts have been treated (see Box 65.4). Teach women to follow the U.S. Preventive Services Task Force (2022) recommendations on Pap and HPV testing:

- If 21 to 29 years old, get a Pap test every 3 years.
- If 30 to 65 years old, get:
  - A Pap test every 3 years, or
  - An HPV test every 5 years, or
  - A Pap test and HPV test together (called co-testing) every 5 years
- If older than 65, ask the health care provider whether Pap tests and HPV tests can be stopped.

Vaccination to protect patients against HPV is one of the most important interventions available, especially for MSM. Teach patients about the various vaccinations available (Table 65.2), and encourage them to be immunized.

CHLAMYDIA INFECTION

Pathophysiology Review

Chlamydia trachomatis is an intracellular bacterium and the causative agent of cervicitis (in women), urethritis, and proctitis. It

---

TABLE 65.2 Human Papillomavirus (HPV) Vaccines

Vaccination	Prevention Type	Sex Assigned at Birth and Age Recommended
Gardasil 9 (available in the United States and Canada)	Cervical, vulvar, vaginal, anal, oropharyngeal, and other head/neck cancers caused by HPV types 16, 18, 31, 33, 45, 52, 58 Cervical, vulvar, and anal precancerous or dysplastic lesions caused by HPV types 6, 11, 16, 18, 31, 33, 45, 52, 58 Genital warts caused by HPV types 6, 11	United States: • Males and females 9–45 yr Canada: • Males 9–26 yr; can be administered to men aged 27 and older based on ongoing risk of exposure to HPV • Females 9–26 yr; can be administered to women aged 27 and older based on ongoing risk of exposure to HPV
Cervarix (available in Canada)	Cervical disease, precancerous cervical lesions, and anogenital cancers caused by HPV types 16, 18	Males 9–26 yr Females 9–26 yr; can be administered to women aged 27 and older based on ongoing risk of exposure to HPV

NOTE: The status of Gardasil in Canada is "Canceled Post Market" as of publication; Gardasil 9 in Canada remains "Marketed."
Data from Centers for Disease Control and Prevention (CDC). (2021). *Human papillomavirus (HPV) vaccination: What everyone should know.* https://www.cdc.gov/vaccines/vpd/hpv/public/index.html; Government of Canada. (2021). *Human papillomavirus vaccine: Canadian immunization guide for health professionals.* https://www.canada.ca/en/public-health/services/publications/healthy-living/canadian-immunization-guide-part-4--active-vaccines/page-9-human-papillomavirus-vaccine.html#p4c8a3.

invades the epithelial tissues in the reproductive tract. The incubation period ranges from 1 to 3 weeks, but the pathogen may be present in the genital tract for months without producing symptoms.

C. trachomatis is reportable to local health departments in all states. In the United States, it is the most frequently reported bacterial sexually transmitted **infection** (CDC, 2022b). Diagnosed cases continue to increase yearly, which reflects more sensitive screening tests and increased public health efforts to screen high-risk people. Because it is frequently asymptomatic, the estimated incidence is about double what is reported.

👤 PATIENT-CENTERED CARE: HEALTH EQUITY

Chlamydia Rates

Significant imbalances in **health equity** exist between racial/ethnic groups. In 2020, chlamydia rates were six times higher in Black people versus White people, and also were high in prevalence in men who have sex with men (MSM) (CDC, 2022b) Advocate for all patients who may need screening for chlamydia based upon your assessment.

Interprofessional Collaborative Care
Recognize Cues: Assessment

As with all interviews concerning *sexuality,* use a nonjudgmental approach and provide privacy and confidentiality. Obtain a complete history, including a genitourinary system review, psychosocial history, and sexual history (see Box 65.2). In particular, ask about:

- Presence of symptoms, including vaginal or urethral discharge, dysuria (painful urination), pelvic **pain,** and any irregular bleeding (for women)
- A history of sexually transmitted diseases (STIs)
- Whether current or past sexual partners have had symptoms or a history of STIs
- Whether the patient has had a new partner, or multiple sexual partners
- Whether the patient or a current or recent partner has had unprotected intercourse

👤 PATIENT-CENTERED CARE: GENDER HEALTH

Urethritis in Men

Ask men about dysuria, frequent urination, or discharge, which may indicate urethritis. Patients with chlamydia may report a mucoid discharge that is more watery and less copious than gonorrheal discharge. Some men have the discharge only in the morning on arising. Complications of untreated chlamydia in men include epididymitis or epididymo-orchitis and sexually acquired reactive arthritis.

Men may report penile discharge, urinary frequency, and dysuria. In contrast, many women have no symptoms. Those with symptoms may report mucopurulent vaginal discharge (typically yellow and opaque), urinary frequency, and abdominal discomfort or **pain.** Cervical bleeding, from infected, fragile tissue, may present as spotting or bleeding between menses and frequently after intercourse. Complications of **infection** with chlamydia include salpingitis (inflammation of the fallopian tubes), pelvic inflammatory disease (PID), and **reproduction**

problems, including infertility, ectopic pregnancy, and complications with a newborn that is delivered. These health problems are discussed in detail in maternal-child textbooks.

Diagnosis is made by sampling cells from the endocervix, urethra, or both, easily obtained with a swab. Because chlamydiae can reproduce only inside cells, cervical (or host) cells that harbor the organism (or parts of it) are required in the sample. Tissue culture obtained from the cervical os during the female pelvic examination or from male urethral examination obtained by swabbing has been replaced by genetic tests. Nucleic acid amplification tests (NAATs) are the most common method of detecting chlamydia in endocervical samples, urethral swabs, and urine. Samples can be obtained by swab by the examining clinician or by a patient-collected swab or urine specimen. Retesting after 3 months is advised to detect repeat **infection** (Workowski et al., 2021).

All sexually active women 25 years old or younger and all women older than 25 years with a new partner, multiple partners, a partner with other concurrent partners, or a partner with an STI should be screened annually for chlamydia (Workowski et al., 2021). Routine screening is also recommended for men who have sex with men (MSM) (Workowski et al., 2021).

Take Actions: Interventions

Drug Therapy. The treatment of choice for chlamydia infections is doxycycline. Alternate drug treatments include azithromycin (usually given in a single dose at the time of the initial visit with the health care provider) and levofloxacin. The one-dose course, although more expensive, is preferred because of the ease in completing the treatment. Directly observing the patient taking the medication in the health care setting will assure you of adherence.

Sexual partners should be treated and tested for other STIs. Expedited partner therapy (EPT), or patient-delivered partner therapy, shows signs of reducing chlamydia **infection** rates (Workowski et al., 2021). EPT involves treating sexual partners of patients diagnosed with chlamydia infection or gonorrhea by providing prescriptions or medication to the patient, which they can take to their partner(s), without the partner(s) needing to be examined by a provider of care. Evidence shows that when the patient gives the drug to their partner(s), rates of infection decrease, and more partners report receiving treatment (Workowski et al., 2021).

Care Coordination and Transition Management

Self-Management Education. As with all STI diagnoses, patient and partner education is a crucial nursing intervention geared toward effectively treating the condition and reducing the risk of reinfection. Teach about the:

- Sexual mode of transmission
- Incubation period
- High possibility of asymptomatic infections and the usual symptoms, if present
- Need for antibiotic treatment of **infection** and the need to complete all medications, even if feeling better
- Need for abstinence from sexual intercourse until the patient and partner(s) have all completed treatment (7 days from the start of treatment, including if treated with the single-dose regimen)

- Need for all patients to be rescreened 3 months after treatment
  - Women should be rescreened for reinfection 3 months after treatment because of the high risk for PID
  - If patients cannot be rescreened in 3 months, they should be rescreened within 12 months whenever they seek health care
- Need to return for evaluation if symptoms recur or new symptoms develop (most recurrences are reinfections from a new or untreated partner)
- Complications of untreated or inadequately treated *infection,* which may include PID, infertility, ectopic pregnancy, or newborn complications

GONORRHEA

Pathophysiology Review

Gonorrhea is a sexually transmitted bacterial *infection* caused by *Neisseria gonorrhoeae,* a gram-negative intracellular diplococcus. It is transmitted by direct sexual contact with mucosal surfaces (vaginal intercourse, orogenital contact, or anogenital contact) (Rogers, 2023).

The first symptoms of gonorrhea may appear within a week after sexual contact with an infected person. The disease can be present without symptoms and can be transmitted or progress without warning. In women, ascending spread of the organism can cause pelvic infection (pelvic inflammatory disease [PID]), ectopic pregnancy, miscarriage, premature labor or birth, neonate eye infection, ongoing pelvic pain, and sepsis (if left untreated). In men, gonorrhea can cause fertility reduction, proctitis, and sepsis (if untreated).

Interprofessional Collaborative Care

Recognize Cues: Assessment

Establish a trusting relationship and use a nonjudgmental approach to gather complete information. A complete history includes a review of the genitourinary system, and collecting a sexual history. Sites of sexual exposure or intercourse should be elicited, because gonorrhea can affect the genitals, rectum, and throat. Assess for allergies to antibiotics.

The *infection* can be asymptomatic in both men and women, but women have asymptomatic, or "silent," infections more often than do men. If symptoms are present, men usually notice dysuria and a penile discharge that can be either profuse yellowish-green fluid or scant clear fluid. The urethra, epididymis, seminal vesicles, and prostate can become infected. Men seek curative treatment sooner, usually because they have symptoms, and thereby avoid some of the serious complications.

Women may report a change in vaginal discharge (yellow, green, profuse, odorous), urinary frequency, or dysuria. The cervix and urethra are the most common sites of *infection.*

Anal symptoms may include itching and irritation, rectal bleeding or diarrhea, and painful bowel movements. Assess the mouth for a reddened throat, ulcerated lips, tender gingivae, and lesions in the throat. Fig. 65.8 shows common sites of gonococcal infections.

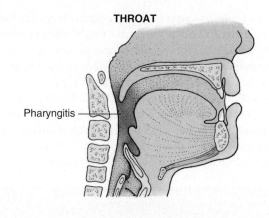

THROAT

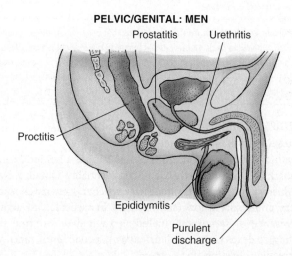

PELVIC/GENITAL: MEN

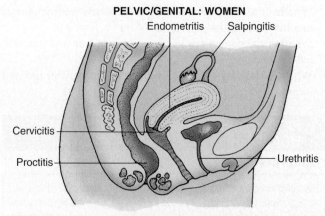

PELVIC/GENITAL: WOMEN

FIG. 65.8 Areas of involvement of gonorrhea in men and women.

Fever may be a sign of an ascending (PID or epididymitis) or systemic (disseminated gonococcal) *infection.* Symptoms may also include shoulder, wrist, or lower extremity pain, and a rash.

Clinical symptoms of gonorrhea can resemble those of chlamydia *infection* and need to be differentiated. Nucleic acid amplification tests (NAATs) are the most common type of testing for the initial microbiologic diagnosis of gonorrhea; culture is also used when antibiotic resistance is suspected (Ghanem, 2022). During examination, the health care provider can swab the male urethra or female cervix to obtain specimens.

Patient-collected pharyngeal, rectal, urine or vaginal swabs can also be used to diagnose gonorrhea, allowing for testing without a full examination (Ghanem, 2022).

All patients with gonorrhea should be tested for syphilis, chlamydia, hepatitis B and hepatitis C, and HIV infection and, if possible, examined for HSV and HPV because they may have been exposed to these STIs as well. Sexual partners who have been exposed in the past 30 days should be examined, and specimens should be obtained.

Take Actions: Interventions

Uncomplicated gonorrhea is treated with antibiotics. Chlamydia *infection*, which is four times more common, is frequently found in patients with gonorrhea. Because of this, patients treated for gonorrhea should also be managed with drugs that treat chlamydia infection.

Drug Therapy. Drug therapy recommended by the CDC for uncomplicated gonorrhea of the pharynx, cervix, rectum, or urethra is IM ceftriaxone in a single dose at the time of visit. A co-infection with chlamydia is treated also with doxycycline. Alternative treatments include gentamicin plus azithromycin (both in a single dose at the time of visit), or cefixime in a single dose (Workowski et al., 2021).

A test-of-cure is not required for treatment of uncomplicated urogenital or rectal gonorrhea treated with ceftriaxone or one of the alternative treatments; patients with oropharyngeal gonorrhea treated with any alternative treatment should be advised to return for a test-of-cure in 14 days (Workowski et al., 2021). Advise any patient to return for a follow-up examination if symptoms persist after treatment. Reinfection is usually the cause of these symptoms.

Sexual partners must be educated about the *infection* and treated (not just evaluated) to prevent reinfection. Although the best treatment for gonorrhea is injected ceftriaxone, expedited partner therapy (EPT) is still available in the form of oral cefixime (plus oral doxycycline for people without a documented chlamydia test) or oral azithromycin (Workowski et al., 2021).

Gonorrhea *infection* can become disseminated, requiring hospitalization for initial drug therapy and testing for endocarditis and meningitis (Workowski et al., 2021). If symptoms resolve within 24 to 48 hours, the patient may be discharged to home to continue oral antibiotic therapy while recovering.

Self-Management Education. Teach the patient about transmission and treatment of gonorrhea. Explain that the use of medication to treat chlamydia *infection* at the same time is important, as the likelihood of coinfection is high. Discuss the possibility of reinfection, including the risk for pelvic inflammatory disease (PID) in women (see discussion of PID later in this chapter).

Instruct patients to abstain from sexual activity until the antibiotic therapy is completed and they no longer have symptoms. Reinforce the need to always use condoms. Explain that gonorrhea is a reportable disease.

Patients with gonorrhea (or any other STI) may have feelings of fear or guilt. They may be concerned that they have contracted other STIs or consider the disease a religious or spiritual punishment for their sexual behaviors. Such feelings can impair relationships with intimate partners. Encourage patients to express their feelings, and offer other information and professional resources to help them understand their diagnosis and treatment. Ensure privacy during your discussion, and maintain confidentiality of personal health information.

Mpox

Mpox is a poxlike disease that is part of the virus family that causes smallpox; however, mpox is rarely fatal (CDC, 2022a). Formerly known as monkeypox, the terminology was updated in November 2022 to "mpox"; both terms were used simultaneously for one year as the phrase "monkeypox" was phased out (World Health Organization, 2022b).

In 2022, a global outbreak of mpox occurred with the primary mode of transmission being through intimate contact. Although this condition is not traditionally considered a sexually transmitted infection (STI), at the time of publication, evidence showed that 98% of individuals infected via the most recent outbreak were gay or bisexual men, with 95% of transmission occurring via sexual contact (Thornhill et al., 2022).

Pathophysiology Review

The virus responsible for mpox can enter through the oropharynx or nasopharynx; it can also be spread intradermally, or through oral, anal, or vaginal sex (Moore et al., 2022). Once inside the body, the virus replicates at the entry site and then moves to the local lymph nodes. The initial viremia and incubation period of 7 to 14 days leads to viral spread, and the second viremia includes 1 to 2 days of fever and lymphadenopathy, followed by the eruption of lesions in the oropharynx and skin that continue to expand over the body (Moore et al., 2022).

Interprofessional Collaborative Care
Recognize Cues: Assessment

Ask patients about travel to endemic areas, as well as whether they have had sexual contact with anyone potentially infected. Assess for fever, myalgias, fatigue, headache, and lymphadenopathy. Assess skin lesions, which are usually firm and 2 to 10 mm in size, for which stage they are currently in. Mpox usually progresses in 1- to 2-day increments from a macular eruption to papules, vesicles, and then pustules (Moore et al., 2022). Following a 5- to 7-day pustular phase, crusting takes place over the next 1 to 2 weeks, with full resolution in 3 to 4 weeks following the onset of symptoms (Moore et al., 2022).

Take Actions: Interventions

Remind patients that the risk for contracting mpox is higher for men who have sex with men (MSM), for those who engage in sex with multiple partners, and for those who have casual sex (especially without condoms) (Hill, 2022). Teach that at the onset of symptoms, patients should isolate and contact their primary health care provider to be seen (Hill, 2022).

Treatment for mpox is supportive in nature. Teach patients to avoid contact with others, to wear a mask, and to keep lesions covered as much as possible (Moore et al., 2022). Remind patients that they are contagious until the crusts fall off the mpox lesions.

Immunization can be administered for mpox before or within 4 days following exposure (CDC, 2023e). For patients who have already been exposed, known as postexposure prophylaxis (PEP) (CDC, 2023e), getting the vaccine quickly after exposure can serve to reduce the symptoms associated with the virus.

Two current vaccinations are available in the United States: Jynneos and ACAM2000. Jynneos is approved as a smallpox and mpox vaccination; ACAM2000 is approved as a smallpox vaccination with expanded access for vaccination against mpox.

Jynneos is to be given to people 18 years of age and older who are at high risk to contract mpox; it is administered in two intramuscular doses, 4 weeks apart (Bavarian Nordic A/S, 2023).

Administration of ACAM2000, a live virus vaccine, requires special training to deliver the vaccine percutaneously with a bifurcated needle (Military Health Services, 2023). Videos showing how to administer this vaccination are available via the CDC website. Teach patients to take precautions to avoid spreading the vaccine virus during this time.

✴ INFECTION CONCEPT EXEMPLAR: PELVIC INFLAMMATORY DISEASE

Pathophysiology Review

Pelvic inflammatory disease (PID) is an acute syndrome resulting in tenderness in the tubes and ovaries (adnexa) and, typically, dull pelvic *pain*. Some women experience only mild discomfort or menstrual irregularity, whereas others have acute *pain*, which can affect their gait. Others experience no symptoms at all (i.e., so-called "silent" or "subclinical" PID).

This infectious process involves movement of organisms from the endocervix upward through the uterine cavity into the fallopian tubes (CDC, 2021b). Usually multiple pathogens are involved in the development of PID. Sexually transmitted organisms are most often responsible, especially *C. trachomatis* and *N. gonorrhoeae* (Ross & Chacko, 2022). Bacterial vaginosis is also a common causative agent (Ross & Chacko, 2022).

The spread of *infection* to other organs and tissues of the upper genital tract occurs from direct contact with mucosal surfaces or through the fimbriated ends of the tubes to the ovaries, parametrium, and peritoneal cavity (Fig. 65.9). This may involve one or more pelvic structures, including the uterus, fallopian tubes, and adjacent pelvic structures. The most common site is the fallopian tube (salpingitis).

Complications of PID include chronic pelvic pain, infertility, risk for ectopic pregnancy, tubo-ovarian abscess (TOA), a serious short-term condition requiring hospitalization in which an inflammatory mass arises on the fallopian tube, ovary, and/or other pelvic organs, and (rarely) fatal intra-abdominal sepsis (Ross & Chacko, 2022). Additionally,

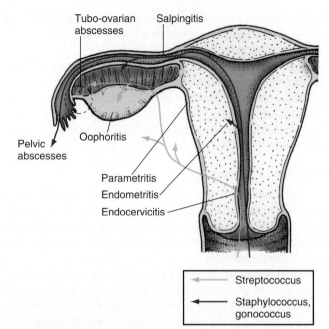

FIG. 65.9 The spread of pelvic inflammatory disease.

perihepatitis—inflammation of the liver capsule and peritoneal surfaces of the anterior right upper quadrant—occurs in some women with PID (Ross & Chacko, 2022). This condition is characterized by right upper quadrant pain with a pleuritic component (often the right shoulder), fever, chills, nausea, and vomiting.

Infections can be spread during sexual intercourse, during childbirth (including the postpartum period), and after abortion. *Sepsis and death can occur, especially if treatment is delayed or inadequate.*

Interprofessional Collaborative Care
Recognize Cues: Assessment

History. Obtain a complete history of the symptoms plus menstrual, obstetric, sexual, and family history. Inquire about any previous episodes of pelvic inflammatory disease (PID) or other sexually transmitted infections (see Box 65.2). Assess for contraceptive use, a history of reproductive surgery, and other risk factors previously discussed. Ask the patient whether sexual abuse has occurred. If so, encourage her to discuss what happened and whether she was seen by a health care provider.

Many of the same factors that place women at risk for STIs also place them at risk for PID, including having multiple sexual partners, practicing inconsistent use of condoms, and having a history of sexually transmitted infections.

Physical Assessment/Signs and Symptoms. One of the most frequent symptoms of PID is lower abdominal or pelvic *pain*. Conduct a complete pain assessment. Other symptoms include irregular vaginal bleeding (spotting or bleeding between periods), dysuria (painful urination), an increase or change in vaginal discharge, dyspareunia (painful sexual intercourse), malaise, fever, and chills.

Observe whether the patient has pain with movement. She may bend forward to guard the abdomen. She may find it difficult to independently get onto the examination table or stretcher. Assess for lower abdominal tenderness, possibly with rigidity or rebound tenderness. A pelvic examination by the health care provider may reveal yellow or green cervical discharge and a reddened or friable cervix (a cervix that bleeds easily). Diagnostic criteria for PID are listed in Box 65.5. The diagnosis of PID is based on health history, physical assessment, and laboratory tests. Imaging studies and laparoscopy are not generally used to make the diagnosis.

Psychosocial Assessment. The woman with symptoms of PID may be anxious and fearful of the examination and unknown diagnosis. She may need reassurance and support during the examination because of pelvic *pain.* Explain what is taking place in real time to help promote understanding.

Because PID is often associated with an STI, the woman may feel embarrassed or uncomfortable discussing symptoms or history. She may also experience complicated feelings and emotions related to sexual partners, or fear of whether she will be able to bear children after this diagnosis. Use a nonjudgmental approach, and encourage expression of feelings and concerns. Assessing the patient's level of concern is important, as a referral to a mental health professional for ongoing care may be helpful. See the box titled Interprofessional Collaboration: Psychosocial Concerns and STIs.

BOX 65.5 Diagnostic Criteria for Pelvic Inflammatory Disease (PID)

Minimum Criteria for Initiating Empiric Treatment for Pelvic Inflammatory Disease

For women experiencing pelvic or lower abdominal pain, treatment should be initiated if **one or more** of the three minimum criteria are present during pelvic examination:
- Cervical motion tenderness
- Uterine tenderness
- Adnexal tenderness

Additional Criteria to Increase the Specificity of the Diagnosis of PID
- Oral temperature >101°F (>38.3°C)
- Abnormal cervical mucopurulent discharge or cervical friability
- Abundance of white blood cells (WBCs) on saline microscopy of vaginal fluids
- Elevated erythrocyte sedimentation rate
- Elevated C-reactive protein
- Laboratory documentation of cervical infection with *Neisseria gonorrhoeae* or *Chlamydia trachomatis*

More Specific Criteria for Diagnosing PID, Warranted in Selected Cases
- Histopathologic evidence of endometritis on endometrial biopsy
- Transvaginal sonography or MRI demonstrating thickened, fluid-filled tubes with or without free pelvic fluid or tubo-ovarian complex, or Doppler studies suggesting pelvic infection
- Laparoscopic findings consistent with PID

Data from Center for Surveillance, Epidemiology, and Laboratory Services, Centers for Disease Control and Prevention (CDC), & U.S. Department of Health and Human Services. (2021). *Sexually transmitted infections treatment guidelines, 2021. MMWR Recommendations and Reports 2021, 70* (No. RR-4): 1-192.

INTERPROFESSIONAL COLLABORATION
Psychosocial Concerns and STIs

The patient with psychosocial concerns that may have arisen due to a sexually transmitted infection may benefit from referral to a mental health professional. These individuals can help the patient work through emotions that can accompany an STI, including feelings of embarrassment, betrayal, anger, or fear, or concerns about infertility or **reproduction** implications.

These members of the interprofessional team hold master's or doctoral degrees; they help patients adjust to life changes through education and support. Advance practice nurses who specialize in this capacity are psychiatric–mental health nurse practitioners who can also diagnose mental health conditions and prescribe drug therapy, in addition to providing counseling.

According to the Interprofessional Education Collaborative (IPEC) Expert Panel's Competency of Roles and Responsibilities, using the unique and complementary abilities of other team members optimizes health and patient care (IPEC, 2016; Slusser et al., 2019).

Laboratory Assessment. The health care provider obtains specimens from the cervix, urethra, and rectum to determine the presence of *N. gonorrhoeae* or *C. trachomatis.* The white blood cell (WBC) count may be elevated but is not specific for PID. A sensitive test that detects human chorionic gonadotropin (hCG) in urine or blood should be performed to determine whether the patient is pregnant (Pagana et al., 2022). Microscopic examination of vaginal discharge is done to evaluate for the presence of WBCs.

Other Diagnostic Assessment. Abdominal *ultrasonography* may be used to determine any presence of appendicitis or tubo-ovarian abscesses (TOAs), which need to be ruled out when the diagnosis of PID is made. Ultrasound can be used to visualize the upper genital tract. CT or MRI can be helpful in determining whether there is gastrointestinal pathology (Ross & Chacko, 2022).

Analyze Cues and Prioritize Hypotheses: Analysis

The priority collaborative problems for a patient with pelvic inflammatory disease (PID) are:
1. *Infection* due to invasion of pelvic organs by sexually transmitted pathogens
2. *Pain* due to infectious process

Generate Solutions and Take Actions: Planning and Implementation
Managing Infection and Pain

Planning: Expected Outcomes. The patient with PID is expected to experience resolution of the *infection,* be free of abdominal *pain,* and prevent reinfection.

Interventions. Interprofessional collaborative care includes antibiotic therapy and self-management measures. Uncomplicated PID is usually treated on an ambulatory care basis. The CDC recommends oral and/or parenteral antibiotics for PID

(CDC, 2021c). The CDC (2021c) recommends hospitalization for the patient with PID if:

- A surgical emergency (e.g., appendicitis) has not been excluded as a diagnosis
- The patient is pregnant
- She cannot follow or tolerate treatment as an outpatient
- There is severe illness, nausea and vomiting, or high fever
- A tubo-ovarian abscess (TOA) has been diagnosed
- There has been no clinical response to earlier oral antimicrobial treatment

Inpatient therapy involves a combination of several IV antibiotics until the patient shows signs of improvement (e.g., decreased pelvic tenderness for at least 24 hours). Most commonly, a combination of ceftriaxone, doxycycline, and metronidazole is used (Workowski et al., 2021). Alternate treatments include the use of cefotetan and doxycycline, or cefoxitin and doxycycline. Oral antibiotics are continued at home until the course of treatment has lasted 14 days.

Patients who can be treated on an ambulatory basis may be prescribed IM or oral therapy, depending on the degree of severity of PID diagnosed. Most commonly, IM ceftriaxone and PO doxycycline are given (Workowski et al., 2021).

Antibiotic therapy relieves *pain* by destroying the pathogens and decreasing the inflammation caused by *infection.* Other measures to treat pain include taking mild analgesics and applying heat to the lower abdomen or back. As with any infection, encourage the patient to increase the intake of fluids and eat nutritious foods that promote healing. Teach the patient to rest in semi-Fowler's position, and encourage limited ambulation to promote gravity drainage of the infection, which may help relieve **pain.**

⚠ NURSING SAFETY PRIORITY

Action Alert

Instruct patients being treated for PID on an ambulatory care basis to avoid sexual intercourse for the full course of antibiotic treatment, until their symptoms have resolved, and until their partner(s) has been treated for any STIs (Workowski et al., 2021). Teach them to check their temperature twice daily and to report any increase in temperature to their health care provider. Remind them to be seen by the health care provider within 72 hours from the start of antibiotic treatment and then 1 and 2 weeks from the time of the initial diagnosis.

Laparoscopy can confirm the presence of PID, but it is uncommonly performed for this purpose alone (Ross & Chacko, 2022). It is more frequently performed if the patient has not responded to outpatient treatment and the health care provider is considering alternative causes for symptoms, or if the patient's symptoms are not improving or are worsening after 72 hours of inpatient treatment (Ross & Chacko, 2022). Before surgery, provide information about the procedure. After surgery, care is similar to that of any patient after laparoscopic abdominal surgery (see Chapter 9). One difference is that she may have a wound drain for drainage of abscess fluid if an abscess was removed during the procedure. Observe, measure, and record wound drainage every 4 to 8 hours as ordered.

Care Coordination and Transition Management

Home Care Management. Remind the patient how to identify symptoms of persistent or recurrent *infection* (persistent pelvic *pain*, dysmenorrhea, low backache, fever), and teach about the importance of completion of treatment, rest, and healthy nutrition. Parenteral antibiotic therapy may be given at home, but usually the health care provider changes the treatment regimen to oral antibiotics before hospital discharge (Box 65.6). If parenteral therapy is continued, collaborate with the home health care nurse to arrange for services.

Self-Management Education. Teach the patient with PID to see their primary health care provider for follow-up to confirm that the *infection* has resolved, yet to report any signs and symptoms of a recurrent *infection* right away. Home care for the patient who had laparoscopic surgery is discussed in Chapter 9.

NCLEX Examination Challenge 65.2

Physiological Integrity

The nurse is caring for a client diagnosed with pelvic inflammatory disease (PID). Which of the following client statements demonstrates an understanding of oral antibiotic drug therapy? **Select all that apply.**

A. "I will finish the antibiotics even if I feel better."
B. "I can resume sexual intercourse tomorrow."
C. "I can chew on calcium carbonate tablets if this medication makes me feel nauseated."
D. "I have to see the health care provider a month after finishing this medication."
E. "I can take this medication with food or on an empty stomach, depending on how I feel."

BOX 65.6   Patient and Family Education

Oral Antibiotic Therapy for Sexually Transmitted Infections and Pelvic Inflammatory Disease

- Take medicine for the number of times a day that it is prescribed and until it is completed, even if you begin to feel better.
- Antibiotics can be taken on an empty stomach or with food depending on which drug was prescribed. Follow the instructions of your health care provider.
- Do not take antacids containing calcium, magnesium, or aluminum, such as calcium carbonate tablets, with your antibiotics. They may decrease the effectiveness of the antibiotic.
- Your sexual partner must be treated if you have a sexually transmitted infection (STI). Expedited partner therapy is one way to ensure that partners are treated.
- Do not have sex until after you and your partner complete your antibiotic therapy. Wait 7 days to resume intimacy if treatment was delivered in one dose.
- Drink at least 8 to 10 glasses of fluid a day while taking your antibiotics.
- Be sure to return for your follow-up appointment after completing your antibiotic treatment.
- Call if you have any questions or concerns.

Teach the patient to contact her sexual partner(s) for examination and treatment. All sexual partners should be treated for gonorrhea and chlamydia *infection* regardless of whether they have symptoms. Remind the patient about follow-up care, and counsel her about the complications that can occur after an occurrence of PID, including recurrence, chronic pelvic *pain,* ectopic pregnancy, and infertility.

Teach about the use of condoms, which can provide contraception, protect against STIs, and decrease the risk for future episodes of PID. Help the patient understand that having sexual intercourse with multiple partners increases the risk for recurrent episodes. Remind her to use a new condom with each sexual encounter. Douching has also been suggested as a risky behavior for development of PID and/or infection with chlamydia or *N. gonorrhoeae.*

Psychosocial concerns may require counseling. A patient who has PID may exhibit a variety of feelings (guilt, disgust, anger) about having a condition that may have been transmitted to her sexually. These feelings may affect her relationship with significant others and future sexual partners. She may also have concerns about future fertility if PID has damaged or scarred the fallopian tubes and other organs involved in *reproduction.* Provide nonjudgmental emotional support and allow time for her to discuss her feelings. Collaborate with a mental health care provider as needed as a longer-term method of support for the patient.

Health Care Resources. The cost of antibiotics for patients with PID and other STIs may be a concern for those who are uninsured, underinsured, or impoverished. Nonjudgmentally ask the patient directly if she can pay for the drug and follow-up visits. Collaborate with the case manager or social worker, as these professionals can help to locate free or reduced-cost drugs and community resources for women who cannot afford them.

If infertility is a result of PID, the patient may need referral to a clinic specializing in infertility treatment and counseling. She can also contact infertility support groups, which exist in many local communities.

Evaluate Outcomes: Evaluation

Evaluate the care of the patient with PID based on the identified priority patient problem(s). The expected outcomes include that the patient should:
- Experience resolution of the *infection*
- Report or demonstrate that *pain* is relieved or reduced and that she feels more comfortable
- Articulate a plan for ensuring treatment of her partner, obtaining antibiotics, and returning for follow-up care

GET READY FOR THE NEXT-GENERATION NCLEX® EXAMINATION!

Essential Nursing Care Points

Health Promotion/Disease Prevention	Chronic Disease Care
• Teach people how to avoid contracting or transmitting a sexually transmitted infection (STI) by using condoms and dental dams. • Teach about the availability of expedited partner therapy.	• Remind patients with STIs such as genital herpes and HIV that the infection can still be transmitted even while undergoing treatment. • Provide ongoing care to patients with secondary or tertiary syphilis.
Regenerative or Restorative Care	Hospice/Palliative/Supportive Care
• Recognize that patients with pelvic inflammatory disease (PID) may require urgent or lifesaving care. • Teach patients to complete antibiotic therapy even if they begin to feel better. • Provide therapeutic communication and a nonjudgmental presence when caring for patients with an STI.	• Refer patients with tertiary syphilis to supportive care resources, palliative care, or hospice as appropriate.

Mastery Questions

1. A client scheduled for a Pap smear tells the nurse that a small blister on her labia several months ago resolved spontaneously. Which action would the nurse take *first*?
   A. Collect a sexual history.
   B. Prepare for the Pap smear.
   C. Notify the health care provider.
   D. Gather supplies for antibiotic injection.

2. A 43-year-old female client who has never been vaccinated against human papillomavirus (HPV) asks about receiving this immunization. When the client reports being sexually active with multiple partners, which nursing response would be appropriate?
   A. "I can begin the immunization process for you today."
   B. "You will need three doses of this vaccination due to your age."
   C. "It would be better for you to limit your number of sexual partners."
   D. "HPV vaccination is only intended for younger children and adolescents."

NGN Challenge 65.1

The nurse is reviewing the flow sheet for a 33-year-old client in the emergency department with abdominal and pelvic pain, fever, and cervical motion tenderness who is awaiting admission. The nurse reviews the previous nurse's notes in the electronic health record and the vital signs completed by assistive personnel (AP).

Highlight the findings that would require **immediate** follow-up.

NURSING FLOW SHEET

Time	0313	0546	0710
Temperature	99.1°F (37.3°C)	99.6°F (37.6°C)	101.8°F (38.8°C)
Heart rate	82 beats/min	96 beats/min	110 beats/min
Respiratory rate; SpO₂	20 breaths/ min; 98%	18 breaths/ min; 97%	20 breaths/ min; 97%
Blood pressure	120/76 mm Hg	128/78 mm Hg	134/94 mm Hg

0313: Alert and oriented × 4; CN intact; PERRLA; equal movement and grasp all 4 extremities. Reports increasing abdominal and pelvic pain that began a week ago. States that when pain began, it was very mild and she thought she had a virus, but pain has continued to increase to the point that it is now rated at 7 on a 0-to-10 scale. Has not eaten anything unusual; denies diarrhea and nausea. Denies headache, chest pain, or changes in breathing. Emergency health care provider performed pelvic examination; cervical motion tenderness and scant yellow vaginal discharge noted. Transvaginal ultrasound ordered. Orders received for pain medication.

0422: Transported to sonography.

0546: Back from sonography. Pain rated at 6 on a 0-to-10 scale. Transvaginal ultrasound results received, showing enlarged ovaries and uterus with indistinct borders. Communicated findings to emergency health care provider, who reviewed the report and diagnosed pelvic inflammatory disease (PID). Orders received for antibiotic therapy, further pain medication, and admission to medical-surgical unit.

NGN Challenge 65.2

The nurse has documented an assessment for a 23-year-old client who is seeing the primary health care provider today for a routine women's health examination.

History and Physical	Nurses' Notes	Vital Signs	Laboratory Results

October 1
Height: 67 in (170.2 cm); weight: 224 lb (101.6 kg). VS: T 98.8°F (37.1°C); HR 72 beats/min; RR 18 breaths/min; BP 136/92 mm Hg. SpO₂ 99% on RA. Here for regular annual gynecologic examination. History of mild hypertension and hypercholesterolemia controlled by medication. Client reports getting consistent readings of 130s over 90s when she takes her blood pressure at home. Denies leg swelling, shortness of breath, chest pain, or pressure. Reports becoming sexually active in the past 18 months with 2 different partners; states she is monogamous with current partner but is concerned because "sometimes I feel like I have bumps, burning, and itching" in and around the vaginal area. States that these symptoms come and go intermittently every few months. Sometimes the area is clear, and sometimes she can see small red lesions if she uses a mirror for visualization. Health care provider in to see patient.

Complete the diagram by selecting from the choices below to specify what potential condition the client is likely experiencing, **2** nursing actions that are appropriate to take, and **2** parameters the nurse should monitor to assess the client's progress.

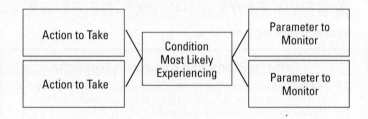

Actions to Take	Potential Conditions	Parameters to Monitor
Reassure that intermittent burning and itching are normal.	HIV infection	Red blood cell count
Encourage discussion of symptoms with her partner.	Hepatitis B infection	Frequency of symptom occurrences
Teach that infection can be transmitted even if symptoms subside.	Genital herpes infection	Urinalysis every 6 months
Request prescription for oral antifungal medication.	Pelvic inflammatory disease	Adherence to antiviral treatment
Refer to psychiatric–mental health nurse practitioner.		Repeat Pap test next month

REFERENCES

Albrecht, M. (2022a). Epidemiology, clinical manifestations, and diagnosis of genital herpes simplex virus infection. *UpToDate*. Retrieved May 29, 2023, from https://www.uptodate.com/contents/epidemiology-clinical-manifestations-and-diagnosis-of-genital-herpes-simplex-virus-infection.

Albrecht, M. (2022b). Treatment of genital herpes simplex infection. *UpToDate*. Retrieved May 29, 2023, from https://www.uptodate.com/contents/treatment-of-genital-herpes-simplex-virus-infection.

American College of Obstetricians and Gynecologists. (2023). *How to prevent sexually transmitted infections (STIs)*. https://www.acog.org/womens-health/faqs/how-to-prevent-stis.

American Sexual Health Association. (2023). *Herpes*. https://www.ashasexualhealth.org/herpes/.

Bartz, D. (2023). Pericoital (on demand) contraception: Diaphragm, cervical cap, spermicides, and sponge. *UpToDate*. Retrieved May 31, 2023, from https://www.uptodate.com/contents/pericoital-on-demand-contraception-diaphragm-cervical-cap-spermicides-and-sponge.

Bavarian Nordic A/S. (2023). *Package insert – Jynneos*. https://www.fda.gov/media/131078/download.

Burchum, J., & Rosenthal, L. (2022). *Lehne's pharmacology for nursing care* (11th ed.). St. Louis: Elsevier.

Carusi, D. (2023). Condylomata acuminate (anogenital warts): Treatment of vulvar and vaginal warts. *UpToDate*. Retrieved May 29, 2023, from https://www.uptodate.com/contents/condylomata-acuminata-anogenital-warts-treatment-of-vulvar-and-vaginal-warts.

Centers for Disease Control and Prevention (CDC). (2021a). *Genital herpes – CDC detailed fact sheet*. https://www.cdc.gov/std/herpes/stdfact-herpes-detailed.htm#ref2.

Centers for Disease Control and Prevention (CDC). (2021b). *Pelvic inflammatory disease (PID)—CDC fact sheet*. https://www.cdc.gov/std/pid/stdfact-pid-detailed.htm.

Centers for Disease Control and Prevention (CDC). (CDC). (2021c). Sexually transmitted diseases treatment guidelines—2015. *Morbidity and Mortality Weekly Report Recommendations and Reports*, *70*(4), 1–192.

Centers for Disease Control and Prevention (CDC). (2022a). *About monkeypox*. https://www.cdc.gov/poxvirus/monkeypox/about.html.

Centers for Disease Control and Prevention (CDC). (2022b). *Chlamydia—CDC fact sheet*. https://www.cdc.gov/std/chlamydia/stdfact-chlamydia-detailed.htm.

Centers for Disease Control and Prevention (CDC). (2022c). *Genital HPV infection—fact sheet*. https://www.cdc.gov/std/hpv/stdfact-hpv.htm.

Centers for Disease Control and Prevention (CDC). (2022d). *How to use condoms and other barriers*. https://www.cdc.gov/condomeffectiveness/index.html.

Centers for Disease Control and Prevention (CDC). (2023a). *2022 national notifiable conditions*. https://ndc.services.cdc.gov/search-results-year/.

Centers for Disease Control and Prevention (CDC). (2023b). *Interim clinical considerations for use of JYNNEOS and ACAM2000 vaccines during the 2022 U.S. Mpox outbreak*. https://www.cdc.gov/poxvirus/mpox/clinicians/vaccines/vaccine-considerations.html.

Centers for Disease Control and Prevention (CDC). (2023c). *Sexually transmitted diseases*. https://www.cdc.gov/std/default.htm.

Centers for Disease Control and Prevention (CDC). (2023d). *Syphilis*. https://www.cdc.gov/std/syphilis/.

Centers for Disease Control and Prevention (CDC). (2023e). *Vaccination*. https://www.cdc.gov/poxvirus/mpox/interim-considerations/overview.html.

Cleveland Clinic. (2023). *Estrogen*. https://my.clevelandclinic.org/health/body/22353-estrogen.

Curry, K., Chandler, R., Kostas-Polston, E. A., Alexander, I., Orsega, S., & Johnson-Mallard, V. (2022). Recommendations for managing sexually transmitted infections: Incorporating the 2021 guidelines. *The Nurse Practitioner*, *47*(4), 10–18.

Ghanem, K. (2022). Clinical manifestations and diagnosis of Neisseria gonorrhoeae infection in adults and adolescents. *UpToDate*. Retrieved May 29, 2023, from https://www.uptodate.com/contents/clinical-manifestations-and-diagnosis-of-neisseria-gonorrhoeae-infection-in-adults-and-adolescents.

Hicks, C., & Clement, M. (2022a). Syphilis: Epidemiology, pathophysiology, and clinical manifestations in patients without HIV. *UpToDate*. Retrieved May 29, 2023, from https://www.uptodate.com/contents/syphilis-epidemiology-pathophysiology-and-clinical-manifestations-in-patients-without-hiv.

Hicks, C., & Clement, M. (2022b). Syphilis: Screening and diagnostic testing. *UpToDate*. Retrieved May 29, 2023, from https://www.uptodate.com/contents/syphilis-screening-and-diagnostic-testing.

Hill, B. (2022). The 2022 multinational monkeypox outbreak in non-endemic countries. *British Journal of Nursing*, *31*(12), 664–665. https://doi.org/10.12968/bjon.2022.31.12.664.

Hoke, T., et al. (2022). Internal (formerly female) condoms. *UpToDate*. Retrieved May 29, 2023, from 5-29-23 https://www.uptodate.com/contents/internal-formerly-female-condoms.

Indiana Department of Health. (2021). *STDs and men who have sex with men*. https://www.in.gov/health/hiv-std-viral-hepatitis/files/MSM-in-Indiana-Fact-Sheet-2021.pdf.

Interprofessional Education Collaborative. (2016). *Core competencies for interprofessional collaborative practice: 2016 update*. https://ipec.memberclicks.net/assets/2016-Update.pdf.

Military Health Services. (2023). *Smallpox*. https://health.mil/Military-Health-Topics/Health-Readiness/Immunization-Healthcare/Vaccine-Preventable-Diseases/Smallpox-ACAM2000.

Moore, M., Rathish, B., & Zahra, F. (2022). Mpox (Monkeypox) [Updated 2022 Nov 30]. In: *StatPearls [Internet]*. Treasure Island, FL: StatPearls Publishing; 2023 Jan-. Available from: https://www.ncbi.nlm.nih.gov/books/NBK574519/.

National Cancer Institute. (2023). *HPV and cancer*. https://www.cancer.gov/about-cancer/causes-prevention/risk/infectious-agents/hpv-and-cancer.

Pagana, K. D., Pagana, T. J., & Pagana, T. N. (2022). *Mosby's manual of diagnostic and laboratory tests* (7th ed.). St. Louis: Elsevier.

Palefsky, J. (2022). Human papillomavirus infections: Epidemiology and disease associations. *UpToDate*. Retrieved May 29, 2023, from https://www.uptodate.com/contents/human-papillomavirus-infections-epidemiology-and-disease-associations.

Pourmand, A., & Marcinkowski, B. (2022). Recognizing human trafficking victims as patients in the emergency department. ACEP Now. https://www.acepnow.com/article/recognizing-human-trafficking-victims-as-patients-in-the-emergency-dept/.

Rapoza, S. (2022). Sex trafficking: A literature review with implications for health care providers. *Advanced Emergency Nursing Journal*, *44*(3), 248–261.

Rogers, J. L. (2023). *McCance and Huether's Pathophysiology: The biologic basis for disease in adults and children* (9th ed.). St. Louis: Elsevier.

Ross, J., & Chacko, M. (2022). Pelvic inflammatory disease: Clinical manifestations and diagnosis. *UpToDate*. Retrieved May 29, 2023, from https://www.uptodate.com/contents/pelvic-inflammatory-disease-clinical-manifestations-and-diagnosis.

Slusser, M., Garcia, L., Reed, C., & McGinnis, P. (2019). *Foundations of interprofessional collaborative practice in health care*. St. Louis: Elsevier.

Thornhill, J., et al. (2022). Monkeypox virus infection in humans across 16 countries – April-June 2022. *The New England Journal of Medicine*. https://doi.org/10.1056/NEJMoa2207323. https://www.nejm.org/doi/full/10.1056/NEJMoa2207323.

U.S. Department of Health and Human Services (USDHHS), Office of Disease Prevention and Health Promotion. (2023). *Healthy people 2030*. https://www.healthypeople.gov/.

U.S. Preventive Services Task Force. (2022). *Cervical cancer: Screening*. https://www.uspreventiveservicestaskforce.org/uspstf/draft-update-summary/cervical-cancer-screening-adults-adolescents.

Workowski, K., et al. (2021). Sexually transmitted infections treatment guidelines, 2021. *Morbidity and Mortality Weekly Report Recommendations and Reports, 70*(No. RR-4), 1–192.

World Health Organization. (2022a). *Sexually transmitted infections*. https://www.who.int/news-room/fact-sheets/detail/sexually-transmitted-infections-(stis).

World Health Organization. (2022b). *WHO recommends new name for monkeypox*. news.un.org/en/story/2022/11/1131082#.

Page numbers followed by *b* indicates boxes, *f* indicates illustrations, and *t* indicates tables.